P9-DHT-899

ELSEVIER

evolve

∴ *To access your Student Resources, visit:*

http://evolve.elsevier.com/Edmunds/NP/

Student Resources

- **Appendix: Economic Foundations of Prescriptive Authority**
  Provides an understanding of basic economic principles and explains how they influence prescribing practice and drug use.

- **Bonus Reference Tables**
  More than 30 additional tables, organized by chapter and offering valuable information and enrichment.

- **Drugs@FDA—A Catalog of FDA-Approved Drug Products**
  A comprehensive and up-to-date database of FDA drug approvals and withdrawals.

- **Patient Teaching Guides**
  A collection of Gold Standard© patient handouts, covering the drugs most commonly prescribed in primary care, are ready to print for use in clinical practice.

- **Resources for Patients and Providers**
  Annotated references to journal articles, websites, and other key resources.

- **WebLinks**
  Organized by chapter, websites have been chosen to supplement the content of the textbook.

http://evolve.elsevier.com/Edmunds/NP/

THIRD
EDITION

Pharmacology for the Primary Care Provider

Marilyn Winterton Edmunds, PhD, ANP/GNP
Adjunct Faculty
Johns Hopkins University, School of Nursing
Baltimore, Maryland

Maren Stewart Mayhew, MS, ANP/GNP
Nurse Practitioner
Beltsville, Maryland

with Christopher Bridgers, PharmD
Clinical Pharmacist
Saint Joseph's Hospital of Atlanta
Atlanta, Georgia

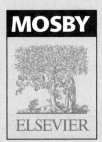

MOSBY

ELSEVIER

11830 Westline Industrial Drive
St. Louis, Missouri 63146

PHARMACOLOGY FOR THE PRIMARY CARE PROVIDER, 3rd edition   ISBN: 978-0-323-05131-6

Copyright © 2009 by Mosby, Inc., an affiliate of Elsevier Inc.

All rights reserved. No part of this publication may be reproduced or transmitted in any form or by any means, electronic or mechanical, including photocopying, recording, or any information storage and retrieval system, without permission in writing from the publisher. Permissions may be sought directly from Elsevier's Rights Department: phone: (+1) 215 239 3804 (US) or (+44) 1865 843830 (UK); fax: (+44) 1865 853333; e-mail: healthpermissions@elsevier.com. You may also complete your request on-line via the Elsevier website at http://www.elsevier.com/permissions.

Notice

Knowledge and best practice in this field are constantly changing. As new research and experience broaden our knowledge, changes in practice, treatment and drug therapy may become necessary or appropriate. Readers are advised to check the most current information provided (i) on procedures featured or (ii) by the manufacturer of each product to be administered, to verify the recommended dose or formula, the method and duration of administration, and contraindications. It is the responsibility of the practitioner, relying on their own experience and knowledge of the patient, to make diagnoses, to determine dosages and the best treatment for each individual patient, and to take all appropriate safety precautions. To the fullest extent of the law, neither the Publisher nor the Authors assumes any liability for any injury and/or damage to persons or property arising out of or related to any use of the material contained in this book.

The Publisher

Previous editions copyrighted 2004, 2000

Library of Congress Cataloging-in-Publication Data

Edmunds, Marilyn W.
    Pharmacology for the primary care provider / Marilyn Winterton Edmunds, Maren Stewart Mayhew, with Christopher Bridgers. – 3rd ed.
        p.; cm.
    Includes bibliographical references and index.
    ISBN 978-0-323-05131-6 (pbk.: alk. paper) 1. Pharmacology. 2. Primary care (Medicine) I. Mayhew, Maren Stewart. II. Bridgers, Christopher. III. Title.
    [DNLM: 1. Pharmacology. 2. Drug Therapy. 3. Pharmacology, Clinical. 4. Primary Health Care. QV 38 E24p 2009]
    RM301. 28. E34 2009
    615' 1–dc22   200803515

Acquisitions Editor: Kristin Geen
Developmental Editor: Lauren Lake
Publishing Services Manager: Jeff Patterson
Project Manager: Jeanne Genz
Design Direction: Ellen Zanolle

Printed in the United States of America

Last digit is the print number: 9 8 7 6 5 4 3 2

Working together to grow
libraries in developing countries

www.elsevier.com | www.bookaid.org | www.sabre.org

ELSEVIER   BOOK AID International   Sabre Foundation

Contributors

Ivy M. Alexander, PhD, C-ANP
Associate Professor and Director
Yale University School of Nursing
Adult Nurse Practitioner
Yale University Health Services
New Haven, Connecticut

Bonnie R. Bock, BSN, MS, CRNP
Goucher College
Baltimore, Maryland

Jan DiSantostefano, MS, NP
SAS Institute, Inc.
Cary, North Carolina

James D. Hoehns, PharmD, BCPS
Associate Professor (Clinical)
University of Iowa College of Pharmacy
Iowa City, Iowa
Research Director
Northeast Iowa Family Medicine Residency
Waterloo, Iowa

Clair L. Kaplan, RN/MSN, APRN(WHNP), MHS, MT(ASCP)
Assistant Professor of Nursing
Yale University
School of Nursing
New Haven, Connecticut

Jane Kapustin, PhD, CRNP
Assistant Professor and
Adult NP Program Director
University of Maryland, Baltimore
Baltimore, Maryland
Nurse Practitioner
Joslin Diabetes Center
University of Maryland Medical Systems
Baltimore, Maryland

Laura Miller, MSN, FNP, C-ANP
Richmond Health Center
Richmond, California

Elizabeth A. Monson, BSN, MS, ANP
University of Maryland Medical Center
Baltimore, Maryland

Sandi M. Nettina, MSN, APRN-BC, ANP
Clinical Instructor
Johns Hopkins University
School of Nursing
Baltimore, Maryland
Nurse Practitioner
Department of Family Practice
Columbia Medical Practice
Columbia, Missouri

Jessica Purcell, PharmD, MPH
Pharmacy Resident
University of Iowa
Iowa City, Iowa
Pharmacy Resident
Northeast Iowa Family Medicine Residency
Waterloo, Iowa

Kenneth Saffier, MD
Contra Costa Regional Medical Center
Martinez, California

Laurie Scudder, MS, NP
Clinical Assistant Professor
George Washington University
Washington, DC
Pediatric Nurse Practitioner
School Based Health Centers
Baltimore, Maryland

Janet S. Selway, DNSc, CRNP
Instructor
Johns Hopkins University
Baltimore, Maryland
Nurse Practitioner
Johns Hopkins Hospital
Department of Surgery
Baltimore, Maryland

V. Inez Wendel, MS, ANP, GNP
Geriatric Nurse Practitioner
Johns Hopkins University
Baltimore, Maryland

Theresa Pluth Yeo, PhD, CRNP
Adjunct Assistant Professor
Thomas Jefferson University
School of Nursing
Philadelphia, Pennsylvania
Nurse Practitioner
Thomas Jefferson University Hospital
Philadelphia, Pennsylvania

Reviewers

Cathleen Ahern, RN, PMHNP
Oregon Health & Science University
Portland, Oregon

Deborah H. Allen, MSN, RN, FNP, APRN-BC, AOCNP
The Preston Robert Tisch Brain Tumor Center
Duke University
Durham, North Carolina

Anne Bateman, EdD, APRN-BC
University of Massachusetts–Worcester
Graduate School of Nursing
Worcester, Massachusetts

Kathryn Baxter, MS, FNP, CWOCN
Assistant Professor of Clinical Nursing
Colon and Rectal Surgery Group
College of Physicians and Surgeons
Columbia University
New York, New York

Lora Beebe, PhD, APRN-BC
University of Tennessee
Knoxville, Tennessee

Susan E. Bennett, RN, MSN, APN-C
University of Missouri–Kansas City
Kansas City, Missouri

Kathryn A. Blair, PhD, APRN-BC, FNP
Univeristy of Colorado–Colorado Springs
Colorado Springs, Colorado

Margaret T. Bowers, MSN, APRN-BC
School of Nursing
Duke University
Durham, North Carolina

Christine Wanich Bradway, PhD, RN
Assistant Professor of Gerontological Nursing
School of Nursing
University of Pennsylvania
Philadelphia, Pennsylvania

Susan A. Bruce, MS, ANP
University at Buffalo
Buffalo, New York

Reamer L. Bushardt, PharmD, RPh, PA-C
Assistant Professor and Director
Physician Assistant Program
Medical University of South Carolina
Charleston, South Carolina

Pamela Z. Cacchione, PhD, APRN-BC
School of Nursing
Doisy College of Health Sciences
Saint Louis University
St. Louis, Missouri

Kimberly M. Campbell, RN, MSN, ARNP
Northern Kentucky University
Highland Heights, Kentucky

Ramona G. Chinn, PhD, APRN-BC
School of Nursing
University of Hawaii
Honolulu, Hawaii

Wendy Sue Clark, RN, MSN
University of Saint Francis
Fort Wayne, Indiana

Mary Anne Blum Condon, RN, CNP, PhD
Decker School of Nursing
Binghamton University
Binghamton, New York

Kathryn Jones Cooper, RN, MSN, ACNP, APRN-BC
Assistant Professor
Union University Germantown
Germantown, Tennessee

Lisa A. Cranwell-Bruce, RN, MS, FNP-C
Georgia State University
Atlanta, Georgia

Leslie Louise Davis, RN, MSN, ANP-C
Clinical Associate Professor
School of Nursing
University of North Carolina at Chapel Hill
Chapel Hill, North Carolina

Mary P. Donovan, ANP, ACNP, DNP
School of Nursing
Columbia University
New York, New York

Sharon Dudley-Brown, PhD, APRN, BC, FNP
Associate Professor
School of Nursing
The Catholic University of America
Washington, District of Columbia

Gina Duggar, ANP, MSN, APRN-BC, AOCNP
Nell Hodgson Woodruff School of Nursing
Emory University
Atlanta, Georgia

Nancy J. Fishwick, PhD, APRN-BC
School of Nursing
University of Maine
Orono, Maine

Cynthia E. Fitzgerald, PhD, RN, ARNP
Gonzaga University
Spokane, Washington

Elizabeth E. Fuentes, MS, RN, FNP-C
Associate Clinical Professor
FNP Program Coordinator
Texas Woman's University
Dallas, Texas

Linda H. Garrett, DSN, APRN-BC, FNP, LNC, SANE
Coordinator, Nurse Practitioner Programs
East Tennessee State University
Johnson City, Tennessee

Theresa N. Grabo, PhD, APRN-BC
Associate Professor
Director of Graduate Programs
Binghamton University
Binghamton, New York

Sheila Grossman, PhD, APRN-BC, FNP
Professor and Director
Family Nurse Practitioner Track
School of Nursing
Fairfield University
Fairfield, Connecticut

Elaine Brooks Harwood, MSN, RN, APRN-BC
Clinical Assistant Professor
Coordinator, Adult Nurse Practitioner Program
The University of North Carolina at Chapel Hill
Chapel Hill, North Carolina

Dalice L. Hertzberg, RN, MSN, APRN-BC
Instructor
Department of Pediatrics
School of Medicine
University of Colorado at Denver Health Sciences Center
Denver, Colorado

Kim Hudson-Gallogly, MS, RNC, WHNP
North Georgia College and State University
Dahlonega, Georgia

Laima M. Karosas, PhD, APRN
Quinnipiac University
Hamden, Connecticut

Marye Dorsey Kellermann, RN, MSN, CRNP
Associate Professor
Coppin State University
Baltimore, Maryland

Maripat D. King, RN, MSN, ACNP-BC
Clinical Instructor
University of Illinois at Chicago
Chicago, Illinois

Patricia Biller Krauskopf, PhD, RN, CFNP
Associate Professor and Coordinator
Family Nurse Practitioner Track
Shenandoah University
Winchester, Virginia

Kathleen M. Lamaute, EdD, APRN-BC, FNP
Faculty
South University
West Palm Beach, Florida

Patricia Lange-Otsuka, EdD, APRN-BC, MSN, CNE
Interim Dean and Professor of Nursing
School of Nursing
Hawaii Pacific University
Kaneohe, Hawaii

Karen C. Lyon, PhD, APRN, CNS, CNOR, CNAA
University of Texas at El Paso
El Paso, Texas

Liz Macera, PhD, NP-C
University of California at San Francisco
San Francisco, California

Lynda A. Mackin, PhD, APRN-BC
Associate Clinical Professor
University of California at San Francisco
San Francisco, California

Kathleen McGrath, RN, MS, CPNP
Advanced Practice Nurse
Golisano Children's Hospital
University of Rochester Medical Center
Rochester, New York

Beverly Monti, DNP(c), MSN, FNP
Veterans Administration Loma Linda
   Healthcare Systems
Loma Linda, California

Patrick J. M. Murphy, PhD
Assistant Professor
College of Nursing
Seattle University
Seattle, Washington

Marie Napolitano, PhD, RN, FNP
Oregon Health & Science University
Portland, Oregon

Angela Mary Nelson, RN, MSN, CCRN, ACNP
Assistant Professor, Clinical Nursing
Columbia Presbyterian Medical Center
Columbia University
New York, New York

Joshua J. Neumiller, PharmD
College of Pharmacy
Washington State University
Spokane, Washington

Anne P. Odell, PhD, FNP
Assistant Professor
School of Nursing
Azusa Pacific University
Azusa, California

Karen Koozer Olsen, PhD, FNP-CS, FAANP
Professor
Texas A&M University-Corpus Christi
Corpus Christi, Texas

Carrie F. Palmer, MSN, RN, ANP, CDE
School of Nursing
University of North Carolina at Chapel Hill
Chapel Hill, North Carolina

Sabita Persaud, PhD, RN
Assistant Professor
Bowie State University
Bowie, Maryland

Sandra Pfanz, DrPH, APRN-BC
Associate Professor/Director, FNP Program
Saint Xavier University
Certified Adult Nurse Practitioner
University of Illinois Medical Center
Chicago, Illinois

Valeria Ramdin, PhD(c), MS, RN-BC
Northeastern University
Boston, Massachusetts

Ginger Raterink, DNSc, ANP-C
University of Colorado at Denver Health
   Sciences Center
Denver, Colorado

Kris Robinson, PhD, FNP-BC
The University of Texas at El Paso
El Paso, Texas

Nancy Jex Sabin, RN, MS, FNP
Clinical Assistant Professor
Hahn School of Nursing and Health Science
University of San Diego
San Diego, California

Deborah A. Sampson, PhD, APRN, FNP
Assistant Professor
School of Nursing
University of Michigan
Ann Arbor, Michigan

JoAnne M. Saxe, RN-C, MS, ANP
Adult Nurse Practitioner Program
Department of Community Health Systems
School of Nursing
University of California at San Francisco
San Francisco, California

Marlene Gail Smith Sefton, PhD, APN, CFNP
University of Illinois at Chicago
Chicago, Illinois

Barbara Sheer, DNSc, FNP-C, FAANP
Associate Professor
University of Delaware
Newark, Delaware

Sharon Souter, PhD, RN
Patty Hanks Shelton School of Nursing
Abilene, Texas

Dawn Salpaka Stone, MN, RN, ANP
Associate Professor
College of Graduate Nursing
Western University of Health Sciences
Pomona, California

Cheryl Swayne, RN, C, MN, FNP
Associate Professor
Northern Kentucky University
Highland Heights, Kentucky

Anne C. Thomas, PhD, APRN-BC, ANP, GNP
Assistant Professor
School of Nursing
University of Michigan
Ann Arbor, Michigan

Barbara Todd, MSN, CRNP, APRN-BC, FAANP
University of Pennsylvania
Philadelphia, Pennsylvania

Charlotte Torres, EdD, RN, FNP-C
Professor of Clinical Nursing
School of Nursing
University of Rochester
Rochester, New York

June A. Treston, MSN, CRNP
Associate Program Director
Family Health Practitioner Program
University of Pennsylvania
Philadelphia, Pennsylvania

Mary Ann Troiano, RN, MSN, FNP
Assistant Professor
Monmouth University
West Long Branch, New Jersey

Gwyn M. Vernon, MSN, CRNP
University of Pennsylvania
Philadelphia, Pennsylvania

Lynn Davis Waits, RN, MSN, FNP-C
Georgia College and State University
Milledgeville, Georgia

James Whyte IV, ND, MSN, ARNP
College of Nursing
Florida State University
Tallahassee, Florida

Lynn Wimett, RN, MS, APN, EdD
Regis University
Denver, Colorado

Jacki S. Witt, JD, MSN, RNC, WHNP
University of Missouri–Kansas City
Kansas City, Missouri

Concetta L. Zak, DNP, MBA, APRN-BC
University of Illinois at Chicago
Chicago, Illinois

Preface

As the title proclaims, this text is written for all types of primary care providers but with a particular emphasis on new drug prescribers, particularly nurse practitioners and physician assistants. Our goals are to present comprehensive information on the drugs most commonly prescribed in primary care practice, and to do it in a concise and easily digestible manner.

As in the previous two editions of *Pharmacology for the Primary Care Provider*, the Third Edition assumes that the reader has a strong grasp of biochemical principles and clinical practice, and it therefore focuses on the basic information that every prescriber must know. Unlike many pharmacology text books and drug prescribing texts, this book does not attempt to cover every drug, nor every facet of the drugs included. With the multitude of drug information that is easily available, it is not necessary to repeat information about all those drugs in this text.

This is a unique text that mirrors how clinicians really practice. Research has indicated that most clinicians have a small basic list of drugs that they prescribe and about which they have mastered the details. They know when the patient does not fit the drug profile, and they know when they need to consider drugs not on the prescribers' list.

This book follows this same format by highlighting the most common or important drug in a category (often found on the list of the Top 200 Drugs) and providing detailed information about that drug. All other drugs in the category then are compared with the key drug, and only information that is new, different, or very important about the additional drugs is presented for comparison and mastery. This text relies heavily on the most important basic concepts that clinicians must master about a drug category.

Especially for new prescribers, the goal is mastery of basic information about the drug category and a small number of key drugs.

Many features of this text are designed to aid the practitioner in decision making and practice:

- Drug tables at the beginning of each chapter outline the classifications of drugs discussed in that chapter and identify the key drugs to be mastered.
- The Top 200 Drugs prescribed in the United States are identified in the table by the icon ☀.
- Complete discussions on drug action and drug treatment principles are presented for every drug category.
- Clinical Alerts, highlighted by the icon ☄, impart essential information that primary care providers must remember so they can avoid serious problems. The Alerts include cautions for prescribing, information about drug interactions, or warnings about particularly ominous adverse effects of which the clinician should be aware.
- Clinical Guidelines, Evidence-Based Recommendations, and Cardinal Points of Treatment are included for all drug categories. These help direct clinical decision making and are based on a variety of sources.
- Patient Education sections in every chapter provide effective patient teaching about medications to help ensure patient compliance.
- Patient Variables sections alert the provider to special considerations that are based on age, pregnancy, race, and other factors.

No part of the health care delivery system changes faster than the pharmacologic component. New information is discovered every day. Sometimes we discover that beliefs we have about drug use are incorrect, and new strategies are required. For example, we have made changes in the use of hormones to treat women with menopausal symptoms because of new adverse effects that were found. New products go on the market almost daily. What we know or don't know about these products affects the care we provide. Clinicians must stay up-to-date on new information if they are to give safe and effective care.

Using the most recent information is not the exclusive domain of research-based academicians but is the foundation of accepted health care practice for all primary care practitioners. To help the clinician stay current, several continuously updated sources are provided, free of charge, with purchase of this text. In addition to the readings and references listed in the back of this book, instructors and students who purchase the text will be given access to the Evolve Resources to Accompany *Pharmacology for the Primary Care Provider*, Third Edition. This website, which is an invaluable resource for continuing education, contains the following:

- Bonus reference tables that provide enrichment information not covered in the text are available on the website.
- An entire chapter on drug economics has been moved from the book to the Evolve website.
- Resources for patients and providers that were formerly located at the end of every chapter are now available on the website.
- More than 1100 WebLinks arranged by chapter are available on the website and should prove helpful to both provider and patient.
- A link to the FDA's *Catalog of FDA-Approved Drug Products* is provided on the website.

Of additional interest for the instructor, the Evolve Resources website provides the following: a free 300-question test bank and an electronic image collection that offers more than 120 full-color illustrations. Also, 20 Archie animations illustrate the specifics of use of various drugs. PowerPoint lecture slides that can be used to teach each chapter are also included.

The advent of evidence-based medicine has changed how we think about pharmacotherapeutics. It is important to learn what really works as opposed to what has been done traditionally. Research will have a direct impact on what we do. Therefore, this book teaches providers how to think about drug use through discussion of evidence-based medicine studies, appraisal of clinical guidelines and protocols, and consideration of role studies conducted to examine how professionals actually prescribe medication and how critical decisions can and should be made.

NEW TO THE THIRD EDITION

This Third Edition reflects the most current thoughts and trends in primary care. Several chapters have been reordered, expanded, or pared down; however, the most dramatic changes are seen within the chapters themselves. The website links to clinical guidelines, the focus on evidence-based practice, and the focus on cardinal points of treatment all should help to assure the new prescriber that the drugs he or she is prescribing are the ones that should be used. Information about key drugs is often expanded, and any redundant information about related drugs has been eliminated. This text follows The Joint Commission (TJC) guidelines in discussing dosages and time schedules and tries to highlight critical information that the clinician must master.

ORGANIZATION

Part One contains chapters on essential concepts for the prescription of medications.
- Unit 1 describes primary health care providers and the various dimensions of their role. It also covers the legal parameters and professional role implementation of prescriptive authority and explains what we know about different types of primary health care providers.
- Unit 2 is one of the most important in the whole text. It focuses on the pharmacokinetics and the pharmacodynamics of various drugs. Specific factors are considered in terms of prescribing drugs to geriatric, pediatric, and pregnant patients.
- Unit 3 discusses some of the things that underlie the "art" of prescribing, including the therapeutic relationship between drug prescriber and patient. Practical tips on writing prescriptions are explored, and principles of evidence-based medicine, clinical guidelines, critical decision making, and patient education are discussed.

Part Two contains 12 discrete units that discuss well known drug categories and the common primary care conditions for which they are used. Chapter text and drug monographs are arranged for easy readability and ready reference in this consistent and logical manner:

Drug Overview
Indications
Therapeutic Overview
Mechanism of Action
Standardized Guidelines, Evidence-Based Recommendations, and Cardinal Points of Treatment
Treatment Principles, Nonpharmacologic and Pharmacologic
How to Monitor
Patient Variables
Patient Education
Specific Drugs (beginning with key drugs when relevant and then considering different or especially important information about other drugs in the category)

THE FUTURE

Pharmacology for the Primary Care Provider, Third Edition, provides that strong basic knowledge of pharmacology that every care provider needs. The text summarizes extremely complex information in a deceptively simple format and in a manner that only expert clinicians can provide. Students will appreciate the clear and simple explanations. Mastery of these foundational principles, basic protocols, and key drug monographs will prepare primary care clinicians for the realities of daily practice. We invite you to enjoy it, learn from it, carry it with you into the clinical area as you begin to practice, and use the resources provided to both deepen and expand your pharmacologic arsenal.

As you gain experience with this text, we welcome your comments. As you mature and grow in your role as a primary care clinician, we hope that you will help us progress in our role as educators. It is a cooperative relationship.

ACKNOWLEDGMENTS

We would like to acknowledge the contributions of authors for the first edition. Their original work is foundational to the changes that were made for second and third editions. Those original authors include the following:

Susan E. Appling, RN, MS, CRNP; JoAnne T. Baker, RN, MSN, FNP; Elizabeth Blair, MSN, CS-ANP, CDE; Bonnie R. Bock, RN, BSN, MS, CRNP; Alice M. Brazier, MS, CRNP, GNP; James Cawley, MPH, PA-C; Susan E. Childs, RN, MS, CRNP; Sandra L. Cotton, MS, C-ANP; Christy L. Crowther, RN, MS, CRNP; Charles E. Daniels, RPh, PhD, FASHP; George DeMaagd, PharmD, BCPS; Gloria A. Deniz, RN, MS, ARNP; Jan DiSantostefano, MS, CRNP; Susan Waldrop Donckers, RN, EdD, CS, FNP; Michael Dreis, PharmD, MPH; Diane Fatica, RN, MSN, FNP; Kathleen Ryan Fletcher, RN, CS, MSN, GNP; Annette Galassi, RN, MA, CANP, AOCN; Susanne Scharnhorst Gibbons, ANP, GNP, MS; Cynthia Knoll Grandjean, RN, MGA, MSN, NP; Catherine Hagan, MSN, RN, CNS; Major Nancy (Jo) Heisterman, BS, FNP; Linda C. Hersey, MS, CRNP; James D. Hoehns, PharmD, BCPS; Karen Huss, RN, DNSc, CANP, FAAN; Pamela Lynn Jamieson, RNC, MS, NP; Bonnie Kohl, RN, MS, CRNP; M. Lauren Lemieux, MS; Marilyn Little, BS, MS, CS; Jennifer Loud, MSN, CRNP; Karen MacKay, MD; Douglas Matthews, MS, CRNP; Elaine McIntosh, RN, CS, FNP; Patricia C. McMullen, CRNP, MS, JD; Carolyn S. Melby, DNSc, CRNP; Karen L. Minor, RN, MS, CRNP; Maureen Moriarty-Sheehan, RN, MS, CRNP; Candis Morrison, PhD, ACNP; Kathleen Murphy, RN, MS, CRNP; Julie C. Novak, DNSc, RN, CPNP; Katherine M. O'Rourke, MSN, FNP; Katherine M. Pabst, CRNP, MPH; Julianne B. Pinson, PharmD; Stevelynn J. Pogue, MSN, RN, CS, A/GNP, ET; Barbara E. Pokorny, MSN, RN, CS; Jacqueline Rhoads, PhD, RN, CCRN, ACNP, CS; Laurie Scudder, MS, PNP; Diane C. Seibert, BSN, MS, CRNP; Janet S. Selway, MS, CANP, CPNP; Leslie K. Serchuck, MD; Amy B. Sharron, MS, RN, CS, GNP; Laura E. Shay, MS, CANP; Donna M. Thompson, RN, MS, APRN; Laura Keiler Topper, RN, MS, NP; Jan Wemmer, MS, CRNP; Inez Wendel, MS, CRNP; David S. Wing, BBP, MSc; Theresa Pluth Yeo, MSN, MPH, CRNP; and Linda R. Young, PharmD.

Additionally, we want to express our appreciation for the personal stimulation we have received from the many nurse practitioners, physician assistants, nurse midwives, nurse anesthetists, PharmD professionals, physicians, and medical students with whom we have worked over the past few years. They have asked challenging questions and have been clear about the need for a good text in which basic medical content is integrated with pharmacologic principles and nursing approaches. Some of these individuals have been willing to step forward to write that content, and we are grateful for their wisdom, their knowledge, and their assistance.

And finally, we are deeply grateful for the help of the editorial, production, and design staff at Elsevier and specifically wish to thank Lee Henderson, Kristin Geen, Maureen Iannuzzi, Lauren Lake, Jacqueline Twomey, and Jeanne Genz. As always, none of this work would have been possible without the tolerance and support of our very patient families. Maren wishes especially to thank Bill, and Marilyn is indebted to Cliff and her loving children, who all are so tolerant of the tasks we undertake.

A Note to the Student of Primary Care

Begin this text with the chapters in the first unit. Reread the chapter on pharmacokinetics and pharmacodynamics on a regular basis. It is one of the most important chapters in the book, and it is impossible to master these principles in a single reading. Don't expect to memorize everything. This book will be something you want to refer to often in the clinical area as you begin to practice. Try to understand the principles that are being presented, and find examples in your own patients that illustrate them.

As you gain experience with this text, we welcome your comments. As you mature and grow in your role as a primary care clinician, we hope that you will help us progress in our role as educators. It is a cooperative relationship.

Marilyn Winterton Edmunds, PhD, ANP/GNP
Maren Stewart Mayhew, MS, ANP/GNP

Contents

evolve http://evolve.elsevier.com/Edmunds/NP/

Prescriptive Authority and Role Implementation: Tradition vs. Change

INCREASED FOCUS ON PRIMARY CARE

Primary care as a concept involves the provision of integrated, accessible health care services by clinicians who are accountable for addressing "personal health care needs, developing a sustained partnership with patients, and practicing in the context of family and community" (Vaneslow et al, 1995). It is generally agreed that providing health care includes one or more of the following functions: assessing health status, promoting healthy lifestyles, identifying/diagnosing normal and abnormal conditions, determining the causes of abnormal conditions, providing referral to health care specialists, selecting appropriate therapeutic measures, implementing treatment, and supervising or monitoring the patient on an ongoing basis. These tasks are commonly referred to as *prevention, diagnosis, prescription,* and *treatment.* They describe professional behavior that involves deciding what is wrong with a patient and then choosing among available therapeutic options to prescribe and implement a course of treatment. Traditionally, these behaviors have been the exclusive domain of the physician and, to a lesser extent, the dentist, until 1965, when other nonphysician provider roles began to emerge.

TRADITIONAL PROVISION OF PRIMARY CARE

Physicians clearly are the most numerous primary care providers and their prescriptive practice has influenced all other clinicians who gain prescriptive authority. States first began to enact medical practice acts in the 1920s to protect the public safety. Before that time, the quality of medical education and the competency of physicians were variable. Medical practice acts granted title protection to those individuals who called themselves physicians and identified what requirements must be met for that title to be given. Although other categories of health care professionals were certainly in existence at that time, physicians were the first health care practitioners to gain legislative recognition of their practice (Starr, 1982). The statutory definitions initially created by physicians for the scope of their practice were extremely broad. In an exhaustive study of regulatory restrictions on new types of health care providers, Safreit (1992) provided an example (NC Gen. Stat No. 90-18 [1983]) of one state's definition of physician or surgeon as follows:

> Any person...who shall diagnose or attempt to diagnose, treat or attempt to treat, operate or attempt to operate on, or prescribe for or administer to, or profess to treat any human ailment, physical or mental, or any physical injury to or deformity of another person.

Because of the way in which the medical practice acts were written, physicians emerged with an exclusive right to practice that gave them a preeminent position in a hierarchy of healing occupations. Designating physicians as the only providers with diagnostic and treatment authority was intended to protect the public. However, the breadth of the medical practice acts, combined with provisions making it illegal for anyone not licensed as a physician to carry out any acts included in the definition, made it difficult for other health care workers to describe their contributions. All other health care providers, including groups such as nurses and nurse-midwives, had to redefine their tasks or functions as separate from the all-encompassing medical scope of practice. They then had to seek legislative recognition of their own professional roles, no matter how traditional or longstanding their activities might have been (Safreit, 1992).

Dominance of the physician in the health care hierarchy created a virtual monopoly in health care. The medical sociology and professionalization literature is filled with extensive analyses of the factors that led to the development of the cultural, economic, political, and social authority and dominance of the physician, especially the growth and power of organized medicine (Freidson, 1970a, 1970b; Starr, 1982).

Having obtained the exclusive right to practice, however, physicians also recognized their need for the services of other practitioners of healing, who were "useful to the physician and necessary to his practice" (Safreit, 1992), even if it required giving up some of their monopolistic control. A noted medical sociologist who has traced the professionalization of physicians notes that to solve this dilemma, physicians extended their right to practice to a right from the state to control the activities of other occupations, "so as to limit what they could do and to supervise or direct their activities" (Freidson, 1970a). In doing so, the profession was able to establish organizational structures that preserved a distinct sphere of professional dominance and autonomy (Safreit, 1992).

The role of the physician has changed dramatically during the past 50 years. Driven by new technology, new procedures, and new medications, physicians have been attracted into specialty practice in greater numbers, leaving primary care positions vacant. Medicare reimbursement has fueled the growth of tertiary care.

The emergence of nonphysicians who claimed preparation for and the desire to provide primary care services came at a time when there was a shortage of primary care services. The emergence of this new group challenged the professional control by physicians, the organizations that have consolidated their authority, and the legislation designed to protect and preserve that position.

Beginning in 1992, the Physician Payment Review Commission recommended radical changes in Medicare reimbursement methods. This shift directly increased financial reimbursement to clinicians who were providing primary care and thus indirectly created an incentive to attract more providers into primary care. The hope was that the numbers and types of providers would be more evenly aligned with the numbers and types of patients who require health care.

Medical schools began to place greater emphasis on preparing primary care clinicians. Teaching methods shifted from the acute care model to include a greater focus on primary care. The hospitalist emerged as a specialist, thus relieving the primary care physician of the need to provide in-hospital care. Reimbursement began to reward the general practitioner. All of these changes have resulted in qualified success, bringing increased credibility and recognition to primary care providers; however, the number of specialists remains disproportionate.

Notwithstanding the longstanding precedent for physicians to provide primary care, there remained a disparity in the ability of physicians to meet the primary care needs of the populace. Nonphysician providers began to fill that niche with increasing success. The nonphysician providers who emerged during the 1960s and 1970s were well accepted by their patients; delivered high-quality, cost-effective care; and generally increased the access of patients to health care (OTA, 1986). These providers continued to work cooperatively with physician providers, most often in joint practices.

IMPORTANCE OF PRESCRIPTIVE AUTHORITY IN HEALTH CARE DELIVERY

Medications are powerful weapons against disease. Pharmaceutical companies add many new drugs every year to the nation's pharmacopoeia. Thousands of new drugs, including many new drugs for children, are in the research and development pipeline and are providing a new armamentarium for clinicians to use in treating patients with chronic disease.

RESEARCH ON PRESCRIPTIVE PRACTICE OF PHYSICIANS

Physicians and dentists are the professionals who traditionally have been given the undisputed right to prescriptive authority. The prescriptive practice of physicians in primary care practice has been thoroughly documented by the pharmaceutical industry. What medications physicians order and how many prescriptions are written are closely monitored. Studies have not only evaluated basic prescribing practices but have analyzed the effects that multiple variables have on prescribing habits. While the prescriptive behavior of physicians may not be the gold standard of primary care practice, it has been the only standard and their strengths and weaknesses bear exploration by other groups seeking prescriptive authority. Some of the key findings are briefly presented here.

The National Ambulatory Medical Care Survey (Cherry & Woodwell, 2002) collected data on drugs most frequently used in office-based practice and found that 64.21% of all office visits resulted in the generation of at least one prescription. The top five categories of prescriptions were antidepressants, nonsteroidal antiinflammatory agents, antihistamines or bronchodilators, antihypertensives, and antihyperlipidemics. During the past 20 years, these categories have remained relatively consistent, although antimicrobial drugs have now fallen from the top five. In the 2000 National Ambulatory Medical Care Survey (Cherry & Woodwell, 2002), researchers examined physician prescribing in general and in family practice. They found that for those patients who made an office visit, 33.9% did not receive any prescription; however, 28% received one prescription, 16.1% received two, 8.8% received three, 4.9% received four, 3.2% received five, and 5.3% received six. The percent of visits involving medications ranged from 78.8% for internists to 29.9% for general surgeons. General and family practice physicians deal with medications in 76.3% of visits.

Many more studies have examined the types of medications prescribed, and over the years, patterns have changed. Stolley and Lasagna (1969) found that 95% of all physicians prescribed one or more medications to a patient with a common cold, and more than 60% of these prescriptions were for antibiotics. In 1972, a computerized retrieval system examined 20,000 prescriptions and found that antibiotics topped the list of most frequently prescribed medications, followed by tranquilizers, nonnarcotic analgesics, oral contraceptives, and antitussives (Stolley et al, 1972b). In 1974, researchers found sedatives and hypnotics heading the list (21%), and antibiotics (15%), antihistamines (8%), dermatologic preparations (6.6%), and cardiovascular drugs (6.5%) accounted for the top five classifications (Rosenberg et al, 1974). As the years progressed, sedatives, tranquilizers, and hypnotics began to decline in popularity (DeNuzzo, 1981; Knoben & Wertheimer, 1976; Rossiter, 1983). The 2000 National Ambulatory Medical Care Survey, which was released by the Centers for Disease Control and Prevention (Cherry & Woodwell, 2002), shows that the top categories of drugs are very similar to those reported 20 years earlier. However, antibiotic categories have become antimicrobial, accounting for the change in prescribing due to AIDS. The most frequently prescribed drug in 2000 was Claritin, followed by Lipitor, Synthroid, Premarin, and amoxicillin. Acetaminophen was the generic substance most frequently prescribed. The survey documented a 21% increase over the past several years in the percent of office visits in cases in which cardiovascular-renal drugs, such as angiotensin-converting enzyme inhibitors, β-blockers, or antihypertensive medications, were prescribed. Between 1997 and 2000, a 25% increase in percentage of visits occurred in cases in which a hormone was prescribed, whereas the increase in the percent of metabolic/nutrient drug visits rose by 41%. The report suggested that these changes reflect the drug use patterns of the health-conscious baby boomers and the growing number of seniors whose chronic conditions can be treated by the wide variety of medications on the market today. Of note is that in the latest findings presented in the 2004 report, antidepressants are the most widely prescribed drugs. Analysis of the 2003–2004 Ambulatory Medical Care medication data reveals that the top 50 drugs were dominated by six therapeutic classes: pain relievers, cardiovascular-renal drugs, respiratory tract drugs, CNS drugs, hormones, and antimicrobials (USDHHS, 2006).

Less research has been conducted on the appropriateness of physician prescriptive practices, although the literature suggests that some physicians may write prescriptions for problems that might well respond to many nonpharmacologic treatments (Avorn et al, 1991).

The pharmaceutical industry has expended considerable research dollars to try to determine how best to influence prescribers to adopt a particular drug. When a new drug product is developed, research suggests that the rate of adoption by prescribers may be divided into five profiles: innovators, early adopters, early majority, late majority, and laggards. Although the speed at which prescribers adopt the drug varies, the individuals within each profile all go through a four-step process—awareness of the new drug, interest, evaluation, and trial—that leads to adoption.

Denig and Haaijer-Ruskamp (1992) described an "evoked set" that includes a small number of possible treatments (typically containing all therapies, including nondrug therapies) that a physician might consider for a specific condition. Clearly, if a therapy is unfamiliar or unknown, it will not be included in the physician's evoked set. The evoked set for all possible medical problems makes up the "total drug repertoire" or "therapeutic armamentarium" and, on average, includes 144 drug preparations per physician. Researchers have concluded that over a 12-month period, physicians write 5.4% of prescriptions for new drugs, and that 42% of the time, this product replaces a drug that was previously part of the repertoire. "Once a product is part of the evoked set, it has a propensity to be prescribed through habit rather than through active problem-solving" (Groves et al, 2002). So prescribers both adopt and relinquish drugs in their therapeutic armamentarium. This change in the product choice comes as innovation is diffused or communicated through certain channels over time among the members of a social system. Burban, Link, and Doucette (2001) suggested that the factors that influence new drug adoption are the perceived attributes of the innovations, communication channels used to discuss these attributes, the nature of the social system, and physician characteristics.

Other studies over the years have attempted to predict which variables most strongly affect prescribing habits. Younger physicians and specialists tend to prescribe more appropriately and to prescribe fewer medications (Miles & Roland, 1975; NCHS, 1983a; Stolley et al, 1972a, 1972b). Stolley et al (1972b) also noted that generally the more appropriate prescriber was the one who was in a large group practice and who used physician consultants and journal articles to guide pharmacologic decision making. Miller (1973, 1974), Smith (1977), and Stolley & Lasagna (1969) identified multiple variables that may influence drug prescribing. Colleagues, pharmaceutical representatives, journal articles, the *Physicians' Desk Reference*, medical meetings, and journal advertising were reportedly the primary sources of information about medications and therapeutic regimens.

In a summary of recent literature, it has been suggested that financial ties to drug companies may influence physicians' prescribing judgments. One study found that physicians who requested specific additions to a hospital pharmacy were substantially more likely to have met with drug company representatives or to have accepted money from drug companies. However, physicians may not recognize the potential influence of drug companies on their behavior. One study of primary care physicians said that they placed little weight on drug advertisements (68%), pharmaceutical representatives (54%), and patient preference (74%), and that they relied heavily on academic sources for drug information. Yet the study found that commercial rather than scientific sources of drug information dominated drug information materials.

Guidelines issued by the U.S. Food and Drug Administration (FDA) in 2001 prompted the American Medical Association and the Pharmaceutical Manufacturers and Researchers of America (PhRMA) to issue ethical guidelines that clarify the appropriate relationship between pharmaceutical companies and drug prescribers. These guidelines forbid pharmaceutical companies from giving to prescribers non-patient care–related items exceeding $100 in value; they also clarify the role that pharmaceutical companies can and cannot play in the continuing education of provider groups.

PROBLEMS IN THE PRESCRIBING PRACTICE OF PHYSICIANS

Difficulties documented over the years in prescribing have been remarkably consistent. The conclusions of numerous studies suggest the following:

1. Problems are created because of physician failure to keep abreast of changes. Information about new products and new research findings diffuse slowly into practice. Typically, many physicians have been wary about suggestions for change in their practices until they have seen evidence of safety and utility, especially for medications. Physicians in solo or isolated practice often fail to realize that they are out of step with other general practices because they may not have an opportunity for daily critical debate and exchange among colleagues. Few physicians have had sufficient time to keep up-to-date on new materials and instead rely on drug advertisements and pharmaceutical representatives for information. Most information in pharmacology textbooks is outdated before it is printed. New methods of staying up-to-date will be required for safe practice. Use of the Internet, medical journals on CD-ROM, and evidence-based medicine reports, along with the ability to obtain specialist consultations through Telehealth, will dramatically affect how providers obtain and use information, and whether it will make a difference in their practice.

2. Pharmaceutical companies influence practice and provide drug samples. When the bulk of information coming to a physician is provided through biased marketing sources, physicians may have a difficult time evaluating the relative merits of competitive products (Smith, 1977; So, 1998). Intervention by the FDA over the years has limited the amount and type of pressure that drug detail representatives can exert directly on physicians to encourage them to use their products. Requirements for more balanced presentations of information about diagnostic and treatment methods have helped to upgrade the quality of valid information given to physicians. Current PhRMA guidelines are a step in the right direction but remain voluntary.

3. Lack of time has become a major factor in all medical practices. The emphasis on making money in many health maintenance organizations has led to decreased time for patient encounters, leading to inadequate history taking, failure to clearly define the problem, and an overreliance on drug therapy (Avorn et al, 1998).

4. Consumers provide pressure to prescribe medications. Although the interest of consumers in their health

care is usually a positive trait, the demand of patients on the physician to "do something" has translated into an increased insistence by the consumer on being given a prescription. This pressure has increased as a result of the widespread use of Direct-to-Consumer advertising on TV and in lay magazines. Giving in to these pressures has resulted not only in a society of individuals who tend to take a pill for everything but also in the widespread overuse of antibiotics, thus contributing to the problems caused by drug-resistant organisms. In an FDA survey of physicians' prescribing behavior, physicians reported an increase in the number of patients who ask them to prescribe specific drugs. They reported that in 41% of cases, they had to spend time correcting misconceptions of the patient; in 26% of cases, the drug was not needed; and in 9%, the patient wanted the drug rather than another therapy that was ordered. More revealing was the research that showed that when patients asked for a specific prescription, most of the time they received it (Aiken, 2003).

5. Prescriptions are often illegible. Pharmacists report great difficulty in accurately reading the writing of many physicians. This has led to major errors in dispensing of medications as they try to determine what the physician might have written. Use of preprinted prescription pads, fax machines, and computer-generated forms will help to decrease these problems. A steady trend is to require electronically generated prescriptions if reimbursement is to be provided.

6. Providers may fail to detect or anticipate drug interactions. Modern research on the liver has revealed the presence of the cytochrome P450 enzyme system. Lack of provider awareness about the influence of different drugs on these pathways has made many medications ineffective. Many online and PDA programs have the potential to alert the provider to these types of conflicts. Five million times last year, one of the nation's largest real-time computer systems alerted American pharmacists that prescribed drug combinations could trigger potentially lethal drug interactions. The prescription warning system issues 45 million alerts annually. Many warnings are issued for drug interactions that have been well described in the professional literature. An even greater challenge is the growing use of OTC and herbal products; most often, the patient's physician is unaware of this usage, and many of these products do interact with prescription drugs.

SUMMARY

Because physicians and dentists were the only major health care providers with prescriptive authority for many years, much of what we know about prescriptive behavior is based on their patterns. Thus, the practice characteristics of other health care practitioners inevitably will be compared with those of physicians whether physician practices are adequate or not. Rigorous methods have not yet been implemented to examine whether physician performance consistently correlates with approved therapeutic practice. New types of health care providers insist that their prescriptive practices should not be compared with those of physicians, but that all providers should be held to a standard of approved therapeutic practice. These standards of care are just beginning to be defined and are being driven by the concepts of evidence-based medicine.

The bulk of primary care medicines will continue to be prescribed by physicians. What physicians prescribe and how effective they are in choosing the appropriate medication will continue to be important information pertaining to all prescribers with prescriptive authority. The challenge for new health care providers is to learn from the experience of these traditional health care prescribers.

evolve   A continually updated list of useful WebLinks may be found in the Evolve Resources at http://evolve.elsevier.com/Edmunds/NP/

Historical Review of Prescriptive Authority: The Role of Nurses (NPs, CNMs, CRNAs, and CNSs) and Physician Assistants

MARILYN WINTERTON EDMUNDS and JAMES CAWLEY

OVERVIEW

Traditionally, prescriptive authority has been the domain of physicians and dentists. The impact of physician prescriptive authority and primary care practices on other types of providers is important. Research on the practices of nonphysician providers has demonstrated conclusively that they are qualified to provide primary care. Although physicians have a broader education than other types of health care providers such as nurse practitioners and physician assistants, the extent of education required to provide primary care services is not clear. It appears that many physicians may be overeducated to provide primary care, and other clinicians might be just as competent in delivering primary care (Safreit, 1992), leaving physicians to care for patients with more complicated conditions that clearly require an extensive breadth of education. Some nonphysician providers, such as doctors of pharmacy (PharmDs), have added diagnostic and assessment skills to their pharmacology knowledge, making them valuable contributors to the health care team yet not challenging the overall clinical role of physicians.

Because of the importance of medications in treating primary care problems and in providing the full scope of health care services required by the typical primary care patient, all providers must be able to prescribe medications. This is especially true in rural areas, where only one provider may be available. However, it is just as true where many providers are competing with each other and trying to make a living. If meeting patients' needs is the primary focus in the provision of primary care services, then providers should not be artificially restricted from meeting as many needs as possible (Safreit, 1992).

As newcomers, advanced practice nurses, physician assistants, PharmDs, optometrists, and others have had to carve out their prescribing role legally over time and separately in each state. The largest new groups to assume prescriptive authority in the past 50 years have been the nurse practitioners and the physician assistants. Obtaining prescriptive authority was one of the major benchmarks achieved by these new provider groups as they developed their new roles. If one is to understand some of the problems faced by these providers today, one must learn about the history of how their prescriptive authority came to be. To trace the progress of prescriptive authority for these two groups, let us examine their experiences separately because their progress in obtaining prescriptive authority has followed different pathways. Of necessity, this review relies on many historical articles, as well as the classic research and literature that have documented progress in this area.

For many years, the boundaries of nursing practice have been carefully constrained by state nurse practice acts that maintained that "nurses do not treat, diagnose, nor prescribe" (Kelly, 1974). However, the 1960s saw a critical mass of bored, talented nurse clinicians, whose substantial scientific education had been underused, and whose ideas about making changes in their role were spurred on by the consciousness raising of the feminist movement. This happened at a time when other health care personnel were being pulled into the Vietnam War and concern had arisen about how primary health care could continue to be delivered (Edmunds, 2000).

This time was formative for the nurse practitioner (NP) movement. Although some educators decried the NP movement as a cause designed to encourage nurses to leave nursing to become handmaidens to physicians (Rogers, 1972), many nurses and some nursing leaders believed that this role would breathe new life into the profession of nursing (Ford, 1979).

The NP role and the physician assistant (PA) role paralleled each other in development during the mid 1960s. The two roles were initiated as the result of different factors but were fueled by the desire of medics and nurses in Vietnam to continue to practice in an expanded role in the health care field once they returned home. The role of NPs was developed from the traditional nursing foundation; however, the PA role was defined under the guidance and advocacy of the medical profession. These two routes led to somewhat different experiences in role development and role outcome.

The expanded role of the nurse did not begin with NPs. CNMs and CRNAs had already established their own, very clearly defined roles several decades earlier. The CNS trend in educational preparation grew out of the increased use of registered nurses in high-technology cardiac units, intensive care units, and dialysis units in hospitals at about the same time that the NP role was being initiated in the primary care setting.

What all of these roles had in common was that in each case, clinicians assumed some of the functions traditionally reserved for physicians. As such, they came to be known as *advanced practice roles*.

THE PRESCRIPTIVE AUTHORITY OF NURSES

Changes in Roles for Nurses: When and Why

Advanced practice nurses (APNs) were referred to by a variety of titles, the most lasting of which were *midlevel providers, nonphysician providers*, and *physician extenders*. The first educational programs for providers who sought these new roles had varying names and curricula, awarded different credits, and prepared graduates who exhibited varying skills and competencies.

In contrast to NPs with their primary care focus, CNSs were educated for and practiced primarily in acute inpatient settings and specialty units. As such, although their practice was certainly advanced, they were not responsible for initiating the medical diagnosis and treatment of patients but were true experts in nursing care (Lewis, 1970). They provided advanced consultation and education and conducted research about specific patient problems. This group was frequently the most highly educated of the advanced practice nursing groups in that a master's degree was almost mandatory for entry into the training. However, because they do not directly generate revenue, their role has been difficult to maintain.

Initially, it was unclear whether there would be jobs for any of these nurses with advanced diagnostic and therapeutic training. It was also unclear if they could legally perform some of the tasks that they had been taught to perform. However, the educational programs that were eventually established were highly selective of their students and demanding in their requirements. Students were not allowed to graduate unless they could demonstrate a high degree of competence. Students were typically experienced nurses who were determined to practice nursing in a different way and wanted to make a difference. They were assertive and creative, and they were risk takers (Edmunds, 1978). Because of this combination of experience, competence, and assertiveness, these nurses earned support from patients and grudging acceptance from their physician colleagues.

Although all expanded nursing roles enjoyed an uneasy relationship with medicine during the early phase of their professional development, many physicians assisted in role development by teaching in educational programs and hiring the new types of providers. These physicians clearly came to respect and support the accomplishments of nurses in the advanced practice role. Early antagonism changed to tolerance or acceptance. Then, in the 1990s, new sources of hostility developed among physicians who had once been supportive. The American Medical Association (AMA) began urging physicians to consciously limit further "erosions of their turf" legislatively and professionally, and to view nurses with expanded roles who wanted direct reimbursement for their services as true competitors for patient loyalty and money (Safreit, 1992).

Nevertheless, because of growth in acceptance of the NP role and passage of legal authorization for expanded nursing practice, educational programs thrived. The certificate programs that developed to prepare NPs gave way to university programs, with the understanding that NP education should be attained at the graduate level if it was going to withstand the criticism of physicians. Over time, universities felt the demand from more students who sought entry into NP programs. This led to the development of a multitude of master's degree programs with varying curricula, different standards, and questionable competencies. By 1995, with sudden media attention growing out of health care reform debates, congressional recognition of the NP role, and increased professional visibility for NPs, many other graduate nursing programs were emptying as students rushed to become NPs. This included many of those nurses with preparation as CNSs, who were now seeking retraining as NPs. Capitalizing on increased demand, many facilities changed their admission standards to take advantage of the growing number of NP applicants, some of whom had never even practiced as nurses before they elected to take on this new role. This action by universities did not always consider the market's limited ability to provide a sufficient number of teachers or to hire the increased number of NP students.

In 1996, the American Association of Colleges of Nursing (AACN) released a document called *The Essentials of Master's Education for Advanced Practice Nurses*. The ensuing discussion and acceptance of recommendations in the *Master's Essentials* curriculum led to the notion that almost all nurses with a master's degree were APNs. Thus, the term *advanced practice nurse* lost its ability to denote the CNS, CRNA, CNM, or NP whose role had overlapped so much with traditional physician practice. To distinguish themselves from the now generic title of *advanced practice nurse* used by all nurses with master's degrees, those who assumed tasks usually performed by physicians were referred to by many as APNs, and those in business and industry were described as "nurses with diagnosing and prescribing authority."

Clearly, all advanced practice roles have survived for longer than 40 years because the clinicians who have practiced within them were competent (Brown & Grimes, 1995; OTA, 1986). Patients liked the blend of nursing with the expanded assessment and treatment skills of the new providers. The weight of evidence indicates that "within their areas of competence, NPs and CNMs provide care whose quality is equivalent to that of care provided by physicians. Moreover, NPs and CNMs are more adept than physicians at providing services that depend on communication with patients and preventive actions. ... Patients are generally satisfied with the quality of care provided by NPs ... and CNMs, particularly with the interpersonal aspects of care" (OTA, 1986).

These new providers offered enhanced access to acceptable care, increased productivity, and cost-effective alternatives (OTA, 1986). These behaviors, combined with successful legislative efforts within each state to legally authorize the expanded practice of nurses, ensured survival and growth of the role.

One component of role function, however, with which each of these groups had to grapple was prescriptive authority. Different from CNMs or CRNAs, most NPs thought that they could not fully implement their role or provide services that patients required without being able to prescribe medications (Safreit, 1992). The need for CRNAs and CNMs to have prescriptive authority was less clear. Additionally, some aspects of CNS practice began to move away from hospital-based acute care services and to look increasingly like NP primary care practice. These nurses also desired prescriptive authority. So, these groups of nurses were required to amend the nurse practice acts in all 50 states to obtain broader authority in their new roles and to gain specific authorization to "treat, diagnose, and prescribe." Every state has since addressed this issue, with great variability in the legislation passed. Opening up a nurse practice act for revision was essential but often led to unwanted and unwarranted interpretation or regulation.

LEGAL FOUNDATION OF PRESCRIPTIVE AUTHORITY FOR NURSES IN ADVANCED PRACTICE ROLES

Federal and state statutes and administrative law define control of drugs, including the act of prescribing. How these three elements work together to protect the public has evolved over time. Early regulatory precedents that gave primary prescriptive authority to physicians became a barrier to change for those new health care providers who sought prescriptive authority (Safreit, 1992; Sutliff, 1996).

Role of the Federal Government

Before the turn of the century, no laws were in place to govern the use of drugs. A myriad of elixirs, tonics, and pills that contained any combination of drugs, including opium and cocaine, were sold freely to anyone who was willing to pay the price. It was not until 1906 that the federal government enacted the first law, the Food and Drug Act, which prohibited adulterated or misbranded food or drugs from interstate commerce (Nielsen, 1992).

However, true drug safety was not effectively addressed until 1938, when the U.S. Congress passed the Food, Drug, and Cosmetic Act (21 U.S.C. 301 et seq.), which required drugs to be appropriately tested for safety and labeled with adequate directions for use. However, the explosion of new drug development in the 1940s made the labeling provision difficult to achieve. Thus, the Durham-Humphrey Amendment of 1951 was implemented, creating a separate category of drugs, known as *legend drugs*. Drugs were considered to be legend drugs if they bore the legend, "Caution: Federal law prohibits dispensing without a prescription" (21 U.S.C. 353). These drugs did not require specific package labeling but instead required medical supervision for their sale and use. This act also instituted the process whereby the pharmacist dispensed legend drugs after first obtaining a written prescription from an authorized prescriber (Nielsen, 1992).

The other major piece of federal legislation that affected drug regulation was the Comprehensive Drug Abuse Prevention and Control Act of 1970. This act limited prescribing, dispensing, manufacturing, and distribution to those individuals who were registered with the Drug Enforcement Administration (DEA), an agency of the Department of Justice. It also classified narcotics and other drugs such as depressants and stimulants by their abuse potential, with differing levels of control assigned to each class (Nielsen, 1992). Thus, some legend drugs were further categorized as controlled substances (see Chapter 10 for a classification of controlled substances) and were placed under additional restrictions.

As noted, the DEA *will* register individuals who may prescribe narcotics and other controlled substances. However, registration depends on state authority to prescribe controlled substances. Only health care providers who are granted authority to prescribe controlled substances may be registered by the DEA and receive a DEA number. Consequently, only nurses working in states that grant authority to prescribe controlled substances may receive a federal DEA number. The cost for a DEA number is high and is site specific, so nurses may pay a lot of money if they work in more than one place.

State Control of Prescriptive Privileges

Although the federal government has taken broad control over drug regulation, it has no control over who may prescribe, dispense, or administer drugs (Buppert, 1999). This role belongs solely to the states and is generally addressed in the statutes, rules, and regulations that outline the licensure and scope of practice of specific health care providers. The state law that enables nurses to practice nursing is a legal statute titled the Nurse Practice Act. Nurses are individually licensed by each state in which they practice.

In their efforts to protect a vulnerable and possibly ill-informed public in need of health care, every state has enacted licensing laws for health care providers. If people do not have the information or the ability to make safe judgments about the qualifications and abilities of providers, the state serves as a proxy to gather this information through licensing. Although the state establishes a list of minimum requirements that one must meet to be licensed within that state, meeting these requirements does not necessarily guarantee that the provider is competent. Thus, licensure as a mechanism to protect the public has not been conclusively demonstrated (Bullough, 1980).

Boards of nursing have been somewhat perplexed about how to make certain they are protecting the public safety when the nursing role has changed so dramatically over time. In 1985, the National Council of State Boards of Nursing (NCSBN) adopted a position paper on advanced clinical practice that called for regulations to be adopted within each state that mandates a minimum of master's preparation in a clinical nursing practice specialty, to serve as the basis for advanced clinical nursing practice. NCSBN also mandates recognition of national certification to identify nurses for advanced clinical nursing practice. However, it is clear that use of a national certification examination (established to provide professional recognition) to obtain a license to practice within an individual state is fraught with its own problems (Edmunds, 1992).

Whether traditional registered nurse licensure adequately protects the public when a nurse moves into an expanded role, or whether a second license should be given, is a matter that is still being discussed (Klein, 2007). Nurses with advanced education want legislative parity with physicians, who are not required to obtain additional licenses if they are professionally credentialed in another specialty.

As a result of all these factors, wide variability is seen among states relative to who may prescribe and under what conditions prescriptive authority is granted. In addition, the degree of prescriptive autonomy and authority constantly evolves as new laws are passed and regulations are promulgated.

In their seminal studies, Fink (1975) and, later, Trandel-Korenchuk and Trandel-Korenchuk (1978) attempted to categorize the variations in prescriptive authority allowed in different states as they related to NPs. Essentially, two types of prescriptive authority are afforded to NPs: delegable authority and authority legislated by nursing statutes or regulations. *Delegable authority* requires the nurse to perform under the direction of a physician, mandates the initial physician-patient relationship, and is legally based in medical practice acts. Delegable prescriptive authority can be further delineated into three subtypes: (1) physician determination of patient-specific medications and authorization of the nurse to prescribe accordingly for that patient, (2) standing order/protocols that serve as instructions for prescribing, and (3) renewal of prescriptions by the nurse, based on prescriptions initially ordered by the physician. Without delegated authority, the nurse cannot legally prescribe medications under any circumstances but can recommend nonprescription medications. Although these categories were defined in the 1970s, they are still relevant today, and these differences help to explain some of the barriers to prescriptive authority that have been faced by NPs.

Prescriptive authority has been legislated by the state nurse practice act or by rules and regulations proposed by state boards of nursing and, at times, by medical and pharmacy boards. Two types of prescriptive authority are permitted in nursing legislation. The first type, *dependent authority*, requires that the physician retain ultimate authority through countersignature of prescriptions and/or by a written agreement between the NP and the physician that outlines the need for NP chart review, discussion, and so forth, with the physician collaborator (Bell, 1980). This mode is similar to the delegated authority concept described previously and is practiced in many states. Conversely, *independent authority* allows the NP to prescribe alone. Independent authority may still be restricted, for example, by excluding controlled substances or by limiting drugs to those listed in a formulary.

AN OVERVIEW OF THE PRESCRIBING OF ADVANCED PRACTICE NURSES

Clinical Nurse Specialists

DEFINITION AND SCOPE OF PRACTICE. The clinical specialist in nursing practice is a nurse who, through study and supervised clinical practice at the graduate level (master's or doctorate), has become expert in a defined area of knowledge and who practices in a selected clinical area of nursing (American Nurses Association, 1980).

The role of the CNS embodies a unique combination of tasks. The specialist is prepared to serve as an expert in clinical practice, an educator, a consultant, a researcher, and, often, an administrator. "The boundaries of the specialty are defined by the phenomena of interest to the CNS. These phenomena may change, reflecting the needs of society, and may therefore cause the boundaries to expand" (Sparacino et al, 1990).

EDUCATIONAL PREPARATION AND CERTIFICATION. CNSs constitute a diverse group of nurses whose main commonalities are having a specialty practice and a master's degree. Almost all other components of their program title, curriculum, specialty area, extent of clinical practice, and competency vary according to the philosophy of the university, the individual strengths of the faculty, and the practice site.

Originally perceived as experts in nursing who would provide direct clinical services to patients in tertiary settings and would help other nurses to develop skills in caring for patients with specific problems, CNSs have had their role variously interpreted and accepted (Riehl & McVay, 1973). West Coast hospitals generally have interpreted the CNS role as providing direct one-on-one specialty care to patients and teaching other nurses how to do the same. These nursing roles often became integral to meeting the needs of the institution. East Coast CNSs more frequently define the role as advocating for a particular specialty, such as geriatrics or diabetes, or providing administrative, educational, consultative, or research services within an acute care setting. Because many of the important contributions to patient care that CNSs have made were not billable services for the hospital, CNSs usually were salaried employees and did not bill for their services, thus were not revenue generators. However, they often commanded some of the highest salaries. This made them vulnerable to staffing cuts (Edmunds, 1992). Thus, this role was perceived as a luxury for an institution and often was the first position to be eliminated during times of fiscal austerity.

Many CNSs have had difficulty in finding employment that allows them to use their expertise and education. Their excellent contributions to increasing the quality of nursing care have often been undervalued. Lack of job security and lack of recognition, coupled with the growing demand for NPs, have driven many CNSs into the NP role. This has resulted in virtual NP cannibalization of the CNS role in some geographic areas (Carr, 1996). However, because of the critical care background common to many CNSs, these NPs have begun to return to the hospital in the developing role of acute care NP.

Nurses who electively sit for national certification in a specialty most closely resemble their physician colleagues who become board certified in a particular specialty. This type of certification professionally recognizes the nurse as an expert. This scenario differs from that of other nursing groups such as NPs, who often are required by the state to obtain national certification to be licensed for entry into practice.

STATUS OF PRESCRIPTIVE AUTHORITY. CNSs who were hospital based had no need for prescriptive authority. However, as CNSs left the acute care area to take specialty practice into the home or community, they had an increasing desire to be able to write prescriptions so they could meet the needs of their patients. Currently, CNSs have some form of prescriptive authority in 30 states; in eight of these states, this authority is restricted to those clinical specialists in psychiatric/mental health.

In almost all states in which CNSs have obtained prescriptive authority, this has occurred because they formed coalitions with other APNs and were granted prescriptive authority through those coalitions. In many states, CRNAs, CNMs, NPs, and CNSs all are defined by legislative statute as APNs, and legislation has been written to grant prescriptive authority to APNs—not to individuals with different titles within that category. Because of this, many CNSs acknowledge that they have piggybacked on the efforts of other advanced practice nursing groups within the state to obtain prescriptive authority. In no states have CNSs obtained prescriptive authority while other nurses were denied those privileges (Pearson, 2007). This trend is likely to continue.

No identifiable research studies have focused on CNS prescribing practices. Without research that documents the safety and accuracy of CNS prescriptive authority, few conclusions may be drawn about their practices.

Certified Registered Nurse Anesthetists

DEFINITION AND SCOPE OF PRACTICE. The CRNA is a licensed registered nurse with advanced specialty education in anesthesia who, in collaboration with appropriate health care professionals, provides preoperative, intraoperative, and postoperative care to patients and assists in the management and resuscitation of critical patients in intensive care, coronary care, and emergency situations. Nurse anesthetists are certified after the successful completion of credentials and state licensure review and a national examination directed by the Council on Certification of Nurse Anesthetists (CCNA) (1998). They develop their specialty in anesthesia by completing a graduate curriculum that emphasizes the development of critical judgment and critical thinking. "They are qualified to make independent judgments relative to all aspects of anesthesia care based on their education, licensure, and certification. As clinicians, they are legally responsible for the anesthesia care they provide" (AANA, 1992; AANA website, 2007).

Nurse anesthetists have been providing anesthesia services in this country for longer than a century. Working in conjunction with anesthesiologists, surgeons, and, where authorized, podiatrists, dentists, and other health care providers, nurse anesthetists administer approximately 65% of all anesthetics given each year in the United States. They are found in every setting in which anesthesia is provided and work with every age group and every type of patient. They use the full gamut of anesthesia techniques, drugs, and technology and are the sole anesthesia providers in more than 70% of rural hospitals (AANA website, 2007).

EDUCATIONAL PREPARATION AND CERTIFICATION. Early nurse anesthetists faced a challenge to the legality of their practice when they were charged with illegally practicing medicine in Kentucky (1917) and California (1936). Landmark decisions in these cases established that CRNAs were practicing nursing and not medicine. Today, more than 31,000 CRNAs are practicing throughout the 50 states (AANA website, 2007).

The common denominator for all CRNAs is that they are "anesthesia specialists with a generic foundation in professional nursing" (AANA, 1990). Accredited programs throughout the United States and Puerto Rico have gradually moved to master's degree graduate level education, and half of these programs are located within schools of nursing. Some CRNAs continue to see themselves as nurses, whereas many believe that they have "left nursing" to become specialists in administering anesthesia.

The Council of Accreditation (COA) of Nurse Anesthesia Educational Programs establishes program curricula and accreditation standards for all programs. The educational curriculum consists of 24 to 36 months in an integrated program of academic and clinical study, with COA requiring at least 30 credit hours of formalized graduate study in advanced anatomy, physiology, pathophysiology, biochemistry, physics related to anesthesia, advanced pharmacology, research methodology and statistical analysis, and principles of anesthesia practice. It should be noted that most programs require 45 to 65 credit hours, not 30, in science courses (AANA, 1997).

Students also gain clinical experience by completing residencies in which they are closely supervised as they learn anesthesia techniques, provide anesthesia care to patients, and begin to apply knowledge to clinical problems. COA requires each student to complete a minimum of 450 cases,

and most programs provide about 1000 hours of hands-on clinical experience (AANA, 1997).

Graduates of accredited nurse anesthesia educational programs must meet all requirements prescribed by the COA before they can take the national examination for certification. Passage of this rigorous examination qualifies the graduate for certification as a nurse anesthetist. Every 2 years, the CRNA must meet certain practice and continuing education requirements for recertification (AANA, 2007). As a group, CRNAs are the highest paid of all expanded practice roles with nursing preparation.

AANA (2007) maintains that the CRNA scope of practice includes, among other things, the following:

- Performing and documenting a preanesthetic assessment and evaluation of the patient, including requesting consultations and diagnostic studies; selecting, obtaining, ordering, and administering preanesthetic medications and fluids; and obtaining informed consent for anesthesia
- Developing and implementing an anesthesia plan
- Selecting, obtaining, and administering the anesthetics, adjuvant and accessory drugs, and fluids needed to manage the anesthetic
- Facilitating emergency treatment and recovery from anesthesia by selecting, obtaining, ordering, and administering medications, fluids, and ventilatory support
- Implementing acute and chronic pain management modalities
- Responding to emergency situations by providing airway management, administering emergency fluids and drugs, and using basic or advanced cardiac life support techniques (AANA, 2007)

The 2006 recertification handbook of the CCNA provides the content outline for examination questions used in the national examination (Box 2-1). Approximately 30% of the total questions on the examination are related to the areas of basic science and pharmacology (CCNA, 2006).

STATUS OF PRESCRIPTIVE AUTHORITY FOR THE CRNA. The increasing use of CRNAs in chronic pain clinics and hospice sites has raised the question of whether some CRNAs need prescriptive authority. Whether or not they are providing primary care, CRNAs have been included, often by default, in state legislative efforts directed toward gaining prescriptive authority for other nursing groups.

The federal definition of *prescription* is an order for medication that is dispensed to or for an ultimate user; the definition does not include an order for medication that is dispensed for immediate administration to the ultimate user. Therefore, an order to dispense a drug immediately to a patient who is in bed in a hospital is *not* a prescription (21 CFR 1300.01[b][35]).

Because of this definition, the traditional practice of nurse anesthetists, which involves ordering and directly administering controlled substances preoperatively, intraoperatively, and postoperatively, does not constitute "prescribing" under federal law. Therefore, CRNAs engaged in traditional practice do not need prescriptive authority or an individual DEA registration number to do so (Tobin, 2007). CRNAs engaged in traditional anesthesia practice have no need for a DEA number. However, if the state grants prescriptive authority to CRNAs, and they elect to use

BOX 2-1   Recommended Course Content and Program Competencies in Pharmacotherapeutics for Family Nurse Practitioner (FNP) Programs

RECOMMENDED PHARMACOLOGY COURSE CONTENT

1. Basic principles
   a. Pharmacokinetics—absorption, distribution, metabolism (biotransformation), excretion, bioequivalence, volume of distribution, clearance, half-life, steady state, dosing considerations, therapeutic drug monitoring
   b. Pharmacodynamics—dose-response relationships/therapeutic index, structure-activity relationships, receptors, agonists/antagonists, signaling mechanisms
   c. Adverse drug reactions
   d. Drug interactions—drug-drug; drug-food; drug-disease
   e. Special populations—pregnant mothers, nursing mothers, neonates/children, elderly
   f. Special considerations—self-treatments, alternative therapies, cost, cultural influences, gender, illness, poisoning, abuse, dependence, proper drug administration, genetic and racial effects
   g. Professional roles
   h. Other sources of drug information, evaluation of information, evaluation of drug production/promotion; clinical investigational drug research; patient education, adherence, and participation; monitoring drug effects
2. Prescription writing
   a. Legal considerations
   b. Ethical considerations
   c. Modes of transmitting prescriptions
   d. Minimizing errors
   e. Controlled substances
3. Pharmacotherapeutics of drug groups
   a. Drugs used to manage bacterial, fungal, parasitic, and protozoal infections—cell wall–cell membrane inhibitors, protein synthesis inhibitors, nucleic acid synthesis inhibitors, immunizations, other antiinfective agents
   b. Drugs used to manage cardiovascular conditions—diuretics, angiotensin-converting enzyme inhibitors, centrally acting antihypertensives, adrenergic inhibitors, β-blockers, α-blockers, vasodilators, calcium channel blockers, nitrates and nitrites, cardiac glycosides (digoxin), antiarrhythmics, antihyperlipidemics
   c. Drugs used to manage blood conditions—iron preparations, vitamin B_{12}, folic acid, erythropoietin, anticoagulant agents, antiplatelet agents
   d. Drugs used to manage neuropsychiatric conditions—antiseizure agents, antiparkinsonian agents, antipsychotic agents, mood stabilizers, anxiolytics, hypnotics, dementia drugs, psychostimulants, antidepressants, appetite suppressants, autonomic nervous system drugs
   e. Drugs used to manage pain and inflammatory conditions—opioids, NSAIDs, other agents used to treat pain, anti-gout drugs, muscle relaxants, antimigraine drugs, local and topical anesthetics, nonnarcotic analgesics
   f. Drugs used to manage respiratory conditions—bronchodilators, NSAIDs, corticosteroids, mast cell inhibitors, antihistamines, decongestants, antitussives, antibacterial agents
   g. Drugs used to manage gastrointestinal conditions—H_2 blockers, proton pump inhibitors, antacids, cytoprotectants, antimicrobial agents, anticholinergic agents, laxatives, antidiarrheals, antiemetics, colorectal treatments, stool softeners, prokinetic agents, prostaglandin analog, antiflatulents, emetics
   h. Drugs used to manage endocrine conditions—antithyroid agents, thyroid agents, gonadal hormones, contraceptive agents, pancreatic hormones, diabetic agents, glucocorticoids, antiosteoporosis agents
   i. Drugs used to manage genitourinary conditions—bladder inhibitors, bladder stimulants, prostatic agents, antibacterial agents
   j. Drugs used to manage dermatologic conditions—antibacterials, antifungals, antivirals, ectoparasiticides, sunscreen agents, acne preparations, antiinflammatory agents, antipruritics, prohirsutics, emollients, astringents
   k. Drugs used to manage electrolyte and nutritional conditions—vitamins, minerals, electrolytes, appetite stimulants
   l. Drugs used to manage substance abuse and dependency—smoking cessation aids, alcohol and other drug deterrents

END-OF-PROGRAM COMPETENCY REQUIRED OF FNP GRADUATE

1. Integrates knowledge of pharmacokinetic processes of absorption, distribution, metabolism, and excretion, as well as factors that alter pharmacokinetics, into drug, dosage, and route selection
2. Integrates knowledge of drug interactions in safe prescribing and monitoring practice
3. Detects actual and potential significant drug reactions and intervenes appropriately
4. Incorporates bioavailability and bioequivalence principles into drug selection
5. Prescribes based on appropriate indications for pharmacotherapeutic agents
6. Prescribes therapeutic agents to treat individuals with specific conditions based on factors such as pharmacokinetics, cost, genetic characteristics, etc.
7. Analyzes the relationship between pharmacologic agents and physiologic/pathologic response when prescribing drugs
8. Educates clients about expected effects, potential adverse effects, proper administration, and costs of medication
9. Selects/prescribes correct dosages, routes, and frequencies of medications based on relevant individual client characteristics (e.g., illness, age, culture, gender, and illness)
10. Monitors appropriate parameters for specific drugs

BOX 2-1   Recommended Course Content and Program Competencies in Pharmacotherapeutics for Family Nurse Practitioner (FNP) Programs (Continued)

11. Writes and transmits proper prescriptions that minimize risk of errors
12. Adheres to ethical and legal standards of pharmacotherapeutics
13. Incorporates strategies to improve client adherence to prescribed regimens

14. Consults appropriately when she or he recognizes limitations in knowledge of pharmacotherapeutics
15. Applies current drug information to pharmacotherapeutics
16. Involves client in decision-making process regarding therapeutic intervention, including self-treatment

---

From NCSBN et al (National Organization of Nurse Practitioner Faculties): *Curriculum guidelines and regulatory criteria for family nurse practitioners seeking prescriptive authority to manage pharmacotherapeutics in primary care, summary report, 1998,* HRSA 98-41, Washington, DC, 1998. U.S. Department of Health and Human Services.

prescriptive authority in their practice, they then are subject to DEA registration requirements.

In some states, CRNAs thought that restrictions might be placed on implementation of their role if they were not granted full prescriptive authority. Generally, CRNAs attempt to choose policy or legislative solutions that have the least potential to restrict their practice. Therefore, CRNA groups attempting to determine whether they need prescriptive authority within their states often summarize their arguments as discussed in the following paragraphs.

Possible Benefits of Prescriptive Authority for the CRNA. Acquiring prescriptive authority may enhance professional autonomy and independence, may reduce fears of surgeons about their liability for CRNA practice, may open up future opportunities in pain management clinics, may help reduce bureaucratic red tape, and may resolve issues related to the need for co-signatures.

Possible Disadvantages of Seeking Prescriptive Authority. If lack of prescriptive authority is not really a problem, why raise the issue in other people's minds? If CRNAs introduce legislation for prescriptive authority and this legislation does not pass, does it diminish the implicit authority or perceived competency of CRNAs in the minds of legislators? Is it possible to get legislation passed without making some other compromises that would be troublesome, such as restrictive protocols?

The American Society of Anesthesiologists (ASA) opposes the granting of prescriptive authority to CRNAs, and it has been suggested that they may galvanize other groups against CRNA incursion into this area (Tobin, 2007).

The view of the AANA has been that, whether or not CRNAs need prescriptive authority, independent prescriptive authority enhances the role and so is desirable. It also may alleviate confusion about the exact nature of the authority of CRNAs. However, prescriptive authority is not viewed as an essential component without which they cannot practice (Tobin, 2007). State CRNA chapters vary in their perceived need for prescriptive authority and in terms of their evaluation of the political and professional environment that might bring success to those who seek such authority.

Currently, five states grant independent prescriptive authority to CRNAs (Alaska, New Hampshire, Wyoming, Montana, and Washington). In 19 other states and the District of Columbia, some type of prescriptive authority has been linked to physician control (Tobin, 2007).

Certified Nurse-Midwives

DEFINITION AND SCOPE OF PRACTICE. Nurse-midwifery practice is the independent management of women's health, with a particular focus on pregnancy, childbirth, the postpartum period, care of the newborn, and the family planning and gynecologic needs of women. The CNM practices within a health care system that provides consultation, collaborative management, or referral as indicated by the health status of the client. Certification as a CNM requires education at the postgraduate level in nursing or an allied professional health care field (ACNM, 1992).

The philosophy of the ACNM (ACNM, 2007; ACNM website 2007) emphasizes a focus of the midwife on the needs of the individual and the family for care and physical, emotional, and social support, as well as involvement of significant others in this care according to cultural values and personal preferences. The practice of nurse-midwifery, which is delivered throughout the life span, advocates nonintervention in the normal processes of reproduction and development, as well as health education for women throughout the childbearing cycle. Midwifery has expanded to include gynecologic care of well women throughout the life cycle. Nurse-midwives provide this comprehensive health care, most frequently in collaboration with other members of the health care team.

Women have always taken responsibility for the delivery of children. With the passage of the first medical practice acts in the 1920s, midwives suddenly found themselves directly opposed by obstetricians and legally outside the laws that physicians had crafted. This led to the expansion of formal academic midwifery programs and the requirement for midwives to obtain legal authorization for their services.

In 1963, only 275 nurse-midwives were practicing in the United States. By 2007, that number had increased to more than 7000 CNMs (ACNM website, 2007). Traditionally, CNMs find most of their clients among the indigent, who fear and cannot afford hospital-based obstetric care. Many of these clients have used lay midwives and view birthing as a natural process that should occur under the supervision of women. While continuing to provide care to underserved populations, CNMs now also provide care to women from all cross sections of the country (ACNM, 1997d).

The number of CNM-attended births has increased every year since 1975—the first year that the National Center for Health Statistics began to collect data. In 1998, the most current year for which data are available from the National Center for Health Statistics, 277,811 CNM-attended births occurred in the United States, accounting for 9% of all vaginal births reported that year (ACNM website, 2002).

In addition to more traditional health care settings, some CNMs choose to provide home birth services or work in birthing centers with other CNMs. A collaborative team of CNMs and physicians offers women a combination of primary and preventive care, along with specialized services as needed. The degree of collaboration with physicians depends on the medical needs of the individual woman and the practice setting. Of all visits to CNMs, 90% are made to obtain primary preventive care (70% for care during pregnancy and after birth and 20% for care outside of the maternity cycle). Nurse-midwives on average devote about 10% of their time to direct care of birthing women and their newborns (ACNM website, 2007).

Since the formal inception of the CNM role, extensive research has documented their positive contributions to maternal and fetal care (ACNM, 2007; Clark et al, 1997; MacDorman & Singh, 1998; Oakley et al, 1995; Rosenblatt, 1997). After controlling for a wide variety of social and medical risk factors, the risk of infant death was found to be 19% lower for births attended by CNMs than for births attended by physicians; the risk of neonatal mortality (an infant death that occurs in the first 28 days of life) was 33% lower, and the risk of delivering a low birth weight infant was 31% lower. Mean birth weight was 37 g heavier for CNM-attended births than for physician-attended births. At the same time, CNMs attended a greater proportion of women who were at high risk for poor birth outcome, including African Americans, Native Americans, teenagers, unmarried women, and those with less than a high school education (MacDorman & Singh, 1998).

CNMs were less likely to (1) use continuous fetal monitoring, (2) induce or augment labor, (3) give epidurals, and (4) perform episiotomies. The patients of CNMs were found to have cesarean section rates of only 8.8% compared with 13.6% for obstetricians and 15.1% for family physicians. As a result, CNMs reportedly used 12.2% fewer resources than did their physician colleagues (Rosenblatt, 1997).

EDUCATIONAL PREPARATION AND CERTIFICATION. The ACNM, as the sole professional organization representing CNMs, has crafted the professional direction for midwives. The organization has issued professional standards, program accreditation, and certification standards and has commissioned research and lobbied legislatively on behalf of CNMs.

The ACNM Certification Council oversees the quality and content of nurse-midwifery education programs. The ACNM document *Midwifery Core Competencies Related to Pharmacology* (2000) notes that "prescribing the appropriate medications and treatments during pregnancy, childbirth, [and] the postpartum period, [and] primary health screening of women, family planning, and/or gynecologic services, and [treatment] during perimenopause and postmenopause is an essential component of midwifery education and practice." This knowledge of medications and treatments includes but is not limited to the use of management techniques and therapeutics, such as complementary therapies for which evidence suggests safety and effectiveness, (1) to facilitate the antepartum period and the progress of normal labor, (2) to promote a healthy puerperium and overall health, (3) to treat essentially healthy women with common health problems and gynecologic problems, (4) to meet family planning needs, and (5) to alleviate the discomforts that commonly accompany aging. CNMs also administer local anesthesia, give drugs as needed for emergency

management of the baby at birth, and are knowledgeable about the pharmacokinetics and pharmacotherapeutics of medications commonly used during pregnancy, labor and birth, the puerperium, and the neonatal period, as well as immunizations and medications frequently prescribed for common health problems, family planning and gynecologic care, and as treatment for perimenopausal and menopausal women (ACNM website, 2007).

Students seeking to become midwives who are not already registered nurses but who possess a bachelor's degree in an allied field may attend graduate level midwifery programs and become credentialed as a certified midwife (CM). The ACNM has defended its policy of accepting nonnurses into their programs based on internal research demonstrating that differences in the educational backgrounds of nurses versus nonnurses have not resulted in differences in certification test results. Analysis of certification examination results reveals that degrees do not enhance the clinical competence of a midwife, and they do reflect the ability of both types of programs to prepare competent beginning midwife practitioners. The pursuit of higher degrees by nurse-midwives is encouraged for the purpose of preparing educators, researchers, and theoreticians, because these roles are important for advancing the profession. In 2006, ACNM took the position that a master's degree will be required by 2010 for entry into the CNM role (ACNM website, 2007).

The ACNM Division of Accreditation establishes the criteria for accreditation of educational programs in nurse-midwifery. All ACNM DOA-accredited education programs are affiliated with an accredited university, college, or other institution of higher learning. Currently, 41 ACNM-accredited nurse-midwifery education programs are in place in the United States. Most of these programs offer a master's degree, and four are postbaccalaureate certificate programs. Approximately 68% of CNMs have a master's degree, and 4% have a doctoral degree (ACNM, 2007).

STATUS OF PRESCRIPTIVE AUTHORITY FOR CNMs. Laws and regulations governing the practice of nurse-midwifery are rapidly changing. CNMs are regulated on the state level; therefore, how these professionals practice and interact with other health care professionals, such as physicians, can vary from state to state (ACNM, 2000).

Certified nurse-midwives are legislatively authorized to practice in all 50 states and U.S. territories. In most states, the regulatory agency for the practice of nurse-midwifery is the state board of nursing. As of January 2007, the ACNM website reported that eight states had given limited prescriptive authority to CNMs, 12 states allowed for no prescription of controlled substances, 7 states viewed prescriptive authority as a delegated medical act, and 2 states had regulations pending. Significant overlap in these numbers was noted, with many states reporting limited prescriptive authority and an inability to prescribe controlled substances.

Nurse Practitioners

DEFINITION AND SCOPE OF PRACTICE. Although the term *nurse practitioner* has been debated and criticized because of its similarity to the term *licensed practical nurse*, this title has earned a high degree of acceptability among legislators, educators, and researchers, who now recognize that a different type of nursing service is provided by this group of nurses. Nurse practitioners are those registered nurses who have completed an advanced educational program, usually a graduate master's degree or a post-master's certificate program, that has prepared them to assume responsibility for the health care needs of individuals. This responsibility includes assessment of client status, diagnosis of common acute and chronic problems, and management of care. Most programs have a primary care focus, which implies a continuing health care relationship over an extended period as the nurse listens to, teaches, and negotiates with the patient on how best to maintain health. The 1990s saw growth of the acute care NP, whose role developed following legislation that decreased the number of hours that physicians could work in a week, and after changes in medical school curriculum moved more physicians into the primary care role and away from hospital care. Hospitals have hired an increasing number of acute care NPs over the past 10 years. Acute care NPs have been shown to be a positive addition to many ICUs and specialty services within the hospital setting. Their advanced didactic and clinical training paired with their nursing focus has resulted in a holistic approach to the treatment of acutely ill patients. Although they were initially hired to replace house staff following the Bell Commission recommendations, studies have shown that use of an NP model in the acute care setting results in improved patient outcomes when compared with the use of residents and interns who rotate on a monthly basis through various ICUs and specialty services (Kleinpell & Gawlinski, 2005). In both primary care and acute care, the NP is part of the larger health care team and works collaboratively with other health care personnel in providing care.

The care focus of the NP clearly dictates the curriculum, skills, and focus of the practitioner. In most states, the scope of practice for the NP has been limited to provision of primary care for the age group (pediatrics, geriatrics, adult) or specialty (women's health) for which the NP was prepared.

EDUCATION AND CERTIFICATION. The first NP program began as a pilot study at the University of Colorado. It was the brainchild of Dr. Loretta Ford, RN, and a physician colleague, Dr. Henry Silver. They believed that specially trained master's-prepared nurses could deliver much of the care in pediatric primary care. Their success was touted in many journal articles but was only a step ahead of efforts by other nurses in the country who were, at the same time, seeking to expand their practice. Nurses responded quickly to this new concept. Nurses who felt their skills and knowledge had been underused, as well as those who were dismayed by the lack of recognition, pay, and authority of the registered nurse, flocked to continuing education programs that were set up to accommodate the demand. New programs to educate NPs ranged from 1 week to 18 months. All were unique in design but depended heavily on physician teachers and preceptors. Continuing education programs provided a way for talented nurses from diploma and associate's degree programs to receive this preparation (as they were excluded from participation in the master's programs that were slower to develop). The first 10 years of the NP movement were characterized by so much diversity that a great deal of confusion was seen in the nursing and medical communities about the two different educational entry levels—the continuing education certificate and the master's degree. This caused conflict within the nursing community and made the new role vulnerable to charges from other disciplines that some clinicians were not as well prepared as

others. This educational schism was mended with the agreement by accrediting agencies that all NPs should be master's prepared.

MOVES TO STANDARDIZE CURRICULAR CONTENT. As NP programs became more widely established, it was clear that greater consistency among educational programs would be mandatory if the role was to survive. More careful scrutiny of the preparation of NPs propelled discussions among faculty about what should be done to ensure high-quality programs.

In 1988, the National Organization of Nurse Practitioner Faculties (NONPF) published *Guidelines for Family Nurse Practitioner Curricular Planning*. This was followed in 1990 by *Advanced Nursing Practice: Nurse Practitioner Curriculum Guidelines*, which were prepared to identify essential curriculum content for all NP educational programs. This work was expanded in 1993 and 1994 with the documents *Primary Care Nurse Practitioner Graduate Outcomes* and *Model Program Standards for Nurse Practitioner Programs*. All of these documents circulated within educational groups but did not have a significant impact on the exploding number of curricula. No accreditation of NP programs was available, apart from that granted every 8 years by the National League for Nursing as part of general school of nursing accreditation. In 1995, NONPF issued the publication *Advanced Nursing Practice: Curriculum Guidelines and Program Standards for Nurse Practitioner Education*. This document finally began to attract attention.

During that same year, the AACN began a 2-year effort to establish and define appropriate graduate level nursing curricula. While working in conjunction with NONPF and including many of their recommendations for NP education, AACN issued *The Essentials of Master's Education for Advanced Practice Nursing* (AACN, 1996). All of these documents were written in an attempt to promote standardization of educational requirements essential for the preparation of fully qualified NPs. In April 2002, *Nurse Practitioner Primary Care Competencies in Specialty Areas: Adult, Family, Gerontological, Pediatric, and Women's Health* (USDHHS, 2002) was published; it was updated in 2006. This document has solidified efforts to define and standardize primary care competencies for NPs.

Based on this document, NP curricula assume a bachelor's of science (BS) level foundation of nursing courses and usually experience as a registered nurse. Master's level courses provide as core content advanced courses in physiology, pathophysiology, epidemiology, pharmacology, physical assessment, and diagnosis and management. Additional courses are required to supplement a curricular emphasis on pediatrics, geriatrics, women's health, or another clinical focus. All programs require 500 to 1000 hours of supervised clinical experience as part of the curriculum. Early programs were research focused, and most required a master's thesis or a scholarly paper. The emphasis on evidence-based practice is growing; however, fewer programs today require a formal thesis to demonstrate mastery of the research process (USDHHS, 2006).

With the use of these materials, as of 2002, NPs were expected to master seven domains of competency:
- Management of patient health/illness status
- NP–patient relationship
- Teaching/coaching functions
- Professional role

- Management and negotiation of health care delivery systems
- Monitoring and ensuring quality in health care practice
- Cultural competence (Viens, 2003)

Many of the nurses who wished to become NPs had practiced in critical care areas in the hospital and wanted to return to those settings. This led to the development of acute care nurse practitioner programs, standardized outcome criteria, and certification programs for these individuals.

The educational programs that have been developed for NPs at the master's level are very credit heavy. Most nurses upon graduation assume significantly more professional responsibility. This expanding role of the NP across a variety of settings has led to the development of a clinical doctoral program in nursing at many universities. The AACN now advocates that the entry level for all advanced practice nurses should be the practice doctorate (AACN, 2004).

FAMILY NURSE PRACTITIONER PHARMACOLOGY CURRICULUM RECOMMENDATIONS. Concurrent with attempts to standardize the general NP curriculum, an NONPF task force developed *Curriculum Guidelines and Criteria for Evaluation of Pharmacology Content to Prepare Family Nurse Practitioners for Prescriptive Authority and Managing Pharmacotherapeutics in Primary Care* (NONPF, 1997). This is now available as *Curriculum Guidelines and Regulatory Criteria for Family Nurse Practitioners Seeking Prescriptive Authority to Manage Pharmacotherapeutics in Primary Care* (Yocom et al, 1999). The pharmacotherapeutic preparation of NPs had been one of the most variable components of curricula. A few programs accepted whatever courses nurses had taken in their undergraduate program, whereas other programs required 6 to 7 hours of biochemistry and advanced pharmacology taken with medical students. With more states passing legislation for NP prescriptive authority, NPs wanted to be well prepared for the legal and professional responsibilities associated with writing prescriptions. The move to more clearly specify content in the area of pharmacotherapy was intended to help dispel any criticism that NPs might not have received adequate preparation to prescribe.

CREDENTIALING. As each state determines the requirements for recognizing NPs, differences in scope of practice are evident among the states, although the discrepancies have narrowed over the years. All states have enacted new legislation, have more broadly interpreted their nurse practice acts, or have instituted greater clarity of the NP role through written rules and regulations. Some states require a second license for all those taking on the diagnosing and prescribing roles; other states have required nurses to pass a national certification examination in their area of specialty to obtain state licensure as advanced practice clinicians (Buppert, 1999).

Certification examinations in other health care disciplines are constructed to provide professional recognition to outstanding clinicians. However, NP certification examinations often have been required by the states as a way of attaining entry into practice for the novice and not the peer-recognized clinical expertise of the expert (Bosma, 1997). Most states are moving to require national certification as a minimum requirement for authorization to practice in an advanced practice role. The American Nurses Credentialing Center (ANCC) and the American Academy of Nurse Practitioners (AANP) have developed certification examinations across several specialties over the years. Three other certifying bodies limit their examinations to a selected specialty of NPs. Each certifying agency evaluates the individual NP program curriculum to establish the eligibility of the applicant to sit for a national examination.

Different from PAs, CNSs, CRNAs, and CNMs, NPs have not had a single major professional organization to take the lead in establishing standards, policy, and certification requirements. During early role development, NPs were unable to unite under the umbrella of the American Nurses Association and so fractured into different specialty groups. Each group looked after its own interests. By 1994, 14 major professional organizations had been formed for NPs, with 5 groups offering certification examinations and no groups offering program accreditation. Perceived variability was noted among the certification examinations. Since that time, all credentialing groups have implemented strategies to enhance the psychometric quality of their examinations and to meet similar standards.

Currently, no national policy on NP certification or second licensure is in place (Klein, 2007). In some states, national certification is not required. For those who have passed the examination, the meaning of the credential is more ambiguous than for board-certified physicians. Movement by the NCSBN to set up an interstate compact, whereby states agree to recognize RNs and APNs licensed in other participating states, may lead to more uniform requirements over time and may decrease the disparity in obligations and privileges for nurses from state to state. The compact for APNs is just being instituted, and very few states are currently enrolled.

STATUS OF PRESCRIPTIVE AUTHORITY FOR NPs. Over the past three decades, NPs have steadily gained prescriptive authority on a state-by-state basis through legislative and/or administrative changes in the laws that govern their practice. An annual state survey of NP regulation clearly illustrates the wide variation among states (Phillips, 2007)

All states and the District of Columbia now have granted some form of prescriptive authority to NPs. Five states and the District of Columbia (Arizona, DC, Montana, Oregon, Washington, and Wyoming) have granted full independent prescriptive authority to write prescriptions for all classifications of medications, including controlled substances; thus, no physician-mandated involvement or delegation of prescription writing is required. NPs in 47 states can prescribe all medications, including controlled substances, but require some degree of physician involvement or delegation of prescription authority, and some states limit the quantities prescribed or place other restrictions on the prescribing practices of NPs. In four states (Alabama, Florida, Hawaii, and Missouri), NPs may not prescribe controlled substances but may write prescriptions for legend drugs. In 42 states, the NP prescriber's name must appear on the medication label, whereas in 6 states, the name of the NP is not permitted on the label (Pearson, 2007; Phillips, 2007). Georgia was the last state to grant prescriptive authority. Because of continuing restrictions from the Board of Medicine and delays in enacting regulations, NPs in Georgia are still unable to prescribe medications.

Variability within these categories also exists. The degree of physician involvement may range from a loose collaborative practice agreement with limited oversight to strict physician supervision and review of prescriptive practices. Educational requirements for prescriptive practice also vary widely, with some states requiring only graduation from an approved educational program and/or passage of a certifying examination, whereas others may mandate attendance at yearly continuing education courses or passage of a required pharmacology course (Pearson, 2007).

Protocols, formularies, guidelines, and algorithms developed by various regulatory boards, including the boards of nursing, medicine, and pharmacy, also control the prescriptive practices of NPs in different states. Finally, freedom to prescribe controlled substances varies not only across states but also across the various schedules of controlled substances (Buppert, 1999).

Prescriptive authority within the United States is primarily controlled and regulated by state legislatures and regulatory bodies. They determine the types of drugs to be prescribed, the degree of prescriptive authority to be granted, the regulatory bodies involved in controlling prescriptive practice, and the educational standards that must be met to obtain prescriptive privileges. Changes to prescriptive practices occur through the coordinated efforts of health care providers and other interested groups in working with legislators. Over the years, all 50 states have required consumer, health care provider, legislator, and regulatory body interactions to craft a prescriptive practice environment designed to meet the needs of consumers. How well this has been done and how well the resultant regulations address the concerns of all are variable. The primary differences among states include the degree of professional autonomy or independence recognized by each state and the range of drugs from which NPs are permitted to select.

Safreit, in her exploration of the NP literature from a legal and regulatory vantage point (1992), concluded the following:

> Organized medicine has played a central role in shaping the states' current provisions for APN prescriptive authority. Consistently, individual physicians and medical associations have lobbied against any legislative efforts to acknowledge prescriptive authority as part of the APN's scope of practice. Organized medicine's position on this issue is reflected in the recently adopted AMA state model legislation on the "Regulation of Prescription-Writing Authority of Nurse Practitioners." … [In effect] the model legislation envisions direct physician supervision of the NP, as well as limitations upon the types of drugs the NP may select and the types of patients the NP may prescribe for.
>
> (SAFREIT, 1992)

Although the AMA, the American Academy of Pediatrics, and the American Association of Family Physicians have developed positions designed to control the practice of advanced practice nurses, greater cooperation is seen in other spheres. In 2006, a group of six organizations (including the National Council of the State Boards of Nursing Inc and the Federation of State Medical Boards of the United States Inc) came to an agreement on five assumptions about scope of practice that legislators should use in contemplating changes in scope of practice among health care professionals (NCSBN, 2006). These assumptions, if followed, should provide a rational way for different health care professions to

cooperate in the care of patients. These assumptions include the following:

- The purpose of regulation—public protection—should have top priority in scope of practice decisions, rather than professional self-interest.
- Changes in scope of practice are inherent in our current health care system.
- Collaboration between health care providers should be the professional norm.
- Overlap among professions is necessary.
- Practice acts should require licensees to demonstrate that they have the requisite training and competence to provide a service.

PRESCRIBING CONTROLLED SUBSTANCES

Federal policy has established that only health care providers who are granted prescriptive authority to prescribe controlled substances by the state can be registered by the DEA to obtain DEA numbers. Controversy surrounding the ability of NPs to obtain DEA numbers came to the forefront in 1991, when the DEA published proposed rules and regulations requiring health care providers to have "plenary" (defined as independent) authority to prescribe controlled substances. NPs lacking plenary authority would be defined as *affiliated practitioners* and would be required to use the DEA number of their physician supervisor, with a suffix attached to indicate their affiliated status.

As a result, NPs in many states found that the statutes and regulations governing their practice did not grant independent authority to prescribe controlled substances. For instance, in states that allowed NPs to prescribe controlled substances but required them to use protocols or to establish a written agreement with a physician, NPs were considered to have derived or dependent authority as delegated by physicians and were not considered to have independent authority. According to the DEA, those NPs could not obtain their own federal DEA number.

This action of the DEA created barriers to practice. For instance, the DEA recommendation that an NP should share the DEA number of his or her collaborating physician posed a legal dilemma. NPs who worked with more than one physician also faced logistical issues. In states where NPs were found to lack independent authority, efforts to change these proposed DEA regulations or to establish independent authority within state statutes/regulations were initiated (Buppert, 1999). For example, Maryland NPs responded by writing letters of opposition to the DEA, requested a state attorney general's opinion regarding the status of independent prescriptive authority for NPs practicing in the state, and, finally, supported efforts to clarify statutory language in Maryland regarding independent NP practice.

In response to these and other efforts, the DEA amended the proposed rules and, in June 1993, presented a final rule titled *Definition and Registration of Mid-Level Practitioners (MLPs)* (21 CFR Parts 1301 and 1304 or 58 FR 31171). The specific wording is found in the June 1, 1993, *Federal Register,* and the rule amends Title 21 of the Code of Federal Regulations Parts 1301 and 1304. This rule provided for the registration of all MLPs, including NPs who were authorized by state law to prescribe controlled substances. To differentiate MLPs from other registered providers, the letter M precedes any DEA numbers issued to MLPs. In this way, the DEA has set NPs and other MLPs apart from traditional DEA registrants such as physicians. The DEA considered this necessary because

> ...the controlled substance authority granted to MLPs varies not only from state to state, but often from MLP to MLP within a state at the discretion of the board or of a collaborating physician. The different format registration number serves as an indicator to pharmacists and wholesalers to be alert to the probability that the MLP's controlled substance authority may be subject to specific state restrictions.
>
> (58 FEDERAL REGISTER 31171)

Publication of this rule did not address two ongoing issues in many states related to the inappropriate use of DEA numbers. First, selected insurance companies require all prescriptions to include the prescriber's DEA number as a unique identifier for tracking and billing. Second, some pharmaceutical companies require providers to include their DEA numbers when accepting drug samples. These instances of inappropriate DEA number use have frustrated providers who normally would not find it necessary to obtain a DEA number because their practices do not require controlled substance prescribing.

DISPENSING PRIVILEGES

Traditionally, pharmacists dispense medication based on a prescription from an authorized prescriber. Federal law addresses the labeling and packaging requirements that must be followed. It does not exclude specific prescribers from dispensing medication. Currently, NPs in all states may receive and/or dispense pharmaceutical samples. However, dispensing is often limited to specific sites or circumstances (Pearson, 2007). For instance, in some states, NPs may be able to dispense only samples of medications or may be limited to dispensing at sites located far from pharmacies or within specific types of clinics. Only a few states, such as New Mexico and Arizona, allow unrestricted dispensing of medications.

Prescriptive issues still remain. The question of whether a prescription written by an NP can be filled by a central distribution pharmacy located in a state other than the one in which the NP is licensed had not come up at the time current laws governing pharmacy and pharmacists were written. Therefore, no laws specifically address this issue. The FDA has issued but has not enforced guidelines stating that if a state recognizes a licensed prescriber and no specific regulation is against it, pharmacists in other states should recognize it as legal and fill an out-of-state prescription. However, many of these mail order pharmacies refuse to recognize the legitimacy of an NP prescription. As more and more health plans direct their members to use online or out-of-state mail order pharmacies to fill prescriptions, this is becoming a major problem when the pharmacies refuse to recognize NP prescriptions and delay patients of NPs from receiving needed medications. A search of relevant regulations suggests that only Texas pharmacy law may have some restrictions on whether pharmacists may fill an out-of-state prescription. NPs as individuals and as groups are petitioning both the FDA and the Federal Trade Commission (FTC) for support in requiring pharmacies to follow the previously established regulations and guidelines (see Table 2-1 for nursing summary).

RESEARCH ON THE PRESCRIPTIVE PRACTICES OF ADVANCED PRACTICE NURSES: NPs, CNMs, CRNAs, AND CNSs

Limitations on prescriptive practice can effectively restrict the public's access to affordable and comprehensive primary care delivered by diagnosing and prescribing nurses. Yet, despite the impact that prescriptive privileges can have on access to care, a paucity of research exists on prescriptive practice. What research has been conducted has most often focused on NPs who believed that not having prescriptive authority restricted their ability to deliver needed care.

The first studies of NP prescriptive practices were performed in the early 1980s. One of the largest studies was undertaken by the state of California in 1981 in an effort to guide future legislative initiatives surrounding prescriptive authority for NPs and other midlevel providers. After the prescriptive practices of more than 400 providers at 261 ambulatory practice sites in many underserved areas were evaluated, overwhelming support was revealed for prescriptive authority for NPs and other midlevel providers. All supervising physicians thought that the providers were competent prescribers, and 99% thought they made correct diagnoses. Patient acceptance was also high at 97%. Cost-effectiveness was evaluated as well, and it was found that an additional $2.5 to $3 million would be necessary to provide the same level of patient services if additional time had to be purchased from traditional providers such as physicians. Furthermore, clinic administrators believed that medical services would be sharply curtailed or completely eliminated for significant population groups should prescriptive privileges be denied (Houghland, 1982).

A variety of studies over the intervening years have documented the gradually increasing prescription rate of NPs, particularly expanding the numbers and types of medications for which prescriptions were written (Table 2-2). Scudder (2006) collected data from a national sample of NP attendees at a series of national NP conferences over a 10-year period. The Scudder data, based on a sample of 1399, show the medications currently ordered by this sample of NPs to be fairly consistent with other studies of prescriptive practice of NPs over time (Woodwell, 1997). The Scudder data also demonstrate that NPs frequently recommend OTC products. A total of 93.7% of NPs recommend at least 1 OTC product per day, and 67% recommend 1 to 25 OTC products per day. Seventy-three percent of individuals in the sample had their own DEA number, 11% used a physician's DEA number, and 16% did not prescribe drugs that require a DEA number. (In 10 years, the number of NPs with their own DEA number grew from 33% to 73%. The relatively large number of NPs who do not prescribe drugs requiring a DEA number is not to be interpreted as meaning that those NPs cannot obtain DEA numbers. A large number of NPs who work in employee health, occupational health, or pediatric clinics report that they have relatively low requirements for controlled substances, or they may be in the military or the U.S. Public Health Service and are exempt from DEA registration.) The data also documented that nearly 96% of patients were treated with little or no NP consultation with physicians (Scudder, 2006).

TABLE 2-1   Summary of Pharmacology Preparation and Status of Prescriptive Authority for Diagnosing and Prescribing Nurses

	Nurse Practitioners (NPs)	Certified Nurse-Midwives (CNMs)	Certified Registered Nurse Anesthetists (CRNAs)	Clinical Nurse Specialists (CNSs)
Pharmacology preparation	Pharmacology included in various nursing certificate and master's degree programs; move to require all NPs to have MS degree; NONPF has guidelines for standard NP curriculum; recommendations for FNP pharmacology course content; *Master's Essentials* document specifies advanced pharmacology course; certification exams have pharmacology content, but many exams are available and they vary in quality; exams are not mandatory for all NPs; programs not preaccredited; nursing programs accredited every 8 years by NLN as part of general nursing school reaccreditation	Pharmacology included in various nursing and non-nursing graduate and certificate programs; core competencies described but programs left to determine the content and format of pharmacology content; certification exam has pharmacology content but exam is not mandatory; all programs must be ACNM accredited before students may be admitted and reaccredited on a regular basis; faculty must ensure that students meet competencies for program to retain accreditation	Pharmacology included in various nursing and non-nursing programs; standards and guidelines for accreditation of NA programs describe expectations regarding use of pharmacology in practice, but individual programs are free to determine how to meet those standards; certification exam has pharmacology content and most graduates take the exam; programs must be accredited by AANA before students may be admitted and reaccredited on a regular basis; faculty must ensure that students meet competencies for program to retain accreditation	Pharmacology taught in various nursing master's degree programs; nursing programs accredited every 8 years by NLN as part of general school reaccreditation; advanced pharmacology course recommended by *Master's Essentials* document; content varies widely in practice and by program and specialty; some pharmacology on national certification exams but exam is elective
Status of prescriptive authority	50 states and DC with prescriptive authority with varying levels of restriction	51 jurisdictions with prescriptive authority (including Washington DC, Guam, and American Samoa) with varying levels of restriction	4 states with independent authority; 18 states and DC with dependent authority	30 states with prescriptive authority with varying levels of restriction; in 8 states, authority limited to psychiatric/mental health CNS

TABLE 2-2   Medication Categories Prescribed by Nurse Practitioners (NPs)

Medication Category	1996*	2004*
Antiinfectives	81.4%	89.6%
Diuretics and cardiac agents	60.8%	67.1%
Respiratory	71.3%	76.2%
CNS	41.8%	44.7%
Gastrointestinal	70.0 %	74.5%
Hormones, including OCPs	59.0%	65.5%
Antiinflammatories, analgesics, antipyretics, steroids	80.1%	88.0%
Topicals	74.3%	83.4%
Antineoplastics	4.6%	4.8%
Vitamins, nutritional	59.9%	68.3%

Note: Percents do not total 100 because each NP had multiple responses.
Adapted from Scudder L: Prescribing patterns of nurse practitioners, *J Nurse Practitioners* 2:98-106, 2006; and Edmunds MW, Scudder LC: *Annual descriptive survey of prescriptive practices of nurse practitioners, 1996-1998*, Columbia, MD, 1999, NPAI.

These several studies conducted over the years are remarkably consistent in their findings. NPs tend to order medications appropriate to their preparation as primary care providers and for patients across the age span. NPs are shown to consistently order fewer prescriptions than are ordered by physicians (Woodwell, 1997). A synthesis of the most recent prescribing data suggests that the degree of prescriptive autonomy granted by legislative statutes and administrative regulations has great variability among states, and that overly restrictive regulations harness NP productivity and prevent NPs from making the full contribution to health care for which they are educated (Lugo et al, 2007). Even with severe restrictions, the types and numbers of prescriptions remain relatively stable across regulatory environments, with significant variation noted only in the method used to generate a prescription. Thus, it is difficult to justify imposing strict regulatory limitations on NP prescribing (Safreit, 1992). This conclusion has been shared by an increasing number of state legislative bodies despite consistent attempts by the medical profession to block legislative advances in prescriptive authority.

BARRIERS TO PRACTICE FOR NURSES IN THE DIAGNOSING AND PRESCRIBING ROLES

Four major problems have persisted that prevent the full implementation of APN roles:

1. Regulatory irregularity among the states in authorizing practice continues to be a major problem for a profession that is fairly mobile. The differences in definitions, standards, and scope of practice and restrictions defined by a

nurse practice act vary from state to state and impose difficulties on health professionals as they move to a new state, practice in neighboring states, or provide services over the Internet. The NCSBN has instituted an interstate nursing compact that would help solve some of these problems. A multistate license would allow a nurse to practice in all states that sign on to an agreement, so that separate licensure for the nurse would not be required in each state (Sharp, 1997). Requirements for a second license for APNs have been discussed for years (Edmunds, 1992) and continue to remain an issue (Klein, 2007; Robinson et al, 1996; Sharp, 1997).

2. Antagonism has increased among organized medical groups competing with APNs for patients. A fairly large group of very experienced CNMs and NPs, some with 40 years of experience, now exists. These nurses are ready to be more independent and want to receive direct reimbursement for the care they provide; they do not want to remain salaried employees of the physician. These nurses have made major contributions to the services of many hospitals and practices, but most have not participated in the financial rewards. Lack of direct reimbursement to NPs for their services has been tied to conflict over who is designated as a primary care provider. For many years, NPs were designated as primary care providers for Medicaid patients (the poor) and for children in school-based clinics. However, with recent linkage of Medicare reimbursement and managed care panel status to the primary care provider designation, physicians are rethinking whether NPs should be able to get direct reimbursement rather than having all reimbursement money go through them (Edmunds, 2000).

3. The growing number of NP graduates, some without previous nursing experience, is of concern to those NPs already in clinical practice. The profusion of NP programs, the reduced faculty numbers, and difficulty in obtaining adequate clinical experiences for all students mandate careful consideration of the quality and competency of student educational preparation. Although quality is always important for individuals, it is also essential for the collective, because charges of malpractice for one may affect the ability of many NPs to practice. Competency is imperative because malpractice insurance companies who have charged nurse practitioners the same low rates for insurance as nurses have discovered that if NPs do many of the same things as physicians, they probably should be charged the same rates for malpractice insurance (Miller, 2006). An escalation of rates would force many NPs from the market.

4. As a way of generating huge revenues, the AMA has sold personal information regarding member and nonmember physicians to pharmaceutical companies for many years. Pharmaceutical companies use this information to help track through pharmacies the numbers and types of medications physicians prescribe and to design specific marketing strategies that are based on physician prescribing behaviors (Barclay, 2007). NPs have been unable to obtain equivalent prescriber numbers and so do not participate in the research that underlies this type of data collection. Although NPs would not be any happier than physicians to have their personal information sold, lack of participation in this system has made it difficult for NPs to have

comparable documentation of what medications they prescribe and the safety and competency with which they provide it.

5. Federal Pharmaceutical Drug Manufacturers Association (PDMA) legislation mandates that every year pharmaceutical companies must validate that all health care providers with whom they leave drug samples are licensed prescribers and are legally eligible to receive drug samples. This information is readily available for physicians (through the purchase of information licensed by the AMA and other validation companies) but is difficult to obtain for nurses. Additionally, because NPs do not have independent prescriptive authority in all states but often have delegated prescribing authority, an NP may not be validated in those states without validating the physician with whom they practice. Drug representatives seek to obtain validation information from NPs before they can leave samples, including information about their physician colleague. Some NPs do not understand that this is a federal mandate, and that the pharmaceutical companies are trying to find a way to give them information that the boards of nursing do not make available. If NPs refuse to give the information, then drug representatives have no recourse, and the NPs do not get drug samples for their patients (Edmunds, 2006).

PRESCRIPTIVE AUTHORITY AND THE PHYSICIAN'S ASSISTANT

Over more than 40 years of clinical practice, physician assistants (PAs) have gained considerable legitimacy and widespread acceptance as a profession in the American health care system. In 1965, new state health occupation regulatory acts became necessary with the introduction of PAs to allow them to perform tasks that were traditionally included in the domain of medicine. With nearly all states now legislating prescriptive authority to PAs, an estimated 95% of clinically active PAs have some authority to prescribe (Wing et al, 2004). Legislative and regulatory changes in state medical practice acts made to accommodate PA practice included defining the required qualifications for occupational licensure or certification, defining scope of practice, developing supervisory stipulations, establishing board representation and governance policies, creating professional disciplinary standards, and granting prescribing authority. Often, acts authorizing prescribing authority for PAs were the most difficult to obtain; they typically required separate legislation.

Acceptance of PAs by U.S. physicians, patients, and other health care professions has grown steadily. PAs have proved to be safe and effective health care providers (Hooker & Berlin, 2002; OTA, 1986). PAs demonstrate versatility across clinical practice settings and are employed in private medical offices, teaching and community hospitals, managed care delivery systems, and other health care settings. The medical generalist orientation of PAs allows them to assume functions effectively—not only in primary care roles, but also in inpatient care services and medical specialty practices. Increasingly, PAs are assuming roles in specialties and subspecialties (Cawley & Hooker, 2006).

Prescribing authority for PAs was won through legal and political maneuvering on a state-by-state basis over the past four decades. It has been a long but successful trip to increased recognition of the skills and contributions of the PA.

Overview of the PA Role

PAs are health care professionals who practice medicine under physician supervision. As members of the health care team, PAs provide a broad range of medical diagnostic, therapeutic, and preventive care services. PAs are qualified by formal education and are authorized by national certification to exercise a designated level of autonomy in performing clinical responsibilities within their scope of practice and supervisory relationship. PA clinical practice spans primary care and specialty care roles in a wide range of medical practice settings in rural and urban areas. In addition to their clinical roles, PA professional responsibilities may include providing health care services that complement physician services, such as health promotion and disease prevention, and/or assuming educational, research, and/or administrative duties (Cawley, 2002; Hooker & Cawley, 2003; Jones & Cawley, 1994).

All states have specific requirements for the PA who is seeking entry into practice. Typically, individuals must be graduates of a PA educational program accredited by the Accreditation Review Commission for the Physician Assistant (ARC-PA), and nearly all states require that they possess certification from the Physician Assistant National Certifying Examination (PANCE), the national certification examination administered by the National Commission on Certification of Physician Assistants (NCCPA).

PA educational programs comprise intensive 2- to 3-year biomedical curricula emphasizing a primary care/medical generalist approach. Nationally, PA educational programs do not award a single academic credential, although there has been a marked trend toward the master's degree. Traditionally in PA education, the competency-based model of PA qualification for medical practice has been demonstrated by completion of an approved educational program and receipt of national board certification, rather than by a process tied to a specific academic degree. This format has gained acceptance among medical licensing boards and occupations regulators, but pressure for a standard academic degree awarded for PA education has increased in recent years. Thus, a PA may receive an associate's, a bachelor's, or a master's degree for completion of a PA educational program. In 2007, 135 ARC-PA–accredited PA educational programs were available—an increase from 107 in 1998. More than 100 programs, many of which have been implemented during the past decade, now award the master's degree. A shrinking number of programs continue to award the bachelor's degree or a certificate or an associate's degree. PA programs, which are sponsored by universities, academic health centers, medical schools, teaching hospitals, and colleges, graduate approximately 4700 students annually (Simon & Link, 2006).

The mean length of PA training is 26 months and resembles a shortened version of medical school. Education typically is conducted in two phases—didactic and clinical. PA didactic training usually comprises 10 to 12 months of academic coursework with instruction in (1) the basic sciences—anatomy, physiology, biochemistry, microbiology, pathology, and pharmacology, and (2) the basic clinical sciences—history taking and physical examination, behavioral science, clinical medicine, and diagnosis, including pharmacologic aspects of patient management.

Because knowledge of pharmacology is a required component of practice for a PA, ARC-PA–accredited PA programs must include formal course instruction in basic and clinical pharmacology. ARC-PA standards mandate that PA programs must teach "the principles of clinical pharmacology and medical therapeutics appropriate to the medical therapy for common problems in clinical practice" (ARC-PA, 2006). PA clinical rotations and preceptorships stress the appropriate use of drugs and medications as part of patient care management. A national survey of PA educational programs in 1998 revealed that the typical PA student received an average of 78 hours of instruction in pharmacology, with a range of 28 to 128 hours (Simon & Link, 1998). The University of Utah has developed a model clinical therapeutics curriculum that is used by a number of PA programs.

The national certifying examination for PAs, the PANCE, comprises a written multiple-choice question component, with test item content and scoring standards developed by the National Board of Medical Examiners (NBME). The NCCPA has administered this examination since 1973, and NCCPA certification is required for PA qualification in 49 states. More than 92% of the 60,000 PAs in active clinical practice in 2007 held NCCPA certification (AAPA, 2006).

PANCE question item content assumes that PAs possess academic and clinical training in patient pharmacologic management. On any given PANCE administration, 32% to 38% of the examination items relate to pharmaceutical aspects of patient care management (National Commission on Certification of Physician Assistants, 1996). To meet requirements for continuing certification, NCCPA mandates that PAs must obtain 100 hours of continuing medical education (CME) hours annually and must be recertified by formal examination (the Physician Assistant National Recertifying Examination [PANRE]) every 6 years. Nineteen states require PAs to maintain ongoing NCCPA certification, and a number of states have similar CME requirements for PAs to maintain state licensure. Some states require PA to obtain specific CME credits in pharmacologic patient management prior to being granted prescribing authority.

Legal Foundation of PA Prescriptive Authority

Working with supervising physicians, PAs perform a wide range of delegated medical diagnostic and patient management tasks required in primary care and specialty practice settings, including prescribing medications. Although their clinical practice duties overlap considerably with those of physicians, PAs work in a dependent practice mode.

Initial PA statutes took a delegatory or a regulatory direction. Some states passed PA statutes that were broad in nature. On a fundamental level, they simply affirmed the notion of physician task delegation without providing any specific delineation of the performance of those tasks (delegatory model). Other states enacted laws that accepted the principle of physician task delegation as the basis of PA practice but went further in placing certain stipulations on PA scope of practice and medical task performance (regulatory model). The clear pattern among most states has been toward the regulatory model (Gara & Davis, 2003). State regulatory agencies now tend to recognize prescribing activities of PAs within circumscribed boundaries as an essential component of their modern practice roles (Hansen, 1992; Sekscenski et al, 1994).

Approval of PA prescribing authority has been controversial in some states. In a comparative analysis of state regulatory experiences and policy approaches authorizing PA prescribing, Cohen (1996) found that experiences and policy varied widely. Prescribing was a particularly troublesome barrier to PA practice effectiveness in states such as Maryland and Ohio. A key determinant in the outcome of whether prescriptive authority would be granted was the position of the involved stakeholder groups (medical societies, nursing groups) (Cohen, 1996).

A major aspect of treatment that has limited PA practice is lack of full prescriptive authority. When legally authorized, the privilege of prescribing is usually a restricted one. Because medication is the most frequently employed treatment in medical care, the absence of this privilege limits the scope of medical practice; it restricts where and how PAs can practice. For years, the issue of prescribing privilege was a significant concern of the PA profession. Resolution of prescribing has assured physicians, managers, administrators, and policy makers in the larger health care community about PA safety and effectiveness in that PAs are less costly substitutes for physicians in a variety of clinical situations.

Statutes authorizing state medical and health occupation boards to regulate medical practitioners constitute the legal basis for PA prescribing activities. Typical state regulatory acts establish PAs as the agents of their supervising physicians, and PAs maintain direct liability for the services they render to patients. Supervising physicians define the broad parameters of PA practice activities and the standard to which PA services are held and are vicariously liable for services performed by their PAs.

The legal basis of PA practice is predicated on the doctrine of *respondeat superior*, which affirms and defines the authority of a licensed physician to delegate medical tasks to a qualified health professional working in that practice. A key stipulation is that the physician must appropriately supervise PA practice activities and must assume liability for any adverse actions (Hooker & Cawley, 2003). State health occupations regulatory policy emanating from this tenet has evolved with the stipulation that physician–PA practices should be required to appropriately define the clinical role, activities, prescribing activities, and terms of supervision of the PAs employed (Gara & Davis, 2003).

Most states in which PAs are legally authorized to prescribe have constraints on their prescribing. Such constraints may include the following:

- A physician co-signature is required within a given time frame on an order for inpatient medical or therapeutic orders. (There is a trend to do away with co-signature requirements because in most cases, these have been shown to be unwieldy to enforce and do not enhance patient safety.)
- Limitations are placed on the categories of medications that may be prescribed, that is, drugs delineated in a specific formulary or medication list.
- FDA Schedule II agents (i.e., those defined by the Controlled Substances Act as having the potential for abuse) are excluded from prescriptive authority.
- Prescribing authorization is granted only when drug treatment protocols are used.
- Limitation is placed on the quantities of drugs that may be prescribed by PAs; a few states have limited prescribing

authority to specific medical practice settings (Ohio, Maryland) or to an outpatient or nonhospital setting.

Among the states with prescribing regulations in place, most now grant PAs prescribing privileges for Schedule II through Schedule IV drugs in addition to "prescription legend" drug preparations. Schedule I drugs are not relevant to this discussion because it is illegal for licensed practitioners in the United States to prescribe these drugs. The prescribing privilege for Schedule II drugs is a limited one in about six states. In the other states, the prescribing privilege applies to Schedule III through Schedule V drugs, including prescription legend drugs, with some restrictions by various states on prescribing Schedule III drugs.

Drug preparations referred to as *prescription legend drugs* can be prescribed by PAs with prescribing privileges. PAs also may prescribe OTC medications and drug preparations that do not, by law, require the written order of a licensed prescriber.

History of PA Prescriptive Authority Among States

The first statute authorizing prescribing privileges for PAs was passed in Colorado in 1969. That statute stipulated that graduates of the University of Colorado Child Health Associate Program (one of the first academic health center–based PA programs offering a focus in pediatrics) could prescribe medications without immediate consultation from a supervising physician, provided that the latter subsequently approved the prescription. New York authorized PA prescribing privileges in 1972; later, Maine, New Mexico, North Carolina, Oklahoma, and Kansas followed. By 1979, PA prescribing privileges had been granted in 11 states. The preponderance of states passed PA prescribing authority in the 1980s and 1990s.

Currently, PAs are recognized as health care practitioners authorized to perform physician-delegated medical diagnostic and therapeutic tasks (diagnosis, testing, treatment, and follow-up of patients) by professional licensing boards in all 50 states, Guam, and the District of Columbia. Mississippi in 2000 was the last state to formally recognize PA practice. The website of the AAPA has a table listing that outlines the dimensions of prescriptive authority on a state-by-state basis. This website is updated regularly to reflect changes in prescriptive authority.

All except one state (Indiana) has authorized the supervising physician to delegate prescriptive responsibility to PAs, and 40 states include controlled substances in that authorization. Although some states initially required that PAs use the supervising physician's DEA registration number when prescribing controlled medications, all states that allow PA prescribing of controlled substances now authorize PAs to obtain their own DEA registration. Since 1997, the DEA has required that PAs who prescribe should obtain a DEA number, and virtually all state regulations contain that specific requirement.

PAs are authorized by statute or regulation to prescribe in the aforementioned states, as well as in Guam, the District of Columbia, and most federal facilities, including the military, state and federal correctional institutions, and the Veterans Administration. Box 2-2 lists the details on prescriptive authority among the different states. In most states, PAs are authorized to write prescriptions if the supervising physician

BOX 2-2 Common State Requirements for Physician Assistant (PA) Prescriptive Authority

- Co-signature requirements
- Restriction to formulary; exclusionary formulary
- Controlled substances (Schedule II medications)
- Restriction by practice setting
- Required practice guidelines/management protocols
- Educational requirements
  - Minimum academic degree
  - Continuing medical education

agrees to delegate this responsibility. In general, PAs are authorized to sign prescriptions using their own names and prescription pads that bear the names of themselves and the supervising physician. Often, this permission must be explicit and must be provided in writing. PA laws and/or regulations dealing with prescribing typically indicate which types of medications a PA may prescribe, usually meaning limited to noncontrolled substances or including controlled substances. In some instances, a formulary limits the types of medications that the PA may prescribe. In 44 states, the PA can prescribe controlled substances. Among these states, 29% percent permit PAs to prescribe Schedules II through V, occasionally with a limitation on the supplies of Schedule II drugs.

The authority to dispense medications is also regulated by the state. Pharmacists typically have strongly defended their rights in terms of dispensing and insist that prescribing and dispensing activities be separately regulated. In 28 states, physicians have the authority to delegate dispensing privileges to PAs. PAs dispense medications from office supplies in some practices, most commonly those set in rural clinics or in states that do not specifically prohibit dispensing. In most jurisdictions, giving patients drug samples that have been supplied by a drug company is not the same as dispensing (Gara & Davis, 2003).

PAs prescribe in a wide variety of settings, yet only a small quantity of empirical data on how and when PAs prescribe has been gathered. Studies of patient expectations and satisfaction levels affirm the notion that PAs are expected to perform prescribing activities as part of their role in patient management. One survey administered to PAs working in states with prescriptive authority found that 90% of PAs included prescriptive authority as part of their authorized clinical duties (Willis, 1990).

Nationwide, PAs are estimated to manage more than 221 million patient visits and to write 278 million prescriptions yearly. This amounts to nearly 10% of all prescriptions written annually (AAPA, 2006a). Among the medications most commonly prescribed by PAs are antihypertensives, cholesterol-lowering agents, bronchodilators/respiratory therapy agents, agents to treat diabetes, gastrointestinal medications, and oral contraceptives.

Sixty percent or more of PAs have reported prescribing urinary/vaginal agents, upper respiratory medications, gastrointestinal agents, antiarthritic anti-gout agents, and analgesics. The mean number of prescriptions written by each PA was 50 per week (AAPA, 2006a).

In 2007, the 49 states with PA prescribing privileges (only Indiana lacks prescribing authority) encompassed more than three fourths of the practicing U.S. PAs, covering approximately 75% of the total U.S. population. New York has long permitted physicians to delegate prescribing privilege to the PAs they supervise.

PA professional practice activities, including prescribing activities, tend to be closely regulated by health occupations licensing agencies, most commonly boards of medicine. In some instances, PA and other health occupation regulation is assigned to boards of professional regulation, education, or the healing arts. In 11 states, specific PA licensing boards are in place.

Organized medicine has also played a pivotal role in state regulation of PA practice. Physicians wrote many of the early PA laws because no PAs were available to write them. As the profession grew, predictable strife over how PAs would fit into the health care system was noted. In some states, organized medicine was the state PA chapter's strongest ally; in others, it was their most significant opponent.

In many states, the state medical society is regarded as the voice of medicine. As state legislators considered bills that modified PA regulation and delegated scope of practice, they commonly asked, "What's the medical society's position on this bill?" During the past decade, state medical societies have shown an increased willingness to work as colleagues with PA state societies on health law issues. Today, 42 state PA organizations have sustained relationships with their respective state medical societies (Davis, 2002). This increased level of communication has had a positive impact on the development of state laws and regulations governing PA practice.

Policies of organized medicine on the national level have also played a significant role in state regulation of PA practice over the past 10 years; this is the result of stable and productive relationships with physician leaders. In 1995, the AMA issued guidelines that offered a framework for physician–PA practice; these were adopted as policy by many state medical societies and were used as a default position by others (Davis, 2002).

Research on Prescriptive Practices of PAs

In general, there is a paucity of empirical data on the prescriptive practices of PAs. The only significant study on NPs and PA prescribing was undertaken in a large health maintenance organization. In this study of primary care providers, the annual rate of prescribing was higher for NPs than for adult care physicians by 4%, and PA rates were higher than those for the same cohort of physicians by 9%. Some of the differences could be explained by the type of care that was provided: NPs were providing a large percentage of wellness care for patients, PAs saw more acute problems than chronic ones, and physicians managed more complex patients (Cipher et al, 2006).

Cipher and colleagues (2006) analyzed data from the National Ambulatory Medical Care Survey from 1997 through 2003 and found that prescribing patterns among PAs, NPs, and primary care physicians were similar. The characteristics of all patients seen were similar in terms of geographic region of visit, age, and gender but differed by ethnicity and race. An NP or a PA was the provider of record for 5% of the primary care visits in the National Ambulatory Medical Care Survey (NAMCS) database. The three clinician types were likely to write at least one prescription for

70% of all visits, and the mean number of prescriptions was 1.3 to 1.5 per visit (range, 0 to 5) depending on the provider. PAs were more likely to prescribe a controlled substance for a visit than was a physician or an NP (19.5%, 12.4%, and 10.9%, respectively). Only in nonmetropolitan settings did differences emerge. NPs who worked in rural areas wrote significantly more prescriptions than did physicians and PAs (Cipher et al, 2006).

Legislative Progress

Overly restrictive legal stipulations on prescriptive authority have kept PAs from completely implementing their roles in many settings. Barriers to prescriptive authority increase the costs associated with PA utilization if a physician must also be consulted and may deter PAs from practicing in certain states and/or serving medically needy populations. Inconsistency in state medical practice acts, lack of prescriptive authority, and the absence of Medicare and private third-party reimbursement that affects many rural ambulatory practice settings have been shown to restrict PA utilization (Hansen, 1992). The AAPA has developed model guidelines for state practice acts governing PA practice and prescribing activities to try to enhance PA practice flexibility and standardization among states (AAPA, 2006a).

On the public policy level, barriers to practice that once existed now have largely been resolved. The medical, legal, and economic factors that formerly presented obstacles to PAs in performing the full range of clinical tasks for which they are both educated and certified no longer exist in most instances. States, through their health occupation licensing boards, have considerable control over the qualification requirements and practice activities of PAs, as well as those of physician and other nonphysician health providers such as NPs. State authority in regulating PA and NP health providers permits boards to define provider scope of practice, determine physician supervisory requirements, authorize prescribing activities, and establish and enforce standards of professional conduct and disciplinary procedures.

A number of clinical practice factors have been identified for which PAs could be better used in health service delivery (Hansen, 1992). For example, with the growing need for more providers to care for geriatric and nursing home care patients, nonphysicians were viewed as playing an increasingly important role in service delivery. However, a recent review of the PA and nonphysician literature on their utilization in geriatric care settings shows that they are not being used as anticipated because of the many legal and regulatory barriers that limit what nonphysician providers can do, including restrictions on prescribing authority (Sekscenski et al, 1994).

Delegation of prescribing authority to PAs has been viewed by some physicians as empowering PAs in establishing patient relationships and reducing the power of the physician in that same relationship (Hooker & Cawley, 2003). Whether this desire to retain the sole privilege of prescriptive authority arises from the traditional power of the role or from economic or political factors, physicians have been reluctant to share this prescriptive prerogative with newcomers to health care. Regardless of the preparation of the new providers, it is difficult to make changes in the status quo. That so many states have been willing to permit delegation of this authority to PAs and other nonphysician providers attests to the success that nonphysicians have exhibited in drug prescribing. In fact, no suggestion can be found in the research literature that nonphysicians do not perform well in meeting the medication requirements of patients (OTA, 1986).

A number of reasons have been advanced as to why state regulatory agencies have limited the prescribing privilege of PAs. One reason, cited early in the development of the PA role, is that PAs were not sufficiently trained to be competent prescribers. Further, because the agencies that regulate PA practice historically have comprised largely physicians, concern has arisen about the potential of increased legal liability of supervising physicians associated with the practice of the PA. Physician reluctance can also come from various cultural and/or gender biases. Another possible reason why these agencies may limit or deny prescribing privileges to PAs is the opposition of other health care professionals (namely, nurses and pharmacists) (Cohen, 1996).

Another possible reason for limiting prescribing privilege is largely economic. The initial purpose for developing the PA role was to alleviate a shortage of physician services. In more recent years, and with the advent of a more abundant supply of physician services, the distinction between whether PAs complement physician services or are alternatives for physician services is less clear. The latter quandary over role function implies that PAs are currently viewed as being in competition with physicians for patients (Grumbach & Coffman, 1998). In fact, PAs maintain they do not compete with physicians but instead work with physician practices to enhance and expand medical care services.

ACKNOWLEDGMENTS

The author James Cawley acknowledges the contributions of Howard Cohen, JD, MA; Roderick Hooker, PhD, PA-C; David Mittman, PA; and Nicole Gara in the preparation of the PA information included in this chapter.

evolve A continually updated list of useful WebLinks may be found in the Evolve Resources at http://evolve.elsevier.com/Edmunds/NP/

evolve http://evolve.elsevier.com/Edmunds/NP/

General Pharmacokinetic and Pharmacodynamic Principles

A *drug* is any substance that is used in the diagnosis, cure, treatment, or prevention of a disease or condition (McKenry et al, 2005). This is a general definition that is not very useful because of the great diversity of characteristics and actions of drugs. To be more precise, *pharmacokinetics* is the study of the action of drugs in the body, including the processes of absorption, distribution, metabolism, and elimination. It may be thought of as what the body does to the drug. *Pharmacodynamics* is the study of the biochemical and physiologic effects of drugs on the function of living organisms and of their component parts (Brunton et al, 2005). It includes consideration of the mechanisms of drug action and may be viewed as what the drug does to the body.

These concepts are essential to an understanding of the prescribing role. Although many readers of this text may have had extensive experience in administering drugs, mastery of the content in this chapter is mandatory before moving to the more advanced role of drug prescriber. This chapter therefore is one of the most important in the book and presumes an extensive understanding of the scientific principles of biochemistry, anatomy, physiology, and pathophysiology. The information in this chapter is necessary for the provider to progress from memorizing drug names (an increasingly difficult task) to understanding the process of drug utilization and being able to generalize from basic principles. It will be important to read this chapter more than once and to try to apply the principles to specific drugs. Not everything can be absorbed in one sitting.

A good understanding of physiology is necessary before one can understand the mechanisms of drug actions. The reader may find it useful to review relevant physiology before undertaking the study of a class of drugs. This chapter attempts to express clearly and simply some of the more complex principles of pharmacokinetics. Definitions or concepts that are important in the understanding of pharmacotherapeutics are emphasized. It is written at a deceptively simple level to help clinicians clearly understand major concepts that are commonly overlooked or those that are skimmed quickly but never really mastered.

DRUG NOMENCLATURE

Drugs have three names: chemical name, generic name, and trade, or brand, name. The *chemical name* describes the drug's chemical composition and molecular structure. The *generic name*, or *nonproprietary name*, is the official name assigned by the manufacturer with the approval of the U.S. Adopted Name Council (USAN) and is the name listed in pharmacology reference books (McKenry, et al, 2005). The *trade name*

is the patent name given to the medicine by the company that is marketing the drug. If more than one company manufactures the drug, then the drug will have more than one trade name, thus adding to the confusion. Trade names are usually simpler and easier to remember than generic names because drug companies want you to remember their name and to use their drug. The generic name often will identify the type of drug that it is and thus will reveal the therapeutic effect. For example, it is important to identify a β-blocker by the similar sounding generic names, such as atenolol, metoprolol, or propranolol, vs. learning the trade names (Tenormin, Lopressor, and Inderal, respectively). Providers should refer to drugs by their generic names when communicating with patients and other health care providers. This is very important with OTC medications because the contents of trade name products may vary.

PHARMACOKINETICS

Pharmacokinetics focuses on the processes concerned with absorption, distribution, biotransformation (metabolism), and excretion (elimination) of drugs (Figure 3-1).

Absorption

Absorption describes how the drug leaves its site of administration. The bioavailability of the product is what is most important clinically. *Bioavailability* is how much of the drug that is administered reaches its site of action (Brunton et al, 2005). The fraction of the drug that reaches the systemic circulation is called the *f value*. After a solid or liquid drug has been orally ingested, the drug must break up (disintegrate) and then become soluble in body fluids (dissolution) before the process of pharmacokinetic absorption begins (Stringer, 2005).

Bioequivalence is an issue with generic vs. trade drugs. *Bioequivalence* means that two drug products (1) contain the same active ingredients; (2) are identical in strength or concentration, dosage form, and route of administration; and (3) have essentially the same rate and extent of bioavailability (Brunton et al, 2005). Although a generic drug may have the same amount of drug, because of variability in the way the medication is manufactured, slightly more or less drug may be bioavailable. Legally, the drug must be ±20% of the proprietary drug. This variance becomes a concern with certain drugs, especially when the therapeutic window is narrow (e.g., Lanoxin vs. digoxin). Avoiding variation and complying with preferred drug formularies are the major reasons for ordering "Dispense as written" trade name prescriptions.

	Absorption	Distribution	Biotransformation	Elimination
SITES	Gut ⟶ Plasma	Plasma ⟶ Tissue	Liver	Kidney
CONCEPTS	Bioavailability	Volume of distribution	Enzyme inhibition/ induction First-pass effect	Clearance Half-life Steady state Linear/nonlinear kinetics
	Factors: Drug characteristics Blood flow Cell membrane	Phases: 1. Blood flow from site of administration 2. Delivery of drug into tissues at site of drug action	Phase 1: Oxidation Cytochrome P450 Phase 2: Glucuronidation	

FIGURE 3-1   The process of pharmacokinetics.

FACTORS THAT AFFECT ABSORPTION. Four primary factors must be considered in evaluating drug absorption: drug characteristics, routes of administration, blood flow, and cell membrane characteristics.

Drug Characteristics. The following list includes some general drug characteristics relevant to all routes of administration. (Other factors are discussed under the specific route of administration.)

- *Formulation of the drug*—influences dissolution rate of solid form of drug
- *Concentration of the drug*—the higher the concentration, the more quickly the drug is absorbed
- *Lipophilic drug formulations are more readily absorbable*—Nonionized drugs are more lipid soluble and may readily diffuse across cell membranes. Ionized drugs are lipid insoluble and nondiffusible.
- *Acidic drugs become nonionized in the acidity of the stomach and then diffuse across membranes*—Basic drugs (alkaloids) tend to ionize and are not well absorbed in the stomach, but they may be better absorbed in the small intestine. A change in the pH of the stomach will affect the absorption of many drugs (Katzung, 2006).

Routes of Administration. The complexity of routes of administration and delivery systems has increased greatly. The most common routes for giving medications include oral (PO), topical (TOP, TD), subcutaneous (SubQ), intramuscular (IM), intravenous (IV), and rectal (PR). Other less commonly used routes include intradermal (ID), sublingual (SL), buccal, intraarticular, inhalation, intravaginal, ophthalmic, and aural.

Oral. Oral ingestion is the most common method of drug administration. It is the most convenient and the most economical route; it is also the safest. However, disadvantages of oral administration include the following:

- Poor gastrointestinal absorption may occur because of the physical characteristics of the drug.
- Irritation to the gastrointestinal mucosa may result in ulceration or emesis.

- Destruction of drugs may occur because of digestive enzymes and low gastric pH.
- Interactions may occur between the drug and food or other substances in the gastrointestinal tract.

Many variations are available in oral drug formulations (listed in order from the fastest absorption rate to the slowest absorption rate) including liquids, elixirs, syrups, suspensions, solutions, powders, capsules, tablets, coated tablets, enteric-coated tablets, and slow-release formulations (Brunton et al, 2005; Katzung, 2006).

Controlled-release preparations are designed to provide slow, uniform absorption of a drug (usually with a short half-life) over a long time, usually from 8 to 12 hours. These work with varying degrees of success. Some formulations are provided in a wax matrix that is not absorbed but is excreted in the feces (Brunton et al, 2005). Patients may become concerned about the appearance of this substance in the feces unless the clinician mentions this.

Sublingual Preparations. Some drugs that are nonionic and have high lipid solubility are readily absorbed by the oral mucosa. When drugs are absorbed orally, they must pass through the liver before they are distributed to the rest of the body. Many drugs are extensively metabolized on this first pass, allowing little of the drug to remain active. Drugs absorbed sublingually are advantageous because they avoid the first-pass phenomenon; therefore, the drug will reach the site of action quickly. Sublingual nitroglycerin is an example of a drug that needs to work quickly (chest pain).

Topical. Few drugs easily penetrate intact skin. Lipid-soluble drugs may not be absorbed because the skin acts as a lipid barrier. However, other types of solutions may be absorbed. Skin that is not intact will absorb drugs more readily. Thus, it is important to apply topical medications to intact, healthy skin to ensure the correct absorption. Mucous membranes also readily absorb drugs more readily than intact skin because of increased vascularity. Topical administration has the same advantage of avoiding the first-pass metabolism of the drug through the liver (Brunton et al, 2005).

Rectal. Medications that cannot be given orally often can be given rectally. Rectal medications usually are given when the patient is vomiting or unconscious. One advantage is that less first-pass metabolism of the drug through the liver occurs for rectal than for oral preparations. However, rectal absorption tends to be more inconsistent and less complete than oral absorption, and some drugs may cause rectal irritation. It is not always necessary to have a specially formulated rectal preparation (Edmunds, 2005). For example, oral timed-release morphine tablets will be absorbed rectally and are useful when the patient is unable to take an occasional oral dose of pain medicine.

Inhalation. Drugs can be given by nasal spray for local topical absorption through mucous membranes or by inhaler or nebulizer for pulmonary absorption. Pulmonary absorption uses a large surface area, making absorption rapid. Inhalation delivers the medication directly to the desired site of action, forcing particles of drugs down into the pulmonary system. This also avoids first-pass metabolism in the liver. The disadvantages of inhalation therapy include problems associated with regulating the exact dosage and the fact that many patients experience difficulty in self-administering a drug via inhaler.

Ophthalmic. Drops or ointments may be prescribed for the eye. These should be instilled into the pouch of the lower eyelid and should not be applied directly to the eye surface itself. Anything formulated for use on the eye can be used anywhere else in the body (Edmunds, 2005).

Blood Flow. Circulation at the site of administration is important in the drug absorption process. Decreased circulation (as seen in congestive heart failure) will result in decreased drug absorption (Katzung, 2006). For example, insulin injected into a thigh muscle, followed by exercise, will produce more rapid absorption of the insulin than occurs without exercise.

Cell Membrane Characteristics. When drugs are absorbed, they pass through cells, not between them; therefore, the drug must pass through the cellular wall or membrane. The structure of the cell membrane influences this process (Figure 3-2). The cell membrane is composed of a two-molecule layer of lipids that contain protein molecules between the lipids. It also contains carbohydrate molecules that are attached to the outer surface of the membrane. The proteins can be integral (in which case they go through the membrane) or peripheral (in which case they are attached to the surface of the membrane) (McCance & Huether, 2007). Integral proteins act as structural channels for the transportation of water-soluble substances (ions) or as carrier proteins in active transport. Peripheral proteins are enzymes. Glycoproteins may be antigenic sites in immune reactions or drug receptors. The pores permit the passage of small water-soluble substances such as water, electrolytes, urea, and alcohol (Brunton et al, 2005).

Drugs cross membranes via passive diffusion or active transport. *Passive diffusion* involves the random movement of drug molecules from high to low concentrations. *Active transport* moves molecules that are moderately sized, water soluble, or ionic across cell membranes. In active transport, these molecules form complexes with carriers for transport through the membrane and then dissociate from them. Active transport requires expenditure of energy and can occur against the concentration gradient (Stringer, 2005) (Figure 3-3).

In passive diffusion, the drug molecule penetrates along a concentration gradient as a result of its solubility in the lipid layer of the membrane (Figure 3-4). This transfer occurs in proportion to the magnitude of the concentration gradient across the membrane. The higher the concentration, the more rapid is the diffusion across the membrane. If the drug is not an electrolyte, a steady state is attained when the concentration of free drug is the same on both sides of the

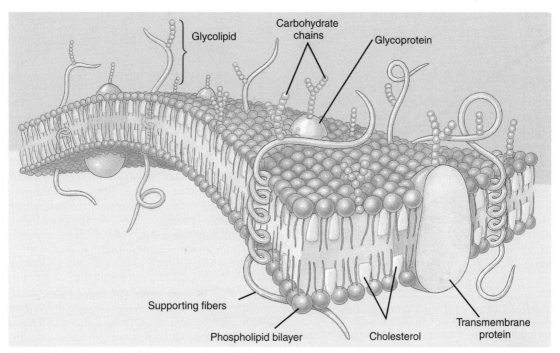

FIGURE 3-2 Cell membrane structure. The lipid bilayer provides the basic structure and serves as a relatively impermeable barrier to most water-soluble molecules. (Modified from Thibodeau GA, Patton KI: *Structure and function of the human body,* ed 13, St Louis, 2008, Mosby.)

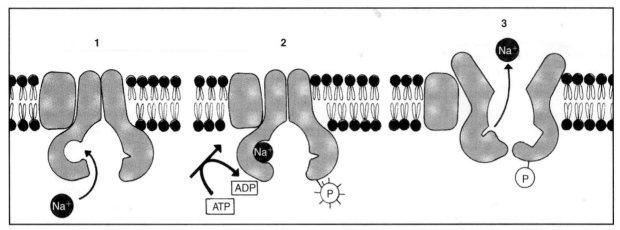

FIGURE 3-3   Active mediated transport. Metabolic energy is necessary for the active transport of many substances, including Na⁺ (Modified from Alberts B et al, editors: *Molecular biology of the cell,* ed 3, New York, 1994, Garland.)

membrane. If the drug is an ionic compound, the steady-state concentration will depend on the difference in pH across the membrane (Brunton et al, 2005).

Whether the drug is lipophilic or hydrophilic affects absorption across cell membranes. Lipids pass through membranes better than hydrophilic molecules do. However, most cell membranes are permeable to water by diffusion or by hydrostatic or osmotic differences across the membrane (Stringer, 2005). The water may carry with it small water-soluble substances such as urea.

The pH of a drug also affects diffusion. Nonionized drugs are more lipid soluble and may readily diffuse across cell membranes. Ionized drugs are lipid insoluble and nondiffusible.

Acidic drugs such as aspirin become nonionized in the acidic environment of the stomach and thus can diffuse across the membranes (DiPiro et al, 2005; Stringer, 2005). A change in the acidity of the stomach, as occurs with antacids, will affect absorption of drugs. Basic drugs such as alkaloids ionize in the stomach and are not well absorbed. These drugs are better absorbed in a less acidic environment such as the small intestine.

Active transport is a process used in the cell in three situations: when a particle is going from low to high concentration, when particles need help entering the membrane because they are selectively impermeable, and when very large particles enter and exit the cell. In order for active transport to occur, different types of pumps assist in the process.

- ABC class pumps transport small molecules across membranes. They consist of two transmembrane domains, and two ATP binding domains. ABC pumps are involved in the transport of small molecules, phospholipids and lipophilic drugs in mammalian cells. In bacteria they transport amino acids, sugars and peptides.
- P-class pumps uses ATP to transport ions against a gradient. They are phosphorylated during transport, which is different from the other classes of active transport pumps. Some examples of P-class pumps are the sodium-potassium pump, calcium transport in muscle cells and the hydrogen-potassium pump in the apical membrane of the stomach.
- The AV-class proton pump moves protons from one side of a membrane to the other and uses ATP as the source of energy. V-class proton pumps are a type of ATPase. They use the energy released by the hydrolysis of ATP to move protons against their concentration gradient.
- F-class proton pumps have also been identified and are the subject of new research.

Distribution

Distribution is the transport of a drug in body fluids from the bloodstream (at the site of absorption) to various tissues in the body. The pattern of distribution depends on the pharmacokinetic activity of different types of tissue and the different physicochemical properties of drugs (Brunton et al, 2005). Drugs vary in their ability to move into various body compartments (e.g., brain, fat, lung, eye). The best way to know

High-solute concentration	Lipid bilayer	Low-solute concentration
Extracellular fluid		Intracellular fluid
Hydrophobic molecules	O₂ CO₂ N₂	
Small, uncharged molecules	H₂O Urea Glycerol	
Large, uncharged molecules	Glucose Sucrose	
Ions	H⁺Na⁺ HCO₃⁻K⁺ Ca⁺⁺Cl⁻ Mg⁺⁺	

FIGURE 3-4   Passive diffusion. Oxygen, nitrogen, water, urea, glycerol, and carbon dioxide can diffuse readily down the concentration gradient. Macromolecules are too large to diffuse through pores in the plasma membrane. Ions may be repelled if the pores contain substances with identical charges. (From McCance KL, Huether SE: *Pathophysiology: the biologic basis of disease in infants and children,* ed 5, St Louis, 2005, Mosby.)

how much of a given drug gets into a particular body compartment is to consult standard reference texts. Because blood is an easily accessible body fluid, blood concentrations often are studied to determine how they relate to drug concentrations in other body compartments. The dose-related effects of a drug are then correlated with a given blood concentration or range of concentration. Once a relationship has been established, blood concentrations can be used to monitor therapy.

Distribution consists of two phases. The first involves movement from the site of administration into the bloodstream. Delivery of the drug into the tissue at the site of action is the second phase of distribution (Katzung, 2006).

The volume of distribution (Vd) is a concept that is useful when one seeks to understand where the drug goes once it is absorbed. *Volume* of distribution is a description of the amount of space into which a drug can be spread or distributed. It is the calculated volume or size of a compartment necessary to account for the total amount of drug in the body if it were present throughout the body at the same concentration found in the plasma (Brunton et al, 2005). Because most drugs are not equally distributed, this is a theoretical concept and not a real volume. It is, however, useful in predicting drug concentrations, understanding how well a drug is absorbed into tissues, and understanding whether it will be accumulated in the tissues. If a drug has a small volume of distribution, it stays in the central compartment and is not widely distributed. If the drug has a large volume of distribution, it is found widely throughout the body. The larger the Vd, the more drug is in the tissue. Because we are able to measure the amount of drug in the bloodstream only through serum levels, calculation of the volume of distribution allows us to estimate or predict the concentration of drug in the tissue (Stringer, 2005). The Vd may be calculated by examining the following relationships:

If

$$\text{Concentration of drug in blood} = \frac{\text{Dose}}{\text{Vd}}$$

then

$$\text{Vd} = \frac{\text{Dose}}{\text{Concentration}}$$

This means that the Vd is equal to the dose of drug in the body divided by the concentration in the blood (Brunton et al, 2005).

Water-soluble drugs have a Vd that is similar to the plasma volume because they are distributed into the blood. The plasma volume for a normal adult is about 3 to 5 liters. Lipophilic drugs have a larger Vd. The total fluid volume in the body is about 40 liters for a 70-kg (150-lb) person. Because the Vd of a lipophilic drug can exceed this volume, it is important to remember that this calculation is of a hypothetical volume, not a real volume. It is the volume that would be required to contain the entire drug in the body if the drug were distributed in the same concentration as in the blood or plasma (Brunton et al, 2005).

Factors that affect the volume of distribution include plasma protein binding, obesity, edema, and tissue binding. Therefore, the Vd for a given drug can change as a function of the patient's age, gender, disease, and body composition.

Geriatric patients often have relatively less muscle and more fat, placing them at risk for accumulation of lipophilic drugs in the adipose tissue. If these patients lose weight and take the same dose, they could become toxic. This can be a particular problem with lipophilic benzodiazepines. In these patients, water-soluble drugs have a smaller Vd, resulting in increased blood concentrations. This effect is even greater if the patient is dehydrated. An example of a drug that may cause this problem is gentamicin. In addition, excess fluid in the interstitial spaces, such as is seen with edema, will affect the distribution of water-soluble drugs.

Any alteration in the normal muscle-to-fat ratio will change the Vd of a drug. In obesity, lipophilic drugs are distributed into adipose tissue and tend to accumulate. Thus, little drug is available elsewhere to produce an effect. For example, phenobarbital is fat soluble. The drug may become trapped in the fatty tissue, causing low blood levels of phenobarbital. Fat-soluble drugs are slowly released from the fat into the bloodstream, so they have a longer duration of action. This factor also may prolong the duration of side effects or may affect dosing schedules.

Drugs that are highly protein bound (>90%) have a volume of distribution that is about the same as the amount of plasma. This is a small volume of distribution. An example would be the thyroid hormones. If the patient has a decreased serum albumin, more active drug is available for protein-bound drugs. If two protein-bound drugs are used, the most tightly protein-bound drug will tend to displace the other. Examples of these drugs include furosemide and the cephalosporins (Brunton et al, 2005; DiPiro et al, 2005).

Another common change that may affect the distribution of drugs in older adults is a decrease in serum albumin. Albumin concentrations decrease slightly with age in most elderly patients, although significant changes that may affect drug therapy may be seen in the chronically ill or malnourished elderly patient (Bourne, 2007). Albumin is the most common protein that binds to various acidic drugs. Significant decreases in albumin may result in a greater free concentration of highly protein-bound drugs. Box 4-3 lists some drugs that have significant protein binding, which may result in greater free concentrations when albumin is significantly reduced. Generally, drugs that are highly protein bound to albumin should be prescribed in reduced doses for patients with low serum albumin values (Bourne, 2007). A practical example of the clinical significance of this relationship can be described with the anticonvulsant phenytoin. In an elderly patient with a low serum albumin concentration (normal, 3.5 to 5 mg/dl), the phenytoin level reported from virtually all laboratories is the bound concentration. In a hypoalbuminemic individual, this value may appear normal or even subtherapeutic. This is because of the greater amounts of "free" or nonbound phenytoin that are getting into the tissue and acting at the receptor level but are not portrayed in the total serum level. The actual level may be much higher or even in the toxic range. Treatment decisions with older adults should not be based solely on drug levels. Treatment decisions must be based on consideration of both patient characteristics and drug levels.

Other protein changes also may have an influence on drug therapy. Patients with acute disease, such as myocardial infarction, respiratory distress, or infectious insult, for example, may experience increases in α_1-glycoprotein, an acute phase reactant protein. This may result in the increased binding of weakly basic drugs, including propranolol or lidocaine, and a less-than-normal response to therapy. Data are lacking concerning the real significance of changes in α_1-glycoprotein and drug therapy in the elderly (DiPiro et al, 2005).

Some drugs have an affinity for specific tissues. This affinity becomes useful when patients with certain infections are under treatment. For example, ciprofloxacin and tetracycline have an affinity for bone.

It is not generally necessary to calculate Vd when drugs are used. However, it is an important concept to understand when one is administering a drug, and it may influence the dosage or choice of a drug. Always consider where the drug will go and how much will get to the target organ or tissue.

The distribution of drugs from the bloodstream to the central nervous system is different than that through other cell membranes. The endothelial cells of the brain capillaries do not have intercellular pores and vesicles. Passive distribution of hydrophilic drugs is restricted. However, lipophilic drugs will easily pass the blood-brain barrier, limited only by cerebral blood flow (Brunton et al, 2005). Highly fat-soluble drugs also cross the blood-brain barrier easily and are likely to cause central nervous system side effects such as confusion and drowsiness.

Biotransformation (Metabolism)

Biotransformation is the chemical inactivation of a drug through conversion to a more water-soluble compound that can be excreted from the body. Biotransformation occurs primarily in the liver, but it also may be found in the lungs and in the GI tract. It involves two major steps in enzyme activity. Phase I makes the drug more hydrophilic through oxidation, reduction, or hydrolysis. Minor changes in the structure of the drug make it more hydrophilic but allow it to maintain all or part of its pharmacologic activity. The cytochrome P450 enzyme system is a part of phase I. Phase II is called *glucuronidation*. It involves *conjugation*, or attachment of particles to the molecule, making it a highly water-soluble substance with little or no pharmacologic activity (Brunton et al, 2005). If blood flow to the liver is decreased, drugs will be metabolized more slowly, leading to a longer duration of action.

Lipophilic drugs pass easily through membranes, including renal tubules, making them difficult to excrete. Biotransformation changes a lipophilic drug that is active and transforms it into a hydrophilic inactive compound that is readily excreted. However, metabolites occasionally have biologic activity or toxic properties (Figure 3-5).

PHASE I: OXIDATION OR REDUCTION OF DRUGS. Phase I involves oxidation or reduction—hydrolysis reactions that make drugs more water soluble so they can be excreted. During this phase, perhaps as many as 40 different P450 enzymes present in the liver may be available to participate as catalysts in the oxidation of drugs. It appears that the metabolism of most drugs can be accounted for by a relatively small subset of these enzymes, with probably half attributed to CYP 3A4. The P450 enzyme system is a topic that is rapidly gaining expanded attention, and new information is becoming available constantly.

The cytochrome P450 enzyme system operates throughout the body. It is concentrated in the liver, intestine, and lungs. The P450 enzyme system resides in the ribosomes, which are sacs in the endoplasmic reticulum. It is named P450 because this is the length of the wave of light that these enzymes absorb. Chemically, the enzyme is a glycoprotein or a sugar plus a protein. Many of the proteins contain heme, hence the name *chrome*. This family of enzymes is divided into groups according to similarity. At least 40 major groups have been identified in humans so far. The major groups named 1, 2, 3, and 4 are known to be involved in drug interactions. These major groups are further divided into groups by their chemical structure, named A, B, and C. The A, B, and C groups are then divided into subgroups named 1, 2, 3, etc. The groups most important in human drug interactions are as follows: CYP 2D6, CYP 3A3/4, CYP 1A2, CYP 2C9/10, and CYP 2C19. In the groups with 3/4 and 9/10, the two are so close in structure that they are difficult to differentiate and have very similar actions (Dresser et al, 2000; Lim et al, 2005; Zhou et al, 2004, 2005).

Advances in technology have resulted in an explosion of information concerning the cytochrome P450 isoenzymes and increased awareness of life-threatening interactions with such commonly prescribed drugs as cisapride and some antihistamines. Knowledge of the substrates, inhibitors, and inducers of these enzymes assists one in predicting clinically significant drug interactions.

The P450 enzyme system is not the same in every individual. Each person receives genetic material that determines individual variations in the enzyme system; this is called *genetic polymorphism*. Thus, individual differences and racial and gender differences occur. These are not yet well known or understood. Patients express their enzyme system in different ways. This explains why different patients react differently to a drug. For example, some patients metabolize codeine (CYP 2D6) quickly and need larger doses, whereas other patients metabolize it slowly and need less.

The essential facts to master about the P450 enzyme system are that there are six primary enzymes that account for

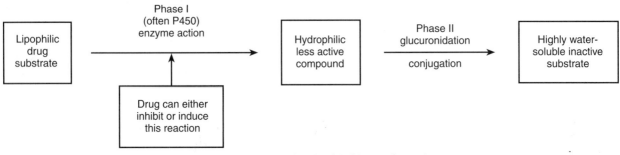

FIGURE 3-5 Processes involved in biotransformation.

the metabolism of nearly all clinically important drugs, and that two of these systems are critically important for drug metabolism (Table 3-1).

CYP 3A4 is an enzyme needed for metabolism of many drugs such as antihistamines, antibiotics, lipid-lowering drugs, antihypertensives, protease inhibitors, and azole antifungals. This system is used in the metabolism of approximately 50% of all clinically useful medications. These enzymes are the most abundant and clinically significant. (In *CYP 3A4*, the notation *CYP* indicates that the property is part of the cytochrome P450 system; *3* indicates the family; *A* indicates the subfamily; and *4* indicates that it is the fourth enzyme in that subsystem.)

The CYP 2D6 enzyme looks different and is different. It metabolizes selective serotonin reuptake inhibitors (SSRIs), pain relievers, β-blockers, and other drugs. This enzyme metabolizes about 30% of all clinically useful medications, is the second most abundant, and participates in converting codeine to morphine.

Of the other four enzymes, the most notable features of each are as follows:
- CYP 2C19—metabolizes proton pump inhibitors, NSAIDs, and β-blockers
- CYP 2C9—metabolizes sulfonylureas, NSAIDs, (S)-warfarin, and sildenafil citrate (Viagra)
- CYP 1A2—metabolizes acetaminophen, (R)-warfarin, theophylline, caffeine, diazepam (Valium), and verapamil
- CYP 2E1—metabolizes acetaminophen, ethanol, inactivation of toxins, and dextromethorphan

A drug can be a *substrate* or one that is affected by alteration of its enzyme metabolism. A drug can also be the one that causes the alteration in the enzyme metabolism of another drug by being an *inhibitor* or an *inducer*. The cytochrome P450 enzyme system may speed up a reaction because it causes the drug to change to a more hydrophilic substance. Any drug that causes the enzyme to metabolize more slowly or decreases the capacity of the enzyme pathway is called an *inhibitor*. For example, if a patient on fluoxetine (Prozac) takes warfarin, the fluoxetine inhibits the P450 enzyme system from metabolizing warfarin and may produce an exaggerated therapeutic response (bleeding). A drug that causes the enzymes to metabolize the substrate more quickly is called an *inducer*. These types of drugs increase enzyme activity by increasing the number of CYP 450 enzymes. Any drug can be involved in this process in two ways. It can be the drug or substrate that is being acted upon, or it can be the inhibitor or inducer that is acting on the enzyme to increase or decrease enzyme conversion of the substrate drug into an inactive compound. The same drug can be both a substrate and an inducer or inhibitor (Brunton et al, 2005). For example, carbamazepine is an auto inducer—it induces its own metabolism. It is the enzyme system, *not* the drug that is being induced or inhibited (see Figure 3-5 to examine these relationships).

A drug can inhibit an enzyme pathway through two mechanisms. The first is competition. This is not usually a problem. If it occurs, it occurs immediately. Most inhibition is metabolic. The inhibitor drug decreases the production of the enzyme. It shrinks the enzyme pathway. This is not an immediate reaction; it may take anywhere from 24 hours up to a week to see the effect, depending on the half-life of the drug (Brunton et al, 2005). From a pharmacokinetic standpoint, the major effects of drug–drug interactions are understood in terms of causing a high or low plasma and tissue level of the drug.

Enzyme induction is much less common than inhibition. These drugs make the pathway work quickly, causing the substrate drug to be deactivated more rapidly. This will lower the level of the drug in the body. The clinically important inducers are anticonvulsants. All anticonvulsants should be considered as possible inducers. Evaluation of these drugs is particularly important when they are being added to a patient's medication regimen.

In addition to cytochrome P450, oxidation of drugs and other xenobiotics can be mediated by non-P450 enzymes, the most significant of which are flavin monooxygenase, monoamine oxidase, alcohol dehydrogenase, aldehyde dehydrogenase, aldehyde oxidase, and xanthine oxidase. Drug oxidation catalyzed by some of these enzymes may often produce the same metabolites as those generated by P450; thus, drug interactions may be difficult to predict without a clear knowledge of the underlying enzymology. Although oxidation catalyzed by non-P450 enzymes can lead to drug inactivation, oxidation may be essential for the generation of active metabolites that create drug action (Brunton et al, 2005).

PHASE II: BIOTRANSFORMATION. Phase II or biotransformation consists of conjugate reactions in which a compound is added to the drug. These reactions bind a chemical group to the drug compound via a covalent linkage. The chemical groups added to the drug are generally highly polar, or ionized. This makes them water soluble and generally inactive. However, a few of these conjugate compounds are active (Brunton et al, 2005).

First-Pass Effect. When a medication is taken orally, it passes from the intestine directly to the liver by way of the hepatic portal blood flow (via the portal vein). Many drugs, such as nitroglycerin and estrogen, are extensively metabolized to inert compounds when they first pass through the liver. Because of this, very large amounts of the drug must be given for a sufficient dose to remain after the first pass through the liver. This is known as the first-pass effect (Stringer, 2005). It is why these drugs are often given via an alternative route, such as sublingual or topical, to avoid the liver on the first pass. Alternative route dosing also makes it possible to give a smaller amount of the drug and have it be effective.

Prodrug. A *prodrug* is a chemical that is pharmacologically inactive. It is biotransformed into a biologically active metabolite in the body. The angiotensin-converting enzyme inhibitor enalapril is an example of a medication that must be transformed from a prodrug to the biologically active metabolite (Brunton et al, 2005). This activity may be reduced in congestive heart failure if the liver is congested, thus delaying treatment of the patient with heart failure.

Elimination

Elimination is the process by which drugs and their metabolites are removed from the body. The liver and the kidney are the two major organs responsible for elimination.

Most elimination occurs through excretion by the kidneys. The processes involved in renal elimination consist of glomerular filtration, tubular secretion, and partial reabsorption. In glomerular filtration, the drug enters the renal tubule by filtration. However, whether this occurs depends on the amount of protein binding because a drug does not filter into the tubule if it is bound to a protein. This action also depends on the rate of glomerular filtration, which in turn depends on the kidney function and cardiovascular status of the patient (Figure 3-6).

Active, carrier-mediated tubular secretion is responsible for adding some organic anion and cation molecules to the

TABLE 3-1   Examples of Clinically Relevant Drugs Metabolized by Various CYP Enzymes

CYP Enzyme

Substrates	1A2	2B6	2C8	2C19	2C9	2D6	2E1	3A4, 5, 7
	clozapine	bupropion	—	Proton pump inhibitors:	NSAIDs:	β-Blockers:	acetaminophen	Macrolide antibiotics:
	cyclobenzaprine	cyclophosphamide		omeprazole	diclofenac	S-metoprolol	chlorzoxazone	clarithromycin
	imipramine	efavirenz		lansoprazole	ibuprofen	propafenone	ethanol	erythromycin
	mexiletine	ifosfamide		pantoprazole	piroxicam	timolol		NOT azithromycin
	naproxen	methadone		rabeprazole	Oral hypoglycemic	Antipsychotics:		telithromycin
	riluzole			Antiepileptics:	agents:	haloperidol		Antiarrhythmics:
	tacrine			diazepam	tolbutamide	risperidone		quinidine
	theophylline			phenytoin	glipizide	thioridazine		Benzodiazepines:
				phenobarbitone	Angiotensin II	aripiprazole		alprazolam
				amitriptyline	blockers:	codeine		diazepam
				clomipramine	NOT candesartan	dextromethorphan		midazolam
				cyclophosphamide	irbesartan	duloxetine		triazolam
				progesterone	losartan	flecainide		Immune modulators:
					NOT valsartan	mexiletine		cyclosporine
					celecoxib	ondansetron		tacrolimus (FK506)
					fluvastatin naproxen	tamoxifen		HIV protease inhibitors:
					phenytoin	tramadol		indinavir
					sulfamethoxazole			ritonavir
					tamoxifen			saquinavir
					tolbutamide			Prokinetic:
					torsemide			cisapride
					warfarin			Antihistamines:
								astemizole
								chlorpheniramine
								Calcium channel blockers:
								amlodipine
								diltiazem
								felodipine
								nifedipine
								nisoldipine
								nitrendipine
								verapamil
								HMG-CoA reductase inhibitors:
								atorvastatin
								cerivastatin
								lovastatin
								NOT pravastatin
								simvastatin
								aripiprazole
								buspirone
								gleevec
								haloperidol (in part)
								metadone
								pimozide
								quinine
								NOT rosuvastatin
								sildenafil
								tamoxifen
								trazodone
								vincristine,5,7

INHIBITORS	cimetidine fluoroquinolones fluvoxamine ticlopidine	thiotepa ticlopidine	gemfibrozil montelukast	fluoxetine fluvoxamine ketoconazole lansoprazole omeprazole ticlopidine	amiodarone fluconazole isoniazid	amiodarone bupropion chlorpheniramine cimetidine clomipramine duloxetine fluoxetine haloperidol methadone mibefradil paroxetine quinidine ritonavir	disulfiram	HIV protease inhibitors: indinavir nelfinavir ritonavir amiodarone NOT azithromycin cimetidine clarithromycin diltiazem erythromycin fluvoxamine grapefruit juice itraconazole ketoconazole mibefradil nefazodone troleandomycin verapamil
INDUCERS	tobacco	phenobarbital phenytoin rifampin	—	—	rifampin secobarbital	—	ethanol isoniazid	carbamazepine phenobarbital phenytoin rifabutin rifampin St. John's wort

From Flockhart D: *Cytochrome P450 drug-interaction table*, Division of Clinical Pharmacology, Indiana University Department of Medicine, 2007 (Available at http://medicine.iupui.edu/flockhart/table.htm).

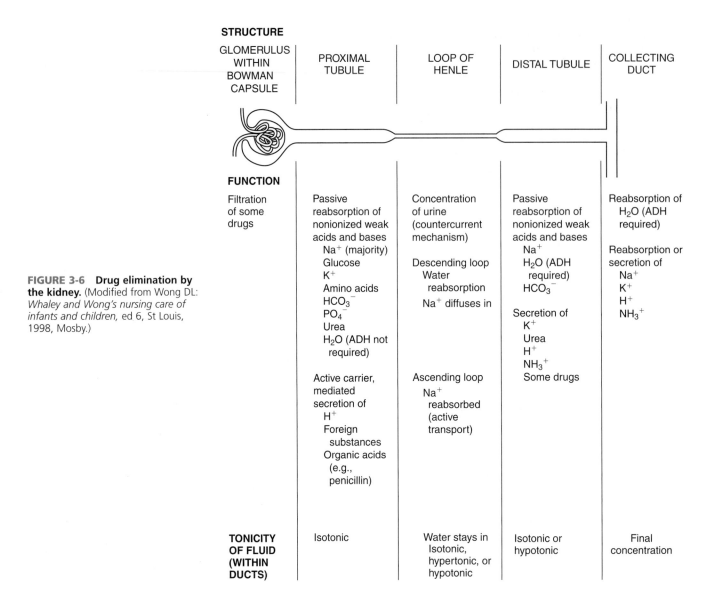

STRUCTURE				
GLOMERULUS WITHIN BOWMAN CAPSULE	PROXIMAL TUBULE	LOOP OF HENLE	DISTAL TUBULE	COLLECTING DUCT
FUNCTION				
Filtration of some drugs	Passive reabsorption of nonionized weak acids and bases Na$^+$ (majority) Glucose K$^+$ Amino acids HCO$_3^-$ PO$_4^-$ Urea H$_2$O (ADH not required) Active carrier, mediated secretion of H$^+$ Foreign substances Organic acids (e.g., penicillin)	Concentration of urine (countercurrent mechanism) Descending loop Water reabsorption Na$^+$ diffuses in Ascending loop Na$^+$ reabsorbed (active transport)	Passive reabsorption of nonionized weak acids and bases Na$^+$ H$_2$O (ADH required) HCO$_3^-$ Secretion of K$^+$ Urea H$^+$ NH$_3^+$ Some drugs	Reabsorption of H$_2$O (ADH required) Reabsorption or secretion of Na$^+$ K$^+$ H$^+$ NH$_3^+$
TONICITY OF FLUID (WITHIN DUCTS)	Isotonic	Water stays in Isotonic, hypertonic, or hypotonic	Isotonic or hypotonic	Final concentration

FIGURE 3-6   **Drug elimination by the kidney.** (Modified from Wong DL: *Whaley and Wong's nursing care of infants and children,* ed 6, St Louis, 1998, Mosby.)

proximal renal tubule. The carrier systems are fairly nonselective and organic ions compete for transport. Thus two drugs may compete for the same active transport carriers, and their excretion will be slowed (Brunton et al, 2005). Although it may be difficult to predict the result, a drug can be both secreted and actively reabsorbed. Penicillin is an important example of this process.

Once the drug has been excreted via active transport in the proximal tubule, weakly acidic or alkaline molecules may undergo passive reabsorption. How much is reabsorbed depends on the pH of the urine. Alkalinization of the urine will increase the excretion of acidic molecules. Acidification of the urine will increase the excretion of basic molecules. Clinical alteration of the pH of urine will hasten the excretion of some drugs, as in the case of drug poisoning or drug toxicity (DiPiro et al, 2005).

If the glomerular filtration rate in the kidneys is reduced, the drug remains in the blood longer. In patients with kidney damage, it is necessary to calculate an estimated creatinine clearance to modify the dosage of medication necessary. This is calculated with the following formula:

$$\text{Creatinine clearance} = \frac{\text{Weight (kg*)} \times (140 - \text{Age [in years]})}{72 \times \text{Serum creatinine (mg/dl)} (\times 0.85)\dagger}$$

Drugs and their metabolites may be excreted through fecal and respiratory routes, through breast milk, and in other ways. The fecal route is often clinically significant. Drugs are metabolized in the liver, and the metabolites are excreted in the bile. These metabolites are reabsorbed into the blood and then are excreted in the urine or, less commonly, are simply excreted in the feces. Excretion from the liver into the bile is accomplished by active transport systems, which are limited in the quantity of metabolites they can excrete (Stringer, 2005). Different drugs may compete for transport. This competition may slow down the excretion of certain drugs; steroids provide an example of competition that slows excretion.

The respiratory route is an important route of excretion in anesthetic gases. Excretion in breast milk is important, not for the quantity excreted, but because of the effect it may have on

*Lean body weight may reflect creatinine production more accurately.
†In females, multiply value × 0.85.

a nursing infant. Other routes such as perspiration, saliva, tears, hair, and skin are not usually clinically significant.

Clearance is loosely defined as a measure of the rate at which the drug is removed from the body (Stringer, 2005). The body can eliminate the drug only if the drug is in contact with the eliminating organ. If a drug is being stored in adipose tissue, it cannot be cleared from the body. Thus, volume of distribution affects the clearance of a drug and hence the half-life.

Specifically, clearance is defined as the volume of plasma from which all drug is removed in a given time. It is measured as volume divided by time:

$$\text{Clearance} = \frac{\text{Rate of removal of drug (mg/min)}}{\text{Plasma concentration of drug (mg/ml)}}$$

This formula yields milliliters of plasma that has had the drug removed from it in the specified amount of time (1 minute). *Total body clearance* is the sum of clearances from the various metabolizing and eliminating organs (Stringer, 2005).

Steady state means there is a stable concentration of the drug, or the drug is being administered at the same rate at which it is being eliminated. This is fairly simple with a continuous infusion of drugs. With intermittent administration of medication, the frequency and amount of the drug must be adjusted to achieve steady state. Parkinson's medications such as carbidopa/levodopa (Sinemet) often require adjustment for both the amount and the interval of dosing to achieve therapeutic levels without reaching toxic levels. Patients who are eliminating a drug more slowly than normal will need smaller doses than will patients who are eliminating the drug normally.

PLASMA CONCENTRATION–TIME CURVE. The plasma concentration–time curve (Figure 3-7) illustrates what happens when a single dose of a drug is given. The time between when the drug is given and when it first takes effect is the *latent period. Onset of action* is the time it first takes effect. When the drug no longer has an effect, this is known as *termination of action.* The *duration of action* is the period of time during which the drug has its effect. The *minimal effective concentration* is the lowest level of concentration that produces the drug effect. The *peak plasma level* is the highest level the drug reaches. If the concentration is high enough to cause adverse drug reactions, this level is known as the *toxic level.* The *therapeutic range* is the area between the minimal effective concentration and the toxic concentration.

FIRST-ORDER/LINEAR KINETICS. The concept of *half-life* is an important one to understand. The half-life of a drug is the amount of time required for the amount of drug in the body to decrease by one half. This is a significant factor in accumulation and elimination of drugs. It depends on clearance and volume of distribution. When a patient is given a drug on a regular schedule, the drug will continue to accumulate until steady state is achieved (Stringer, 2005) (Figure 3-8). The half-life of a drug listed in reference books is an approximation of what the most likely or usual half-life will be in a normal, healthy adult. However, much individual variation occurs and is based on factors that affect volume of distribution and elimination. Half-life is useful for estimating the amount of time it takes to reach a steady state of a drug after a dosage regimen is started. Steady state is reached after 4 to 5 half-lives, which represents 94% to 97% of the eventual steady state. Half-life also can be used to estimate the amount of time it takes to eliminate a drug from the body after it has been discontinued. Again, after 4 to 5 half-lives, about 94% to 97% of the drug will have been eliminated from the body (Brunton et al, 2005). Of course, there is always a difference between the absolute (or theoretical) steady state and what is seen in fact for each patient.

Drugs with short half-lives include ibuprofen and the benzodiazepine lorazepam. Examples of drugs with long half-lives are anticoagulants, diazepam, digoxin, and fluoxetine (Prozac). Drugs with long half-lives must be closely monitored because toxic effects or adverse reactions may last a long time.

In linear or first-order kinetics, drug concentration is increased or decreased in a linear fashion, depending on dosage,

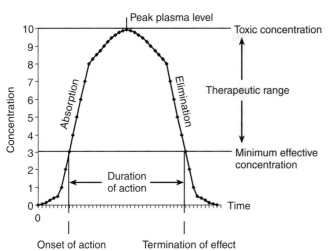

FIGURE 3-7 **Plasma concentration–time curve with single dose of drug.**

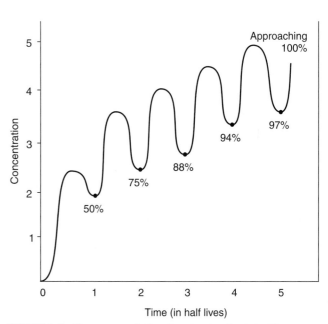

FIGURE 3-8 **Drug accumulation time to steady state.** The line shows concentrations of drugs in the body. (Modified from Hardman JG, Limbird LW et al, editors: *Goodman and Gilman's pharmacological basis of therapeutics,* ed 10, New York, 2001, McGraw-Hill.)

clearance, volume of distribution, and half-life. The drugs appear and disappear from plasma, depending on concentration. However, the percent of drug eliminated is constant.

Average concentration when the steady state is attained during intermittent drug administration may be calculated as follows:

$$\text{Concentration} = \frac{\text{Drug availability} \times \text{Dose}}{\text{Clearance} \times \text{Time}}$$

NONLINEAR KINETICS. Nonlinear kinetics, or zero-order kinetics, is more complicated. In this case, elimination does not depend on the dose or concentration of a drug. The amount of drug eliminated is constant. The drug is removed by saturation of a function, such as protein binding (limiting the amount of protein available for binding), hepatic metabolism (limiting the amount of enzyme causing metabolism), or active renal transport (limiting the amount of carrier). The half-life of the drug depends on the concentration (DiPiro et al, 2005; Stringer, 2005).

Phenytoin is a clinically important example of nonlinear kinetics because of both protein binding and hepatic metabolism. As phenytoin is absorbed, it is bound to plasma protein. When a regimen is started, most of the drug is bound to protein, leaving little free drug. However, as the proteins reach saturation, suddenly a much greater percentage of the absorbed drug is not protein bound and is free drug. When the proteins are saturated, suddenly the free drug, measured as a serum drug level, rises rapidly. A narrow therapeutic window makes toxicity a frequent problem. When the amount of drug concentration exceeds the ability of the liver to metabolize the drug, nonlinear kinetics occurs (DiPiro et al, 2005). Again, the body has a finite ability to produce enzymes that metabolize the drug. Once the body is working at capacity, any additional drug will accumulate and cause toxicity. Another example of a drug that follows nonlinear kinetic principles is theophylline. Drugs that follow nonlinear kinetics are far more difficult to maintain in the therapeutic range and must be monitored closely for toxicity.

PHARMACODYNAMICS

Pharmacodynamics is the study of the biochemical and physiologic effects of drugs and the mechanisms of their action (Brunton et al, 2005). A concise definition of pharmacodynamics to be remembered is "the effect of the drug on the body."

Mechanisms of Drug Action

Most drugs act on the body via chemical reactions with some large molecular component of the organism. The drug alters the function of the component, thereby causing biochemical and physiologic changes that are characteristic of the response to the particular drug. The drug interacts with a chemical receptor (Katzung, 2006). The concept of drug receptors explains the mechanisms of action.

DRUG RECEPTORS. A *receptor* is the component of the organism that binds to a ligand and produces a change in function within the body. Drugs, neurotransmitters, and hormones are known as *ligands*. Figure 3-9 shows three types of cellular receptors. In general, drugs produce their effects by interacting with a receptor. This concept sounds obvious, but it is important to understand how drugs accomplish what they do. An example is a hormone molecule. Figure 3-9 shows three types of cellular receptors. Drugs generally do not create an effect by themselves but through a receptor. The site at which a drug acts depends on localization of the specific receptors (McCance & Huether, 2007). This concept too sounds obvious, but again it is important to understand how drugs accomplish what they do.

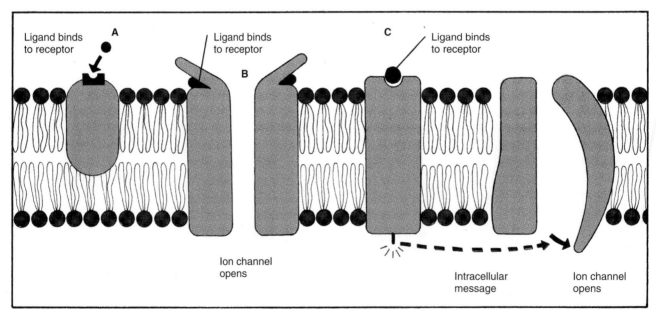

FIGURE 3-9   Cellular receptors. A, Plasma membrane receptor for a ligand on the surface of an integral protein. **B** and **C,** A neurotransmitter can exert its effect on a postsynaptic cell by means of two fundamentally different types of receptor proteins: channel-linked receptors and non–channel-linked receptors. Channel-linked receptors are also known as ligand-gated channels. (**A** is from Huether SE et al: *Understanding pathophysiology,* ed 5, St Louis, 2005, Mosby; **B** and **C** are modified from Alberts B et al, editors: *Molecular biology of the cell,* ed 3, New York, 1994, Garland.)

Most drug receptors are proteins. Some of the most clinically important receptors are cellular proteins, whose normal functions are to be receptors for bodily (endogenous) regulatory molecules (McCance & Huether, 2007). Examples of such molecules are hormones and neurotransmitters. Receptors can be enzymes that are chemical in nature (making it easy for reactions to occur) but that are not totally used up in the reaction. Enzymes free themselves and then continue to be available for reactions with other substrates.

The lock-and-key model of drug–receptor interaction states that the drug molecule must fit into a receptor much the way a key fits into a lock (Figure 3-10). *Drug affinity* is the propensity of a drug to bind or attach itself to a given receptor site. Two types of drug–receptor interactions can occur: agonist and antagonist. An *agonist* is a drug that has affinity for and stimulates physiologic activity at cell receptors normally activated by naturally occurring substances. An *antagonist* is a drug that inhibits or counteracts effects produced by other drugs or eliminates undesired physiologic effects caused by illness. An antagonist may work competitively, with an affinity for the same receptor site as an agonist; or it may be noncompetitive, in which case it inactivates the receptor so that the agonist cannot be effective at any concentration.

ACTIONS OF DRUGS NOT MEDIATED BY RECEPTORS.

Some drugs interact with small molecules or ions that are found in the body. For example, antacids neutralize gastric acid in the stomach. Other drugs have structures close enough to normal biologic chemicals that the body may incorporate them into cellular components; thus, function may be altered. Examples of this type of activity include purines that are incorporated into nucleic acids and are useful in treating cancers and viruses. Recombinant DNA also may serve in this manner, while working with new drugs or being used in new treatment regimens.

Agonist: Chemical fits receptor site well; chemical response is usually good.

Antagonist: Drug attaches at drug receptor site but then remains chemically inactive; no chemical drug response is produced.

Partial agonist: Drug attaches at drug receptor site but only a slight chemical action is produced.

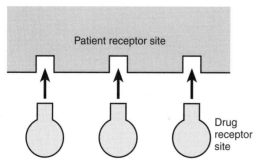

FIGURE 3-10   Drug receptor sites. (From Edmunds MW: *Introduction to clinical pharmacology,* ed 4, St Louis, 2003, Mosby.)

QUANTIFYING THE DRUG–RECEPTOR INTERACTION.

Attempts to quantify the drug–receptor interaction involve calculating the concentration of dose-response relationships. Agonist drug interactions with a receptor are reversible. The amount of effect depends on how many receptors are occupied or are being acted on by the drug. Efficacy is a drug's ability to produce a therapeutic or intended effect. *Free drug* is the amount of drug in the body that is able to bind the receptor (i.e., drug not bound to plasma proteins) (Stringer, 2005). *Potency* is the dependency of effect on its concentration. A drug is more potent than another if less drug is needed to achieve the desired effect. An antagonist will bind to a receptor to inhibit the action of a drug but has no intrinsic action of its own. Inhibition is competitive if it can be overcome by the increased concentration of the agonist. A noncompetitive antagonist prevents the action of the agonist at any concentration.

Adverse Drug Reactions and Side Effects

Adverse drug reactions (ADRs) or events (ADEs) are defined by the World Health Organization as "a response to a drug that is noxious and unintended and occurs at doses normally used for man for prophylaxis, diagnosis, or therapy of disease, or for the modification of physiologic function" (Esch et al, 1971). Essentially, an *adverse event* is any undesirable experience associated with the use of a drug or medical product in a patient. Adverse reactions include any response to a drug that is unfavorable or unintended and that occurs at doses used in humans for prophylaxis, diagnosis, or therapy of disease or for modification of physiologic function (FDA, 1990). This is different from a *side effect*, which is an additional effect, desirable or undesirable, of a drug that is not the primary purpose of giving the drug. For example, an adverse reaction could be the development of a pancytopenia from taking chloramphenicol. A side effect might include photosensitivity caused by tetracycline taken for acne. An unfavorable reaction would be one that is noxious, hurtful, not wholesome, or damaging to tissue. These types of reactions may occur immediately or may take weeks or months to develop, such as the hirsutism, "buffalo-hump," and gynecomastia seen after long-term steroid use.

The incidence of adverse drug reactions has been estimated at around 28%, accounting for about 3% to 6.7% of all hospital admissions (Hanlon et al, 2006). Adverse reactions may be classified into three distinctive types of reactions: (1) an inherent pharmacologic effect of a drug, that is, an excessive degree of the desired effect or an unintended side effect, for example, hypoglycemia seen with insulin use; (2) an allergic reaction, manifested by typical signs and symptoms of an immunologic response; or (3) a local irritant effect characterized by inflammation.

Serious ADEs are defined by the FDA as events caused by a drug that result in a patient's death, hospitalization, or disability, or that cause a congenital abnormality or a life-threatening event, or require an intervention to prevent permanent damage. It has been estimated that each year more than 770,000 people in the United States who are hospitalized experience ADRs at a rate that has increased by 15% over the past several years, costing major hospitals up to $5.6 million per year (Bond & Raehl, 2006). This estimate does not include ADRs that result in admissions, malpractice, and litigation costs, or the costs of injuries to patients. The annual costs of national hospital expenses to treat patients who experience ADRs during hospitalization are estimated to be between $1.56 billion and $5.6 billion. Although published reports indicate that thousands of deaths occur each year as a result of medical error, the true numbers of deaths attributed to ADRs is unknown (Kohn et al, 2001). In a meta-analysis examining the incidence of ADRs in U.S. hospitals, fatal ADRs were found to be one of the four to six leading causes of death (Bond & Raehl, 2006; Lazarou et al, 1998). Publication of studies such as these has led to additional research on the problem. The broad scope of the problem was brought to public attention in 1999 by a report issued by the Institute of Medicine (IOM), *To Err Is Human: Building a Safer Health System* (Kohn et al, 2000).

Most adverse drug reactions are nonallergic. They may result from overdosage, if biotransformation or excretion of normal doses is impaired, or if intake of medication is excessive. They might be a side effect reflecting an unavoidable nontherapeutic effect of the drug. A paradoxical effect or an effect opposite to that expected may develop. Drug interactions may occur, or an idiosyncratic reaction may result from unusual resistance to large doses or unexpected responses to ordinary or even low doses (Gomes & Demoly, 2005).

Most ADRs occur as a result of extension of the desired pharmacologic effects of a drug, often due to variability in the pharmacokinetics and pharmacodynamics seen among patients. Drugs such as warfarin and digoxin are at higher risk for causing ADRs, particularly because of their narrow therapeutic index when toxicity can occur at drug concentrations at or near the upper end of the therapeutic range. Elderly and pediatric patients are also highly vulnerable because drug absorption and metabolism are more variable and less predictable in both of these groups. Some research suggests that numbers of ADRs per patient in both the pediatric age group and in the elderly are higher compared with the middle age range, with the highest rates of ADRs occurring in octogenarians at a rate of 60 ADRs/10,000 people (Young et al, 1997). Elderly patients with comorbidities who are taking multiple medications, those who have a history of ADRs, and those with a reduced capacity to eliminate medications are at high risk for ADRs (Young et al, 1997). Exposure to toxic chemicals throughout the lifetime can have neurologic modulating effects that may last a lifetime. As people age, a decreasing trend in hepatic metabolizing capacity can affect their ability to clear medicines and chemicals assimilated from the environment. This trend, along with decreased urinary clearance, may cause prolonged retention of chemicals in the body. Research has demonstrated that the half-life of drugs processed by hepatic P450 enzymes or through renal elimination is 50% to 75% longer in those older than 65 than in other adults. Common liver and kidney diseases may further decrease drug and chemical clearance from these organs. The polypharmacy that is common among elderly patients may increase the likelihood of drug interactions in the body and potentiating side effects. The nervous system also undergoes changes with aging, including neural loss, altered neurotransmitter and receptor levels, and decreased adaptability to changes initiated by xenobiotics, making the patient more susceptible to neurologic changes (Ginsberg et al, 2005).

In women, a few pharmacokinetic differences can contribute to ADRs. The menstrual cycle and menopausal status can affect the metabolism of some drugs, as can the effects of supplemental estrogen or estrogen-progesterone combinations.

An important consideration in women is the influence of a drug on the effectiveness of oral contraception.

Over-the-counter medications, herbal medications, and oral contraceptive pills (OCPs) often are overlooked when one is taking a medication history in patients; a careful inventory of all medications taken by patients should be performed so harmful drug interactions can be avoided (Osterberg & Blaschke, 2007) (Table 3-2).

If a suspected adverse drug reaction occurs, it is important to confirm and document the reaction.

The key questions that should be answered include the following (Osterberg & Blaschke, 2007):

- Has the observed reaction been previously documented to be due to the drug taken by the patient?
- Is the time course of the reaction consistent with the time(s) of drug administration?
- Could this reaction be due to another clinical condition in the patient?
- Did the reaction improve when the drug was discontinued?
- If not discontinued, did the reaction resolve?
- If the dose was reduced but not discontinued, did the reaction resolve?
- If an antidote was given, did the patient's condition improve?
- Did the reaction recur when (if) the drug was administered again?
- Was the dose appropriate for the patient in terms of age or organ function?

Many significant drug–drug interactions can be understood in terms of cytochrome P450 reactions. However, drug–drug interactions are more complex for at least two reasons. First, some drug–drug interactions can be attributed to pharmacokinetic differences resulting from other enzymes such as

TABLE 3-2 Risk Factors for Developing Adverse Drug Reactions

Provider	Activities That Increase Risk of Drug Reactions
Prescriber	Duplication of medications
	Unclear directions
	Incomplete drug history
	Inappropriate dosing (no age adjustments)
	No follow-up
Pharmacist	Automatic refills
	Prescription errors
	Failure to review medication profile
	Lack of appropriate patient education
Patient	Use of over-the-counter drugs
	Incomplete knowledge of drug history
	Use of alcohol
	Use of multiple pharmacies with no coordination of drugs
	Use of multiple providers
	Poor compliance: drug overuse or underuse

monoamine oxidases, flavin-containing monooxygenases, uridine-5-diphosphate (UDP)–glucuronosyl transferases, and sulfotransferases. These and other drug-metabolizing enzymes also show the characteristics of induction and inhibition by drugs that are associated with P450s, although most have not yet been studied as extensively (Zhou et al, 2005). The other aspect of drug–drug interactions is that some of these are probably pharmacodynamic instead of pharmacokinetic; this occurs when drugs compete for binding to a receptor directly related to the pharmacologic response.

Common drug interactions may be described as summative (when the combined effects of two drugs produce a result that equals the sum of the individual effects of each agent, such as is seen with colestipol plus lovastatin); synergistic (when the combined effect of two drugs is greater than the sum of each individual agent acting independently, as is seen with hydrochlorothiazide [HCTZ] with angiotensin-converting enzyme inhibitor); or potentiating (when one drug increases the effect of the other drug, such as when probenecid inhibits the clearance of penicillin from the body, thereby increasing its effect). These effects may occur rapidly (within 24 hours) or may be delayed for days or weeks (Zhou et al, 2005).

The clinician should always evaluate the risk versus benefit of any possible combination of drugs. The first evaluation is the possibility of a serious drug–drug interaction. Approximately 5% of all drug–drug interactions are clinically significant (Bond & Raehl, 2006). Is the possible reaction serious? Is it reversible? Second, the therapeutic window of the drug in question is important. If the drug has a narrow therapeutic window, then the risk of a drug–drug interaction is greater. Third, consider the time course of the drugs involved. A drug with a long half-life will cause a longer adverse reaction than one with a short half-life. Multiply the half-life of the drug that is being affected by 4 to 5 times, and this will tell you when you will achieve a new steady-state drug level. Fourth, the age of the patient is important. Although most research has been done on adults, adults are the least likely to have drug interactions. Extremes of age—old or young—predispose a patient to adverse reactions. Fifth, coexisting morbidity is also an important factor. Patients with a seizure disorder, cardiovascular disease, or HIV or other infection are at risk for drug interactions. Patients with cardiovascular disease are at extra risk because they often have poor perfusion of the liver, and this affects enzyme action. Also, these patients are usually on several drugs that may have P450 interactions, such as antiarrhythmics and calcium channel blockers (DiPiro et al, 2005; Gomes & Demoly, 2005).

In general, if in doubt, anticipate that the new drug will interact with the drugs the patient is already taking if there is some commonality, such as CYP metabolism or agonist/antagonist issues. When adding a drug to a patient's regimen, the practitioner should always consult a comprehensive drug reference for any known drug–drug interactions. Further, the practitioner should review the profile of the drug for side effects that would be additive to existing therapy, CYP 450 enzyme metabolism, administration issues, and so forth. These factors can hinder optimal care and compliance of the patient. When monitoring drug therapy, it is essential for the clinician to counsel the patient regarding specific signs and symptoms that might accompany a drug–drug interaction or side effects. If recommended, the dosage of one medicine may have to be adjusted when another is added (Brunton et al, 2005).

Certain categories of medications are more likely to be involved in important P450–drug interactions. Some of the most important drug categories involved in drug–drug interactions because of the P450 system are the following:

- Many antibiotics present a risk. Erythromycin is both a substrate and an inhibitor. Many newer quinolones are inhibitors. For example, these antibiotics may inhibit the metabolism of theophylline.
- The azole antifungals are inhibitors.
- Drugs for HIV metabolism are susceptible to induction and inhibition.
- The nonsedating antihistamines are inhibitors. Terfenadine was a very potent inhibitor and was taken off the market because of interactions with several antiinfectives. The other antihistamines have far fewer inhibitor effects.
- The anticonvulsants can be both inhibitors and inducers.
- The metabolism of oral contraceptives can be induced. By induction, the oral contraceptive is metabolized more quickly, leaving less drug in the system and causing the patient to be at higher risk for pregnancy. If a woman on birth control pills takes an antibiotic, she should use a barrier contraceptive for the month she is taking the antibiotics and for 1 week longer.
- Many antidepressants, such as fluoxetine and nefazodone, are inhibitors and substrates.
- Among the cardiovascular drugs, antiarrhythmics may be inhibitors and substrates. Calcium channel blockers are both inhibitors and substrates. Several β-blockers are substrates. All statins are substrates or inhibitors. For example, losartan is a substrate.
- Codeine is a substrate whose metabolism may be induced/inhibited.
- Warfarin is a substrate drug whose metabolism is induced/inhibited by many drugs. It has a very narrow therapeutic window with potentially serious side effects. Extensive information should be collected about any drug added to a patient on a warfarin regimen. International Normalized Ratio (INR) times should be followed closely (even in the absence of drug–drug interactions).
- Cimetidine is an inhibitor of several isoenzyme pathways.
- Cyclosporine is a substrate whose metabolism can be inhibited by many drugs.
- The benzodiazepines can be a substrate whose metabolism is induced or inhibited.
- Caffeine is a substrate.
- Grapefruit juice inhibits the cytochrome P450 enzyme system in the intestine, allowing better absorption of a drug. Drinking large amounts of grapefruit juice can increase the level of certain drugs up to threefold. The cause and mechanism of this are not completely known.
- The effect of herbal medicines is unknown. Anecdotal evidence of drug interactions has been obtained but no scientific evidence. To be safe, assume that herbal medicines are active in the enzyme system, and discourage their use in a patient with risk factors for drug interactions.
- Vitamins, including the antioxidants, are not significant inducers or inhibitors.

In the future, new immunostimulation therapy probably will affect the P450 enzyme system, generally acting as an inhibitor.

See Box 3-1 for a complete listing of known reactions related to the P450 system.

BOX 3-1   Known Cytochrome P450 Enzyme Reactions With Drugs

CYTOCHROME 1A2 ISOENZYMES

Substrates	Inhibitors	Inducers
amitriptyline	cimetidine	phenobarbital
caffeine	ciprofloxacin	phenytoin
clomipramine	clarithromycin	rifampin
clozapine	enoxacin	ritonavir
cyclobenzaprine	erythromycin	
desipramine	fluvoxamine (potent)	**Smoking/polycyclic Aromatic**
diazepam	grapefruit juice	**Hydrocarbons**
haloperidol	isoniazid	
imipramine	ketoconazole	
(R)-warfarin	levofloxacin	
tacrine	norfloxacin	
theophylline	omeprazole	
zileuton	paroxetine	

CYTOCHROME 2C ISOENZYME

Substrates	Inhibitors	Inducers
amitriptyline	amiodarone 2C9	carbamazepine
clomipramine	chloramphenicol 2C9	phenobarbital
diazepam 2C9	cimetidine 2C9	phenytoin
imipramine	fluconazole	rifampin
losartan 2C9	fluoxetine	
omeprazole	fluvastatin	
phenytoin 2C9	fluvoxamine 2C9, potent	
(S)-warfarin 2C9	isoniazid	
tolbutamide	ketoconazole (weak)	
topiramate 2C9	omeprazole 2C9, 2C19	
	sertraline	
	topiramate 2C19	
	zafirlukast 2C9	

CYTOCHROME 2D6 ISOENZYMES

Substrates		Inhibitors	Inducers
amitriptyline	maprotiline	carbamazepine	amiodarone
bisoprolol	meperidine	phenobarbital	cimetidine
chlorpromazine	methadone	phenytoin	clomipramine
clomipramine	methamphetamine	rifampin	desipramine
clozapine	metoprolol	ritonavir	fluoxetine
codeine	mexiletine		fluphenazine
cyclobenzaprine	morphine		haloperidol
desipramine	nortriptyline		mibefradil
dexfenfluramine	oxycodone		paroxetine
dextromethorphan	paroxetine		propafenone
donepezil	perphenazine		quinidine
doxepin	propafenone		ritonavir
fenfluramine	propranolol		sertraline
flecainide	risperidone		thioridazine
fluoxetine	thioridazine		
fluphenazine	timolol		
haloperidol	tramadol		
hydrocodone	trazodone		
imipramine	venlafaxine		

BOX 3-1   Known Cytochrome P450 Enzyme Reactions With Drugs (Continued)

CYTOCHROME 3A4 ISOENZYMES

Substrates		Inhibitors	Inducers
alfentanil	ketoconazole	amiodarone	carbamazepine
alprazolam	lansoprazole	cannabinoids	dexamethasone
amitriptyline	(minor)	clarithromycin	ethosuximide
amlodipine	lidocaine	erythromycin	phenobarbital
astemizole	losartan	fluconazole	phenytoin
atorvastatin	lovastatin	fluoxetine	primidone
busulfan	mibefradil	fluvoxamine	rifabutin
cannabinoids	miconazole	grapefruit juice	rifampin
carbamazepine	midazolam	indinavir	troglitazone
cisapride	navelbine	itraconazole	
clindamycin	nefazodone	ketoconazole	
clomipramine	nelfinavir	omeprazole (slight)	
clonazepam	nicardipine	metronidazole	
cocaine	nifedipine	mibefradil	
cyclobenzaprine	nimodipine	miconazole	
cyclophosphamide	nisoldipine	nefazodone	
cyclosporine	ondansetron	nelfinavir	
dapsone	paclitaxel	norfloxacin	
dexamethasone	pravastatin	quinine	
dextromethorphan	prednisone	quinidine	
diazepam (minor)	quinidine	ritonavir	
diltiazem	quinine	saquinavir	
disopyramide	rifampin	sertraline	
donepezil	ritonavir	troleandomycin	
doxorubicin	(R)-warfarin	zafirlukast	
dronabinol	saquinavir		
erythromycin	sertraline		
estrogens, OBC	tacrolimus		
ethosuximide	tamoxifen		
etoposide	temazepam		
felodipine	terfenadine		
fentanyl	testosterone		
fexofenadine	triazolam		
ifosfamide	verapamil		
imipramine	vinblastine		
indinavir	vincristine		
isradipine	zileuton		

Finally, the activity of specific metabolizing enzymes is selectively affected in individuals with liver disease. The enzyme CYP 2C19 is more sensitive than CYP 2D6. Any recommendations for modification of drug dosage in the presence of liver disease should be based on knowledge of the particular enzyme involved in metabolism of the drug. Much of this information has yet to emerge from ongoing studies (Dresser et al, 2000; Lim et al, 2005).

For the clinician to conclude that a patient is having an adverse reaction to a drug, causality must be demonstrated. This may be done sequentially by (1) examining the chronologic relationship between the adverse reaction and the drug administration, (2) seeing resolution of the adverse reaction once dose has been decreased or discontinued (dechallenge), and (3) seeing recurrence of symptoms after readministration of the agent (rechallenge). In consultation with a specialist, a patient should be rechallenged to confirm causality only when it is imperative to use that particular drug (FDA, 1990). It is obvious that most clinicians must balance the strict documentation of causality with what is practical. This is often determined by how essential the drug is for patient therapy.

In most cases, an adverse reaction is not confirmed strictly because the adverse reaction is a known response pattern of the drug or may be measured by physiologic effects (i.e., blood pressure, laboratory abnormality, serum drug concentration). Occasionally, a patient reaction will be classified as an adverse reaction if it seems unrelated to the patient's concomitant diseases, clinical status, or other therapies (past or present).

Adverse reactions also may be classified by severity. With mild reactions, the patient may experience signs or symptoms, but they are easily tolerated. They often do not require treatment. Moderate reactions produce enough discomfort to interfere with usual activity and require treatment. Severe adverse reactions may incapacitate the patient or may interfere with the patient's ability to work or complete activities of daily living. They even may be life threatening or may contribute to the death of the patient. Although the rate of severe drug reactions may be 5% to 10% of all those reported, FDA records show that the elderly have an increased risk for severe adverse reactions, with patients older than 60 years of age accounting for nearly half of adverse drug reaction–associated deaths (Hanlon et al, 2006; Kvasz et al, 2000). These types of reactions often require hospitalization, intensive medical care, and longer than 15 days for recovery. Severe adverse reactions also may be associated with production of congenital anomalies. See Box 3-2 for some of the drugs commonly implicated in serious adverse effects.

Serious adverse reactions should be voluntarily reported to the FDA Medical Products MedWatch Reporting Program by calling 800-FDA-1088 (or 800-4USP-PRN) or by faxing to 800-FDA-0178 (or 301-816-8532). The FDA uses reports from health professionals and manufacturers to identify problems involving products already on the market. The agency evaluates the seriousness of the health hazard, takes corrective actions, and communicates those actions to the health professional community. Corrective actions may include the

FDA's requiring manufacturers to add new information to the labeling of a product. If a serious warning is required to ensure the continued safe use of a product, the FDA may require the warning to be displayed in heavy type and boxed text at the beginning of the package insert (the "black box"). Finally, the FDA may require a manufacturer to recall or withdraw a product because of a serious problem. Product withdrawals can mean that marketing of the product may be stopped permanently (FDA, 1990).

Drug Interactions

FOOD AND DRUG INTERACTIONS. Because many medications are administered orally, the potential for interaction with food is high. Taken together, food and drugs may alter the body's ability to utilize a particular food or drug. Some of these interactions may result from activation of the P450 enzyme system or from competition with receptor sites. Monoamine oxidase inhibitors (MAOIs) are some of the drugs most noted for drug–food interactions because they cannot be taken with aged cheese or many processed foods. Because both OTC and prescription drugs may interact with food, some principles that are important to stress with every patient include the following:
- Cigarettes can diminish the effectiveness of medication or can create other problems with particular drugs by increasing metabolism.

BOX 3-2   Drugs Associated With Serious Adverse Effects

HEPATOTOXIC DRUGS

acetaminophen	gold compounds
4-aminoquinolines	halothane
amiodarone	isoniazid
anabolic steroid agents	ketoconazole
antithyroid agents	mercaptopurine
asparaginase	methotrexate
azlocillin	methyldopa
carbamazepine	mezlocillin
carmustine	naltrexone
contraceptives (estrogen)	phenothiazine
dantrolene	phenytoin
daunorubicin	piperacillin
disulfiram	plicamycin
divalproex	rifampin
erythromycin	sulfonamides
estrogen DES, conjugated	tetracycline
etretinate	valproic acid

NEPHROTOXIC DRUGS

acyclovir	methotrexate
aminoglycoside antibiotics	methoxyflurane
amphotericin B	neomycin
analgesic combinations	NSAIDs
capreomycin	penicillamine
captopril	pentamidine
cisplatin	plicamycin
cyclosporine	rifampin
demeclocycline	streptozocin
edetate calcium disodium	sulfonamides
enalapril	tetracyclines
gold compounds	vancomycin
lithium	

OTHER TOXICITIES

Anaphylaxis: penicillins, heparin, aspirin, parenteral iron, dextran
Asthma: aspirin, ibuprofen
Blood dyscrasias: chloramphenicol, anticonvulsants, penicillins, hydralazine, sulfonamides, anticancer drugs
Damage to eighth cranial nerve: furosemide, aspirin and other salicylates, vibramycin, gentamicin
Eye damage: topical corticosteroids, ethambutol, thorazine, chloroquine
Peripheral neuritis: isoniazid, vincristine, hydralazine, ethambutol

Modified from McKenry LM, Salerno E: *Mosby's pharmacology in nursing*, ed 22, St Louis, 2006, Mosby; Hardman JG, Limbird LW et al, editors: *Goodman and Gilman's pharmacological basis of therapeutics*, ed 10, New York, 2001, McGraw-Hill; and Katzung BG: *Basic and clinical pharmacology*, ed 8, Norwalk, Conn, 2000, Appleton & Lange.

- Caffeine, which is found in coffee, tea, soft drinks, chocolate, and some medications, can also affect the action of some drugs.

See Table 3-3 for specific information concerning food–drug interactions that should be communicated to patients.

ALCOHOL–MEDICATION INTERACTIONS. Alcohol is another product with vast potential for interactions with drugs. In an alert distributed by the National Institute on Alcohol Abuse and Alcoholism (1995), it was estimated that alcohol–medication interactions may be a factor in at least 25% of all emergency department admissions (Weathermon & Crabb, 1999). An unknown number of less serious interactions go unrecognized and unrecorded.

It has been estimated that approximately 70% of the adult population consumes alcohol at least occasionally, and up to 10% of people may drink daily. Research also suggests that about 60% of men and 30% of women have had one or more adverse alcohol-related life events. These figures together with the facts concerning the substantial numbers of people who take medications suggest that some concurrent use of alcohol and medications is inevitable (Weathermon & Crabb, 1999).

One segment of the population at particular risk for alcohol–drug interactions consists of the elderly, who take 25% to 30% of all prescription medications. Elderly individuals are more likely to experience medication side effects than are younger persons, and these effects tend to be more severe with advancing age. Among persons age 60 years or older, 10% of those in the community and 40% of those in nursing homes fulfill criteria for alcohol abuse (Weathermon & Crabb, 1999).

How Alcohol and Drugs Interact. Both drugs and alcohol travel through the bloodstream to exert the desired effects on the body. With alcohol, the site of action is the brain; therefore, intoxication occurs until the alcohol has been finally metabolized and eliminated, principally by the liver.

The extent to which an administered dose of a drug reaches its site of action is described in terms of its availability. Alcohol can influence the effectiveness of a drug by altering its availability NIAAA, 1995). Typical alcohol–drug interactions include the following (Weathermon & Crabb, 1999):

- An acute dose of alcohol (a single drink or several drinks over several hours) may inhibit a drug's metabolism by competing with the drug for the same set of metabolizing enzymes. This interaction prolongs and enhances the drug's availability, potentially increasing the patient's risk of experiencing harmful side effects from the drug.
- In contrast, chronic (long-term) alcohol ingestion may activate drug-metabolizing enzymes, thus decreasing the drug's availability and diminishing its effects. After these enzymes have been activated, they remain so even in the absence of alcohol, thereby affecting the metabolism of certain drugs for several weeks after cessation of drinking. Thus, a recently abstinent chronic drinker may need higher doses of some medications than are required by nondrinkers to achieve therapeutic levels.
- Enzymes activated by chronic alcohol consumption transform some drugs into toxic chemicals that can damage the liver or other organs.
- Alcohol can magnify the inhibitory effects of sedative and narcotic drugs at their sites of action in the brain.

To add to the complexity of these interactions, some drugs affect the metabolism of alcohol, thus altering its potential for intoxication and the adverse effects associated with alcohol consumption.

The Institute on Alcohol Abuse and Alcoholism Alert is precise in summarizing common drug–alcohol interactions. See Table 3-4 for these interactions.

OVER-THE-COUNTER DRUG INTERACTIONS WITH PRESCRIPTION DRUGS. When patients are taking prescription medications, the additional use of OTC products may become a problem. Although specific drugs should be evaluated for their potential OTC interactions, it is important to be aware of common interactions (Table 3-5). Patients should always read the label of OTC products because common drug interactions are listed in the "Warning" section on those labels. Patients who experience a side effect after taking an OTC medicine for a common ailment should discontinue the product at once and consult a health care provider for guidance.

HERBAL PRODUCT INTERACTIONS WITH PRESCRIPTION DRUGS. Estimates of concurrent use of complementary and alternative medicine (CAM) products with allopathic medicine may vary from 39% to as high as 46% of patients, depending upon the population (Saw et al, 2006). The significance of herb–drug interactions varies, but it is essential to recognize that any interaction has the potential to cause harm. Some prescription drugs that are of the greatest concern, such as anticoagulants or antiplatelet medications, are those that have a narrow therapeutic window. Top-selling herbal drugs such as ginkgo, ginseng, and garlic are known to interact with anticoagulants or antiplatelet drugs. Chamomile, Dong quai, Dan shen, and ginger also may adversely interact with these drugs. It is of particular concern that most patients who are taking both prescription and CAM products do not report this to their health care providers (Saw et al, 2006).

PRECIPITATION OF GENETIC DISORDERS. Each person has a specific genetic composition that may be activated in the P450 enzyme system during metabolism. However, other underlying genetic disorders may be precipitated by medications. Specific metabolic defects in genetic disorders have been discovered, and the increased availability of laboratory studies necessary to make a specific diagnosis has made it possible for providers to be more specific in diagnosis. More widespread exposure of populations to drugs has revealed hitherto unsuspected errors of metabolism. New knowledge has indicated how patients with certain genetic disorders may be treated by drugs and has also expanded the list of medications that might precipitate problems. See Table 3-6 for a list of medications implicated in precipitating or exacerbating genetic disorders (McKenry et al, 2005). Research has also clarified that individual variation in how individuals handle some medications (requiring larger or smaller doses) is probably related to the P450 enzyme system and not to other hidden genetic defects.

DRUG EFFECTS ON LABORATORY TESTS AND BLOOD SUBSTANCES. Although medications exert a therapeutic effect, they also may have unintended consequences on other natural substances in the blood or may alter various laboratory tests. Clinicians should be aware of these changes as they interpret laboratory values and attempt to monitor drug action.

TABLE 3-3   Common Food–Drug Interactions

Medication Category	Common Medication Examples	Interactions and Instructions to Patients
ANTIINFECTIVES		
Penicillins: used to treat a wide variety of infections	amoxicillin (Trimox, Amoxil); ampicillin (Principen, Omnipen); penicillin V (Veetids)	Amoxicillin and bacampicillin may be taken with food; however, absorption of other types of penicillins is reduced when taken with food. Avoid acidic fruit juices, citrus fruits, and acidic beverages such as cola drinks. The antibiotics are acid labile (reduce absorption). Take drug 1 hr before meals (AC) or 2 hr after meals (PC).
Cephalosporins	cefaclor (Ceclor, Ceclor CD); cefadroxil (Duricef); cefixime (Suprax); cefprozil (Cefzil); cephalexin (Keflex, Keftab)	Take on an empty stomach 1hr AC or 2 hr PC meals. Can be taken with food if severe GI upset.
Tetracyclines: used to treat a wide variety of infections	tetracycline HCl (Achromycin V, Sumycin), doxycycline (Vibramycin); minocycline (Minocin)	These drugs should not be taken within 2 hr of eating dairy products such as milk, ice cream, yogurt, or cheese, or of taking calcium or iron supplements. Calcium forms complex with the drug, resulting in reduced absorption of the antibiotic. Take 1 hr AC or 2 hr PC.
Erythromycin or macrolides: used in treating skin and ear infections	erythromycin (E-Mycin, Ery-Tab, ERYC); erythromycin and sulfisoxazole (Pediazole); azithromycin (Zithromax); clarithromycin (Biaxin)	Erythromycins vary in their reactions with food. Avoid meals, acidic fruit juices, citrus fruits, and acidic beverages such as cola drinks. The antibiotics are acid labile (reduce absorption). Take drug 1 hr AC or 2 hr PC.
Sulfonamides: used to treat stomach and urinary tract infections	sulfamethoxazole and trimethoprim (Bactrim, Septra)	Avoid alcohol because the combination may cause nausea. Take on an empty stomach if possible.
ANTIFUNGALS		
	ketoconazole (Nizoral); itraconazole (Sporanox) griseofulvin (Grifulvin V)	Avoid taking these medications with dairy products or antacids. Avoid drinking alcohol or using medications or food that contain alcohol for at least 2 days after taking ketoconazole. This may produce a disulfiram-type reaction.
Methenamine: used in treating urinary tract infections	methenamine (Mandelamine, Urex)	Cranberries, plums, prunes, and their juices help the action of this drug. Avoid citrus fruits and citrus juices. Eat foods with protein, but avoid dairy products.
Nitroimidazole: used to treat intestinal and genital infections caused by bacteria and parasites	metronidazole (Flagyl)	Do not drink alcohol while using this drug; it will cause stomach pain, nausea, vomiting, headache, flushing, or redness of the face. It may produce a disulfiram-type reaction
Quinolones	ciprofloxacin (Cipro); levofloxacin (Levaquin); ofloxacin (Floxin)	Take on an empty stomach 1 hr AC or 2 hr PC meals. Can be taken with food if severe GI upset. Avoid calcium-containing products and vitamins and minerals that contain iron and antacids because these significantly decrease drug concentrations. Taking with caffeine products may increase caffeine levels and produce excitability and nervousness.
CARDIOVASCULAR DRUGS		
Diuretics: eliminate water, sodium, and chloride	furosemide (Lasix); triamterene-hydrochlorothiazide (HCTZ) (Dyazide, Maxzide); triamterene (Dyrenium); bumetanide (Bumex); metolazone (Zaroxolyn); HCTZ (Esidrix, HydroDIURIL)	Diuretics vary in their interactions with nutrients. Loss of potassium, calcium, and magnesium occurs with some diuretics. May require potassium supplement. With some loop diuretics, potassium loss is less significant.
Nitrates: relax veins and/or arteries to reduce work of the heart	nitroglycerin (Nitro, Nitro-Dur, Transderm-Nitro); isosorbide dinitrate (Isordil, Sorbitrate)	Use of sodium (salt) should be restricted for medication to be effective. Use with alcohol may drastically lower blood pressure. Check labels on food packages for sodium.
Antihypertensives: relax blood vessels, increase the supply of blood and oxygen to the heart and lessen its workload; may regulate heartbeat	β-blockers: atenolol (Tenormin); metoprolol (Lopressor); propranolol (Inderal); nadolol (Corgard); ACE inhibitors: captopril (Capoten); enalapril (Vasotec); lisinopril (Prinivil, Zestril); quinapril (Accupril); moexipril (Univasc)	Use of sodium (salt) should be restricted for medications to be effective. Check labels on food packages for sodium. Alcohol and propranolol combination may dramatically lower blood pressure. ACE inhibitors: food can decrease absorption. ACE inhibitors may increase the amount of potassium. Avoid eating large amounts of foods high in potassium.
Anticoagulants: prolong clotting of the blood	warfarin (Coumadin)	Moderation in consumption of foods high in vitamin K is recommended because vitamin K produces blood-clotting substances. Such foods include beef liver; green leafy vegetables such as spinach, cabbage, cauliflower, and Brussels sprouts; potatoes; vegetable oil; and egg yolk. High doses of vitamin E (400 IU or more) may prolong clotting time.

TABLE 3-3   Common Food–Drug Interactions (Continued)

Medication Category	Common Medication Examples	Interactions and Instructions to Patients
Antihyperlipidemics: HMG-CoA reductase inhibitors or "statins" lower cholesterol	atorvastatin (Lipitor); fluvastatin (Lescol); lovastatin (Mevacor); pravastatin (Pravachol); simvastatin (Zocor)	Mevacor should be taken with the evening meal to enhance absorption. Avoid large amounts of alcohol because these may increase risk of liver damage.
CENTRAL NERVOUS SYSTEM DRUGS		
Analgesics/antipyretics	acetaminophen (Tylenol, Tempra)	Take on an empty stomach for more rapid relief because food may slow the body's absorption of the drug. Concurrent use with alcohol can increase the risk of liver damage or GI bleeding.
Antianxiety drugs	lorazepam (Ativan); diazepam (Valium); alprazolam (Xanax)	Use with caffeine may cause excitability, nervousness, and hyperactivity and may lessen the antianxiety effect. Use with alcohol may impair mental and motor functions.
Antidepressants	paroxetine (Paxil); sertraline (Zoloft); fluoxetine (Prozac)	Avoid concurrent use with alcohol. These medications can be taken with or without food.
Analgesics/narcotics	codeine with acetaminophen (Tylenol No. 2, 3, 4); morphine (Roxanol, MS Contin); oxycodone with acetaminophen (Percocet, Roxicet); meperidine (Demerol); hydrocodone with acetaminophen (Vicodin, Lorcet)	Do not consume alcohol because of additive CNS depression. Use caution when motor skills are required.
lithium carbonate: regulates changes in chemical levels in the brain	Various names	Follow the dietary and fluid intake instructions of health care provider to avoid very serious toxic reactions.
MAOIs: act as antidepressant	phenelzine (Nardil); tranylcypromine (Parnate)	A very dangerous, potentially fatal interaction can occur with foods that contain tyramine, a chemical in alcoholic beverages, particularly wine, and in many foods such as hard cheeses, chocolate, beef or chicken livers, sour cream, yogurt, raisins, bananas, avocados, soy sauce, yeast extract, meat tenderizers, sausages, and anchovies. Patient may develop severe headache, nosebleed, chest pain, photosensitivity, or severe hypertension with hypertensive crisis.
Sedative-hypnotics	Various names	Do not use alcohol with any sleep medications. Oversedation occurs.
GASTROINTESTINAL DRUGS		
Antacids, antiulcer medications, histamine blockers: work to reduce acid in the stomach	cimetidine (Tagamet); famotidine (Pepcid); ranitidine (Zantac); nizatidine (Axid)	Follow specific diets given by health care provider. Avoid large amounts of caffeine; dairy products such as milk or cream may increase acid secretion if calcium carbonate is used as a calcium supplement
Laxatives: stimulate intestine, soften stool, add bulk or fluid to stool	Various names	Excessive use of laxatives can cause loss of essential vitamins and minerals and may require replenishment of potassium
MUSCULOSKELETAL DRUGS		
Aspirin: used to reduce pain, fever, and inflammation*	aspirin (Bayer, Ecotrin)	Because aspirin can cause stomach irritation, avoid alcohol. To avoid stomach upset, take with food. Do not take with fruit juice. Buffered or enteric-coated aspirin may also reduce GI bleeding.
NSAIDs: used to relieve pain and reduce inflammation and fever	ibuprofen (Advil, Motrin); naproxen (Anaprox, Aleve, Naprosyn); ketoprofen (Orudis); nabumetone (Relafen)	These drugs should be taken with food or milk because they can irritate the stomach. Avoid taking with the types of foods or alcoholic beverages that tend to irritate the stomach.
Indomethacin: used to reduce pain, swelling, joint pain, and fever in certain types of arthritis and gout	Indocin	This drug should be taken with food because it can irritate the stomach. Avoid taking with the types of foods or alcoholic beverages that tend to irritate the stomach.
Piroxicam: used to reduce pain, swelling, stiffness, joint pain, and fever in certain types of arthritis	Feldene	This medication should be taken with a light snack because it can cause stomach irritation. Avoid alcohol because it can add to the possibility of stomach upset.

*Many over-the-counter cold remedies contain aspirin in combination with other active ingredients.

Table continued on following page

TABLE 3-3   Common Food–Drug Interactions (Continued)

Medication Category	Common Medication Examples	Interactions and Instructions to Patients
Corticosteroids: used to provide relief to inflamed areas; lessen swelling, redness, itching, and allergic reactions	methylprednisolone (Medrol); prednisone (Deltasone); prednisolone (Pediapred, Prelone); cortisone acetate (Cortef)	Take with food or milk to decrease GI distress. Avoid alcohol because both alcohol and corticosteroids can cause stomach irritation. Also avoid foods high in sodium (salt). Check labels on food packages for sodium. Take with food to prevent stomach upset.
Codeine narcotic: used to suppress cough and relieve pain; often with ASA or acetaminophen	aspirin with codeine, Tylenol with codeine	Do not drink alcohol with this medication because it increases the sedative effect. Take with meals, small snacks, or milk because this medication may cause stomach upset.
RESPIRATORY DRUGS		
Antihistamines: used to relieve or prevent symptoms of colds, hay fever, and other types of allergy; act to limit or block histamine	brompheniramine (Dimetane, Bromphen); chlorphenira-mine (Chlor-Trimeton, Teldrin); diphenhydramine (Benadryl, Banophen); clemastine (Tavist); fexofenadine (Allegra); loratadine (Claritin); cetirizine (Zyrtec); astemizole (Hismanal)	Avoid taking with alcoholic beverages because antihistamines combined with alcohol may cause drowsiness and slowed reactions. Take prescription antihistamines on an empty stomach to increase their effectiveness.
Bronchodilators: used to treat the symptoms of bronchial asthma, chronic bronchitis, and emphysema; these medicines relieve wheezing, shortness of breath, and dyspnea; they work by opening the air passages of the lungs	theophylline (Slo-bid, Theo-Dur, Theo-Dur 24, Uniphyl); albuterol (Ventolin, Proventil, Combivent); epinephrine (Primatene Mist)	Avoid eating or drinking large amounts of food or beverages that contain caffeine because both bronchodilators and caffeine stimulate the CNS. High-fat meals may increase the amount of theophylline in the body, and high-carbohydrate meals may decrease it. The effect of food on theophylline products varies.

Modified from McKenry LM, Salerno E: *Mosby's pharmacology in nursing,* ed 22, St Louis, 2006, Mosby; National Consumers' League: *Food drug interactions,* Washington, DC, 1999, National Consumers League.

Tables 3-7 and 3-8 describe some of these common chemical interactions. Medications also may dramatically change the color of urine or feces. These changes are so startling that the patient should be warned to expect them. In most cases, the color changes are otherwise insignificant (McKenry et al, 2005).

CHRONOTHERAPY. Research has demonstrated the increased efficacy of certain treatment regimens when correlated with the circadian rhythm. The circadian clock controls rhythms in endocrine gland secretion, metabolic processes, and behavioral activity. Cyclic variations caused by these processes often are demonstrated by normal temperature changes throughout the day. Certain diseases, such as asthma, angina, diabetes mellitus, and hypertension, fluctuate according to the circadian cycle. Chronotherapy attempts to correlate the peak of drug activity with when it is needed by the body. Some drugs, such as Coumadin, growth hormone, antibiotics, theophylline, antianginals, vasoactive drugs, immunologic drugs, antihistamines, hypnotics, and analeptic drugs, are particularly affected by circadian rhythm. Clinicians are just beginning to understand that when a drug is administered makes a great deal of difference in its action. For example, secretion of catecholamines increases early in the morning as the patient awakens. Catecholamines cause an increase in heart rate, contractile force, cardiac output, and systolic blood pressure, and this places stress on the heart (Berne & Levy, 1998). It is important that any antihypertensive medication is given at a therapeutic level during this time. If a nitroglycerin patch is removed at bedtime, it leaves the patient with low drug levels in the morning at a time when the heart is at increased risk for an anginal episode.

Toxicities and Overdosage

Although changes in patient health, compliance factors, and overaggressive therapy may occasionally lead to overdosage, the most frequent cause of drug toxicity is accidental overdosage. Patients who repeat doses because they cannot remember whether they took their medications, because of confusion over proper dosages, or because of failure to make needed modifications may experience drug toxicity, particularly with those medications with narrow therapeutic margins. Patients at either end of the age spectrum are particularly susceptible to high accumulation of medications because of their relative distribution of muscle, bone, and adipose tissue (McKenry et al, 2005). With OTC products such as ibuprofen and acetaminophen, the dosage for small infants, children, and adults varies dramatically. The suggested amount may not always seem logical; however, the wrong drug dosage may prove lethal. Additionally, even well-maintained patients may become intolerant of their medications if they become dehydrated.

Some of the earliest signs of toxicity may be subtle. For example, the first signs of digoxin toxicity may include feelings of fatigue and heaviness of the legs. Malaise, slight confusion, lack of appetite, inability to concentrate, mild weakness, and changes in sleeping patterns are all easy to overlook unless the clinician has some index of suspicion that toxicity may be a factor.

Unfortunately, a relatively high number of cases of overdosage or poisoning occur when children inadvertently take medication while unsupervised. Little children may open pill containers left at bedsides or in bathroom cupboards and may confuse the pills with candy. Even vitamins and iron may prove lethal to small children. Despite a national campaign

TABLE 3-4 Specific Drug–Alcohol Interactions

Drug Interaction	Physiologic Result
Anesthetics	Chronic alcohol consumption increases the dose of propofol (Diprivan) required to induce loss of consciousness. Chronic alcohol consumption increases the risk of liver damage that may be caused by the anesthetic gases enflurane (Ethrane) and halothane (Fluothane).
Antibiotics	With acute alcohol consumption, some may cause nausea, vomiting, headache, and possibly convulsions; among these antibiotics are furazolidone (Furoxone), griseofulvin (Grisactin and others), metronidazole (Flagyl), and the antimalarial quinacrine (Atabrine). Acute alcohol consumption decreases the availability of isoniazid in the bloodstream, whereas chronic alcohol use decreases the availability of rifampin.
Anticoagulants	Acute alcohol use enhances the availability of warfarin, thereby increasing the patient's risk for life-threatening hemorrhage. Chronic alcohol consumption reduces the availability of warfarin, thereby lessening protection in blood clotting disorders.
Antidepressants	Alcoholism and depression are frequently associated, leading to a high potential for alcohol–antidepressant interactions. Alcohol increases the sedative effect of tricyclic antidepressants, such as amitriptyline, thereby impairing the mental skills required for driving. Acute alcohol consumption increases the availability of some tricyclics, potentially increasing their sedative effects; chronic alcohol use may increase the availability of some tricyclics and may decrease the availability of others. A chemical called *tyramine,* found in some beers and wine, interacts with some antidepressants, such as MAOIs, and one drink may produce a dangerous rise in blood pressure.
Antidiabetic medications	Acute alcohol use prolongs and chronic alcohol consumption decreases the availability of tolbutamide (Orinase). With other drugs, antidiabetic medications may produce symptoms of nausea and headache such as those described for metronidazole.
Antihistamines	Alcohol may intensify the sedation caused by some antihistamines or may cause excessive dizziness and sedation in older persons.
Antipsychotic medications	Acute alcohol use increases the sedative effect of these drugs, resulting in impaired coordination and potentially fatal breathing difficulties, and may result in liver damage.
Antiseizure medications	Acute alcohol increases the availability of phenytoin (Dilantin) and the risk of side effects. Chronic drinking may decrease phenytoin availability, significantly reducing the patient's protection against epileptic seizures, even during a period of abstinence.
Antiulcer medications	Cimetidine (Tagamet) and ranitidine (Zantac) may increase the availability of a low dose of alcohol under some circumstances.
Cardiovascular medications	Acute alcohol use interacts with some drugs to cause dizziness or fainting on standing up. These drugs include nitroglycerin, reserpine, methyldopa, hydralazine, and guanethidine. Chronic alcohol use decreases the availability of propranolol, potentially reducing its therapeutic effect.
Narcotic pain relievers	The combination of opiates and alcohol enhances the sedative effect of both substances, thereby increasing the risk of death from overdose. A single dose of alcohol can increase the availability of propoxyphene, potentially increasing its sedative side effects.
Nonnarcotic pain relievers	Some of these drugs cause stomach bleeding, particularly in the elderly, and inhibit blood clotting; alcohol can exacerbate these effects. Aspirin may increase the availability of alcohol, heightening the effects of a given dose of alcohol. Chronic alcohol use activates enzymes that transform acetaminophen into chemicals that can cause liver damage, even when used in small amounts.
Sedatives and hypnotics	Benzodiazepines that are sedating may cause severe drowsiness with alcohol, thus increasing the risk of all accidents, especially in the elderly. Low doses of flurazepam (Dalmane) interact with low doses of alcohol to impair driving ability, even when alcohol is ingested in the morning. The combination of alcohol and lorazepam may result in depressed heart and breathing functions. Acute alcohol consumption increases the availability of barbiturates, prolonging their sedative effects. Chronic alcohol consumption decreases barbiturate availability through enzyme activation. In addition, acute or chronic alcohol consumption enhances the sedative effect of barbiturates at their site of action in the brain, sometimes leading to coma or fatal respiratory depression.

From Institute on Alcohol Abuse and Alcoholism: *Alert on alcohol and medication interactions,* No. 27 PH355, Washington, DC, January 1995, Institute on Alcohol Abuse and Alcoholism.

to child-proof homes, the number of children who die each year as a result of drug overdosage is far too high.

It also cannot be ignored that some patients, for a variety of reasons, deliberately overdose on medications. Some of these episodes are true suicide attempts; others represent actions that occur because of alcoholic confusion or attempts to gain chemical "highs" that go wrong.

The medication overdose treatment advice in the *Physicians' Desk Reference* (a source frequently consulted for overdosage information) is not accurate and should not be used. Therefore an immediate call to the pharmacist at the local or regional poison control center (Box 3-3) will yield superior information for clinicians who seek to respond to possible or confirmed cases of drug overdosage. Other information may be obtained by consulting the pharmaceutical manufacturer of the drug.

Risk-Benefit Ratio

Every type of drug therapy carries a risk that may be worth taking if the benefits exceed the predictable morbidity and mortality rates of the therapy itself. This is fairly simple to determine for short-term therapy in which results are quickly seen, or the therapy can be terminated if toxicity becomes evident. Risks and benefits are more complicated to calculate for long-term therapy because the results may not be seen until after months or years of treatment. With long-term care, it is more difficult for the clinician to determine whether therapies should be terminated if some toxicities develop because the amount of good that is sacrificed is not always clear, especially to the patient. For example, methotrexate is an agent that is highly toxic to the bone marrow and the liver,

TABLE 3-5   Common OTC Drug Interactions With Prescription Products

Type of OTC Product	Prescription Interactions
Acid (reduces H$_2$ agonists)	This may interact with theophylline, warfarin, or phenytoin
Antacids	If antacid contains aluminum, calcium, or magnesium, it has high potential for drug interaction.
Antiemetics	Do not use with sedatives or tranquilizers. May also be a problem in patients with asthma, glaucoma, or enlarged prostate gland
Antihistamines	These may interact with antidepressants, alcoholic beverages, sedatives, or tranquilizers.
Cough products	If product contains dextromethorphan, it must not be taken with an MAOI.
Nasal decongestants	Do not use with MAOIs, sedatives, tranquilizers, or products with diphenhydramine. If patient is taking antihypertensives or antidepressants, he should not take a nasal decongestant without provider consultation.
Menstrual products	For products that contain caffeine, limit the use of foods or beverages that contain caffeine. If product contains ammonium chloride, do not use in patients with kidney or liver disease.
Nicotine replacement products	These may interact with antidepressants or asthma medications, requiring dosage adjustments.
Pain relievers	If product contains aspirin or salicylate, do not use with anticoagulants. Use care if patient has diabetes, gout, or arthritis. Limit alcohol to fewer than three drinks per day.
Sleep aids	Avoid sedatives, tranquilizers, MAOIs. Avoid alcoholic beverages.
Weight control aids	Do not use with cough/cold or allergy medication that contains any form of phenylpropanolamine. This ingredient also should not be used in patients under treatment for high blood pressure, eating disorders, depression, heart disease, diabetes, or thyroid disease.

Modified from National Consumers League: *Food drug interactions,* developed jointly by the American Pharmaceutical Association, U.S. Food and Drug Administration, Food Marketing Institute, and National Consumers League, 1989.

but it offers substantial hope in preventing joint destruction in patients with rheumatoid arthritis. When methotrexate is properly administered and closely monitored, the risk is slight compared with the potential for joint preservation (DiPiro et al, 2005). However, vitamin D therapy for rheumatoid arthritis is not recommended because the morbidity is far greater than any modest expected benefit.

Unsuccessful and even dangerous therapies were given for decades before the medical profession realized that they did more harm than good. Increasingly, information summarized from research studies on the practice of evidence-based medicine will help to define benefit and risk more clearly in the future. Large-scale randomized controlled trials of drugs will continue to provide data about whether drugs should be

TABLE 3-6   Medications Implicated in the Precipitation of Genetic Disorders

Medication or Drug	Genetic Disorder Stimulated
Anesthetic agents	Sickle cell anemia (hemoglobin S)
atropine, homatropine, ephedrine, other mydriatics or anticholinergics	Angle-closure glaucoma
Barbiturates, aminopyrine, sulfonamides, griseofulvin, hexachlorobenzene, meprobamate, chlordiazepoxide	Acute intermittent porphyria
Corticosteroids	Primary open-angle glaucoma
Levodopa	Huntington's chorea
Oral contraceptives	Dubin-Johnson syndrome
primaquine, other oxidant drugs	Glucose-6-phosphate dehydrogenase (G6PD) deficiency
Salicylates, menthol, corticosteroids	Crigler-Najjar syndrome
Sulfonamides, nitrites, acetanilides	Erythrocyte diaphorase deficiency
Sulfonamides, sulfones	Hemoglobin H, hemoglobin Zurich

Information from DiPiro JT et al, editors: *Pharmacotherapy: a pathophysiologic approach,* ed 5, Norwalk, Conn, 2002, Appleton & Lange; Hardman JG et al, editors: *Goodman and Gilman's pharmacological basis of therapeutics,* ed 10, New York, 2001, McGraw-Hill; and Katzung BG: *Basic and clinical pharmacology,* ed 8, Norwalk, Conn, 2000, Appleton & Lange.

TABLE 3-7   Selected Drug Interference With Laboratory Tests

Drug	Test	Method	Possible Result
acetaminophen	Blood glucose	Glucose oxidase/peroxidase	False decrease
	Pancreatic function testing	Bentiromide	False increase
	Serum uric acid	Phosphotungstate uric acid test	False increase
Anticonvulsants	Thyroid tests	Protein-bound iodine (PBI)	False decrease
Antihistamines	Skin testing	Allergen extracts	False negatives
Antimuscarinic, atropine	Urine test	Phenolsulfonphthalein (PSP) excretion test	False decrease
Ascorbic acid (megadoses)	Occult blood in stool		False negative
	Liver test, LDH and serum	Autoanalyzer	Interference
	Urine glucose	Glucose oxidase test	False decrease
Cephalosporins	Blood glucose	Ferricyanide test	False negative with cefuroxime
	Antiglobulin test	Coombs' test, direct	False positive in neonates when mother received before delivery
	Urine glucose	Copper sulfate test (Benedict's or Fehling's)	False positive or negative
	Bleeding time (coagulation)	Prothrombin time (PT)	Increase or prolonged time
Coffee, tea, cola drinks, chocolate, acetaminophen	Theophylline test for patients taking aminophylline, oxtriphylline, theophylline	Spectrophotometric	False increase
NSAIDs	Urinary bile	Diazo tablets	False positive with mefenamic acid capsules (Ponstel)
	Urinary 5-hydroxyindoleacetic acid (5-HIAA) and urinary steroid determinations	Various assays	False increase

Modified from McKenry LM, Salerno E: *Mosby's pharmacology in nursing,* ed 22, St Louis, 2006, Mosby.

used and what degree of risk the patient may be facing with their prescription.

The risk-benefit ratio expresses the amount of "acceptable" risk of adverse reaction or treatment failure that a patient may face in taking a drug versus the calculation of its potential benefit. It is generally estimated for each drug. The patient and the provider together must determine the degree of risk that will be tolerated. This will probably depend on the severity of the disease for which the patient is being treated.

Design and Optimization of Dosage Regimens

CALCULATING THE THERAPEUTIC INDEX. The decision to use pharmacologic therapy requires the clinician to determine what degree of drug effect is desirable and achievable. If some effect of the drug can be measured easily (e.g., blood pressure for an antihypertensive medication), this can guide dosage. The medication can be adjusted up or down to achieve the optimal dosage in both a practical and sensible manner. However, often it is not possible to measure drug effect so simply. The clinician will have to establish some decision rules about how often to change dosage and by how much. Alternatively, some drugs have very little dose-related toxicity, and maximum efficacy is usually desired. For these drugs, doses well in excess of the average required will both ensure efficacy and prolong drug action.

The therapeutic index, a measure of drug safety, is calculated by dividing the toxic (or lethal) dose by the therapeutic (or effective) dose:

$$\text{Therapeutic index} = \frac{LD_{50}}{ED_{50}}$$

where LD_{50} is the toxic or lethal dose in 50% of the population, and ED_{50} is the effective or therapeutic dose in 50% of the population.

Response of the patient to the drug may be increased by factors that cause higher blood concentrations of a drug or by factors that make the patient more sensitive to a given blood concentration.

The therapeutic response is monitored by examining the index of therapeutic effect to determine whether the therapeutic goal has been attained (e.g., an infection has been suppressed). It should be discriminating and should be practical to measure. The index of toxic effect may also be measured. Again, the measurement should discriminate, it should be sensitive to detect toxicity promptly, and it should be practical to measure.

The concept of therapeutic window is not the same as therapeutic index. The therapeutic window describes the range between the lowest therapeutic concentration and the beginning of toxicity (Figure 3-11). Some drugs have a very

TABLE 3-8   Selected Drug Effects on Specific Blood Substances

Drug	Effect on Blood Chemicals
All drugs	Possible increase in SGOT, SGPT
aminoglycoside	Possible increase in SGOT/SGPT, BUN, bilirubin; possible decrease in K$^+$, Na$^+$
Anticonvulsants	Possible increase in glucose
Antidepressants	Possible increase or decrease in glucose
β-blockers	Possible increase in K$^+$, SGOT/SGPT, uric acid, BUN
carbamazepine	Possible increase in SGOT/SGPT, BUN, bilirubin
carbidopa/levodopa	Possible increase in SGOT/SGPT, BUN, bilirubin
Cephalosporins	Possible increase in PT, increase in SGOT/SGPT
cinoxacin	Possible increase in SGOT/SGPT, BUN
cisplatin	Possible increase in uric acid, BUN; possible decrease in K$^+$
diflunisal	Possible decrease in uric acid
Diuretics (loop)	Possible increase in glucose, uric acid, BUN; possible decrease in K$^+$, Na$^+$
Diuretics (thiazide)	Possible increase in glucose, uric acid, bilirubin; possible decrease in K$^+$, Na$^+$
Diuretics (potassium sparing)	Possible increase in glucose, K$^+$, uric acid, BUN; possible decrease in Na$^+$
mefenamic acid	Possible increase in PT
methyldopa	Possible increase in K$^+$, Na$^+$, SGOT/SGPT, uric acid, BUN, bilirubin
norfloxacin	Possible increase in SGOT/SGPT, BUN
NSAIDs	Possible decrease in glucose
propoxyphene	Possible increase in SGOT/SGPT
penicillin G-K	Possible increase in K$^+$
Injectable	Almost all increase SGOT/SGPT.
azlocillin	Possible increase in Na$^+$, bilirubin; possible decrease in uric acid
carbenicillin	Possible increase in Na$^+$
mezlocillin	Possible increase in Na$^+$, bilirubin
piperacillin	Possible increase in Na$^+$, bilirubin
ticarcillin	Possible increase in Na$^+$, bilirubin; possible decrease in uric acid
prazosin	Possible increase in Na$^+$
rifampin	Possible increase in SGOT/SGPT, uric acid, BUN, bilirubin
trimethoprim	Possible increase in SGOT/SGPT, BUN, bilirubin
tetracycline	Possible increase in BUN (except for doxycycline, minocycline), bilirubin
valproic acid	Possible increase in SGOT/SGPT, bilirubin

Modified from McKenry L, Tessier E, Hogan MA: *Mosby's pharmacology in nursing,* ed 22, St. Louis, 2006, Mosby.

BOX 3-3   Poison Control Centers

American Association of Poison Control Centers Certified Regional Poison Centers provides a list of centers with routine and emergency telephone numbers. Changes are made frequently to these listings. Contact the American Association of Poison Control Centers at 202-362-7217 for updated information.

narrow therapeutic window, making patient monitoring especially important.

Several different strategies may be used to determine how much medication should be used. These include determining a target level, maintenance dosing, and loading dose; individualizing therapy; and performing therapeutic drug monitoring.

Target Level. In target level dosing, a desired or target steady-state concentration of the drug (usually in plasma) is identified, and a dosage is computed that is expected to achieve this value. Drug concentrations are subsequently measured, and dosage is adjusted if necessary to approximate the target more closely. This type of dosing is advisable when the effects of a drug are difficult to measure (or if the drug is given for prophylaxis). Target level dosing is also used when toxicity and lack of efficacy are potential problems, or when the therapeutic window is very narrow. All of these situations require careful titration of dosages (Brunton et al, 2005; DiPiro et al, 2005).

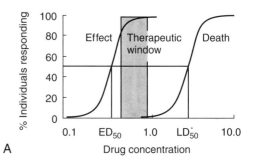

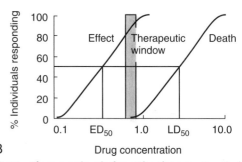

FIGURE 3-11   Therapeutic window. The therapeutic window compares the range of effective drug concentration versus the safety of the drug. Note that the drug in **A** has a much wider therapeutic window than the drug in **B,** even though both drugs have the same therapeutic index. ED, Effective dose; LD, lethal dose. (From Stringer JL: *Basic concepts in pharmacology,* ed 2, New York, 2000, McGraw-Hill.)

When target level dosing is used, the therapeutic objective must relate to an established blood serum therapeutic range, such as that seen with theophylline or digoxin levels. The lower limit of the therapeutic range appears to be approximately equal to the drug concentration that produces about half of the greatest possible therapeutic effect. The upper limit of the therapeutic range is fixed by toxicity, not by efficacy. Usually the upper limit of the therapeutic range is such that no more than 5% to 10% of patients will experience a toxic effect (DiPiro et al, 2005). These figures are highly variable; however, the target usually is chosen as the center of this therapeutic range.

Maintenance Dose. Most drugs are administered as a continuous infusion or as a series of doses designed to maintain steady-state concentration of the drug in plasma and to keep it within a given therapeutic range. To achieve the maintenance dose, the rate of drug administration is adjusted such that the rate of input equals the rate of loss. If the clinician knows the clearance and availability for that drug in a particular patient, the appropriate dose and dosing interval may be calculated to achieve the desired concentration of the drug in plasma (Brunton et al, 2005).

Loading Dose. If the target concentration of a dose must be met rapidly, a "loading dose"—a dose or a series of doses—is given at the onset of therapy. This may be desirable if the time required to attain steady state through administration of the drug at a constant rate (4 to 5 elimination half-lives) is long relative to demands of the condition for which the patient is being treated. This is commonly seen with antiarrhythmic drugs when the effect of the drug is required immediately. Because loading doses tend to be large and often are given parenterally and rapidly, they can be particularly dangerous if toxic effects occur as a result of actions of the drug. An overly sensitive individual may be exposed abruptly to a toxic concentration of a drug. If the drug involved has a long half-life, it may take a long time for the concentration to fall if the level achieved is excessive (Brunton et al, 2005).

Individualizing Dose. Information about the patient also helps in tailoring the dosage. Calculation of the glomerular filtration rate and creatinine clearance may be required to determine dosage in individuals with kidney disease. Adjustments in dosage to compensate for liver damage may be necessary. Comorbidity and the concurrent use of other medications, food, or alcohol may also require dosage modifications to achieve the desired level in the patient.

Therapeutic Drug Monitoring. Therapeutic drug monitoring involves measuring serum drug levels in patients receiving drugs with a narrow therapeutic window, to maximize efficacy and minimize toxicity (Brunton et al, 2005; Katzung, 2006). Some of the most commonly administered drugs that must be closely monitored through serum blood levels include theophylline, phenytoin, carbamazepine, digoxin, and aminoglycoside antibiotics.

In monitoring serum drug levels, it is important to consider the time of sampling of the drug concentration. If intermittent dosing is used, the concentration of drug measured in a sample taken at virtually any time during the dosing interval will provide information about drug toxicity and may be used to confirm other clinical findings that suggest toxicity (DiPiro et al, 2005; Katzung, 2006). However, serum drug levels used to measure drug concentration for the purposes of adjusting the dosage regimen must be taken at specified times to reflect accurate levels.

Drug levels vary dramatically throughout the dosing cycle because the blood level rises and falls throughout the day, as in a trough. If a blood sample is taken shortly after the drug is administered, the level may be uninformative or even misleading. Levels may be very high but not reflective of toxicity; conversely, levels may be low because distribution is delayed relative to changes in plasma concentration (Brunton et al, 2005; Katzung, 2006). When the goal of measurement is adjustment of dosage, the sample should be taken well after the previous dose is given. As a rule of thumb, one should test just before the next planned dose, when the concentration is at its minimum level. However, this does not provide relevant information about drugs that are nearly completely eliminated between doses. For individuals with renal failure, in whom concerns about drug accumulation are high, determination of both maximum and minimum concentrations is recommended.

Before taking a serum sample, it is also important to consider whether the patient has reached steady-state concentrations. Steady state usually is achieved after 4 to 5 half-lives have passed. If a sample is obtained too soon after dosage is started, it will not accurately reflect clearance. Yet, for toxic drugs, if one waits until the drug is at steady state, the level may already be within a toxic range. The protocol in *Goodman & Gilman's* (Brunton et al, 2005) suggests that when it is important to maintain careful control of concentrations, one may take the first sample after 2 half-lives (as calculated and expected for the patient), assuming that no loading dose has been given. If the concentration already exceeds 90% of the eventual expected mean steady-state concentration, the dosage rate should be halved, another sample obtained in another 2 half-lives, and the dosage halved again if this sample exceeds the target. If the first concentration is not too high, one proceeds with the initial rate of dosage. Even if the concentration is lower than expected, one usually can wait until steady state is achieved in another 2 half-lives and then can proceed to adjust dosage. (Computer programs are available for the management of particularly difficult drug level calculations.) Table 3-9 shows the best time to draw blood levels for several different medications.

PRACTICAL APPLICATION OF PHARMACOKINETICS AND PHARMACODYNAMICS TO DRUG PRESCRIBING

When the underlying scientific principles inherent in pharmacokinetics and pharmacodynamics are applied, some very practical suggestions can be made for rational drug therapy:

- *Always try nonpharmacologic therapy first.* Continue it even after a medication has been started.
- *Use a drug only when clearly indicated for a specific purpose.* It may be difficult for a provider to resist prescribing a medication for every symptom that annoys the patient, particularly when the patient is demanding resolution or relief. Well-directed advice and sound instructions often substitute for medication.
- *Use only one drug whenever possible.* Many patients with chronic disease who take numerous medications may need

TABLE 3-9   Therapeutic Ranges of Serum Drug Concentrations for Selected Drugs

Drug	Serum Concentration (Therapeutic Level, mcg/ml Unless Otherwise Indicated)	Time to Draw Blood Samples (Hours After Last Dose)
ANTIBIOTICS		
amikacin (Amikin)	15-25	Obtain peak and trough levels: draw peak 15-30 min after intravenous (IV) dose or 1 hr after intramuscular (IM) dose; trough 5 min before next dose.
gentamicin (Garamycin)	4-10	
netilmicin (Netromycin)	6-10	
tobramycin (Nebcin)	4-10	
ANTICONVULSANTS		
carbamazepine (Tegretol)	4-12	Steady state 1-2 weeks
ethosuximide	10-100	Steady state 10-30 days
phenobarbital	10-40	Steady state 1-2 weeks
phenytoin (Dilantin)	10-20	Steady state 2-3 days
primidone (Mysoline)	5-12	Steady state 1-2 days
valproic acid (Depakene, Depakote)	50-100	Steady state 1-2 days; then draw sample before next dose
ANTIDEPRESSANTS		
lithium	0.6-1.4 mEq/L	Steady state 3 weeks; draw before next dose
CARDIOVASCULAR		
digoxin (Lanoxin)	0.9-2 ng/nl	Steady state 1 week; draw before next dose, at least 6 hr after last dose
lidocaine (Xylocaine)	1.5-5	Steady state 6-12 hr; draw any time during infusion
procainamide (Pronestyl)	4-10	Steady state 12-24 hr; draw before next dose
quinidine (various)	3-6	Steady state 1.5 days; draw before next dose
RESPIRATORY		
theophylline (various)	10-20	Steady state in 1-2 days in adults; up to 1 week in neonates; IV: draw any time; oral; draw before next dose

From McKenry LM, Mosby'sSalerno E: *Mosby's pharmacology in nursing,* ed 22, St Louis, 2006, Mosby.

to have the drugs stopped and reevaluated. Elderly patients, in particular, may have been on drugs almost forever, and nobody has ever thought to stop them. They may have had an acute illness that required additional medications or higher dosages that are no longer required. Some patients become very attached to particular drugs and do not want to stop them.

- *Use lowest effective dose.* If dosage is titrated up to a higher level and no additional benefit is seen, titrate it down to the previous dose. This saves money and decreases the risk of adverse effects. Drug reactions are often dose related and may be prompted by the philosophy that if a little bit is good, an added amount will do no harm and may ensure success.
- *Start low and go slow.* Usually, change dosage by no more than 50% and no more often than every 3 to 4 half-lives. This usually means no change for 1 to 2 weeks after a dose is started.
- *Simplify the regimen whenever possible.* Give the fewest doses and at the most convenient hours of the day to improve compliance.

- *If possible, use the side effect profile of one drug to treat other symptoms.* For example, if a patient has depression and insomnia, use trazodone or mirtazapine, which may be sedating, instead of sertraline (Zoloft) or fluoxetine (Prozac), which are most commonly associated with insomnia.
- *Monitor closely for therapeutic effects.* Although drug levels may be evaluated as appropriate, trust your observation of the patient's clinical response more than the blood level. For example, the therapeutic level of phenytoin is usually between 10 and 20 mcg/ml. However, elderly patients often do best on a drug level of 8 mcg/ml. Drugs that are given over prolonged periods are more apt to produce adverse reactions; thus, the dosage must be carefully monitored and reduced at the first sign of difficulty.
- *Keep good patient records.* A history of allergy, recent hepatitis, renal insufficiency, smoking, alcoholism, or other comorbidity helps to alert the health care provider that the patient may be at greater risk for developing adverse reactions or drug–drug interactions.

TABLE 3-10 Electronic Media Sources With Current Drug Information

Title	Address	Description
FDA Human Drugs Page	www.fda.gov/cder	Extensive library of information specific to drugs; regulatory guidance
Food–Drug Interactions	http://www.niaaa.nih.gov/Publications	National Institute on Alcohol Abuse and Alcoholism: extensive discussion of interaction between food and different medications
Med Files	www.geocities.com/HotSprings/2255/drugs.html	Comprehensive listing of medical/pharmaceutical information
Rx List	www.rxlist.com	Top 200 drugs; detailed database on prescriptions
Up-to-Date	www.uptodate.com	Comprehensive evidence-based clinical information resource; extensive drug database (LexiComp); available on the Web, desktop, and PDA; content strenuously reviewed, comprehensive, and concise

- *Be particularly careful with some drugs that are highly associated with adverse effects.* Insulin, steroids, and many drugs used in chemotherapy and AIDS treatment are good examples. Prescription of these drugs mandates that the health care provider offer extensive education to the patient and the family if the drugs are to be used safely.

- *Always keep drug interactions and adverse effects in mind when evaluating the patient.* They are the rule rather than the exception. When using drugs with a great potential for adverse reactions, careful monitoring may prevent serious problems. Pancytopenia need not occur if leukopenia is detected early; deafness will not result if signs of eighth nerve impairment are promptly investigated. It is not just luck that allows the health care provider to help the patient avoid problems with drug therapy.

- *Finally, stay up-to-date.* Many journals hold articles for 6 to 12 months before publication; most textbooks are in production for longer than a year after they are submitted for publication. Thus, these sources of information may be outdated before they are even printed. New research findings should constantly be consulted and evaluated; valid findings should be incorporated into practice. In this age of electronic information dissemination, the standards of practice may be expected to shift to incorporate more new knowledge than was ever available before. Thus, it is imperative for clinicians to find ways to update their knowledge on a regular basis.

Many publishers of pharmaceutical information have realized that information about new products and new recommendations must reach health care providers in a timely manner. Publishers of several of the most comprehensive drug texts have developed methods for accomplishing this. *Facts and Comparisons* (J. B. Lippincott) allows readers to subscribe to a monthly update service for their text, as well as providing content on disk and CD-ROM. *Clinical Pharmacology* from Gold Standard and Elsevier is an electronic drug information reference for health care professionals that can be accessed online, on CD-ROM, or on PDA.

The Internet is becoming the biggest source of online information about drugs. Electronic databases linked to universities or pharmaceutical companies contain the latest information about drugs in terms of FDA approval and marketing. Table 3-10 lists some of the best and most user-friendly sites currently available to update drug information.

evolve A list of pharmaceutical company websites can be found on the Evolve Learning Resources website.

SUMMARY

Current drugs provide health care providers many options for medications they may use, alone or in combination. These drugs represent real opportunities to cure disease, resolve symptoms, and improve quality of life for patients. More information about how the agents work, ways to increase their effectiveness, and the risks inherent in their use is discovered every day. Used wisely and thoughtfully, medications are wonderful assets to the health care provider's treatment armamentarium; used unwisely, they may cause even greater difficulties and distress for both the patient and the provider.

evolve A continually updated list of useful WebLinks may be found in the Evolve Resources at http://evolve.elsevier.com/Edmunds/NP/

4 Special Populations: Geriatrics

BARBARA RESNICK and MARILYN WINTERTON EDMUNDS

Over the past century, the number of older adults has increased more than 10-fold and continues to increase. In the year 2000, approximately 35 million people were age 65 or older (National Center for Health Statistics, 2007). Women who reach age 65 can expect to live an additional 19 years, and men at age 65 can expect to live an additional 16 years. Because the length of life has increased, older adults are living longer with chronic illnesses (Ray & Street, 2005). Specifically, nearly 60% of older African American adults have high blood pressure, and a growing share of elderly African Americans, Hispanics, and Native Americans have diabetes.

Older adults make up 14% of the population yet account for 30% of medication expenditures. Up to 82% are taking at least one drug (Frankfort et al, 2006). Among a national sample of 2950 older adults, 12% took 10 medications daily and 23% were taking 5 prescription medications (Frankfort et al, 2006). The most common drug classes used are cardiovascular, analgesic, and central nervous system drugs (Passarelli et al, 2005). In addition, these individuals may add supplements, vitamins, and various home remedies to the regimen. Research has suggested that it is the number of pills a patient takes every day rather than the number of medications taken that is correlated with adverse drug reactions (ADRs) (Cramer, 2002). Because of a variety of issues, including limited knowledge of the impact of specific drugs on older adults, multiple medication use, and normal age- and disease-associated changes, older adults are at increased risk of experiencing ADRs (Bourne, 2007). It is essential for the health care provider to consider these issues before prescribing medications for this population.

Elderly patients are often affected by polypharmacy, both because they see multiple prescribers and because they self-treat with OTC medications. It is estimated that more than 40% of OTC drugs are purchased by people in this same age group. Despite the fact that older adults constitute a major group of drug users, most drug studies are performed on individuals 55 years of age or younger. It is essential for the health care provider to consider these issues before prescribing medications for this population.

FUNCTIONAL ASSESSMENT

Functional assessment is the core concept of geriatrics. When one is evaluating elderly patients, it is important to assess their ability to function in addition to what medical illnesses they may have. Classic assessment tools include Katz's Activities of Daily Living (ADLs) to assess mobility and the Folstein Mini-Mental Status Examination (MMSE) to assess cognitive function. Once medications have been started, it is essential to evaluate for the efficacy of drugs and for ADRs. Evaluation also must include any changes in the functional status of the patient that may result from medications. Common expressions of functional decline include weight loss, decline in mobility, incontinence, and falls (Gallo et al, 2006).

PHARMACOKINETIC CHANGES THAT AFFECT DRUG THERAPY

Pharmacokinetics refers to the way that drugs are absorbed, metabolized, distributed, and eliminated from the body. Although these processes are variable from patient to patient, the aging patient undergoes changes in some of these areas that may significantly affect the way a drug is handled by the body. Consideration of each of these processes when one prescribes drug therapy in the elderly can prevent inappropriate dosing and can prevent ADRs and their complications for patient care. Changes in the ways in which the body handles medications are behind the dosing advice to "Start low and go slow!" in the elderly.

Absorption

The overall significance of changes in the absorption of drugs with aging is not completely clear. There appears to be little, if any, significance in the amount of drug absorbed when drugs are passively absorbed. However, some reduced absorption has been noted in older adults for some compounds that are actively absorbed such as galactose, calcium, thiamine, and iron (Bourne, 2007). Physiologic changes that affect the GI tract include a reduction in acid output and the subsequent alkaline environment. These changes affect drugs such as B_{12} that require an acid medium for absorption, although this has not been well documented. Reductions in blood flow, enzyme activity, gastric emptying, and bowel motility may support the delay in absorption of some drugs, although such reductions probably have minimum, if any, effect on the extent of absorption.

Further support for the insignificance of these physiologic changes is based on the fact that most drugs are absorbed via passive diffusion. Because the GI tract has such a large surface area, the extent of absorption of most drugs is not affected. Nonionized forms of a drug (i.e., those that are more lipid soluble) are more readily absorbed than ionized forms. If a drug such as an antacid is administered, the GI pH will be raised and the absorption of acidic drugs may be delayed or decreased. Compounds such as iron or calcium and certain vitamins that depend on active transport mechanisms and thus the delivery of oxygen for absorption may be affected by decreased blood flow in the aging patient's GI tract (Burton et al, 2005).

BOX 4-1	Examples of Drugs That Distribute into Body Water or Lean Body Mass

digoxin	cimetidine
lithium	gentamicin
meperidine	phenytoin
theophylline	

Data compiled from Burton ME et al: *Applied pharmacokinetics and pharmacodynamics: principles of therapeutic drug monitoring (applied pharmacokinetics and pharmacodynamics)*, ed 4, Baltimore, 2005, Lippincott Williams & Wilkins; Duthie EH et al: *The practice of geriatrics*, ed 4, Philadelphia, 2007, Saunders.

BOX 4-2	Examples of Lipid-Soluble Drugs

diazepam	thiopental
chlordiazepoxide	Antipsychotics
flurazepam	Antidepressants

Data compiled from Burton ME et al: *Applied pharmacokinetics and pharmacodynamics: principles of therapeutic drug monitoring (applied pharmacokinetics and pharmacodynamics)*, ed 4, Baltimore, 2005, Lippincott Williams & Wilkins; Duthie EH et al: *The practice of geriatrics*, ed 4, Philadelphia, 2007, Saunders.

A change in the rate of absorption may also occur as the result of alterations in motility and in the rate of gastric emptying. Some of these may be caused by disease processes (e.g., CHF, GI tract disease), but more often, these problems are produced by the actions of medications themselves. Cathartics can increase GI motility and thereby increase the rate at which another drug passes through the GI tract. This can be a problem for enteric-coated products. Similarly, anticholinergics decrease motility and metoclopramide stimulates motility, thereby altering the rate of drug absorption with some medications (e.g., ethanol, levodopa, tetracycline, acetaminophen). Food can delay or reduce the absorption of certain drugs, particularly antibiotics.

Distribution

The distribution of drugs in the body, which is dependent on the chemical composition of the agent involved, may be affected by the aging process. As individuals age, the decline in total body water and lean body mass may affect drugs that are distributed into these areas (Box 4-1). Changes in total body water and lean body mass may result in limited distribution of drugs into these areas. Unadjusted dosing can result in increased serum concentrations, leading to an enhanced effect or toxicity.

Specifically, as we age, decreased lean body mass usually is coupled with an increase in total body fat. Changes in body fat are reported as increasing from 18% to 36% in males and from 33% to 48% in females from the ages of 15 to 60 years. The increase in body fat can result in an increase in the volume of distribution of lipid-soluble drugs, leading to drug accumulation and the potential for toxicity. For example, certain drugs such as diazepam and chlordiazepoxide have a higher volume of distribution than do other anxiolytics such as lorazepam and oxazepam because of the lipid solubility of the former two drugs. Box 4-2 lists additional examples of lipid-soluble drugs that may require downward adjustments in dose and slowly titrated increases if used in the elderly. The risk of accumulation and toxicity is a real concern with high doses of these agents in the elderly (Bigos et al, 2006; Burton et al, 2005).

Another common age change that affects the distribution of drugs in older adults is a decrease in serum albumin. Albumin concentrations decrease slightly with age in most elderly patients, although significant changes that may affect drug therapy may be seen in the chronically ill or in malnourished elderly patients (Bourne, 2007). Albumin is the most common protein that binds to various acidic drugs. Significant decreases in albumin may result in a greater free concentration of highly protein-bound drugs. Box 4-3 lists some drugs that have significant protein binding, which may result in increased free concentrations when albumin is significantly reduced. Generally, drugs that are highly protein bound to albumin should be prescribed in reduced doses for patients with low serum albumin values (Bourne, 2007). A practical example of the clinical significance of this relationship can be described with the anticonvulsant phenytoin. In an elderly patient with a low serum albumin concentration (normal, 3.5 to 5 mg/dl), the phenytoin level reported from the laboratory will reflect both the bound and free concentrations and, in a hypoalbuminemic individual, may appear normal or even subtherapeutic. This occurs because of the greater free amounts of phenytoin that are getting into tissue and acting at the receptor level but are not portrayed in the total serum level. The actual level may be much higher or even in the toxic range. Treatment decisions for older adults should not be based solely on drug levels but must be reached after consideration of both patient characteristics and anticipated drug levels.

Other protein changes may also have an influence on drug therapy. Patients with acute disease, such as a myocardial infarction, respiratory distress, or infection, for example, may experience increases in α-1-glycoprotein, an acute phase reactant protein. This may result in the increased binding of weakly basic drugs, including propranolol or lidocaine, and a less-than-normal response to therapy. Data on the real significance of changes in α_1-glycoprotein and drug therapy in the elderly are lacking (Bigos et al, 2006; Burton et al, 2005).

BOX 4-3	Sample Drugs With High Binding Affinity to Albumin

phenytoin	theophylline
warfarin	phenobarbital
naproxen	Antidepressants

Data compiled from Burton ME et al: *Applied pharmacokinetics and pharmacodynamics: principles of therapeutic drug monitoring (applied pharmacokinetics and pharmacodynamics)*, ed 4, Baltimore, Lippincott Williams & Wilkins, 2005; Duthie EH et al: *The practice of geriatrics*, ed 4, Philadelphia, 2007, Saunders.

Biotransformation (Metabolism)

Numerous age-related changes in hepatic structure and function have been described, although liver function seems to be well maintained in old age. Few consistent and reproducible observations and a lack of correlation between structural and functional data characterize the present state of our knowledge. In contrast to renal clearance, no equally reliable method of estimating hepatic drug clearance has been developed. The contribution of age to altered drug clearance in the elderly is difficult to assess because drug interactions, numbers and types of drugs taken at a time, underlying disease, and increased interindividual variability are superimposed on the aging process. A decline in liver volume and blood flow and a reduction in in vitro and in vivo metabolic capacity have been shown in older subjects; these events explain the physiologic basis for reduced hepatic drug clearance in this age group.

The significance of hepatic blood flow changes may be seen with drugs that have a high first-pass metabolism or a high extraction ratio in the liver. These drugs are considered to have flow-limiting metabolism. When flow is reduced, as may occur with aging, less drug is metabolized and increased amounts may be present in active form in the blood. When drugs with first pass metabolism are prescribed for the elderly, lower doses may be necessary. Examples of drugs that have high extraction ratios are listed in Box 4-4 (Bigos et al, 2006; Burton et al, 2005).

Other hepatic changes that occur with age that may affect the metabolism of drugs include changes in specific pathways or types of metabolism. The purpose of drug metabolism is generally to make drugs more water soluble for elimination. Phase I metabolism can be described as involving preparatory processes whereby minor molecular modifications are made to drugs. Phase I includes oxidation reduction, demethylation, and hydroxylation. Phase I metabolism is more likely to decrease with age than is phase II metabolism. Drugs that are metabolized by phase I metabolic pathways, including cytochrome P450 (CYP450) enzyme systems, may accumulate in the older adult. Such drugs should be used cautiously and at lower doses in the elderly. Examples of drugs that undergo phase I metabolism include lidocaine, phenytoin, propranolol, and theophylline. If possible, the use of alternative agents within a class of drugs that are metabolized differently (e.g., phase II) should be considered. If these drugs are prescribed in the elderly, lower doses should be used, and patients should be monitored for adverse effects. Examples of drugs whose clearance depends on phase I metabolism are listed in Box 4-5. Drugs that are metabolized by phase II metabolic processes, including conjugation, acetylation, sulfonation, and glucuronidation, show no reported change in clearance with aging (Burton et al, 2005).

Drugs that are metabolized by the liver may undergo reduced metabolism with aging because of changes within the liver itself or changes caused by other disease states. Aging influences associated with declining liver mass, as well as decreased hepatic blood flow, altered nutritional status, other physiologic changes, and diseases such as CHF, may result in the loss of hepatic reserve. Consequently, patients are at increased risk of adverse effects because of competition for the same metabolic enzymes when drugs are added to the existing regimen (Bigos et al, 2006; Burton et al, 2005). Drug substances that are metabolized and excreted by the liver should be used at a starting dose that is 30% to 40% less than the average dose used in middle-aged adults (Wynne, 2005).

Elimination

Longitudinal studies reflect a great degree of variability in renal function changes with aging. Age-related changes in renal function are the single most important physiologic causative factor in ADRs. Biologic changes that occur in the aging kidney include decreases in the number of nephrons; decreases in renal blood flow, glomerular filtration rate, and tubular secretion rate; and increases in the number of sclerosed glomeruli. In addition, atherosclerotic changes and declining cardiac output decrease renal perfusion by 40% to 50% between the ages of 25 and 65 years. The end result of these changes is noted in creatinine clearance, which is reported to decrease by 10% for each decade after age 40 (Bigos et al, 2006).

In addition to the normal reduction in renal function that may occur with aging, chronic diseases including CHF, liver disease, and acute urinary retention from benign prostatic hyperplasia—conditions that lead to dehydration—can also affect renal function and further complicate the required dosing. Creatinine is a muscle byproduct that is almost exclusively removed by the kidney, making it an excellent marker by which to measure renal clearance. Daily creatinine is related to age and serum creatinine concentrations. A drug's clearance is the amount of blood from which a drug is cleared per unit time. Although creatinine clearance is used to measure renal function, it is important to note that this is only an estimated value. Numerous formulas are available that can be used to

---

BOX 4-4	Sample Drugs With High Liver Extraction Ratios or First-Pass Effect
lidocaine	verapamil
meperidine	Estrogens
morphine	Nitrates
propranolol	Barbiturates
metoprolol	(e.g., phenobarbital)

Data compiled from Burton ME et al: *Applied pharmacokinetics and pharmacodynamics: principles of therapeutic drug monitoring (applied pharmacokinetics and pharmacodynamics)*, ed 4, Baltimore, 2005, Lippincott Williams & Wilkins; Duthie EH et al: *The practice of geriatrics*, ed 4, Philadelphia, 2007, Saunders.

BOX 4-5	Sample Drugs That Undergo Phase I Metabolism
diazepam	piroxicam
flurazepam	quinidine
chlordiazepoxide	barbiturates

Data compiled from Burton ME et al: *Applied pharmacokinetics and pharmacodynamics: principles of therapeutic drug monitoring (applied pharmacokinetics and pharmacodynamics)*, ed 4, Baltimore, 2005, Lippincott Williams & Wilkins; Duthie EH et al: *The practice of geriatrics*, ed 4, Philadelphia, 2007, Saunders.

calculate the creatinine clearance values, many of which may overestimate or underestimate the patient's true creatinine clearance. Creatinine clearance is measured by collecting urine for 24 hours. This, unfortunately, may not be practical in many institutions; therefore, we calculate estimated creatinine clearance. In older adults, creatinine clearance calculations may be especially inaccurate because these individuals have very little muscle mass and produce very little creatinine. A patient's serum creatinine may be reported as low, for example, 0.5 mg/dl (normal, 0.6 to 1.2 mg/dl), thus reflecting good excretion of creatinine. This information can be highly deceptive and often leads to overestimation of renal function when used with various available formulas. When renally excreted drugs are prescribed for the elderly, calculated creatinine clearance should be used to estimate renal function. Lower drug doses or longer intervals between dosing should be used when renal impairment is evident. Table 4-1 lists drugs that depend on the kidneys for elimination and that therefore may require dose adjustments in the elderly (Burton et al, 2005).

A formula that is commonly used to calculate estimated creatinine clearance is the Cockcroft-Gault equation. Unfortunately, the Cockcroft-Gault equation is noted to overestimate glomerular filtration rate. A simple modification of the Cockcroft-Gault equation has been recommended (Oo & Hill, 2002). This replaces the serum creatinine value with 1 mg/dl if the value is less than 1 mg/dl.

$$\text{Men: Creatinine clearance} = \frac{\text{Weight(kg*)} \times (140 - \text{Age in year})}{72 \times \text{Seruim creatinine (mg/dl)}}$$

$$\text{Women: Creatinine clearance} = \frac{\text{Weight(kg*)} \times (140 - \text{Age in year})}{72 \times \text{Seruim creatinine (mg/dl)} (\times 0.85)\dagger}$$

Creatinine clearance can also be estimated with the use of a variety of computer programs. (Quartarolo et al, 2007). Other kidney changes that occur with aging include a decrease in renal concentrating ability and renal sodium conservation, which may be a factor in patients who are taking high-dose diuretics.

In summary, it is recommended that when drugs are prescribed for older adults, a lower dose than is normally indicated should be the starting dosage and the dosage should be titrated up slowly (Bourne, 2007; Burton et al, 2005).

PHARMACODYNAMIC CHANGES IN THE ELDERLY THAT MAY AFFECT DRUG THERAPY

Pharmacodynamic changes are defined loosely as changes in concentration-response relationships or receptor sensitivity. Pharmacodynamic changes in the elderly may be due to changes in receptor affinity or number or to changes in hormonal levels. The impact of drugs that affect the central nervous system (e.g., benzodiazepines, anesthetics, metoclopramide, narcotics) and the cardiovascular system (e.g., β-blockers, calcium channel blockers, diuretics) is frequently altered in older adults. The physiologic changes associated with aging and the altered homeostatic mechanisms in the elderly may cause an increased sensitivity to

---

*Lean body weight; may reflect creatinine production more accurately.
†In women, multiply the value × 0.85.

TABLE 4-1   Sample Drugs That May Require Dose Adjustment in the Elderly Because of Renal Impairment

Drug Class	Drug Names
Antibiotics	Aminoglycosides, e.g., gentamicin, tobramycin, amikacin
	sulfamethoxazole, trimethoprim
	β-Lactams: cephalosporins (most), imipenem, ticarcillin
	tetracycline
	vancomycin
	aztreonam
	ciprofloxacin, norfloxacin
	nitrofurantoin
Antivirals	amantadine, rimantadine
Antineoplastics	methotrexate, bleomycin, nitrosourea, cisplatin
Antifungals	amphotericin B, fluconazole
	acyclovir, famciclovir
Analgesics	Opiate analgesics, e.g., meperidine, morphine
Cardiac medications	β-Blockers, e.g., atenolol, nadolol
	digoxin
	procainamide, bretylium
	Angiotensin-converting enzyme inhibitors, e.g., captopril, lisinopril, and others
	Other antihypertensives, e.g., clonidine
	Diuretics, e.g., thiazides, furosemide, spironolactone
Ulcer medications	Histamine$_2$ blockers: cimetidine, ranitidine, famotidine
Psychoactive medications	lithium, atypical antipsychotics, antipsychotics
Other agents	allopurinol, acetazolamide, chlorpropamide, gold sodium thiomalate, metoclopramide

Data compiled from Burton ME et al: *Applied pharmacokinetics and pharmacodynamics: principles of therapeutic drug monitoring (applied pharmacokinetics and pharmacodynamics)*, ed 4, Baltimore, 2005, Lippincott Williams & Wilkins; Duthie EH et al: *The practice of geriatrics*, ed 4, Philadelphia, 2007, Saunders.

---

specific drugs. Table 4-2 lists common age-associated changes and the medications that are affected by them. This increase in sensitivity may be the result of changes that occur in the drug receptors as the result of aging, or it may be caused by reduced reserve capacity in the aged patient. Results of these receptor changes include greater sensitivity to or intensity of drug action and a greater duration of drug action (Bourne, 2007).

The body system most significantly affected by increased receptor sensitivity is the central nervous system, wherein

TABLE 4-2   Age-Related Changes That Influence Drug Response

Age-Related Changes	Drugs Affected by Changes or That Exacerbate Changes
Orthostatic hypotension	Phenothiazines, tricyclic antidepressants
Bowel and bladder problems: Urinary retention, constipation, prostatic hypertrophy	Anticholinergics
Impaired thermoregulation	Phenothiazines, alcohol, aspirin
Reduced cognitive function	Any psychoactive medication
Postural stability impaired	Alcohol, diuretics, anticholinergics, antihypertensives
Glucose intolerance	Glucocorticoids, insulin

increased sensitivity to numerous drugs is evident (Bigos et al, 2006). Factors that may contribute to this greater sensitivity include a decrease in the number of neurons, a decrease in cerebral blood flow, and an increase in permeability of the blood-brain barrier. In the central nervous system, inhibitory and excitatory pathways are delicately balanced to modulate cognition. With aging, a selective decline occurs in some pathways, while others are preserved (Bigos et al, 2006).

Drugs with anticholinergic side effect profiles are often used in the elderly (Table 4-3), and these drugs are commonly associated with central and peripheral adverse effects. Commonly reported adverse side effects include sedation, confusion, orthostatic hypotension, constipation, dry mouth, urinary retention, tachycardia, and blurred vision (Bourne, 2007; Handler et al, 2006). The increased incidence of these events with aging may be the result of a decrease in the neurotransmitter acetylcholine, which is associated with the aging process (Hartikainen et al, 2007). This greater sensitivity to anticholinergic side effects includes a greater risk of dizziness and subsequent falls and fractures, along with loss of cognitive performance

TABLE 4-3   Categories of Anticholinergic Drugs That Can Cause Adverse Effects in Elderly Patients

Drug Class	Drug Names
Antispasmodics	belladonna, dicyclomine, propantheline
Antiparkinsonian agents	benztropine, trihexyphenidyl
Antihistamines	diphenhydramine, chlorpheniramine, hydroxyzine
Antidepressants	amitriptyline, imipramine
Antiarrhythmics	quinidine, disopyramide
Neuroleptics	thioridazine, chlorpromazine
Over-the-counter agents	Cold remedy products, antidiarrheals, doxylamine

Data compiled from Burton ME et al: *Applied pharmacokinetics and pharmacodynamics: principles of therapeutic drug monitoring (applied pharmacokinetics and pharmacodynamics)*, ed 4, Baltimore, 2005, Lippincott Williams & Wilkins; Duthie EH et al: *The practice of geriatrics*, ed 4, Philadelphia, 2007, Saunders.

(Bourne, 2007; Duthie et al, 2007). Drugs with anticholinergic effects should be avoided if at all possible in the elderly. If these are used, one should consider using doses that correspond to roughly half the normal dose (Bourne, 2007; Handler et al, 2006).

Benzodiazepines such as diazepam, alprazolam (Xanax), flurazepam, and lorazepam, among others, have an increased pharmacodynamic effect in elderly patients. Benzodiazepine-induced psychomotor impairment may include ataxia, delayed reaction time, increased body sway, and decreased proprioception (Bourne, 2007).

Changes in responsiveness to other parts of the central nervous system can also affect the patient's response to drug therapy. A decline in the neurotransmitters norepinephrine and dopamine has been reported in the elderly. The decline in dopamine may lead to an increased sensitivity to dopamine-blocking agents (e.g., neuroleptic agents; structurally similar agents, including metoclopramide) (Bourne, 2007).

The cardiovascular system is another body system in which pharmacodynamic changes can result in greater sensitivity (Bourne, 2007) or, in a few cases, loss of sensitivity to cardioactive drugs. Orthostatic hypotension occurs more commonly in the elderly because of the loss of baroreceptor response and the failure of cerebral blood flow autoregulation; it can be aggravated by drugs with sympatholytic activity (Box 4-6). Consequences of orthostatic hypertension in the elderly include dizziness and an increased risk of falls and fractures. Medications that cause orthostatic changes probably should be used with caution in the elderly, and lower doses should be prescribed.

Other cardiovascular changes that occur in the aging patient that may be influenced by drug therapy include a decrease in resting heart rate and a decrease in cardiac output in response to exercise. Drugs that may affect cardiac output include calcium channel blockers and β-blockers; their use should be monitored carefully, especially in patients with a history of systolic dysfunction (Egger et al, 2005). Positive inotropic agents such as digoxin have an increased effect in elderly patients because of their greater sensitivity to the drug, which predisposes them to a greater risk of toxicity.

Although many drugs have been reported to produce an enhanced response in the elderly, a few have elicited a decreased response. β-blockers reportedly produce a lesser

BOX 4-6   Examples of Drugs That May Cause Orthostatic Hypotension in the Elderly

Antihypertensives
Anticholinergics
Phenothiazines
Antidepressants (e.g., amitriptyline, trazodone)
Diuretics
Vasodilators (e.g., nitrates, alcohol)

Data compiled from Burton ME et al: *Applied pharmacokinetics and pharmacodynamics: principles of therapeutic drug monitoring (applied pharmacokinetics and pharmacodynamics)*, ed 4, Baltimore, 2005, Lippincott Williams & Wilkins; Duthie EH et al: *The practice of geriatrics*, ed 4, Philadelphia, 2007, Saunders.

response in the elderly, suggesting that changes occur within the receptors themselves or in response to elevated plasma norepinephrine levels as aging progresses. With an increased focus on improving outcomes in patients with CHF, numerous researchers are examining the effects of β-blockers in reducing blood pressure in the elderly and are seeking to explain why some of these medications may seem to be less effective in elderly than in younger patients (Duthie et al, 2007).

Anticoagulant drugs that may produce a greater response or effect in the elderly are those that reflect an intrinsic, age-related change in receptor sensitivity. Drugs such as warfarin and heparin may produce an exaggerated response in the elderly patient, possibly because of a decrease in clotting factors with age or because of protein-binding changes (Bourne, 2007). These agents should initially be dosed lower in the elderly patient and should be monitored carefully for an appropriate response.

Because of the physiologic changes that are noted in elderly patients and the potential problems that may result from pharmacologic therapy, treatment regimens for elderly patients must begin with nonpharmacologic strategies. A basic focus on diet, hydration, exercise, and weight loss often forms the foundation for any other successful intervention and reduces the numbers of medications that might be required for concurrent problems. Although this is an obvious and fundamental principle in the care of the elderly, the utility of these goals may often be overlooked as providers rush to treat.

COMMON CONCERNS RELATED TO MEDICATION USE IN OLDER ADULTS

Adverse Drug Reactions

An ADR is any response that is unintended and undesired and that occurs at normal recommended dosages. The reaction may be idiosyncratic or pharmacologically predictable. It is important for the clinician to learn how to prevent ADRs because they represent the fourth leading cause of death in the United States, ahead of pulmonary disease, diabetes, AIDS, pneumonia, accidents, and automobile deaths. Finally, the rate of ADRs increases exponentially when a patient is taking four or more medications (Jacubeit et al, 1990).

Efforts to reduce polypharmacy are important, but for many patients, the number of medications cannot be reduced without causing harm. That is why an understanding of the basis for drug interactions is important. This will allow health care providers to make the most appropriate choices when prescribing and to avoid preventable ADRs.

Cumulative side effects of medications taken concurrently increase the risk for adverse reactions. ADRs are more common in older adults, and it is anticipated that many of these reactions are not identified by older adults, who assume that the problems are normal age changes. Medication use in elderly patients increases their risk for ADRs and potentially serious consequences, including falls. The rate of ADRs in the elderly is higher than that in younger adults (Grady, 2006). The body systems most frequently associated with ADRs in the elderly are the cardiovascular system and the CNS.

The most important class of drug interactions involves the cytochrome P450 microsomal enzyme system, which handles a variety of xenobiotic substances (Egger et al, 2005). The potential is real for interactions between these enzymes and calcium channel blockers, β-adrenergic-blocking agents, angiotensin-converting enzyme inhibitors, and angiotensin receptor blockers. No interactions with diuretic antihypertensives have been observed because these drugs are renally eliminated and are more vulnerable to drug interactions that occur in the kidney.

Most medications taken by older adults are self-administered, and this fact has implications for recognition, underreporting, and the mortality statistics associated with ADRs. Specifically, what happens in the purview of a person's private dwelling regarding medication use is much less known or controllable than what occurs in hospital, long-term care, or other institutional settings. The overwhelming majority of elders live in the community, and the prescriber must keep this in mind when working with them. A study that examined drug prescribing for community-dwelling elderly patients (Handler et al, 2006) concluded that nearly 25% were taking inappropriate medications, and this placed them at increased risk for ADRs. ADRs can mimic many clinical syndromes in the geriatric patient. The importance of monitoring for ADRs cannot be overemphasized. ADRs may be associated with drug interactions; this is a theoretically preventable drug-related problem in patients taking multiple drugs. Drug reactions occur in up to 24% of institutionalized elderly patients and may be even more frequent in community-dwelling elderly patients, who often self-medicate with numerous OTC drugs. Drug interactions and ADRs can have serious consequences for the elderly and can increase both morbidity and mortality in this most vulnerable population (Barry et al, 2006).

Certain drugs commonly cause ADRs in the elderly, and these drugs should be used with caution. They include digoxin, anticoagulants, NSAIDs, systemic corticosteroids, diuretics, β-blockers, methyldopa, clonidine, benzodiazepines, calcium channel blockers, and sedative-hypnotics. Table 4-4 describes the ADRs that are most likely to occur when these drugs are used. Newer drugs and drug groups must likewise be used cautiously in older adults.

Specifically, the treatment of depression with selective serotonin reuptake inhibitors (SSRIs) is common among older adults (Spina & Scordo, 2002). When using these drugs, clinicians should consider the possibility of the serotonin syndrome. (Serotonin syndrome most often occurs when two drugs that affect the body's level of serotonin are taken together at the same time. The drugs cause too much serotonin to be released or to remain in the brain area and may produce a life-threatening condition.) SSRIs have a high potential for pharmacokinetic interactions because of their selective effects on CYP isoenzymes. Therefore, these agents should be closely monitored or avoided in elderly patients treated with substrates of these isoforms, especially those with a narrow therapeutic index. On the other hand, citalopram and sertraline exhibit low inhibitory activity for different drug-metabolizing enzymes and appear particularly suitable in an elderly population.

Polypharmacy

Many older adults need a variety of medications. The highest prevalence of medication use is among women 65 years of age and older. Among a national sample of 2950 older

TABLE 4-4   Adverse Drug Reactions Commonly Caused in Older Adults

Drug	Likely Adverse Reaction
Tricyclic antidepressants	Urinary incontinence
Antiparkinsonian agents Diuretics Sedative-hypnotics Antihistamines	Urinary retention
Antianxiety agents β-Blockers Antihypertensives: methyldopa, clonidine, reserpine digoxin	Depression
diuretics Sedative-hypnotics Benzodiazepines Nonsteroidal antiinflammatory drugs cimetidine Narcotics Alcohol	Delirium
Sedative-hypnotics Alcohol Antihypertensives Antiparkinsonian agents Narcotics Nitrates Diuretics Neuroleptics	Increased risk for falls
Tricyclic antidepressants quinidine Antihistamines bethanechol propantheline	Constipation

adults, 12% took 10 medications daily and 23% took 5 prescription medications (Frankfort et al, 2006). In general, older adults account for 13% to 14% of the total population; they use one fourth of OTC drugs and up to one third of prescribed medications. The average older adult uses 4.5 prescription medications and 2 OTC medications each day. In addition, these individuals may add supplements, vitamins, and various home remedies to the regimen. Moreover, many of these drugs are inappropriately prescribed (Baier, 2007; Laroche et al, 2006; Sloane et al, 2002). Those who are 85 years of age or older are at even greater risk of polypharmacy (Bigos et al, 2006).

Numerous studies document the use of multiple medications that are inappropriately prescribed for the elderly (Baier, 2007; Sloane et al, 2002). Patients visit multiple prescribers who are often unaware of what other prescribers have given them. They self-treat with OTC medications and CAM. They trade medications with others and take their medications irregularly to save money.

Use of multiple medications increases the risk of drug–drug interactions, ADRs, and potential exacerbation of medical problems. In a study of older adults admitted into acute care facilities with CHF (Grady, 2006), polypharmacy was reported to be one of the direct causes of disease exacerbation. In their classic 1995 study, Leape et al. estimated that drug–drug interactions accounted for 3% to 5% of preventable ADRs (Leape et al, 1995). However, the explosion of

knowledge regarding the P450 enzyme system in the liver has allowed clinicians to develop a new understanding about drug combinations that may be problematic (see Chapter 3), and automated computer alerts regarding drug interactions help to limit some of these problems.

The Beers criteria (Beers, 1997), which are explicit although not evidence-based guidelines, are among the most commonly used techniques for assessing the appropriateness of drugs that are prescribed for the elderly. Many drugs that are at high risk for producing ADRs in the elderly, and those that are less likely to produce severe ADRs have been identified with the use of these criteria (Molony, 2004). A positive correlation has been noted between ADRs and drug prescribing practices that fail to comply with the Beers criteria. The Beers criteria, in fact, may be used by clinicians to predict the occurrence of ADRs, particularly among those elderly patients who are taking fewer than five drugs (Chang et al, 2005) (Box 4-7). Efforts to reduce polypharmacy are important, but for many patients, the number of medications cannot be reduced without causing harm. That is why it is important for clinicians to attain an understanding of the basis for drug interactions. This will allow us to make the most appropriate choices when prescribing and to avoid preventable ADRs.

CAM is increasing in popularity in the United States. These products are not rigidly regulated, and it is therefore difficult to assess the likelihood of drug–drug interactions, toxic effects, or side effects. Moreover, these interactions/reactions to CAM are not anticipated by many individuals. In a study (Saw et al, 2006) of older adults undergoing preoperative screening, it was noted that almost half (42.7%) used CAM, 20% used CAM that resulted in anticoagulation, 14% used CAM that altered blood pressure, and 7% used CAM that had other cardiac effects. Older adults must be educated about the potential drug interactions and side effects of CAM, and providers must be alerted to the prevalent use of these products among this population. Most of these individuals did not tell their health care providers that they were using herbal products (Saw et al, 2006).

To help decrease the risk of multiple medication use, software programs are available to help older adults monitor their medication regimens for possible interactions. The specific outcomes of these types of interventions in decreasing the risk of polypharmacy are under evaluation. The trend, however, is to continue to encourage both older adults and their health care providers to consider the potential risk of multiple medications and to use only those medications that are necessary.

Adherence With Drug Regimen

Adherence is defined as the extent to which a patient follows a planned medical regimen. *Adherence* and *concordance* are the terms used to replace the term *compliance*. Drug nonadherence takes many forms, including deliberate omission of a medication, unintentional and intentional overdosing, errors in dosing frequency, use of medications other than as the provider intended, incorrect mode of administration, and use of drugs prescribed for another individual. Nonadherence may be deliberate or unintentional. Compliance with medications is low when patients are in denial regarding the nature/severity of their condition; when medications are prescribed for preventative reasons for conditions that are symptomless; when patients

---

BOX 4-7 Sample Medications That Require Lower Dosages Because of Decreased Clearance in the Elderly

DECREASED RENAL CLEARANCE IN THE ELDERLY

Aminoglycosides
vancomycin
Fluoroquinolones
Penicillins
imipenem
digoxin (limit dose to 0.125 mg/day, consider every other day)
ACE inhibitors
β-Blockers (atenolol, nadolol)
sotalol
glyburide
ranitidine, cimetidine, famotidine
lithium

DECREASED HEPATIC CLEARANCE IN THE ELDERLY

Benzodiazepines
Calcium channel blockers
lidocaine
phenytoin
celecoxib (Celebrex)
theophylline
imipramine or desipramine, trazodone
isoniazid
procainamide

MEDICATIONS TO AVOID IN PATIENTS OLDER THAN 65: SHORT LIST (THE BEERS LIST)

Sedating antihistamines (e.g., diphenhydramine)
Sedative-hypnotics (e.g., diazepam)
Sedating antidepressants (e.g., amitriptyline)
Antispasmodics (e.g., oxybutynin, dicyclomine)

MEDICATIONS TO AVOID IN PATIENTS AGE OLDER THAN 65: LONG LIST

Anticholinergic agents
Sedating antihistamines (Benadryl, Periactin, Atarax)
ticlopidine
methyldopa
reserpine
disopyramide (Norpace)
meperidine (Demerol)
propoxyphene (Darvon)
Barbiturates (e.g., Fiorinal, Nembutal, Seconal)
Benzodiazepines (Librium, Valium, Dalmane, Halcion)
  • Use benzodiazepines with caution.
  • Use shorter-acting agents (e.g., Ativan, Restoril).
  • Use low doses (<3 mg Ativan; <15 mg Restoril).

INCREASED RISK OF PHYSICAL PERFORMANCE DECLINE

Meprobamate
Sedating antidepressants (Elavil, Doxepin, Imipramine)
Amitriptyline is highly anticholinergic.
Alternatives for pain: Pamelor, Neurontin, Lyrica
methylphenidate (Ritalin)
Antiemetics (Phenergan, Tigan)
GI antispasmodics (e.g. Donnatal, Bentyl, Levsin)
Antidiarrheals (Lomotil)
Urinary antispasmodics (Ditropan)
Nonsteroidal antiinflammatory drugs (NSAIDs)
Especially avoid Indocin, Toradol, Ponstel, and Feldene.
  • Limit to low dose, short duration, short half-life.
Skeletal muscle relaxants (e.g., Flexeril, Soma)

From Gray SL et al: Benzodiazepine use and physical performance in community-dwelling elders, *J Am Geriatr Soc* 51:1563-1570, 2003; Curtis LH et al: Inappropriate prescribing for elderly Americans in a large outpatient population, *Arch Intern Med* 164:1621-1625, 2004; Williams CM: Using medication appropriately in older adults, *Am Fam Physician* 66:1917-1924, 2002; Fick DM et al: Updating the Beers criteria for potentially inappropriate medication use in older adults: results of a US consensus panel of experts, *Arch Intern Med* 163:2716, 2003.

feel no benefit from taking the medication; when patients do not believe that the medication will affect their condition; when no immediate consequences result from not taking the medication; and when patients feel that the short-term disadvantages of the medication (such as side effects) outweigh its long-term benefits (APhA, 2003).

It is essential to explore with the older individual what he or she is actually doing with regard to daily medication use and then compare this against the "prescribed" medication regimen. Patients should bring all medicines with them to office visits. Allow and encourage the individual to explain reasons for any deviations, and provide clarification if there has been some confusion about how to take a specific medication. Box 4-8 provides a listing of some of the commonly identified reasons for drug nonadherence. Address each of these potential reasons and help the

patient come up with a reasonable solution to facilitate future adherence. Simple techniques such as writing out, in large print, daily medications; filling daily medication boxes for those with cognitive impairment; and/or changing to a generic (i.e., less expensive) drug option may resolve problems with adherence.

Some of the essential aspects of prescribing that will enhance patient adherence to the regimen include the following:

• Use nondrug treatment whenever possible; do not substitute a drug for effective social care measures.
• Prescribe the lowest feasible dose (often less than half the usual adult dose).
• Prescribe the smallest number of medications with the simplest dose regimens.
  • Once daily is best.
  • Time doses to mealtimes.

BOX 4-8   Common Reasons for Drug Noncompliance

- Cost of medications
- Complicated schedule
- Unrealistic schedule
- Impaired cognition and judgment
- Unpleasant side effects
- Lack of knowledge related to NEED and purpose of medication
- Denial of problem for which treatment is being prescribed
- Fear of drug side effects or exacerbation of other problems
- No perceived response/effect for drug treatment

- Provide simple verbal and written instructions for every medication, including what it is for.
- Be aware that presenting symptoms may result from existing medications.
- Regularly review chronic treatment; it may be possible to stop medications or to reduce the dose when necessary.
- Establish partnerships to ensure compliance.
  - Patient
  - Family (educate on indications and adverse effects)
  - Pharmacists
  - Home health aides
- Use devices that facilitate taking of medication.
  - Use pill boxes and pill calendars.
  - Label containers with large type.
  - Pill containers should open easily.
- Keep accurate medication list.
- Ensure easy access to medications.
- Affordability
- Medication delivery
- Evaluate for patient factors that affect compliance.
  - Dementia
  - Major depression

Both prescribers and patients should keep a written list of all current medications. This list can be used as a tool for discussion of any issues that the patient may have with his medicines. This will allow the clinician to remember to provide consistent teaching about drug therapy at every office visit. Some data indicate that nonadherence is often the result of a lack of understanding from the patient's perspective regarding the purpose, dosing regimen, and anticipated therapeutic effects of the drug. Without adequate teaching, the drug may simply be stopped by the patient (Bourne, 2007).

Costs of Medications

Prescription drugs represent a significant out-of-pocket cost for older adults. More than 15% of the older adults who use prescription medications are unable to pay for them. Not all patients participate in Medicare Part D, which offers prescription coverage for some medications. The lack of uniformity in what is covered by the different groups that offer Plan D benefits and the costs involved have created broad dispari-

ties that have frustrated and upset many elderly patients and have caused Congress to continue to examine this program closely. Medicaid does cover prescription drugs listed on state Preferred Drug Formularies for those individuals who qualify. In addition, pharmacy assistance, a state-run program to provide prescription drug services for those who do not qualify for Medicaid, is available in some states. Box 4-9 provides examples of ways in which drug costs can be controlled. It is essential to consider the cost benefit for drugs prescribed by examining findings from randomized clinical trials and sophisticated cost analyses.

PROCESS MODEL OF PRESCRIBING FOR THE ELDERLY

Christianes' consideration of a systematic method of helping providers evaluate choices when prescribing drugs for elderly patients led to the development of a specific model that is still relevant today (Troupin, 2001). This model consists of a few basic questions that include the following.

Why Use a Drug?

This question is meant to prompt the clinician to review what clinical indication(s) is being addressed by the prescription. Associated questions should focus on whether there is a clear link between the drug being considered and the disease entity being treated, and whether other, nonpharmacologic means are available to address the condition. Too often, clinicians do not consider whether the condition definitively requires a medication. It should be determined if the goal of medication therapy is to cure, to manage future risks associated with the condition, or to provide comfort for the patient. (Patient comfort, achieved through direct relief of symptoms or through acknowledgment of the patient's pain, is always a desired goal.) Therapies should be recommended to improve, maintain, or stabilize functionality. All too often, elders are placed on medications without clear indication, to treat "symptoms of aging" rather than a specific diagnosis, and without *objective functional or other baseline* data that can be used to determine further dosage adjustments. Hence, when the medication begins to interact with other drugs, to affect comorbid conditions adversely, or to reduce function, the prescriber lacks sufficient information to make appropriate clinical decisions. The clinician should obtain appropriate baseline data by administering Katz ADLs, Barthel's Index of Activities of Daily Living, the Patient Health Questionnaire Nine-Symptom Depression Checklist (PHQ-9; Pfizer Inc, New York, NY), MMSE, or whatever test is appropriate to the clinical situation that

---

BOX 4-9   Techniques to Decrease Costs for Prescription Medications

- Check on drug costs before prescribing, and search for the lowest cost alternative within drug groups.
- Use generics when possible.
- Start with small quantities of new prescriptions (starter dosing with 1-week supply).
- Use the lowest dose necessary to achieve the desired effect.
- Eliminate all unnecessary medications.

will help to reveal functionality prior to implementation of therapeutics and during regular intervals thereafter.

Whatever the situation, the intent of drug therapy should be clearly determined. This is where the art is needed in providing care—the interface between knowing patients and knowing medicine. "There can occasionally be prescribing decisions made which aren't perfectly rational, but which make sense in the context of a particular patient." This model states that regardless of the reason a patient receives therapy, the reason(s) should be clearly identified (Troupin, 2001).

Why Should This Particular Drug Be Used?

In the best of situations, the prescription of a drug should be based on the best available evidence from peer-reviewed, randomized, controlled trials conducted in patient populations with similar age, sex, and disease state characteristics as those of the patient. Decisions should be made with the use of statistically significant outcomes data that show proven clinical and quality-of-life benefits. The reality is that these data often are not available in a perfect combination of content and relevance. But when such information is available, it should be considered the "gold standard" for decision making. Other factors that enter into the prescribing decision include practice matters such as availability, cost, and dosing schedules. All of these factors influence whether the patient will adhere to the therapy once it is prescribed.

After a therapy is selected, the next question should be addressed.

Why Should This Drug Not Be Used?

This question again should prompt a review of the potential contraindications, side effects, and toxicities, and other reasons why this drug might not be a good therapeutic choice for the patient. The drug should be specifically evaluated with respect to past and current medical problems in a given patient that could influence the risks or benefits of a particular therapy. For example, some drugs have a very narrow therapeutic window that may necessitate additional monitoring or may predispose to a high rate of complications. With study, perhaps a comparable drug can be selected to minimize these risks (Troupin, 2001).

Finally, it is necessary to consider a review of all potential drug–drug interactions and herb–drug interactions for patients who take a variety of prescribed and OTC therapies. Much of the drug interaction information in the literature has been generated by single drug–drug profiles. This means that the information may not be helpful when patients are taking three or five or even eight drugs, as is common in elderly patients. Therefore, what we know about drug–drug interactions for many elderly patients is incomplete.

Although they are somewhat time consuming, these steps provide a rational path by which the safety and benefit of pharmacotherapies can be maximized in middle-aged or older patients, while known or potential risks are minimized. If this approach is made part of standard practice, the time should be budgeted to support this model of care. Christianes maintains that this model should be used in an expanded format in two specific situations: (1) when one is assuming care of a new patient—start with a thorough review of his current therapies; and (2) when a patient returns for a follow-up visit after hospitalization—a careful evaluation should be done. Often, medications are prescribed in the hospital for symptom relief or as standard as-needed therapies. If not reviewed, these may become routine medications solely because the drugs were never reevaluated (Troupin, 2001). Clearly, other signs, symptoms, or events serve as "red flags" for the prescriber to indicate that drug therapy should be reevaluated in elders. For instance, the patient experiences weight loss >5% of baseline, abrupt change in medical condition, abrupt change in functionality, a new pain syndrome, recent hospitalization or surgery, instability of medical conditions, care provided by a new home care provider, transfer to a new living environment (long-term care [LTC] or assisted living), and so forth. Under these situations, the process model should be used in an expanded form. The intent is to help the prescriber become proactively aware of circumstances in which reduced dosages may be necessitated or an increased number of ADRs may occur.

Drug therapy is seen as almost mandatory in the elderly patient. Thinking clearly about what may be required to enhance or preserve the health of the elderly and avoiding the development of additional symptoms is a special challenge for those who work with geriatric patients.

evolve A continually updated list of useful WebLinks may be found in the Evolve Resources at http://evolve.elsevier.com/Edmunds/NP/

5 Special Populations: Pediatrics

The dramatic decrease in infant mortality rates throughout the twentieth century has paralleled the development of improvements in the prevention, diagnosis, and treatment of pediatric problems; the introduction of better technology; and the increasingly effective use of pharmacologic products. Because children are subject to many of the same diseases as adults, they sometimes are treated with the same drugs and biologic products as adults. However, use of these drugs to treat children is rarely based on evidence-based medicine.

The preparation of valid and generalizable knowledge about drug use in children has been problematic at best. Few clinicians want to experiment with children; few parents would knowingly allow their infants or small children to participate in research studies that would entail risk of any kind. As a result, many drugs are currently labeled with the comment, "Safety and efficacy not established for children." Many of the initial data about drug use in children were based on first-hand observations by clinicians who tried drugs even when no guidelines were available to assist them. What these clinicians quickly determined was that children are not just small adults who require smaller doses. Health care providers who do not learn that lesson are likely to create problems for themselves and for their patients (Cuzzolin et al, 2006).

What has been determined is that one third of drugs tested separately in children under the FDA Pediatric Exclusivity Program had different effects than they did in adults; some were more toxic, and others were completely ineffective (Li et al, 2007). "Seventy-five percent of drugs used in kids have never been tested in this population, yet they are used in kids every day. Kids are our therapeutic orphans" (Li et al, 2007).

PHARMACOKINETICS OF DRUG THERAPY IN INFANTS AND CHILDREN

Determining how to give medications to children involves having an especially good understanding of the various physiologic factors that may be affected by these drugs. The growing but immature child is a dynamic and changing entity whose unique characteristics must be understood if errors are to be avoided. The practitioner must remember that information must be mastered for each of the age groups that make up the pediatric category: preterm infants (gestational age younger than 36 weeks), neonates (30 days old and younger), infants (1 to 12 months), toddlers (1 to 4 years), children (5 to 12 years), and adolescents (12 years and older). Fundamental to this understanding is knowledge of the unique pharmacokinetic variables that may be encountered in pediatric dosing for each of these groups. In recognizing the maturational disparities among children of the same age, developmental differences are further compounded by the

same qualities that affect therapeutic response in adults, such as disease, environment, and genetic traits. Consequently, when compared with adults, a wider range of responses to a particular drug treatment can be expected in a population of children; in fact, the same child's response to a regimen can change rapidly during a single treatment course.

Experts generally agree that devising a therapeutic regimen is most difficult for the youngest patients, particularly neonates. Signs of efficacy or toxicity are difficult to recognize, and newborns are the least able to withstand adverse effects. Neonates often experience the greatest number of therapeutic errors.

Drug Absorption

Many expect drug absorption in infants and children to follow the same basic principles as in adults. However, three factors tend to be especially important in children. First, the physiologic status of the infant or child determines blood flow at the site of parenteral drug administration. Factors that may reduce blood flow to muscular or subcutaneous tissues include cardiovascular shock, vasoconstriction caused by sympathomimetic agents, and heart failure. Under these conditions, absorption of any medications injected into intramuscular or subcutaneous tissue would be reduced. In premature infants with little muscle mass, perfusion to these areas and the resulting absorption are extremely irregular. In larger children, more rapid absorption occurs from the deltoid muscle than from the vastus lateralis muscle, whereas medications are absorbed the slowest from the gluteal muscles (AAP, 1997). Peripheral vasomotor instability, thermal instability, and reduced muscular contractions in premature infants compared with other children and adults also influence drug absorption from intramuscular sites. Toxic drug concentrations may be provoked if perfusion to intramuscular or subcutaneous tissues suddenly increases, promoting greater absorption of medication and increasing the amount of drug that enters the circulation. Drugs that have narrow therapeutic margins, such as anticonvulsants, cardiac glycosides, or aminoglycoside antibiotics, are particularly good examples of drugs with which toxicity may be encountered when absorption is variable (Burton et al, 2005).

Second, for neonates, another factor in absorption is the changing status of GI function. In the first weeks of life, the intestine is highly permeable and premature babies may absorb substances that cannot penetrate the more mature intestine. The presence of amniotic fluid in the stomach ensures an alkaline pH during the days after birth. (Although neonates quickly develop an acidic gastric environment, they do not produce normal levels of gastric acid until somewhere between the ages of 3 and 7 years.) During the neonatal period, the absorption of orally administered members of the penicillin family is enhanced, as is the absorption of carbamazepine suspension, diazepam, and digoxin. Both increased production of gastric acid and slow or varying peristalsis through the GI tract create situations in which orally administered drugs may be partially or totally inactivated by the low pH of gastric contents. Acid-labile drugs, such as ampicillin, nafcillin, and penicillin, develop higher serum concentrations in the presence of higher gastric acid, whereas lower serum concentrations may be found with phenobarbital, phenytoin, and acetaminophen (Levine et al, 2000). Drug absorption may be delayed or increased to a greater extent than anticipated because of the absence of intestinal flora, reduced enzyme function, delays in gastric emptying, deficient transport mechanisms across neonatal intestinal membranes, or slow GI transit. The stomach begins to empty more quickly once the infant is 6 to 8 months old. At that time, GI transit may become faster and more unpredictable. Low concentrations of bile acids and lipase may decrease the absorption of lipid-soluble drugs. The activity of pancreatic enzymes is decreased in neonates and infants up to 4 months of age (Koren & Cohen, 2006). These factors are particularly important to remember when one is contemplating the administration of a sustained-release agent. If the drug passes through the GI tract rapidly, absorption will be insufficient and a subtherapeutic dose will be delivered. Rectal suppositories generally should be avoided for drug administration, primarily because children may not retain the dosage form long enough to receive the entire dose.

Because so little research has been conducted on oral vs. intravenous administration, differences in the bioavailability of drugs through different routes of administration in premature infants are poorly understood. If a drug is poorly absorbed from the GI tract of an adult, absorption may be much more efficient in a premature child because of the delayed emptying. The one common finding of most studies is that drug absorption varies widely; the younger the child, the more erratic may be the absorption (Burton et al, 2005).

Third, the skin of premature and newborn infants has a greater ability to absorb some chemicals because of increased hydration and increased permeability, resulting from underdevelopment of the stratum corneum in the epidermal barrier. The transdermal route may be used therapeutically in selected infants to reduce the unpredictability of some oral and intramuscularly administered medications, such as theophylline. However, commercially available transdermal dosage forms are not intended for pediatric patients and would deliver doses much higher than those needed for infants and children. Rubbing the drug into the skin, incorporating the drug in an oily vehicle, and using an occlusive dressing sometimes by wrapping the infant in plastic wrap may increase cutaneous absorption of topical products (Edmunds, 2005). Children have the potential for increased absorption through the skin because their skin is thinner and more sensitive—thus allowing for greater penetration—particularly if the skin is damaged or an occlusive dressing (even a diaper) is applied over the medication. Factors that increase transdermal drug absorption also increase the risk to the infant of toxic effects following topical use of drugs, as well as such items as hexachlorophene soaps, boric acid, powders, or rubbing alcohol (Gilman, 1990). Both clinicians and parents should remember that small

children can ingest a topical drug by sucking or licking it off of an accessible patch of skin.

Drug Distribution

Drug distribution as a process is determined by two factors: (1) the physicochemical properties of the drug itself (i.e., the molecular weight, etc.), which do not vary, and (2) the physiologic factors specific for the patient, including total body water, extracellular water, protein binding, and pathologic conditions that modify physiologic function, all of which vary widely in different patient populations (Nahata, 2002).

The distribution volumes of drugs vary in the child as the body composition changes through growth and development. The neonate has a higher proportion of its body weight in the form of water than does the adult, who has 50% to 60% of body weight in water. Small premature neonates may have 85% of their body weight as water, with 40% of that amount as extracellular water, whereas the normal full-term neonate usually has only about 70% body weight as water. Because many drugs are distributed throughout the extracellular water space, the volume or size of the extracellular water compartment may be important in determining the concentration of drug at the receptor sites. This is an especially important consideration because many neonates diurese heavily in the first 24 to 48 hours of life, and many important drugs are water soluble (Koren & Cohen, 2006; Nahata, 2002). Water-soluble drugs, such as the aminoglycoside antibiotic gentamicin, will be distributed more widely in the body, resulting in lower serum levels. To compensate, a higher dosage is necessary.

Another variable that affects drug distribution in premature infants is a reduced percentage of fat. Premature infants may have 1% of body weight in fat compared with 15% in normal full-term infants (Yaffe & Aranda, 2004). Organs that ordinarily would accumulate high concentrations of lipid-soluble drugs in adults and older children may not accumulate as much in infants. Early on, when the proportion of body fat is small, lipid-soluble drugs such as vitamins A and E do not distribute as well, provoking higher drug concentrations in the serum. In such cases, the dosage may have to be reduced to avoid toxicity. In older children, the alterations in body fat associated with obesity and extreme emaciation obviously affect fat storage of drugs just as they do in adults.

In addition to fat, selected drugs are stored to a smaller extent in other tissues. For example, the tetracyclines chelate with calcium and so have a high affinity for the rapidly growing teeth and bones of infants and young children (Kleigman et al, 2007).

Drugs are not distributed uniformly throughout the body. For example, drug distribution to the central nervous system is small, and movement through the brain's rich blood supply is unique. Drugs must move from the bloodstream across the blood-brain barrier. Because certain drugs, such as highly lipid-soluble drugs (e.g., tetracycline, diazepam), readily penetrate the central nervous system, there is no absolute barrier. However, the blood-brain barrier is encountered when drugs that are moving from the blood across the capillary endothelium are restricted by the close approximation of the glial cells with the capillary endothelium. Also, drug access to the cerebrospinal fluid is limited by the epithelium of the choroid plexus (Kleigman et al, 2007).

In premature infants, incomplete glial development enhances permeability of the blood-brain barrier and permits drugs and bilirubin to enter the central nervous system more readily. Poorly lipid-soluble drugs such as gentamicin and penicillin may then cross the blood-brain barrier when administered in large doses, when administered via rapid intravenous infusion, or when administered to neonates with renal failure. The permeability of the blood-brain barrier in infants and children of all ages is increased in meningitis, brain tumors, and cranial trauma. In these conditions, drugs that do not ordinarily enter the central nervous system may do so without difficulty (Yaffe & Aranda, 2004).

Some drugs are reversibly bound to plasma proteins (usually albumin), fat, bone, or other tissues. Diazepam, digoxin, furosemide, and warfarin are examples of drugs that are highly bound to plasma albumin. When bound, these tissue-bound drugs are not free to gain access to receptor sites and thus are pharmacologically inactive. Some tissue-bound drugs are released when plasma concentrations fall; thus, these tissues are said to act as drug storage depots (Burton et al, 2005).

Plasma protein binding in neonates is comparatively low because of decreased plasma protein concentration, lower binding capacity of protein, decreased affinity of proteins for drug binding, and competition for certain binding sites by endogenous compounds. Because of this, the concentration of free drug in plasma is increased and exerts powerful pharmacologic effects that can result in greater drug effect or toxicity. Acidosis, cold stress, and hypoglycemia in the neonate may produce free fatty acids that act to displace drugs from plasma albumin-binding sites (Burton et al, 2005). However, because drugs bound to plasma proteins cannot be eliminated by the kidneys, an increase in free drug concentration may also increase its clearance (Nahata, 2002).

In the neonate, bilirubin, maternal hormones, and other endogenous substances also occupy available plasma protein-binding sites. Sulfonamides, furosemide, large doses of vitamin K, and sodium benzoate given to the mother during labor or delivery, or passed to the baby through breastfeeding, may compete with serum bilirubin for binding to albumin. If these drugs are given to a neonate with jaundice, they can displace bilirubin from albumin. Because of the greater permeability of the neonatal blood-brain barrier, substantial amounts of bilirubin then could enter the brain and cause kernicterus. Additionally, as the serum bilirubin rises for physiologic reasons or because of a blood group incompatibility, bilirubin displacement of a drug from albumin can substantially raise the free drug concentration. This might occur without altering the total drug concentration and would result in a greater therapeutic effect or toxicity at normal concentrations (Koren & Cohen, 2006).

The decreased capacity for plasma protein binding of drugs can increase their apparent volumes of distribution. The clinical implications of this action are that to obtain a therapeutic serum concentration of many drugs, premature infants will require a larger loading dose than that required for older children and adults (Burton et al, 2005).

Finally, certain drugs distributed in the breast milk of breastfeeding mothers may pose problems for infants. The American Academy of Pediatrics (AAP) updates its classic statement every few years and lists drugs that should be avoided by the mother during pregnancy and breastfeeding if at all possible and the effects of drugs on infants. Drugs that are absolutely contraindicated during breastfeeding include bromocriptine, cimetidine, clemastine, cyclophosphamide, ergotamine, gold salts, methimazole, phenindione, and thiouracil (AAP, 2001).

Drug Metabolism

The biotransformation of drugs into usable substances in the body involves chemical reactions that convert a drug to an inactive or a less active compound. These metabolic reactions usually produce metabolites that are less lipid soluble and more readily eliminated than are highly lipid-soluble compounds. Not all metabolites are pharmacologically inactive. Active metabolites are excreted unchanged or undergo additional metabolic reactions. Poorly absorbed lipid-soluble drugs, such as the penicillins, are not metabolized but are excreted unchanged (Burton et al, 2005).

In general, drug metabolism in infants is substantially slower than that in older children and adults. The newborn's kidneys are immature, and because most drug metabolism takes place in the liver, the fact that the P450-dependent mixed-function oxidases and the conjugating enzymes of infants are only 50% to 70% of adult values is an important consideration in the treatment of children (Leeder et al, 1997). Different enzymes are present in varying amounts, but the capacity to increase production of all enzymes continues until the third or fourth year of life. For example, the glucuronidation pathway is undeveloped in infants, but the sulfation pathway is relatively well developed and may compensate for deficits in the other pathway in the presence of some drugs (Gupta & Waldhauser, 1997; Rane, 2004).

Given neonates' decreased ability to metabolize drugs, they may be at increased risk for adverse effects because of slow clearance rates and prolonged half-lives, particularly in drugs given over long periods. One of the earliest cases in which serious adverse effects were observed in neonates following administration of a drug that had not been adequately studied in pediatric patients was the development of "gray baby syndrome" after treatment with the antibiotic chloramphenicol. After 23 deaths in neonates, it was determined that the immature livers of these infants were unable to clear chloramphenicol from the body, allowing toxic doses of the drug to accumulate (Levine et al, 2000). These facts make it essential for the clinician to consider the maturation of the infant when evaluating whether to administer drugs metabolized in the liver. Conversely, some drugs that a mother might take would induce the fetal hepatic enzymes to mature early. This would result in faster metabolism of certain drugs, with less therapeutic effect and lower plasma drug concentrations. One of the drugs that might cause this action is phenobarbital (Koren & Cohen, 2006). By the first birthday, the liver's metabolic capabilities are not only mature but more vigorous than those of an adult, probably because the child's liver has a greater volume per kilogram of body weight. Although this phenomenon is probably most apparent between the ages of 2 and 6 years, it continues until approximately 10 to 12 years of age so that certain drugs may need to be given in higher dosages or more often. An example of this is theophylline. A child between 1 and 9 years of age with asthma might require markedly higher doses of theophylline on a weight basis compared with an adult (Burton et al, 2005).

Although most drug metabolic reactions occur in the liver, the GI tract, kidney, and plasma may also biotransform some drugs. The extent of use of these alternate forms of metabolism is usually identified in pharmacokinetic tables, and these forms account for only a small percentage of drug metabolism.

Excretion

As with metabolism, the growth and maturity of the child's organs have a significant effect on the elimination of drugs. Difficulty in excreting drugs that results from incomplete development of the fetal renal excretion system, including reduction in glomerular filtration, tubular secretion, and tubular reabsorption, is gradually resolved with increased gestational age but may still be markedly decreased at birth and may only slowly develop to capacity over the first year of life.

For the first few days of life, the glomerular filtration rate (GFR) of a neonate may be at only 30% to 40% of the adult rate. This rate may be even lower in premature babies. As the child grows and matures, the clearance rate improves, even during the first week of life. By the end of the third week of life, GFR is usually 50% to 60% of the adult value and may reach the adult value by 6 months (Burton et al, 2005).

This developmental process has implications for drug clearance, particularly for common drugs such as penicillin, aminoglycosides, and digoxin, for which rates may fall to 17% to 34% of the adult clearance rate. If a child is ill enough to require these drugs, its GFR may not improve as predicted during the first weeks and months of life. This will necessitate adjustments in dosage and dosing schedules. The child will require more vigilant monitoring, and appropriate dosages should be calculated based on plasma drug concentrations determined at intervals throughout the course of therapy (Koren & Cohen, 2006).

Changes in urinary pH may also affect the rate at which a drug is excreted. Ammonium chloride, ascorbic acid, and other drugs that acidify the urine increase the rate at which pseudoephedrine, meperidine, quinidine, and other weak bases are excreted. Sodium bicarbonate and other drugs that alkalinize the urine increase the rate at which phenobarbital, aspirin, nitrofurantoin, and other weak acids are excreted. Although increasing the rate at which a drug is excreted shortens its effect, decreasing urinary excretion increases the drug's duration of action (Yaffe & Aranda, 2004).

EFFECT OF DISEASE ON DRUG PROCESSES IN CHILDREN

Drugs generally produce their effects by combining with an enzyme, cell membrane, or other cellular component. The cellular component, or receptor, with which the drug combines has a chemical or structural affinity for a highly specific drug. Investigators have reported that receptors are present and functional in young children, and the degree of receptor response appears to correlate with birth weight (Yaffe & Aranda, 2004). However, requirements for larger doses of medications such as digoxin for infants and children have been attributed to a greater affinity of the child's developing myocardial digoxin receptors for digitalis derivatives (Burton et al, 2005). Other examples include the increased sensitivity of neonates to curare and atropine and their heightened resistance to succinylcholine, both of which result from immature development of receptors for these drugs.

The liver and kidney play major roles in the metabolism and excretion of drugs. Thus, diseases of either of these organs often affect drug action. Drug metabolism is a complex function of the liver that varies because of modifications in hepatic blood flow, extraction capacity of the drug from the blood, and serum drug binding. Both type and severity of liver disease may alter all of these factors. Shifts to different metabolic pathways within a diseased liver may sometimes compensate for damage to one part; therefore, it is sometimes difficult to predict how drug metabolism will be altered in illness.

Drugs can be divided into two categories on the basis of hepatic extraction characteristics. The first category consists of drugs with a high hepatic extraction ratio (>0.7), whose clearance will be affected by blood flow. Drugs such as lidocaine, morphine, and propranolol have high extraction ratios, and, if given to patients with cirrhosis and congestive heart failure, the clearance of such drugs is decreased. The second category includes drugs with a lower extraction ratio (<0.2) and a low affinity for plasma proteins. The action of these drugs would be influenced more by hepatocellular function and less by changes in hepatic blood flow or plasma protein binding. Examples of these drugs include acetaminophen and theophylline. Most of the information about the effects of liver damage on drug metabolism comes from studies on adults; how this information relates to children is unclear. What has been determined is that careful monitoring is needed to avoid toxic reactions in children with liver damage (Burton et al, 2005).

In cases of renal failure, again, the major information on drug clearance comes from studies on adults. Renal clearance of drugs is directly proportional to the GFR as measured by endogenous creatinine clearance tests. The increased numbers of fatty acids associated with renal impairment may also displace drugs from protein-binding sites. The decrease in plasma albumin that accompanies the nephrotic syndrome reduces the number of available binding sites; consequently, extensively bound drugs would achieve higher plasma concentrations (Burton et al, 2005). Attention to the pharmacokinetic data on drugs eliminated by the kidney is required in children, particularly for those drugs with narrow therapeutic margins and for drugs that produce few observable, measurable clinical responses.

Other disease conditions may also affect drugs. Cystic fibrosis appears to be associated with a requirement for increased doses of drugs. Patients with hypoxemia, critically ill patients with severe head trauma, and those with a variety of GI diseases all may require dosage adjustments for a variety of medications (Kleigman et al, 2007). Again, the adjustments required often have been based on clinical anecdotes and have not been confirmed by valid research studies.

CHOOSING A DRUG REGIMEN

The goal of pediatric drug therapy is to obtain the desired therapeutic response without adverse effects. Although most drugs are not labeled for pediatric use, few are absolutely contraindicated. When children become critically ill, medications perhaps considered risky for use may be required. Case studies of these treatment decisions provide important information for clinicians. Some of the drugs that should be avoided in children include the following:
- Tetracycline—stains the permanent teeth when administered to children younger than 9 years
- Codeine and dextromethorphan—poor antitussives for infants who are vulnerable to respiratory depression. CYP

2D6 converts codeine to morphine, and this enzyme is not developed in very young babies.

- Aspirin—associated with Reye's syndrome
- Valproic acid—higher incidence of liver toxicity in children younger than 2 years

ADVERSE DRUG REACTIONS IN CHILDREN

The potential for drug–drug interactions and adverse effects is increased in very ill children and infants. Children may be exposed to drugs likely to cause adverse reactions in three major ways: (1) transplacentally, when the drug is administered to the mother during pregnancy and delivery; (2) through direct administration of the drug to the child; and (3) by ingestion of the drug in breast milk after the drug has been administered to a nursing mother (AAP, 2001). These three periods are the only stages in life during which one is exposed to and affected by drugs administered to another person—the mother (Gupta & Waldhauser, 1997).

The incidence of adverse reactions in pediatric patients is unknown. Because of the fragility of young children and the complexity of their illnesses, their pharmacotherapy is frequently complicated by misadventure and adverse drug reactions that are unavoidable or difficult to assess. However, studies generally have found the rate of adverse reactions to be equal to that in adults. This rate may be as high as 5.8% of drugs administered to children, although the rate is higher if the child is hospitalized rather than ambulatory (Hansten & Horn, 2007). Because of their differences in morphology and in disease processes and treatments, young children experience a different range of adverse drug reactions. These reactions may not necessarily be predictable from the adult experience. Adverse drug reactions may have profound immediate, delayed, and long-term implications for the neurologic and somatic development of children (Gupta & Waldhauser, 1997).

Drugs that affect the fetus transplacentally are discussed in detail in Chapter 7 on pregnant and breastfeeding women. The effects of adverse reactions from drugs administered during labor and delivery usually are easily noted and short-lived. Central nervous system depression in the newborn may result from analgesics or anesthetics. Excessive uterine stimulants are associated with anoxic encephalopathy, whereas excessive intravenous fluids may cause convulsions or electrolyte disturbances (Burton et al, 2005). Any drugs given to a premature infant or neonate while the liver is immature may potentially cause adverse reactions. The persistence of maternal hormones and drugs in the newborn's bloodstream increases the risk of such interactions. (See section on metabolism in Chapter 3 on pharmacokinetics.)

With younger children, it may be difficult to distinguish whether the child is having an adverse reaction, is experiencing symptoms of the underlying illness (Gupta & Waldhauser, 1997), or is having a paradoxical reaction to a drug (such as hyperactive behavior with antihistamines or chloral hydrate and sleepiness with stimulants like Ritalin). Over-the-counter preparations (particularly antihistamines and adrenergic drugs found in various cough syrups, cold remedies, decongestants, and nose drops) also may provoke adverse reactions in pediatric patients. A broad spectrum of reactions may be seen, varying from minor hypersensitivity reactions to more serious problems with alterations in growth or damage to anatomic or physiologic systems, along with numerous other problems (Hansten & Horn, 2007). A list of adverse effects associated with commonly prescribed drugs is found in Table 5-1.

CALCULATIONS OF PEDIATRIC DOSAGES

Simple approximated reduction in the adult dose is not a safe or effective way of calculating pediatric doses of many medications because of differences in pharmacokinetics in infants and children. The package insert provided by the manufacturer is the best source for pediatric dose recommendations. These recommendations are usually stated in milligrams per kilogram or per pound so the clinician is required to calculate the actual dose to be given. Special formulations for children may be confusing. For example, acetaminophen drops for infants are three times as concentrated as the oral liquid for children. This type of confusion caused inadvertent overdosing of cough and cold products for children under the age of 2 years and eventually led to their withdrawal from the market.

The Joint Commission's National Patient Safety Goals and Medication Management Standards Sentinel Event Alert in early 2008 concluded that current procedures using age or pounds for calculating drug dosages for children should be changed in order to reduce the risk of medication errors in children. All children of the same age are not the same size, so formulas that use age in their calculation should no longer be used.

Thus, two new recommendations regarding pediatric dosages have broad implications for change. First, The Joint Commission now recommends that all pediatric patients should be weighed in kilograms, and that the use of kilograms should become the standardized weight used for prescriptions, medical records, and communication. Pediatric patients are not to be given drugs classified as high risk until the patient has been weighed, unless it is a true emergency. Second, in addition to using pediatric-specific medication formulations and concentrations when possible, prescribers are asked to write out how they arrived at the proper dosage, as dose per weight, so that the calculation can be double checked by a pharmacist, a nurse who is giving the drug, or both.

The pediatric dosage rule based on kilograms (Clark's Rule) should dictate future drug dosage orders. This rule is shown as:

$$\text{Adult dose} \times \frac{\text{Weight (kg)}}{70} = \text{Child's dose}$$

Calculations of dosage based on weight are conservative and tend to underestimate the required dose. A technique that more closely approximates the recommended dosage is based on body surface area (BSA). If manufacturers recommend that BSA should be used for calculating the medication dosage, a nomogram for calculating a child's BSA (Figure 5-1) may be included in the package. The reliability of the BSA method rests on the accuracy with which the BSA is calculated. Critics of the method maintain that the errors inherent in determining BSA make this method less reliable than dosage based on accurate weights.

When the prescribed drug has a wide therapeutic index and is dosed on a per-kilogram basis, weight can be estimated within 10% of the patient's actual weight without greatly

TABLE 5-1   **Drugs Associated With Specific Adverse Effects in Infants and Children**

Drug	Adverse Effect
Iodides, corticosteroids	Acne
Penicillins, heparin, aspirin, parenteral iron, dextran preparations	Anaphylaxis
aspirin, bethanechol, Mucomyst inhalation, epinephrine inhalation	Asthma
Barbiturates, minocycline, phenytoin, amikacin, streptomycin	Ataxia
chloramphenicol, anticonvulsants, penicillins, hydralazine, sulfonamides, anticancer drugs	Blood dyscrasias
Penicillins (especially ampicillin), allopurinol, anticonvulsants, nitrofurantoin, sulfonamides, phenobarbital, anticancer drugs	Cutaneous eruptions
furosemide, aspirin and other salicylates, vibramycin, gentamicin (auditory and vestibular)	Damage to the eighth cranial nerve
Sodium and potassium penicillin salts; diuretics, salicylates, ammonium chloride, sodium bicarbonate, potassium chloride	Electrolyte disturbances
tetracycline, hexachlorophene, phenothiazine	Exaggerated sunburn
Topical corticosteroids, ethambutol, thorazine, chloroquine	Eye damage
Antihistamines, atropine, and other anticholinergic agents	Hallucinations
atropine, bulk-forming laxatives, diphenoxylate	Ileus, intestinal obstruction
isoniazid, rifampin, erythromycin estolate, acetaminophen, sulfonamides, methyldopa, chlorpromazine	Liver damage
penicillamine, trimethadione, probenecid	Nephrotic syndrome
isoniazid, vincristine, hydralazine, ethambutol	Peripheral neuritis
Penicillins, lead, salicylates, outdated tetracyclines, cephaloridine, anticonvulsants, gentamicin, streptomycin, amikacin, neomycin, kanamycin	Renal damage
Antihistamines, nasal decongestants, bronchodilators, central nervous system stimulants	Restlessness, agitation, insomnia, excessive crying
Anabolic steroids, adrenocorticosteroid, psychotropic drugs, central nervous stimulants, vitamins given in excess	Suppression of growth
Tetracyclines in children under 8 years	Temporary suppression of bone growth
carbenicillin, clindamycin, clofibrate, gold preparations, griseofulvin, iron	Unpleasant taste, altered taste sensation

influencing the final dosage. Once a patient weighs 40 to 50 kg (88 to 110 lb), it is time to switch to an adult dose. It is mandatory for the clinician to look at weight-based dosage calculations repeatedly. If the calculated dosage exceeds the usual adult dosage, recheck your numbers. Remember, sometimes a child's dosage will exceed an adult's because of his faster metabolic rate.

Another common source of error in children's dosage is failure to divide the total daily per-kilogram dose by the number of doses to be given in a day, thereby mistaking it for an individual dose that needs to be repeated.

Pediatric Formulation Variables

The form in which a drug is manufactured and the way in which the parent gives the drug to the child determine the actual dose to be administered. Most oral drugs in soluble solutions are readily absorbed from the GI tract. Solid oral dosage forms (i.e., tablets, capsules, and powders) cannot cross the GI membrane until they have been dissolved in the GI fluids. If dissolution is extremely slow, a portion of the drug will be lost in the feces (Gupta & Waldhauser, 1997). A slow dissolution rate increases drug exposure to gastric acid,

thereby increasing the risk of degradation. Some drugs, such as erythromycin estolate, are esters that cannot be absorbed until they have been converted by intestinal enzymes. Infants with immature intestinal enzyme function may be unable to convert these drugs; thus, they may be lost in the feces (Burton et al, 2005).

Many drug preparations for children are provided in the form of elixirs or suspensions. Elixirs are alcoholic solutions in which the drug molecules are dissolved and evenly distributed. No shaking is required, and unless some of the vehicle has evaporated, the first dose from the bottle and the last dose should contain equivalent amounts of drug (McKenry & Salerno, 2006).

Suspensions contain nondissolved particles of drug that must be distributed throughout the vehicle by shaking. If shaking is not thorough each time a dose is given, the first doses from the bottle may contain less drug than the last doses, with the result that less than the expected plasma concentration of the drug may be achieved early in the course of therapy. This will result in decreased drug effectiveness. Conversely, toxicity may occur late in the course of therapy, when unexpectedly high doses are given. This

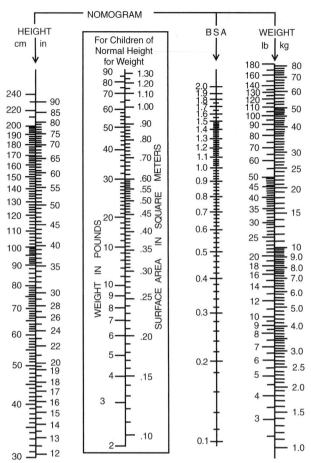

FIGURE 5-1   Body surface area (BSA) is indicated where the straight line that connects height (on the left) and weight (on the right) intersects the BSA column or, if the patient is larger than average size, by weight alone (enclosed area). (Modified from data by Boyd E, West CD. In Behrman RE et al: *Nelson textbook of pediatrics,* ed 18, Philadelphia, 2007, Saunders.

uneven distribution is a potential cause of inefficacy or toxicity in children who are taking phenytoin suspensions (Edmunds, 2005).

Health care personnel or parents who crush or mix medication with other products may increase drug palatability but make changes that affect the pharmacokinetic properties of the drug. It is particularly common for parents to mix medication with infant cereal, applesauce, or even formula. (This is a problem because there can be no guarantee that the child will eat or swallow all of the food.) Thus, it is essential that the prescriber know the form in which the drug will be dispensed and that he provide proper instructions to the pharmacist and to the patient or parent (McKenry & Salerno, 2005). Timed-release oral drugs are specially formulated to promote slow absorption over a period of several hours, when a prolonged duration of action is desirable. Some Dilantin capsules and antihistamine combination products are available as timed-release products for children. Evidence suggests that these products are often erratically absorbed and may be susceptible to changes in gastric pH and GI motility (McKenry & Salerno, 2005).

Difficulties in intramuscular absorption caused by decreased muscle mass and poor blood flow have already been discussed; however, it should also be mentioned that drugs in aqueous vehicles are rapidly absorbed from the muscle.

Other drugs in poorly soluble vehicles that are incompletely absorbed include digoxin, diazepam, and phenytoin. In fact, not only are some of these drugs painful when administered intramuscularly, but often they precipitate at the injection site and are gradually redissolved or are removed by phagocytosis. Other poorly absorbed drugs include ampicillin, cephradine, and dicloxacillin (Yaffe & Aranda, 2004).

Administration of medication through buccal and sublingual routes avoids drug destruction by GI fluids and the liver. However, the effectiveness of this form of delivery depends on whether the child is old enough to keep the drug in contact with the absorbing membrane, and whether he can refrain from swallowing or chewing the tablet until it is completely dissolved. Because most drugs administered by these routes produce an unpleasant taste and mild irritation (Edmunds, 2003), even older children may not be able to cooperate with this route of administration.

Pediatric suppositories and rectal solutions are common forms of drug administration, particularly for neonates. However, absorption in older children is very slow and highly unreliable and may produce substantial bowel irritation. Although it is difficult to control the amount of medication that is actually absorbed, this route avoids destruction of the medication by GI products and the liver. The presence of feces in the bowel limits absorption, presumably by limiting drug access to the absorbing membrane. Drug absorption is terminated if the child defecates (Edmunds, 2003). Additional research on rectal administration suggests that aminophylline retention enemas permit better dosage control than is achieved when the same drug is administered as a rectal suppository, and that inflammation of the colon increases the amount of hydrocortisone absorbed as a retention enema (McKenry & Salerno, 2005).

The pulmonary epithelium and the respiratory tract mucosa allow rapid passage of volatile liquids, gases, aerosol preparations, and isoproterenol. Although pulmonary dosage is irritating to the mucosa and difficult to regulate, the rich blood supply, extensive absorbing surface area, and high permeability of the respiratory tract aid in the absorption of large amounts of medication. If the child is able to hold his breath after aerosol nebulization, effective dosage may be achieved. Otherwise, medication may be lost when it goes into the mouth and is swallowed and excreted (Edmunds, 2003).

Many drugs used in pediatric patients are not available except in injectable form. Drugs such as atropine, digoxin, epinephrine, morphine, phenobarbital, and phenytoin must be diluted, and a dosage must be used that is smaller than that intended for adult patients. Dilution of some products may alter the bioavailability or compatibility of drugs. If multiple drugs are administered through the same site, additional problems of drug interactions may be seen. Children may develop toxicity from some ingredients used in drug preservatives or stabilizers (Edmunds, 2003). Errors that occur in the calculation of the parenteral dosage, the dilution of the product, or even the administration of very small dosages may produce potentially dangerous consequences.

Ophthalmic absorption of medication is promoted by measures that increase the amount of drug that the eye can retain, and that increase the length of time the drug is in contact with the absorbing membrane. Thus, ointments that cover the eye with an oily film provide higher dosages than ophthalmic drops (Edmunds, 2003). Little children are usually very intolerant of eye drops, and efforts to get a little child to hold his head back during instillation, to close his eyes, or to refrain from blinking are rarely successful. Ocular inflammation or injury decreases the blood–aqueous humor barrier, thereby increasing absorption of many ophthalmic drugs (Burton et al, Laso et al, & Parker et al, 2005). Ophthalmic absorption is so great that in premature babies the extent of absorption could potentially lead to systemic toxicity.

Nasal solutions often are well absorbed across the nasal and sinus mucosae. However, infants and young children are likely to swallow these preparations, even when the child's head is held in the lateral head low position.

STATUS OF DRUG DOSING AND POLICY REGARDING CHILDREN

An area of considerable attention, research, and change is that involving research on drug dosing for children. In 1995, the AAP reported that for only a small proportion of all drugs and biologic products marketed in the United States were clinical trials performed in pediatric patients, and most marketed drugs were not labeled for use in pediatric patients or for use in specific pediatric age groups. An FDA survey similarly concluded that for most products indicated for diseases occurring in both adults and children, little information about pediatric use was provided in the labeling (Banner, 2002; Cuzzolin et al, 2006). For vaccines and antibiotics, pediatric use information is generally adequate, but many drugs used in the treatment of both common childhood illnesses and more serious conditions carry little information about use in pediatric patients. Data on the pharmacokinetics, pharmacodynamics, efficacy, and safety of drugs in infants and children are even more difficult to find. For example, an FDA report demonstrates that less than half the drugs approved for treatment of HIV infection or accompanying opportunistic infections carry any pediatric safety or effectiveness information (Cuzzolin et al, 2006). For drugs that do have pediatric information, the data are often incomplete and are limited to certain pediatric age groups. Pediatric labeling is also particularly inadequate for such drug classes as antidepressants, antihypertensives, antirheumatic drugs, medications to treat GI problems, steroids, prescription pain medications, and drugs to treat ulcerative colitis (Cuzzolin et al, 2006).

Many of the drugs and biologic products most widely used in pediatric patients carry disclaimers stating that safety and effectiveness in pediatric patients have not been established (Cuzzolin et al, Atzei et al, and Fanos et al, 2006). Clearly, the term *children* as used in much of the pharmaceutical literature refers to a group with widely differing members. Thus, safety and effectiveness information about some of these group members may not be valid for other group members, and attempts to generalize from one category to another may result in drug errors. The unique differences in neonatal, as opposed to adolescent, drug response are obvious, but subtle changes in the response to drugs occur throughout the total growth and developmental cycle.

An evaluation of available pharmacologic recommendations for children reveals that for some pediatric age groups, information is particularly sparse. For example, for most drug classes, almost no information is available on use in patients younger than 2 years of age. The FDA compiled a list of the 10 drugs that were most widely prescribed for pediatric patients, on an outpatient basis, based on 1994 data from IMS America, Ltd, a research firm that provides data on prescription drug use. These drugs included albuterol inhalation solution, Phenergan, ampicillin injections, Auralgan otic solution, Lotrisone cream, Prozac, Intal, Zoloft, Ritalin, and Alupent syrup. In each case, the drug label lacked any use information for the age group for which the drug was prescribed, or the information was inadequate. These 10 drugs were prescribed more than 5 million times in 1 year for pediatric patients in age groups for which the label carried a disclaimer or lacked adequate use information (Cuzzolin et al, 2006).

evolve For information on the 10 drugs most widely prescribed for pediatric patients, see the Evolve website.

The absence of pediatric labeling information may sometimes require the provider who is caring for children to choose between prescribing drugs without well-founded dosing and safety information and using other, potentially less effective therapies. Inadequate pediatric labeling thus exposes children to the risk of unexpected adverse reactions or treatment that is less than optimal. Even after a drug has been used in pediatric patients for some time, and clinical experience with the drug is substantial, directions for safe and effective use in pediatric patients are not provided on the label (Cuzzolin et al, 2006).

Children were formerly viewed as a population entirely distinct from adults, in whom the safety and effectiveness of a drug had to be established entirely independently. The reality of drug use has made a difference. It has become increasingly accepted that children may be considered a demographic subpopulation with many similarities to the adult population. In some cases, drugs and biologic products behave similarly in demographic subgroups, including age and gender subgroups, even though some variations in pharmacokinetics may be seen. The FDA reported in the *Federal Register* (59 FR 64240, December 13, 1994) that adequate and well-controlled trials in children may not be needed to establish pediatric use information.

Clearly, some difficulties are associated with testing of drugs in the pediatric population. These include, among others, ethical issues surrounding difficulty in recruiting study patients, obtaining informed consent for tests not directly of benefit to the child, use of placebo controls in a vulnerable population, and possible discomfort and risk to the child. Because of these problems, researchers who wish to conduct studies that include children have had difficulty receiving approval from many institutional review committees (Nahata, 2002). Failure to conduct pediatric testing may therefore deprive pediatric patients, in some cases, of significant therapeutic advances. *Therapeutic orphans* is the term that was coined to refer to drugs that lack sponsorship for use in children.

Although use of a particular drug in children is no longer considered a new indication (with the exception of specific pediatric indications), additional information on pediatric patients is needed if appropriate dosing recommendations are to be provided. The correct pediatric dose cannot necessarily be extrapolated from adult dosing information using an equivalence based on weight milligrams per kilogram (mg/kg) or on body surface area (mg/square meter [m^2]). Because potentially significant differences in pharmacokinetics may alter a drug's effect in pediatric patients, dosing is much less precise.

The effects of growth and development of various organs, maturation of the immune system, alterations in metabolism throughout infancy and childhood, changes in body proportions, and other developmental changes may result in significant differences in the doses needed by pediatric patients and adults (Nahata, 2002). For example, studies have shown that fentanyl, a potent opioid widely used in the anesthetic management of infants and small children but not labeled for use in pediatric patients younger than 2 years of age, exhibits differences in clearance between the neonatal period and 2 or more months of age, resulting from improving hepatic blood flow and hepatic microsomal maturation (Koren, 2001). Comparable doses in adults and neonates (calculated on a mcg/kg basis) produce a twofold to threefold higher plasma concentration in neonates. Again, development of the gray baby syndrome after chloramphenicol was administered to infants with immature livers was directly related to decreased metabolism of this drug by the glucuronyl transferase that could convert it to the inactive glucuronide metabolite. Pharmacokinetic differences of this type demonstrate the importance of studying the pharmacokinetics of a drug in pediatric patients and in different ages before children are widely exposed to it.

Inadequate dosing information may cause pediatric patients to be exposed to dangerously high doses or to ineffective treatment. This dramatically increases the probability of adverse reactions. Cases in which inadequately studied drugs have resulted in serious adverse effects in pediatric patients include teeth staining from tetracycline, kernicterus from sulfa drugs, withdrawal symptoms following prolonged administration of fentanyl in infants and small children, seizures and cardiac arrest caused by bupivacaine toxicity, development of colonic stricture in pediatric patients with cystic fibrosis after exposure to high-dose pancreatic enzymes, and hazardous interactions between erythromycin and midazolam (Nathan et al, 2003).

Other factors also may interfere with the appropriate drug dosing of children. Many drugs widely prescribed for infants and children are not available in a suitable dosage form for children. Examples include phenobarbital, acetazolamide, and rifampin. When these products are altered to be given to children through dilution or reformulation, questions must be raised about their stability and compatibility. The problems associated with intravenous infusion of medications are compounded by the need for low fluid volumes and by limited access to intravenous sites (Nahata, 2002). Failure to develop a pediatric formulation may deny pediatric patients access to important therapeutic advances or may require pediatric patients to take the drug in homemade or poorly bioavailable formulations (Cuzzolin et al, 2006).

The absence of pediatric testing may thus result in less than optimal treatment for many pediatric patients (AAP, 1997). Although significant progress has been made in the area of pediatric pharmacokinetics over the past several decades, few studies have correlated pharmacokinetics with pharmacodynamics.

In late 1994, the FDA amended its regulations governing the content and format of labeling for human prescription drug products. The final rule revised the current "Pediatric Use" subsection of the professional labeling requirements for prescription drugs to provide for the inclusion of more complete information about use of a drug in the pediatric population (ages birth to 16 years). The final rule, which applies to prescription drug products, including biologics, recognized several methods of establishing substantial evidence to support pediatric labeling claims. This includes, in certain cases, relying on studies carried out in adults. This final rule also requires that if no substantial evidence supports any pediatric use or use in a particular pediatric population, the labeling shall state this. Drug company sponsors are required to reexamine existing data on their products to determine whether the "Pediatric Use" subsection of the labeling for drugs already being marketed can be modified based on already adequate and well-controlled studies in adults. In such cases, the FDA will have concluded that the course of the disease and the positive and negative effects of the drug are sufficiently similar in the pediatric and adult populations to allow extrapolation from adult efficacy data to pediatric patients. Other information supporting pediatric use must ordinarily include data on the pharmacokinetics of the drug in the pediatric population for determination of appropriate dosage. In some cases, companies will be required to submit a supplemental application to comply with new drug labeling requirements, to show that the drug can be used safely and effectively in pediatric patients.

The specific labeling required by the FDA under the "Pediatric Use" subsection of the labeling says as follows:

> The safety and effectiveness of (drug name) have been established in the age groups to (note any limitations [e.g., no data for pediatric patients under 2, or only applicable to certain indications approved in adults]). Use of (drug name) in these age groups is supported by evidence from adequate and well-controlled studies of (drug name) in adults with additional data (insert wording that accurately describes the data submitted to support a finding of substantial evidence of effectiveness in the pediatric population).
>
> (U.S. FDA, 1994)

If appropriate, under the Clinical Pharmacology, Contradictions, Warnings, Precautions, and Dosage and Administration sections, additional and specific information might be provided as a "Pediatric Use" subsection.

After looking at all drugs for which at least 50,000 prescriptions/year are used in pediatric patients, the FDA compiled a list of drugs for which additional pediatric information could produce health benefits in the pediatric population. Drugs with "meaningful therapeutic benefit" over existing treatments and those that are widely used in pediatric populations are now required to undergo specific pediatric studies, which should be completed by the drug manufacturing company before they may be marketed (FDA, 1994). The new rules for testing were designed to provide more pediatric use information in the labeling of drugs. This will help practitioners to obtain reliable information on which they can base decisions to prescribe a drug for use in pediatric patients. It is not intended to limit the manner in which a practitioner may prescribe an approved drug.

Overall, tremendous progress has been made over the past decade in the area of collecting information about drug prescribing in children. FDA regulations have continued to upgrade the extent of labeling of drugs with pediatric information, and substantial progress has been made.

In 1997, the Pediatric Exclusivity Program approved by Congress authorized the FDA to grant 6-month extensions of marketing rights when pharmaceutical companies complete FDA-requested pediatric trials. The indications studied included asthma, tumors, attention-deficit/hyperactivity disorder, hypertension, depression/generalized anxiety disorder, diabetes mellitus, gastroesophageal reflux disease, bacterial infection, and bone mineralization. One third of the drugs tested had different effects in children than in adults. Of 59 drugs, 12 were found to be ineffective in children, 5 required dosing changes, and trials in 9 resulted in new safety information for children. Since the program began, 300 drug studies in children have resulted in 122 drug labeling changes for pediatric use. Of note is the "black box" warning that was added to certain antidepressants and a drug for hepatitis because pediatric studies indicated increased risk for suicidal thoughts or behavior (Li et al, 2007).

SPECIAL COMPLIANCE PROBLEMS IN CHILDREN

Compliance may be more difficult to achieve in pediatric patients than in other individuals because it involves not only the parents' conscientious efforts to follow directions but also such practical matters as measuring errors, spilling, and spitting out. For example, because the measured volume of "teaspoons" ranges from 2.5 to 7.8 ml (Burton et al, 2005), parents should obtain a calibrated medicine spoon or syringe from the pharmacy for dosing small children. These devices improve the accuracy of dose measurements and simplify administration of drugs to children.

When one is evaluating compliance, it is often helpful to ask if an attempt was made to give another dose of medicine after the child spilled part of what was offered. Parents may not always be able to say with confidence how much of a dose the child actually received. Parents must be told whether to wake the baby for his every-6-hour dose day or night. These matters should be discussed and made clear, and no assumptions should be made about what the parents may or may not do. Compliance problems frequently occur when antibiotics are prescribed to treat otitis media or urinary tract infection and the child feels well after a few days of therapy. Parents may also feel that the child is well and may stop giving the medicine, even though it was prescribed for 10 or 14 days.

This common situation should be anticipated so that parents can be told why it is important to continue the medicine for the prescribed period even if the child seems to be "cured."

Practical and convenient dosage forms and dosing schedules should be chosen to the extent possible. The easier it is to administer and take the medicine and the easier the dosing schedule is to follow, the more likely it is that compliance will be achieved.

Consistent with their ability to comprehend and cooperate, children should be given some responsibility for their own health care and for taking medications. This should be discussed in appropriate terms with both the child and the parents. This is particularly true with chronic problems such as asthma, diabetes, and arthritis. Possible adverse effects and drug interactions with over-the-counter medicines or food also should be discussed. Whenever a drug does not achieve its therapeutic effect, the possibility of noncompliance should be considered. Ample evidence suggests that when noncompliance with the prescribed regimen is a big factor in a child's not getting well, parents' or children's reports about their compliance may be grossly inaccurate. Random measurement of serum concentrations and pill count may help to disclose noncompliance (McKenry & Salerno, 2005). Computerized pill containers that record each lid opening have been shown to be very effective in measuring compliance.

SUMMARY

Working with children is a rewarding experience. However, the clinician's responsibility for accuracy and careful monitoring and record keeping is even greater with children than with other patient populations. Their physical and developmental immaturity often presents a vulnerability and risk that allow little margin for error.

evolve A continually updated list of useful WebLinks may be found in the Evolve Resources at http://evolve.elsevier.com/Edmunds/NP/

Neonate 130 days

6 Special Populations: Pregnant and Nursing Women

Providing drug therapy to pregnant or lactating women poses a unique challenge for health care practitioners. Because these patients represent a state of duality, the clinician who prescribes a drug for them must always consider the impact of that treatment on the developing fetus or infant. Hence the benefit of any drug to a pregnant patient must be carefully weighed against the potential teratogenic risk to the fetus. In the lactating mother, the choices between premature weaning (before the age of 1 year), temporarily interrupting breastfeeding, or breastfeeding while taking medication must be carefully weighed against the benefits of breastfeeding and the deleterious effects of early weaning. Because controlled clinical trials cannot be conducted in pregnant women, literature support of current practice is based on historical data, case reports, and animal research trials. Much of the literature in this area is based on case reports and drug research, but it may not be evidence based in nature (AAFP, 2002; AAP, 2001; Spencer et al, 2001).

During pregnancy, the clinician must be aware of the changing physiologic characteristics of the patient throughout gestation, as well as those of the growing fetus. Additionally, although multiple factors may affect the teratogenicity of a drug, one of the most important is the timing of the drug exposure. Three stages of development are generally considered when the teratogenic potential of a drug is assessed (Briggs et al, 2005; Koren, 2006): the 2 weeks after conception and before implantation (the *preimplantation phase*), the embryonic period (weeks 3 through 8), and the fetal period (weeks 9 through delivery). In the past, clinicians have overestimated the ability of the placenta to protect the fetus and in fact, the term *placental barrier* is a misnomer in that the placenta allows the crossing of most drugs and dietary substances.

For the breastfed infant, the provider must understand the dynamics between the mechanisms of the drug's entry into mother's milk and what happens once the infant ingests it, taking into account the infant's age, health status, and ability to metabolize and excrete the medication. Primarily, medication transfers into human milk through a concentration gradient that allows passive diffusion of free (non–protein-bound) and nonionized medication. Different choices and greater caution may be needed in infants younger than 1 week old, premature infants, and compromised infants with health problems because they may have a lessened ability to tolerate, metabolize, or excrete medications. Finally, more medication transfer occurs during the early postpartum period because of large gaps between the mammary alveolar cells, but less transfer occurs during the weaning process because of a decrease in the milk supply caused by nursing sessions that are shorter or fewer (Koren, 2006; Spencer et al, 2001).

Overall, what the mother consumes is also consumed by the fetus or infant, with the exception of large organic ions such as heparin and insulin. In fact, virtually all (99%) drugs cross the placenta, and most medications penetrate human milk to some degree (Hale, 2008; Shephard & Lemire, 2007). Ideally, the pregnant or lactating woman should take as few drugs as possible, although exposure is usually more significant for the developing fetus than for the breastfeeding infant. Usually breastfeeding infants have less exposure because the concentrations of most medications in human milk are extraordinarily low, and with few exceptions, the dose delivered to the nursing infant is subclinical (Hale, 2008). Frequently, however, some form of drug therapy is necessary to treat the physiologic and hormonal changes that occur during pregnancy and postpartum, symptoms produced by the expanding uterus or functioning breast, and/or concomitant illnesses such as asthma, upper respiratory infection, epilepsy, or diabetes mellitus. Clinicians in the primary care setting should anticipate such complaints and should be prepared to treat patients appropriately.

Unfortunately, despite the obvious need for drug therapy and the prevailing apprehension about using drugs in these special populations, clinicians may not be aware of information that is available to help them make astute clinical decisions. Because of the medicolegal implications of treating pregnant women and infants, pregnant women have been excluded from most clinical drug trials. Hence, evidence is insufficient regarding the safety and efficacy of many drug therapies during pregnancy. Notably, very few drugs have been granted FDA approval for use during pregnancy, and drugs that can be used during lactation are just being categorized. Thus, drugs for pregnant or lactating patients must be selected based on safety data derived from animal research and clinical data generated from case reports, retrospective case-control trials, and personal experience. What's more, during lactation the care given to mothers may be confounded by breastfeeding misinformation. Consequently, to provide the most astute and contemporary care, those who treat the breastfed infant or the pregnant mother may have to consult the most accurate and up-to-date resources available. This includes using both telephone consultations and Internet resources for assistance in choosing the most appropriate medication (Box 6-1).

BOX 6-1 Sources of Information on Potential Teratogens

COMPUTERIZED DATABASES

American Academy of Pediatrics. Available at www.aap.org

The Organization of Teratology Information Services (OTIS). Available at www.otispregnancy.org

Repro-Tox, Columbia Women's Hospital, Washington, DC, 202-293-5138

Teratology Information System (TERIS), Department of Pediatrics, University of Washington, Seattle, Washington

TOXLINE, National Library of Medicine, Bethesda, Maryland

CURRENT PREGNANCY EXPOSURE REGISTRIES

www.fda.gov/womens/registries/registries.html

LACTATION

Breastfeeding and drugs information, University of California San Diego, 900-226-7536

Hale T: *Medications in mothers' milk*, ed 12, Oklahoma City, OK, 2008, Hale Publications.

Tom Hale's lactation registry:
   http://neonatal.ttuhsc.edu/lact/html/drug_entry.html
   http://neonatal.ama.ttuhsc.edu/lact/
   http://neonatal.ama.ttuhsc.edu/lact/html/lactation_registry.html
   www.ibreastfeeding.com

Lawrence R: *Breastfeeding: a guide for the medical professional*, St Louis, 1999, Mosby.

Newman J, Pitman T: *Dr. Jack Newman's guide to breastfeeding*, Toronto, 2000, HarperCollins Publishing.

DEPRESSION

Pregnancy and depression information. Available at www.pregnancyanddepression.com

Registry for bupropion exposure. Available at www.pregnancyregistry.gsk.com/bupreg.pdf

evolve Please also see the supplemental tables on the Evolve Resources website.

DRUGS IN PREGNANT WOMEN

Incidence

Although the ideal condition may be the avoidance of any medications or chemicals during pregnancy, research has demonstrated that 90% of pregnant women have or develop medical problems that require them to take more than one prescription drug during pregnancy (Shephard & Lemire, 2007). Studies have shown that the average patient uses five to nine different drugs during pregnancy; 4% of pregnant women take more than 10 drugs during pregnancy; and 65% of women admit to self-administration of drugs during pregnancy. Additional research has demonstrated that the extent of fetal exposure to drugs may be vastly underestimated; patient medical charts reveal less than one fourth of the drugs actually consumed by the patient (Briggs et al, 2005; Koren, 2006).

PRINCIPLES OF TERATOLOGY: INCIDENCE AND TYPES OF MALFORMATIONS

The desire for a healthy baby is universal. Mothers cannot help but worry about the health of their unborn child. Regardless of the mother's concerns, many factors not under her control may influence the outcome of the pregnancy. Information about the thalidomide tragedy in the early 1960s, fueled by regulatory agencies, lawyers, and the public, has stimulated an intense search for the origin, prevention, and treatment of congenital malformations (Briggs et al, 2005). However, although vigilance in this area has been heightened, most knowledge about the effect of different drugs on the fetus comes from the experience and observation of clinicians—not from scientific research.

Congenital malformations occur in many different forms, and their incidence varies widely. The incidence of major malformations in the general population is usually quoted as 2% to 3%, or 20 to 30 per 1000 live births. This translates into 200,000 birth defects annually (Schardein & Macina, 2006). Major malformations are those that are incompatible with survival (e.g., anencephaly) or that require major surgery for correction (e.g., cleft palate, congenital heart disease). If minor malformations are included (e.g., ear tags, extra digits), the rate of occurrence may be as high as 10% (Briggs et al, 2005). Congenital malformations account for about 14% of all infant deaths. Problems that arise during fetal development or within 1 month after birth account for two thirds of all infant mortality in this country (Schardein & Macina, 2006).

Although much attention has been paid to the causes of obvious physical deformities, growing research suggests that concern should extend to events beyond the narrow limit of congenital anatomic malformations. Evidence suggests that future intellectual, social, and functional development of the unborn child also may be adversely affected. In particular, toxic manifestations of intrauterine exposure to drugs may be subtle, unexpected, and delayed.

Common lore blames drug exposure of the pregnant mother for any type of fetal damage that occurs. However, less than 5% of congenital malformations are probably related to drugs (Briggs et al, 2005). Only 19 drugs or groups of drugs have been identified as probable teratogenic agents in humans (Table 6-1). This contrasts with the almost 1000 teratogens that have been identified for laboratory animals (Schardein & Macina, 2006). This public misperception probably grew from media attention that surrounded the extreme fetal deformities that occurred as part of the thalidomide tragedy of the 1960s.

Thalidomide

Thalidomide is a central nervous system depressant that was used as a sedative-hypnotic agent and to reduce the nausea and vomiting of pregnancy. As many as 10,000 children were reportedly deformed as the result of use of this drug in as many as 30 countries, although the confirmed number is closer to 8000. The thalidomide episode focused the attention of both the scientific community and the lay community on the question of safe drug use in pregnant women. This drug was said to increase the rate of dysmelia by 80%, up to a rate of about 3:1000 to 5:1000 births. The reported malformations resulted when thalidomide was taken on days 21 to 36 after conception (days 34 to 50 postmenses). The risk that a woman will have a malformed child following thalidomide ingestion has been

TABLE 6-1   Drugs Considered to Be Teratogenic in Humans

Drug	Major Defects
ACE inhibitors	Fetal renal dysplasia, fetal limb contractures, craniofacial deformities, hypoplastic lung development, fetal skull ossification defects
Antithyroid compounds, iodine	Hypothyroidism, goiter, scalp defects

Antibiotics
    Aminoglycoside
    Tetracycline
Cephalosporins (cefaclor, cephalexin, cephradine)
	Ototoxicity, eighth nerve
	Staining of teeth, hypoplasia enamel, inhibition of bone growth
	Possible minor abnormalities

Anticancer agents methotrexate	Polymorphic Multiple congenital anomalies, cranial and malformation of extremities
Androgenic hormones	Masculinization, clitoromegaly, labial fusion
isotretinoin, etretinate	Structural anomalies 25%; mental retardation 25%; craniofacial, cardiac, thymic, CNS abnormalities; ear, mouth, and eye abnormalities; great vessel transposition of heart, ventricular septal defect
thalidomide	Severe limb, ear abnormalities

Antiepileptics
    phenytoin
 	
    lamotrigine
    primidone
    tegretol
    valproic acid
    carbamazepine
	Double risk malformations: cleft lip, palate, cardiac
	Fetal hydantoin syndrome: craniofacial, appendicular, cardiac, and skeletal, motor, and mental deficiency
	Congenital anomalies and seizure disorders
	Microcephaly, cardiac, facial, mental deficiency
	Dysmorphic
	Neural tube defect, spina bifida, facial defects
	Craniofacial, digital, neural tube defects

Coumarin anticoagulants	Nose, skeleton, CNS, ophthalmologic abnormalities, mental retardation
Alcohol	Fetal alcohol syndrome: facial, microcephaly, mental retardation, CNS dysfunction
Methadone	Facial, cardiac, urogenital, mental, and speech impairment
diethylstilbestrol (DES)	Uterine adenosis, cancer in females, accessory gonadal lesions in males
penicillamine	Skin hyperelasticity
Vitamin A analogues	Craniofacial, cardiac, CNS, thymic, mental retardation
Cocaine	Cardiovascular, CNS, neurologic defects

From Schardein JL, Macina OT: *Human developmental toxicants: aspects of toxicology and chemistry,* New York, 2006, CRC; Gabbe SG et al: *Obstetrics—normal and problem pregnancies,* ed 5, New York, 2007, Churchill Livingstone, Inc.

estimated to range from 2% to 25%, and retrospective analysis suggests that the mortality rate is 45%. Today, much controversy surrounds thalidomide research in women affected by human immunodeficiency virus and rheumatoid arthritis (Schardein & Macina, 2006; Shephard & Lemire, 2007).

Determinants of Teratogenicity

The most important determinant of the teratogenicity of an agent is the timing of the drug exposure (Figure 6-1). Exposure to drugs during the preimplantation phase results in an all-or-none effect: The affected cells either die or are described as undifferentiated, or *totipotential*, meaning that if one cell is damaged, another can assume its function (Briggs et al, 2005; Schardein & Macina, 2006). During this period, no malformations can be induced because there is no cell differentiation to allow any selective toxic reaction. Exposure to a teratogen may be lethal to the ovum, or the ovum may regenerate completely after exposure to a sublethal dose. Thus, exposure during this time may kill the conceptus, and the patient may not realize that she is pregnant; however, if the pregnancy continues, the risk of congenital anomalies is not increased (Briggs et al, 2005).

The most critical period in which drug exposure should be avoided is the *embryonic period* (weeks 3 through 8), during which major organogenesis occurs and the risk of inducing major malformations is greatest. The damage induced by a drug administered during this period will depend on what organ systems were forming during the time of exposure. Because many organ systems form in parallel, multiple congenital defects may result from one drug exposure. The classic teratogenic period in humans lasts from 31 days after the last menstrual period through 10 weeks from the last menstrual period (Briggs et al, 2005), which corresponds to the period of organogenesis (14 to 56 days).

After embryogenesis occurs, the organ structures continue to grow and mature physiologically during the *fetal period* (weeks 9 through term). During the fetal period (57 days to

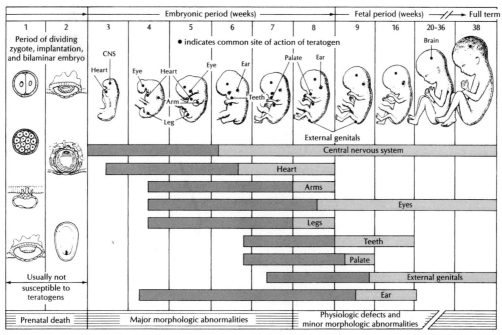

FIGURE 6-1   Critical periods in human development. Periods most susceptible to teratogenesis are indicated in black; less sensitive stages are shown in white. (From Moore K: *Before we are born: basic embryology and birth defects,* ed 5, Philadelphia, 1998, Saunders.)

term), major malformations are not likely to occur, yet organ systems formed during the embryonic period may be damaged by exposure during the second or third trimester (Schardein & Macina, 2006; Shephard & Lemire, 2007; Weiner & Buhimschi, 2003) and anomalies are more likely to involve functional aspects such as mental development and reproduction or fetal growth. Thus, exposure to a teratogen during this period may result in intrauterine growth retardation, and, because the central nervous system continues to develop throughout gestation, exposure may cause mental retardation or subtle, delayed behavioral effects.

The placenta plays an important role in determining the teratogenic potential of a drug, primarily by allowing drugs to reach the fetus but perhaps also by allowing for the biotransformation of drugs before they reach the fetal circulation. The surface area of the placenta increases during gestation, while placental thickness decreases. Both of these structural changes favor the transfer of chemicals to the fetus (Briggs et al, 2005). In fact, as was stated earlier, nearly all drugs readily cross the placenta, reaching fetal concentrations of 50% to 100% of those in the maternal circulation. Primarily, the physiologic processes that govern the passage of drugs across the placenta are the same as those that apply to the passage of drugs across any lipid membrane. Once the drug has crossed the placenta, it is in the fetal circulation. Several other physicochemical properties affect the rate and/or extent of placental transfer, including lipid solubility, protein binding, and pH of the mother and fetus (Briggs et al, 2005). Currently, little is known about the contribution of the placenta to the metabolism of drugs that pass through it. However, metabolic inactivation of drugs by the placenta appears to be of less clinical concern than is the potential for the placenta to

metabolize less active compounds to toxic metabolites (Koren, 2006).

Several other factors that illustrate the principles of teratology include the following (Briggs et al, 2005; Schardein & Macina, 2006):

- *Maternal-fetal genotype*—Maternal absorption, metabolism, and distribution, placental transfer, and fetal metabolism characteristics unique to each maternal-fetal pair as a result of genetic heterogeneity influence fetal susceptibility to a potential teratogen. This is easy to understand when clinicians observe that for the same teratogen, some individuals will prove especially susceptible, whereas others will be unusually resistant.

- *Dose-response relationships*—The amount of medication taken often correlates with the observed response. Aberrant development may range from no effect at low doses to organ-specific malformations at intermediate doses to embryo-fetal toxicity at high doses. The extent of damage is also influenced by the stage of development and the route of administration.

- *Specificity of agent*—The extent of adverse environmental influences on developing tissues depends heavily on the agent involved. Some agents have greater teratogenic potential than others, resulting in part from factors such as drug dosage, maternal metabolism, and placental transfer.

- *Drug interactions*—Two teratogens administered separately may have a very different effect when given together. Induction or inhibition of enzyme systems and competition for binding sites caused by the two drugs may influence the levels of unbound and active teratogens.

Finally, the response of the fetus to an administered medication tends to differ from that of the mother. This may result from increased blood-brain permeability and the immaturity of liver enzymes in the fetus.

Determining the Teratogenic Potential of Drugs

In general, animal models predict poorly whether a drug or chemical is a human teratogen, and it is extraordinarily difficult to directly extrapolate findings in animals to pregnant women (Schardein & Macina, 2006). As clinicians gain experience with a drug, case reports may provide the first evidence that an agent is teratogenic in humans. Although human investigations are necessary to demonstrate that an agent is teratogenic, such studies are not informative until the agent has already damaged many children (Schardein & Macina, 2006). For the best sources of information on potential teratogens, to report or investigate an exposure, or to obtain a list of current pregnancy exposure registries, see Box 6-1.

Counseling Pregnant Patients About Drug Use

The safe use of a drug in a single pregnancy or even in a large number of pregnancies does not ensure that the drug is safe in all pregnancies (Briggs et al, 2005). Very few drugs can be declared "safe in pregnancy." The present state of knowledge does not allow prediction with any degree of certainty as to when a particular drug will prove teratogenic to a particular fetus. References can describe only relative risks for a specific population—not specific risks for specific patients (Briggs et al, 2005). To help quantify the measure of risk that a drug presents to the fetus, the FDA developed a classification scheme to aid in the selection of drug therapy for pregnant women, and all drugs must be labeled with an FDA pregnancy category rating (Table 6-2). See *evolve* for content updates.

Additionally, several textbooks and computer online services are available to assist clinicians in determining the teratogenic potential of a drug. Several sources of information can be used to help the clinician determine whether an agent has known teratogenic potential. However, for most drugs, the information needed to make such a determination is insufficient. Ultimately, the decision about whether to prescribe a drug to a pregnant woman should be made only after a thorough discussion has taken place between the patient and her health care provider.

The benefits of the drug to the mother must be weighed against the risk potential to the developing fetus.

The ideal time to counsel women regarding drug use during pregnancy is before conception because the critical time for problems to occur is before the woman knows she is pregnant. More and more women seek information from their health care providers before conception, hoping to prevent possible adverse effects. Clinicians should stress medication use for preventative purposes, as medically indicated, and only for those medications thought to be safe for continued use during pregnancy.

When a clinician discovers that a pregnant woman has been exposed to a dangerous drug, it is important to provide the patient with as much information as possible. First, determine whether the fetus was exposed during organogenesis; if so, refer the patient for a detailed ultrasonogram and to a perinatologist. If the exposure occurred outside organogenesis, then ordering an ultrasonogram to reassure the mother is an option. With drugs that have a high potential for fetal damage, the patient should be encouraged to make a thoughtful decision regarding whether to continue the pregnancy (Friedman & Polifka, 2007; Schardein & Macina, 2006) (Box 6-2).

COMMON CONDITIONS REQUIRING TREATMENT DURING PREGNANCY

Physiologic Changes

The physiology of pregnancy differs substantially from what is thought of as normal, and profound changes occur throughout gestation. As the uterus grows from the beginning of gestation to the end of pregnancy, it progressively occupies more room in the abdomen, pressing the digestive organs and diaphragm up toward the lungs.

Despite the many physiologic changes that occur during pregnancy that could theoretically affect absorption, bioavailability of the drug during pregnancy does not appear to be altered. Maternal blood volume increases by 30% to 40% (500 to 1800 ml) to support the requirements of the developing fetus. This may lead to decreased plasma concentrations of

TABLE 6-2   Pregnancy Category Ratings

Category	Description
A	Adequate, well-controlled studies in pregnant women have not shown an increased risk of fetal abnormalities. The possibility of fetal harm appears remote.
B	Animal studies have revealed no evidence of harm to the fetus; however, no adequate and well-controlled studies in pregnant women have been conducted. *Or* Animal studies have shown an adverse effect, but adequate and well-controlled studies in pregnant women have failed to demonstrate a risk to the fetus.
C	Animal studies have shown an adverse effect, and no adequate and well-controlled studies in pregnant women have been conducted. *Or* No animal studies have been conducted, and no adequate and well-controlled studies in pregnant women have been conducted. Give drugs only if the potential benefit justifies the potential risk to the fetus.
D	Studies, adequate well-controlled or observational, in pregnant women have demonstrated a risk to the fetus. However, the benefits of therapy may outweigh the potential risks. Give only if the drug is needed for a life-threatening situation or a serious disease for which safer drugs cannot be used or are ineffective.
X	Studies, adequate well-controlled or observational, in animals or pregnant women have demonstrated positive evidence of fetal abnormalities. Use of the product is contraindicated in women who are or may become pregnant.

From Meadows M: Pregnancy and the drug dilemma, *FDA Consumer Magazine,* 2001. (Available at www.fda.gov/fdac/features/2001/301_preg.html#categories)

BOX 6-2 Counseling Pregnant Patients Who Have Ingested Medications or Chemicals

INFORMATION TO OBTAIN FROM THE PATIENT

Name(s) of the drug(s) or chemical(s) involved

Exact exposure date(s)

Exact date of the first day of the last menstrual period, to determine what organs were being formed during exposure(s)

Exact amount(s) to which the patient was exposed

INFORMATION TO GIVE TO THE PATIENT

From 2% to 3% of all pregnancies result in major malformations. This is the expected natural incidence.

Drugs or chemicals may cause 4% to 5% of major malformations. Caffeine, nicotine, and alcohol in substantial quantities may be harmful, and their use should be stopped.

From 20% to 25% of all pregnancies are spontaneously terminated by completely undetermined factors.

Abortions are rarely indicated following exposure to drugs, chemicals, or environmental pollutants.

some drugs. Decreased albumin and α_1-acid glycoprotein concentrations during pregnancy will result in decreased protein binding for highly bound drugs. For drugs metabolized by the liver, this can result in misinterpretation of total plasma concentrations of low extraction ratio drugs and overdosing of high extraction ratio drugs administered by nonoral routes. Renal clearance and the activity of the CYP isozymes—CYP3A4, 2D6 and 2C9, and uridine 5′-diphosphate glucuronosyl transferase—are increased during pregnancy. In contrast, CYP1A2 and 2C19 activity is decreased (Anderson, 2006).

Renal function improves during gestation because renal plasma flow increases by 30% and the glomerular filtration rate (GFR) increases by as much as 50%. Because of this improved renal filtration, serum urea, creatinine, and uric acid levels usually are decreased in pregnancy. Cardiac output increases by as much as 32% because of an increased heart rate (up 10 to 15 bpm) and increased stroke volume (Ilett & Hale, 2002).

Not all changes in the system are positive to the mother. During pregnancy, a hypercoagulable state develops, with increased levels of fibrinogen and of factors VII, VIII, IX, and X. And, because bowel tone and gastrointestinal peristalsis decrease, constipation may become a problem for the pregnant women. Pregnant women also have a high incidence of heartburn because of decreased gastrointestinal motility, increased estrogen and progesterone that decreases lower esophageal sphincter tone, and the increased pressure of the growing uterus on the abdomen (Ilett & Hale, 2002).

Nausea and Vomiting

Nausea and vomiting, common symptoms during pregnancy, often are regarded as an unpleasant but normal part of pregnancy during the first and early second trimesters. Nausea and vomiting of pregnancy (NVP) occur in approximately 75% to 80% of pregnant women. NVP is self-limiting, typically starting 2 to 3 weeks after a missed menstrual period and continuing from the 8th to the 12th week of pregnancy. It is usually worse in the morning before the mother gets out of bed. The exact etiology and pathogenesis of NVP are poorly understood and are most likely multifactorial. Some theories for the etiology of NVP involve psychological predisposition, evolutionary adaptation, hormonal stimuli, increased levels of human chorionic gonadotropin (hCG), and/or increased levels of progesterone associated with decreased gastric emptying, and *Helicobacter pylori* infection. Treatment ranges from dietary and lifestyle changes to vitamins, antiemetics, and hospitalization for intravenous therapy. Treatment generally begins with nonpharmacologic interventions; if symptoms do not improve, drug therapy is added. Although NVP has been associated with a positive pregnancy outcome, the symptoms can significantly affect a woman's life, both personally and professionally. Given the substantial health care costs, as well as the indirect costs, and the potential decrease in quality of life due to NVP, providers must acknowledge the impact of NVP and provide appropriate treatment (Badell et al, 2006).

Although NVP most frequently is self-limited, approximately 1% to 3% of pregnant women may experience severe nausea and vomiting, defined as hyperemesis gravidarum. This condition, which affects 3.5 of 1000 infants, is debilitating and can result in significant weight loss, electrolyte imbalance, ketosis, dehydration, and malnutrition. Overall, treatment of NVP should depend on the severity of symptoms, the impact of symptoms on a woman's quality of life, and the safety of the fetus. Treatments range from dietary and lifestyle changes to vitamin supplementation, antiemetic therapy, and hospitalization. Treatment generally begins with nonpharmacologic interventions; drug therapy is added if nausea or vomiting does not improve. Such patients often require hospitalization for the administration of intravenous fluids and electrolytes, antiemetics, and sedation. Additionally, treatment with corticosteroids has been found to be effective (Safari et al, 1998).

Formal evaluation is limited regarding the agents used to treat NVP. Currently, no drug has been approved by the FDA for treating NVP, and no standard treatment protocol exists. Considering the available pharmacologic and nonpharmacologic approaches to NVP, health care providers should understand that adequate treatment often involves a balance between nonpharmacologic and pharmacologic options.

Benedictine (10 mg doxylamine/10 mg pyridoxine) was used for NVP in an estimated 10% to 25% of pregnant women in the United States from 1958 to 1983. In the 1960s, numerous birth defects (limb deformities, cleft palate, pyloric stenosis) associated with the use of Benedictine were reported worldwide (Schardein & Macina, 2006). However, the product has been studied since then, and those results have been refuted. Doxylamine and pyridoxine now carry a category B and A rating, respectively. Although the company voluntarily removed the branded product from the market in 1983, the active ingredients are available in other countries on a nonprescription basis (e.g., Unisom nighttime sleep aid, vitamin B_6), or the product can be prescribed and compounded.

Management of mild to moderate NVP begins with nonpharmacologic steps before medication use is prescribed. Usual products recommended for the treatment of nausea and vomiting include multivitamins and pyridoxine (vitamin B_6), a water-soluble B-complex vitamin and a necessary coenzyme in the metabolism of lipids, carbohydrates, and amino acids. Pyridoxine can be taken alone or with doxylamine for the treatment of NVP. If given alone, the dosage should be oral pyridoxine 25 mg every 8 hours or 75 mg/day.

A few antihistamines have been studied for the treatment of NVP. Meclizine, dimenhydrinate, and diphenhydramine have been used alone to treat NVP. In general, antihistamines directly inhibit the action of histamine at the histamine$_1$ (H_1) receptor and indirectly affect the vestibular system, thereby decreasing stimulation of the vomiting center. In addition, muscarinic receptor inhibition may play a role in antihistamine antiemetic activity. No correlation exists between the sedative or local anesthetic effect of an antihistamine and its efficacy as an antiemetic.

No specific dosing guidelines for pregnant women have been made available to health care providers; hence, standard adult dosages are recommended, that is, diphenhydramine 25 to 50 mg orally every 4 to 6 hours, or 10 to 50 mg intravenously or intramuscularly every 4 to 6 hours as needed; meclizine 25 mg every 4 to 6 hours as needed; and dimenhydrinate orally or rectally 50 to 100 mg every 4 to 6 hours as needed.

A number of dopamine antagonists can be used for the treatment of NVP. During nausea and vomiting, dopamine receptors in the stomach mediate inhibition of gastric motility and may provide a site of action for antiemetic dopamine receptor antagonists. Dopamine, specifically at the dopamine$_2$ (D_2) receptors, is also implicated in emetic signaling through the chemoreceptor trigger zone. The three main classes of dopamine receptor antagonists are phenothiazines, butyrophenones, and benzamides. Low doses of phenothiazines antagonize the interaction of dopamine with D_2 receptors to exert an antiemetic effect. Phenothiazines used in the treatment of NVP include prochlorperazine and promethazine. Metoclopramide, a benzamide, is a strong central and peripheral D_2 antagonist. It exerts modest antiemetic effects by enhancing lower esophageal sphincter tone and decreasing transit time through the upper gastrointestinal tract (Badell et al, 2006).

No specific dosing guidelines for these agents are available for pregnant women. Possible regimens are those established for adult patient populations, including promethazine 12.5 to 25 mg every 4 to 6 hours orally or rectally as needed, prochlorperazine 5 to 10 mg orally or 10 to 25 mg rectally every 6 hours as needed, or metoclopramide 5 to 10 mg orally or intravenously every 6 hours as needed.

Because of the effectiveness of serotonin antagonists in patients with chemotherapy-induced nausea and vomiting, physicians have begun to prescribe ondansetron 8 mg orally every 12 hours as needed for NVP. Serotonin antagonists exert their effects at the 5-hydroxytryptamine$_3$ (5-HT$_3$) receptors both centrally and peripherally. This diffuse block works at the small bowel, vagus nerve, and chemoreceptor trigger zone, providing decreased stimulation of the medullary vomiting center.

Corticosteroids have been evaluated for the treatment of severe NVP and hyperemesis gravidarum. Although a precise dosage has not been established for corticosteroids in the treatment of hyperemesis gravidarum, a possible regimen is oral or intravenous methylprednisolone 48 mg/day given in three divided doses for 2 to 3 days. If no response is seen within 3 days, the treatment should be stopped. If symptoms have not improved within 72 hours of the start of corticosteroid treatment, response beyond that time is not likely. Otherwise, the dosage may be tapered appropriately over 1 to 2 weeks. For women with recurrent vomiting, the tapered dosage may be stopped and the lowest effective dosage continued for up to 6 weeks. Corticosteroids should not be administered beyond this period for treatment of NVP because of maternal side effects (Badell et al, 2006).

Table 6-3 contains a list of common antiemetics and other drugs used during pregnancy.

General Information on Infections in Pregnant Women

The need for antimicrobial therapy in the pregnant woman requires confrontation of the potential risks of antibacterial agents for the developing fetus and the mother. The literature in this field is sometimes contradictory. Extensive clinical experience shows that penicillins, cephalosporins, and erythromycin (except erythromycin estolate) can be considered safe for the developing fetus and for the pregnant woman. Nitrofurantoin is a valid antibacterial option in pregnancy, except near or at term. Isoniazid, ethambutol, and rifampin should be used for the treatment of tuberculosis in pregnancy, but attention must be paid to the potential toxicity of isoniazid for the mother. For several other antimicrobial agents (aminoglycosides, fluoroquinolones, newer macrolides, metronidazole, rifampicin, vancomycin), a potential teratogenic or toxic risk has been documented in animal or human studies; however, their use during pregnancy is justified when no safer alternative is available. A few antibacterials should be absolutely avoided in pregnancy: tetracyclines, cotrimoxazole, and chloramphenicol according to a teratogenic risk or a toxic risk for the fetus or the mother, and clindamycin according to its high risk-benefit ratio. The safety data on many other antibacterials, including carbapenems, ketolides, and streptogramins, during pregnancy are very limited or lacking. More data on the risks of antibacterial agents are needed to discern optimal therapy for bacterial infection during pregnancy (Nahum et al, 2006; Nardiello et al, 2002).

Significant pharmacokinetic changes occurred during pregnancy for the penicillins—the fluoroquinolones and gentamicin—indicating that dosage adjustments may be necessary for these drugs. With the exception of chloramphenicol, all of these antibiotics are considered compatible with breastfeeding (Nahum et al, 2006).

See Table 6-3 for an evaluation of different medications that may be used.

SPECIFIC INFECTIONS OF CONCERN
Urinary Tract Infection

Bacterial infections of the urinary tract constitute the most common medical complication of pregnancy (Shephard & Lemire, 2007). Pregnancy itself does not cause a major increase in the acquisition of bacteria, but it sets the stage for the urinary colonization established before pregnancy to lead to symptomatic infection and subsequent invasion of the kidney.

Factors that increase the incidence of urinary tract infection in all women compound the normal physiologic changes in the pregnant woman and increase the potential for infection. Some

TABLE 6-3　Recommended Drugs for Common Problems During Pregnancy

Clinical Condition	Recommended Drugs
Nausea and vomiting	Antihistamines 　dimenhydrinate (Dramamine) B 　diphenhydramine (Benadryl) B in third trimester 　meclizine (Antivert, Bonine) B Phenothiazines 　promethazine (Phenergan) C 　prochlorperazine (Compazine) C 　doxylamine C 　metoclopramide (Reglan) B 　phosphorated carbohydrate solution (Emetrol G) 　pyridoxine (vitamin B_6) A
Infections	Penicillins B Cephalosporins B (avoid cefaclor, cephalexin, cephradine)
Cardiovascular	Alpha-adrenergic receptor agonists 　methyldopa (Aldomet)—B: Usually safe but benefits must outweigh the risks. Usually drug of choice. 　labetalol (Normodyne, Trandate)—C: Safety for use during pregnancy has not been established. 　pindolol (Visken)—B: Usually safe but benefits must outweigh the risks. 　metoprolol (Lopressor, Toprol XL)—C: Safety for use during pregnancy has not been established. Calcium channel blockers 　nifedipine (Adalat, Procardia)—C: Safety for use during pregnancy has not been established. Centrally acting alpha-adrenergic agonists 　clonidine (Catapres)—C: Safety for use during pregnancy has not been established. Diuretics 　hydrochlorothiazide (Esidrix, HydroDIURIL [B])—D (expert analysis): Safety for use during pregnancy has not been 　　established. 　furosemide (Lasix)—C: Safety for use during pregnancy has not been established. Vasodilators—decrease peripheral resistance by inducing vasodilation 　nitroprusside (Nitropress)—C: Safety for use during pregnancy has not been established. 　hydralazine (Apresoline)—C: Usually safe but benefits must outweigh the risks.
Anticonvulsant (for eclampsia)	Anticonvulsants—administered to prevent seizures in severe preeclampsia or eclampsia 　phenytoin (Dilantin)—D: Unsafe but benefits may outweigh risks. 　magnesium sulfate (Bilagog)—A: Safe in pregnancy.
Acne	Topical benzoyl peroxide—C Topical clindamycin—B
Constipation	Bulk-forming laxatives (e.g., Metamucil, Citrucel, Perdiem)—C:　Colace (docusate)—C: May be used later in pregnancy with less risk.
Heartburn/gastroesophageal reflux disease	MgAl combination antacids prn (Milk of Magnesia)
LICE Head lice Pubic lice Scabies	H_2 antagonists ranitidine, cimetidine—B permethrin 1% cream rinse (Nix)—B permethrin 1% cream rinse (Nix) or pyrethrins with piperonyl butoxide—B permethrin 5% cream (Elimite)—B

Gabbe SG et al: *Obstetrics—normal and problem pregnancies,* ed 5, New York, 2007, Churchill Livingstone, Inc.

of these factors include history of previous urinary tract infection, structural abnormalities in the urinary tract, and long periods of inactivity or sitting.

For women at risk for recurrent urinary tract infection, prevention and treatment begin with nonpharmacologic therapy: forcing fluids, wearing cotton underpants, avoiding bubble baths and pantyhose, and taking frequent breaks from sedentary activities to walk around. Choice of an antibiotic agent in pregnancy must be influenced by the potential for the agent to injure the mother and/or her developing fetus. The agents considered safe and thus the most widely used in pregnancy are the penicillins and the cephalosporins. The sulfonamides may displace bilirubin from albumin-binding sites and consequently have been associated with hyperbilirubinemia when administered near term. Nitrofurantoin is contraindicated near term because of the risk of hemolytic anemia. The sulfonamides and nitrofurantoin, however, have been used safely in pregnancy when precautions are taken to discontinue before 36 weeks.

Sexually Transmitted Diseases

Intrauterine or perinatally transmitted STD can have severely debilitating effects on pregnant women, their partners, and their fetuses. All pregnant women and their sex partners should be asked about STDs, counseled about the possibility of perinatal infection, and ensured access to treatment, if needed.

Centers for Disease Control and Prevention (CDC) policy is that all pregnant women in the United States should be tested for HIV infection as early in the pregnancy as possible.

A serologic test for syphilis should be performed on all pregnant women at the first prenatal visit. In populations in which use of prenatal care is not optimal, rapid plasma reagin (RPR) card test screening (and treatment, if that test is reactive) should be performed at the time a pregnancy is confirmed. Women who are at high risk for syphilis, live in areas of high syphilis morbidity, are previously untested, or have positive serology in the first trimester should be screened again early in the third trimester (28 weeks of gestation) and at delivery. All pregnant women should be routinely tested for hepatitis B surface antigen (HBsAg) during an early prenatal visit (e.g., first trimester) in each pregnancy, even if they have been previously vaccinated or tested. All pregnant women should be routinely tested for *Chlamydia trachomatis*. All pregnant women at risk for gonorrhea or living in an area in which the prevalence of *Neisseria gonorrhoeae* is high should be tested at the first prenatal visit for *N. gonorrhoeae*. All pregnant women at high risk for hepatitis C infection should be tested for hepatitis C antibodies at the first prenatal visit. Evaluation for bacterial vaginosis (BV) might be conducted during the first prenatal visit for asymptomatic patients who are at high risk for preterm labor (e.g., those who have a history of a previous preterm delivery) (Wokowski & Berman, 2006). Based on the results of these tests, the mother and perhaps the infant will require treatment.

Because of substantial geographic variation in drug strains and drug-resistant organisms, recommended antibiotics may vary and may change for STDs. STDs in pregnancy may require special care. The clinician should consult the latest recommendations from the CDC on treating each type of STD in a pregnant woman (Barkley, 2007; Wokowski & Berman, 2006).

Asthma

Retrospective studies suggest that in about one third of women with asthma, asthma becomes worse during pregnancy; in one third, it becomes better, and in one third, it remains unchanged (Namazy & Schatz, 2005). In women whose asthma becomes worse during pregnancy, peak severity occurs at 29 to 36 weeks of gestation. Asthma becomes less severe during the last 4 weeks of pregnancy. Wheezing during labor and delivery is uncommon, occurring in only 10% of women and usually responding to inhaled bronchodilator therapy. The change in the severity of asthma during pregnancy is sometimes dramatic and tends to be consistent in subsequent pregnancies.

Poorly controlled asthma has been shown to have an adverse effect on the fetus, resulting in perinatal mortality, increased prematurity, intrauterine growth retardation, low birth weight (LBW), and neonatal hypoxia. Risks to the mother of uncontrolled asthma during pregnancy include preeclampsia, gestational hypertension, hyperemesis gravidarum, vaginal hemorrhage, and preterm labor. However, when asthma is well controlled, an increased risk of poor outcome is not apparent (NIH, 1993).

In published studies, no significant relationships were found between adverse perinatal outcomes and the use of inhaled β-agonists, inhaled corticosteroids, theophylline, or cromolyn-nedocromil. An observed increased risk of preterm and LBW infants was associated with oral corticosteroid use. To date, no asthma medications have been proved to be teratogenic, and it is clear that the greater risk to the fetus is uncontrolled asthma (Namazy & Schatz, 2005). Thus, the pregnant patient who is asthmatic may continue to take the same asthma medications that she was taking before she became pregnant. Although the fetus may exhibit physiologic response to the medications, in most cases, the effect on the developing fetus is negligible. The primary care practitioner should examine the risk categories of various medications to maximize the risk-benefit ratio.

Women with severe or uncontrolled asthma are at higher risk for pregnancy complications and adverse fetal outcomes than are women with well-controlled asthma. Recent evidence-based guidelines have concluded that it is safer for pregnant women with asthma to be treated pharmacologically than for them to continue to have asthma symptoms and exacerbations. According to the Asthma and Pregnancy Working Group (APWG) of the National Asthma Education and Prevention Program, optimal treatment of asthma during pregnancy includes the treatment of comorbid allergic rhinitis (AR), which can trigger or aggravate asthma symptoms. In general, treatment of both asthma and AR during pregnancy should follow the same stepwise approach that is used in the general population (Yawn & Knudtsen, 2007). In general, second-generation antihistamines are more potent, have a longer duration of action, and produce minimal sedation. The American College of Obstetricians and Gynecologists and the American College of Allergy, Asthma and Immunology (ACOG-ACAAI) have recommended consideration of cetirizine and loratadine, preferably after the first trimester, for pregnant women who need maximal topical therapy and cannot tolerate chlorpheniramine or tripelennamine (ACOG-ACAAI, 2000). ACOG-ACAAI based this statement on reassuring animal data for these second-generation antihistamines, which carry a Pregnancy B rating, and the fact that they are associated with fewer anticholinergic and sedative effects. The Yawn and Knudtsen (2007) article contains detailed charts that list the tetragonic potential for common asthma and allergy drugs.

Epilepsy

In pregnant women with epilepsy who are being treated with antiepileptic drugs (AEDs), careful clinical management is vital because seizure frequency can change during pregnancy. During pregnancy, seizure activity increases in 40% of women, decreases in 10%, and does not change in 50%. Both seizure activity and AED treatment can have consequences for the developing fetus. Although the management of epilepsy during pregnancy is beyond the expertise of the primary care provider, some risk-benefit details are available, along with other information that the clinician may want to be aware of and/or use to provide anticipatory guidance to women of childbearing age.

First, anticonvulsant use during pregnancy has resulted in several "syndromes" and is associated with an increased incidence of malformation, at two times the normal rate (Schardein & Macina, 2006). Therefore, 8 to 12 months before conception, referral to a neurologist is warranted to discuss a 6-month or longer drug-free trial vs. monotherapy at the lowest effective dose to minimize teratogenicity. Once pregnant (planned or unplanned), the benefit-risk ratio favors continued use of the woman's current anticonvulsant(s). Changing her medication at this point is contraindicated because it is usually too late to prevent teratogenicity, and seizure control is imperative. During pregnancy, an increase in medication may be needed; therefore, drug levels should be monitored frequently both during pregnancy and for 2 to 3 months postpartum, when the need may decrease. Failure to adequately control seizures may lead to status epilepticus, which is associated with 33% maternal and 50% fetal mortality rates (Pennell, 2006).

As was noted previously, renal blood flow and glomerular filtration increase during pregnancy as a function of increased cardiac output; in addition, plasma volume, extravascular fluid, and adipose tissue increase to create a larger volume of distribution. The level of serum albumin decreases, which reduces drug binding, increases the free fraction, and increases drug clearance. These pharmacokinetic alterations can affect AED concentrations and are most important for AEDs that are highly protein bound, hepatically metabolized, or renally cleared. Both total and free levels of highly protein-bound AEDs, including phenytoin and valproate, should be monitored.

Lamotrigine metabolism and clearance increase during pregnancy, and an understanding of the effect of pregnancy on lamotrigine concentrations is particularly important because this drug is being used increasingly in women who are considering pregnancy. Women treated with AEDs during pregnancy should have their drug levels monitored throughout pregnancy and should have their doses adjusted accordingly. The frequency of monitoring depends on the particular AED, with more frequent monitoring required for lamotrigine (Pack, 2006). Complications of epilepsy and AED treatment include stillbirth, prematurity, low birth weight, major and minor malformations, and cognitive delay later in life. Certain AEDs have more adverse effects than others. Data from some prospective studies indicate that phenobarbital and valproate are associated with significant increases in major malformations, and retrospective studies show lower verbal IQs and a greater need for extra assistance in school for children whose mothers received valproate during pregnancy (Pack, 2006). Monitoring of AED levels and dosage adjustment are warranted throughout pregnancy.

Second, maternal folic acid deficiency is induced by anticonvulsants (especially valproic acid, phenytoin, and phenobarbital), which reduce gastrointestinal absorption or increase hepatic metabolism of the vitamins with consequent increased risk of neural tube defects. Therefore, folic acid supplementation is crucial, and recommendations vary from 1 to 5 mg/day (Briggs et al, 2005).

Finally, anticonvulsant use (especially phenobarbital and phenytoin) is also associated with hemorrhagic disease of the newborn. This may be caused by decreased vitamin K–dependent clotting factors (Briggs et al, 2005; Montouris, 2005). Maternal prophylactic oral vitamin K (10 to 20 mg/day) beginning at 36 weeks and newborn prophylaxis with the routine 1 mg given immediately after delivery have been recommended to counteract these effects. In the postpartum period, breastfeeding is recommended; however, differential transfer of individual AEDs occurs in breast milk, and the infant should be observed clinically (Pack, 2006). Breastfeeding may prevent withdrawal symptoms in the infant. Risks and benefits should be discussed with the infant's mother.

Diabetes

Diabetes occurs in 4% of U.S. pregnancies, of which 3% are insulin-resistant (i.e., adult-onset) diabetes, and 90% are gestational diabetes mellitus (GDM) (ADA, 2006). The strong correlation between the level of maternal hyperglycemia and adverse pregnancy outcome has been well established. Therefore, the major imperative in the management of diabetes in pregnancy is to decrease the glucose level to near normoglycemic values (Murphy et al, 2007). Achieving normoglycemic values during pregnancy requires close surveillance and meticulous care, which is paramount to achieving optimal mother-infant outcomes. Pregnancy outcomes for women with type 1 diabetes remain poor with increased risk of major congenital malformation, stillbirth, premature delivery, and perinatal death compared with the background maternity population (Murphy et al, 2007).

During pregnancy, the mean percentage increase in insulin requirement throughout pregnancy is 114%, compared with a 50% increase in insulin levels in normal pregnancy. It is influenced by prepregnancy maternal weight, weight gain at 20 to 29 weeks, and duration and type of diabetes. During the postpartum period, a precipitous decrease in insulin requirements occurs; thereafter, the insulin requirements gradually increase to prepregnancy levels or slightly higher over the next 5 to 7 days. From 35% to 50% of women with GDM will develop non–insulin-dependent diabetes mellitus within 15 years after delivery. Breastfeeding lowers insulin requirements for some mothers; some even experience a complete remission that may last throughout lactation and/or for several years, thus delaying or reducing the risk of subsequent diabetes (ADA, 2006; Murphy et al, 2007).

Pregnant women with diabetes mellitus should be treated with insulin (pregnancy category B), exercise, and diet. Gestational diabetic patients should be treated with diet and exercise, with insulin added as needed. Although oral agents are available, some are pregnancy category D, and although those in category B are being researched, evidence to support their use during pregnancy is insufficient. Hence today, diet, exercise, and insulin therapy as needed remain the gold standard of care.

Improved blood glucose control in the first 7 weeks following conception reduces congenital malformation, perinatal mortality, and premature delivery.

Women with diabetes who are planning a pregnancy are recommended to take folic acid 5 mg daily, from before conception until 12 weeks of gestation (Murphy et al, 2007).

Hypertension

Hypertension is the second leading cause of maternal death in the United States (after embolism) and is a major cause of stillbirth and neonatal mortality; BP monitoring should be maintained closely. In normal pregnancy, systolic and diastolic pressures decrease by about 5 to 10 mm Hg by the middle of pregnancy; they then gradually increase to starting levels at term. Hypertension may, of course, precede pregnancy, but it more commonly develops during pregnancy, in which case it may be classified as gestational hypertension or preeclampsia. In both cases, BP levels can change very quickly: The increase in BP rarely starts before 20 weeks but may be a major problem by the third trimester (24 to 36 weeks). Official U.S. guidelines on the management of high BP during pregnancy have been published by the working group of the National High Blood Pressure Education Program and were most recently revised in July of 2000 (Pickering, 2005). Preeclampsia may be one of the last areas for which increased attention is focused on diastolic pressure. It has been proposed that hypertension of pregnancy should be principally defined in terms of diastolic pressure (Cooper et al, 2006; Friedman, 2006).

Hypertension due to preeclampsia complicates about 5% of all pregnancies, 10% of first pregnancies, and at least 20% of pregnancies in women with a history of chronic hypertension. It is the third leading cause of maternal mortality and is characterized by visual disturbances such as scintillations and scotomata, headache, and epigastric pain due to hepatic inflammation and swelling; quickly increasing or nondependent edema may be a signal of emergent preeclampsia. However, the signal theory of edema was removed from most diagnostic criteria for preeclampsia (Cooper et al, 2006). Symptoms appear only during pregnancy or the early puerperium. The condition most frequently appears during the 20th to 24th week of gestation and disappears within 40 days postpartum.

Preconceptually choosing a medication that is first line during pregnancy may be wise. It is interesting to note that in the first trimester, some mothers experience a lowering of blood pressure and are able to discontinue their medication (Gibson, 2002). If, however, diastolic blood pressure is greater than 110 mm Hg or systolic blood pressure is greater than 160 mm Hg, regardless of the type of hypertension, treatment is imperative because these values have been associated with an increased risk of intrauterine growth restriction and placental abruption. Finally, patients should be closely monitored for adequacy of treatment to decrease risk to both mother and fetus (Working Group, 2001). Most women with chronic hypertension in pregnancy have stage 1 or 2 hypertension (defined as systolic blood pressure of 140 to 179 mm Hg, or diastolic blood pressure of 90 to 109 mm Hg) and are at low risk for cardiovascular complications within the short time frame of pregnancy. Among women with stage 1 or 2 preexisting essential hypertension and normal renal function, most pregnancies have good maternal and neonatal outcomes. These women are candidates for nondrug therapy because, to date, no evidence suggests that pharmacologic treatment results in improved neonatal outcomes. Because blood pressure usually falls during the first half of pregnancy, hypertension may be easier to control with less or no medication.

The value of continued administration of antihypertensive drugs to pregnant women with chronic hypertension continues to be an area of debate. Although it may be beneficial to reduce the blood pressure of the mother with hypertension, lower pressure may impair uteroplacental perfusion, thereby jeopardizing fetal development (Working Group, 2001).

ACE inhibitors, angiotensin receptor blockers (ARBs), and statins are contraindicated during the first trimester of pregnancy. These should be stopped before the time of conception and should be replaced by safer alternatives such as methyldopa, labetalol, or extended-release nifedipine (Murphy et al, 2007).

Depression

Mothers with severe depression may be at risk of harming themselves and/or their infant; this, of course, includes suicide and infanticide. Additionally, parenting and infant development are known to be adversely affected by maternal depression (Spencer et al, 2001). In a 1998 review of prospective controlled studies, both tricyclic antidepressants (TCAs) and selective serotonin reuptake inhibitors (SSRIs) were found to be potentially associated with the risk of minor physical

anomalies, neonatal complications, and prematurity yet were relatively safe during pregnancy (Gentile, 2006). Subsequently, in 2000, a meta-analytic review of epidemiologic studies found that fluoxetine was not associated with the risk of any measurable teratogenic effects during the first trimester of pregnancy (Koren, 2006). Research is ongoing in this area, and further assistance in determining the risk-benefit ratio may be found at the "Pregnancy and Depression" website (www.pregnancyanddepression.com), which lists many past and current studies. A final resource is the American Academy of Pediatrics 2000 statement that outlines the risks of several psychotropic medications used during pregnancy for depression, as well as for other psychiatric illnesses. Although each case should be assessed individually and the risk-benefit ratio should be thoroughly discussed with the mother, it seems that generally, the benefits of these medications outweigh the risks, particularly if the mother's disease is severe or if she relapses with discontinuation of medication (Gentile, 2006). When medication is necessary, it is prudent to prescribe the minimum effective dose. Because withdrawal syndromes have been observed in nonbreastfed infants postpartum (especially with TCAs), consider encouraging breastfeeding or halving the dose 1 week before delivery (Gentile, 2006).

FDA guidelines for assessing the category of risk for various medications are listed in Table 6-4.

Although the category C medication bupropion may seem a logical first choice, it is important to note that it is assigned category C only because no human studies have been conducted; thus, its safety remains untested.

According to the Evidence-Based Medicine Working Group of the AAFP, the SSRIs—specifically, fluoxetine and sertraline—and the TCAs have been found in studies to be safe and effective in reducing the symptoms of depression.

Epidemiologic studies with paroxetine have shown an increased risk of congenital heart malformation in the form of atrial and ventricular septal defects. Paroxetine carries

TABLE 6-4 Risk Categories for Select Antidepressants

Medication	Brand Name	Pregnancy Risk Category
bupropion	Wellbutrin	C
desipramine	Norpramin	C
doxepin	Sinequan	C used systemic; B used topically
mirtazapine	Remeron	C
nefazodone	Serzone	C
SSRIs:	SSRIs:	C
fluoxetine	Prozac	C
sertraline	Zoloft	C
trazodone	Desyrel	C
venlafaxine	Effexor	
amitriptyline	Elavil	D
imipramine	Tofranil	D
nortriptyline	Pamelor	D
paroxetine*	Paxil	D

Modified from Brundage SC: Preconception health care, *American Family Physician* 65(12): 2507-2514, June 15, 2002. Copyright © 2002 American Academy of Family Physicians. All rights reserved.

*The American College of Obstetricians and Gynecologists (ACOG) recently warned against use of paroxetine in pregnancy because of unpublished reports of a high rate of cardiac malformations.

a category D pregnancy risk factor. However, most data on antidepressants have not shown that they increase the risk of major malformation, although one study showed that fluoxetine was associated with a greater risk of minor malformation.

Evidence is conflicting regarding the association between antidepressants and perinatal complications such as preterm delivery. Several, although not all, studies have reported an increased risk of premature birth among pregnant women who are taking fluoxetine.

A withdrawal syndrome or neonatal toxicity, described as transient jerky movements (possibly seizures), respiratory distress, and feeding difficulties have been reported in some babies born to mothers who are taking antidepressants. This has prompted labeling changes for antidepressant medications that warn of potential neonatal complications.

Studies evaluating long-term neurodevelopmental outcomes in children exposed to antidepressants in utero have not demonstrated a deficit in language, behavior, or IQ.

Although SSRIs (fluoxetine and sertraline) and TCAs are considered safe and effective according to the AAFP review, SSRIs tend to be associated with fewer side effects and are often considered first-line medications. That being said, the ACOG has not issued a practice guideline on antidepressant use during pregnancy. Therefore, critical to the management and treatment of depression during pregnancy is the individualized assessment and weighing of the risks and benefits of serious depression vs. treatment options.

Many women are taking medication for depression before becoming pregnant and use the preconception visit as the time to discuss with their provider whether the need for medication is likely to be sustained during pregnancy. Abrupt discontinuation is not recommended, and many clinicians suggest that women at high risk for serious depression during pregnancy might best be served by continuing medication throughout pregnancy (Dolan, 2005).

During lactation, sertraline (Zoloft), paroxetine (Paxil), and TCAs (amitriptyline [Elavil], nortriptyline [Pamelor], and desipramine [Norpramin]) are a few preferred agents; fluoxetine must be used prudently, if at all, because of its long half-life (Gentile, 2006). TCAs have a greater number of maternal side effects, especially drowsiness, but no side effects have been reported in infants, and after a moderate dose of 75 mg, the drug was essentially undetectable in the infant's serum (Hale, 2008). Several studies of sertraline generally have confirmed that the transfer of it or its metabolite is minimal and attainment of significant plasma levels in infants is remote when the maternal dose is less than 150 mg. Furthermore, only one ostensible infant side effect (benign neonatal sleep) has been reported, and this resolved independently (Hale, 2008). Studies of paroxetine generally conclude that infant serum levels are for the most part undetectable, and no infant side effects have been reported (Hale, 2008). It has been suggested that mothers treated with fluoxetine during pregnancy should be transitioned to sertraline or paroxetine after the time of delivery (Spencer et al, 2001). To limit exposure to fluoxetine in this scenario, one strategy would be to discontinue fluoxetine 1 week before delivery and then switch to sertraline or paroxetine shortly after delivery. Alternatively, the mother could be continued on fluoxetine while closely observing the infant and, at about 6 weeks, measuring infant serum levels of fluoxetine and norfluoxetine (Gentile, 2005, 2006; Spencer et al, 2001).

Other Disorders

Pregnant or lactating women have the same problems as nonpregnant women. When symptoms are mild, treatment may be forgone. However, alternative treatment is not always effective, and pharmacologic preparations may be required.

KNOWN HAZARDS TO MOTHERS AND THEIR CHILDREN

Extensive medical literature describes the negative effect on people of the use of alcohol, nicotine, caffeine, cocaine, and marijuana. (See summaries of the literature in major texts, including Briggs et al, 2005.) However, increasing attention has been paid to these and other products and to their effects on pregnancy, the unborn fetus, the neonate, and the breastfed infant. Emerging research suggests that the negative effect during pregnancy is more extensive than was commonly believed. Effects on the breastfed infant from maternal use of these substances vary from minimal or none to significant morbidity, making them contraindicated during breastfeeding. The following sections outline what is known about these common substances (Briggs et al, 2005; March of Dimes website, 2007).

Isotretinoin (Accutane)

Isotretinoin, which is used to treat severe recalcitrant nodular acne, is commonly prescribed in the United States. Isotretinoin must not be used by female patients who are or may become pregnant. To determine whether a woman is a candidate for isotretinoin, the clinician must determine that the woman is not breastfeeding or pregnant, is reliable in understanding and implementing instructions, is able to understand how to prevent pregnancy, and, if currently or potentially sexually active, is able to comply with using two types of contraception. Prior to use, it must be confirmed that the woman had an initial negative pregnancy test along with a second negative test taken on the fifth day of the first menses after isotretinoin treatment had begun, and thereafter ongoing negative monthly pregnancy tests. There is an extremely high risk that severe birth defects will result if pregnancy occurs while one is taking isotretinoin in any amount, even for a short time. Any fetus exposed during pregnancy may be affected. No accurate means can be used to determine whether an exposed fetus has been affected. Because of this toxicity, isotretinoin can be marketed only under a special restricted distribution program called *iPLEDGE* (https://www.ipledgeprogram.com/). Under this program, prescribers must be registered and activated through the iPLEDGE program and can prescribe isotretinoin only to registered patients who meet all requirements of iPLEDGE. Isotretinoin can be dispensed only by a pharmacy registered and activated with iPLEDGE. Registered and activated pharmacies can receive isotretinoin only from wholesalers who are registered with iPLEDGE.

Isotretinoin is contraindicated during lactation because it is likely significantly secreted in human milk with subsequent potential treatment risks.

Vaccinations

The rubella vaccine is a commonly prescribed potential teratogen. In the sexually active woman with a negative rubella titer, it is prudent to administer while on the menses and with a negative pregnancy test or immediately postpartum. She should not become pregnant for at least 2 months (Lawrence & Lawrence, 1999). When indicated, the high-risk breast-feeding mother should be vaccinated for rubella regardless of the age of the infant (Hale, 2008). Otherwise, lactating mothers of normal healthy infants may receive the immunization when the child is 1 year or older (Zip, 2006).

Caffeine

In 1980, the FDA removed caffeine from the list of compounds generally regarded as safe, citing animal evidence that caffeine caused birth defects, fetal death, and decreased birth weight. High doses (25 to 30 cups of coffee in humans) in rats caused skeletal defects, missing digits, and growth retardation. Smaller amounts (2 or 3 cups of coffee in humans) caused delayed bone development (Briggs et al, 2005).

Since then, additional studies have refuted the reported association between caffeine and birth defects. At least 15 studies have been published associating the consumption of caffeine-containing beverages during pregnancy with reproductive outcomes. Although caffeine does not appear to be teratogenic in humans, whether it causes spontaneous abortion or low birth weight remains controversial, largely because of limitations in the studies performed to date (Schardein & Macina, 2006).

What is known about the effects of caffeine? The amount of caffeine in an average cup of coffee (about 1.4 to 2.1 mg/kg) is safely below the amount that induces congenital defects in animals. Quantities in tea and soft drinks are even smaller. At present, there is new evidence that suggests that there is a higher incidence of miscarriage in women who drink caffeine. There is no evidence that suggests that pregnant women should avoid caffeine completely. However, they should be encouraged to limit their intake to moderate use (about 2 to 4 caffeine-containing beverages per day) because caffeine may exert a small but measurable effect on fetal growth (Schardein & Marcina, 2006).

Breastfeeding mothers are encouraged to limit their intake to the equivalent of less than 5 cups of coffee or to less than 16 oz per day of chocolate (theobromine) because although the milk levels are low, it can accumulate in the infant, causing symptoms of caffeine excess (AAP, 2001).

Alcohol

Alcohol is a known teratogen, and its use is contraindicated during pregnancy (Cone-Wesson, 2005). It is estimated that 65% of mothers in the United States continue to drink some alcohol during pregnancy, thus exposing their fetus. The result is that as many as 5% of all congenital anomalies may be attributed to prenatal alcohol exposure (Schardein & Macina, 2006). Drinking rates during pregnancy are significantly higher among women of lower socioeconomic status, those using other illicit drugs, and teenagers.

Among alcoholic women who drink during pregnancy, about 30% to 40% of their offspring will have fetal alcohol syndrome (FAS) (Briggs et al, 2005). This syndrome is associated with altered morphogenesis, growth deficiency, and mental retardation. FAS was described more than 30 years ago, but its presence has often been overlooked by clinicians.

In the United States, FAS is generally estimated to occur in 1:1000 to 3:1000 live births. The incidence among children born with only partial expression of FAS may be as high as 3:1000 to 5:1000. The average IQ of children with FAS is 68, or mildly retarded (Cone-Wesson, 2005). FAS now surpasses Down syndrome and spina bifida as the leading cause of mental retardation in the United States (Briggs et al, 2005). Many other children will show milder effects, including growth retardation and neurologic defects. Significantly higher perinatal mortality, lower birth weight, and lower IQ, not necessarily concurrent with the full syndrome, all have been reported from studies of children of alcoholic mothers (Shephard & Lemire, 2007).

The quantity and chronicity of exposure are correlated with increased damage to the fetus. FAS is associated with the mother's consuming the equivalent of 90 ml of absolute alcohol/day (six mixed drinks, six 4-oz glasses of wine, or six 12-oz beers) throughout pregnancy. LBW occurs in infants with as little as 30 ml absolute alcohol daily (Briggs et al, 2005). However, infants born to mothers who consumed an average of fewer than two drinks daily have the same rate of malformation as those born to abstinent mothers. The impact of a single drinking binge is unknown (Shephard & Lemire, 2007). Despite this research, a specific safe level of alcohol consumption has not been established.

During lactation, occasional moderate use of alcohol (a drink or two) is acceptable (AAP, 2001). Ideally, to prevent or minimize alcohol exposure, the mother will breastfeed her infant just before drinking, will drink with a meal to slow absorption, and then will wait at least 2 to 3 hours before breastfeeding again. Heavy or daily ingestion of more than two drinks daily has been associated with psychomotor delay and decreased linear growth (Hale, 2006). The possible risks of frequent or heavy ingestion should be discussed with the mother. If she is unable to abstain from daily or heavy ingestion, then a discussion about minimizing infant exposure and/or weaning is necessary (Hale, 2006). While the mother is intoxicated, breastfeeding should be delayed until the euphoric effects have dissipated. For each missed feeding during this period, the mother should pump and discard to remain comfortable and maintain milk supply.

Nicotine and Smoking

Cigarette use by pregnant women in urban regions generally has been found to range from 22% to 28% (SAMHA, 2006). Because of the significant numbers of women who smoke during pregnancy, smoking is among the most widely researched topics in teratology. Smoking has not been linked to congenital malformation but is associated with physical and intellectual growth retardation (SAMHA, 2006).

How do clinicians help the mother who smokes? First, it is important to assess the level of risk. Clearly, the effects are dose related to the number of cigarettes smoked per day; therefore, a reduction in smoking will decrease the risk of fetal retardation.

Several studies have reported that the more pronounced effects of smoking on fetal growth occur after the second trimester. Most recent studies, but not all, have reported a significant relationship between lowered birth weight and the amount of second-hand smoke to which the pregnant non-smoking woman may be subjected.

Studies indicate that if pregnant smokers also regularly consume at least one alcoholic drink per day and consume high quantities of caffeine (5 cups of coffee per day), the risk of retarded fetal growth is considerably increased (SAMHA, 2006).

An increase in the rate of spontaneous abortion has been documented among smokers, with relative risks ranging from 1.2% to 1.8%. The greater the amount smoked, the higher is the relative risk. This may result from fetal hypoxia caused by decreased uteroplacental perfusion. Smoking during pregnancy also decreases maternal blood pressure for up to 15 minutes per cigarette smoked, thus decreasing the flow of oxygenated blood from the uterus to the placenta. A link between maternal smoking and asthma has also been described (SAMHA, 2006).

Cocaine

In contrast to some products that have a questionable effect on mother or fetus, cocaine represents a known danger to both. National estimates of fetal cocaine exposure events range from 91,500 to 240,000 (about 4.5% prevalence). Cocaine and its metabolites readily cross the placenta, thereby exposing the fetus (Bauer et al, 2005; Singer et al, 2004). Many adverse fetal outcomes may be blamed on the powerful vasoconstrictive and hypertensive actions of cocaine. These changes may increase the risks of miscarriage, preterm labor, and low birth weight. Although cocaine use is not confined to any socioeconomic group, lack of prenatal care compounds the risk to the fetus and traditionally has been a hallmark of the maternal cocaine abuser (SAMHA, 2006).

A large percent of studies suggests that congenital defects and fetal vascular accident defects are associated with the use of cocaine in pregnancy. Overall, the risk of teratogenicity for the cocaine-exposed fetus is small but still greater than for the overall population. Congenital defects observed include decreased APGAR scores; strokes; congenital heart defects; and genitourinary, limb, facial, and gastrointestinal defects (March of Dimes website, 2008; Shephard & Lemire, 2007). One consistent finding is small head circumference at birth in a fetus who has been exposed to cocaine; this finding often correlates with a small brain, although these babies do seem to have normal intelligence (March of Dimes website, 2008). Other fetal risks associated with cocaine use during pregnancy include intrauterine growth retardation, prematurity, spontaneous abortion, premature rupture of membranes, placenta previa, pregnancy-induced hypertension, abruptio placentae, bradycardia, and neurobehavioral problems.

After delivery, some babies who were regularly exposed to cocaine before birth may exhibit mild behavioral disturbances or may be jittery and irritable. They may startle and cry at the gentlest touch or sound, are difficult to comfort, and may be described as withdrawn or unresponsive. Other cocaine-exposed babies may "turn off" surrounding stimuli by going into a deep sleep for most of the day. Usually, these behavioral disturbances resolve over the first few months of the baby's life (March of Dimes website, 2008).

Several case reports have documented that infants exposed to cocaine via breastfeeding experience typical adverse effects; therefore, use of cocaine is contraindicated during lactation. With one-time exposure, a minimum period of 24 hours of pumping and discarding milk must occur before breastfeeding is resumed (Hale, 2008).

Marijuana

The percent of women reported to use marijuana during pregnancy ranges from 9.5% to 27% (Friedman & Polifka, 2007). Despite concerns about congenital malformations caused by marijuana use during pregnancy, a cause-effect relationship has not been established (March of Dimes website, 2008). Although marijuana has been found to be teratogenic in animals, maternal marijuana use during pregnancy has not been studied extensively. It has not been conclusively demonstrated that marijuana use has any negative long-term effect on fetal growth. Low birth weight and height may result from impaired fetal oxygenation associated with high carbon monoxide levels, rather than from the marijuana itself. Children exposed to marijuana before birth are more likely to have subtle problems that affect their ability to pay attention but do not seem to have lowered IQ (March of Dimes website, 2008). It is contraindicated during lactation as studies show significant absorption and metabolism in infants (Hale, 2008).

DRUGS IN BREASTFEEDING MOTHERS
The Transfer of Drugs

Regardless of the limitations, research is ongoing in the area of lactation, and some data are available on most medications, although this may reflect the findings of small research studies and not evidence-based practice. Most available information has been derived from measurements of drug concentration in milk or clinical observations in breastfeeding infants (Briggs et al, 2005). Many factors affect the excretion of drugs in breast milk, but most are excreted in subclinical amounts. In fact, medications usually are measured in terms of milligrams per liter (mg/L) or micrograms per liter (mcg/L). To provide a prospective, 1 mg/L is the equivalent of 3 drops in 42 gallons, and 1 mcg/L is the equivalent of 1 drop in 14,000 gallons. The average intake of most infants younger than 6 months of age is less than 1 liter per day (Lawrence & Lawrence, 1999). Factors or mechanisms that determine drug entry into breast milk include maternal plasma level (usually the most important factor), amounts of protein binding and lipid solubility, molecular weight, oral bioavailability (expressed as pK_a of the drug), and half-life. The dose of a drug that an infant receives during breastfeeding is dependent on the amount excreted into the breast milk, the daily volume of milk ingested, and the average plasma concentration of the mother. The lipophilicity, protein binding, and ionization properties of a drug will determine how much is excreted into the breast milk. The milk-to-plasma concentration ratio has large intersubject and intrasubject variability and is often not known. In contrast, protein binding is usually known. An extensive literature review was done to identify case reports that included infant concentrations from breastfed infants exposed to maternal drugs. For drugs that were at least 85% protein bound, measurable concentrations of drug in the infant did not occur if no placental exposure was reported immediately prior to or during delivery. Knowledge of the protein-binding properties of a drug can serve as a quick and easy tool by which to estimate exposure of an infant to medication via breast-feeding (Anderson, 2006).

Once the infant has ingested the medicated breast milk, the milk must evade being destroyed in the infant's gut, must be absorbed through the gut wall, and then must avoid being metabolized or stored in the liver before it can establish a plasma level and become bioactive in the infant (Hale, 2008; Spencer et al, 2001). In general, these parameters explain the transfer of drugs; however, the absolute dosage that the infant receives from the breast milk can really be determined only via research that measures actual milk levels (Hale, 2008).

Assessing Risk vs. Benefit

General considerations to ponder before prescribing and to assist the clinician in determining the optimal drug choice and breastfeeding management plan can be viewed in Box 6-3. Also, both the American Academy of Pediatrics and Dr. Tom Hale have assessed many medications and placed them into risk categories (Boxes 6-4 and 6-5). Keeping these details in mind, most medications (over-the-counter or prescribed) are considered safe for the breastfed infant and do not usually necessitate a disruption in breastfeeding. Moreover, medications that are approved for direct use in the infant's age group, including prednisone (up to 80 mg), fluconazole (Diflucan), inhaled albuterol (Proventil), and acyclovir (Zovirax), are also generally considered safe for use in nursing mothers (Tables 6-4, 6-5, and 6-6). Nonetheless, certain

exceptions do exist in classes of medications, particularly among antidepressants, immunosuppressants, and cardiovascular medications (Spencer et al, 2001).

Conversely, exposure to radioactive isotopes, antimetabolites, cancer chemotherapy agents, and a minute number of other medications does necessitate a temporary or permanent interruption in breastfeeding. Drugs of abuse—amphetamines, cocaine, heroin, marijuana, and phencyclidine—are all contraindicated during breastfeeding because they are hazardous to the health of both the nursing infant and the mother. Therefore, the mother must choose between breastfeeding and the drug. Smoking and alcohol present special circumstances that were discussed previously under the section on known hazards to mothers and their children.

Overall, even though available information is limited and there may be risks, it is important to preserve the breastfeeding relationship except in the rare previously mentioned exceptional circumstances. (See Boxes 6-3 to 6-5.)

Management of Interruption or Weaning

"Even a temporary interruption in breast-feeding carries the risk of premature weaning, with the subsequent risks of long-term artificial feeding."
(AMERICAN ACADEMY OF FAMILY PHYSICIANS, 2002)

Any recommendation to interrupt breastfeeding or to commence weaning must clearly outweigh the benefits conferred by nursing. The American Academy of Pediatrics

---

BOX 6-3   Considerations for Use of Drugs During Breastfeeding

1. Avoid using medication when possible, but when indicated, evaluate the infant dose and perform individual risk assessment.
2. Preferred drugs are those for which breastfeeding data are available. Check for alternatives and use the safest drug.
3. For many drugs, a relative infant dose of <10% is considered safe.
4. With dangerous or radioactive compounds, wait 4 to 5 half-lives before resuming breastfeeding (see http://neonatal.ama.ttuhsc.edu/lact/html/radio.html). Discontinuation of breastfeeding for some hours/days may be required, particularly with radioactive compounds. To maintain a full milk supply, mothers should pump both their breasts 8 to 10 times for 15 to 20 minutes with an effective pump and should discard the milk. When possible, suggest that the mother store expressed breast milk in advance.
5. Be cautious during the newborn period because it is generally agreed that medications are more likely to penetrate milk during the neonatal period than during mature milk production. This is particularly true for the first 10 days of life, when apparent large gaps between the mother's alveolar cells permit enhanced access for immunoglobulins and most other drugs.
6. Choose drugs with short half-lives, high protein binding, low oral bioavailability, or high molecular weight. Be cautious with drugs that have active metabolites with longer half-lives or that have long pediatric half-lives. Maternal plasma levels, in conjunction with the degree of protein binding, are usually the most important determinants of milk concentration. Only that which is "freely soluble" in the plasma can transfer into milk.
7. If it is possible that a drug may present a risk to the infant, consider measuring blood concentrations in the nursing infant. Exposure of the infant may be reduced by timing the dosing to occur just after feedings and/or before sleep periods, in conjunction with striving to time feedings just prior to dosing or outside the peak. Use of expressed breast milk from an earlier strategic pumping or substituting formula (as a last resort) for selected feedings is an acceptable alternative.
8. Be cautious with preterm, low birth weight, and ill infants, especially those with liver or kidney disease.
9. Consider the side effects that are mostly likely to occur in the infant, and educate the mother to watch for them. Changes in feeding, stooling, and mental status, behavioral changes, and weakness are the primary side effects that may forewarn of problems.
10. Many drugs are safe in breastfeeding, and the benefits of breastfeeding often outweigh any risks to the infant's well-being.

BOX 6-4   Hale's Lactation Risk Categories

L1: SAFEST

- Drug that has been taken by a large number of breastfeeding mothers with no observed increase in adverse effects in the infant
- Controlled studies in breastfeeding women fail to demonstrate a risk to the infant, and the possibility of harm to the breastfeeding infant is remote; alternatively, the product is not orally bioavailable in an infant.

L2: SAFER

- Drug that has been studied in a limited number of breastfeeding women with no increase in adverse effects in the infant
- And/or the evidence of a demonstrated risk that is likely to follow use of this medication in a breastfeeding woman is remote.

L3: MODERATELY SAFE

- No controlled studies in breastfeeding women show that the risk of untoward effects to a breastfed infant is possible, or controlled studies show only minimal nonthreatening adverse effects.
- Drug should be given only if the potential benefit justifies the potential risk to the infant.

L4: POSSIBLY HAZARDOUS

- Positive evidence of risk to the breastfed infant or to breast milk production has been found, but the benefits from use in breastfeeding mothers may be acceptable despite the risk to the infant (e.g., if the drug is needed in a life-threatening situation or for a serious disease for which safer drugs cannot be used or are ineffective).

L5: CONTRAINDICATED

- Studies in breastfeeding mothers have demonstrated significant and documented risk to the infant based on human experience, or it is a medication that has a high risk of causing significant damage to an infant.
- The risk of using the drug in breastfeeding women clearly outweighs any possible benefit derived from breastfeeding.
- The drug is contraindicated in women who are breastfeeding an infant.

NR: NOT REVIEWED

Milk Levels

These values are averages and may change; different studies report varying results. Consult Dr. Hale's book for more detailed information.

Theoretical Infant Dose

This is the maximum infant dose per kilogram based on current documented milk levels.

BOX 6-5   American Academy of Pediatrics Risk Categories

Compatible—maternal medication usually compatible with breastfeeding

Concern—drugs for which the effect on nursing infants is unknown but may be of concern

Caution/Side Effects—drugs that have been associated with significant effects on some nursing infants and should be given to nursing mothers with caution

Cessation/Temporary—radioactive compounds that require temporary cessation of breastfeeding

Cytotoxic—cytotoxic drugs that may interfere with cellular metabolism of the nursing infant

NR—not reviewed

TABLE 6-5   First and Alternative Choice Agents Used During Lactation by Maternal Ailment

Problem	First Choice	Alternative Choices
Allergic rhinitis	beclomethasone (Beconase) fluticasone (Flonase) cromolyn (NasalCrom)	cetirizine (Zyrtec) loratadine (Claritin) sedating antihistamines
Asthma	cromolyn (Intal) nedocromil (Tilade) albuterol (Proventil) inhaler	fluticasone (Flovent) beclomethasone (Beclovent)
Cardiovascular	hydrochlorothiazide (Oretic) metoprolol tartrate (Lopressor) propranolol (Inderal) labetalol (Normodyne)	nifedipine (Procardia XL) verapamil (Calan SR) hydralazine (Apresoline)
Contraception	Lactational amenorrhea Barrier methods	Nonhormonal IUD Sterilization
Depression	sertraline (Zoloft) paroxetine (Paxil)	nortriptyline (Pamelor) desipramine (Norpramin) amitriptyline (Elavil)
Diabetes	Insulin glyburide (Micronase) glipizide (Glucotrol)	acarbose (Precose) tolbutamide (Orinase)
Epilepsy	phenytoin (Dilantin) carbamazepine (Tegretol)	ethosuximide (Zarontin) valproic sodium (Depakote)
GI Distress	ranitidine, cimetidine	
Infections	Penicillins, gentamicin, erythromycin	Cephalosporins
Pain	ibuprofen (Motrin) morphine/codeine (30 mg) acetaminophen (Tylenol)	hydrocodone (Vicodin)

Data from Spencer JP et al: Medications in the breast-feeding mother, *Am Fam Physician* 64:119-126, 2001; Hale TW: *Medications in mother's milk*, Oklahoma City, OK, 2008, Hale Publications; Briggs GG et al: *Drugs in pregnancy and lactation*, Baltimore, MD, 2005, Williams & Wilkins; Gabbe SG et al: *Obstetrics—normal and problem pregnancies*, ed 5, New York, 2007, Churchill Livingstone, Inc.

TABLE 6-6   Medications for Which the Risks of Weaning Normally Outweigh the Risks of Using Medication While Breastfeeding

Always watch for applicable side effects. The author provides a foundation based on current information for making clinical decisions. Each dyad is unique and must be individually assessed with the most up-to-date and current information.

These agents are also considered compatible with breastfeeding by the American Academy of Pediatrics (AAP), have a Hale rating of L3 (moderately safe), L2 (safer), or L1 (safest), and have had no significant side effects documented to date.	These agents have a Hale rating of L3 (moderately safe), L2 (safer), or L1 (safest) and have had no significant side effects or precautions to date, but they have not been reviewed by the AAP.
acetaminophen (Tylenol) L1	acarbose (Precose) L3
acyclovir (Zovirax) L2	albuterol (Proventil) inhaler L1 (inhaled therapy unlikely to cause side effects)
amoxicillin (Amoxil) L1	amoxicillin with clavulanate (Augmentin) L1
carbamazepine (Tegretol) L2	azithromycin (Zithromax) L2
ceftriaxone (Rocephin) L2	beclomethasone (Vanceril inhaler) L2
cimetidine (Tagamet) L2	cephalexin (Keflex) L1
clindamycin (Cleocin) L2 (vaginal)/L3 (oral)	cetirizine (Zyrtec) L2
erythromycin (E-mycin) L1 (one case of pyloric stenosis linked to ingestion through breast milk)	chlorpheniramine (Chlor-Trimeton) L3
fluconazole (Diflucan) L2 (has an FDA safety profile for neonates 1 day old)	cromolyn sodium (Intal) L1
hydralazine (Apresoline) L2	clotrimazole (Lotrimin) L1
ibuprofen (Advil) L1 (preferred NSAID)	gabapentin (Neurontin) L3 (limited data)
labetalol (Normodyne) L2	gentamicin (Garamycin) L2
loratadine (Claritin) L2	dextromethorphan (DM) L1
methocarbamol (Robaxin) L3 (limited studies)	dimenhydrinate (Dramamine) L2
morphine L3	diphenhydramine (Benadryl) L2
nifedipine (Procardia) L2	famciclovir (Famvir) L2 (acyclovir preferred)
ofloxacin (Floxin) L3 (preferred quinolones; use cautiously)	famotidine (Pepcid) L2 (preferred because of low secretion)
penicillin G L1	guaifenesin (Robitussin) L2
prednisone 80 mg/day used short term	insulin L1
prednisolone (Prelone) L2 if 80 mg/day (for acute use, preferred when dosages of prednisone exceed 20 mg/day)	lansoprazole (Prevacid) L3
propranolol (Inderal) L3 (preferred β-blocker)	meclizine (Antivert) L3
tetracycline (Terramycin) L2 (avoid long-term exposure)	miconazole (Monistat) L2
theophylline (Theo-Dur) L3	montelukast (Singulair) L3 nedocromil sodium (Tilade) L2 nystatin (Mycostatin) L1 omeprazole (Prilosec) L2 (limited studies) permethrin 5% (Nix) L2 prochlorperazine (Compazine) L3 (use with caution) promethazine (Phenergan) L2 (preferred) ranitidine (Zantac) L2 salmeterol (Serevent) L2 (limited studies) tobramycin (Tobrex) L3 tretinoin (Retin-A) (topical) L3 valacyclovir (Valtrex) (prodrug of acyclovir) L1 zafirlukast (Accolate) L3 (>99% protein bound and poorly absorbed with food)

Data from American Academy of Pediatrics Policy Statement: Use of psychoactive medication during pregnancy and possible effects on the fetus and newborn, *Pediatrics* 110:1035-1039, 1997; Hale TW: *Medications in mother's milk,* Oklahoma City, OK, 2008, Hale Publishing; Gabbe SG et al: *Obstetrics—normal and problem pregnancies,* ed 5, New York, 2007, Churchill Livingstone, Inc.

Committee on Drugs periodically publishes a policy statement regarding the transfer of drugs and other chemicals into human milk, but this resource is limited by infrequent updates, omissions, and inadequate details of the medications (Spencer et al, 2001). Although these data are limited, they are helpful in guiding clinicians with day-to-day treatment decisions. To assist in the furthering of knowledge in this field, a lactation registry documents the effects of a wide variety of medications for exposed infants and their impact on maternal lactation, in addition to registering mothers with certain health conditions, including breastfeeding-related problems (Louik et al, 2007) (see Box 6-3).

evolve A continually updated list of useful WebLinks may be found in the Evolve Resources at http://evolve.elsevier.com/Edmunds/NP/

7

Establishing the Therapeutic Relationship

Up to half of all patients with serious chronic illnesses do not take their medication as prescribed and thus fail to derive the expected benefits (Massachusetts Medical Society, 2007). How can this finding be true? Whose responsibility is it when patients fail to comply? What role does the provider play in helping the patient implement the therapeutic regimen or in impeding the process? How can health care providers seek to change this statistic?

Although the health care practices of medicine, nursing, pharmacy, and other related disciplines rest on a scientific foundation, how scientific principles are introduced in the relationship with the patient has everything to do with therapeutic success. Spoken of as the "art" of care, substantial evidence suggests that this component of health care is equally as important as the "science" of health care. This dimension of care is behind the admonitions to "treat the patient, not the laboratory numbers" and to "individualize therapy."

The *therapeutic experiment* is a term that has been in vogue in schools of pharmacy for a number of years. The concept of a therapeutic experiment suggests that to have rational use of drug therapy (which implicitly means the right drug, to the right patient, at the right time, in the proper dosage, by the appropriate route of administration, for the right problem), a therapeutic process must take place.

However, the therapeutic experiment is something that should not be limited to the taking of medications. It is really a concept that may be expanded to apply to the whole gamut of interactions between patient and provider. Basically, what every clinician and every patient wants is to find the best solution for the patient's problems and to establish a cooperative relationship so that the patient will carry out the plan successfully. Although this may seem like a simple objective, it is deceptively complicated.

As patient and provider come together, they bring different knowledge, skills, resources, anxieties, and expectations to the relationship. It is not like a chemical reaction, with a predictable product as a result of their interactions. Each patient is so different that each time therapy is prescribed, it is essentially a therapeutic experiment with that unique patient. It is important to share this attitude of engaging in a therapeutic experiment with the patient at the outset of working together, so that the patient understands the variability of outcomes for each trial.

Patients must understand that many factors lead to the success of a therapeutic regimen. For example, two patients with the same problem both may take the same medication but may have entirely different outcomes. Thus, a continuing relationship with the health care provider is essential in making adjustments to discover the proper therapy for the individual patient.

Pressure was exerted on the faculty of a graduate nursing program by a psychologist who thought that all psychologists should gain prescriptive authority. He suggested that all the faculty had to do was to develop some videotapes for psychologists to view that would teach them how to prescribe medications. "It is as simple as following a recipe," he maintained. Because he had never written a prescription, clearly, he underestimated both the knowledge base and the interpersonal skills required in the process of working with patients through the prescribing process.

ESTABLISHING THERAPEUTIC RELATIONSHIPS IN TREATMENT

The therapeutic experiment is implemented through the relationship established between the health care provider and the patient. This relationship will be therapeutic if it allows the goals of treatment to be met. Therefore, the major task of patient and provider is to establish a long-term relationship so that treatment, including the use of medications, will be implemented appropriately and effectively. It involves a stepwise process—identify a problem, assess it adequately, identify various potential solutions, examine the variables needed to judge the risk-benefit ratio of the solutions, choose the most appropriate solution, and, finally, identify the effects (both beneficial and adverse) that may result from implementation of the chosen solution (see Chapter 9 on making clinical decisions).

Several factors are essential to establishing this therapeutic relationship. These include time, attitude, information, communication, and positive feedback.

Time

Establishing a relationship, particularly with those patients who seek primary care, requires an investment of time. This is especially so with elderly patients. Time is an especially scarce resource in today's managed care environment. Actually, time is a wise investment in cost-effective treatment that is required early in the relationship to assess the patient's status accurately through history taking and listening. Time invested by one consistent provider is required. Continuity of care is essential for collecting additional information and making modifications as the patient exhibits response to the initial therapy. Offices with policies that make it easy for patients and providers to have brief follow-up conversations by telephone, whenever either of them requires it, also help make to relationships more satisfying and successful.

Attitude

How the clinician uses time with the patient and what the clinician says to the patient reflect a basic attitude. This attitude is expressed in the answer to the question, "Who owns the problem?" If the answer is that the patient owns the problem, then care is delivered with the attitude that the health care provider is there to assist the patient in getting or staying well. If the attitude is that the patient has a problem for the provider to solve, then the provider owns the problem and often hastens to solve it. This is an essential concept for clinicians to sort out in their minds because it fundamentally affects how the therapeutic relationship is established and defines the rules for continuing the relationship.

Information

Expert diagnosticians have maintained that the most important part of information gathering is the history. Many formats have been established for collecting needed information about a patient. The open-ended questions of medical and nursing school are almost always abbreviated or reduced to checklists and forms by the experienced clinician in day-to-day clinical practice. It is important to obtain a comprehensive database for patients for whom pharmacologic therapy is anticipated, especially with regard to medications. This type of information often is best obtained by having patients fill out preprinted forms regarding their medication experience. Although it would be ideal to have this information before the first visit with the health care provider, the reality is that a comprehensive history may take several visits to acquire, with the health care provider collecting a little more information with each visit. Using a history-taking form about medications, such as that illustrated in Figure 7-1, helps to standardize the information collected and allows it to be expanded during several succeeding sessions. The information collected should be not only comprehensive but also customized to the patient population (inner city, migrant, elderly) and to the specific problem under evaluation (e.g., cardiovascular, diabetes). If patient medications are to be adequately managed, an updated medication list should be part of every chart (Rooney, 2003) and should be updated routinely with every visit.

Communication

Effective two-way communication between patient and health care provider requires a consistent commitment to respecting the other's role in the relationship. It involves more listening than speaking, but a true exchange of information and ideas is essential.

During the course of therapy, the patient's expectations must be fulfilled. *Transference*, or the subconscious redirection to one person of feelings and attitudes toward others (e.g., parents, authority figures), may further influence the patient's relationship with the health care provider in a positive or negative manner, depending on the patient's previous experiences. All of these factors play a part in establishing honesty and trust in the patient–provider relationship.

Other strategies that have been identified as helpful in establishing a relationship with the patient include the health care provider's friendliness; a positive, confident approach; a thoughtful response to patient complaints; encouraging patient questions; a supportive, nonjudgmental method of eliciting and responding to patient admissions of noncompliance;

and encouraging patients to become actively involved in their own care. Techniques that encourage active patient participation as opposed to provider-dominated decisions, negotiating rather than dictating a treatment plan, and identifying and resolving barriers to compliance are also helpful. Finally, attempting to find congruence between patient and provider in their understanding of a problem and its management and efforts to motivate the patient and increase patient satisfaction are also helpful (Frishman, 2007; Goeman & Douglass, 2007; Swanson, 2003; Wilson et al, 2007).

Some of the specifics of what is communicated to the patient must focus on the therapeutic goals of treatment. When medications are involved, the nature of the experiment with that particular medication and that particular patient should be explored. Clear expectations must be communicated about mutual decision making, taking medications as ordered, returning for monitoring of effectiveness of the intervention, and the need to adjust dosages or medications over time.

Health care providers must refine listening and questioning skills. They must focus first on the patient, then the environment, and then themselves. Specifically, the tasks are to learn to judge the patient's verbal or nonverbal cues to see whether the patient is ready to receive information. Providers should first attend to the physical environment of the discussion (privacy, freedom from distractions). And, finally, they must pay attention to their own mannerisms, tone of voice, and language. They should use active listening with feedback to ensure that the information sent is the same as the information received.

In the classical article by Chessare (1998) on teaching clinical decision making to physicians, the author maintains that after presenting information, the health care provider needs to elicit the patient's preferences for health and other outcomes. For example, it is not enough to give a family the probability that a child will be left with significant morbidity after a potentially life-sustaining procedure. It is also necessary to have the parents consider what the morbidity may mean to them and their child. This discussion should include information on the child's somatic and psychological well-being in the context of family life and the financial repercussions for the family of specific clinical decisions (Chessare, 1998). A prudent course must be charted between creating uncontrolled and unfounded anxieties on the one hand and generating a false sense of equally groundless security and reassurance on the other.

To lead discussions of this type, health care providers will need to understand how framing the problem for a decision maker can affect the decision. Health care providers must know some techniques for helping the patient or family deal with probabilities when making a particularly difficult decision. The provider should elicit preferences from patients and parents regarding the outcomes of medical treatment.

Health care providers also have a societal duty to consider the consequences of decisions made by both patients and themselves for the greater good of the community. For example, parents' decision not to provide immunization for their child because of concerns about adverse reactions places others in the community at risk. When a higher-cost strategy gives no added benefit to the patient, then it is appropriate for the health care provider to use a lower-cost choice. When higher-cost strategies of potential benefit are available, the health care provider must be able to frame decisions for families such that they understand the expected added

Name_____ Address_____ Age_____

Date_____ Provider _____

Updated on:_____ By _____

MEDICATION REGIMEN

Record for all OTC products (nonprescription pain relievers, laxatives, vitamins, ear/eye/nose drops, anti-diarrheals, inhalers, breathing medications, creams, ointments, sleeping pills, cough or cold medications, feminine hygiene medications, etc.) and Rx medications.

	Name of Medication	Strength	Dosage Form	Directions	Purpose	Compliance
Med 1						
Med 2						
Med 3						
Med 4						
Med 5						
Med 6						
Med 7						
Med 8						
Med 9						
Med 10						
Med 11						
Med 12						

Which of the above medications has the patient stopped taking? Why? *Put number next to medication.*
(1) per provider's order (2) side effect (3) didn't think it was important (4) couldn't afford it (5) didn't think it was working (6) ran out and couldn't get refill (7) other_____

Does the patient see multiple health care providers?   Y   N
Does the patient use multiple pharmacies?   Y   N
Is the patient able to read prescription labels?   Y   N
Is the patient able to open childproof caps?   Y   N
Does the patient receive or need assistance with medications?   Y   N   If Yes, describe:_____
_____

History of medication allergy?   Y   N
If yes, medications involved:_____ _____ _____
(1) aspirin (2) sulfas (3) codeine (4) penicillin (5) radiopaque dyes (6) local anesthetics
(7) other (specify)_____
Describe what happened in the allergic reaction(s)_____
_____
_____

Adverse effects (record any major adverse/side effects related to current or past drug therapy):
Medication involved   Description of reaction   Year
_____
_____
_____
_____

FIGURE 7-1 Comprehensive medication evaluation.

SOCIAL HISTORY

What alcoholic beverages does patient drink?

Beverage	How much/day (ounces)?
Wine	_____
Beer	_____
Hard liquor (whiskey, gin, etc).	_____

Does patient smoke tobacco?   Y   N   How many packs/years? _____

How much of the following does the patient drink/day (convert to ounces)?

Beverage	Amount (ounces/day)
Caffeinated coffee	_____
Decaffeinated coffee	_____
Caffeinated tea	_____
Decaffeinated tea	_____
Caffeinated sodas	_____

Has patient ever used or currently uses any of the following drugs?

	Route	Currently using?	Past user?	Date stopped
Heroin				
Cocaine				
Crack				
Marijuana				
Amphetamines				
Depressants/barbiturates				
Other				

SOURCE/PAYMENT OF MEDICATIONS

How does patient obtain medicines? (1) goes to pharmacy to pick up, (2) caregiver goes to pharmacy, (3) pharmacy delivers to home, (4) pharmacy mails to home, (5) other_____

Is it difficult for patient to obtain medicines? Y N Why? (1) can't get out to get them (2) can't get to doctor to get renewed prescriptions (3) can't afford them (4) forget to get them refilled (5) other_____
Are prescriptions filled at more than one pharmacy? Y N Unknown

From what type of pharmacy are prescriptions most frequently obtained? (1) chain (2) supermarket chain (3) independent (4) mail order (5) HMO (6) VA pharmacy (7) other_____

Name of pharmacy_____Phone # of pharmacy_____

Does patient know the pharmacist's name? Y N_____
Does pharmacy have a delivery service available? Y N Don't know
Does patient use it? Y N Is there an extra charge? Y N Don't know
Who assists patient in selection of specific OTC products?
(1) health care provider (2) pharmacist (3) friend (4) relative (5) caregiver (6) no one, patient selects them
(7) other_____

FIGURE 7-1, cont'd   **Comprehensive medical evaluation.**

Continued

How are prescription medications paid for? (1) free at the VA (2) medical assistance card (3) pharmacy assistance card
(4) prescription insurance card (5) cash
Does patient receive a senior citizen discount? Y N
Does patient have a co-payment per prescription? Y N Amount_____

ADMINISTRATION

Who gives patient the medications? (1) patient takes them with no assistance (2) patient takes them with assistance
(3) spouse gives them to patient (4) professional caregiver gives them to patient (5) other gives them to patient_____

Did patient take medication this morning? Y N Don't know
If not, why not? (1) forgot (2) ran out (3) side effects (4) other_____
How often does patient NOT take ANY prescription medications? (1) daily (2) once a week (3) less than once a week
but more than once a month (4) less than once a month

UNDERSTANDING

Does patient seem to understand purpose of medications?	Fully	Somewhat	Not at all
Does patient understand medication schedule?	Fully	Somewhat	Not at all
Is patient aware of expected side effects?	Fully	Somewhat	Not at all
Does patient have an understanding of what effects to report to health care provider?	Fully	Somewhat	Not at all
Does caregiver understand purpose of medications?	Fully	Somewhat	Not at all
Does caregiver understand medication schedule?	Fully	Somewhat	Not at all
Is caregiver aware of expected side effects?	Fully	Somewhat	Not at all
Does caregiver have an understanding of what effects to report to health care provider?	Fully	Somewhat	Not at all

FIGURE 7-1, cont'd Comprehensive medical evaluation.

benefit (Chessare, 1998; Kraetschmer et al, 2006). For example, the family of a patient with tuberculosis might be convinced that it is in the interest of public safety for a judge to put the patient in jail until a supervised course of medication therapy can be concluded rather than allow the patient to remain noncompliant with drug therapy in the community. It is essential for providers to help the patient recognize that other factors, in addition to his own preferences, must be considered in the decision of whether to take medication for a particular problem.

Implicit in the communication process is the guarantee that once data about a problem have been presented clearly to a family, health care providers will do their utmost to provide the best therapy. It is part of the provider's role to avoid strategies that provide no benefit to the patient. Practicing evidence-based medicine leads to cost-effective care because data are sought to validate strategies that lead to the best outcomes.

Providers also do not have the right to withhold effective therapies chosen by the family simply because they are more costly than others. Because managed care is about providing health care within budget constraints, the pressure to contain costs by limiting care is significant in most plans. This is especially true regarding drug therapy. This pressure is strongest in for-profit plans, where breaking even is not enough. It is now also seen with Medicaid patients, for whom drug choices may be severely limited by formularies for less costly, and sometimes less effective, medications. Ethically, providers must refrain from withholding strategies that are marginally superior to others simply because they are too expensive. This is sometimes difficult given the restrictions of some payment plans, but in some situations, to

do otherwise is a violation of the patient–provider relationship (Kraetschmer et al, 2006).

If policies of a managed care organization or other organization would preclude the prescription of recommended therapy, the provider must continue to act as the family's agent and help them obtain the desired care. When the provider cannot support the desires of the patient, he has a duty to make this clear to the patient. If the patient continues to see his desire as appropriate, the provider must assist him in finding another provider (Chessare, 1998; Kraetschmer et al, 2006).

Not only does communication have to be examined from a philosophical or procedural point of view, but specific information must be discussed in the patient encounter. The construction of a diagnostic plan is based on critical decision making. The problem itself must be clearly defined by some clinically measurable, verifiable means, for example, a lump in the breast can be defined as a malignant lesion only after pathologic examination. Only known information can be used to define a problem; no assumptions can be accepted in the problem definition.

The provider's assessment of the patient's history and physical and laboratory information will answer the questions, "What etiology?" "Why now?" and "How severe?" This step allows for further refinement of the problem and speculation as to the probable causes and potential risk to the patient based on information gathered in the database. "What etiology?" suggests potential treatments of a correctable cause; "Why now?" is particularly important in acute exacerbations of chronic disease or detection of immune deficiencies, for it leads to an approach that treats the acute problem and prevents further difficulty. "How severe?" leads to decisions on the rapidity and perhaps the nature of treatment (see Chapter 9 on making clinical decisions).

Next, the therapeutic objective must be clearly defined and stated before treatment is begun. The goal or objective should be (1) realistically attainable with available therapeutic agents, (2) clearly related to the problem as defined and assessed, and (3) measurable.

Finally, the indices of therapeutic effect are determined. These measures of the therapeutic objective should be discriminating, identified, and relevant to the therapeutic objective. Identification of discriminating therapeutic indices allows the practitioner to recognize when the therapeutic objective has been achieved. It is the identification of those subjective and objective parameters that the practitioner will monitor to determine the degree of therapeutic achievement. These are often suggested from well-established clinical guidelines.

If the patient agrees to drug therapy, the provider must offer specific explanations about what medication the patient is to take and why (see Chapter 9 on making clinical decisions). The selected modality should be as specific for the problem and the therapeutic objective as possible. Evidence-based medicine will provide direction about what has proved effective. In the absence of definitive recommendations, agents or modalities will be selected on the basis of cost, efficacy, lowest toxicity, and other patient and drug variables.

Both patient- and agent-related variables must be considered in the final selection and administration of an agent. *Agent-related variables* are defined as those properties of any agent that are characteristic of that agent and that affect its use in a given situation. Examples of this would be chemical properties, formulation, absorption, metabolism and excretion, toxicity, half-life, and bioavailability (see Chapter 3 on pharmacokinetics).

Patient-related variables are defined as those preexisting conditions that in some way alter the expected effects of an agent on the patient, that is, renal function or dysfunction, liver function or dysfunction, age, weight, individual response, concomitant disease, the disease or problem itself, compliance or noncompliance, or allergy. Patient-related variables also may include absolute or relative contraindications for use of an agent in a given patient. An example would be the use of sympathomimetic amines in a hypertensive patient.

Detailed instructions must be given to the patient, preferably in writing, about how to take medication (see Chapter 8 on tips in writing prescriptions and Chapter 10 on design and implementation of patient education). One cannot rationally administer an agent without first understanding variables that affect its administration. Patients should understand what they might expect, both positively and negatively, when taking this medication.

And, finally, patients should understand their responsibility to report back to the provider about how the "experiment" is progressing. Direct observation of the chosen indices of effect and toxicity is the final and most important step in the implementation of the therapeutic experiment in the actual situation. This step involves eliciting subjective and objective data as a follow-up to administration of the agent. Obviously, there is no point in establishing a therapeutic objective unless providers will be able to know when the objective has been achieved, or when a toxic index is being approached.

From the first discussions of therapy, patients must understand the providers' expectations about having them return for laboratory tests and clinic appointments. Again, whether the report is on what patients have done in handling their problems or whether they report back on the success of the provider's plan depends on the attitude that has been established about who owns the problem.

One example of a realistic expectation might be that the patient will bring all medications (current and recently discontinued, prescription and OTC, internal and topical, liquid and solid) with him in a bag for follow-up visits. Reviewing the medications together, validating that the medications were taken as ordered, and noting the number of pills that are left are all important ways in which the provider can assess whether the patient has been compliant.

Positive Feedback

Relationships that acknowledge sacrifice, hard work, and cooperation are likely to thrive. Obstetricians who yell at or scold pregnant women who gain too much weight during their pregnancy finally learned that yelling only drove away the mothers; it did not make them stop eating. Being flexible when possible, accepting occasional lapses in compliance, attempting to understand the patient's point of view, and being appreciative of efforts that are made to change all assist in the development of a trusting relationship. Overly critical or rigid clinicians often create a milieu in which it is difficult for patients to tell them the truth about noncompliance. It then becomes impossible to determine whether the medication is working. This dooms the therapeutic experiment.

FAILURE OF THE THERAPEUTIC RELATIONSHIP

The success of the therapeutic relationship will be measured by the compliance of the patient. Patient noncompliance with medications is a major unresolved problem that health care providers must face. Drug noncompliance may be seen as the inappropriate self-administration of medications (Mochari et al, 2007). This implies that the results of self-administration vary according to the health care provider's advice and cannot be equated with therapeutic effectiveness. However, *noncompliance* really is a neutral term, describing one aspect of patient behavior that may be appropriate or inappropriate to the patient's best interests (Barker et al, 2006).

How does noncompliance begin? Patients often come to a health care provider almost as a last resort, after having tried a number of remedies for symptoms; consulted family, friends, or other authority figures; and developed half-formed or inaccurate models to explain symptoms and illness. Age, sex, race, ethnic background, family, social class, education, past experience, and place in the world will have affected how the patient views the problem and sees the world in general. Although today's patients are more likely to be better informed about medical care than patients were in the past, they also are more likely to be skeptical of the medical profession. They may have read about successful malpractice suits and medical mistakes, heard about bad experiences in medical care from friends, or have had bad experiences themselves. They may come from a lower socioeconomic class, be less educated, or have different value systems than the health care provider. They may have underlying fears and concerns and certain expectations for the visit but may be reluctant to express them for fear of being thought foolish (Barker et al, 2006). Direct-to-consumer advertising may have led to self-diagnosis and expectations about therapy.

Although health care providers may make diagnoses and prescribe effective treatments, they may not detect or allay the patients' underlying concerns or meet the patients' expectations for the visit. Providers may make false assumptions that the patients' value systems are like their own.

Noncompliance continues as a growing concern for practicing clinicians. The National Library of Medicine PubMed Database includes more than 55,900 articles related to compliance, representing only a portion of the published literature. The average compliance rate for a prescribed treatment regimen has been estimated at 50%; compliance rates for chronic therapy and asymptomatic diseases were even lower (Massachusetts Medical Society, 2007; Swanson, 2003).

If medication is involved in the treatment plan, the provider's goal is simply "to get every patient to purchase, take, continue, report back, [and] identify what helps and what hinders." Problematic behavior can be exhibited as overutilization or underutilization of medication. *Overutilization* describes patients who take one or more medications at a higher dose or frequency than prescribed. It also describes patients who take medications from several different providers who are unaware of the other medications the patient is taking, whether prescription drugs or OTC products (Briesacher et al, 2007).

Underutilization includes taking medications at lower doses or at less frequent intervals than prescribed. If a patient does not fill a prescription or stops taking the medication without authorization by the physician, this is considered underutilization. Other examples might include when patients cut their pills in half to stretch out the supply of costly medications. In another scenario, with antibiotic therapy, patients feel better in 3 days and stop taking the medication (Briesacher et al, 2007).

Noncompliant behavior leads to no benign consequences. Overutilization of medications places a person at greater risk for adverse effects. Underutilization of medicines may result in therapeutic failure, leading to an increase in disease severity. In either case, a higher rate of hospitalization and increased costs for medical care may result. A meta-analysis of seven research studies demonstrated that an overall hospitalization rate of 5.5% might be attributed to noncompliance. This percentage equals 1.94 million annual hospital admissions, at a cost of $8.5 billion (Driscoll et al, 2007). Noncompliance by patients with cardiovascular disease, a particularly prevalent problem, has been estimated to be a factor in 125,000 deaths and several hundred thousand hospitalizations a year. The calculated cost to society is over $1.5 billion in lost earnings, resulting from lost workdays (Bangalore et al, 2007; Charles et al, 2003; Simmons & Dubreuil, 2007).

Noncompliance with efficacious therapeutic regimens may thwart the goals of both provider and patient in reducing suffering, preventing illness, improving functional status, and increasing longevity. If the extent of the patient's noncompliance is hidden from the provider, poor outcomes may be mistakenly attributed to inadequate dosage, failure of the regimen itself, or incorrect diagnosis. Any of these conclusions could lead to inappropriate action by the health care provider during later patient visits (Barker et al, 2006).

Most studies of factors associated with compliance are described in small cross-sectional reports, making inferences of causality subject to error. However, an increasing number are prospective. Most studies of compliance have involved hospital-based patients, leaving questions about their general applicability, but when ambulatory patients have been studied, results tend to be similar. Numerous studies have been undertaken to evaluate the short-term effectiveness of various interventions designed to improve patient compliance. These studies have consistently found that patients are unfamiliar with their prescribed medications and how to take them (Charles, 2003; Graney et al, 2003; Marple et al, 2007; Simpson et al, 2003), and that patients make errors when taking medications 25% to 59% of the time (Barker et al, 2006). The research literature (Bagchi et al, 2007; Bezie et al, 2006; Marple et al, 2007; Massachusetts Medical Society, 2007) suggests that there are six major risk factors for noncompliance:

1. Noncompliance rates tend to be higher for preventative care than for treatment of established illnesses. It has also been demonstrated that there is better compliance for medications perceived to be important, such as cardiac or diabetic agents, than for those that are seemingly less important, such as antacids or mild analgesics.
2. Noncompliance increases in extent with the duration of therapy, such as is seen in chronic diseases such as diabetes, hypertension, epilepsy, and depression.
3. Noncompliance is highest for regimens that require significant behavioral change, such as smoking cessation or weight loss.
4. Noncompliance often results from a poor understanding of instructions.
5. Noncompliance increases with the complexity of the treatment regimen, that is, when many drugs are taken concurrently and/or when drugs must be taken at frequent intervals.
6. Noncompliance increases when unpleasant side effects occur.

Clearly, patients who are symptomatic are more likely to be compliant than those who are not, especially if the symptoms are relieved by treatment recommendations. It is surprising that such sociodemographic variables as gender, race, education, occupation, income, and marital status usually do not correlate with compliance behavior (Charles et al, 2003). People who have a stable support system and a stable family situation tend to be more compliant.

Although it is generally accepted that older people are more likely to be noncompliant, the bulk of the early research literature indicates that aging does not affect compliance with prescribed medications. Elderly individuals may have fewer daily distractions in their lives, enabling them to concentrate on their medication regimens. This is in contrast to middle-aged and younger patients who are involved in their careers and other activities, causing them to forget about their medications. Elderly patients, however, have been shown to have difficulty in opening childproof medication containers and may have greater difficulty in reading or understanding instructions, and this may adversely affect compliance (Piette et al, 2005).

Unfortunately, identifying the noncompliant patient is very difficult. Studies have shown that physicians tend to overestimate patient adherence to treatment regimens. Studies on specific factors related to compliance have found no relationship with gender, socioeconomic status, or education (Driscoll et al, 2007; Gardiner & Dvorkin, 2006; Mochari et al, 2007).

So, how can health care providers better identify and improve compliance in their patients? An early study in Great Britain claims that the assumption behind the terms *compliance* and *adherence* in medicine taking suggest patient fault and should be abandoned in favor of the term *concordance*. This term, they suggest, expresses a therapeutic alliance between the prescriber and the patient, describing a negotiated agreement that may even be an agreement to disagree (Wilson et al, 2007).

Concordance, as a process, imposes new responsibilities on both parties. Patients must take a more active part in the consultation process, and prescribers must communicate the evidence to enable patients to make an informed decision about diagnosis and treatment and benefit and risk. Prescribers should know and accept patients' choices while continuing to negotiate the treatment as part of an ongoing consultation process.

Effective communication practices must extend beyond those used in the patient–provider therapeutic relationship to include the family and the pharmacist.

Primary communication among pharmacist, patient, and provider takes place through the prescription. At the very least, when pharmacists dispense prescriptions, they have the opportunity to detect miscommunications or unfounded expectations, to validate why the medication is being prescribed, and to clarify or reinforce health care prescribers' instructions. Reinforcement through repetition is an effective strategy in achieving compliance (Mochari et al, 2007).

However, pharmacists may assist the provider and the patient in many other ways. A growing number of pharmacists use computers to establish and maintain patient profiles. The computer alerts the pharmacist when patients refill their prescriptions too soon, identifying possible overutilization. The pharmacist's regular review of patient profiles also permits identification of underutilization by patients who are not regularly refilling their prescription. Writing complete information on the prescription about how the patient should be taking the medication gives pharmacists valuable information that will assist them in helping the patient be more compliant.

At visits, the clinician should assess whether patients are able to open their medication bottles easily, read the label correctly, and tolerate the dosage. They should detect patient fears about developing an addiction to the drug, often a particularly insidious but unfounded concern. They also have an opportunity to counsel patients, no matter how well educated, who believe they will "outgrow" their need for insulin, high blood pressure medication, or thyroid medication.

Confusion about therapeutic regimens frequently occurs following transition times such as discharge from an emergency department, hospital, or long-term care facility. These times often are associated with the addition of new prescriptions or a change in prescriptive regimen. One study found that 47% of emergency department visits led to the prescribing of at least one additional medication, and in 10% of those visits, the new medication added a potential adverse interaction. Because health care providers who see patients in these settings usually are not the patients' primary care providers, special care should be taken by the primary care provider on the next visit to review prescriptions. Patients may not understand if they are supposed to use the old medications as well as the new ones, make substitutions in product, or just make changes in dosage (Turnbough & Wilson, 2007).

Another factor that influences compliance is the issue of higher drug prices. The high cost of medication continues to be an important factor in determining whether some patients will have a prescription filled (Massachusetts Medical Society, 2007). It is difficult for the provider to learn about the cost of these medications, particularly because there may be substantial variability in price, depending on where the prescription is filled. Providers periodically should take the time to contact several community pharmacists for cost information before prescribing new products. Also, a good relationship with pharmacists will encourage them to alert health care providers to the price differential between new drugs and similar older drugs that may be as effective and much less costly.

SUMMARY

Concordance between provider and patient is the key to therapeutic relationships. In seeking concordance, the problems associated with medicine taking have been remarkably absent from almost all public discussion about the benefits and expectations of contemporary medicine. Further research is needed into the beliefs that people hold about medicines and about their motivation and reaction to information giving and to the behavior of health care workers, family members, and friends. Ongoing work on developing interventions to modify medicine-taking behavior should continue.

Efforts to secure appropriate medicine taking among patients must be based not on manipulation but on strengthening patients' understanding and control over their illnesses and treatment. With new medicines, features such as combination products, modified (sustained-release) formulations, high-dose short courses, improved tolerability, design characteristics, alternative delivery systems, and linking of administration to circadian rhythms may be designed to overcome difficulties posed by noncompliance.

Providers should consider reevaluating medicines that are now in use to gauge their robustness in terms of the relationship between dose and effect. Continuing research will be required to explore the effects of containers, labeling, and other information giving, and how they facilitate or limit medicine taking.

Patients want more information on medicines, and giving them greater control over treatments received may change compliance. Although establishing a therapeutic relationship is essential, at the other end of the spectrum are all the new electronic and communications media, such as telephone help-lines, information on the Internet, and use of PDAs and other interactive electronic devices that are consulted increasingly by patients. The importance of information sources that do not involve face-to-face communication with health care professionals is growing rapidly.

Primary care providers must take care to focus not simply on seeking to achieve better compliance but on empowering patients to take part in concordant partnerships with all health care providers, so that their medicine-taking decisions are as informed as possible by scientific evidence and consonant with their own perceptions and wishes.

evolve A continually updated list of useful WebLinks may be found in the Evolve Resources at http://evolve.elsevier.com/Edmunds/NP/

8 Practical Tips on Writing Prescriptions

Many sources describe the importance of prescriptive authority for full implementation of the health provider's role; however, very few texts describe the mechanics and technicalities of the actual process. Students of all disciplines with prescriptive authority admit to extreme anxiety in writing their first prescriptions. They are concerned about not only what they write, but how they write it. However, most clinicians describe learning this process on the job, under the tutelage of another clinician or preceptor, often while under extreme pressure to master other skills. Casual observation of prescriptions submitted to a pharmacy reveals the wide array of formats used in writing prescriptions, some leading to a greater chance for errors than others. Research also shows that, similar to writing a check, the format with which one begins is often the format that persists, even if it is not the best.

WHO MAY WRITE PRESCRIPTIONS?

State law identifies those health care providers who are authorized to write prescriptions. This fact accounts for the substantial state-by-state variation in prescriptive authority. Traditionally, physicians have had full prescriptive authority, dentists and podiatrists have had prescriptive authority for a limited formulary, and veterinarians have had the ability to prescribe, dispense, and administer medications. State laws have been amended in every state to provide prescriptive authority to certain other providers, such as doctors of osteopathy, NPs, and PAs. This authority may be granted directly to these providers or indirectly through delegated authority from a physician (see Chapters 1 and 2 for information on nurses and PAs). Each state determines the qualifications and credentials that are essential for a provider to obtain prescriptive authority; these may include specific courses in pharmacology before prescriptive authority is granted, as well as ongoing requirements for continuing education in pharmacology.

The exact extent of prescriptive authority is also determined by the state. This includes the types of drugs that the provider is authorized to prescribe. Over-the-counter medications require no state authorization. Indeed, these medications often are initiated and controlled by patients. Drugs that require a prescription include legend drugs and controlled substances. *Legend drugs* include the vast majority of medications, such as those given for hypertension, diabetes, or asthma. If a state determines that providers may write prescriptions for controlled substances, it also establishes a mechanism for monitoring that activity, such as granting the provider a number or putting the provider on an approved list. Once he has received documentation of this authority from the state, the health care provider is eligible to apply to the federal Drug Enforcement Administration (DEA) for a federal DEA number to be used on all prescriptions for controlled substances.

The DEA oversees controlled substances. This agency attempts to limit professionals who may prescribe controlled substances to those who are authorized and competent to do so, and to monitor the activity of such individuals to make certain they are in conformance with federal law. Such monitoring is essential because of the potential for misuse and abuse of these substances by both patients and providers. The DEA does not define who is to receive DEA numbers but relies on the states for this information (U.S. Department of Justice, DEA, 2006). States issue a state-controlled substance license. This number seems to have little purpose other than to document for the DEA that the applicant is recognized as a prescriber within the state and is eligible for the federal DEA number.

The health care provider who seeks a federal DEA number may obtain an application by calling 202-307-7255; by going to the DEA website at www.DEADiversion.usdoj.gov; or by writing the Drug Enforcement Administration Registration Division, Washington, DC 20537, and submitting the appropriate information and fees. Fees are sufficiently high to deter casual acquisition. Providers must indicate on the application the specific schedules of drugs that they are authorized by the state to prescribe. Nonphysician prescribers are required to fill out a specific addendum to the DEA application to validate state authority to engage in the prescription of controlled substances. DEA numbers issued to "midlevel providers" begin with the letter M, followed by a number that corresponds to the first letter of the last name (i.e., E for Edwards) and a computer-generated sequence of numbers. Physician and midlevel practitioners' manuals, available by special request, contain essential rules and regulations related to use or misuse of the DEA number. If applicants meet the DEA requirements, they are issued a number linked to their place of employment. One exception is that military and U.S. Public Health Service physicians are exempt from registration. This number is valid for 3 years and then may be renewed. This federal number is also reported to the state and is included in the materials distributed to pharmacists within that state (U.S. Department of Justice, DEA, 2006).

DRUG SCHEDULES

Federal statute has established five schedules of controlled substances, ranked in order of their abuse potential and in inverse proportion to their medical value. A complete list of controlled substances may be obtained by writing to Superintendent of Documents, U.S. Government Printing Office, Washington, DC 20402, or by consulting the website for this office. The drugs in these schedules are revised periodically by the DEA as circumstances warrant.

Drugs in Schedule I have the highest potential for abuse, and their use is limited to research protocols, instructional purposes, or chemical analysis. Ongoing research may eventually establish a medical role for some of these substances under selected circumstances. On the other end of the spectrum, Schedule V drugs are available by prescription or may be sold over the counter in some states, depending on state law (U.S. Department of Justice, DEA, 2006). See Table 8-1 for a sample Schedule of Controlled Drugs.

Controlled drugs often have restrictions on the number of refills permitted. When they are dispensed to a patient via prescription, the label of any controlled substances under Schedule II, III, or IV must contain a symbol that designates the schedule to which it belongs and the following warning: "Caution: Federal law prohibits the transfer of this drug to any person other than the patient for whom it was prescribed." Internet and mail-order pharmacies may not fill prescriptions for controlled substances.

Classification of drugs into these schedules is flexible. Thus, any drug can be placed under control, upgraded or downgraded, or possibly even removed from control over time. For example, new information might cause a change in schedule classification, or epidemic abuse of an uncontrolled drug may cause it to be added to the controlled substance list.

COMPONENTS OF THE TRADITIONAL PRESCRIPTION

Although state law may mandate the specifics of what is required on a prescription, there is general agreement about some things that should be included, whether required by law or not. Most states insist that the hospital name or the imprinted name of the prescriber, along with credentials, address, and telephone number, must be preprinted on the prescription pad for controlled substances but not for noncontrolled drugs. It is important, however, for the pharmacist to be able to easily contact the prescriber. In institutions where there are many prescribers, an institutional prescription pad may allow the prescriber to use a number rather than having all prescriber names printed on the pad. Prescriptions must be preprinted, typed, or written in ink and must be signed by an authorized prescriber to be valid. See a good example of a prescription see Figure 8-1.

TABLE 8-1 Federal Schedule of Controlled Drugs

	Substance Characteristics	Type of Restriction	Examples
I	High abuse potential No currently accepted medical use For research, instructional use, or chemical analysis only	Approved protocol necessary	heroin, marijuana, LSD, peyote, mescaline, psilocybin, methamphetamine, acetylmethadol, fenethylline, tilidine, dihydromorphine, methaqualone
II	High abuse potential Currently accepted for medical use as narcotic, stimulant, or depressant May lead to severe psychologic and/or physical dependence	Written prescription only No refills Emergency dispensing without written prescription permitted Container must carry warning label	morphine, codeine, hydromorphone (Dilaudid), methadone, Pantopon, meperidine (Demerol), cocaine, oxycodone (Percodan), oxymorphone (Numorphan), amphetamine (Dexedrine), methamphetamine (Desoxyn), phenmetrazine (Preludin), methylphenidate (Ritalin), amobarbital, phenobarbital, secobarbital, fentanyl (Sublimaze), sufentanil, etorphine hydrochloride, phenylacetone, dronabinol, nabilone
III	Less abuse potential than drugs in Schedules I and II Currently accepted for medical use and includes compounds that contain limited quantities of certain narcotic and nonnarcotic drugs May lead to physical dependence or high level of psychologic dependence	Written or oral prescription required Prescription expires in 6 months No more than 5 prescription refills Container must carry warning label	Derivatives of barbituric acid except those that are listed in another schedule, glutethimide (Doriden), nalorphine, benzphetamine, chlorphentermine, clortermine, phendimetrazine, paregoric and any compound, mixture, preparation, or suppository dosage form that contains amobarbital, secobarbital, or pentobarbital
IV	Low abuse potential relative to Schedule III substances Currently accepted for medical use May lead to limited physical or psychologic dependence	Written or oral prescription required Prescription expires in 6 months No more than 5 prescription refills Container must carry warning label	barbital, phenobarbital, methylphenobarbital, chloral hydrate, ethchlorvynol (Placidyl), ethinamate (Valmid), meprobamate (Equanil, Miltown), paraldehyde, methohexital, phentermine, chlordiazepoxide (Librium), diazepam (Valium), oxazepam (Serax), clorazepate (Tranxene), flurazepam (Dalmane), clonazepam (Klonopin), prazepam (Verstran), alprazolam (Xanax), halazepam (Paxipam), temazepam (Restoril), triazolam (Halcion), lorazepam (Ativan), midazolam (Versed), quazepam (Dormalin), mebutamate, dextropropoxyphene dosage forms (Darvon), and pentazocine (Talwin-NX)
V	Low abuse potential relative to Schedule IV substances Currently accepted for medical use; consists primarily of preparations of certain narcotic and stimulant drugs generally for antitussive, antidiarrheal, and analgesic purposes Have less potential for physical or psychologic dependence	May require written prescription or may be sold over-the-counter Check state law	buprenorphine and propylhexedrine

From U.S. Department of Justice, DEA: *Prescribers' manual*, Washington, DC, 2006, U.S. Department of Justice.

Robert Jones, M.D., ABFP	Jean Fairway, ANP	1155-3
DEA NO.	DEA NO.	

Dan Smith, M.D.
DEA NO.

Bonnie Brown, ANP
DEA NO.

Lois Lane, PNP
DEA NO.

STEVENS FOREST PROFESSIONAL CENTER, SUITE 109
OAKLAND MILLS, 9650 SANTIAGO ROAD, COLUMBIA, MD 21045
PHONE: 997-5333

NAME   AGE

ADDRESS   DATE

Rx: tetracycline 250 mg

Sig: i̇ capsule po 1h ac or 2 h pc tid × 10 days
            for soft tissue infection

D: 42 capsules please

VOLUNTARY FORMULARY PERMITTED

REFILLS   GENERIC SUBSTITUTION   ☐ YES   ☐ NO   M.D.

FIGURE 8-1 **Common components of a prescription.**

Is there one correct way to write a prescription? Yes. And it should be followed consistently and without deviation each time a prescription is written. It contains the components as identified in the sections on top portion, middle portion, and bottom portion that follow.

Top Portion

The top portion of the preprinted prescription form contains the patient's name, address, and age or birth date. The patient's weight also may be included here when relevant. The date on which the prescription is written is required.

- *Name and address of the patient*—Most states require the address if the prescription is written for a controlled substance. It is always a good idea to include the address on a prescription; this will help the pharmacist to make certain that the correct person is picking up the drug.
- *Date that the prescription is written*—By law, a patient usually has up to 120 days to fill a prescription for a controlled or a noncontrolled drug. Medicaid or Medical Assistance prescriptions often must be filled within a shorter period, usually 10 days, although states may vary on their specific practices. The date on the prescription helps the pharmacist to determine if the patient waited too long to fill the prescription. Some patients hold a prescription in case they need it at another time. This is equivalent to giving patients an inappropriate ability to diagnose and prescribe for themselves in the future.
- *Age and weight of the patient*—The pharmacist needs this information to assess the accuracy of the prescription as written. Dosage modifications based on age and weight may be suggested or validated by the pharmacist with this information, particularly for pediatric and geriatric patients.

Middle Portion

The middle portion of the prescription, the part that is individualized for each patient, contains five main items:
1. *Superscription*—The symbol "Rx" from the Latin recipe meaning "take," is included.
2. *Inscription*—Drug ingredients and their quantities, strength, or concentration are specified.
3. *Drug*—The full name of the medication is written clearly and specifically. Do not use abbreviations (Koczmara et al, 2006). If handwriting legibility is an issue, print or type the information required. There must be no question as to the meaning of what is written. Some pharmaceutical companies supply preprinted pads for certain prescriptions, reducing the chance for error (and encouraging the prescribing of their product) (Jayawardena et al, 2007; Mills, 2007; Varkey et al, 2007).
4. *Strength or concentration*—The dose of the medication to be dispensed must be specified.
5. *Signature*—This usually is indicated by an "S," representing the Latin *signa*, which means "mark." Other individuals use "Sig." which means, "Directions for use." Thus, the signature includes instructions to be placed on the outside of the package to direct the patient how and when to take the medicine and in what quantities. The signature component of the prescription should not be confused with the prescriber's signature that is placed at the bottom of the form. It is especially important to be complete in writing instructions for how the medication should be taken.

First, it is important for the patient to understand how to take the medication. The prescription should be specific about this and should not just indicate, "Take as directed."

Research has shown that failure to write instructions clearly is responsible for many of the medication errors that patients make. Patients often do not understand instructions, become confused over time, or fail to make changes when therapy is modified (Aspinall et al, 2007). The imprecision of poorly written directions can also influence a patient's ability to comply. To improve patient recall and reduce administration errors, patients require explicit directions. A high percentage of reported administrative errors result from the direct failure of patients to comprehend the directions on the prescription label (Cohen, 2007). In one study, when given a prescription for tetracycline 250 mg with the directions, "Take 1 capsule every 6 hours," only 36% of 67 participants interpreted the directions to mean around the clock, for a total of 4 doses in 24 hours. Approximately 25% would have been noncompliant by omitting the late-night dose because they would have divided the day into three 6-hour periods while they were awake. Although in this instance, the pharmacist has adequate information to counsel the patient, the example demonstrates the importance of prescription writing and labeling (Aspinall et al, 2007).

Second, clarity and precision in writing instructions also help the pharmacist. Federal regulations now mandate that pharmacists must provide education and counseling to patients regarding their medication. Having specific information about why the patient is taking the medication and how the patient should take the medication allows the pharmacist to help reinforce the provider's directions, discover errors in the writing or the filling of the prescription, and obtain feedback about how patients think they should take the medication. Given the growing number of new drugs on the market, the importance of identifying the symptom, indication, or intended effect for which the medication is being prescribed becomes more important and can be added in just a few words, for example, "for nausea," "at headache onset," etc. This additional information allows the pharmacist who is dispensing the prescription to help assess compliance and reinforce the provider's instructions. An example of this can be seen with propranolol, which may be used to treat several different problems. It would be nonsensical for a pharmacist to explain how important it is for a patient to take the medication to control high blood pressure when the patient is being treated for migraine headaches. Knowing the intent of the treatment will aid the pharmacist in communicating with the patient and providing feedback to the provider (Bernstein et al, 2007).

Finally, specific instructions on the container assist the prescriber in reviewing medications ordered by other prescribers. Patients should always bring all medications that they take with them to each office visit. Errors may be detected more easily when instructions on each container are examined. The number of tablets/capsules/teaspoons is designated by small roman numerals, for example, one = *i*, two = *ii*, three = *iii*, etc. Examples of signatures might include the following: "Take i tablet 1 hour before eating or 2 hours after eating 3 times a day," "Mix i teaspoon in a full glass of orange juice to be taken morning and evening," or "Take ii capsules with food each morning." See Table 8-2 for examples of abbreviations commonly used in prescribing medications.

- *Subscription*—The pharmacist is instructed on how to compound the medicine. Although compounding pharmacies still exist, the advent of modern pharmaceutical

TABLE 8-2   Abbreviations Commonly Used in Prescription Writing

Abbreviation	Meaning
sig	Directions for use
qAM	Every morning
bid	Two times daily while awake
tid	Three times daily while awake
qid	Four times daily while awake
q8h	Every 8 hours around the clock
ac	Before meals
pc	After meals
hs	At hour of sleep or bedtime
tsp	Teaspoon
prn	As needed

packaging and unit dosing means that this component of the prescription usually is met by specifying the dosage form (capsule, tablet, liquid, suspension, cream, ointment) and the amount to be dispensed. The prescriber may specify that the product is to be taken PO, IV, IM, etc. (Bridge, 2007). The abbreviation "D" preceding the amount to be dispensed is used to indicate "Give."

- *Quantity or volume*—This indicates how much medication is to be dispensed. Order enough for the standard course of the medication or enough to last until the next scheduled visit. Order standard volumes when writing for liquids. The *Physicians' Drug Reference* or package insert lists standard volumes under "How Supplied." Sometimes, the volume or number of doses that may be ordered is limited by how much will be paid for by a prescription reimbursement plan.

- *To summarize*—In writing this part of the prescription, the first line usually contains the drug name and strength. The second line contains the instructions for taking the drug. The third line tells the pharmacist how much and in what form the medication should be dispensed.

Bottom Portion

The bottom portion of the preprinted prescription form contains other standard information. The number of refills and the prescriber's signature and credentials are required. If a controlled substance is prescribed, the federal DEA number is also to be listed. Finally, some prescriptions include a box that should be checked if generic substitution is authorized.

- *Refills*—This section indicates to the pharmacist and to the patient whether this drug may be refilled. Refills are not permitted on Schedule II drugs. On other scheduled drugs, a maximum of five refills or a 6 months' supply is allowed, whichever comes first. On nonscheduled legend drugs, individual states set limits on the maximum number of refills allowed by law. Medicare, Medical Assistance (Medicaid), and insurance plans often limit the number of medications that may be dispensed per prescription. The prescriber should always indicate the number of refills permitted or should write "NO REFILL" to discourage the patient from entering a number. If it is left blank, the pharmacist will have to contact the prescriber by telephone should a patient request a refill.

- *Provider signature*—Most states require that the prescriber's name must be legibly printed, stamped, or typed following the prescriber signature. Any credentials required by the state should appear after the signature.
- *DEA number*—Federal law requires that this number must appear on all prescriptions for controlled substances. (It may appear at the top or the bottom of the prescription form, as dictated by state law.) In most states, hospital house staff members who are not licensed within the state may use the hospital DEA number when writing outpatient prescriptions for Schedule III to V drugs. Most states do not recognize a hospital DEA number for Schedule II drugs on outpatient prescriptions. To reduce exposure of the prescriber's number, DEA numbers should not be used for identification or other purposes and should not be pre-printed on the prescription form.
- *Generic substitutions*—The provider should indicate whether or not the medication ordered may be dispensed through a generic substitution. Through efforts to decrease cost, this procedure is becoming more common. However, providers must evaluate the bioequivalence of different generic products if substitution is permitted. If you do not wish a generic substitution, be sure to write "Dispense as written" or "Brand medically necessary."

ELECTRONIC DRUG PRESCRIPTIONS OR E-SIGN

In 2000, President Clinton signed the Electronic Signatures in Global and National Commerce Act, known as "E-Sign." This new law affects state and federal requirements related to prescriptions. The importance of the law is that although it does not require individuals to use or accept electronic records or signatures, it does give those records and signatures legal enforceability when they are used.

The E-Sign Act states that electronic records and electronic signatures that are used in any transaction "in or affecting interstate or foreign commerce" have the same legal effect as their paper and handwritten counterparts. E-Sign then, effectively voids requirements that prescriptions be written on paper or printed as a hard copy. Furthermore, E-Sign does away with state and federal requirements that prescriptions be "hand signed" or signed by the practitioner "in writing" or in the practitioner's "own handwriting." (Regulations of the DEA originally required that a prescription for a Schedule II drug could be filled only upon presentation of a written prescription signed by the practitioner. Under traditional practice, as outlined by the DEA, a Schedule II prescription could be faxed, but the controlled substance would not have been dispensed until the pharmacist had reviewed the written and signed original prescription [Hirsch, 2000; Krohn, 2003].)

E-Sign also makes it clear that any record-keeping requirement related to transactions involving interstate commerce may be met when electronic records are kept. The electronic record must accurately reflect the information to be retained and must remain accessible to all who have a right to see the information. An electronic record that meets these two criteria satisfies the requirement that the "original" record must be kept. All state and federal agencies were required to revise their laws based on this statute. State and federal agencies also may specify performance standards related to the retention of electronic records and signatures, such as standards that ensure accuracy, record integrity, and access to retained records. E-Sign specifically and emphatically prohibits the reimposition of tangible or paper record requirements (except for compelling law enforcement or national security reasons) (Hirsch, 2000; Krohn, 2003).

DRUG PRESCRIBING ETIQUETTE

Many policies for prescription writing have come from tradition, common sense, or institutional practice. A search of the literature produces very few answers about how to handle specific problems or what is universally deemed appropriate. However, prescribers encounter "policies" frequently as they try to care for their patients. In one research study of the prescription-writing behavior of internal medicine and family practice residents, 85% of respondents reported that they had written prescriptions for nonpatients. Using answers based on what they would do in specific vignettes, under certain circumstances, up to 95% of residents would write a prescription for an individual who is not their patient (e.g., a sibling). Thirteen percent of residents believed that some ethical guidelines on prescription writing activity exist. Only 4% of residents reported that they were aware of federal or state laws that address the appropriateness of physician prescription writing for nonpatients. None of the residents were able to describe the circumstances that make prescription writing for nonpatients illegal or unethical based on legal statutes or ethical guidelines, respectively. Because practice habits are established during completion of the educational program and initial clinical experience, it is important that all drug prescribers learn about the ethical, legal, and liability implications of writing prescriptions (Aboff et al, 2002).

New prescribers will learn quickly that there are some acceptable and some less than acceptable prescribing behaviors:

- Federal law stipulates that providers may not write prescriptions for narcotics for themselves or their family members. There is no written prohibition against providers writing prescriptions for other nonnarcotic controlled substances for themselves or their family members. However, it is considered a lack of good judgment to do so, unless there are no other providers in the area. A person who is sick enough to require this type of drug probably needs the evaluation of someone besides a family member.
- If a provider consistently writes prescriptions for controlled substances for family members, the pharmacist would probably call to discuss this with the provider. There is no law that requires pharmacists to do so; it would simply be a courtesy to let providers know that their behavior does not fit within the norm. However, the DEA, which also closely monitors controlled substance prescription writing, would likely initiate an investigation if prescribing to family came to their attention.
- Health maintenance organizations (HMOs), particularly in the western part of the United States, have begun to closely monitor the prescribing practices of their provider

employees. Prescriptions written for family members in these plans may not qualify for reimbursement under this more closely restricted supervision. This would be particularly true for providers such as dentists who write prescriptions for hormone replacement therapy or oral contraceptives for their wives or anyone else. This would be perceived as exceeding their scope of authority.

- Prescriptions that are refilled frequently, although the patient is not required to return to the provider for evaluation of response, stimulate questions in the minds of pharmacists about the therapeutic goal.
- Providers often have large caches of drug samples, some of which they trade or share with other providers who might not ordinarily have access to those products. This practice is on the margin of legality and, if known, might prompt an investigation.
- It is risky to write a prescription without seeing a friend. Remember, if the patient is not in the practice, the provider is still legally responsible for whatever he accepts responsibility for doing. Friendship should not enter into this very serious professional responsibility. If something seems out of the norm, stay away from it; this is a good rule for a provider to follow, especially if he is new to the prescribing role.
- Controlled substances must be returned to a "reverse distributor"—someone who is authorized to accept outdated controlled substances. Review the information from the DEA on how to return medications (U.S. Department of Justice, 2006).

AVOIDING MISTAKES

It is infrequent that one encounters a provider who approaches writing prescriptions casually. However, concern about not making a mistake is not all that is required to avoid problems. Clearly, the most important factor required for safe prescription writing is an adequate knowledge base on the part of the provider (Cohen, 2007). Good intentions do not compensate for a lack of knowledge. Because numbers and types of drugs are some of the most frequently changing components of any part of health care, prescribers must keep up-to-date. Prescribers often continue to prescribe the same medications in the same ways as when they were students. With the continual growth in pharmacologic knowledge, this may be not only limiting, but dangerous (Grissinger, 2007).

An influx of new drugs places additional demands on the prescriber. Research by pharmaceutical researchers (Groves et al, 2002) has demonstrated that most physicians have a "total drug repertoire" that contains an average of 144 drug preparations. These drugs constitute a number of "evoked sets"—a pooling of different sets that contain the small number of possible treatments that a provider might consider for different conditions. The drugs in these "evoked sets" parallel the life cycle of a drug on the market—introduction, growth, maturity, and decline. Marketing firms try to influence the rate of "diffusion" of information about their products while drugs are under development by sending product information to providers. Recently, they also have focused on direct-to-consumer advertising to draw attention to new products. Whether or when a provider adds or drops a drug to his "evoked set" depends on whether he is an "innovator, early adopter, early major-

ity, late majority, or laggard." Groves et al found that 5.4% of new prescriptions written over a 12-month period were for a drug newly adopted by that physician within the previous 12 months. Furthermore, when a new prescription was written, 42% of the time this was done to replace a drug that was part of the repertoire (Groves et al, 2005).

The 1999 Institute of Medicine report "To Err Is Human" estimated that medication errors account for 7000 deaths per year; this led to the House Commerce Subcommittee on Health and Environment hearing on this problem in February of the year 2000. This report is filled with descriptions of errors in health care, including what caused them and what might be done. Virtually every health-related organization has devoted newsletters, websites, or journal articles to the issue of medication errors within their discipline or organization.

Research studies have shown that errors in writing prescriptions are fairly common, and that they occur at a rate of 14% to 40%, depending on the study and the variables examined (Aspinall et al, 2007; Devine et al, 2007; Grissinger, 2007). In one study of physician behavior, the most frequent errors included ordering of nonformulary drugs and erroneous or unspecified dosage strength. No difference in error rate was noted among physicians who had completed various levels of training. Other studies documented errors in drug use, some of which could be reduced by adding the patient's diagnosis to the prescription to stimulate questions about the appropriateness of the drug selected (Hustey et al, 2007; Koczmara et al, 2006; Mann et al, 2007). One particularly large study cited specific factors associated with errors such as not noting a decline in renal or hepatic function that requires alteration of drug therapy; ignoring patient history of allergy to the same medication class; using the wrong drug name, dosage form, or abbreviation for both brand and generic names; incorrect dosage calculations; and atypical or unusual and critical dosage frequency considerations. In this same study, the group of factors most commonly associated with errors consisted of those related to knowledge and the application of knowledge related to drug therapy (30%); knowledge and the use of knowledge regarding patient factors that affect drug therapy (29.2%); use of calculations, decimal points, or unit and rate expression factors (17.5%); and nomenclature factors (incorrect drug name, dosage form, or abbreviation) (13.4%) (Cohen, 2007). A 2005 study that evaluated the types of medication errors that occur in a pediatric emergency room found that 59% of prescriptions contained errors. Minor omissions represented the most common error (62%), followed by incomplete directions (23%), dose/directions errors (6%), and unclear quantity to dispense (5%). The number of errors was inversely related to the years of experience of the prescriber (Taylor et al, 2005).

What we have learned is that medication errors result from single or multiple breakdowns in a system's continuum of diagnosing an ailment, planning a therapeutic regimen, prescribing and dispensing drugs, and administering the drug. Many errors are attributable to the failure to disseminate drug knowledge.

What leads to other common errors in prescription writing? One study suggests that some conditions are more likely to produce prescribing errors: those related to the work environment (workload, caring for other providers' patients, hurried prescribing), those related to the team (incomplete written communication, verbal orders), and those related to the individual (hunger, tiredness, knowledge deficit). Staffing shortages, poor work environment, low morale, inexperience, excessive tasks, absence of protocols, unhelpful patients, complex diseases, and language or communication problems are also contributing factors (Dean, 2002).

Certainly the failure to write clearly and specifically causes many problems. Analysis has shown that 80% of the errors due to illegible handwriting are caused by only a few providers (Slomski, 2007). Pharmacists may inadvertently substitute drugs because of a combination of illegible handwriting on the prescription and the pharmacist's misinterpretation of other clues that might have prevented the errors (Cohen, 2007). Individuals who cannot or do not write clearly may want to print in block capital letters rather than use cursive writing. Occasionally, a prescriber's handwriting is so poor that, to avoid problems, he has rubber stamps made or uses preprinted pads for the prescriptions that he often writes. Increasingly, offices are using computers to electronically transmit prescriptions to pharmacies, thus reducing illegibility problems. E-prescribing has been touted as a way to improve patient safety through generation of legible, accurate prescriptions that have been checked for harmful interactions (Krohn, 2003). These systems are promising yet not widespread enough to currently make a difference.

Many other errors occur through carelessness or inattention on the part of either the prescriber or the pharmacist. Regulations to restrict the numbers of hours that hospital house staff practice are aimed at helping health care providers to be more alert when they work, including when they are writing prescriptions.

Labeling the prescription with the exact times of day the medication is to be taken, such as 6:00 AM, 12:00 PM, 6:00 PM, and 12:00 AM, may reduce some medication errors. Providers should keep in mind that patients will be more compliant if the regimen complements their daily schedule, and if the instructions are easily understood. To improve patient understanding, instructions should be written on the bottle and on an instruction sheet in large enough print for someone who is visually impaired (Cohen, 2007). It is also important to educate each patient aggressively about the names and purposes of all prescription drugs. This helps reduce errors by making the patient a partner in the process.

Based on a survey of successful malpractice lawsuits involving medications, Buppert (2006) suggests some specific things that should be done to reduce the potential for problematic prescriptions:

- Write clearly, or invest in an electronic prescription transmission system.
- When a patient has disclosed suicidal ideation, write for no more than a 7-day supply of any medication that could be lethal if taken all at once.
- Warn patients of side effects.
- Discontinue a medication when it causes a cautioned side effect.
- Get informed consent when a drug can cause permanent side effects and less risky alternatives are available.
- If you are prescribing differently from the directions on the drug manufacturer's package insert (i.e., "off-label"), document the rationale for deviating from the package insert instructions, and be prepared to prove that the standard of care supports the alternative prescribing regimen.

- When a medication is known to cause some adverse effects after long-term use, avoid using the drug for long-term therapy, or monitor carefully for the onset of potential problems.
- Ask, listen, and alter the plan.

Table 8-3 describes some other specific errors and how they might be avoided.

ADMINISTRATIVE CONCERNS

Formularies

In an effort to reduce costs and channel prescriptions to a smaller number of total drugs, a growing number of organizations have established drug formularies. Many managed care organizations, HMOs, private insurance plans, and state Medicaid programs, as well as federal Medicare programs, the Veterans Administration, and the military, have created their own formularies to meet the specific needs of their patient populations. Although some health care providers object to placement of any limitations on the drugs they may prescribe, this is a growing trend throughout the nation. Pressure is also put on pharmaceutical companies to provide drugs to some programs at a greatly reduced rate if they wish to have their products appear on the approved formulary list. How the formularies are established, how inclusive they are, and how regularly they are updated based on the latest scientific care guidelines are the factors that determine whether the institutional formulary will be an asset or a liability for the provider. A formulary may restrict providers from using those agents with which they are most comfortable or have the broadest experience. The most frequent complaint against formularies is that they are slow to accept and add new and effective drugs.

As a cost-cutting mechanism, some pharmacies order medications in large doses and then split them. This practice of drug division, by cutting or by weight, leads to inaccuracies in dosage. Prescribers should confirm that the pharmacies they work with do not participate in this risky practice (Bachynsky et al, 2002; Rosenberg et al, 2002; Teng et al, 2002).

Medicaid

To write prescriptions for patients on Medicaid (or Medical Assistance, as it is known in many states), the prescriber must be an authorized Medicaid prescriber. Individuals who apply to the state will be issued a Medicaid provider number to be used on all prescriptions. This number may be different from the Medicaid render number (the number of the person who actually delivers the care to the patient) and the Medicaid reimbursement number (the number of the person who will receive reimbursement for the service). In some situations, all numbers will be for the same provider; in other cases, particularly large institutions, the numbers will all be different.

Medicaid prescriptions are filled only from a Medicaid prescription form provided by the state for that purpose. After filling in the authorized prescriber number, the prescriber should check to see if the patient's Medicaid card is up-to-date before writing the prescription. Each eligible patient must have a separate card.

Because Medicaid is a joint state and federal program, each state has its own specific requirements regarding Medicaid policies. Most states have a Medicaid formulary that identifies a circumscribed number of drugs that will be covered under Medicaid. Many new medications, expensive

TABLE 8-3   Errors Commonly Made in Writing Prescriptions

Common Error	Solutions
Patients may fail to recognize that they have two prescriptions for the same medication, especially when some drugs may be listed according to generic name and some according to trade name.	Use nonproprietary names when ordering and always use the same drug name when writing a prescription; avoid the chance that the patient may take one "digoxin" tablet per day and one "Lanoxin" tablet per day; add patient diagnosis to prescription.
Confusion of look-alike drugs	Watch for drugs that are similar in spelling: acetohexamide vs. acetazolamide, hydralazine vs. hydroxyzine. Watch for other minor differences: chloroquine HCl vs. chloroquine phosphate, quinidine sulfate vs. quinidine gluconate. Drug names should never be abbreviated.
Errors in dosage strength or concentration	Decimal points may be difficult to see: Use 50 and not 50.0; use 0.5 and not .5. Solid dosage forms often come in a variety of strengths; liquid preparations, particularly for infants and children, are sometimes available in different concentrations. It is dangerous to request a drug by volume without specifying the concentration, particularly for children; order the standard volumes listed in texts or package inserts when writing for liquid antibiotics; for children, have a system of systematic double-checking of accuracy of prescriptions. Pharmacists may ask patients to turn in old containers when new products are ordered; this provides a double-check on accuracy and on what the patient is taking.
Patients fail to understand how to take medication.	Never write "take as directed"; be specific about what you want the patient to do.
Use of misleading abbreviations in writing prescriptions:	
tid vs. q8h	Clarify the difference between q8h and tid: tid means while awake.
hs: hour of sleep or take at bedtime	What if the patient takes a midday nap or works nights? Clarify sleeping habits.
ac or pc: before or after meals	What if patient eats more than three meals/day?
× 3d	Does this mean for 3 days or for three doses?
qd	Means every day but is often mistaken for qid, four times a day
u = units	Avoid using u as an abbreviation for unit; 4 u of regular insulin may be read as 40 units.
tsp = teaspoonful	The amount of drug varies a good deal depending on the specific teaspoon that is being used; this is not a good term to use when ordering a drug whose exact dosage is important.
prn = as needed	Patients should have a very clear idea about when they "need" the drug; place limits on the numbers of pills taken, e.g., "take 1 tablet every 4 hours as needed." Do not write "refill prn"; it means *refill indefinitely* and few prescriptions should be given that latitude.
Patient altering of prescription to increase number of refills or number of pills	Write "one refill" and not "1 refill" to avoid tempting patients to change it to "4 or 10 refills." Many prescribers draw a tight circle around the number of pills to be dispensed so that patients may not insert a 1 in front of the number or zeroes after the number, or the provider may write "ten" instead of 10 to limit tampering with the number.

Data from Cohen, 2007.

trade name products, or drugs designated as "less than effective" by the FDA have been omitted from these formularies. With the slowing economy and the tremendous financial pressures experienced by states, additional cuts were initiated in 2003 by the establishment of state "Preferred Drug Formulary" lists that reduced the authorized drug lists to around 100 drugs—omitting many of the more expensive trade name drugs. Payment will not be made for drugs outside the formulary unless a waiver stipulating that the treatment is medically necessary or life sustaining has been obtained before the prescription is submitted for filling. Many drugs that have gone from legend to over-the-counter still have some dosages that are available by prescription so that Medicaid or insurance coverage will apply. It is standard among most states that Medicaid prescriptions must be filled within 10 days, and the maximum number of refills is two. (Birth control pills often may be filled for a maximum of six cycles.) The prescription usually may not be written for more than a 100-day supply of drug. (This includes the initial prescription and two refills.)

Out-of-State Prescriptions

Patients should be cautioned to get prescriptions filled before they leave the state, or they should verify that there will not be a problem getting them filled in the state to which they are going. Some states prohibit pharmacists from filling prescriptions written in another state or may have regulations that do not allow them to fill prescriptions if they were written by a PA or a nurse practitioner NP. However, many states have no specific laws regarding the filling of prescriptions written out of state. Regardless of the law, pharmacists may refuse to fill any prescription about which they have suspicions. This is particularly true of prescriptions for controlled substances.

More and more, out-of-state prescriptions are becoming a factor for prescribers to consider. The population is mobile. People both move frequently and travel throughout the country or the world on business. Patients may cross state lines to receive care at the nearest facility. Children may leave home to go to universities in other states. Some prescription plans are centralized, with all prescriptions being filled in a central place in the country and mailed to the enrolled member. Advances in telehealth may make the distance between prescriber and patient less important but may create the need for different types of licensing, monitoring, and law.

Another recent trend has been for insurance plans to direct their members to send prescriptions to out-of-state mail order or Internet pharmacies, where costs may be less. Many of these large "virtual pharmacies" have refused to recognize legal prescriptions written by providers who are not physicians. The resolution of this problem has been a focus of national NP groups (Edmunds, 2003a).

A substantially different problem is for patients to use the Internet to obtain medications without a prescription, or without seeing a physician. This practice is illegal, and any drugs purchased over the Internet, particularly those coming in from outside the country, are subject to monitoring and seizure by the FDA in conjunction with other federal agencies. Many of the drugs available outside the United States are counterfeit drugs, and their purity, safety, and efficacy are not guaranteed. Until recently, the United States has been able to limit the use of these drugs through tight federal control. The use of the Internet for ordering makes control of these products more and more problematic (Edmunds, 2003b) (see www.FDA.gov/oc/buyonline).

Prescriptions by Telephone Orders

When traditional prescriptions are used, except for prescriptions for Schedule I and II drugs, any prescriptions may be sent via telephone to a pharmacy. (E-prescriptions may be sent for all scheduled medications.) Most states provide that in an emergency situation, the pharmacist may dispense a limited amount (usually not more than a 48-hour supply) of a Schedule II drug on the verbal order of a provider. The provider then must make sure that the pharmacy has a written prescription to cover that order within 72 hours.

A common practice in some busy offices is for lay personnel such as receptionists, rather than nurses, to call the pharmacy with a telephone prescription order. This does not remove the provider's legal responsibility for the accuracy of the order. Thus, providers who call in their own telephone orders to the pharmacy maintain some control over their liability. In some states, it is prohibited by state law for providers to delegate this responsibility to another person.

Prescription Refilling Policy

Many prescriptions allow the patient to obtain refills to the original order. If refills are left on the original prescription, the pharmacy may fill them. In most states, a prescription is valid for a year after it is written (6 months for Schedule III to V prescriptions), regardless of the number of refills on the prescription. After this time, a new prescription must be obtained from the health care prescriber.

If no refills are remaining on the prescription, or if the original prescription does not have refills, then the prescriber who wrote the original prescription may authorize additional refills if appropriate. State regulations vary, and the prescriber should confirm who can approve the refill, who can receive that approval, and how that information is conveyed. In most instances, a refill authorization must be received from the prescriber or from a designated agent of the prescriber, usually someone employed to transmit a prescription drug order on behalf of the prescriber (Jolowsky, 2007).

State laws also dictate how information can be transmitted, who can receive this information, and what documentation is required. A pharmacist is allowed to receive the information, and in some states, this authority is extended to pharmacy interns and technicians. If received audibly, the information must be put into writing. Most states allow facsimile copies for prescriptions and renewals; this is viewed as medical information transferred between health care professionals. It is the pharmacist's responsibility to ascertain the validity of the information.

The patient's medical record at the office should document that refills of the prescription are authorized. This information is conveyed, via the presigned order form, to the pharmacy. It is then the responsibility of the pharmacist who is accepting and filling the prescription to use judgment to ensure the validity of the information (Jolowsky, 2007).

Dispensing of Medications

The actual provision of medication to the patient from an office or store supply is called *dispensing*. This is different from administering medication, the process commonly performed by registered nurses wherein a pharmacist dispenses the medication and the nurse physically sees that the medication is taken by the patient. Some state laws allow for limited dispensing of medications, usually in the following two situations.

Drug sampling is a type of limited dispensing. Pharmaceutical company field representatives leave medications with health care providers with prescriptive authority who have authorization to receive them. Because of the Pharmaceutical Drug Manufactures Act of 1988, which was passed to decrease provider abuse of sampled drugs, drug field representatives are not authorized to leave samples with any prescriber unless it can be validated that the individual is a legal prescriber. The state boards of medicine give validation companies information about physician prescribers every year and "validate" that they are licensed prescribers. The situation is more complex for nonphysician prescribers. For example, in many states, NPs do not have independent prescriptive authority but have delegated authority established through a collaborative agreement with a physician. In those states, a validation company not only must ensure that the practitioner is a licensed prescriber but also must obtain the name of the physician with whom they have a collaborative agreement. This information must come from an authoritative agency, usually the board of nursing. In many states, the boards of nursing cannot or will not give validation companies this information. In attempting to be compliant with Prescription Drug Marketing Act (PDMA) regulations and provide samples to NPs, companies have attempted to have NPs fill out a form that asks for information about their license and collaborating physician. If NPs are willing to fill out the forms, they are being given drug samples. Many NPs refuse to sign these forms, not understanding why they are being asked to do so (Esat, 2003). In some states, however, NPs are authorized to accept and distribute samples by the written rules and regulations that govern NP prescriptive authority.

Medication packets with a few doses, primarily of a medication that is new to the market, are given to providers to encourage them to try the product so they can gain experience with it and then recommend it to their patients. Multiple problems with both the process and the theory behind drug sampling have led to a decline in this process over the years.

Limited dispensing of medications is legal in emergency facilities and is confined to the dispensing of one or two doses of specific medications required in emergency situations. A few doses of narcotic analgesics or antibiotics are the most frequently dispensed drugs in these settings.

Drug Substitution by the Pharmacist

When prescribers write a prescription using a product's trade name, the question of generic substitution arises. In states where generic substitution is automatically allowed, or where prescription or insurance plans require generic substitution whenever possible, the pharmacist will have to determine whether there is an acceptable generic substitute for an ordered medication. In many situations, pharmacists may dispense the generic substitute without notifying the health care provider. They should, however, notify the patient, pass along cost savings to the patient, and indicate the substituted brand on the original prescription and the prescription drug label. If a prescriber is concerned about the bioequivalence of a particular medication or for patient compliance reasons, the prescriber may write "Do not substitute" or "Dispense as written" on the original prescription, if no change from what is written is desired.

PREVENTING PROBLEMS IN DRUG USE

The health care prescriber faces three common problems in the process of providing medications: the abusing patient, the abusing health care provider, and the financially needy patient.

Most health care prescribers will, at some point in their practice, encounter drug-seeking patients. These often include "professional" patients who have become addicted to narcotics or well-intentioned individuals who are misusing drugs. In either case, the provider's index of suspicion should be aroused, particularly about the need for controlled substances, when a patient (1) asks for narcotics by name, indicating that they are the only thing that will relieve the problem; (2) carries copies of abnormal laboratory tests, electrocardiograms that document a myocardial infarction, or other documents that support subjective complaints of pain; or (3) calls frequently seeking refills or increasingly larger amounts of medication because he lost or spilled the medicine.

Validation of suspicious behavior of a patient may be confirmed in talking with the pharmacist. Attempts to refill prescriptions early, change prescriptions so that more drug will be dispensed, and use multiple providers to obtain prescriptions for the same drugs are all indications that the patient has a problem. Sometimes, pharmacists have received alerts from other pharmacists or hospitals that a particular patient is in the area telling a particular story. This type of cooperation and sharing of information helps assist health care providers in avoiding traps or prevents them from being taken in by a scam artist.

Providers who are feeling increasingly uncomfortable about patient drug requests should carefully confront patients about their observations. They also should offer support and assistance if the patient inappropriately relies on medications. They should not continue to provide prescriptions to the patient. Providers who feel that they cannot continue to meet the needs of a patient have a responsibility to help that patient find another health care provider.

Occasionally, a pharmacist or a health care provider will discover that a patient has obtained a prescription pad and is writing his or her own prescriptions. This or any other type of illegal behavior must be reported immediately to the police.

The same problems occur when health care providers encounter professional colleagues whose behavior seems inappropriate. When the possibility exists that the health care provider may be involved in drug abuse or misuse, gentle confrontation is essential. These individuals should be referred to the relevant medical, nursing, or pharmacy boards for impaired provider counseling. This is an effective way of acknowledging problems and still remaining in good professional standing so that a license to practice is not permanently sacrificed.

The final type of prescribing problem concerns patients who really need medications but cannot afford to buy them. Many pharmaceutical companies provide medications for people in need, apart from their drug sampling program to providers. NeedyMeds is an Internet site that contains information on patient assistance programs offered by pharmaceutical manufacturers. It provides listings on more than 125 companies and 800 drugs. The site (www.needymeds. com) provides an alert service so that users will know whenever changes are made to the database.

GOOD COMMUNICATION AND DEVELOPING A POSITIVE RELATIONSHIP WITH THE PHARMACIST

The specialized knowledge and watchful eye of the pharmacist may be an important resource for the primary care provider. Establishing a personal relationship with the pharmacists most likely to fill the prescriber's prescriptions helps the provider to create a team with the goal of eliminating errors and increasing patient satisfaction with medications.

Pharmacists are particularly aware of changing drug formulations in over-the-counter products. Because of this, they are able to guide primary care providers in the most effective over-the-counter products to recommend to patients. Pharmacists also tend to be aware of which diseases are endemic in the community and what medications seem to be most effective in controlling them. As pharmacology specialists, they often should be consulted when one is selecting drug therapy for a difficult case. Finally, pharmacists may provide the one centralized source of oversight of the many prescriptions that patients receive from different providers. In this capacity, pharmacists who use sophisticated software are often the ones who detect or prevent drug interactions or overdosages, and who discover contraindications.

It is true that in the past an adversarial role developed between some pharmacists and new nonphysician prescribers in some states. However, as new prescribers have demonstrated their competence and willingness to be part of a responsible health care team, most pharmacists have become very supportive and helpful to these new prescribers. What little research has been conducted in this area demonstrates that very few pharmacists report problems with prescriptions written by nonphysicians. The most successful prescriber–pharmacist relationships are built on mutual respect for each other's skills and knowledge.

Many primary care providers who are new to an area or new to the prescriber role would do well to visit their local pharmacies and meet the pharmacists who work there. Providing some written material about who they are and about their background, education, credentials, and clinical interests may be important in establishing a positive relationship. Initiating consultation with pharmacists, making time to answer their questions, being receptive to suggestions, and expressing appreciation for assistance are essential in establishing a relationship that will result in the best care for the patient. Pharmacists often hear what patients say about their office visits. Thus, they may be a valuable source of information about patient understanding and acceptance of the care they have received and their willingness or ability to comply with ordered therapy. All of this feedback is available if a good relationship is established.

The prescription is a formalized communication between the prescriber and the pharmacist. Although a prescription contains the very formulaic information required by law, there is no reason why specific directions or concerns for the pharmacist about the medication cannot be written on the prescription. An example might be particular concerns about drug bioequivalence of generic agents and a note asking that the same generic agent be used each time the prescription is filled, or a note asking the pharmacist to tell the patient that the prescription cannot be refilled until the patient returns to the provider for further evaluation.

SUMMARY

Writing a prescription may be stressful at first, until the format is ingrained in the student's mind. The most important factors to consider are the accuracy and appropriateness of the prescription, not the format. When the health care provider works together with the pharmacist, a relationship may be established that will benefit all individuals involved.

evolve   A continually updated list of useful WebLinks may be found in the Evolve Resources at http://evolve.elsevier.com/Edmunds/NP/

Treatment Guidelines and Evidence-Based Decision Making

9

CRITICAL DECISION MAKING

One of the writers to dominate the field of critical thinking, Eddy, observed that the quality of health care is determined by two main factors: the quality of the decisions that determine what actions are taken, and the quality with which those actions are executed—what to do and how to do it. If the wrong actions are chosen, no matter how skillfully they are executed, the quality of care will suffer. Similarly, if the correct actions are chosen but the execution is flawed, the quality of care will suffer (Eddy, 1990). Health care requires clinicians who can make decisions autonomously. It is therefore essential that health care providers consciously strive to develop effective problem-solving and decision-making skills (Edwards, 2007).

In the past, how did students learn to make clinical decisions? The traditional educational approach in all health care disciplines until the last decade was an implicit apprenticeship model, in which health care providers follow the actions of attending physicians or preceptors with little attention to the mechanics of the diagnostic and treatment strategies. Thus, the quality of the learning is often highly dependent on the influence of the mentor.

Diagnostic reasoning is an important part of the health provider's role. It is not uncommon in the first diagnosis and management class in medical school to find students absolutely silent when they hear the first discussions about how to make a diagnosis "You mean that is how you arrive at a diagnosis? Your best guess?!" Some clinicians also comment, "I must have missed something. It has to be more precise than that."

Clinical decision making has components of judging and evaluating, but decision making implies not just contemplation but also action based on choices. Certainly part of the process of decision making is *critical thinking*, a term that has been in vogue for many years in nursing. However, implicit in the process of decision making is establishing goals and taking risks beyond what is thought of as critical thinking.

The intrusion of insurance plans, restricted formularies, and managed care into clinical practice means that resources for health care clinicians are restricted. The presence of many patients without any insurance or who are underinsured affects clinical decision making in a practice. Ordering multiple tests to rule in or rule out various disease states is not an option. More than ever before, health care providers must learn critical thinking skills in making proper clinical judgments. So the question becomes, "How do we individually and collectively ensure that higher-level thinking is engaged for health care problem solving?" (Ellerman et al, 2006).

CRITICAL THINKING

Benjamin S. Bloom's seminal work in 1956 on the original taxonomy of educational objectives for the cognitive domain does not contain the term *decision making*. However, each of the two higher cognitive domains—synthesis and evaluation—contains verbs that involve planning, composing, designing, constructing, creating, setting up, organizing, appraising, evaluating, comparing, revising, and assessing—all components of the decision-making process as recognized in the 2000 revision of that taxonomy (Anderson et al, 2000).

Much of the initial research about critical thinking in clinical settings was completed in the 1980s and 1990s by nurses. Much of the early work was conducted by nursing faculty as they prepared for National League for Nursing program accreditation. This early work by nurses and not by physicians informs the literature on critical thinking. These early writers agree that critical thinking involves dimensions of logic, problem solving (Beyer, 1985), and scientific inquiry and might be defined as "careful, deliberate, goal directed thinking based on principles of science and the scientific method" (Bandman & Bandman, 1995). Clearly, the construct of critical thinking is not a set body of knowledge but rather a nonlinear dynamic process (Jacobs et al, 1997; Videbeck, 1997); it is not an outcome.

Watson and Glaser (1964) dominated the literature about critical thinking in nursing, arguing that it has two basic components: knowledge and an attitude of inquiry. *Knowledge* includes knowledge of the domain-specific subject matter and knowledge of specific mental operations or critical thinking skills. *Attitude* denotes frame of mind or an attitude of inquiry, curiosity, and willingness or desire to examine and explore the problem. This component is uniquely developed in each individual and results from the health care provider's personality and culturally determined behavioral norms.

However, knowledge and an attitude of inquiry alone do not capture true critical thinking. The thinker must critically appraise knowledge. This component of thinking allows the thinker to apply, synthesize, and evaluate what is known and, as such, brings critical thinking into the highest cognitive domain. This process of critical thinking is outlined in Figure 9-1.

As can be seen from this figure, the clinician's knowledge is key. Clearly, the beginning student or novice will have less knowledge than the expert. This is particularly true in clinical practice fields like medicine and nursing. However, health care provider students do not have minds as empty as blank pages. They have information from previous courses and experiences. RNs returning for nurse practitioner (NP)

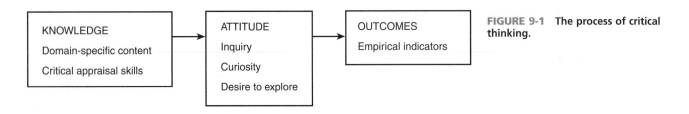

FIGURE 9-1   **The process of critical thinking.**

education may have had years of successful clinical practice. Many older students have had other careers before they turned to health care. All these students have some knowledge but need additional information that is evaluated and then organized so it becomes usable. Early researchers suggested that the mind might be thought of as a series of matrices in which information is stored. The matrix is entered and information retrieved as the individual recognizes patterns, sees similarities, recognizes what is important, generalizes, and uses common sense (Elstein et al, 1990).

Beginners have inconsistent information. Recognition of their lack of knowledge dictates the organization of the curriculum. For example, advanced pharmacology content is wasted in the first semester before students master components of health assessment, physiology, and other basic information about diagnostic or treatment methods that will give important context to their drug knowledge.

Research into the critical thinking that a clinician uses in diagnostic reasoning and problem solving suggests two different theories of clinical expertise. The first theory proposes that experts perform better than novices because they have better problem-solving strategies. The alternative theory suggests that experts perform better because they have more knowledge. Current evidence in the literature supports the latter position—that clinical expertise is largely a function of domain-specific knowledge (Elstein et al, 1990; Lange et al, 1997). For example, several researchers have found that the diagnostic strategies used by experts and novices are very similar. Norman and colleagues suggest that experts do not possess any innate or learned advantage in problem-solving techniques. Rather, experts solve problems better because they know more in their domains than novices do, and problem-solving expertise generalizes somewhat within a domain of medical knowledge (e.g., rheumatology) but does not necessarily generalize to other domains (e.g., pulmonary, cardiology) (Norman et al, 1985). This early research has now been substantiated by additional clinical research (Cockcroft, 2007; Crespo et al, 2004; Hadley et al, 2007; Hobgood et al, 2005).

There is no ideal way to think. Thinking processes differ among individuals. The literature suggests that it is possible to facilitate the development of cognitive skills in clinical decision making, but overall, little information is available on how the cognitive skills associated with decision making may be stimulated and, in particular, how the characteristics of critical thinkers may be fostered.

Some examples might prove instructive. In the clinical setting, one wise clinician sends beginning students into the room to begin to interview the patient and then has them report back after they have obtained only the chief complaint. Then, using patient age and gender and the chief complaint, students are asked to generate a differential of all the things that might be responsible for causing the chief complaint. The faculty member helps students with limited knowledge add to their database of possible differentials by assisting them to stretch their thinking. Students then return to the patient with a systematic plan of questioning, which involves asking about all the possible elements on the differential, to rule them in or rule them out. This is a different way of teaching students to think and to organize information, rather than having them ask all the general questions in a standard comprehensive history. Through this method, one also teaches students an expectation about broader thinking and systematic questioning.

In other situations, schemata, algorithms, or mental models have been used in decision making. These are all abstract representations of information gained from experience, and they assist us in understanding the world and the reality in which people exist (Terry et al, 2007). The foundational research of Benner (1984) and Benner and Tanner (1987) emphasizes the place of experience in the quality of thinking.

Although much of critical thinking and clinical decision making may be related to natural curiosity and intelligence, some attributes (steps or tools) tend to make thinking more complete. Myrick and Yonge (2002) describe the importance of preceptor questioning in helping students think critically. If clinicians have knowledge, then it is important to observe what they do with that knowledge so one can determine the extent of critical thinking that is taking place. Some observable behaviors of critical thinkers have been identified as the ability to do the following:

- Distinguish between observation and inference and facts and claims
- Determine the reliability of a claim or source
- Evaluate the accuracy of statements
- Differentiate relevant from irrelevant data
- Differentiate between warranted and unwarranted claims
- Recognize ambiguous or equivocal claims/arguments
- Discern inconsistencies in reasoning
- Identify an argument's strength
- Draw inferences

An additional way of determining whether critical thinking has taken place is to look at the outcomes of the critical thinking process (Box 9-1).

Lack of knowledge, problems in attitude, and flaws in critical appraisal may result in defective thinking. For example, one may have good knowledge of a subject but may be inflexible or unwilling to consider other options or points of view. Likewise, the individual may have curiosity, motivation, and interest but may lack the knowledge necessary to develop alternatives and to consider options (Riddell, 2007; Seldomridge & Walsh, 2006; Turner, 2007).

BOX 9-1 Empirical Indicators of Critical Thinking

SYNTHESIS OF RELEVANT INFORMATION

Obtains data from all sources
Distinguishes relevant from irrelevant data
Validates data obtained
Identifies missing data

PREDICTION OF OUTCOMES

Predicts multiple outcomes
Recognizes ramification of actions

EXAMINATION OF ASSUMPTIONS

Recognizes assumptions
Detects bias
Identifies unstated assumptions

GENERATION OF OPTIONS

Recognizes relationships of action or inaction
Transfers thoughts and concepts to multiple settings
Develops alternate courses of action

IDENTIFICATION OF PATTERNS

Identifies relationships/patterns
Recognizes logical inconsistencies or fallacies
Pinpoints generalizations
Develops plan of action consistent with a model and/or
    seeks alternative models

CHOICE OF ACTIONS

Determines a choice of action
Evaluates the effects of own actions
Evaluates the soundness of conclusions
Measures worth of action to client/society

From Jacobs PM et al: An approach to defining and operationalizing critical thinking, *J Nurs Educ* 36:19-22, 1997.

DECISION MAKING

In exploring how people make decisions, nursing has focused almost exclusively on the process of critical thinking, whereas the medical literature is filled with research on diagnostic and clinical decision making. Reports suggest that in most medical schools, when clinical reasoning is taught, this is provided as an add-on and is not continued as an integral component of the rest of the courses. Because of this lack of curricular integration, one of the early writers on medical decision making concluded that special courses in clinical reasoning appear to have a marginal effect (Chessare et al, 1996). The general focus of most medical curricula is on acquisition of knowledge; how to search for and critically evaluate evidence is a skill that is generally addressed superficially, if at all.

Some of the research findings of the past 20 years about decision making of nurses are provocative. Findings suggest that many nurses are action oriented, resulting in a focus on action rather than on analysis of all relevant data. A study based on NP students found that they often attempted to formulate a diagnosis too early in the decision-making process. Almost all of the NP students had practiced as staff nurses in acute care settings, where rapidly formulating a diagnosis was important. Although that manner of clinical decision making was successful for experienced clinicians, for inexperienced NP students, formulating hypotheses too early often resulted in incomplete assessments (Lipman & Deatrick, 1997). Thus, skills that had helped students as RNs were counterproductive in the new role without a broader knowledge base.

Research suggests that much of the confusion that is seen in some NP students early in their program can be attributed to a reworking of decision-making and critical-thinking skills. The NP program asks students to take their existing domain-specific knowledge, in which they have "expert" skills, and use it to process information in new ways and to exhibit different behaviors. It appears that asking them to do this temporarily suspends use of their previously learned skills. (Another explanation proposed for this phenomenon is that NPs are inhibited by their return to a setting in which they must undergo intense scrutiny of their performance by preceptors/faculty members as they attempt to use newly acquired knowledge and skills [Roberts et al, 1997].) What some faculty members have begun to accept is that combining a nursing education foundation with advanced medical information may require a paradigm shift for the student, prompting reorganization of existing knowledge and critical thinking skills and not just the addition of new knowledge. In this paradigm shift, NP students must move to a new developmental stage that allows them to recognize the limitations of their existing knowledge and must learn how to acquire needed knowledge to assume increased responsibility for their own judgment and decisions. Simply put, the problem for NP students is probably the result of "taking an expert and asking [him] to be a novice again" (Roberts et al, 1997).

The medical literature abounds with reports on decision making and the development of diagnostic skills. One of the best authors to bring together the various theories and ideas has been Eddy (1990, 2005, 2007). He suggests that, in general, the goal of a health care decision maker is to choose an action that is most likely to deliver the outcomes the patient wants. Eddy goes on to identify the two main steps involved in making a clinical decision. First, the outcomes of the different options must be estimated; then, the desirability of the outcomes of each option must be compared. "The first step involves collecting and analyzing whatever evidence exists regarding the benefits, harms, and costs of each option. Because the available evidence is virtually never perfect or complete, this step will also involve some subjective judgment" (Eddy, 2005). For example, should a patient with a prostatic mass continue to be monitored, have chemotherapy, or undergo surgery?

The resulting estimates of that analysis then form the basis for the second step. Three types of comparisons are required in the second step: (1) The benefits of a practice must be compared with the harms (e.g., risks, side effects, inconvenience, length of disability, anxiety), (2) the health outcomes must be compared with the costs, and (3) if it is not possible to do everything because of limited resources, the amount of benefit gained and the resources consumed must be compared with those of other options so that priority will be given to options that have the highest yield (Eddy, 2005) (Figure 9-2).

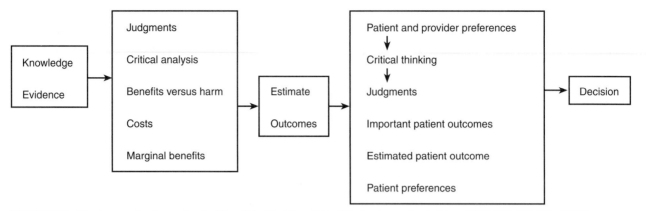

FIGURE 9-2   The two main steps of a decision. (Modified from Eddy DM: Anatomy of a decision, *JAMA* 263:441-443, 1990.)

No matter how explicitly, how consciously, or how correctly each of these steps is performed, these factors must be considered every time a decision is made regarding a health practice. This is true whether the decision is made by an individual clinician, whether a group of health care providers are recommending a guideline for a group of patients, or whether third-party payers are setting coverage policy. To appreciate this, imagine trying to advise a patient regarding the merits of a health practice without considering any evidence of its effects or the magnitude of the benefit or harm caused by the practice, and without caring whether the benefit outweighs the harm.

Anyone who makes a responsible decision regarding a health practice must have some idea, however uncertain, of the evidence that justifies its use, of its consequences, and of its desirability. It is important to separate the decision-making process into these two steps for several reasons. Specifically, Eddy's two steps involve different thought processes, have different anchors, and might be performed by different people. In addition, different degrees of agreement about the results can be expected. The first step is to agree on the facts. The anchor is empirical evidence. The process is a scientific one that involves experiments, analysis of evidence, and forecasting. The required skills are analytic. Finally, assuming there is some evidence to evaluate, it should be possible to get reasonable, open-minded people to agree on the results of this step (Eddy, 2005).

This is where evidence-based medicine (EBM) is to play a role. Essentially, this is the *science* of medicine. It is clear that step one, as so clearly articulated by Eddy, resembles very much the model of critical thinking so dominant in the nursing literature. The terminology and the focus may be a little different from each other, but the basic components of domain-specific knowledge and an attitude of evaluation, along with critical analysis of the data, are embedded in step one of clinical decision making.

Returning to Eddy's model, the second step is to clarify the personal values or preferences of the patient. The move to managed care and the recognition that the patient has rights as a consumer of care with resultant restriction on resources have served to highlight the necessity of joint decision making between the patient and the clinician. The thought process is not analytic but personal and subjective—it is an appeal not to the left side of the brain, but to the right side of the brain, or even the gut. Different people can properly have different preferences. There is no single correct answer, and there is no obligation that everyone must agree (Eddy, 2007).

Now, we are getting to the *art* of medicine.

To the extent that science is involved in this step at all, it is the science of discovering peoples' preferences—through polls, questionnaires, and focus groups—that is involved. Perhaps most important, the people whose preferences count are the patients, because they are the ones who will have to live (or die) with the outcomes. Others might intervene if an individual's decision is based on inaccurate information (e.g., insistence on antibiotic therapy for a viral upper respiratory tract infection), is illegal (e.g., drug abuse), or harms a public interest (e.g., refusal of control measures for an infectious disease), or when the patient is not competent enough to make a decision. However, assuming these complications do not apply, it is the patient's preferences that should determine the decision (Eddy, 2007).

In one of the classic research studies of how expert clinicians make clinical diagnoses, Elstein and colleagues (1990) proposed that expert physicians generate specific diagnostic hypotheses well before the time that they gather most of the data for a particular case. Rather than progressively and systematically converging on a diagnosis through a series of constraining questions, experienced physicians appear to leap directly to a small array of provisional hypotheses very early in their encounter with the patient. These provisional hypotheses are generated out of the physicians' background knowledge of medicine, including their range of specific experiences, in conjunction with the problematic elements recognized in the early stages of encounter with the patient.

The physicians in the Elstein study were considered expert clinicians by their peers. They were not novices but had a substantial body of domain-specific knowledge. In this study, four components of the process of hypothesis generation emerged. Although these are described serially, it is likely that some of them occur together. The components are as follows:

- Attending to initially available cues
- Identifying problematic elements from among these cues and searching long-term memory
- Generating hypotheses and suggestions for further inquiry
- Informally rank-ordering hypotheses according to the physician's subjective estimates

Rank ordering is based on the physician's evaluation of probability (estimates closely approximate the population base rate for a disease), seriousness (life-threatening or incapacitating conditions are ranked higher than their population base rate warrants), treatability (a treatable problem is ranked higher so that any treatment that might possibly be helpful will not be overlooked), and novelty (the uniqueness of the problem keeps the physician interested in the case and ensures that unlikely avenues are explored, thus protecting the patient from the physician's premature closure on a more generally probable hypothesis that, in a particular case, might be in error) (Elstein et al, 1990).

The work of Benner (1984) remains one of the foremost accomplishments in describing the passage of a nurse from novice to expert and in detailing the ways in which nurses with varying levels of experience function. Benner's (1984) seminal work describes the process of skill acquisition by nurses, indicating a developmental approach to decision making, commencing with decision analysis and progressing to hypothetical-deductive reasoning, with the eventual emergence of the expert who functions at an intuitive level. Later, Benner and Tanner (1987) examined the effects of intuition on an expert nurse's ability to make clinical decisions. They identified the following six key aspects of intuitive judgment:

1. Pattern recognition—recognition of relationships
2. Similarity recognition—recognition of relationships despite obvious differences
3. Commonsense understanding—having a deep understanding of a given entity
4. Skilled know-how—ability to visualize a situation
5. Sense of salience—ability to recognize what is important
6. Deliberative rationality—ability to anticipate events

These six aspects are seen to work in synergy in expert practice and not as solo components of behavior. These aspects are remarkably similar to the reported ways in which hypotheses are generated by expert physicians (Elstein et al, 1990).

It is clear, then, that the realities of how nurses and physician experts make clinical decisions are quite similar and may vary from the model of what might be the ideal, as proposed by Eddy. Clearly, the extent of knowledge of the clinician makes a difference, as does the experience of the clinician. However, in view of the switch to a deeper consideration of EBM, the conclusions of clinicians and their behavior, even if they are experts, will increasingly have to be validated by supporting evidence.

In teaching critical decision making, the new guiding principle for teacher–learner interactions might be embodied in the question, "What's the evidence?" This new guiding principle must permeate didactic lectures, discussions on rounds, and case-based sessions. New curricula must foster the development of analytic skills in a more purposive manner (Chessare et al, 1996). Some of the specific competencies that should be taught are summarized in Table 9-1.

It seems clear that diagnostic errors may occur among both experts and novices as a result of inadequate information processing. In Kassirer and Kopelman's important work (1989), diagnostic errors were classified into four major types:

1. Faulty hypothesis triggering
2. Faulty context formulation
3. Faulty information gathering and processing
4. Faulty verification of diagnoses

Faulty hypothesis triggering may occur when the clinician fails to consider appropriate initial hypotheses or fails to revise hypotheses to reflect new information. Faulty context formulation may occur when a clinician has different goals than the patient has for a clinical encounter. For instance, a clinician may fail to deal with all problems important to the patient when the pressure to see other patients places constraints on the clinician's time. Faulty gathering and processing of information may occur when clinicians fail to order appropriate tests, or when they misinterpret the predictive value of findings or test results. Finally, faulty verification may occur when clinicians fail to collect enough evidence to confirm a diagnosis adequately or to rule out competing diagnoses.

It also must be acknowledged that diagnostic errors can result because the information-processing capacities of both experts and novices are limited. The short-term memory capacity of the human information-processing system is considerably less than its capacity for long-term memory storage. Thus, unstructured inputs of large amounts of information can quickly overload the system. Even in simple medical cases, the range of facts to be considered is large compared with the number of items (typically five to seven) about which humans can simultaneously think. "Provisional diagnoses or hypotheses formed early in the patient encounter serve as organizers or bases for chunking in data collection, keeping to a manageable number of categories under which information is filed" (Elstein et al, 1990). This strategy of organizing large numbers of facts into smaller numbers of clusters leads to the development of automatic, well-learned

---

TABLE 9-1   Specific Curricular Content to Enhance Critical Analysis for Problem Solving

General Content to Be Included in Curricula	Specific Content
Basic tools of clinical epidemiology	Rates, incidence, prevalence, risk assessment, diagnostic test characteristics, and reproducibility of diagnostic information
Rules of evidence and research methods	Knowledge of research methods and assessment of causality, demonstrated knowledge of the hierarchy of research designs to avoid bias and confounding, and the strengths and weaknesses of each design
Hypothetical-deductive reasoning process	The science of decision making and the hypothetical-deductive reasoning process
Biases and heuristics	Learning about incumbent biases and mental shortcuts of heuristic thinking
Uncertainty and probabilistic thinking	Ways to minimize error in judgment and probabilistic thinking
Incorporating the patient's values into medical decisions	Decision analysis
Medicine for populations	Policy analysis, cost-effectiveness analysis

Modified from Chessare JB et al: Impact of a medical school course in clinical epidemiology and health care systems, *Med Teach* 18:233-227, 1996.

information management processes (Allen et al, 2004; Young et al, 2007). In diagnostic reasoning, these clusters of information may assume the form of causal models that are based on pathophysiologic relationships, epidemiologic principles, or schematic algorithms. However, although such heuristics may simplify diagnostic decision making, they also may lead to diagnostic errors (Kempainen et al, 2003).

The main sources of error in medical decision making correspond to the two main steps in Eddy's (1990) model: "A decision can be flawed either if there is a misperception of the outcomes or if there is a misperception of the values that patients place on the outcomes." Most misperceptions result from failure of critical thinking. See Table 9-2 for a summary of common misperceptions that distort clinical decision-making accuracy.

Effective clinical decision making avoids flaws in the evaluation of outcomes or in patient preferences. Attention to three principles is helpful. First, decisions should be based on outcomes that are important to all patients. The health outcomes that patients experience and care about are primarily reduction in pain and avoidance of anxiety, disfigurement, disability, and death. These health outcomes are not the same as other outcome measures, such as statistics (e.g., the prevalence of a problem), intermediate biologic outcomes (e.g., the cell type of a cancer), or test results (e.g., serum cholesterol level). These other outcome factors may influence the effectiveness of an intervention and may help forecast health outcomes, but by themselves, "they cannot be experienced by a patient and should not be the basis for a decision. The logic for this principle is straightforward; the ultimate purpose of all medical practice is to maintain and improve the health of patients. The only way to achieve this is to focus on the outcomes they can experience and care about health outcomes" (Eddy, 2007).

Second, the effects of a decision on patient outcome should be estimated as accurately as possible, given the available evidence. As has been stated before, estimates of outcome should be based on evidence. All the pertinent evidence should be evaluated and critically analyzed with appropriate analytic methods, and decisions should not be affected by personal or professional biases. This is the information that clinicians should present to patients in a meaningful and understandable manner (Eddy, 2007).

The third principle is that the preferences assigned to the outcomes of an intervention should reflect as accurately as possible the preferences of the specific person who will receive the outcomes—that is, not just what is generally perceived to be the best outcome but the wishes of the specific patient. This may be accomplished only when the clinician has taken sufficient time to understand the values and wishes of the patient. If a patient chooses to delegate the decision to the provider or to someone else, the values of the other person inevitably replace those of the patient and will determine what will happen to the patient. This is a weighty responsibility (Eddy, 2007).

One way to clarify the appropriateness of a decision is to confirm that the goals of the patient and those of the clinician are congruent and appropriately defined (Fraenkel & McGraw, 2007). A goal consists of cognitive expectancies that organize the relationship between perception of the environment and development of the intention to act (Bandura, 1986). On another level, provider goals should not conflict. For clinicians, if

TABLE 9-2   Sources of Error in Clinical Decision Making

Sources of Error	Examples
Misperception of the outcomes	Important outcomes may be ignored. Extraneous outcomes might be included. Available evidence regarding outcomes may be incomplete. Existing evidence might be overlooked. Evidence might be misinterpreted. Reasoning might be incorrect. Personal experiences might be given undue weight. Reliance on wishful thinking might occur.
Misperceptions of patients' preferences	Patient might misunderstand outcomes. The measure of the effect might be misleading. The outcomes might be presented or framed in different ways, leading to different conclusions. The patient might not be consulted at all. Health care providers might project their own preferences onto the patient.
Logical flaws in thinking and evaluating	
Type of evidence available for determining intervention	"If there is no direct evidence from randomized, controlled trials, intervention should not be used."
Degree of certainty regarding existence of an effect	"The P value is only .1 which is not statistically significant. The intervention should not be used."
Seriousness of the outcome	"If the outcome without treatment is very bad, we have to assume that the treatment might work."
Need to do something	"This intervention is all that is available."
Novelty or technical appeal of an intervention or treatment	"This machine takes such a pretty picture it must have some use."
Other factors	Pressure from patient, family, the press, the courts; the amount of paperwork; personal financial interests

Modified from Eddy DM: Anatomy of a decision, *JAMA* 263:441-443, 1990.

the dual goals of diagnosing and treating the disease itself and diagnosing and treating the patient's responses to health problems are incongruent, the result may be flawed information processing.

Critical Decision Making Regarding Pharmacologic Therapy

Decision making is on a higher cognitive plane than critical thinking—which is primarily a process. Decision making requires not only critical thought but sometimes a degree of courage to take a position and take action. Both diagnostic and treatment plans arise from the decision that is made.

Not all clinical decisions are critical. In the course of caring for a patient, a multitude of decisions must be made. Some change the course of the patient's health irrevocably, for example, a decision as to whether the patient should undergo chemotherapy or a decision about specific types of surgery. Some of the decisions are clearly those that must be made by the health care provider, for example, tests that are essential. However, most of the decisions should be made by the patient. The effective therapeutic relationship involves negotiation between the health care provider and the patient to arrive at the most acceptable course.

Many systems have been developed during the past decade to organize clinical decision making into a simpler, more systematic process. Clinical guidelines, algorithms, and EBM are all designed to specify the critical decisions that must be made with regard to a particular process or procedure.

Some pharmacology texts suggest that all drug decisions are critical. However, sometimes drugs are virtually identical, and it does not matter which drug is selected. Sometimes patients have a preference for the taste of a certain product, cost may be a factor, the number of doses required per day may be associated with compliance, or patients may be reluctant to make a change. Sometimes decisions that are critical for one patient because of age, comorbidity, or other patient variables are not critical for another patient without those limitations. For example, a drug that produces impotence may be unacceptable to a 40-year-old married man, but for a particular 70-year-old widower, impotence may not be an issue. However, the clinician cannot generalize these preferences.

What decisions are absolutely essential for every patient? Analysis of current pharmacologic texts, journal articles, and contemporary research suggests that for every patient, at least five critical clinical decisions must be made by the provider who contemplates drug therapy. Some of these decisions seem obvious. However, they are rarely written down as maxims. See the critical decision-making algorithm in Figure 9-3.

CONFIRM THE DIAGNOSIS. This suggestion seems obvious but failure to do this accurately has led clinicians to mistakenly assume that epigastric burning is esophageal reflux and to order, incorrectly, a trial of proton pump inhibitors. The patient in actuality was presenting with signs of coronary artery disease. Thus, an incorrect diagnosis led to incorrect treatment.

The clinician should determine whether nonpharmacologic regimens should be continued, or whether it is time to add pharmacologic intervention. This mandates that providers have the commitment to try nonpharmacologic regimens and should not automatically resort to writing a prescription the first time a patient complains. It also requires that the

clinician is kept abreast of alternative medicine approaches used by clinicians and patients for the purpose of delaying prescription use. Research confirms that this critical decision is often eliminated because of the desire on the part of both provider and patient to do something—even if it is not the right thing (Hobgood et al, 2005).

DETERMINE THAT A MEDICATION WILL BE PRESCRIBED AND THEN DETERMINE HOW AGGRESSIVE THE THERAPY IS GOING TO BE. It is also important for the clinician to determine whether the selected regimen is safe in this particular patient situation. Treatment selection must be individualized. Making these determinations requires the prescriber to define the clinical goal clearly. The goal must be shared by the patient. Therefore, whether the goal is curative or palliative, and whether it involves symptom reduction or prevention, it must be clearly articulated. Once the goal is specified, then patient and drug variables such as the age of the patient, the presence of smoking or allergy, comorbidities (particularly those that affect the renal, hepatic, or immunologic system), other medications that are being taken, the severity of the disease, the risk-benefit ratio, and the cost of the product must be evaluated. It is extremely important that the medication regimen that the patient is currently using for other diagnoses be factored into the decision-making tree. For instance, Bactrim DS and the statin classes can increase INR times in a patient who is on Coumadin.

SELECT THE DRUG AND START IT. Sometimes there is a standard first-line drug. Sometimes there are many options from which to select. The effect of the medication and the timing of taking it within the patient's life are very important to explain. For instance, Sinemet is impeded by the ingestion of protein foods, and cruciferous vegetables add to the effect of Synthroid. Asking questions about care provided to the patient by other health care providers is vital to the safe prescription of drugs. Often, reports are not received from specialists or walk-in clinics that the patient may have used. Concomitant prescriptions for other drugs (even those used recently, such as vitamin E, which can increase INR times) may prove hazardous to patient care.

DETERMINE THE EFFECTIVENESS OF THE PRESCRIBED DRUG ONCE THE PATIENT BEGINS TO TAKE THE PRODUCT. Evaluation of drug effectiveness varies by drug, so the appropriate time interval must be selected. For selective serotonin reuptake inhibitors and some antihypertensive agents, it may take several weeks for effectiveness to be determined. Antibiotics probably should produce changes in patient status within 48 to 72 hours. Critical elements include therapeutic effects and the presence of adverse or toxic effects. These should be communicated in writing to the patient by the pharmacist or the clinician. Be certain that the patient can read and understand the instructions. A clinic-appointed interpreter should be provided to assist non–English-speaking clients.

Based on evaluation of the patient's reaction to the medication, the clinician will decide to (1) continue the medication because it is doing what it should, or because it is partially working and should be given more time, (2) modify the regimen in some way (another medication added

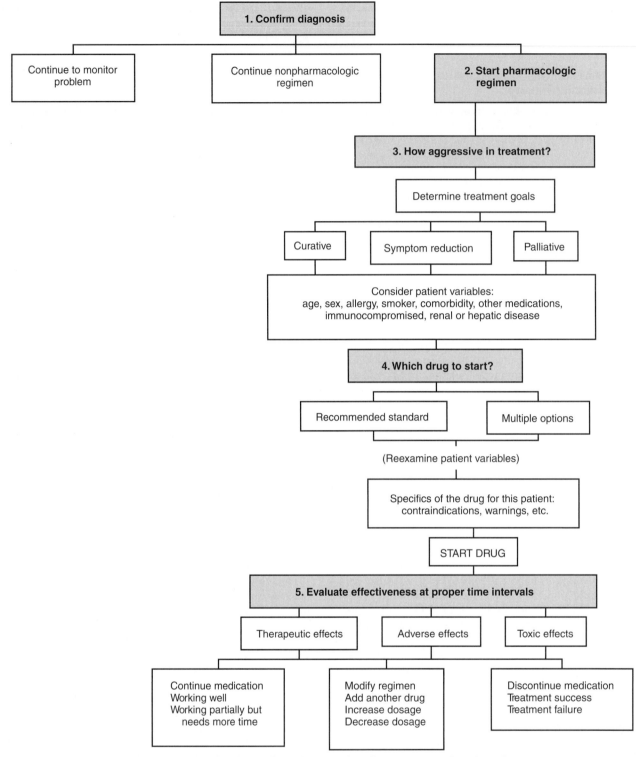

FIGURE 9-3   Critical decision-making algorithm for all patients regarding drug therapy.

or dosage increased or decreased), or (3) discontinue the medication because the therapeutic objective has been reached and the medication is no longer needed, or the medication was a treatment failure and should be stopped.

The processes of critical thinking and of clinical decision making converge in the decision to begin to prescribe medication for a patient. How earnestly decision makers strive to advance their knowledge of drugs, how critically they evaluate

the literature, and how attentive they are in developing a therapeutic relationship with the patient to determine values and preferences will ultimately influence the accuracy of the decisions that are made. Access to the latest drug information through palm pilot use and incorporation of knowledge gained from Web-based information systems for clinicians are indispensable to today's clinician. Thus, good research and a knowledge base of drugs, excellent communication skills with the patient, and incorporation of state of the art resources will improve health outcomes jointly held by the patient and the care provider.

New Products: How to Determine Which Drugs to Prescribe

With all the new drug products that are entering the market, how does the clinician stay current with what he might be prescribing? It may take time and effort to learn them, but several guidelines developed by Philip Mohler (2006) should prove helpful:

- Is the new product clearly more efficacious than existing drugs? In some cases, the medical literature can be helpful to the clinician in answering this question. In many cases, it may be difficult to compare the efficacy of a new drug vs. that of older "standard" products because new drugs often are tested only against placebo. Meta-analyses and other systematic reviews may be helpful to the clinician in answering these questions. Ample time and careful investigation are needed.

- Does the new dosage or the formulation of an older product offer significant advantages? Again, this requires research. Scrutinize new drugs that end with XL, CR, ER, SR, or XR. Does the drug offer clinically relevant new efficacy, safety, or adherence benefits, or is it simply a "me too" product?

- What does the new drug cost? Clinicians often do not know the costs of the prescriptions they are writing for their patients. However, the use of expensive prescriptions often is correlated with the fact that many new prescriptions never get filled. As the numbers of patients who are uninsured or underinsured continue to grow, it is critical for providers to know what the prescriptions cost and to communicate with patients about their ability to pay for them.

- Is the new drug safe for this particular patient? This also may be difficult to evaluate. Proceed slowly: See what 6 to 12 months of postmarketing experience reveals in terms of both efficacy and side effects. Weigh carefully the risks associated with a new drug against its value for a specific patient.

When discussing new drugs with pharmaceutical representatives, the clinician should ask about direct comparison head-to-head studies with older, standard drugs in comparable doses. Also, one should ask for the absolute risk reduction (not relative risk reduction), the number needed to treat, and the size of the clinical trial. For your decision making, use excellent unbiased resources such as *The Prescriber's Letter, The Medical Letter,* Epocrates, knowledgeable colleagues, and local pharmacists and pharmacologists (Mohler, 2006).

EVIDENCE-BASED MEDICINE

Training for Uncertainty

Renée C. Fox, noted medical sociologist, has suggested that one of the major tasks of health care providers as they begin to train for their health professional role is training for uncertainty. She suggests that everyone must deal with two basic types of uncertainty. The first results from incomplete or imperfect mastery of available knowledge. No one can have at his command all skills and all knowledge of the lore of medicine. The second depends on limitations in current medical knowledge. There are innumerable questions to which no clinician, however well trained, can as yet provide answers. A third

source of uncertainty derives from the first two. This consists of difficulty in distinguishing between personal ignorance or ineptitude and the limitations of present medical knowledge. It is inevitable that every clinician must constantly cope with these forms of uncertainty, and that grave consequences may result if he is not able to do so (Fox, 1957).

In the past, these uncertainties have presented difficult challenges for health care providers that will be made more difficult by the plethora of knowledge that is now available every day. How does one discover what is known? Formerly, clinicians read textbooks, attended lectures, and learned beside other, more seasoned clinicians, who served as mentors and role models. These practices established lifelong patterns for clinician learning and forever influenced how they practiced.

How does one gain mastery of the information that is known? Although most health care providers take seriously their responsibility to keep current with new research, they simply do not have the time. Given the large number of journals that are being published and the wealth of available website information, a casual calculation for clinicians in general medicine is that they would have to read 19 articles per day, 365 days per year, to stay current. This is an impossible feat; most health care providers have less than an hour per week to devote to reading medical journals (Young et al, 2007).

Today, Fox's two questions have become even more important and even more challenging to answer. Available information about various clinical topics is growing exponentially every day and may have a dramatic impact on how clinicians practice. New research findings that shed light on physiology, pathophysiology, disease management, diagnostic technique, and pharmacology chip away at the "received view," often changing the very foundation of practice. A growing group of scientists are studying the process of information diffusion to learn how what is known becomes communicated to relevant individuals, and how it may be translated into usable information. Studies of information diffusion are essential if efforts to assist individuals overwhelmed with the burgeoning knowledge of today are to be enhanced. Indeed, one of the major challenges that clinicians face today is how to sort through all the information that is available, how to organize it, and how to retrieve the important and valid information that is essential to their practice (Shuval et al, 2007).

The Internet has both helped and hindered this process of information retrieval. Large medical databases are being created by many different groups. Depending on group goals, these databases do help in organization and retrieval of information. However, the quality of data varies widely, and evaluating data is a daunting task. Some of the information is superb; other information is methodologically flawed and cannot be accepted as proven fact. One recent search in the National Library of Medicine PubMed database on the topic of cytochrome P450 metabolism produced 26,980 citations for a restricted 2-year search. Another crucial task today involves evaluating the quality of what is reported before it can be incorporated into practice.

Health care practice has changed so profoundly that this event can appropriately be called a *paradigm shift.* A way of looking at the world that defines both legitimate problems and the spectrum of evidence that may bear on their solution is called a *scientific paradigm.* When limitations or defects in an existing paradigm are widely apparent to such a degree that the paradigm is no longer useful in solving problems, the paradigm is challenged and gradually is replaced by a new way of looking at the world. The new way of looking at health care decision making, called *EBM*, varies so dramatically from the traditional way of thinking about health care decisions that it may be said to represent a paradigm shift.

The Traditional Decision-Making Paradigm

Details about EBM are outlined most precisely in the foundational explanatory article written by the Evidence-Based Medicine Working Group (1992), "Evidence-Based Medicine: A New Approach to Teaching the Practice of Medicine." In this article, components of both the traditional paradigm and of the new paradigm were articulated.

As was noted, the following traditional paradigm assumptions about the knowledge required to guide clinical practice have been in place:

- Unsystematic observations from clinical experience are a valid way of building and maintaining one's knowledge about patient prognosis, the value of diagnostic tests, and the efficacy of treatment.
- The study and understanding of the basic mechanisms of disease and pathophysiologic principles are sufficient guides for clinical practice.
- The combination of thorough traditional medical training and common sense is sufficient to allow one to evaluate new tests and treatment.
- Content expertise and clinical experience form a sufficient base from which valid guidelines for clinical practice can be derived.

According to this paradigm, clinicians have a number of options when making clinical decisions. They can reflect on their own clinical experience, reflect on the underlying biology, go to a textbook, or ask a local expert. Upon examination of these assumptions, it is clear how the notion developed that the best education would be tied to the best teachers in the best schools. Learning at the footstool of good clinicians or experts was important. This paradigm also implies that many opportunities for quality learning are available at these institutions but are not available to those who are educated in other institutions.

Additionally, the tradition has been that reading the introduction and discussion sections of a paper could be considered an appropriate way of gaining relevant information from a current journal. Physicians' research efforts often consisted of flipping through journals and reading the last five sentences of the conclusion of each study, as time permitted.

The traditional paradigm of decision making places a high value on traditional scientific authority and adherence to standard approaches. Answers frequently are sought through direct contact with local experts or through reference to the writings of international experts (Steinberg & Luce, 2005).

What Is Evidence-Based Health Care?

Evidence-based health care (EBHC) has become a popular term for providers and may be described as a paradigm shift in both practice and teaching. In reality, EBHC represents an evolution of focus on critically appraising available evidence that had been in progress for many years; this requires the increased use of randomized clinical trials and the promulgation of rigorous clinical guidelines (Steinberg & Luce, 2005). "Long-established methods of care and practice have fallen as a result of being submitted to this rigorous process,

and clinicians who learned standards of treatment as recently as just a few years ago are finding it necessary to re-learn diagnostic priorities and management protocols that had become second nature" (Scudder, 2006). EBM is a decision-making framework that facilitates complex decisions across different and sometimes conflicting groups. In EBM, research and other forms of evidence are considered on a routine basis in making health care decisions. With the use of computer technology to classify, categorize, compare, and analyze content in large databases, the diffusion of knowledge about best practices into clinical care is finally possible.

Researchers and physicians at the Department of Clinical Epidemiology and Biostatistics at McMaster University in Ontario, Canada (www.hiru.mcmaster.ca/ceb), coined the term *evidence-based medicine*. Its core idea was that clinicians should consider the effectiveness and harm associated with different interventions before they are implemented. The department helped clinicians accomplish this by publishing a series of articles and a textbook and has held annual workshops to teach physicians how to quickly find, evaluate, and extract critical information from medical studies. By now, virtually every major medical, nursing, dental, and pharmacy school has incorporated EBM into its curriculum to some extent (Steinberg & Luce, 2005).

EBM may be defined as the purposeful, conscientious, explicit, and judicious use of the current best evidence in making decisions about the care of individual patients. The key phrase is "making decisions." EBM represents a shift in the way that health care providers and researchers use medical research to make decisions. It formalizes some of the critical thinking and clinical decision-making processes that have already been discussed.

In their seminal article, the EBM Working Group (1992) specifies the assumptions of the new EBM paradigm:

> Clinical experience and the development of clinical instincts (particularly with respect to diagnosis) are a crucial and necessary part of becoming a competent clinician. Many aspects of clinical practice cannot, or will not, ever be adequately tested. Clinical experience and its lessons are particularly important in these situations. At the same time, systematic attempts to record observations in a reproducible and unbiased fashion markedly increase the confidence one can have in knowledge about patient prognosis, the value of diagnostic tests, and the efficacy of treatment. In the absence of systematic observation, one must be cautious in the interpretation of information derived from clinical experience and intuition, for it may at times be misleading.
>
> The study and understanding of basic mechanisms of disease are necessary but insufficient guides for clinical practice. The rationales for diagnosis and treatment, which follow from basic pathophysiologic principles, may in fact be incorrect, leading to inaccurate predictions about the performance of diagnostic tests and the efficacy of treatments.
>
> Understanding certain rules of evidence is necessary to correctly interpret literature on causation, prognosis, diagnostic tests, and treatment strategy.
>
> (EVIDENCE-BASED MEDICINE WORKING GROUP, 1992)

It follows from these assumptions that clinicians should regularly consult the original literature. They should be able to critically appraise the methods and results sections to evaluate information important in solving clinical problems and providing optimal patient care. It also follows from a close examination of existing literature that "clinicians must be ready to accept and live with uncertainty and to acknowledge that management decisions are often made in the face of relative ignorance of their true impact" (EBM Working Group, 1992).

The new paradigm puts a much lower value on both written and personal authority. The underlying philosophy of EBM is that health care providers "can gain the skills to make independent assessments of evidence and thus evaluate the credibility of opinions being offered by experts" (EBM Working Group, 1992). The decreased reliance on authority does not imply rejection of what can be learned from colleagues and teachers, whose experience has provided them with skills and insight into methods of history taking and physical examination, as well as diagnostic strategies. The knowledge gained from years of practice can never be acquired solely from formal scientific investigation. A final corollary of the new paradigm is that providers whose practice is augmented by and based on an understanding of the research will provide superior patient care.

The EBM Working Group (1992) suggests that EBM training focuses primarily on the development of research skills and use of the *critical appraisal exercise*. At the general research and database level, this critical appraisal exercise works by converting complex information from literally thousands of individual studies into user friendly risk estimates through the following four main steps:

1. *Defining an answerable and structured question about the target population, outcomes, and intervention or exposure*—A focused clinical question should clearly address problems in the areas of therapy, diagnosis, cause, and prognosis.
2. *Searching the published literature for sources of data that might answer the question*—Beginning in 2001, PubMed (www. PubMed.org), the search engine from The National Library of Medicine's Medline, implemented changes through a new search filter in the Clinical Queries section that allows users to easily retrieve systematic reviews and evidence-based clinical practice guidelines. Medline's index includes important evidenced-based materials, including the Cochrane Database of Systematic Reviews, The American College of Physician's Journal Club, and articles from the journal *Clinical Evidence* and other sources, providing a powerful research tool for the researcher or clinician. (When searching PubMed, use the controlled vocabulary, referred to as *Medical Subject Headings,* or *MeSH,* to index references. Most unsuccessful searches are the result of failure to use this MeSH terminiology. The MeSH database can be found on PubMed by clicking on the word MeSH from the side bar on the home page [Doig & Simpson, 2003; Scudder, 2006].)
3. *Appraising or evaluating the data for methodologic rigor and relevance to the question*—Critically appraise studies to determine their validity and applicability. A well-recognized hierarchy of clinical research methods has emerged with well-designed and executed randomized controlled trials considered to be the gold standard, with the least susceptibility to bias. Concerns about bias increase in the following order with other types of study designs: nonrandomized controlled trials, prospective or retrospective cohort studies, cross-sectional studies, case-control studies, case series and registries, and case reports (Scudder, 2006; Steinberg & Luce, 2005). In addition to noting the research method, be sure that the evidence is applicable to the particular patient population; studies conducted in a specific patient group may not be generalizable to others.
4. *Describing and analyzing study data to answer the question posed.*

EBM does depend on the clinician's having a strong traditional knowledge base. A sound understanding of epidemiology and pathophysiology is necessary to interpret and apply the results of clinical research. The patients for whom clinicians provide care may differ substantially from those included in an EBM research study. Understanding the underlying pathophysiologic processes allows the clinician to better judge whether research results are applicable to the patient at hand or are not generalizable. Having a strong foundation in science also helps the clinician to conceptualize and remember information about different clinical problems.

EBM emphasizes that research must be a part of every major medical decision. In an attempt to solve the time constraint problem, EBM provides methods, strategies, and technologies that make it possible for health care workers to quickly find the most relevant and reliable research (Schmidt & Brown, 2007). Closer consideration of EBM as a way of making decisions undermines the assertion of some clinicians that nonphysician providers, who do not have the same clinical education as physicians, cannot develop the same clinical database as physicians. Nonphysician providers may not need the same education as physicians if they have the skills needed for retrieval and evaluation of scientific information. In fact, health care providers who have graduated from master's degree programs or doctoral programs may have an advantage over other types of health care providers because they may already have strong research and critical appraisal skills that were developed during the research or dissertation component of their programs.

In teaching about EBM, criteria may be developed to help students evaluate other types of research. Table 9-3 provides criteria that may be helpful in evaluating different types of studies. As learning becomes more sophisticated, additional criteria can be introduced. For example, EBM teaches students to evaluate trials based in part on whether they are randomized. Randomized trials are considered the most reliable. Students must learn to appreciate methodologic merit without discarding all findings if the study is not randomized. Students must learn how to arrive at the strength of inference associated with a clinical decision. EBM also has influenced the development of clinical guidelines. Some practice guidelines have begun to be categorized into one of three types. Type A guidelines are supported by randomized trial, type B guidelines are supported by trials other than randomized trials, and type C guidelines are not clearly supported. Teachers can point out instances in which criteria can be violated without reducing the strength of the inference (Scudder, 2006).

Scudder (2006) suggests that implementing an evidence-based change in practice may be simple or difficult, depending on the magnitude of the change and the institution in which the change is being made. It is important to consider instituting an evaluative process that will provide feedback about how well a change is working in your own patient population. Notwithstanding the evidence, the art of providing care must not be ignored. Change must be integrated with patient preferences and the provider's clinical expertise. Is this new treatment or diagnostic method both applicable and acceptable to your patients? Can your patient adhere to

TABLE 9-3   Suggested Criteria for Analysis of Diagnosis, Treatment, and Review Articles

Type of Study	Analysis Criteria
Diagnosis studies	Has the diagnostic test been evaluated in a patient sample that included an appropriate spectrum of mild and severe, and treated and untreated disease, plus individuals with different but commonly confused disorders? Was an independent, blind comparison made vs. a "gold standard" of diagnosis?
Treatment studies	Was the assignment of patients to treatment randomized? Were all patients who entered the study accounted for at its conclusion?
Review articles	Were explicit methods used to determine which articles should be included in the review?

Modified from Stevens L: Evidence-based medicine, *Med Net* 4:5-11, 1998.

this change? Or, in other words—If your patient care plan is not broken, should you fix it because the evidence says you should? (Scudder, 2006)

evolve   For further information on the use of EBM, see the supplemental tables on the Evolve Learning Resources.

Growth of Evidence-Based Medicine as a Decision-Making Process

In an ideal world, during an actual patient encounter, a health care provider would use a terminal in the examining room or a handheld PDA to review research before arriving at solutions to problems. The most important aspect of EBM is that the research that health care providers review should be related to specific problems on which the providers are working, and that this review should be done quickly and efficiently.

Much of the process of teaching EBM involves helping clinicians hone their computer database search skills. The process of defining the problem, locating the information needed to solve the problem, and selecting the most relevant and reliable research findings requires skills not previously emphasized in the clinical curricula.

Key to the development and greater use of EBM is the greater availability of computers and increased use of the Internet. Many articles have been published about EBM that include instructions on how to access, evaluate, and interpret the medical literature. Curricular revisions have been suggested for teaching programs. Proposals have been put forward to help clinicians use the principles of clinical epidemiology in everyday clinical practice (Shuval et al, 2007). The format used in writing textbooks has begun to change; a rigorous review of available evidence is included, as are the methodologic criteria used to evaluate the validity of the clinical evidence and the quantitative techniques used to summarize the evidence (Flores-Mateo & Argimon, 2007). Several medical journals have revised the abstract format for their articles, incorporating material in the abstract about methods and design to help assist readers in article evaluation. Practice guidelines are now being developed that are based on rigorous methodologic review of the available evidence, and ethical guidelines for professional continuing education suggest greater reliance on EBM in content presentations.

Barriers to the Implementation of Evidence-Based Decision Making

Despite the advantages that are touted by some, EBM has not been universally applauded. Both antipathy and skepticism toward EBM may result from doubt about whether EBM can ever truly be applied in day-to-day practice. Some clinicians react negatively to the process because the name implies that what physicians did previously was not evidence based. Other emotional barriers to the acceptance of EBM may be based on the following facts:

- *New providers start with rudimentary critical appraisal skills and the topic may be threatening to them.*
- *People like quick and easy answers*—Cookbook medicine has its appeal. Critical appraisal involves additional time and effort and may be perceived as inefficient and distracting from the real goal (to provide optimal care for patients).
- *For many clinical questions, high-quality evidence is lacking*— If such questions predominate in attempts to introduce critical appraisal, a sense of futility can result.

Based on the experience of the EBM Working Group (1992), several common misinterpretations of the EBM paradigm have emerged. These are discussed in the following paragraphs.

Evidence-Based Medicine Ignores Clinical Experience and Clinical Intuition

On the contrary, it is important to expose learners to exceptional clinicians who have a gift for intuitive diagnosis, a talent for precise observation, and excellent judgment in making difficult management decisions. The better that experienced clinicians can dissect the process they use in diagnosis and clearly present it to learners, the greater will be the benefit. Institutional experience can also provide important insights. Diagnostic tests may differ in their accuracy, depending on the skill of the practitioner (EBM Working Group, 1992).

Understanding of Basic Investigation and Pathophysiology Plays No Part in Evidence-Based Medicine

The dearth of adequate evidence demands that clinical problem solving must rely on an understanding of underlying pathophysiology. Moreover, a good understanding of pathophysiology is necessary for accurate clarification of clinical observations and for appropriate interpretation of evidence (especially in deciding on its generalizability) (EBM Working Group, 1992).

Evidence-Based Medicine Ignores Standard Aspects of Clinical Training, Such as the Physical Examination

Careful history taking and physical examination provide much, and often the best, evidence for diagnosis and direct treatment decisions. The clinical teacher of EBM must give considerable attention to teaching the methods of history taking and clinical examination, with particular attention to which items have demonstrated validity and to what strategies enhance observer agreement (EBM Working Group, 1992).

It may be observed that five factors influence medical decision making: (1) the patient's situation, (2) the patient's desires and values, (3) the health care provider's values, (4) the health care provider's experience, and (5) evidence from research. EBM plays a role only in the last factor.

Clearly, an escalating movement toward use of more scientific data is emerging as a result of the introduction of clinical practice guidelines, the focus on disease management strategies, the application of quality improvement methods in health care, and the need to translate clinical trial results into actual practice. Many of these trends are driven by health economic factors. Increasingly, practice guidelines are not written by groups of gray-haired academicians in rooms but instead are based on EBM data and are designed to help clinicians evaluate the reliability of the guidelines.

Does Evidence-Based Medicine Improve Patient Outcomes?

Whether EBM will succeed in becoming the dominant philosophy in clinical decision making rests on whether patients cared for in this fashion enjoy better health. "This proof is no more achievable for the new paradigm than it is for the old, for no long-term randomized trials of traditional and evidence-based medical education are likely to be carried out" (EBM Working Group, 1992). What we do have are a number of short-term studies that confirm that the skills of EBM can be taught. Growing research suggests that teaching in this way may help graduates to stay up-to-date.

Health care providers will continue to face a burgeoning volume of literature, increased use of new technologies, deepening concern about escalating health care costs, and growing scrutiny of the quality and outcomes of medical care. In a real sense, whether EBM becomes a mainstream process depends in part on the goals that health care providers have for it. The EBM movement has already influenced how practice guidelines and critical pathways are written. Also, health care clinicians in most major U.S. and British Commonwealth professional schools have learned how to distinguish reliable from unreliable studies and how to search medical databases for data that can be used to solve real-world medical problems. If nothing else, EBM will complement traditional methods of learning and decision making by attempting to lighten the load of clinicians who are trying to keep up with and evaluate published literature in their field.

CLINICAL GUIDELINES

Accepted standards of clinical conduct practice guidelines have proliferated throughout medicine over the past decade. Health care providers are confronted with a plethora of guidelines that have been developed for various purposes by a diverse body of public and private organizations. Practice guidelines that specify how to treat patients with specific medical conditions and how to perform specific procedures have been published in the health care literature. Their use by managed care plans, hospitals, and government programs is expected to affect health care practice substantially in the coming years.

Recommendations for practice in medical textbooks and review articles often do not provide a systematic and careful explanation of the underlying rationale associated with clinical practice guidelines. Review articles often reflect what an author (who may or may not be an expert) believes is proper practice (Eddy, 1990, 2007). Readers of medical textbooks or review articles often do not know to what extent the recommendations are based on science or on personal opinion because the author is not required to perform a systematic literature review or to demonstrate how the recommendations are linked to the science, as is expected with a practice guideline (Woolf, 1995).

Clearly, there are differences between agreed-on, normative practice standards and clinical practice guidelines recommended as the "usual" way to treat patients or guide treatment within a particular institution to achieve cost containment or to enhance efficiency. However, acceptance of clinical practice guidelines may have other consequences such as redefining the scope of practice for the various clinicians involved, serving as a way to pinpoint careless or negligent practice, or making it difficult for providers to practice outside of a clinical guideline. This is a particular problem if clinicians fail to individualize guidelines for specific patients. Guidelines that also mandate when procedures may be performed, lengths of hospital stay, and other practices may affect clinical practice dramatically. Aspects of primary care are logical targets for the development of clinical practice guidelines, and primary care clinicians may now frequently be required to comply with them for reimbursement or legal reasons.

What Are Clinical Practice Guidelines?

Official statements that outline how to prevent, diagnose, and treat specific medical conditions or how to perform certain clinical procedures are called *clinical practice guidelines* (Woolf, 1995). (These also may be called *clinical policies, standards, treatment protocols, practice parameters,* or *appropriateness criteria.*) Clinical practice guidelines are frequently issued by government agencies, medical specialty societies, and other health organizations. These guidelines address specific health problems (such as the 19 clinical practice guidelines from the Agency for Healthcare Research and Quality [AHRQ]), clinical practices, or groups of clinical practices (e.g., *Guide to Clinical Preventive Services,* U.S. Preventive Services Task Force).

Guideline development has been encouraged over the years by changes in the traditional reimbursement mechanisms that have forced health care organizations and providers to seek new ways to control escalating health care costs by reducing practice variances and enhancing the quality of patient care. These acknowledged methods are designed to inform and teach both seasoned and novice clinicians.

Medline searches yield thousands of entries about clinical guidelines. The National Guideline Clearinghouse (www.guideline.gov/) is a comprehensive database for thousands of the most up-to-date clinical practice guidelines. Valid guidelines, when appropriately disseminated and implemented, are purported to lead to changes in clinical practice and improvements in patient outcomes.

> **evolve** For a list of organizations involved in the development of clinical practice guidelines, see the supplemental tables on the Evolve Learning Resources.

Guidelines are more likely to be valid if they are developed with the use of systematic reviews, national or regional guideline development groups (including representatives of key disciplines), and explicit links between recommendations and scientific evidence. Peer review guidelines are another element of the process that may ensure validity. (See Table 9-4 for factors that should be considered when one is evaluating a clinical practice guideline.)

Considerable resources are required to develop evidence-linked guidelines, but this investment can be recouped through relatively small changes in the process or outcome of care. Good leadership and technical support are required for the successful development of clinically valid guidelines, a process that depends on small group procedures of guideline development panels and translation of evidence into recommendations. The process of valid guideline development is certainly an area in which further research is needed.

Process for Guideline Development

One of the best analyses of information on clinical guidelines comes from Woolf (1995). His work suggests that current methods for developing practice guidelines include (1) informal consensus development, (2) formal consensus development, (3) evidence-based guideline development, and (4) explicit guideline development.

Informal consensus development is the most commonly used method. Experts meet to discuss and decide on recommendations subjectively, based on their experience and knowledge. Guidelines produced in this manner without explicit decision rules are often of poor quality. They usually do not include adequate documentation of how conclusions were reached. *Formal consensus development* uses a systematic approach to formally assess expert opinion, reach agreement, and make recommendations. This popular 1970s approach often used a modified Delphi method to arrive at recommendations by scoring the opinions of experts. Both informal and formal consensus development methods describe what experts believe is appropriate based on their own knowledge, research, and experience.

Evidence-based guideline development first appeared in the 1980s. Through this approach, an expert panel follows a systematic research method of gathering relevant studies and reviewing the data. Based on the validity of findings, recommendations are linked directly to scientific evidence of effectiveness. When recommendations are made, rules of evidence are emphasized over expert opinion.

Finally, *explicit guideline development* specifically clarifies recommendations by calculating the potential benefits, harms, and costs of available interventions, estimating the possibility of the outcomes, and comparing the desirability of the outcomes based on patient preferences. These guidelines are based on statistical probability and arise primarily from organizational imperatives.

In both the evidence-based and the explicit approach, the clinician should have a clear understanding of the quality of the evidence on which the recommendations are based and the extent to which the guidelines are based on opinion. Woolf also suggests that four essential steps must be followed in the development of practice guidelines:

1. *Introductory decision making*—This step includes the selection of topic and panel members and clarification of purposes of the clinical practice guideline.
2. *Assessment of clinical appropriateness*—This is accomplished through review of scientific evidence and expert opinion. An extensive literature review of perhaps thousands of articles may be performed to search for relevant research studies. The research is rigorously critiqued, and data may be supplemented by expert opinion when data are lacking.
3. *Assessment of public policy issues*—Resource limitations and feasibility issues are major factors to consider.
4. *Guideline document development and evaluation*—This involves drafting of the document, peer review, and pretesting.

Regardless of the care with which clinical guidelines are developed, it is difficult for participants to define optimal care (Woolf, 1995). This is so in part because science cannot define optimal care with certainty. Data are often lacking in

TABLE 9-4   Factors to Consider When Evaluating a Clinical Practice Guideline

Factors to Consider	Specific Things to Evaluate
Source	Sponsoring organization, federal agency, panel composition
Appropriateness of method	Informal consensus panel, formal consensus panel, evidence-based process, explicit approach
Scientific rigor in evaluation of scientific evidence	Comprehensiveness of literature review, classification of study designs, consideration of sources of bias, methods used for synthesizing results
Use of expert opinion/clinical experience	Qualifications of panel as experts
Decision making	Documentation of rationale, decision rules, link between strength of recommendations and quality of evidence, appropriateness of recommendation language
Public policy issue considerations	Cost-effectiveness considered, health care system constraints recognized
Feasibility issues	Ability for guideline to be implemented; consideration of time, simplicity, medicolegal, and reimbursement issues
Peer review	Groups or individuals who reviewed guidelines and provided feedback
Congruence with other practice guidelines	Presence of conflicting guidelines on the same topic, impact on other general or institutional policies
Timeliness	Recent research findings incorporated
Funding	Did funding source introduce bias into guideline development?

Adapted with permission from Woolf SH: Practice guidelines: what the family physician should know, *Am Fam Physician* 51:1455-1463, 1995. Copyright © 1995; American Acadamy of family Physicians.

medicine, and studies often suffer from design flaws that limit internal and external validity. Subtle aspects of clinical judgment cannot always be measured empirically. Additionally, the process of analyzing evidence and blending it with expert opinion is imprecise.

Techniques used to summarize data, such as meta-analysis and decision analysis, may be inappropriate and so may generate misleading results. Expert panel recommendations may be skewed by panel member biases or distorted by organization politics. "Experts" on the panel may not be representative of all experts on the subject (Woolf, 1995).

Finally, recommendations that may be based on what is best, as defined in the guidelines, may not be appropriate for an individual or a local population. Thus, the patient's medical history, personal circumstances, coexisting illnesses, personal preferences, and biologic variability may indicate that an individual patient is better served by options other than those recommended in the guidelines (Woolf, 1995). Therefore, a central issue that must be addressed in practice guideline development is how to develop guidelines that appropriately allow for variations in clinical populations and practice settings. Despite recognition of this problem, guideline development through its formalistic approach works against incorporating flexibility into recommendations. It is difficult to determine when clinical circumstances vary enough that guideline recommendations should differ, how recommendations should be modified for a specific clinical setting, and whether the benefit associated with such site-specific guidelines justifies the expense of their development. Early research in this area suggests that site-specific guidelines can substantially improve the expected health benefit for the patient and the economic efficiency of practice guidelines.

Limitations in the Use of Clinical Practice Guidelines

Clinical practice guidelines have limitations. This is not a problem as long as guidelines are worded in such a manner that limitations are acknowledged. If guidelines are written so rigidly that they overstate the certainty of recommendations, underestimate the complexity of patient care, or use rigid language to define the certainty of optimal care, "cookbook medicine" occurs. Guidelines that describe treatment without linking it to valid scientific evidence, or that ignore the individuality of patients, restrict the professional intuition of skilled clinicians and mislead students. Thus, sensitivity to these issues and careful crafting of the language of guidelines are paramount in development of the final product.

Another limitation of practice guidelines is the degree of precision with which they are written. Some guidelines have been criticized because they are too vague. Lack of clarity in the recommendations, particularly for diagnostic testing or monitoring, is commonly seen. However, explicit recommendations can be harmful if they are derived arbitrarily, without supporting evidence, or if they provide an unreasonable and expensive standard that attorneys, utilization reviewers, insurance companies, and others might insist must be met. If good evidence suggests that clarity is needed in the recommendations, then it is important to be precise; if evidence is inadequate and explicit language is used simply in the interest of clarity, other possibly appropriate treatments may be precluded (Woolf, 1995).

Using Guidelines to Modify Clinical Practice

When a new guideline appears in a professional journal or text, clinicians should be skeptical about its utility until it has been closely evaluated. The same critical analysis that is used in EBM or that NPs and PAs learn when writing scholarly papers or theses should serve them well in evaluating the scientific rigor on which a guideline is built. The same validity tests and critical thinking that are used by all disciplines in critiquing clinical studies should be applied to analysis of the merits of the clinical guideline. Mossler (1997) describes six half-truths about clinical guidelines:

1. *Guidelines are cookbook medicine*—Evidence-based guidelines require the application of judgment, assessment, and decision making in their use and differ from cookbook medicine, which dictates elements of care.
2. *Guidelines are a legal hazard*—Good guidelines specify good medicine in that they are evidence based and not opinion driven.
3. *Guidelines do not work*—Alone, they do not improve care. They must be incorporated into an organized, systematic approach to reduce variations in practice.
4. *Time and effort should not be wasted on developing guidelines because they are available from other sources*—Internal guideline development introduces many new people to the improvement process and improves their understanding of problems and solutions.
5. *The task of implementing guidelines is the task of getting physicians to use them*—This is only part of the task. A team-oriented attitude is warranted.
6. *Guideline use should be validated by outcomes data*—If *outcomes* means results of improvement processes, then this is true. But if *outcomes* refers to individual adverse events, these data are of little value and this step should not be included as a routine part of the guideline process.

The validity of clinical guidelines should be seriously questioned if inadequate information is provided about how the recommendations were derived. As in any research study, the method should be clearly specified and the participants described. The quality of the scientific arguments used in making the recommendations should be weighed. If they are supported by strong evidence, then compliance with the recommendations should be considered. If evidence is equivocal or weak and the recommendations are based primarily on expert opinion, the personal preferences of the provider and of the patient should influence the decision. Providers have personal views on the relative importance of science and opinion in making practice decisions. Providers who believe that clinical practice should always be based on science will decide not to follow guidelines that do not meet their standards. Those who have confidence in the opinions of experts might be more willing to follow weaker guidelines.

Patient preferences also must be considered if the evidence is not conclusive because patient evaluation of potential benefit and harm can make the same practice acceptable for one patient and inappropriate for another (Barry et al, 1988). Table 9-4 lists factors that should be considered when one is evaluating a clinical practice guideline. Evaluation of these factors will help clinicians determine whether they should or should not change their practice to be in accordance with the recommendations of the guideline.

Clinicians must look beyond the guidelines to consider who is writing the guideline and whether that group has an agenda. Does the organization have a dominant philosophy that might influence the flavor of a guideline? Are the panel members biased? Who funded the expensive research process that underlies most guideline development? When experts or organizations with an interest in a specific clinical problem develop guidelines, examination of the topic may be conducted with a narrow focus and with little concern for other important health problems. The resultant recommendations may be based on the implicit and mistaken assumption that the provider's attention, time, and other resources can be devoted entirely to that problem. Although such an approach comes naturally to topic-oriented experts, such recommendations may be unreasonable for primary care providers, who are responsible for preventing or treating dozens of health problems in every patient.

Some practice guidelines dictate expensive laboratory testing or are so cumbersome that they become unrealistic, potentially harmful, and costly. "The problem of focused preoccupation groups that develop guidelines has been apparent to primary care providers struggling to provide children with universal hepatitis B vaccination, universal lead screening, and universal hearing screening. Each of these initiatives was recommended by groups concerned only with these problems" (Woolf, 1995).

Primary care clinicians will be faced with growing numbers of guidelines and the need to become more sophisticated consumers of practice guidelines. These guidelines should set criteria for accepting recommendations. Those that lack documented methods should receive less attention than those based primarily on science. Evidence-based guidelines often rate the quality of the supporting evidence (such as "good evidence for..." "insufficient evidence to make recommendation," "good evidence to exclude").

Guidelines may be less biased if members of an interdisciplinary body that includes multiple perspectives develop them. Recommendations issued by a specialty society or other organization whose members benefit from the practice may reflect the effect of the recommendations on the specialty and its members. Occasionally, clinical practice guidelines issued by different organizations have contradictory recommendations. In this case, the clinician must critique the methods by which the guidelines were developed. If conflicting groups do not agree on the scientific evidence, the provider should personally examine the critical studies to reach an independent conclusion. If there is no disagreement on the scientific basis for the recommendations, differences in recommendations may occur because of differences in panel member opinions, organizational policies, or writing styles. The clinician will have to come to his own conclusions about what the recommendations should be (Woolf, 1995).

Long-Term Consequences of Clinical Guideline Use

Currently, most practice guidelines are developed entirely on the basis of clinical concerns. Although health economics may have played a major role in the surge in guideline development, most current practice guidelines do not include analyses of cost-effectiveness, although the long-term treatment selected may have considerable financial implications. This often occurs because the clinical experts on such panels lack expertise in economic issues. These experts often recommend against performing diagnostic tests or treatments, not because of cost considerations but rather because of concerns about potential adverse effects or inadequate evidence of benefit. This may not be true for groups that have a strong business interest in controlling costs, such as payers, employers, and health plans.

The increased use of clinical practice guidelines has implications both for public policy and for litigation. Providers are concerned that the introduction of practice guidelines will reduce their clinical decision-making authority, and that their failure to follow clinical practice guidelines will lead to medical liability. Although practice guidelines are an increasing part of medical practice, only limited litigation suggests the extent to which guidelines will be used to set the applicable standard of care.

From a legal perspective, the primary issue is whether practice guidelines will be used to set the standard of care, or whether they will serve as just one more piece of evidence that a jury would consider in determining medical liability. Some writers have suggested that perhaps the courts should admit guidelines into evidence, but that they should not be used as the sole determinant of the standard of care. This approach will surely facilitate health care provider acceptance of guidelines by not imposing liability for failure to follow guidelines without additional evidence to determine the standard of care. Several independent legal reviews have concluded that practice guidelines may be more likely to reduce than to increase malpractice liability (Hirshfeld, 1994).

In theory, it might be assumed that the use of evidence-based guidelines derived from studies of clinical outcomes will improve patient outcomes. However, although interest in clinical guidelines is growing, no documentation shows their effectiveness. Few studies have examined whether guidelines change health care provider practices and patient health. The debate over guideline effectiveness has been hampered by the lack of a rigorous overview. In an examination of 59 published evaluations of clinical guidelines, all except 4 of the studies detected significant improvements in the process of care after guidelines were introduced, and in studies that assessed the outcomes of care, significant improvements were found. However, the extent of these improvements in performance varied considerably.

SUMMARY

To cut through all of the rhetoric written about clinical practice guidelines, it is clear that the development of practice guidelines might both help and harm patients and providers. Guidelines might improve the clinical decision making of health care clinicians by assisting in the education of new clinicians, provide current evidence and expert opinion on important clinical topics, and improve the research focus by identifying gaps in the evidence. However, they have the potential to harm patient care if the recommendations are inaccurate, and if compliance with flawed recommendations is enforced by organizations or courts. Health care providers who practice outside accepted clinical guidelines may risk losing reimbursement for services and precertification for procedures, as well as sacrificing favorable practice insurance. The extent of pressure on health care providers to comply with guidelines is anticipated to increase, and compliance may become a condition for licensure, reimbursement, or avoidance of fines (Woolf, 1995).

Expectations for guidelines remain high because they are one of only a few instruments of health care reform that promise to improve the quality of care while reducing overall health care costs. Thus, efforts to develop guidelines are likely to continue unabated in the foreseeable future. Additional research is needed to compare different methods of developing and disseminating guidelines.

evolve A continually updated list of useful WebLinks may be found in the Evolve Resources at http://evolve.elsevier.com/Edmunds/NP/

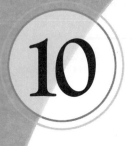

Design and Implementation of Patient Education

MARILYN WINTERTON EDMUNDS and JANN KEENAN

Practitioners educate patients about their disease, their medications, and ways that they can improve their health. When patients accurately understand their medications, adherence and cooperation are enhanced. However, many patients do not understand the written materials given to them to read because of low health literacy. Less than full understanding of health materials and written medical directions inevitably decreases the patient's ability to implement the treatment plan. Greater attention and effort should be taken to ensure that patient education materials are designed so that patients really get the message clinicians want to teach.

THE PROCESS OF PATIENT EDUCATION

Many texts describe the different components of the teaching process in depth (see Resources section on Evolve). Many of the experts on whom current practice is based began writing in the 1980s and the 1990s. Experts (Falvo, 2004; Lorig, 2000; Redman, 2004) agree that the essential items that should be incorporated into teaching include the following:

• *Assess the patient's desire to learn.*

It is beneficial to determine the patient's need to learn. Often, the provider wishes to provide information about a new treatment regimen or medication, or to respond to a patient's direct questions. Just because a provider knows that a patient needs information does not mean that the patient recognizes that need or, in fact, expects to learn from the provider. Patient education cannot be a one-way dispensing of information.

• *The patient must view proposed patient education as relevant.*

A study that examined the information-seeking behavior of individuals regarding their prescriptions (Morris et al, 2006) concluded that patients exhibited one of four distinct types of behavior when receiving drug information. This study suggests that patients gravitate to the information source they feel is most appropriate to them or with which they feel most comfortable (Dandavino et al, 2007).

• *Assess the patient's motivation and ability to learn.*

This requires getting to know patients and evaluating their interest in learning. Educational materials then should be tailored to patients' individual needs, including knowledge, reading ability, beliefs, and experiences, as well as primary language.

• *Negotiate, together, what needs to be taught.*

Formalize this negotiation by writing specific and measurable objectives with the patient ("Learn about adverse effects of the medication" is not measurable; "list five possible adverse effects" is considered a measurable and obtainable objective) (Redman, 2004).

• *Select a teaching method.*

Based on the patient's learning style, methods in which verbal instructions, written materials, audiovisual materials, Internet materials, or a combination are offered may be used. The method and pace of the teaching must be selected for each patient, acknowledging differences in the ways people learn and the rates at which they learn. Different teaching skills may be needed at different times for the same patient. Teaching should be carried out in small segments over several sessions.

• *Evaluate learning.*

Did the patient meet the objectives? Asking the patient to repeat back, return a demonstration, or follow through on a behavior that illustrates how well he has learned the material allows the provider to assess the degree of patient understanding or mastery. You may say, "I want to make sure I was clear with my message. In your own words, explain to me how to take this medicine." Feedback enhances learning. It shows patients the extent of their progress and increases confidence that they can learn the material (Falvo, 2004).

Reinforcement provides rewards for a given behavior and may be positive or negative (Mann et al, 2007; Wolf et al, 2007a). Offering verbal praise or congratulations for good adherence or a change in behavior may be the most effective way. Negative reinforcement or fear arousing may be effective, but it must be used cautiously.

• *Reduce barriers to adherence.*

Evaluation of adherence by an experienced clinician may help him to find ways to eliminate problems with the regimen and facilitate cooperation. The clinician might suggest that the patient should use special pill containers or adjust the medication regimen around his activities, or he might discuss with the patient ways to reduce cost.

• *Combine several methods of teaching to provide optimally effective interventions.*

Use of multiple types of teaching techniques can help the clinician to (1) accommodate different learning abilities or preferences, (2) compensate for low levels of literacy, (3) enhance retention of information, and (4) promote reinforcement.

What Should the Patient Be Taught?

The patient's need for information depends on the disease process, the treatment plan, and the patient–provider relationship. When a patient is first diagnosed with a medical problem, education must start with explaining the pathophysiology in terms the patient will understand and describing what the prognosis might be. It is only when patients understand what has happened to them that they can move on to consider what to do about it.

The initiation of new medication therapy requires fairly extensive teaching. It is clearly not possible to provide all information that patients might need in a single teaching session. Instead, the health care provider should have a plan in mind for the things that need to be covered, and this needs to be shared with patients. Information also should be shared regarding perceptions, expectations, and options (Lorig, 2000; Shapiro et al, 2006) (Box 10-1).

Additional teaching will be required when therapy is changed, medication dosages or schedules are adjusted, or changes in a patient's condition warrant additional modifications to therapy. Teaching then becomes individualized to what the patient requires and thus is packaged in quantities that the patient can handle. Each change offers an opportunity for a short educational session.

The health care provider must be familiar with the legal issues involved in the situation. Patients have the right to obtain information about their diagnosis, treatment, and prognosis. Informed consent is a principle that is implicit in the process of prescribing a medication for a patient. The practitioner has a legal obligation to ensure that patients understand their condition, the treatment proposed, and the risks and benefits of the treatment recommendations. The law requires that the amount and type of information provided to the patient should be "reasonable." It is up to the practitioner to determine what is reasonable for each patient to understand. The accepted standard of care ensures that practitioners are held legally responsible if they fail to advise

---

BOX 10-1   Key Information to Be Provided to Patients About Medications

Drug name (generic and brand)

Intended use and expected action

Route, dosage form, dosage, and specific administration schedule (hours of day to take)

Special directions for storage or preparation of medication

Special directions for administration of medication

Common side effects and serious adverse reactions

What patient should do if side effects occur

Potential drug–drug, drug–food, or drug–alcohol interactions

Prescription refill information

Action to be taken in the event of a missed dose

Special precautions when medication is taken (e.g., driving, actions requiring alertness)

Other information particular to the patient or the drug

When to return to the health care provider

How patients will know that the drug is doing what it should do

From Redman BK: *Advances in patient education*, New York, 2004, Springer; Wolf MS et al: To err is human: patient misinterpretations of prescription drug labeling instructions, *Patient Educ Couns* 67:293-300, 2007.

---

a patient adequately. Notes in the patient record should summarize the topics covered.

Various studies have found discrepancies between the information that clinicians perceive as important and the information that patients desire (Dolan et al, 2004; Safeer & Keenan, 2005; Schillinger et al, 2006; Shershneva et al, 2006). Rare or serious side effects are awkward to discuss. Some health care providers have been reluctant to volunteer in-depth discussion of these topics for fear of frightening patients, believing it may decrease their adherence with treatment. However, Reyes-Ortiz and colleagues (2005) found that seizure patients wanted to receive specific information on potentially serious side effects associated with carbamazepine. Although this information made the patients perceive the drug as risky, no patient refused treatment, and no evidence of a negative reaction was observed after patients had been given extensive information. The authors concluded that patients who are given detailed information may be able to accurately recognize side effects, should they occur.

Although formal teaching is carefully planned, teaching in the clinical areas often occurs in response to a patient's question and is implemented on the spur of the moment without adequate preparation, planning, or overall consideration of what the patient needs to know. Using scientific or professional jargon, providing too much technical detail, or being unnecessarily vague all hinder or destroy the teaching process. Although it is impossible to avoid answering impromptu questions (even if they take the provider by surprise), it is essential to have an overall written plan that will cover what will be taught, how it will be taught, and how the clinician will know when the patient has learned the material. Some hospitals and clinics schedule time for patient teaching, often for groups of patients with the same clinical diagnosis (Falvo, 2004).

As was introduced earlier in the discussion of process, formalization of the teaching–learning experience begins with the writing of specific objectives. Objectives reflect the blend of patient and provider decisions regarding the treatment philosophy, the use of results from research, learner motivation and need to learn, continuity in learning, sequential arrangement of the behavior to be learned, and the priority of learning. Specifically, the objectives must describe new behaviors that will occur because of changes in patients' thinking or understanding. The best objectives are precisely stated by describing the important conditions that surround performance and by specifying the criteria for acceptable performance. These are often based on national recommendations, clinical guidelines, or standard treatment goals for a particular disease or problem (Redman, 2004). Specific goals help to clarify for patients what they are to do (Falvo, 2004). For example, "Blood pressure will decrease to the diastolic reading of less than 95 mm Hg within 3 months" is specific, measurable, and based on national guidelines. As patients and providers craft objectives together, the provider has a chance to evaluate patients' knowledge, understanding, and general motivation to change behavior.

How Will Patient Education Be Accomplished?

Both the content and the process of patient education are important factors for consideration when specific teaching–learning objectives are planned. Many patients are overwhelmed when they first learn that they have a new diagnosis.

Fear and anxiety increase the confusion they often feel and interfere with their learning. Address these anxieties directly ("No, you don't have cancer").

To avoid increasing the stress that patients may feel, teaching should be conducted systematically when the learner is ready to learn. It should be provided in a timely manner, in a quiet and unhurried environment that gives patients a chance to ask questions. It is difficult to fulfill these criteria in today's busy health care system. Educational research has suggested that people are able to remember three major things that they are taught in any one session (Wolf et al, 2007). And they generally remember those things in the order in which they are presented. Providers who accept these premises and develop a teaching plan consistent with them can set aside small periods of time to devote to teaching a few, very specific things. Review on subsequent visits to evaluate learning and retention of information. Then the provider can move on to the next phase of information sharing that has been identified. The patient's family, caregivers, or loved ones might be included in the educational sessions as appropriate and in accordance with HIPAA privacy requirements.

In an effort to specifically improve medication adherence, the literature suggests a variety of strategies for providing patients with information about their medications (Barker et al, 2006; Jafri et al, 2007; Schultz et al, 2004). These strategies include verbal instruction, verbal and written instruction, and/or audiovisual aids. Some CDs, DVDs, and websites on the Internet combine audiovisual and written information in an interactive process.

Verbal education is often provided as one-on-one counseling, particularly when a patient's condition is first diagnosed and when therapy is first being implemented. Verbal instruction provides content and then gives the patient a chance to ask questions. Patients with chronic diseases such as diabetes or hypertension, who have extensive needs for teaching, may come together in small groups for part of their educational experience. Group interaction and observation may actually enhance learning because the context for learning is enhanced.

Written information can be provided in the form of special labels for prescription bottles, patient package inserts, single-page materials developed by individual pharmacists or organizations, and booklets. The health care provider, the health care institution, and professional specialty organizations may prepare and disseminate written information. Regardless of the source, information should be provided to meet specific educational needs and should not be provided to the patient until the patient is ready to receive it.

Audiovisual programs may use CDs or videocassettes. The greater availability of these resources and the wider use of VCRs, DVDs, and CDs in the home have led to the development of lending libraries with information on common topics. Wider availability of personal computers has increased the use of CDs for teaching patients. Use of the Internet to collect information allows patients to select what they want and to download and print it for future reference (Waters et al, 2005; Teasdale & Shaikh, 2006).

Research attention is now focused on the use of computers (Gresty et al, 2007; Kuhl et al, 2006), both to assess and to meet the needs of patients. Research (Koivunen et al, 2007; Navarre et al, 2007) suggests that patients might actually be more comfortable disclosing personal information to a computer than to a human being, even though they know the information will be reviewed by a health care professional. Although many educators initially thought that computers would not be appropriate for audiences with poor literacy skills, research findings have revealed the opposite. Investigators have found that the use of an audio computer-assisted self-interview system may result in more candid reporting of certain health behaviors and may be acceptable to subjects with poor literacy skills (Beranova & Sykes, 2007; Mackenzie et al, 2007).

All teaching methods, with the possible exception of patient package inserts, have been shown to improve knowledge and enhance information retention (Lorig, 2000; Redman, 2004). A combination of verbal and written information, or the use of verbal counseling along with audiovisual aids, is generally superior to the use of traditional written material only. Most patients prefer a combination of written and verbal information, and studies have shown that this approach is most effective in improving knowledge (Redman, 2004). When other criteria (such as efficacy, volume, logistics, and cost) are used to evaluate the best strategy for providing patient education, the preferred method again is to provide information both in writing and verbally. This is especially important for new prescriptions (Davis et al, 2006; Redman, 2004). Providing only written information is usually insufficient for patient education.

Reduced Literacy as a Barrier to Patient Education

Functional health literacy is

> the ability to read, understand, and act on health information. This includes such tasks as reading and comprehending prescription labels, interpreting appointment slips, completing health insurance forms, following instructions for diagnostic tests, and understanding other essential health-related materials required to adequately function as a patient. Functional health literacy varies by context and setting and may be significantly worse than one's general literacy.
>
> (ANDRUS & ROTH, 2002)

An individual may be able to read and understand general materials with familiar content at home or at work but may struggle when presented with medical material of the same complexity that contains unfamiliar vocabulary and concepts. This applies even to well-educated patients. Health literacy includes reading ability, numeracy skills (described as the ability to perform mathematical computations with numbers embedded in printed materials), and comprehension. Some authors suggest that numeracy, or quantitative literacy, may be the most important element of health literacy (Jackson, 2005; Nielsen-Bohlman et al, 2004; U.S. Public Health Service, 2005). For example, this would include reading how many pills one should take and when they should be taken—a skill that is essential for adequate and safe medication administration.

Lack of adequate literacy skills is a major barrier to patients' receiving proper health care. People with low reading levels have problems accessing the health care system, understanding recommended treatments and consent forms, and following the instructions of providers. Patients are routinely expected to read and understand labels on medicine containers, appointment slips, informed consent documents, and health education materials (Buchbinder et al, 2006; Davis et al, 2006). Thus, patients with lower literacy often have poor health outcomes (Weis et al, 2005). The number of years of school completed as reported by patients was four or five levels higher than their actual reading ability, as revealed on the Wide Range Achievement Test (WRAT), a word pronunciation and recognition test (Hironaka & Paasche-Orlow, 2006).

Many of the health educational materials that have been developed for patients by pharmaceutical companies, professional associations, and institutions are not suitable because a serious mismatch is noted between the level at which the patient can read and the level at which the materials are written. Approximately half of the population struggles with basic reading skills, and studies (Jackson, 2005) have found the following to be true:

- 35% of English-speaking patients could not read or understand basic health-related materials (i.e., had inadequate or marginal functional literacy).
- 42% of patients were unable to comprehend directions about taking medication on an empty stomach.
- 60% could not understand a standard consent form.
- 81% of elderly patients (age >60 years) had inadequate functional literacy.

One study (Rogers et al, 2006) of an indigent, uninsured, urban population documented average reading levels that were 4.6 grades below the last grade completed in school, with mean reading comprehension at the fifth grade level. Clearly, literacy problems are very prevalent and so critical that it is understandable that *Healthy People 2010* devoted some of its health communication objectives to this issue (USDHHS, 2002).

Notwithstanding the desire of some providers to develop patient teaching materials, there is no lack of prewritten patient educational materials. Many materials are available for sale, although the investment required to purchase this information for all patients may become prohibitive. In fact, the problem lies not in finding patient education materials but in evaluating their quality, readability, and applicability, particularly because many of them are written at too high a level for patient understanding. Many patient education handouts, such as those available over the Internet, may be modified and customized to the individual patient. However, even a cursory evaluation of these materials reveals that most are written at a higher reading level than is essential for most patients. No commercially available handouts should be used for patients unless they have been carefully assessed for readability. Most will require revision to be acceptable, no matter how "pretty" they look or how much money was spent to prepare them. Information from drug companies must be carefully screened because they often consist of more advertisement than information. Keeping sentences short and choosing simple words makes it much easier to develop reading materials at a simple and straightforward reading level (Redman, 2004).

Developing Written Materials Based on Literacy Requirements

The health literacy problem in the United States is extensive. The mean literacy level in the United States is at or below the eighth grade level (Redman, 2004). One in five adults tested at or below the two lowest levels, as determined by the National Adult Literacy survey. Although these levels are roughly translated to reading at about the fifth grade reading level, most health materials are written at the tenth grade level or above (Schillinger et al, 2006).

To match the learner to the material, teachers must know something about the factors that determine readability. Readability can be predicted in three ways: (1) by the Cloze method, in which every fifth word in a reading passage is removed and the reader is asked to fill in the words based on the meaning of other words in the passage; (2) by the predictability of certain words in reading passages; and (3) by formulas that are based on the length of words and of sentences. These formulas have been validated against reading tests.

Assessing the readability of content that has already been commercially prepared, or that is being developed by the clinician, was formerly a very cumbersome process. Redman (2004) explains three of the methods most commonly used to determine grade level of health care content; all involve counting the number and length of sentences and syllables in words. Computer word processing software now almost universally comes with a program that is used to automatically analyze the reading difficulty of files. However, there has not been good congruence between the computer calculations of readability and those that are done by hand, and many literacy specialists frown on the computer calculations (Redman, 2004). Nevertheless, in a busy clinician's office, using a Microsoft Word command on the Tools toolbar under Spelling gives you statistics for the Flesch readability scale in a quick and easy format.

If clinicians plan to develop their own written materials, they should be familiar with the various readability formulas that are useful for different types of text. For example, the Fry readability formula uses a graph to determine the level of materials from grades 1 through college; however, the standard Fry formula is not useful with passages of fewer than 300 words. Modified Fry tools and a dictionary of words correlated to grade level have been developed that may be used with shorter passages. The FOG readability formula uses number of sentences and number of polysyllabic words and is useful for grade 4 through college. The Flesch formula uses average sentence and word length and is useful for grades 5 through college (see Box 10-2 for an example). The SMOG formula counts the number of sentences and the number of words with three or more syllables and is useful for grades 5 through college. Redman (2004) compared readability formulas with use of the same health educational materials and found that the Flesch, FOG, and Fry formulas correlate highly with each other.

Designing Patient Education Materials

A portion of the overall objectives that are written to ensure that patients understand their health conditions, proper administration of their drugs, and general medical instructions should be covered in the written material given to patients. Particular attention should be paid to including the essential facts that each patient should know about his or her medications.

If only one handout will be prepared for all patients receiving a given drug, the readability should be below the eighth grade level and preferably at the fifth grade level (Cotunga et al, 2005). (By contrast, most patient leaflets included with medicine are written at a tenth to twelfth grade level.) In the ideal world, two or three handouts at different ability levels could be prepared for each drug. In

BOX 10-2   Flesch Readability Formula

1. For short pieces, test the entire selection. For longer pieces, test at least three randomly selected samples of 100 words each. Do not use introductory paragraphs. Start each sample at the beginning of a paragraph.
2. Determine the average sentence length (SL) by counting the number of words in the sample and dividing by the number of sentences. Count as a sentence each independent unit of thought that is grammatically independent, that is, whose end is punctuated by a period, question mark, exclamation point, semicolon, or colon. In dialog, count speech tag (e.g., "he said") as part of the quoted sentence.
3. Determine the word length (WL) by counting all the syllables in the sample as if reading the words aloud. Divide the number of syllables by the number of words in the sample and multiply by 100.
4. These indices then are applied to the formula to compute the reading ease: $RE = 206.835 - 1.015\,SL - 0.846\,WL$, where RE is the reading ease score, SL is the average sentence length in words, and WL is the average word length measured as syllables per 100 words.

INTERPRETATION OF THE FLESCH READING EASE SCORE

Reading Ease	Grade Level	Description of Style	No. Syllables/100 Words	Average Sentence Length
90-100	5	Very easy	123	8
80-90	6	Easy	131	11
70-80	7	Fairly easy	139	14
60-70	8-9	Standard	147	17
50-60	10-12	Fairly difficult	155	21
30-50	College	Difficult	167	25
0-30	College graduate	Very difficult	192	29

From Falvo DR: *Effective patient education: a guide to increased compliance*, ed 3, New York, 2004, Jones & Bartlett; Flesch R: *The art of readable writing*, New York, 1974, HarperCollins; Redman BK: *Advances in patient education*, New York, 2004, Springer.

some communities, handouts in several languages may be needed.

People at all literacy levels prefer simple, attractive materials. Pictures, diagrams, and videotapes help to communicate information to patients, especially those with low literacy skills. Most people, even those who read well, rely on visual cues to reinforce learning.

Oral and visual tools help patients absorb new information, and this increases learning. Supplementing text with pictures helps when one is providing self-care or medication instructions to low literate patients.

GENERAL PRINCIPLES TO USE IN PREPARING PATIENT EDUCATION MATERIALS

- *The goals of the handout should be stated in the material.*
- *Limit content to one or two educational objectives*—List what the reader will learn and do after he has read the information.
- *Emphasize the desired behavior rather than the medical facts*—Patients find it difficult to relate abstract statistics to their own experience.
- *Use clear captions, ample "white space," and photographs or realistic illustrations to attract the reader's attention and to reinforce the message*—Illustrations should depict the desired behavior that you want the patient to adopt.
- *Always avoid medical jargon, and use common words*—Terms should be concrete and familiar to the patient. For example, replace "antithrombotic agent" with "a drug that prevents blood clots."
- *The most readable educational materials are on no more than one page, front and back*—Longer materials can be used as long as they follow basic health literacy principles.
- *The material should include sections of bulleted lists in lieu of exclusively using running text in paragraphs*—Key items or warnings should be highlighted with bullets or icons.
- *The print size should be at least 12 point for body copy for the general public*—Use 14-point typeface if the material is designed for older adults.
- *Written instructions should be interactive*—Practitioners can accomplish this by developing materials that ask patients to do, write, say, or show something to demonstrate their understanding of a concept (Falvo, 2004).
- *Whenever possible, prepare materials in cooperation with patients who have low health literacy skills*—Their input will result in culturally sensitive and personally relevant information.

Writing in an "easy-to-read" style goes beyond writing at the fifth grade reading level or limiting words to three syllables. Individuals should develop materials so their patients not only *can* read the materials but also will *want* to read them. Writing from a positive rather than a negative view helps make materials acceptable. A checklist for assessment of written materials, developed by Jann Keenan, EdS, a health literacy specialist and public health educator, appears in Box 10-3.

Using Multimedia for Patient Education

Audiovisual materials might be reserved for common conditions with lengthy or complex instructions. Videotapes, audiotapes, and slides are available from pharmaceutical manufacturers for products that have complicated interaction, mixing, or administration features. The patient should be allowed time to view the material in a private or semiprivate area and then should be given a chance to ask questions. The provider should reinforce verbally the important points of

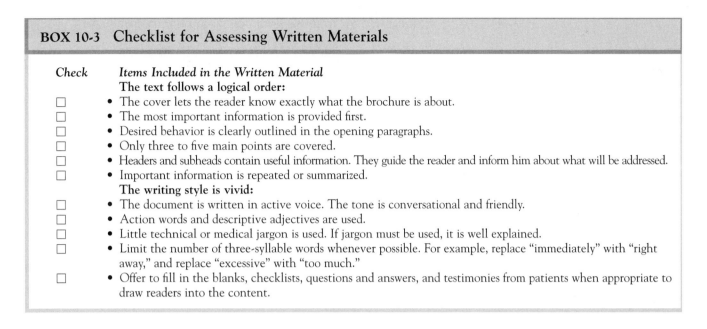

BOX 10-3   Checklist for Assessing Written Materials

Check	Items Included in the Written Material
	The text follows a logical order:
☐	• The cover lets the reader know exactly what the brochure is about.
☐	• The most important information is provided first.
☐	• Desired behavior is clearly outlined in the opening paragraphs.
☐	• Only three to five main points are covered.
☐	• Headers and subheads contain useful information. They guide the reader and inform him about what will be addressed.
☐	• Important information is repeated or summarized.
	The writing style is vivid:
☐	• The document is written in active voice. The tone is conversational and friendly.
☐	• Action words and descriptive adjectives are used.
☐	• Little technical or medical jargon is used. If jargon must be used, it is well explained.
☐	• Limit the number of three-syllable words whenever possible. For example, replace "immediately" with "right away," and replace "excessive" with "too much."
☐	• Offer to fill in the blanks, checklists, questions and answers, and testimonies from patients when appropriate to draw readers into the content.

the videos and should provide additional written materials to support learning.

Intervention studies have examined the feasibility and efficacy of using multimedia presentations of health information to reach audiences with poor literacy skills (DeWalt et al, 2004; Reyes-Ortiz et al, 2005; Weiss et al, 2006; Wolf et al, 2005). The AMC Cancer Research Center examined the use of an interactive computer program to deliver information regarding breast cancer to women with poor literacy skills. In the formative research stages, women reported that they thought the computer would be an appropriate channel by which to receive such information because they could use it at their own pace and could select information that was of greatest interest to them. In addition, they reported that they would want the computer to be located in a kiosk or private area so that others would not see the material they were studying.

PATIENT AND PROVIDER USE OF THE INTERNET FOR EDUCATIONAL PURPOSES. The Internet is becoming a source of up-to-date health information not only for providers but also for patients. Many Internet sites meet the needs of both groups (Boxes 10-4 and 10-5).

Although many commercial websites provide reliable information, others may be more interested in selling something. Commercial sites are identifiable by "com" at the end of their web addresses. The letters "org" denote a nonprofit group, "gov" a government agency, and "edu" an educational entity.

Several studies, including those done by Bussey-Smith and Rossen (2007), indicate that computerized health information is as effective as face-to-face instruction in increasing knowledge. Wolf and colleagues (2004) concluded that knowledge, active coping, information seeking coping, and social support were promoted by patients with HIV/AIDS who used the Internet. Their preliminary findings suggest an association between use of the Internet for health-related information and health benefit among people living with HIV/AIDS.

Patients from many different cultures and demographic backgrounds are searching the Internet (Box 10-6 and Table 10-1). Men are more likely to search online for health information about their own problems; women are more likely to search online for information on behalf of someone else (Bussey-Smith & Rossen, 2007).

EVALUATION OF LEARNING

Patient education in general is designed to change behavior, increase satisfaction, and promote adherence to the medication regimen. When objectives are written specifically, the outcomes of behavior change are clearly articulated. Thus, it should be simple to monitor the extent of learning that has taken place. When blood sugars do not come down and stay down, when blood pressure remains high, when weight is not lost—failure has occurred somewhere in the process. Sometimes the failure occurs right at the beginning of the teaching–learning process because the patient does not accept the provider's recommendations for change or is not ready to change. The goals that are established are meeting the needs of the provider and not the patient. Sometimes the process breaks down when patients do not understand what to do, cannot afford the treatment plan, or lose confidence in their ability to change. Whatever the problem, the health care provider must attempt to discover where the process went wrong (Redman, 2004).

It is important that the patient be engaged during the teaching–learning process. Active participation in learning facilitates retention. The more active the participation is and the more sensory involvement is provided, the more effective is the learning that takes place. Throughout the teaching process, summarize, repeat, and keep it simple. Providers should check for comprehension as they go along. Have the patient repeat important points. It is important not to be threatening or intimidating when quizzing patients on information that has been discussed (Falvo, 2004; Redman, 2004). Then, document in the patient's chart the extent and result of education provided. List the important topics covered, state what written material was given to the

BOX 10-4   Professional Organizations

American Academy of Allergy, Asthma, and Immunology, 611 E Wells St, Milwaukee, WI 53202; Phone: 414-272-6071,
Fax: 414-272-6070, www.infoaaaai.org

American Academy of Dermatology, 930 N Meacham Rd, Schaumburg, IL 60173-4965; Phone: 847-330-0230

American Academy of Family Physicians, 8880 Ward Pkwy, Kansas City, MO 64114; Phone: 816-333-9700,
Fax: 816-333-0303, www.aafp.org/familymed

American Academy of Neurology, 1080 Montreal Ave, St. Paul, MN 55116; Phone: 612-695-1940, www.aan.com

American Academy of Nurse Practitioners, Capitol Station LBJ Building, PO Box 78711, Austin, TX 78711;
Phone: 512-442-4262, Fax: 512-442-6469, www.aanp.org

American Academy of Orthopaedic Surgeons, 6300 N River Rd, Rosemont, IL 60018-4262; Phone: 847-823-7186

American Academy of Pediatrics, 141 Northwest Point Blvd, Elk Grove Village, IL 60007; Phone: 847-228-5005,
Fax: 847-228-5097, www.kidsdocsaap.org; wwwaap.org

American Academy of Physician Assistants, 950 N Washington St, Alexandria, VA 22314-1552; Phone: 703-836-2272

American Association of Nurse Anesthetists, 222 South Prospect Ave, Park Ridge, IL 60068; Phone: 708-692-7050

American Cancer Society, 1599 Clifton Rd NE, Atlanta, GA 30329; Phone: 404-320-3333

American College of Chest Physicians, 3300 Dundee Rd, Northbrook, IL 60062-2348; Phone: 847-498-1400, Fax: 847-498-5460

American College of Emergency Physicians, PO Box 619911, Dallas, TX 75261; Phone: 972-550-0911, Fax: 972-580-2816,
www.acep.org

American College of Gastroenterology, 4900-B S 31st St, Arlington, VA 22206-1656; Phone: 703-820-7400, www.acg.gi.org

American College of Nurse Midwives, 818 Connecticut Ave NW, Ste 900, Washington DC 20005; Phone: 202-408-7050,
Fax: 202-408-0902, www.nurse.org/ACNP/

American College of Nurse Practitioners, 1501 Wilson Blvd, Suite 509, Arlington, VA 22209; Phone: 703-740-2429,
Fax: 703-740-2553

American College of Obstetricians and Gynecologists, 409 12th St SW, PO Box 96920, Washington, DC 20090-6920;
Phone: 202-638-5577, www.acog.com

American College of Physicians, Independence Mall, W 6th St at Race, Philadelphia, PA 19106-1572; Phone: 215-351-2400,
www.acponline.org

American College of Surgeons, 633 St. Clair St, Chicago, IL 60611; Phone: 312-664-4050, Fax: 312-440-7014, postmaster
facs.org; www.facs.org

American Diabetes Association, 1660 Duke St, Alexandria, VA 22314; Phone: (703) 549-1500, www.diabetes.org

American Federation of Home Health Agencies, 1320 Fenwick Ln, Ste 100, Silver Spring, MD 20910; Phone: 301-588-1454

American Gastroenterological Association, 7910 Woodmont Ave, 7th Fl, Bethesda, MD 20814-3015; Phone: 301-654-2055,
Fax: 301-654-5920, www.gastro.org

American Geriatrics Society, 770 Lexington Ave, Ste 300, New York, NY 10021; Phone: 212-308-1414, Fax: 212-832-8646,
infoamgeramericangeriatrics.org/www.american geriatrics.org

American Heart Association, 7272 Greenville Ave, Dallas, TX 75231-4596; Phone: 214-373-6300, www.americanheart.org

American Hospital Association, One N Franklin, Ste 27, Chicago, IL 60606; Phone: 312-422-3000, www.aha.org

American Lung Association, 1740 Broadway, New York, NY 10019-4374; Phone: 212-315-8700, www.lungusa.org

American Medical Association, 515 N State St, Chicago, IL 60610; Phone: 312-464-5000, Fax: 312-464-4623, www.ama-assn.org

American Neurological Association, 5841 Cedar Lake Rd, Ste 204, Minneapolis, MN 55416; Phone: 612-545-6284,
Fax: 612-545-6073, www.lwilkersoncompuserve.com

American Orthopaedic Society, 6300 N River Rd, Ste 727, Rosemont, IL 60018; Phone: 847-698-1694, Fax: 847-823-0536

American Psychiatric Association, 1400 K St NW, Washington, DC 20005; Phone: 202-682-6000, Fax: 202-682-6114,
www.apapsych.org or www.psych.org

American Public Health Association, 1015 15th St NW, 3rd Fl, Washington, DC 20005-2605; Phone: 202-789-5600,
Fax: 202-789-5661, www.apha.org

American Society on Aging, 833 Market St, Ste 511, San Francisco, CA 94103-1824; Phone: 415-974-9600 or 800-537-9728,
Fax: 415-974-0300

American Society of Internal Medicine, 2011 Pennsylvania Ave NW, Ste 800, Washington, DC 20006; Phone: 202-835-2746

American Thoracic Society, 1740 Broadway New York, NY 10019-4374; Phone: 212-315-8700, Fax: 212-315-6498, www.thoracic.org

Arthritis Foundation, 1330 W Peachtree St, Atlanta, GA 30309; Phone: 404-872-71010, www.arthritis.org

Association of Reproductive Health Professionals, 2401 Pennsylvania Ave NW, Ste 350, Washington, DC 20037;
Phone: 202-466-3825, Fax: 202-466-3826, www.arhp.org

Asthma and Allergy Foundation of America, 1125 15th St NW, Ste 502, Washington, DC 20005; Phone: 202-466-7643,
Fax: 202-466-8940, www.infoaafa.org

Gerontological Society of America, 1275 K St NW, Ste 350, Washington, DC 20005-4006; Phone: 202-842-1275

Infectious Disease Association of America, 11 Canal Center Plaza, Ste 104, Alexandria, VA 22314; Phone: 703-299-0200,
Fax: 703-299-0204

National Hospice Organization, 1901 N Moore St, Ste 901, Arlington, VA 22209-1714; Phone: 703-243-5900,
Fax: 703-525-5762, www.nho.org

National Organization of Nurse Practitioner Faculties, One Dupont Circle, NW #530, Washington, DC 20036;
Phone: 202-452-1405, Fax: 202-452-1406, www.nonpfaacn.nche.edu

BOX 10-5   Self-Help Numbers for Patients and Providers

Adoption Center, National: 800-862-3678
Adoption of Special Kids: 415-543-2275
Agent Orange (Veterans Payment Program): 800-225-4712
AIDS Clearinghouse, National: 800-458-5231
AIDS Clinical Trials Information Service: 800-TRIALS-A
AIDS and HIV Hotline, National: 800-342-AIDS, 800-344-7432 (Spanish)
Al-Anon Family Group Headquarters, Inc: 800-344-2666
Alcohol and Drug Information, National Clearinghouse for: 800-729-6686, 800-487-4889
Alcoholism, American Council on: 800-527-5344
Alcoholism and Drug Dependence, National Council on: 800-622-2255
Alzheimer's Association: 800-272-3900
Alzheimer's Disease Education and Referral Center: 800-438-4380
American Liver Association: 800-223-0179
American Red Cross: 202-737-8300
Amyotrophic Lateral Sclerosis Association: 800-782-4747
Anemia Foundation: 800-522-7222
Arthritis Consulting Services: 800-327-3027
Arthritis Foundation: 800-283-7800
Autism Hotline, National: 304-525-8014, 800-428-8476
Battered Women's Justice Project: 800-903-0111
Blind, American Foundation for the: 800-232-5463
Blind Children's Center: 800-222-3566
Blind and Dyslexic, Recordings for the: 800-221-4792
Blind, Guide Dog Foundation for the: 800-543-4337
Blind, Job Opportunities for the: 800-638-7518
Blind, National Office of the: 800-424-8666
Blinded Veterans' Association: 800-669-7079
Blindness, Foundation Fighting (RP): 800-683-5555
Blindness (Prevent Blindness America): 800-331-2020
Brain Injury Association: 202-296-6443
Brain Injury National Foundation: 800-444-6443
Breast Cancer, Y-Me National Organization Hotline: 800-221-2141
Burn Association, American: 312-642-9260
Burn Victim Foundation, National: 800-803-5879
Cancer Foundation, The Candlelighters Childhood: 800-366-2223
Cancer Information and Counseling Line, AMC: 800-525-3777
Cancer Institute, National (Cancer Information Service): 800-4-CANCER
Cancer Research, American Institute for: 800-843-8114
Cancer Society, American: 800-ACS-2345
Cerebral Palsy Association, United: 800-872-5827
Child Abuse and Family Violence, National Council on: 800-222-2000
Child Abuse, National Committee to Prevent: 312-663-3520, 800-422-4453
Child Protection and Custody, Resource Center on: 800-527-3223
Cleft Palate Foundation: 800-242-5338
Cocaine (Phoenix House Foundation): 800-COCAINE, 800-DRUG HELP, 800-262-2463
Craniofacial Association, Children's: 800-535-3643

Crohn's and Colitis Foundation: 800-343-3637
Cystic Fibrosis Foundation: 800-FIGHT-CFU, 800-344-4823
Deaf, Captioned Films and Video Programs for the: 800-237-6213
Deafness Research Foundation: 800-535-3323
de Lange Syndrome Foundation: 800-753-2357
Depressive Illness, National Foundation for: 800-248-4344
Depressive and Manic Depressive Association, National: 800-82-NDMDA
Diabetes Association, American: 800-DIABETES
Diabetes Foundation, American: 800-232-3472
Diabetes Foundation, Juvenile: 800-223-1138
Domestic Violence, National Coalition Against: 303-839-1852
Domestic Violence, National Hotline: 800-799-SAFE
Domestic Violence, National Resource Center: 800-537-2238
Down Syndrome Congress, National: 800-232-NDSC
Down Syndrome Society, National: 800-221-4602
Drug and Alcohol Treatment Routing Service, National: 800-662-HELP (4357)
Drug Dependence, National Council on Alcoholism: 800-622-2255
Drug Information, National Clearinghouse for Alcohol: 800-729-6686
Dyslexia Society: 800-222-3123
EAR Foundation: 800-545-4327
Easter Seal Society: 800-221-6827
Eldercare Locator Information and Referral Line: 800-677-1116
EMERGE (Counseling and Education to Stop Male Violence): 617-422-1550
Epilepsy Foundation, American: 800-332-1000
Epilepsy Information Service: 800-642-0500
Eye Care Project Helpline, National: 800-222-3937
Facial Disfigurement: 800-332-3223
Facial Reconstruction, National Foundation for: 212-263-6656
Family Violence Helpline, National Council on Child Abuse and: 800-222-2000
Genetic Support Groups, Alliance of: 800-336-GENE
Guillain-Barré Syndrome Foundation, International: 610-667-0131
Headache Foundation, National: 800-843-2256
Hearing Aid Helpline: 800-521-5247
Hearing and Communication Handicaps: 800-327-9355
Hearing, Dial-a- (Screening Test): 800-222-EARS
Hearing Information Center: 800-622-3277
Hearing Institute, Better: 800-327-9355
Heart Association, American: 800-242-8721
Hemophilia, National Foundation: 800-42-HANDI
Hepatitis Hotline, American: 800-223-0179
High Blood Pressure Line (National Heart, Lung, and Blood Institute): 800-575-WELL
Hospice International, Children's: 800-242-4453
Hospice Organization Helpline, National: 800-658-8898
Huntington's Disease Society: 800-345-HDSA (4372)
Impotence Information Center: 800-843-4315

BOX 10-5   Self-Help Numbers for Patients and Providers (Continued)

Incontinence Information Center: 800-543-9632
Incontinence, Simon Foundation for: 800-23-SIMON
Interstitial Cystitis Association: 212-979-6057
Juvenile Diabetes Foundation: 800-533-2873
Kidney Foundation, National: 800-622-9010
Kidney Fund, American: 800-638-8299
Kidney Patients, American Association of: 800-749-2257
Knight-Ridder Information, Inc: 800-334-2564
Leukodystrophy Foundation, United: 800-728-5483
Liver Association, American: 800-223-0179
Lung Association, American: 800-LUNG-USA
Lung Line Information Center (National Jewish Center for Immunology and Respiratory Medicine): 800-222-LUNG
Lupus Foundation of America: 800-558-0121
Lyme Disease Foundation: 800-886-5963
Lymphedema Network, National: 800-541-3259
March of Dimes Birth Defects Foundation: 914-428-7100
Marfan Foundation, National: 800-8-MARFAN
Medicare Hotline: 800-638-6833
Mental Health Association, National: 800-969-6642
Mentally Ill, National Alliance for the: 800-950-NAMI
Healthy Mothers, Healthy Babies Coalition: 202-863-2458
Multiple Sclerosis Association of America: 800-833-4672
Multiple Sclerosis Society, National: 800-LEARN-MS, 800-344-4867
Muscular Dystrophy Association: 800-572-1717
Myasthenia Gravis Foundation: 800-541-5454
National Alliance for the Mentally Ill: 800-950-6264
National Drug and Alcohol Treatment Hotline: 800-662-HELP
National Manic/Depressive Association: 800-826-3632
Neurofibromatosis Foundation: 800-323-7938
Obsessive-Compulsive Foundation: 203-878-5669
Optometric Association, American: 314-991-4100
Organ Donation, The Living Bank: 800-528-2971
Organ Donor Hotline: 800-243-6667
Osteoporosis Foundation, National: 800-223-9994
Ostomy Association, United: 800-826-0826
Paget's Disease Foundation: 800-23-PAGET
Panic Disorder Information Helpline: 800-64-PANIC
Paralysis Association, American: 800-225-0292
Parkinson's Disease Association, American: 800-223-APDA (2732)
Parkinson's Disease Foundation: 800-457-6676

Parkinson Foundation, National: 800-327-4545
Planned Parenthood Federation of America: 800-230-7526
Podiatric Medical Association, American: 800-FOOT-CARE
Prevent Blindness America: 800-331-2020
Prostate Information Center: 800-543-9632
Psoriasis Foundation, National: 503-297-1545
Radon (Federal Hot Line): 800-767-7236
Rare Disorders, National Organization for: 800-999-6673
Red Cross, American: 202-737-8300
Rehabilitation Information Center, National: 800-346-2742
Rehabilitation Technology, Center for: 800-726-9119
Respiratory (Lung Line Center): 800-222-5864
Reyes Syndrome Foundation, National: 800-233-7393
Safety Council, National: 800-621-7619
Scleroderma Foundation, United: 800-722-4673
Sexually Transmitted Disease Hot Line, National: 800-227-8922
Sickle Cell Disease Association of America: 800-421-8453
Skin Cancer Foundation: 800-SKIN-490
Sleep Disorders Association, American: 507-287-6006
Social Health Association, American: 919-361-8422
Speech-Language-Hearing Association, American: 800-638-TALK
Spina Bifida Association of America: 800-621-3141
Spinal Cord Injury Association: 800-962-9629
Stroke Association, National: 800-787-6537
Stroke Connection of the AHA: 800-553-6321
Stuttering, National Center for: 800-221-2483
Sudden Infant Death Syndrome (SIDS) Alliance: 800-221-SIDS, 800-638-7437
Tourette Syndrome Association: 800-237-0717
Trauma (American Trauma Society): 800-556-7890
Tuberous Sclerosis Association, National: 800-225-NTSA
Victim Assistance, National Organization of: 202-232-6682
Vietnam Veterans and Their Families, National Information System for: 800-922-9234
Vision and Aging, Lighthouse National Center for: 800-334-5497
Visiting Nurse Preferred Care: 800-426-2547
Wegener's Granulomatosis Support Group, Inc: 800-277-9474
WomanKind: 612-924-5775

patient, and provide an assessment of the patient's level of comprehension and any evidence of the patient's intention to comply.

Specific things that might assist in improving compliant medication-taking behavior for most patients include developing treatment plans that require frequent provider–patient contact; using reminder cards; completing drug evaluation assays; tailoring the therapeutic regimen to the patient's characteristics and environment; providing reinforcement through behavioral feedback that promotes adherence or discourages noncompliant behavior; and enhancing patient involvement in such activities as taking blood pressure at home or establishing therapeutic contracts with the provider (Falvo, 2004; Lorig, 2000). These strategies should be kept in mind when objectives for learning and evaluation of the learning process are crafted.

SUMMARY

Sufficient research has been conducted to demonstrate that patient education is really not an optional activity for the health care provider. Although if has long been recognized as important, patient education often has been omitted because of lack of time, lack of reimbursement, and lack of intrinsic valuing. Patient educational needs were often perceived as

BOX 10-6   Terms Frequently Used in Electronic Communications

BBS: Bulletin Board System; allows users to hold discussions and make announcements that others can read and to which they can respond

Browser: Software for bringing up and displaying Web pages; examples: Netscape Navigator and Microsoft Internet Explorer

E-Mail: Electronic messages sent between or among computers; similar to an electronic telephone

Home Page: Website introductory page

HTML (HyperText Markup Language): Web page format coding system

http (HyperText Transfer Protocol): System of communication rules for the World Wide Web

Hyperlink: Text that can be linked to other text by clicking with a mouse at designated points

Internet: A massive worldwide electronic network composed of smaller computer networks that are linked together

Listserves: Groups of users, usually with a common interest, linked together through the Internet; facilitates rapid delivery of information to everyone and allows queries and responses

Modem: Accessory that connects computers to telephone lines and allows computers to talk to each other

Password: Personal letters or numerals used to identify authorized user access to locked systems

Search Engine: Software programs that search databases or documents for key words or phrases

SMTP (Simple Mail Transfer Protocol): Governs transmission of e-mail through the Internet

URL (Uniform Resource Locator): Internet address of an Internet page; similar to a telephone number, each is unique

Usenet Newsgroups: Electronic discussion groups organized around topics of mutual interest to participants

Virus: A destructive program that invades and infects other programs, causing them to malfunction or self-destruct

www (World Wide Web): Network of electronic sites linked to form a global electronic network for transmitting information in text, graphic, audio, or video formats.

TABLE 10-1   Websites That Offer Information for Navigating the Web

Site	URL Address
Beginners Central	www.northernwebs.com/bc
The Help Web	www.imagescape.com/helpweb
The Internet Learning Tree	world.std.com/-walthowe/ilrntree.html
Internet Starter Kit	ss2.mcp.com/resources/geninternet/frameiskm.html
Internet Web Text Index	www.december.com/web/text
Too Old for Computers?	www.portals.pdx.edu/-isidore/tooold.html
Welcome to Folks Online	www.folksonline.com

needs of the patient and not really as needs that should be met by the health care provider. However, if health care providers are forced to pay attention to the bottom line of health care costs, they can no longer remain so cavalier about a process that may save so much money and bring such great dividends in increased patient awareness. Indeed, providing patient education empowers patients to more fully become partners in establishing and meeting their own health care goals.

evolve A continually updated list of useful WebLinks may be found in the Evolve Resources at http://evolve.elsevier.com/Edmunds/NP/

Dermatologic Agents

DRUG OVERVIEW

Class	Subclass	Generic Name	Trade Name
Topical Corticosteroids (see Table 11-2)			
Immunosuppressive drugs		pimecrolimus	Elidel ✷
		tacrolimus	Protopic
Antiinfectives			
Topical antibiotics		mupirocin ✷	Bactroban ✷
		bacitracin	Bacitracin, Baciguent
		erythromycin	Akne-mycin
		gentamicin	Garamycin
		nystatin ✷	Mycostatin
		polymyxin B sulfate	In Polysporin, Neosporin
Topical antifungals	Azoles	clotrimazole	Lotrimin, Mycelex, Lotrisone
		econazole	Spectazole
		ketoconazole ✷	Nizoral
		miconazole	Monistat-Derm
		oxiconazole	Oxistat
		sertaconazole	Ertaczo
		sulconazole	Exelderm
	Allylamine/benzylamine derivatives	butenafine	Mentax
		naftifine	Naftin
		terbinafine	Lamisil ✷
	Hydroxypyridones	ciclopirox	Penlac, Loprox
	Others	nystatin ✷	Nystatin, Mycostatin
		haloprogin	Halotex
		tolnaftate	Tinactin
		selenium sulfide lotion	2.5% Selsun
Topical antivirals		acyclovir ✷	Zovirax ✷
		penciclovir	Denavir
Scabicides/ pediculicides		crotamiton	Eurax
		ivermectin	Stromectol
		malathion	Ovide
		permethrin	Elimite, Nix
		lindane	Kwell
Acne Preparations			
Antibacterial/ keratolytic		benzoyl peroxide	Benzac (prescription), many brands OTC
		metronidazole	MetroGel
		clindamycin ✷	Cleocin-T
Topical retinoid		tretinoin	Retin-A, Avita
Oral retinoid		isotretinoin	Accutane

Table continued on following page

DRUG OVERVIEW (Continued)

Class	Subclass	Generic Name	Trade Name
Local Anesthetics	Short acting	procaine HCl	Novocain
		chloroprocaine	Nesacaine
	Intermediate acting	lidocaine HCl	Xylocaine
		mepivacaine HCl	Carbocaine HCl
		prilocaine HCl	Citanest
	Long acting	bupivacaine HCl	Marcaine, Sensorcaine
		etidocaine	Duranest
		tetracaine HCl	Pontocaine HCl

✳ Top 200 drug.

INDICATIONS

Topical Corticosteroids

- Inflammatory and pruritic dermatoses that are responsive to corticosteroids, such as psoriasis, eczema, contact dermatitis, and many other dermatoses

Topical Antiinfectives (Antibiotics)

- Infection prophylaxis in minor cuts, wounds, burns, and skin abrasions; aid to healing
- Treatment of superficial infections of the skin caused by susceptible organisms amenable to local treatment

Antifungals

- Superficial fungal infections (see Table 11-4)

Scabicides/pediculicides

- See Table 11-5 for indications.

Topical and Oral Acne Preparations

- Acne vulgaris

Local Anesthetics

- Local anesthetics are indicated for a variety of uses, which include minor surgical procedures, suturing, and relief of itching or pain from wounds, burns, and/or hemorrhoids.
- Local anesthesia does not depress the patient's level of consciousness, which makes its use much safer than general anesthesia. Local anesthetics may be applied as a powder, gel, lotion, ointment, spray, or injection into a small area. If a larger area is required for anesthesia, a nerve trunk (epidural, spinal) or a single nerve may be injected to provide for regional anesthesia. This discussion is not intended as a complete presentation but rather as a brief overview of common local anesthetics used in primary care.
- Local anesthetics may be combined with vasoconstrictors (epinephrine) to prolong action by decreasing systemic absorption. However, at the ends of arteries, such as in the fingers, toes, penis, and nose, vasoconstrictors are not safe for use. In those areas, gangrene may develop because of severe vasoconstriction.
- A number of local agents are used safely on mucous membranes, ulcers, or wounds. If agents are applied to the oral cavity, however, the patient may have difficulty swallowing. Therefore, food should be withheld for at least 1 hour to prevent aspiration. Use with caution in areas of inflammation.
- Do not use if solutions are discolored or if they contain precipitants. If the solution does not contain a preservative, it must be discarded after opening. Because some situations of severe anaphylaxis have resulted from the use of local anesthetics, have resuscitation equipment on hand before use or emergency backup plans when any anesthetic is used. Obtain the patient's prior history of local anesthetic use before administration. Patient or guardian should sign a permission form before consenting to any procedure involving a local anesthetic.

This chapter discusses preparations used for skin, nail, and hair problems. These preparations are used for an extremely large array of dermatologic problems. See each section for more specific indications. General issues in topical medications are discussed; then corticosteroids, antiinfectives, acne medications, and local anesthesia are discussed, each in a separate section. The purpose of this chapter is to discuss the most common of the various available agents. It does not attempt to mention all of the preparations or the myriad indications for these agents. This chapter focuses on the topical use of these products. See appropriate chapters for more information about drugs from specific drug categories.

THERAPEUTIC OVERVIEW OF DERMATOLOGIC AGENTS

Anatomy and Physiology

The primary function of the skin is as a barrier. It functions to protect and thermoregulate. The skin is involved in the immune response, biochemical synthesis, and sensory detection.

The skin's barrier function is compromised when the skin has been damaged, or when inflammation is present.

The skin, the largest organ of the body, consists of three distinct layers: epidermis, dermis, and subcutaneous tissue (Figure 11-1). The epidermis is the outer layer of the skin. The thickness of the epidermis ranges from 0.05 mm on the eyelids to 1.5 mm on the palms and soles. Five layers make up the epidermis. Basal cells form a single layer of cells that make up the innermost layer of the epidermis. These basal cells divide to form keratinocytes. The other layers are formed as keratinocytes change until they migrate to the outer layer to become the major component of the stratum corneum. The stratum corneum provides protection to the skin by acting as a barrier. The thicker the epidermis, the greater is the barrier protection provided.

The dermis, similar to the epidermis, varies in thickness, ranging from 0.3 mm on the eyelid to 3 mm on the back. Three types of connective tissue—collagen, elastic tissue, and reticular fibers—make up the dermis. Different from the epidermis, the dermis is made up of nerves, blood vessels, hair follicles, and apocrine and eccrine glands.

Subcutaneous tissue is the deepest layer. Distribution is dependent on sex characteristics. Age, heredity, and caloric intake also influence distribution. The subcutaneous tissue provides padding and insulation to the underlying structures.

Pathophysiology

Three types of primary skin lesions have been identified: the macule, the papule, and the vesicle. Variations of these lesions are named according to the size of the lesion. Secondary lesions include erosion, ulcer, fissure, crust, lichenification, atrophy, excoriation, scar, and keloid.

When one is describing a skin lesion, it is important to name accurately the type of lesion by using this terminology. Location on the body and pattern of distribution are important. Timing and course should include whether the onset was acute or insidious. Also, the presence of any systemic signs and symptoms should be noted.

MECHANISM OF ACTION

Topicals work by being absorbed into the skin. Their effect is local. The specific mechanisms of action are discussed in each separate section.

Topical preparations are available in a bewildering array of products, including many combination products, steroid products of different strengths, and antiinfectives of every kind. The primary care provider should become familiar with a few products and treatment measures rather than trying to master the complete array. Superficial skin infections and acne are commonly treated in primary care. If the patient does not respond to standard care, he is referred to a dermatologist. Primary care providers should be able to identify suspicious lesions and refer patients promptly to dermatology; such patients frequently require surgical treatment.

Where applicable, specific information regarding standard guidelines, evidence-based recommendations, cardinal points of treatment, pharmacologic treatment, and nonpharmacologic treatment is provided later in the chapter.

Factors That Affect Drug Absorption

Topical therapy is unique because the skin is directly accessible for both diagnosis and therapy. Drugs used to treat skin problems can be applied directly to the site. All topical agents can also be absorbed systemically. Consider the adverse effects of the systemic medication when you are ordering topical agents.

Factors that affect the extent of drug absorption into the skin include the status of the skin, the characteristics of the drug, and the characteristics of the administration vehicle. Absorption is increased when the skin is broken or inflamed. In addition, absorption increases in cases in which skin integrity is compromised or the skin is thinner. Because of the vascular composition of the skin, mucous membranes absorb medication in high concentrations. The vehicle or base affects percutaneous absorption (Table 11-1). The vehicle may hydrate the outer layer of skin by preventing water loss. With improved hydration, the absorption of medication and the depth of penetration are enhanced.

Absorption of topical medications is slow and incomplete compared with drugs given orally. For optimal absorption, apply them to moist skin either immediately after bathing or after wet soaks.

Prescribing the appropriate amount of topical medication is important. Too large a tube may be very costly to the patient, yet a small tube may not include enough medication to cover the entire area. To estimate the amount that should be prescribed, the rule of nines can be used (Figure 11-2).

How Topical Agents Are Used

CREAMS, OINTMENTS, PASTES

1. Take a small amount of cream or ointment into the palm of the hand, and rub the hands together until the medication has a thin sheen.
2. Apply a small amount of ointment or cream as a thin layer to the skin. Excess medication is lost when it rubs off onto the clothing.

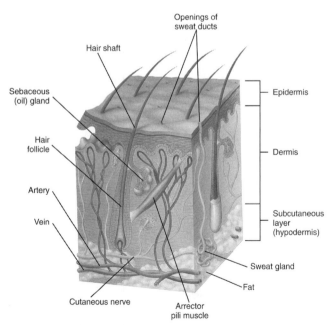

FIGURE 11-1   Structure of the skin. (From Thibodeau G, Patton K: *Anatomy and physiology*, ed 3, St Louis, 1996, Mosby.)

TABLE 11-1   Characteristics of Vehicle of Selected Topical Products

	Creams	Ointments	Gels	Solutions and Lotions	Aerosols
Base	Mixture of several different organic oils and water	Mixture of a limited number of organic compounds consisting primarily of petroleum jelly with little or no water	Greaseless mixtures of propylene glycol, water, and alcohol	Alcohol, water, and some chemicals	Drug suspended in a base and delivered via a propellant (e.g., isobutane, propane)
Color	White, somewhat greasy	Translucent, greasy feeling persists on skin	Clear with a gelatinous consistency	Clear or milky	
Versatility	Most frequent base prescribed, used on nearly all body areas, especially useful in the intertriginous areas (e.g., groin, genital area, axillae)	Greater penetration, useful for drier lesions, enhanced potency	Unpleasant sticky feeling, may be irritating	Most useful for scalp because it penetrates the hair shaft	Useful for applying to scalp via a long probe attached to a can
Miscellaneous	Cosmetically more acceptable; can be drying after prolonged use, best used for acute exfoliative dermatitis	Too occlusive for acute exudative eczematous inflammation; too occlusive for intertriginous areas	Alcohol gels feel cool and are drying; useful in acute exudative inflammation (e.g., poison ivy); nonalcoholic gels are more lubricating and can be useful in drying scalp lesions; useful in scalp areas because other vehicles mat hair	May be drying and irritating when used in intertriginous areas	Convenient for patients who lack mobility and have difficulty in reaching lower legs; useful for moist lesions (e.g., poison ivy)

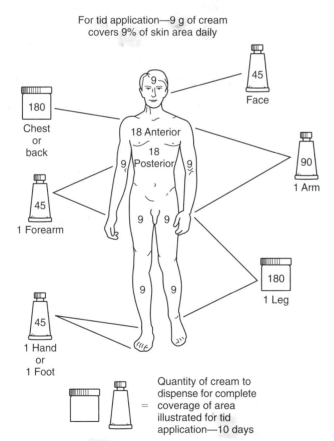

For tid application—9 g of cream covers 9% of skin area daily

Quantity of cream to dispense for complete coverage of area illustrated for tid application—10 days

FIGURE 11-2   Rule of nines to calculate quantity of medication to be dispensed. (From Habif TP: *Clinical dermatology*, ed 4, St Louis, 2004, Mosby.)

3. Apply topical medications with long, downward strokes to the affected areas. Avoid back-and-forth strokes because they may cause irritation of the hair follicles.
4. A tongue blade may be used for the application of topicals in a paste form.
5. Make sure to wash hands after application.

LOTIONS
1. Instruct the patient to shake the container to mix the suspension well.
2. Carefully pour a small quantity of lotion into the palm of the hand.
3. Apply a thin layer to the skin using firm, downward strokes. Avoid using gauze unless the liquid is very thin. Cotton balls should be avoided when medication is applied because they retain the suspended particles of medication.
4. Wash hands after application.

SPRAYS AND AEROSOLS
1. Shake the container well.
2. Direct spray toward the affected body part while holding the container upright 6 to 12 inches away from the body. Avoid spraying into the eyes.
3. At moderate range, spray lightly, covering the surface once.

POWDERS
1. Apply powder lightly to dry skin with gauze or a powder puff as needed.

How to Monitor

- Monitor for therapeutic and adverse effects. See specific classes of drugs for details.

Patient Variables

- Specifics are discussed under each class of drug.
- Geriatric skin is thinner and is more absorbent than the skin of younger adults.
- Children absorb about three times as much as adults do.
- Children younger than 12 years of age generally should not be treated with group I or II topical corticosteroids.
- Pregnant and lactating women need to be especially careful about topical agents that are absorbed systemically. Agents known to be harmful to the fetus include tretinoin, lindane, and podophyllum.

Patient Education

Topical medications come in many forms. Each has an effective and appropriate method of application. Topical medications should be applied thinly or lightly. The application of extra amounts usually does not provide increased benefit. Teach the patient the correct method of application for the particular preparation prescribed.

- Apply a small amount to the affected area two to four times a day.
- These products are for external use only. Do not use in the eyes.
- If the condition does not improve in 3 to 5 days, call the health care provider.
- If the condition worsens, or if a skin reaction develops, discontinue the agent. Wash the affected area and call the health care provider.

Topical Corticosteroids

For a listing, see Table 11-2.

> The most common complication is suppression of the hypothalamic-pituitary-adrenal (HPA) axis, which usually is not associated with symptoms until the steroid is stopped.

THERAPEUTIC OVERVIEW OF TOPICAL CORTICOSTEROIDS

Toxicity to topical corticosteroids, although not common, is the same as the toxicity that occurs when steroids are given systemically. Other common adverse effects include atrophy, striae, telangiectasia, purpura, acne, perioral dermatitis, and steroid rosacea. Glaucoma and cataracts may develop after prolonged use of corticosteroids around the eyes. The risk of side effects is increased when topical corticosteroids are used over a prolonged time, under occlusion, on the face, and on intertriginous locations.

MECHANISM OF ACTION

Topical corticosteroids diffuse across cell membranes and induce cutaneous vasoconstriction commensurate with their potency. This results in a local antiinflammatory effect. The topical route is elected when a local effect is preferred to the systemic effect produced by the same product given orally. Topical corticosteroids inhibit the migration of macrophages and leukocytes into the area by reversing vascular dilation and permeability of small vessels in the upper dermis. See Chapter 50 for further information.

TREATMENT PRINCIPLES

Standardized Guidelines

No general standardized guidelines are found. There are some guidelines for treatment of specific diseases or skin conditions. See www.guidelines.gov for specific conditions. (See Table 11-4.)

Evidence-Based Recommendations

- No specific evidence-based relevant studies have been conducted.

Cardinal Points of Treatment

- Initiate therapy with an agent of the lowest potency needed, and use for as short a time as possible.
- Group I corticosteroids are used for severe dermatoses over nonfacial/nonintertriginous areas such as psoriasis, severe atopic dermatitis, or severe contact dermatitis. They are especially useful over the palms and soles, which tend to resist topical corticosteroid penetration because of skin thickness.
- Preparations of intermediate to potent strength are appropriate for mild to moderate nonfacial/nonintertriginous dermatoses.
- Eyelid and genital dermatoses should be treated with topical corticosteroids of mild strength.
- Preparations of mild to intermediate strength should be considered when large areas are treated because of the likelihood of systemic absorption.
- Treatment should be discontinued when the skin condition has resolved. Tapering the corticosteroid will prevent recurrence of the skin condition. Tapering is best performed by gradually reducing the potency and dosing frequency at 2-week intervals.
- Therapy may be continued for chronic diseases that are responsive to treatment; patients should be monitored for the development of adverse effects and/or tachyphylaxis (rapid development of a decreased response).
- Generic topical corticosteroids are effective for treatment of most skin disorders in the primary care setting. Generic medications often have slightly less potency or vehicles that are less cosmetically appealing, but the substantial cost savings may offset any differences in efficacy or feel.

Pharmacologic Treatment

Topical corticosteroids are ranked according to potency, with group I as the most potent and group VII as the least potent. It is usually sufficient to divide them into high-, medium-, and low-potency groups. Frequently, weaker strengths are used because they are considered to be safer. However, adequate strength is necessary for a therapeutic response. Weak OTC hydrocortisone is not effective against many dermatoses; a medium-strength steroid from class III or IV is often more effective. If the patient does not respond, treatment should be reevaluated.

Potency is the most important variable when a topical steroid is selected. A drug from each potency level should be chosen to meet the prescriptive needs of the patient. The

TABLE 11-2   Topical Corticosteroids Ranked by Potency*

Group	Generic Name	Dosage Form	Strength (%)	Brand Name
I, Very High	clobetasol propionate	Cream, ointment	0.05	Temovate, generic
	betamethasone dipropionate	Ointment	0.05	Diprosone, generic
	diflorasone diacetate	Ointment	0.05	Psorcon E, generic
	halobetasol propionate	Cream, ointment	0.05	Ultravate, generic
II, High	amcinonide	Cream, lotion, ointment	0.1	Amcinonide
	betamethasone dipropionate	Cream	0.05	Diprosone
	betamethasone valerate	Ointment	0.1	Generic
	desoximetasone	Cream, ointment	0.25	Topicort, generic
	diflorasone diacetate	Gel	0.05	Generic
	fluocinolone acetonide	Cream, ointment (emollient base)	0.05	Psorcon E, generic
	fluocinonide	Cream	0.2	Synalar, generic
	halcinonide	Cream, gel, ointment	0.05	Lidex, generic
	triamcinolone acetonide	Cream, ointment	0.1	Halog
		Cream, ointment	0.5	Kenalog, generic
III, Medium	betamethasone dipropionate	Lotion	0.05	Maxivate, generic
	betamethasone valerate	Cream	0.1	Beta-Val, generic
	clocortolone pivalate	Cream	0.1	Cloderm
	desoximetasone	Cream	0.05	Topicort LP, generic
	fluocinolone acetonide	Cream, ointment	0.025	Synalar, generic
	flurandrenolide	Cream, ointment	0.025	Cordran SP (cream), Cordran
		Cream, ointment, lotion	0.05	Cordran
		Tape	4 mcg/cm^2	Cordran
	fluticasone propionate	Cream	0.05	Cutivate, generic
		Ointment	0.005	
	hydrocortisone butyrate	Ointment, solution	0.1	Locoid, generic
	hydrocortisone valerate	Cream, ointment	0.2%	Westcort, generic
	mometasone furoate	Cream ointment, lotion	0.1	Elocon, generic
	triamcinolone acetonide	Cream, ointment, lotion	0.025 or 0.1	Kenalog, generic
IV, Low	alclometasone dipropionate	Cream, ointment	0.05	Aclovate, generic
	desonide	Cream	0.05	DesOwen, generic
	fluocinolone acetonide	Cream, solution	0.01	Synalar, generic
	hydrocortisone	Lotion	0.25	Generic
		Cream, ointment, lotion	0.5	
		Cream ointment, lotion, solution	1	
		Cream, ointment, lotion	2.5	
	hydrocortisone acetate	Cream, ointment	0.5, 1	Cortef, Lanacort 10 Crème, generic

*Range: group I (very potent) to group IV (least potent).

potency of a steroid is not determined by its strength but by vasoconstrictor assays.

 The dose of one steroid does not correlate with the dose of another, that is, diflorasone diacetate (Psorcon) ointment 0.05% is much stronger than hydrocortisone 2.5%.

Vasoconstrictor assays measure skin blanching when an agent is applied to skin under occlusion. A difference in potency may be noted between generic and name brand corticosteroid equivalents. Pharmacists are allowed to substitute generic drugs unless the health care provider requests "No substitutions" or "Brand necessary."

Use low-potency agents in children, on large areas, for mild conditions, and on body sites that are especially prone to steroid damage, such as the face, scrotum, axilla, flexures, and skin folds.

Steroids that are potent are used for severe conditions or on a small area of the body.

Reserve high-potency agents for areas and conditions resistant to treatment with milder agents; these may be alternated with milder agents. Short-term intermittent therapy with the use of high-potency agents may be more effective and may cause fewer adverse effects than continuous treatment with low-potency agents. No fluorinated or high-potency steroid should be used on the face.

For all groups, apply the product sparingly two to four times a day. Adequate results are usually achieved with twice-a-day application and a course of therapy of 2 to 6 weeks. To prevent rebound, do not discontinue treatment abruptly after long-term use of a potent agent. Instead, reduce the frequency of application, or use a lower-potency agent.

When desired results are not achieved, stop therapy for 4 to 7 days, and then resume treatment with a different agent. A more potent steroid may be needed.

Triamcinolone is commonly used because it is available generically and comes in a variety of strengths. Triamcinolone 0.5% is a good product of medium strength that is effective for many rashes seen in the office setting.

GROUP I. Topical corticosteroids in Group I are superpotent agents. The amount of drug applied to the body per day and the duration of treatment must be carefully monitored. Per week, a maximum of 50 g of cream or ointment should be used. The duration of daily use of super-potent topical corticosteroids should not exceed 2 weeks, if possible. A period of a week is needed before a group I topical steroid can be used again. This is called *cyclic* or *pulse dosing*. Diflorasone diacetate can be used under occlusion; betamethasone dipropionate cannot. Occlusive dressings should be used for no longer than 12 hours at a time. Renal suppression, skin atrophy, and other side effects are possible. Patients who use group I topical corticosteroids should be monitored closely for HPA suppression. Prescriptions should limit refills.

GROUP II. These are also considered high-potency corticosteroids. The risk of adverse effects is reduced if these agents are used for less than 6 to 8 weeks, except on the face or areas where opposing skin surfaces touch (e.g., skin folds of the groin, axillae, and breasts).

GROUPS III THROUGH V. These are considered preparations of medium potency. They are the most commonly indicated preparations for skin conditions for which prescription strength corticosteroids are required. They often have different chemical bases. Treatment duration should not exceed 8 weeks (see previous section on Group II).

GROUPS VI AND VII. These preparations of low potency are useful for covering large areas. Group VII agents are generally OTC preparations that are not strong enough to treat many conditions.

How to Monitor

- Reevaluate after about 10 days to determine whether the condition is responding to treatment.
- Monitor for superinfection.
- High-potency topical steroids may require periodic evaluation of HPA axis suppression with the use of morning plasma cortisol, urinary free cortisol, and adrenocorticotropic hormone (ACTH) stimulation tests. If evidence of HPA axis suppression is noted, the health care provider should attempt to withdraw the topical corticosteroid very gradually. Decrease the number of applications or change to the use of a less-potent steroid to begin withdrawing the steroid from the patient.

Patient Variables

GERIATRICS

- Geriatric patients are more susceptible to secondary infection when steroids are used.
- They also are more susceptible to the systemic effects of topically applied medications because their skin tends to be thin.

PEDIATRICS

- Children, in comparison with adults, have a larger skin surface area–to–body weight ratio. They may be more susceptible to topical corticosteroid–induced HPA axis suppression and Cushing's syndrome. In children, symptoms of HPA may include linear growth retardation, delayed weight gain, and low cortisol levels.
- The least-potent steroid that is compatible with effective treatment should be used.
- Potent corticosteroids should not be used to treat diaper dermatoses.

PREGNANCY AND LACTATION

- *Category C:* No reports have described congenital anomalies or adverse effects associated with the use of corticosteroids during pregnancy. The use of group I through III corticosteroids in large amounts and with occlusive dressings for long periods of time has been shown to cause fetal abnormalities in animals, although none have been documented in humans.
- Effects on lactation are not known.
- Corticosteroids absorbed systemically can be detected in breast milk in quantities that are not likely to affect the infant.
- Use with caution.
- These drugs should not be applied to the nipples prior to nursing.

Patient Education

- Do not use for longer than the prescribed length of time.

SPECIFIC DRUGS

CONTRAINDICATIONS

- Allergy to any component in the product
- Primary bacterial infection, such as impetigo, acne, erysipelas, cellulitis, rosacea, or perioral dermatitis

WARNINGS

 HPA axis suppression has occurred. Limit the amount, potency, and length of treatment.

PRECAUTIONS

- Very high-potency or high-potency agents should not be used on the face, under the arms, or in the groin area.
- Care should be taken when applying topical corticosteroid to the eyelids or around the eyes because it may get into the eyes.
- With prolonged use, steroids may cause steroid-induced glaucoma or cataracts.
- Local irritation may develop; discontinue use.
- Skin atrophy is common with higher potency and longer duration of treatment.
- Psoriasis: Do not use as sole therapy in widespread plaque psoriasis.
- Infection: Treating skin infection with topical corticosteroids can worsen the infection.

PHARMACOKINETICS

- Corticosteroids are absorbed through the skin.
- Time to peak concentration is 12 to 24 hours.
- Corticosteroids are protein bound, metabolized by the liver, and excreted in urine and bile.

ADVERSE EFFECTS
  Local

- Itching, burning, erythema, folliculitis, perioral dermatitis, acneiform eruption, dry skin, allergic contact dermatitis, maceration, secondary infection, skin atrophy striae, and telangiectasia. Use of topical corticosteroids under occlusion may cause these adverse effects more frequently.
- With reduction or discontinuation of potent topical corticosteroids, chronic plaque psoriasis may develop into pustular psoriasis. To prevent rebound effects, long-term or potent topical corticosteroids should be discontinued

gradually or the patient switched to a less-potent steroid, to facilitate withdrawal.

Systemic

- Reversible HPA axis suppression may be induced by topical steroids.
- Symptoms of Cushing's syndrome, hyperglycemia, and glycosuria may be induced.

Overdosage

- Topical steroids are absorbed systemically in quantities sufficient to produce systemic complications.

Immunosuppressive Drugs

SPECIFIC DRUGS

pimecrolimus (Elidel), tacrolimus (Protopic)

INDICATIONS

- Short-term and intermittent long-term treatment of mild to moderate atopic dermatitis in nonimmunocompromised patients who are at least 2 years old.

MECHANISM OF ACTION

- Calcineurin inhibitor; blocks production of proinflammatory cytokines by T-lymphocytes and prevents release of inflammatory mediators from cutaneous mast cells and basophils
- Less likely than topical corticosteroids to cause systemic immunosuppression
- Does not cause skin atrophy

WARNINGS

- Black box warnings for potential risk of cancer (skin malignancies and lymphoma) have been issued with this class of drugs. Based on data from animal studies, the case reports, and the pharmacology, these agents may increase the patient's risk of developing cancer. Although this risk is uncertain, the FDA advisory emphasizes that use of these products should strictly follow each product's labeling.
- Long-term safety (longer than 1 year) unknown
- Do not use Elidel in children younger than 2 years of age because its effect on immune system development is unknown.

PRECAUTIONS. An FDA-approved medication guide must be given to the patient when an outpatient prescription (new or refill) is dispensed if the medication is to be used without direct supervision by a health care provider. Medication guides are available at www.fda.gov/cder/Offices/ODS/medication_guides.htm.

PHARMACOKINETICS

- Minimally absorbed through the skin, even when applied to large areas of inflamed skin

ADVERSE EFFECTS

- Transient local irritation with mild to moderate burning, warmth, stinging, itching, and erythema

DOSAGE AND ADMINISTRATION

- Topical calcineurin agents are considered second-line agents in the treatment of atopic dermatitis/eczema. They should be limited to use in patients who have failed treatment with other therapies.
- Apply twice daily until resolved. Do not use with occlusive dressings.

Antiinfectives

TOPICAL ANTIBIOTICS

Mupirocin is the only drug in this class that is used exclusively for topical infection, and it is the only one discussed here in detail. Mupirocin represents a major advance because it allows topical treatment of impetigo. Bacitracin is very effective for most topical infections. Triple antibiotic ointments vary in their composition; usually, they contain neomycin, which causes a greater number of allergic reactions than are produced by other topical agents. See Chapter 57 for information on other drugs in this class.

THERAPEUTIC OVERVIEW OF TOPICAL ANTIINFECTIVES

Most pathogens cultured from infected dermatoses are group A β-hemolytic streptococci, *Staphylococcus aureus*, *Streptococcus pyogenes*, or any of these pathogens in combination. Gram-negative infections of the skin are relatively rare.

MECHANISM OF ACTION

Mupirocin blocks the protein synthesis of bacteria by binding with the transfer ribonucleic acid (tRNA) synthetase.

TREATMENT PRINCIPLES

- Appropriate drug selection depends on diagnosis and culture whenever possible.
- Systemic antibiotics are needed for diffuse impetigo, cellulitis, and other more-than-superficial infections. Apply gauze dressing if indicated.
- Treatment should be reevaluated if no improvement is seen in 3 to 5 days (Table 11-3).

> **Apply with caution to skin with impaired integrity** because this may allow increased systemic absorption of the drug. Combination antibiotic and steroid preparations often are not indicated because topical steroids can impair the body's ability to fight infection.

How to Monitor

- Reevaluate in 3 to 5 days; if no improvement, change treatment.
- Monitor long-term use especially carefully.
- Prolonged use may result in the development of resistant organisms. It may also result in the overgrowth of nonsusceptible organisms, including fungi.
- Topical neomycin is a contact sensitizer, with sensitivity occurring in 5% to 15% of patients. Symptoms include itching, reddening, edema, and failure to heal.

Patient Education

- Cover with sterile bandage, if needed.

TABLE 11-3   Important Characteristics of Topical Antibiotics

Antibiotic	Effective Against	Formulation	Administration
mupirocin	Gram positive	2% cream, ointment	tid
bacitracin	Gram positive	500 units/g ointment	daily to qid
erythromycin	Gram positive	0.5% (ophthalmic), 2% ointment; 2% gel	bid/tid
gentamicin	Gram negative	0.3% ointment (ophthalmic); 0.1% ointment, cream	tid or qid
neomycin	Gram negative	3.5, 5 mg/g ointment; 3.5 mg/g cream	tid
polysporin with neomycin and bacitracin	Gram negative	5000 *or* 10,000 units/g cream, ointment	tid

SPECIFIC DRUGS

See Table 11-3 for dosage and administration recommendations for selected topical antibiotics.

mupirocin (Bactroban)

INDICATIONS

- Impetigo caused by *S. aureus*, β-hemolytic streptococci, and *S. pyogenes*.
- Mupirocin is a naturally occurring antibiotic that is structurally different from other topical antibiotics. Mupirocin is produced by fermenting *Pseudomonas fluorescens*. It is useful against infections caused by *S. aureus*, including methicillin-resistant and β-lactamase–producing strains, *Staphylococcus epidermidis*, *Staphylococcus saprophyticus*, and *S. pyogenes*.

CONTRAINDICATIONS

- Prior sensitization to any of the ingredients
- Use in eyes

WARNINGS

- For external use only
- Deep infection may require systemic antibiotics.
- Use with caution in large or deep wounds, animal bites, or serious burns.

PRECAUTIONS

- Mupirocin has not been formulated for use on mucosal surfaces; intranasal use may produce stinging and drying.
- Polyethylene glycol is a component of the base. It can be absorbed systemically through damaged skin. Because polyethylene glycol is excreted via the kidneys, the product should not be used over large areas in patients with renal failure.

Patient Variables

PREGNANCY AND LACTATION

- *Category B:* Adequate studies on pregnant women have not been performed.

- It is not known whether mupirocin is excreted in breast milk. When a mother is breastfeeding, the use of mupirocin should be temporarily discontinued.

PHARMACOKINETICS

- No measurable systemic absorption occurs.

ADVERSE EFFECTS

- Local adverse effects consist of burning, stinging, or pain (1.5%) and itching (1%).
- Less than 1% of patients have reported rash, nausea, erythema, dry skin, tenderness, swelling, contact dermatitis, and increased drainage.

DOSAGE AND ADMINISTRATION

- A small amount of mupirocin should be applied to the affected area three times a day.
- If no improvement is seen in 3 to 5 days, the treatment should be reevaluated.
- A gauze dressing may be applied over the topical antibiotic.

OTHER DRUGS IN CLASS

Other drugs in this class are similar to the key drug except as follows:

bacitracin (Bacitracin, Baciguent)

- Bacitracin, a polypeptide antibiotic, inhibits streptococci, pneumococci, and staphylococci and other gram-positive organisms.
- Bacitracin is very poorly absorbed through the skin.
- Allergic sensitivity is rare but may develop.

neomycin sulfate (Neomycin, Myciguent) and gentamicin (Gentamicin, G-Myticin, Garamycin)

- Neomycin and gentamicin are aminoglycosides. They are effective against gram-negative organisms such as *Escherichia coli*, *Proteus*, *Klebsiella*, and *Enterobacter* species.
- Neomycin is an ingredient in several triple antibiotic ointments such as Neosporin.
- Gentamicin is more effective than neomycin against *Pseudomonas aeruginosa*, staphylococci, and group A β-hemolytic streptococci.
- In a patient in renal failure, the drug may accumulate, leading to nephrotoxicity, neurotoxicity, and ototoxicity.

polymyxin B sulfate

- Polymyxin B is most effective against anaerobic gram-negative organisms, that is, *Pseudomonas aeruginosa*, *E. coli*, *Enterobacter*, and *Klebsiella* species.
- Gram-positive organisms and most strains of *Proteus* and *Serratia* are resistant to polymyxin B.
- Polymyxin B–induced toxicity may lead to neurotoxicity and nephrotoxicity.
- Hypersensitivity to polymyxin B rarely occurs.

TOPICAL ANTIFUNGALS

See Table 11-4.

Some topical fungal infections are treated topically, others systemically. The systemic antifungals are discussed in Chapter 66. The decision to treat topically or systemically depends on the severity of the infection, the extent of the skin infected, and prior treatment history.

TABLE 11-4   Indications, Patient Variables, and Administration of Antifungals

Medication	Indication	Administration	Pediatric	Pregnancy/ Lactation	Formulation
clotrimazole (Lotrimin, Mycelex)	*T. pedis*	bid, 4 wk	No: <2 yr; 2 to 12 yr with supervision	B/Unknown	OTC and Rx; 1% cream; topical solution, lotion
econazole (Spectazole)	*T. pedis* *T. cruris* *T. corporis* *T. versicolor* Candida *T. cruris* *T. corporis* *T. versicolor* Candida	daily, 1 mo daily, 2 wk daily, 2 wk daily, 2 wk bid, 2 wk bid, 4 wk bid, 4 wk bid, 4 wk —	—	C/Unknown	Rx; 1% cream
ketoconazole (Nizoral)	*T. pedis* *T. cruris* *T. corporis* *T. versicolor* Candida	daily, 6 wk daily, 2 wk daily, 2 wk daily, 2 wk daily, 2 wk	No	C/Unknown	Rx; 2% cream, shampoo
miconazole (Monistat)	*T. pedis* *T. cruris* *T. corporis* *T. versicolor* Candida	bid, 4 wk bid, 2 wk bid, 4 wk daily, 2 wk bid, 2 wk	—	C/unknown	OTC; 2% cream, ointment, powder, spray, spray powder, spray liquid, solution
oxiconazole (Oxistat)	*T. pedis* *T. cruris* *T. corporis* *T. versicolor*	1-2/day, 4 wk 1-2/day, 2 wk 1-2/day, 2 wk daily, 2 wk	No: <12 yr	B/Enters breast milk	Rx; 1% cream and lotion
sertaconazole (Ertaczo)	*T. pedis*	2/day, 4 wk	No: <12 yr	C/Enters breast milk	Rx 2% cream
sulconazole (Exelderm)	*T. corporis* *T. cruris* *T. pedis* *T. versicolor*	1-2/day, 3 wk 1-2/day, 3 wk 2/day, 4 wk 1-2/day, 3 wk	No: <12 yr	C/Enters breast milk	Rx 1% cream
butenafine (Mentax)	*T. pedis* *T. cruris* *T. corporis* *T. versicolor*	bid or daily, 4 wk daily, 2 wk daily, 2 wk daily, 2 wk	No: <12 yr	B/Unknown	Rx; 1% cream
naftifine (Naftin)	*T. pedis* *T. cruris* *T. corporis*	bid, 4 wk bid, 4 wk bid, 4 wk	No	B/Unknown in milk	Rx; 1% cream and gel
terbinafine (Lamisil)	*T. pedis* *T. cruris* *T. corporis*	1-2/day, 1-4 wk 1-2/day, 1-4 wk 1-2/day, 1-4 wk	No: <12 yr	B/Secreted	Rx; 1% cream, 10 mg/g gel
nystatin (Mycostatin)	Candida	2-3/day	—	B/compatible	Rx; 100,000 units/g cream, ointment, powder
haloprogin (Halotex)	*T. pedis* *T. cruris* *T. corporis* *T. manuum* *T. versicolor*	bid, 2-3 wk Intertriginous 4 wk	No	B/Unknown	Rx; 1% cream and solution
tolnaftate (Tinactin)	*T. pedis* *T. cruris* *T. corporis* *T. versicolor*	bid, 2-3 wk bid, 2 wk bid, 2-3 wk bid, 2-3 wk	—	C/Unknown	OTC; 1% cream, solution, gel, powder, spray powder, spray liquid
ciclopirox (Penlac)	Onychomycosis	At bedtime	No	B/Unknown	Rx; 8% topical solution
selenium sulfide (Selsun)	*T. versicolor*	daily, 1 wk	No	C/—	OTC and Rx; 1%, 2.5% lotion/ shampoo, 1% shampoo

—, Not indicated.

THERAPEUTIC OVERVIEW OF ANTIFUNGALS

Fungal infections can affect almost every part of the body. *Tinea* refers to the *Dermatophyte* fungus that is the most common type found in skin and nail infections. Dermatophytes infect and live in the dead keratin of the stratum corneum, hair, and nails. They can affect the skin and mucosal surfaces and can cause internal infection. Another type of fungi is the yeast-like *Candida* species. The most common cause of candidiasis is *Candida albicans*, which causes infection in skin folds and groin, along with red skin and satellite lesions.

Tinea infections are classified by body region.

- *Tinea capitis* is a seborrhea-like scaling of the scalp. It is commonly caused by *Trichophyton tonsurans* and is often seen in children. *T. tonsurans* does not fluoresce under Wood's lamp. A negative potassium hydroxide (KOH) test does not rule out tinea. Diagnosis is made by the brush method of culturing.
- *Tinea corporis* presents as a pruritic, ring-shaped lesion or scaly patches on exposed skin surfaces or the trunk in adults who are caring for children with tinea capitis. Any dermatophyte may cause this, but *Trichophyton rubrum* is the most common. Microscopic examination of scrapings or culture confirms the diagnosis.
- *Tinea cruris* manifests as pruritic erythematous lesions in the groin area, especially in men who are engaging in strenuous physical activity involving large amounts of sweating. Microscopic examination or culture confirms the diagnosis.
- *Tinea pedis* starts as interdigital toe infections that progress from dry scaling to maceration, hyperkeratotic skin, and inflammatory vesicular bullous eruptions. It is the most common tinea infection seen in primary care. Most infections are easily identifiable and are caused by *Trichophyton* and *Epidermophyton* species. KOH reveals hyphae. Culture is diagnostic.
- *Tinea versicolor* or *pityriasis versicolor* presents as pale macules found on the trunk, arms, or neck. It is caused by *Microsporum furfur* (now called *Pityrosporum orbiculare*), a yeast. *Pityrosporum* is part of the normal skin flora, but it may overgrow. KOH reveals large, blunt hyphae and spores. Culture is not useful.
- *Onychomycosis* is fungal infection of the nails. It can be caused by dermatophytes, molds, and *Candida*. Mixed infections are common. Microscopic examination confirms diagnosis.

MECHANISM OF ACTION

See Chapter 66.

TREATMENT PRINCIPLES

Standardized Guidelines

None

Evidence-Based Recommendations

- Topical allylamines and azoles are effective for athlete's foot.
- Oral itraconazole and oral terbinafine are effective for fungal nail infections.
- Oral fluconazole and topical ciclopirox provide modest benefits in fungal nail infection.

Cardinal Points of Treatment

- Apply by gently massaging into affected skin and surrounding area.
- In general, treatment must last long enough for a complete turnover of skin to occur after the symptoms have resolved. If treatment is not carried out long enough, the infection may recur. Some infections require maintenance therapy to prevent recurrence. Several antifungal topical products, such as clotrimazole, are combined with a steroid to relieve itching and inflammation.

  Once these symptoms have disappeared, the steroid combination should be discontinued. Continued use of the steroid antifungal combination may allow development of resistant organisms.

Newer antifungals reach high concentrations in the epidermis and appendages that persist over time, and they have improved the effectiveness of treatments for fungal skin disease, especially of the nails. Ciclopirox is the first topical antifungal to be effective against onychomycosis. However, most antifungals are effective against the common fungal infections. The provider should become familiar with a few agents. Select one of the older agents such as clotrimazole or miconazole that are available in generic form. Terbinafine, a newer, more potent agent (also OTC), is useful because of its shorter duration of treatment. One factor to consider is cost; the older agents are less expensive. Also consider formulation. Decide which formulation would best deliver the medicine to the infection, and choose an antifungal to match. Note that the OTC antifungals come in a wider variety of formulations than do the prescription antifungals. Another factor is prior use of antifungals. Ask the patient whether he has used OTC antifungals before coming to the office. The older antifungals are usually available OTC. If the patient has failed a trial of OTC antifungal, he will probably need a more potent antifungal.

All azoles are equally effective for *T. pedis*. If the patient develops resistance to an azole, an allylamine may be used. Terbinafine, available by prescription, is a popular choice.

How to Monitor

- Monitor for efficacy and secondary infections.
- Onset of improvement is variable, depending on severity of infection, location of infection, and potency of medication used. Improvement may be seen in 1 day or may take as long as 2 or more weeks.

Patient Variables

- Older patients are often susceptible to superinfection.
- See Table 11-4 for pediatrics and pregnancy guidelines.

Patient Education

- Before treatment, wash the skin with soap and water and dry thoroughly.
- When treating athlete's foot, wear well-fitting, ventilated shoes. Change socks and shoes daily.
- Even though symptoms may abate, continue to follow the treatment plan for the prescribed length of time.
- Notify the health care provider if symptoms do not improve in 2 weeks (*T. cruris* and *T. corporis*) or 4 weeks (*T. pedis*).

- Notify the health care provider of any symptoms of irritation at the site of application (e.g., redness, itching, burning, blistering, swelling, oozing). All are possible signs of sensitization.

SPECIFIC DRUGS

econazole (Spectazole), clotrimazole (Lotrimin, Mycelex), ketoconazole (Nizoral), miconazole (Monistat-Derm, Lotrimin AF), Sertaconazole (Ertaczo), butenafine (Mentax), naftifine (Naftin), terbinafine (Lamisil), nystatin (Nystatin, Mycostatin), haloprogin (Halotex), tolnaftate (Tinactin), ciclopirox (Penlac, Loprox), selenium sulfide lotion 2.5% (Selsun)

See Table 11-4 for specifics regarding antifungal medications.

CONTRAINDICATIONS
- Hypersensitivity to any component of the product

WARNINGS
- Not for ophthalmic use

PRECAUTIONS
- For external use only. Avoid contact with the eyes.
- If irritation or sensitivity develops, discontinue use and institute appropriate therapy.

ADVERSE EFFECTS
- Erythema, stinging, blistering, peeling, pruritus, urticaria, burning, and general skin irritation

TOPICAL ANTIVIRALS
SPECIFIC DRUGS

acyclovir (Zovirax), penciclovir (Denavir)

INDICATIONS
- Oral antivirals are indicated for herpes zoster infections (see Chapter 68 for further information on antivirals).
- Drug resistance has occurred with topical and oral treatment.
- Acyclovir
  - Management of episode(s) of herpes genitalis
  - Limited non–life-threatening monocutaneous herpes simplex infections in immunocompromised patients
  - Active against herpes simplex virus (HSV) types I and II, varicella zoster virus, Epstein-Barr virus, and cytomegalovirus
  - *Unlabeled use:* herpes labialis (cold sores)
- Penciclovir
  - Treatment of recurrent herpes labialis in adults
  - Active against HSV

CONTRAINDICATIONS
- Hypersensitivity or chemical intolerance

WARNINGS
- For cutaneous use only; do not use in eyes
- *Pregnancy category B:* enters breast milk/caution advised; American Academy of Pediatrics (AAP) "compatible"
- Safety and efficacy in children not established

PRECAUTIONS
- Do not exceed the recommended dosage and administration.
- No data demonstrate that acyclovir will prevent transmission of infection to other people or will prevent recurrent infection when applied in the absence of signs and symptoms.
- Viral resistance has not been observed, but the possibility exists.

ADVERSE EFFECTS
- Mild pain with transient burning/stinging, pruritus edema, or pain at application site

PATIENT EDUCATION
- For external use only
- Avoid application near the eyes.
- Ointment must thoroughly cover all lesions.
- Use a finger cot or rubber glove to apply ointment to prevent the spread of infection.
- Start as soon as there is suspicion or evidence of infection.
- Acyclovir ointment is not a cure for herpes simplex infection and is of little benefit in treating recurrent attacks.

DOSAGE AND ADMINISTRATION
- Acyclovir: 5% ointment. Apply sufficient amount to cover lesions every 3 hours (six times per day) for 7 days.
- Penciclovir: 1% cream. Apply to every lesion every 2 hours while awake for 4 days. Use on lips and face only.

SCABICIDES/PEDICULICIDES

See Table 11-5.

THERAPEUTIC OVERVIEW OF SCABICIDES/PEDICULICIDES

A mite called *Sarcoptes scabiei* causes scabies, a contagious disease. It is frequently found in individuals who are living in close contact with others and in children. For reasons unknown, black-skinned persons rarely acquire scabies.

The mite has a 30-day life cycle. Within 60 minutes after arriving on the skin, the fertilized female burrows into the stratum corneum, where she lays two or three eggs a day. As the female advances, she leaves behind the eggs and fecal matter. The eggs reach the age of maturity in 14 to 17 days.

TABLE 11-5 Indications for Scabicides and Pediculicides

Medication	Scabies	PEDICULOSIS (LICE)	
		Head Lice	Body Lice
crotamiton	X*		
lindane†	X	X	X
malathion		X	X
permethrin	X	X	X
ivermectin	X	X	X

*Not very effective.
†Indicated only as a second-line drug.

After the mites reach adulthood, they repeat the cycle. The infested person may not experience any symptoms for about 1 month after the initial infestation until the mites increase in number to approximately 20.

Lice cause pediculosis, another contagious disease. They are active and are able to move quickly, leading to rapid transmission to others. They are usually found in overcrowded settings or in populations with inadequate hygiene. Elementary school children are at risk. Shared hats or combs can transmit head lice. Black-skinned persons from all cultures rarely get lice.

Three types of lice can affect humans: *Pediculus humanus* var. *capitis* (head lice), *Pediculus humanus* var. *corporis* (body lice), and *Pthirus pubis* (pubic or crab lice). Head and pubic lice nits can be found on hair shafts. Body lice reside on clothing and appear on the skin only to feed.

Lice feed approximately five times a day, using their mouths to pierce the skin, injecting irritating saliva, and sucking blood. After feeding, they develop their characteristic rust coloring. Hypersensitivity is induced by the saliva, which is injected when they pierce the skin, and possibly by fecal matter. The life cycle is about 1 month. Each day, the female lays about six eggs, which incubate for 8 to 10 days. Lice reach maturity in 18 days.

Scabies are commonly removed by combing the hair with a fine-tooth comb. Heat is known to destroy both eggs and live lice. A variety of non–drug-related therapies have emerged that involve hot air treatments and vacuuming of the hair; these may be helpful adjuvant therapies when used with medications.

TREATMENT PRINCIPLES

Standardized Guidelines

See CDC Recommendations at Workowski KA, Berman SM: Sexually transmitted disease treatment guidelines, 2006, *MMWR Recomm Rep* 55(RR-11):1-94, 2006.

Evidence-Based Recommendations

- Malathion and permethrin are effective for head lice.
- Permethrin is effective in scabies.
- Crotamiton is less effective than permethrin in scabies.
- Oral ivermectin is likely to be beneficial in scabies.

Cardinal Points of Treatment

SARCOPTES (SCABIES)
- First line: Permethrin cream (5%) applied to all areas of the body from the neck down and washed off after 8 to 14 hours or ivermectin 150 -200 mcg/kg orally as a single dose for adults or children,

PEDICULOSIS (LICE)—HEAD
- First line: permethrin 1% to 5%
- Second line: malathion
- Third line: lindane
- Fourth line: ivermectin

PEDICULOSIS—BODY
- First line: permethrin 1% cream rinse applied to affected areas and washed off after 10 minutes or pyrethrins with piperonyl butoxide applied to the affected area and washed off after 10 minutes

- Second line: malathion 0.5% lotion applied for 8 to 12 hours and washed off or ivermectin 0.15 mg/kg minimum to 0.2 mg/kg maximum repeated in 2 weeks
- Elimination of scabies or pediculosis requires attention to details.
- If any step is left out, recontamination is likely. Treat all infected people simultaneously: household members for head lice and sexual partners for body lice.
- Instructions specific to the medication selected must be followed completely. Scrupulous cleaning of the environment is vital. All infected persons must be treated simultaneously.

> **Unless used properly, lindane has a risk of producing neurotoxicity, including seizures. Malathion also has a remote possibility of causing CNS toxicity.**

- Pyrethrins are natural extracts from the flowers of chrysanthemums that are available OTC. Organism resistance to pediculicides is growing. Treatment failures are common. Permethrin is a synthetic compound that is more effective and less allergenic than the natural products. Significant resistance to permethrin 1% has developed recently. Permethrin 5% is more effective. These products are considered very safe when used according to the package labeling.
- Malathion is an organophosphate pesticide. It is probably the fastest killing most ovicidal pediculicide. Disadvantages include the odor and concerns regarding the alcohol vehicle. It is effective against lice resistant to permethrin.
- Lindane is a slow-killing pesticide that is stored in adipose and nerve tissue. Concerns about environmental contamination have arisen. Over the past 20 years, it has become less effective than other treatments.
- Ivermectin is indicated for onchocerciasis (river blindness) and strongyloidiasis. It is used for treatment of head lice when all other therapies have failed. It is not ovicidal, so a second treatment is necessary. It is given by mouth and is not applied topically.

How to Monitor

- Reevaluate 10 days after treatment. Consider retreatment if the condition is not resolved. Look for sources of reinfection.
- In scabies, pruritus may persist for several weeks after treatment and does not necessarily indicate the need for retreatment. Dermatitis may persist for months after treatment. Triamcinolone 0.1% may be used to help with pruritus and dermatitis.
- In pediculosis, if live lice can be found after 1 week, reapply treatment.

Patient Variables

GERIATRICS
- In the elderly patient, fewer cutaneous lesions may occur, but the itching is intense.
- The elderly have decreased immunity, and this may allow greater numbers of mites to survive and multiply.
- In nursing homes, it is possible for all residents to have mites.

PEDIATRICS

- Epidemics are very common in elementary schools.
- Scabies usually is not suspected in an infant; thus, infants may have a more generalized spread over the body than adults. Regional lymph nodes may swell.

> 💣 Because lindane is absorbed through the skin and children have more skin surface area relative to body weight, pediatric patients may end up with higher blood levels of the drug.

- Contraindicated in premature infants because their skin may be more permeable than that of a full-term infant and their liver enzymes may not be fully developed.

PREGNANCY AND LACTATION

- *Category C*: crotamiton, contraindicated topically; lindane, pyrethrins, ivermectin.
- *Category B*: malathion and permethrin
- Lindane is secreted in low concentrations in breast milk.
- Malathion secretion is unknown, but it is absorbed systemically by the mother.
- The implications of permethrin and crotamiton use during lactation are unknown.

Patient Education

- Shake solution well.
- Apply the drug as directed.
- Treatment of all members of the household may be necessary.
- Wash all clothing and bed linen in soap and hot water.
- Nonwashable clothing should be sealed in plastic bags for 48 to 72 hours and then dry cleaned.
- Reapplication is required in 7 to 10 days only if live lice are present.
- Avoid contact with eyes and mucous membranes. Do not apply to inflamed skin. Flush eyes if exposed.
- Discontinue drug use and notify health care provider if itching or skin irritation persists.
- These drugs are intended for external use only; internal ingestion may produce toxicity.
- Oils may enhance absorption. If using oil-based hair products, wash, rinse, and dry hair before applying.
- Use only one application to avoid overdosing.

SPECIFIC DRUGS

See Table 11-6 for pharmacokinetics of selected scabicides and pediculicides.

crotamiton (Eurax)

CONTRAINDICATIONS

- Known sensitivity to any of the components

WARNINGS

- For external use only
- Do not apply to acutely inflamed skin, raw weeping surfaces, eyes, urethral meatus, or mouth.
- Use with caution in children; safety and effectiveness are not established.

ADVERSE EFFECTS. See Table 11-7 for adverse effects of selected scabicides and pediculicides.

OVERDOSAGE. Ingestion of crotamiton causes a burning sensation in the mouth; mucosal irritation of the mouth, throat, and stomach; nausea and vomiting; and abdominal pain.

DOSAGE AND ADMINISTRATION

- For scabies, thoroughly massage lotion into the skin of the whole body from the chin down, paying particular attention to all folds and creases. Wash off after 8 to 12 hours.
- A second application is advisable 24 hours later.
- Change clothing and bed linen the next morning.
- Take a cleansing bath 48 hours after the last application.

lindane (Kwell)

CONTRAINDICATIONS

- Hypersensitivity; seizure disorders, acutely inflamed skin, raw weeping surfaces, or other skin conditions that may increase systemic absorption; crusted (Norwegian) scabies and other skin conditions that may increase systemic absorption (e.g., atopic dermatitis, psoriasis)

WARNINGS

> 💣 Lindane penetrates the skin and has the potential for CNS toxicity; the young are at greater risk for toxicity. Contraindicated in neonates. Use with caution in patients who weigh less than 110 lb (50 kg). Not intended for use in infants.

- Simultaneous application of creams, ointments, or oils may enhance absorption. Do not leave on longer than the recommended time. Be extremely careful not to overdose, especially in children.

TABLE 11-6 Pharmacokinetics of Pediculicides

	Absorption	Time to Peak	Onset of Action	Kill Time in Pediatrics	Ovicidal Activity in Pediatrics, %	Residual Activity in Pediatrics	Application Time in Pediatrics	Metabolism	Excretion
malathion	<10%	1 hr	<1 hr	4.4 min	95	Up to 4 wk	8-12 hr	—	Unknown
permethrin	<2%	7 days	30 minutes	10-15 min	95	Up to 10 days	10 min	Liver	Urine
lindane	<13%,	6 hr	24 hr	190 min	45-70	None	4 min	Stored in fatty tissues, including the brain	Urine over 5 days

TABLE 11-7 Adverse Effects of Selected Pediculicides

Drug	Common Side Effects	Serious Adverse Effects
crotamiton	Skin irritation	Allergic sensitivity
malathion	Skin irritation	Remote possibility of systemic toxicity, abdominal cramps, respiratory distress, muscle paralysis, seizures
permethrin	Pruritus; mild transient burning, stinging, itching	Tingling, numbness, and rash signify more serious problems.
lindane	Skin irritation	In <0.001% of patients, central nervous system effects, dizziness to convulsions; eczematous eruptions

- Although lindane has not shown an increased incidence of liver tumors in mice, other derivatives of hexachlorocyclohexane have demonstrated carcinogenicity.
- Use as second-line drug only.
- Additional restrictions: An FDA-approved medication guide must be distributed when an outpatient prescription (new or refill) is dispensed, when this medication is to be used without the direct supervision of a health care provider. Medication guides are available at http://www.fda.gov/cder/Offices/ODS/medication_guides.htm.

DRUG INTERACTIONS
- No drug interactions have been reported.

OVERDOSAGE
- Overdose or oral ingestion can cause CNS excitation. Seizures may occur if taken in sufficient quantities.

DOSAGE AND ADMINISTRATION
- For *scabies*, with cream and lotion products, apply a thin layer to dry skin and rub in thoroughly. Allow the drug to remain on the skin for 8 to 12 hours, and then remove by thorough washing. Use of 2 oz is sufficient for an adult. Apply the lotion from the neck to the toes. Scabies rarely affects the head of children or adults but this may occur in infants. One application is usually curative. Many patients exhibit persistent pruritus after treatment. Reapplication is not recommended.
- For *pediculosis capitis* and *pubis*, apply the shampoo in sufficient quantity (2 oz maximum) only to thinly cover the hair of the pubic area. Rub into the hair until lather forms (may use small amount of water) and leave in place for 4 minutes. Wash thoroughly and remove nits with nit comb or tweezers. Reapplication is not recommended. Treat sexual contacts concurrently.

malathion (Ovide)
CONTRAINDICATIONS
- Hypersensitivity to any component of the formulation; use in neonates and/or infants

PRECAUTIONS
- Malathion topical agents contain flammable alcohol. Avoid exposing lotion and wet hair to open flame or electric heat, including hair dryers. While applying lotion or while hair is wet, the patient or person applying the lotion should not smoke.
- Exposure to carbamate- or organophosphate-type insecticides or pesticides in individuals using malathion may increase the possibility of increased systemic absorption of these pesticides or insecticides via the skin or respiratory tract.
- Do not use malathion in children younger than 2 years of age.

MECHANISM OF ACTION
- Malathion has lousicidal and ovicidal properties.
- It is an organophosphate pediculicide liquid for topical application to the hair and scalp that acts via cholinesterase inhibition.
- Malathion binds to the hair shaft, thus giving residual protection against reinfestation.

ADVERSE EFFECTS
- Irritation of the scalp can occur.

DRUG INTERACTIONS
- No drug interactions have been reported with malathion lotion. Malathion inhibits cholinesterase; thus, theoretically, a reaction with some aminoglycosides, anesthetics, antimyasthenics, or cholinesterase inhibitors or succinylcholine may occur.

OVERDOSAGE

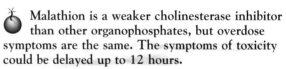

Malathion is a weaker cholinesterase inhibitor than other organophosphates, but overdose symptoms are the same. The symptoms of toxicity could be delayed up to 12 hours.

- The symptoms include abdominal pain, anxiety, unsteadiness, confusion, diarrhea, labored breathing, dizziness, drowsiness, increased sweating, watery eyes, muscle twitching, pinpoint pupils, seizures, and slow heartbeat.

DOSAGE AND ADMINISTRATION
- Sprinkle lotion on dry hair and rub gently until the scalp is thoroughly moistened. Pay special attention to the back of the head and neck.
- Allow the hair to dry naturally; do not use heat; leave uncovered.
- After 8 to 12 hours, wash the hair with a nonmedicated shampoo. Rinse and use a fine-tooth comb to remove dead lice and eggs.
- If required, repeat with second application in 7 to 9 days. Further treatment is generally not necessary.
- Evaluate and treat other family members as needed.
- A recent study found malathion 0.5% one or two 20-minute applications 98% effective.

permethrin (Elimite, Nix)
CONTRAINDICATIONS
- Hypersensitivity to pyrethyroid, pyrethrin, chrysanthemums, or any component of the formulation; lotion is

contraindicated for use in infants younger than 2 months of age

WARNINGS

- Permethrin is associated with carcinogenesis in mice and an increase in pulmonary adenomas and benign liver adenomas.

PRECAUTIONS

- Scabies and head lice infestation may be accompanied by erythema, swelling, and itching; permethrin may exacerbate these problems.

MECHANISM OF ACTION

- Permethrin is a synthetic pyrethrin. It is active against lice, ticks, mites, and fleas.
- It acts on the parasite nerve cell membranes by disrupting the sodium channel current and slowing repolarization, causing paralysis of the pests.

ADVERSE REACTIONS

- Mild, transient symptoms, such as burning, stinging, pruritus, numbness, tingling, erythema, edema, or rash

OVERDOSAGE

- If the drug is swallowed, perform gastric lavage and use general supportive measures.

DOSAGE AND ADMINISTRATION

- For *S. scabiei,* thoroughly massage into the skin from the head to the soles of the feet. Treat infants (2 months or older) on the hairline, neck, scalp, temple, and forehead. Remove the cream by washing after 8 to 14 hours. Usually, 30 g is sufficient for the average adult. One application is curative.
- For *Pediculus capitis,* permethrin 1% (Nix) cream rinse: Use after the hair has been washed with shampoo, rinsed with water, and towel dried. Apply a sufficient volume to saturate the hair and scalp. Allow to remain on the hair for 10 minutes before rinsing off with water. A single treatment eliminates head lice infestation. Combing of nits is not required for therapeutic efficacy but may be done for cosmetic reasons. Resistance to permethrin 1% is increasing. Permethrin 5% (Elimite) topical cream may be applied to clean, dry hair and left on overnight (8 to 14 hours).

Acne Preparations

TOPICAL AND ORAL

DISEASE PROCESS

Acne is a disease that involves the sebaceous glands. Sebaceous glands remain small throughout childhood. At puberty, hormone levels cause increased gland size and sebum secretion. The face, chest, back, and upper arms have the largest and most numerous sebaceous glands. Acne may last for about 8 to 12 years if not treated. Acne is classified as mild (comedonal acne), moderate (papular and pustular acne), and severe (cystic acne). Mild acne consists of more than 20 comedones or fewer than 15 inflammatory papules, or a lesion count of less than 30. Moderate acne includes 15 to 50 papules and pustules with comedones or rare cysts. Total lesion count may range from 30 to 125. Severe acne involves primary inflammatory nodules and cysts. Also present are comedones, papules, and pustules or total lesion count of greater than 125.

Sebum is secreted into the follicular canal. Acne begins with blockage of this canal. Sebum, an irritant fatty acid, causes inflammation and swelling and forms a comedone. *Propionibacterium acnes,* an anaerobe, is a normal skin resident and is the primary contaminant of sebum. *P. acnes* secretes chemotactic factors that attract leukocytes, causing inflammation.

TREATMENT PRINCIPLES

Standardized Guidelines

- Institute for Clinical Systems Improvement (ICSI) Acne Management (2003)

Evidence-Based Recommendations

- Benzoyl peroxide effective for moderate acne
- Topical clindamycin and erythromycin effective for inflammatory lesions in mild, moderate, or severe acne
- Topical tretinoin effective for inflammatory and noninflammatory lesions in mild and moderate acne
- Azelaic acid effective for inflammatory and noninflammatory lesions in mild to moderate acne

Cardinal Points of Treatment

- The effectiveness of treatment depends on the motivation of the patient. If the acne bothers the parent more than it bothers the teen patient, then compliance will be low. The face is usually involved and is exposed for all to see. The trunk may also be affected. Acne has a psychologic as well as a physical effect on the individual; this must be addressed with the patient.
- Treatment depends on the severity of the acne (Table 11-8). Nonpharmacologic treatment addresses contributing factors such as hormones and mechanical causes. Much patient education is needed. Diet is not considered causative in acne, but the patient should avoid foods that trigger an exacerbation.
- In general, topical or oral antibiotics are effective for inflammatory lesions, and topical retinoids are effective for comedonal lesions. In addition to the drugs mentioned in this section, oral contraceptives are commonly used to treat acne in women. Much variation has been noted in response to treatment; different combinations of medications may be tried.

TABLE 11-8 Treatment Sequence for Acne

Severity	First-Line Treatment	Second-Line Treatment	Third-Line Treatment
Mild	Salicylic acid and/or benzoyl peroxide	Topical antibiotics	Topical retinoids azelaic acid
Moderate	Oral antibiotics	Benzoyl peroxide	Topical retinoids or azelaic acid
Severe	Topical or oral antibiotics	Topical retinoids	Isotretinoin

- Usually, 6 to 12 weeks are needed to determine the effectiveness of a treatment. Modification of treatment is often needed. Once the inflammation is under control, medications may be tapered as tolerated.

Pharmacologic Treatment

SALICYLIC ACID. Salicylic acid is available OTC alone and in combination, often with benzoyl peroxide. It is a well-tolerated keratolytic agent that causes less irritation than benzoyl peroxide.

BENZOYL PEROXIDE. Benzoyl peroxide is an oxidizing agent that is bactericidal against *P. acnes*. It is available OTC and in higher strengths by prescription. It may be used with salicylic acid, topical or oral antibiotics, or topical retinoid. The 2.5% concentration of benzoyl peroxide seems to be as effective as higher concentrations but is less irritating. Use water-based, not alcohol-based, preparations to reduce irritation.

ORAL AND TOPICAL ANTIBIOTICS. Many antibiotic topical preparations are used for the treatment of mild to moderate acne. Common topical antibiotics include clindamycin and erythromycin. Both are antibacterial and antiinflammatory. Clindamycin is less irritating. Topical antibiotics are used (1) for mild papular acne, (2) for a patient who refuses or cannot tolerate oral antibiotics, and (3) to wean patients who are under good control from oral to topical preparations (Table 11-9). Topical antibiotics are generally safe and well tolerated. Bacterial resistance can occur. Skin irritation is generally mild.

Oral antibiotics are effective in inflammatory acne. Oral antibiotics may decrease the effectiveness of oral contraceptives. The most commonly used oral antibiotics are tetracycline and erythromycin. Resistance to erythromycin is becoming more common. Tetracycline has antiinflammatory effects and is commonly given at a dose of 500 mg po bid. Other antibiotics used for this condition include doxycycline, minocycline, clindamycin, amoxicillin, and trimethoprim/sulfamethoxazole. These antibiotics are typically given for months at a time. When the skin is clear, taper the antibiotic to the lowest effective dose. Consider topical antibiotics. A recent study has shown that topical and oral antibiotics for acne increase the patient's risk for upper respiratory tract infection.

TOPICAL RETINOIDS. Topical retinoids are generally used as second- or third-line therapy. Topical retinoids are vitamin A derivatives that normalize keratinization. They are very effective for the treatment of comedones and are effective against both inflamed and noninflamed acne lesions. These agents can be used alone or in combination with antibiotics. Their usefulness is limited by irritation.

ISOTRETINOIN. Isotretinoin (Accutane), another vitamin A derivative, is an oral third-line product for severe acne. It has major medical and legal implications, especially when prescribed to females of childbearing age. Isotretinoin is a known teratogen that is available only through a program provided by the manufacturer. Isotretinoin may be prescribed only by a specially trained practitioner. Primary care providers may see patients on isotretinoin for possible follow-up and for other medical problems. The health care provider must be aware of and must understand the potential drug-related severe health problems and common side effects. Isotretinoin is discussed briefly for this purpose. Isotretinoin is extremely expensive, and most insurance programs will not reimburse the patient's cost.

How to Monitor

- Acne may get worse before it gets better. Improvement may not be seen for 4 to 6 weeks. Old lesions may take months to fade. Watch for adverse effects (Table 11-10).
- Improvement is judged by the number of new lesions that form after 6 to 8 weeks of therapy.
- Additional time is required for improvement on the back and chest to be seen.

Patient Variables

PEDIATRICS

- Acne usually begins in puberty. It becomes less active in the late teens.
- Safety and efficacy have not been established in children younger than 12 years of age.
- Isotretinoin may cause premature closure of the epiphyses.

PREGNANCY AND LACTATION

- *Category C:* benzoyl peroxide
- *Category C:* tretinoin
- *Category X:* Isotretinoin is very teratogenic in any amount even for a short period; if pregnancy occurs, abortion must be discussed with the patient.

The effects of these medications during lactation are not known.

RACE. Whites are affected to a greater extent than any other race.

TABLE 11-9   Dosage and Administration of Common Acne Products

Drug	Dosage	Administration
benzoyl peroxide	Start with lowest dosage. Experiment with various bars, creams, lotions. Increase dosage as tolerated.	Cleansers: Wash face once or twice daily. Moisten involved skin areas before application. Rinse well and pat dry. Other dose forms: Apply daily; gradually increase to bid-tid. Apply small amount to affected area. Remove with mild soap and water if excessive stinging occurs. Resume treatment the next day.
tretinoin	Start with 0.025% cream, use smallest amount possible to cover area. Use cream for dry skin, gel (90% alcohol) for excessively oily skin. Maintain dosage until response is seen, then gradually decrease.	Start with test area twice a week; gradually increase area of use and frequency. Frequency of three times a week usually adequate; apply before bedtime. Apply when skin is dry, 20 min after washing. After applying, wash hands.

TABLE 11-10 Adverse Effects of Acne Preparations

Drug	Common Side Effects	Serious Adverse Effects
azelaic acid	Itching, burning, stinging, and erythema	Hypopigmentation, especially with dark skin.
benzoyl peroxide	Excessive drying, peeling, inflammation, swelling, allergic contact sensitization/dermatitis, bleaching of skin or fabric	Excessive scaling, erythema, or edema
tretinoin	Skin irritation	Contact allergy is rare; skin may become inflamed, swollen, blistered, or crusted; increased or decreased pigmentation, increased sun sensitivity
isotretinoin	Dried mucous membranes, nosebleeds (up to 80%), cheilitis (>90%), hand and foot epidermis peel, dry eyes; gastrointestinal effects include dry mouth, nausea, vomiting, abdominal pain, anorexia, weight loss, and inflammation of gums	Central nervous system effects include fatigue, headache, and visual disturbances; myalgia, hypertriglyceridemia, hepatitis, pancreatitis, pseudotumor cerebri

GENDER. Acne affects both males and females. Males frequently have the most severe cases, but the most persistent cases tend to occur in females.

Patient Education

- Current research does not show a link between diet and acne (e.g., that chocolate and French fries increase acne). However, avoid such foods if they are believed to be trigger outbreaks.
- Instruct the patient to wash the face two or three times a day with warm water and a mild soap. Do not scrub the face because this may aggravate the condition.
- Use water-based makeup. Avoid oily moisturizers and skin cleansers.
- Avoid digging and squeezing the comedones. This may aggravate the condition and cause scarring.
- Acne may get worse at the beginning of any treatment for acne. Be patient and continue treatment because this is usually only temporary.
- Be consistent and follow all instructions provided by the health care provider. Notify the health care provider of any problems. The health care provider will determine whether treatment should be discontinued.
- Use mild soap to avoid skin irritation.

SPECIFIC DRUGS

benzoyl peroxide

CONTRAINDICATIONS

- Hypersensitivity
- Cross-sensitivity with benzoic acid derivatives (cinnamon and certain topical anesthetics) may occur.

WARNINGS

- After reports of tumor development in rodents, benzoyl peroxide was downgraded in 1991 by the FDA from category I (safe and effective) to category III (data insufficient to permit classification).
- No evidence suggests that benzoyl peroxide is a tumor promoter in humans.

PRECAUTIONS

- This agent is for external use only. Contact with eyelids, lips, mucous membranes, and highly inflamed or damaged skin should be avoided.

- If accidental contact occurs, rinse with water.
- Discontinue use if severe reaction develops, then institute the appropriate therapy. Product use may be resumed after the reaction clears, with less frequent applications.
- The color of hair and fabric may be lightened as a result of the oxidizing effects of benzoyl peroxide.
- Some benzoyl peroxide products contain sulfites. This may cause allergic reactions, including anaphylactic symptoms and asthmatic episodes. In the general population, the prevalence of sulfite sensitivity is unknown. It is most frequently seen in those patients with asthma.

PHARMACOKINETICS. Benzoyl peroxide is not absorbed systemically.

MECHANISM OF ACTION

- The primary action of benzoyl peroxide is antibacterial, especially against *P. acnes*. It is believed that bacterial proteins are oxidized by the active or free radical oxygen. As the levels of *P. acnes*, lipids, and free fatty acids drop, resolution of acne occurs.
- Benzoyl peroxide has a drying action and removes excess sebum, which leads to desquamation (drying and peeling) of the skin.

ADVERSE EFFECTS. See Table 11-10.

DRUG INTERACTIONS

- Simultaneous use of benzoyl peroxide with tretinoin may increase skin irritation.
- Transient skin discoloration may occur with the simultaneous use of sunscreens that contain *para*-aminobenzoic acid (PABA).

OVERDOSAGE

- Excessive scaling, erythema, and edema are effects of overdosage.
- Treatment involves discontinuing product use and applying cool compresses, emollients, or low-dose topical hydrocortisone.

PATIENT EDUCATION

Avoid the use of other skin irritants such as sunlight, sun lamps, and other topical medications unless approved by the health care provider.

- Read patient instructions included with the product.
- Before use, wash the treatment area and allow it to dry.
- Keep product away from eyes, mouth, and mucous membranes. Rinse with water if contact occurs.
- A transitory feeling of warmth or slight stinging may occur. Expect dryness and peeling. Decrease frequency of use or discontinue if excessive redness or discomfort occurs. Discontinue use and contact health care provider if irritation is excessive.
- Water-based cosmetic use is permissible.

DOSAGE AND ADMINISTRATION. See Table 11-9 for dosage and administration recommendations.

tretinoin (Retin-A Cream, Gel)

- *Unlabeled uses:* topical treatment for different skin cancers and various other dermatologic conditions, to enhance the percutaneous absorption of topical minoxidil and other topical agents, and to improve the appearance of photodamaged skin, especially wrinkling and liver spots

CONTRAINDICATIONS. Hypersensitivity to any component of the product; sunburn

WARNINGS

> **Tretinoin is for external use only. Keep it away from the eyes, mouth, angles of the nose, and mucous membranes. Severe local erythema and peeling at application site may be induced.**

- Use product less frequently or stop use temporarily or completely, if warranted. If applied to reddened skin, a severe local reaction may occur.

PHARMACOKINETICS

- Tretinoin is metabolized by the skin.
- Approximately 5% of the compound is excreted in the urine and feces.

MECHANISM OF ACTION

- Tretinoin promotes and increases cell turnover of both the normal follicle and comedones. Cohesion between keratinized cells is decreased.
- Tretinoin works on the acne precursor lesion, the microcomedones, causing fragmentation and expulsion of the micro plug. Closed comedones are converted into open comedones. With continued use, comedone formation is prevented.

DRUG INTERACTIONS

> **The stratum corneum becomes thin with continual application of tretinoin. This makes the skin more susceptible to irritation from sunburn and sun damage and irritation from wind, cold, or dryness.**

- Cosmetics, astringents, alcohol, and acne soaps that have drying properties and strong concentrations of spices or limes may increase the possibility of interaction with tretinoin.
- Use caution when administering tretinoin with sulfur, resorcinol, benzoyl peroxide, or salicylic acid because significant skin irritation may result.

OVERDOSAGE. Topical tretinoin overdose will lead to severe localized skin irritation.

isotretinoin (Accutane)

INDICATIONS. Severe cystic acne not responding to conventional therapy

WARNINGS

> **Isotretinoin must not be used by females who are pregnant. The risk of a deformed infant is extremely high if pregnancy occurs while the patient is taking isotretinoin in any amount for even a short period of time.**

HOW TO MONITOR

- The primary health care provider may be asked to monitor the patient while on isotretinoin. Patients must be monitored closely, using the following guidelines:
  - Pretreatment: one negative serum pregnancy test prior to initiating treatment; a second test must be performed during the first 5 days of the menstrual period immediately preceding the start of therapy; complete blood cell count (CBC), liver function test, triglyceride level
  - After 2 to 3 weeks of treatment: triglyceride level, then every 4 weeks; for levels exceeding 350 to 400 mg/dl, repeat in 2 to 3 weeks; for levels exceeding 700 to 800 mg/dl, stop medication because of risk for pancreatitis
  - After 4 to 6 weeks of treatment: CBC, liver function
  - A monthly pregnancy test must be performed before the patient receives the refill.

PRECAUTIONS

> **Isotretinoin has the potential for causing many severe health problems. Headaches, which may be indicative of benign intracranial hypertension (especially when combined with minocycline and tetracycline), corneal opacities, decreased night vision, inflammatory bowel disease, hypertriglyceridemia, hepatotoxicity, and musculoskeletal symptoms such as arthralgia may occur. Diabetic patients may demonstrate problems with control of their blood sugar.**

- As with initiation of all acne treatment, the condition may be temporarily exacerbated.

PHARMACOKINETICS. Isotretinoin is metabolized in the liver, and 99.9% binds to the plasma albumin. It is excreted in urine and bile.

MECHANISM OF ACTION. The exact mechanism of action is not known. The drug decreases the amount and composition of the sebum lipid. This reduction is maintained while the patient is taking the drug. After treatment has ended, the composition returns to normal, but production may not return to pretreatment levels.

ADVERSE EFFECTS
- See Table 11-10 for a full list of adverse effects.
- Cheilitis can be handled easily with the use of a petrolatum product such as Aquaphor.
- Dry eyes may make the patient unable to wear contact lenses.

PATIENT EDUCATION. Roche Laboratories' pregnancy prevention program includes a patient qualification checklist, information about treatment, contraception and serum pregnancy testing information, an optional referral form to expert contraception counseling, patient self-evaluation, consent forms, and a follow-up survey.

Local Anesthetics
MECHANISM OF ACTION

Local anesthesia causes loss of sensation by first blocking nerve conduction in the smaller unmyelinated fibers that carry pain, and then progressing to the larger myelinated fibers for pressure and motor function. The extent of anesthesia depends on a variety of factors, including the amount of medication used, body temperature, pH, the amount of protein binding, and dilution by tissue fluids. Local anesthetics work by blocking the flow of sodium ions, thereby preventing depolarization of the nerve fiber and conduction or transmission of the impulse.

Local anesthetics are divided into two groups: esters and amides. Esters are derivatives of *para*-aminobenzoic acid. Hypersensitivity reactions may occur with esters, which are metabolized by hydrolysis. Amides are derivatives of aniline. Allergies to drugs in the amide group are rare. These are metabolized primarily in the liver and then are excreted primarily in the urine as metabolites. These two groups differ in pharmacokinetics, including protein binding, onset, duration, and allergic potential. The amides are generally more useful clinically.

Pharmacokinetics
- Absorption is complete, unless epinephrine is added.
- Onset depends on the type of block, medication, body fluids, pH, and temperature.
- The amides vary in protein binding. Lidocaine and mepivacaine are bound moderately. Etidocaine and bupivacaine are highly bound. The esters are hydrolyzed in the plasma by pseudocholinesterase, and the amides are degraded in the liver by enzymes. Esters are less stable than amides. Esters are metabolized to *para*-aminobenzoic acid, which may cause a severe reaction.
- Peak concentration of the drug depends on the type but is reached in 10 to 30 minutes (Table 11-11).

Patient Variables
- Dosage varies according to the weight of the patient and the site and type of procedure.
- Children and the elderly are especially prone to aspiration when agents are used in the oral cavity.

PREGNANCY AND LACTATION
- *Categories B and C:* See Table 11-11.

HOW TO MONITOR
- Monitor for adverse effects, including cardiac arrhythmias, shock, and/or local reactions.
- Blood pressure, respiratory status, blood flow to the area, ability to swallow, and motor control and sensations also should be monitored.

TABLE 11-11 Pharmacokinetics of Local Anesthetics

Drug	Amide or Ester	Onset of Action	Duration of Action	Protein Bound	Pregnancy Category	How Supplied
SHORT ACTING						
procaine	Ester	2-5 min	15-60 min	5.8%	C	1%, 2%, 10%
chloroprocaine	Ester	6-12 min	30 min	—	C	1%, 2%, 3%
INTERMEDIATE ACTING						
lidocaine	Amide	<2 min	30-60 min	64.3%	B	0.5%, 1%, 2%, 4%, with and without epinephrine
mepivacaine	Amide	3-5 min	45-90 min	77.5%	C	1%, 1.5%, 2%, 3%
prilocaine	Amide	<2 min	60-120 min	55%	B	4% with and without epinephrine
LONG ACTING						
bupivacaine	Amide	5 min	2-4 hr	95.6%	C	0.25%, 0.5%, 0.75% with and without epinephrine
etidocaine	Amide	3-5 min	5-10 hr	94%	B	1%, 1.5% with and without epinephrine
tetracaine	Ester	15 min	2-3 hr	75.6%	C	1%, 2%, 3%

- Patients may need to be placed on cardiac monitors, depending on the type of procedure and agent used.

Patient Education

- Reactions to local anesthetics range from dermatitis to anaphylactic shock.
- The patient may lose all sensation, including the sensations of temperature, pressure, and touch. Protect the area until sensation returns.
- Motor function is lost only if concentrations of the drug are present over time (spinal anesthesia). If regional anesthesia has been achieved, the area of the body must be protected from heat, cold, and pressure because those senses will not be intact.
- Local application to the oral cavity results in a decreased ability to swallow and could result in trauma to the buccal mucosa or tongue.
- Patients should be advised to use topical anesthetics exactly as prescribed. Aerosols should not be inhaled. Provide instruction for rectal applications. If hemorrhoids are bleeding, systemic absorption will be increased. Suppositories should be refrigerated before use and moistened with water or lubricant before insertion.

SPECIFIC DRUGS

Short-Acting Local Anesthetics

procaine (Novocain)

INDICATIONS. Spinal anesthesia primarily

CONTRAINDICATIONS. Hypersensitivity to procaine or other ester-type anesthetics.

WARNINGS

- Have resuscitation equipment on hand during use.
- Effect on fetal development not determined

PRECAUTIONS

- Use with caution in patients with heart block, rhythm disturbances, hyperthyroidism, or other endocrine diseases, or shock.

  > Use lowest dose possible for effective anesthesia, especially in children and in elderly or debilitated patients.

- Consult standard references for exact amount of medication for specific procedure or technique.
- If vasopressor is added, use with caution in patients already on any medication likely to raise pressure, for example, monoamine oxidase inhibitors (MAOIs).

PATIENT VARIABLES
  Pregnancy and Lactation
- Category C

ADVERSE EFFECTS. May provoke CNS and cardiovascular symptoms

OVERDOSAGE
- Hypotension and cardiac arrest are possible.
- Other symptoms include nervousness, dizziness, headache, urticaria, and edema.

Intermediate-Acting Local Anesthetics

lidocaine hydrochloride (Xylocaine with and without Epinephrine)

INDICATIONS
- Lidocaine can be used as a local anesthetic and administered topically in a gel, ointment, spray, lotion, or cream.
- Lidocaine also can be infiltrated into an area for local anesthesia or nerve block.
- Lidocaine has an additional use as an antiarrhythmic, in which case it is administered intravenously by direct injection or by continuous infusion.

CONTRAINDICATIONS. Hypersensitivity to lidocaine or to local anesthetics of the amide group

WARNINGS. Have emergency resuscitation equipment and drugs on hand.

PRECAUTIONS
- Safety of use depends on the proper dose, technique, and rapidity of administration in emergencies.
- Consult standard textbooks for specifics.

PATIENT VARIABLES
  Pregnancy and Lactation
- Category B
- Not known if excreted in human breast milk

OVERDOSAGE
- Reactions are similar to other amide anesthetics and range from CNS manifestations of nervousness and euphoria to twitching, convulsions, and unconsciousness.
- Allergic manifestations include urticaria, edema, and anaphylactoid reactions.
- Cardiovascular reactions include bradycardia, hypotension, and shock.
- Neurologic reactions include loss of sensation or motor control and loss of bowel or bladder function.

Long-Acting Local Anesthetics

bupivacaine hydrochloride (Marcaine with and without Epinephrine)

INDICATIONS
- Dental and oral surgeries, minor surgical procedures, and therapeutic procedures such as joint injections
- Only the lowest concentration recommended for obstetric procedures
- Chemically, product is related to lidocaine but lasts longer.

CONTRAINDICATIONS
- Do not give with known sensitivity to bupivacaine or any other local anesthetic.
- Not used for obstetric paracervical blocks

WARNINGS
- Do not use 0.075% for obstetric anesthesia.
- Use only if resuscitation equipment and drugs are available.
- Do not use with epinephrine if patient is on MAOIs or antidepressants of the amitriptyline or imipramine type because hypotension may result.

- Because results are long lasting, warn patient of inadvertent trauma to lips, buccal mucosa, and tongue.

PATIENT VARIABLES

Pediatrics

- Not recommended for use in children younger than 12 years

Pregnancy and Lactation

- *Category C*

OVERDOSAGE. Same as other amides: CNS, cardiovascular, and allergic symptoms

DOSAGE AND ADMINISTRATION. Dose varies with the procedure, the area required, the patient's condition, vascularity of tissues, and the duration of anesthesia desired. Individualize the dose.

> **evolve** A continually updated list of useful WebLinks may be found in the Evolve Resources at http://evolve.elsevier.com/Edmunds/NP/

Eye, Ear, Throat, and Mouth Agents

DRUG OVERVIEW

Class	Subclass	Generic Name	Trade Name
EYE AGENTS			
Antiinfectives			
Antibiotics	Quinolones	ciprofloxacin ✷	Ciloxan solution
	Aminoglycosides	gentamicin sulfate	Garamycin ointment and solution
		tobramycin	Tobrex ointment and solution
	Sulfonamides	sulfacetamide sodium 10%	Sodium Sulamyd ointment, solution; Bleph-10
	Macrolides	erythromycin ✷	Ilotycin ointment
	Combination	neomycin, polymyxin B, and bacitracin zinc	generic
		gramicidin, neomycin, polymyxin B,	Neosporin ointment
Antivirals		trifluridine	Viroptic solution
NSAIDs		ketorolac	Acular
Histamine H$_1$ Blockers		azelastine	Astelin ✷
Mast Cell Stabilizers		nedocromil	Alocril, Tilade
Steroid antiinflammatory drugs		dexamethasone ✷	Decadron
Glaucoma medications			
Sympathomimetics		brimonidine	Alphagan-P ✷
β-Adrenergic–blocking agents		timolol ✷	Timoptic
Parasympathomimetics (miotics, direct)		pilocarpine	Isopto Carpine, Pilocar, Pilostat
Cholinesterase inhibitors (miotic)		demecarium	Humorsol
Carbonic anhydrase inhibitors		dorzolamide	Trusopt
Prostaglandins		latanoprost	Xalatan ✷
Other Eye Medications			
Sympathomimetics		phenylephrine hydrochloride	Neo-Synephrine
Vasoconstrictors		naphazoline hydrochloride	Naphcon Forte, Opcon

Table continued on following page

DRUG OVERVIEW (Continued)

Class	Subclass	Generic Name	Trade Name
Lubricants		artificial tears	Lacrisert, generic
Anesthetics		proparacaine hydrochloride	Alcaine, Paracain
Diagnostics		fluorescein sodium, proparacaine	Flucaine, Fluoracaine
EAR		hydrocortisone, neomycin sulfate, polymyxin	Cortisporin otic
		ciprofloxacin and hydrocortisone suspension	Cipro HC otic
NOSE			
(See Allergic Rhinitis, Chapter 13)			
THROAT/ORAL			
Antifungals		nystatin ✳	Mycostatin
		clotrimazole	Mycelex
Other		penciclovir	Denavir
		carbamide peroxide	Gly-Oxide Liquid solution 10%
		chlorhexidine gluconate ✳	Peridex

✳ Top 200 drug.

Eye Agents

INDICATIONS

Conjunctivitis

A great many products are available for the eye. Drugs selected for inclusion here are those seen most commonly, and only one representative drug has been chosen for many categories. The drugs featured in this chapter have a wide variety of diagnostic and therapeutic uses. The two eye diseases most commonly seen in primary care that are treated medically are infectious conjunctivitis and seasonal allergic conjunctivitis. Most eye conditions require referral to an ophthalmologist.

THERAPEUTIC OVERVIEW OF EYE AGENTS

Anatomy, Physiology, and Pathophysiology

The eye is protected by the tear film, which covers the cornea and conjunctiva, up to the lid margins; it provides moisture, lubrication, oxygen, and protective chemicals, including cytokines. Tears are regularly distributed over the lens by blinking of the eyelid. Tears drain through the puncta at the lid margins (Figure 12-1), into the lacrimal ducts and sac, then to the nasolacrimal duct and to the nose. Medications in the tears may be systemically absorbed through the nasal and pharyngeal mucosa.

Figure 12-2 shows the internal anatomy of the eye. The conjunctiva covers the inside of the eyelids and the cornea. Aqueous humor is produced by the ciliary body. Excess humor drains through the canals of Schlemm in the trabecular meshwork.

In glaucoma, the intraocular pressure (IOP) is too high, causing injury and death of nerve cells. Reducing the IOP can arrest the progression of the disease. Open-angle glaucoma involves no mechanical obstruction to outflow. In narrow-angle glaucoma, the iris mechanically obstructs outflow.

Disease Process

Conjunctivitis is the most common eye disease. Conjunctivitis can be caused by bacteria, virus, or allergy.

BACTERIAL CONJUNCTIVITIS. Bacterial conjunctivitis is most often caused by *Streptococcus pneumoniae*, *Haemophilus influenzae*, *Staphylococcus aureus*, *Pseudomonas* species, and *Moraxella* species. Gram-negative infections are less common than gram-positive infections. *Haemophilus* is common in children. Chlamydial infection is an important cause of blindness. Bacterial conjunctivitis is often accompanied by large amounts of purulent discharge. Some minor pain may occur, but no changes in vision have been reported. Bacterial conjunctivitis is spread through contact.

VIRAL CONJUNCTIVITIS. Viral conjunctivitis is by far the most common cause of conjunctivitis. It is usually caused by adenovirus type 3, which is commonly called *pink eye* in children, and is extremely contagious; it is spread by touching infected secretions. Duration is from several days to 3 weeks or longer. The eye can be very painful, and pharyngitis, fever, malaise, and preauricular adenopathy may be associated. The conjunctiva is red with large amounts of clear discharge.

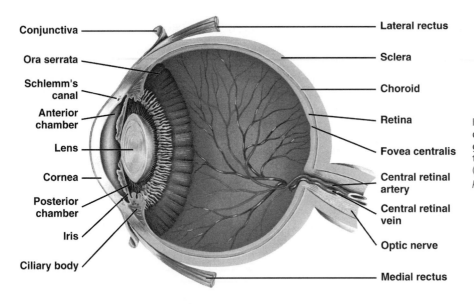

Conjunctiva
Ora serrata
Schlemm's canal
Anterior chamber
Lens
Cornea
Posterior chamber
Iris
Ciliary body

Lateral rectus
Sclera
Choroid
Retina
Fovea centralis
Central retinal artery
Central retinal vein
Optic nerve
Medial rectus

FIGURE 12-1   Lacrimal apparatus. Tears drain through the puncta at the lid margins, into the lacrimal ducts and sac, then to the nasolacrimal duct and to the nose. (From Thibodeau GA, Patton KT: *Anatomy & physiology*, ed 6, St Louis, 2007, Mosby.)

Herpes zoster conjunctivitis usually affects one eye. It is usually accompanied by a vesicular rash distributed along the ophthalmic division of the trigeminal cranial nerve.

ALLERGIC CONJUNCTIVITIS. Allergic conjunctivitis is a common problem for patients with allergies. It is often seasonal but may occur year round with allergies to dust or mold. It presents with itching and tearing and is characterized by "cobblestone" papillae on the upper tarsal conjunctiva.

GLAUCOMA. Glaucoma is another condition that is managed by the ophthalmologist. It is common for a patient to be on two or more medications for glaucoma. The primary care provider must be aware of the possible systemic side effects of eye drops and potential drug interactions.

CONDITIONS THAT REQUIRE ANESTHESIA. Topical anesthetics are used only when eye pain makes it impossible for the practitioner to examine the eye. Topical anesthetics retard corneal healing and may allow a corneal abrasion to progress to a corneal ulcer.

> Anesthetics generally are used only by ophthalmologists. If a patient is using them, he must use great care to avoid injuring the eye.

OTHER EYE PROBLEMS

- Sympathomimetics and vasoconstrictors are OTC agents that are commonly used for relief of red, irritated eyes. Generally, they are safe and effective. However, chronic use is discouraged because of rebound inflammation.
- Ocular lubricants (i.e., artificial tears) are also OTC agents. They are also very safe and effective in relieving irritated eyes. They are used in elderly patients and in those who are on medications that cause dry eyes.
- Fluorescein is used in the primary care setting when the eye is examined for abrasions or foreign bodies. When the strips are used, they should be moistened with sterile water. Place

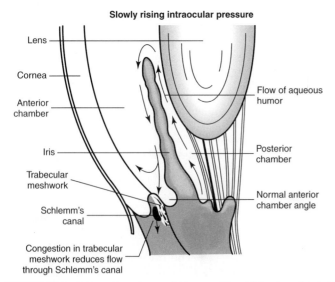

Slowly rising intraocular pressure

Lens
Cornea
Anterior chamber
Iris
Trabecular meshwork
Schlemm's canal
Congestion in trabecular meshwork reduces flow through Schlemm's canal

Flow of aqueous humor
Posterior chamber
Normal anterior chamber angle

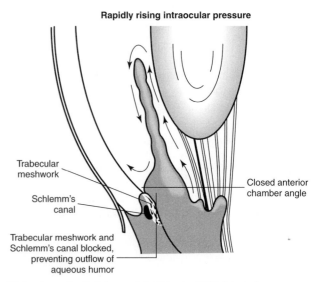

Rapidly rising intraocular pressure

Trabecular meshwork
Schlemm's canal
Trabecular meshwork and Schlemm's canal blocked, preventing outflow of aqueous humor

Closed anterior chamber angle

FIGURE 12-2   Internal anatomy of the eye. (From Thibodeau GA, Patton KT: *Anatomy & physiology*, ed 6, St Louis, 2007, Mosby.)

the moistened strip at the fornix in the lower cul-de-sac close to the punctum of the eye. The patient should then blink several times. Allow a few seconds for staining. An injury will show up as an intense green fluorescent color. Rinse out the eye with sterile irrigating solution.

TREATMENT PRINCIPLES

Standardized Guidelines

- The American Academy of Ophthalmology has Preferred Practice Patterns for many ophthalmology problems. The guidelines for conjunctivitis are reflected in this discussion.

Evidence-Based Recommendations

- Randomized controlled trials have demonstrated no difference in the effectiveness of many antibiotics for bacterial conjunctivitis.

Cardinal Points of Treatment

1. Diagnose the cause of conjunctivitis.
2. Ophthalmic antibiotics are effective for bacterial conjunctivitis and are commonly used to prevent secondary bacterial infection in viral conjunctivitis.

Effective treatment demands accurate diagnosis. Primary care providers collect pertinent information and begin the process of diagnosis. However, many problems require referral to a specialist for care. See Table 12-1 for evaluation and management of potentially serious eye problems.

Ophthalmic solutions are absorbed systemically, and this may pose secondary problems. In general, any adverse reaction that a medication may cause when taken orally can occur when the medication is given as an eye drop. Patient factors that increase systemic absorption include lax eyelids and hyperemic or diseased eyes. Absorption is more of a problem in infants and in the elderly than in other individuals.

TABLE 12-1 Evaluation and Management of Potentially Serious Eye Problems

Complaint or Problem	Suggested Treatment
EMERGENCIES	
Chemical burn	Irrigate eye for 15-20 min; send to emergency department.
Retinal artery occlusion with sudden, painless loss of vision in one eye	Must be seen by specialist within 90 min to preserve vision
"Something in eye"	Check visual acuity in each eye, document findings; if significant loss of vision or blurring, refer patient to specialist. Examine eye for foreign body: Evert eyelid, and if a foreign body is seen, do not irrigate, but flick off with a needle; if fine powder, irrigate. Stain with fluorescein dye to check integrity of epithelial surface; moisten strip if eye is dry, touch strip to inner conjunctival surface, let patient blink, then shine flashlight (blue filter preferred); epithelial break stains green, refer to specialist.
Red eye	Check vision; if vision is decreased, refer to specialist. Check injection, use finger pressure test to determine whether conjunctival or ciliary (Figure 12-3); press lower lid against cornea, draw downward; conjunctiva should blanch; ciliary injection is around the limbus, does not blanch; if ciliary injection, refer to specialist.
CONTACT LENSES	
Symptoms: Lens wearers are at risk for corneal abrasion and infection and for hypoxic corneal injury.	If patient complains of pain, remove contact lens, check for abrasion with fluorescein dye, refer to specialist.
CORNEAL ABRASIONS	
Symptoms: pain, foreign body sensation, photophobia, tearing, or blepharospasm immediately after insertion or removal of contact lens or from direct trauma to the eye from projected particles	Remove contact lens, stain eye with fluorescein dye, remove foreign body if present; topical antibiotic may be required; refer to specialist.
Signs: epithelial defect confirms corneal abrasion; may become infected and progress to corneal ulceration	
HYPOXIC CORNEAL INJURY	
Symptoms: during contact lens wear, blurred vision, conjunctival hyperemia, pain	Remove contact lens, stain with fluorescein dye, evaluate, and refer to specialist if necessary.
Signs: conjuctival hyperemia and ciliary flush, contact lens immobility, diffuse corneal edema; may lead to corneal neovascularization and scarring	
Conjunctivitis	Diagnostic cultures generally not necessary Treat with antibiotics: Use a broad-spectrum drug or one that covers gram-positive organisms; refer if not resolved in 7 days.

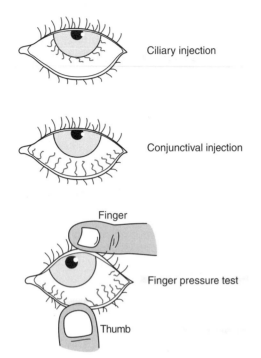

Ciliary injection

Conjunctival injection

Finger

Finger pressure test

Thumb

FIGURE 12-3 Diagnostic technique in determining ciliary or conjunctival injection (see Table 12-1).

The formulation affects absorption by determining the amount of time the medication stays in contact with the conjunctiva. Ointments are more completely absorbed than suspensions; suspensions are more completely absorbed than solutions. Minimize systemic absorption of ophthalmic drops by compressing the lacrimal sac for 3 to 5 minutes after instillation. This retards the passage of drops to other areas of absorption.

Eye drops must be used properly to be effective. One drop of medication is all the eye can retain. Using two drops is wasteful. If more than one drop is used, wait 5 minutes before applying the second drop. Do not use eyecups because of the risk of contamination. See the section on patient education for instructions on how to administer eye medication.

BACTERIAL CONJUNCTIVITIS. Topical ocular antiinfectives are used to treat external bacterial infections of the eye and its adnexa, such as conjunctivitis, corneal ulcer, dacryocystitis, and hordeolum. The usual course of treatment is 3 to 5 days, but treatment may be extended to 7 days. Most antibiotics are effective; the least expensive broad-spectrum agent is usually the preferred treatment. Sulfacetamide sodium, instilled three or four times a day, usually is considered for first-line treatment. If the patient is allergic to sulfa, select another medication that is active against gram-positive bacteria, such as erythromycin. Neosporin is limited by the frequency of allergy to neomycin. The use of topical fluoroquinolones is discouraged by some writers. Gonococcal and chlamydial conjunctivitis is usually treated with systemic antibiotics. See Chapter 57.

⚕ **Prolonged use of topical antibiotics may result in overgrowth of nonsusceptible organisms, including fungi. Ophthalmic ointments may retard corneal wound healing.**

VIRAL CONJUNCTIVITIS

- Viral conjunctivitis is not usually treated with an antiviral. However, specific viral infections caused by such organisms as herpes simplex are treated with antiviral ophthalmic products. Trifluridine should be prescribed only for patients who have been given a clinical diagnosis of herpetic keratitis by an ophthalmologist. Systemic absorption is negligible. Some practitioners routinely treat viral conjunctivitis caused by an adenovirus with topical antiinfectives to prevent secondary bacterial infections. However, this practice is controversial. Some school systems require that a child with pinkeye be treated before returning to school.
- Artificial tears, topical antihistamines, and cold compresses may alleviate symptoms.
- If conjunctivitis is severe or fails to resolve within 3 weeks, the patient should be referred to an ophthalmologist.

ALLERGIC CONJUNCTIVITIS. Any allergic rhinitis should be treated appropriately first, unless the ocular symptoms are severe. If ocular symptoms persist after allergies are adequately controlled, consider treatment. First-line treatment is a topical histamine$_1$ receptor antagonist or a nonsteroidal antiinflammatory agent. Topical mast cell stabilizers have a slower onset of action but are good for long-term treatment. Systemic antihistamines may be useful. Severe allergic conjunctivitis may require topical corticosteroids.

⚕ **Primary care providers should not prescribe steroid eye drops. Steroids should be ordered only after an ophthalmologist has examined the eye with a slit lamp.**

Corticosteroids suppress the body's inflammatory response. They delay healing and may allow bacteria to overwhelm the area and produce serious infection. Steroid eye drops may increase the virulence of a herpes infection and potentiate both fungal and bacterial infections. Long-term use of steroids may lead to glaucoma or cataracts.

How to Monitor

- Monitor for therapeutic effect and for local and systemic adverse effects.

ANTIBIOTICS. Long-term use of topical antibiotic products requires periodic examination for such signs as itching, redness, edema of the conjunctiva and eyelid, or failure to heal. These could be signs of sensitization. In severe cases of infection, examination of stained conjunctival scrapings and culture studies are recommended.

Patient Variables

GERIATRICS

- Older patients are susceptible to systemic effects of topical eye drops. For example, β-blocker eye drops used for glaucoma can exacerbate chronic heart failure.
- Use with caution and monitor closely for adverse reactions.
- No change in dosage is required.

PEDIATRICS, PREGNANCY, AND LACTATION. Table 12-2 lists considerations for ophthalmic drug use in pediatric, pregnant, and lactating patients.

TABLE 12-2   Characteristics of Eye Medications

Medication	Indications/Action	Use in Pediatrics	Use in Pregnancy	Warnings/ Precautions	Common Side Effects	Serious Side Effects
ANTIINFECTIVES					Local discomfort	
ANTIBIOTICS	Bacterial conjunctivitis				Local discomfort	Hypersensitivity
Ciprofloxacin	Gram-positive and gram-negative organisms	>1 yr	C		Local discomfort	Precipitates, hyperemia
gentamicin	Gram-positive and gram-negative organisms	>1 yr	C		Local discomfort	Bacterial and fungal corneal ulcers
tobramycin	Gram-positive and gram-negative organisms	Safe	B		Local discomfort	
sulfacetamide	Gram-positive and gram-negative organisms	>2 mo	C		Local discomfort	Bacterial and fungal corneal ulcers
erythromycin ointment	Gram-positive organisms	Neonates	B		Redness	
Neosporin solution	Gram-positive organisms	No	C		Redness	Sensitivity to neomycin
ANTIVIRAL						
trifluridine	Herpes simplex virus 1 and 2	>6 yr	C		Mild burning, palpebral edema	Hypersensitivity, viral resistance
NONSTEROIDAL ANTIINFLAMMATORY						
ketorolac	Allergic conjunctivitis	>3 yr	C/D (third trimester)	Rheumatoid arthritis, contact lenses	Burning and stinging Superficial keratitis or infection, corneal edema	Hypersensitivity, bleeding Tendency, keratitis, delayed wound healing
HISTAMINE H₁ BLOCKER						
levocabastine, azelastine	Allergic conjunctivitis	>12 yr	C	Contact lenses	Burning and stinging headache, visual, dry mouth, somnolence	Nausea, rash, dyspnea
MAST CELL STABILIZER						
nedocromil	Allergic conjunctivitis	>6 yr	B	Contact lenses	Headache, burning irritation, unpleasant taste	Hypersensitivity, asthma
STEROID						
Dexamethasone	Inflammatory conditions	No	C		Many	Many; see Chapter 50
GLAUCOMA MEDICATIONS						Many systemic
Sympathomimetic						
brimonidine	Decreased production of aqueous humor Increased outflow of aqueous humor	No	B	MAOIs, cardiovascular disease, decreased hepatic or renal function	Pruritus, hyperemia, burning, drowsiness, dry mouth	Hypertension, respiratory, muscle pain, systemic sympathomimetic effects; see Chapter 13

Table continued on following page

TABLE 12-2   Characteristics of Eye Medications (Continued)

Medication	Indications/Action	Use in Pediatrics	Use in Pregnancy	Warnings/Precautions	Common Side Effects	Serious Side Effects
β-Blocker						
timolol	Decreased production of aqueous humor	No	C	Atrioventricular block, CHF, bradycardia, bronchospasm, asthma, COPD, diabetes, hyperthyroidism	Discomfort, blurred vision, rash, dizziness, headache, gastrointestinal upset	Cerebrovascular, respiratory, central nervous system, and others; see Chapter 18
Parasympathomimetic						
pilocarpine	Increased outflow of aqueous humor	No	C	Pupil constriction, retinal detachment, asthma, bradycardia, hypotension	Local irritation, corneal edema, ciliary spasm, miosis, headache, transient night blindness	Systemic β-blocker effects; see Chapter 2
Cholinesterase Inhibitor						
demecarium	Increased outflow of aqueous humor	No	X	Narrow-angle glaucoma, asthma, PUD, bradycardia, hypotension, recent myocardial infarction, epilepsy, parkinsonism	Burning, redness, intense miosis	Iris cysts, systemic anticholinergic
Carbonic Anhydrase Inhibitor						
dorzolamide	Decreased production of aqueous humor	No	C	Sulfa allergy, decreased renal or hepatic, respiratory distress, diabetes	Burning, bitter taste, headache, GI distress, paresthesias, tinnitus, myopia	Hypersensitivity, electrolyte imbalance, nephrotoxicity, blood dyscrasias
Prostaglandin						
latanoprost	Increased outflow of aqueous humor	No	C	Change in pigmented tissue, intraocular inflammation, contact lenses	Blurred vision, burning, stinging, foreign body sensation, itching	Eyelash changes, eyelid skin darkening, iris color change, macular edema
OTHER						
Sympathomimetic						
phenylephrine	Minor eye irritation	<1 yr	C	Headache, dizziness	Excitability, restlessness, palpitations	
Vasoconstrictor						
naphazoline	Redness	No	C	Narrow-angle glaucoma, MAOIs, contact lenses, hypertension, cerebrovascular disease, hyperglycemia, hyperthyroidism	Rebound, floaters, congestion, hypersensitivity	Narrow-angle glaucoma, hypersensitivity, systemic adrenergic effects
Lubricant						
artificial tears	Protection and lubrication	Yes	C	Reevaluate if irritation increases or persists	Transient stinging	
Anesthetic						
proparacaine	Diagnostic procedure	No	C	Cardiac disease, hyperthyroidism	Mild local irritation; protect eye from damage, erosions	Hypersensitivity, systemic toxicity, long-term use: corneal opacities, permanent visual loss

TABLE 12-2 Characteristics of Eye Medications (Continued)

Medication	Indications/Action	Use in Pediatrics	Use in Pregnancy	Warnings/ Precautions	Common Side Effects	Serious Side Effects
Diagnostic						
fluorescein	Diagnosis of abrasion, foreign bodies	No	C	History of hypersensitivity, allergies, or asthma; do not use in patients with soft contact lenses, will cause them to discolor	Burning sensation; temporary stinging	Hypersensitivity, stains contact lenses

Patient Education

- If the patient experiences any reaction, he should discontinue medication and call the provider.
- Some product contents may be absorbed by soft contact lenses. Avoid wearing soft lenses while using medications.
- Store medication as directed on the package.

EYE DROPS
- Wash hands.
- Tilt head backward or lie down and gaze upward.
- Grasp lower eyelid below eyelashes and pull the eyelid away from the eye to form a pouch.
- Place dropper directly over eye. Avoid contact of the dropper with the eye, finger, or any surface.
- Have patient look upward just before applying a drop.
- After instilling the drop, look downward for several seconds.
- Release the lid slowly and close eyes gently. With eyes closed, apply gentle pressure with fingers to the inside corner of the eye for 3 to 5 minutes.
- Do not rub the eye or squeeze the eyelid. Minimize blinking.

OINTMENTS
- Wash hands. Hold ointment in hand for a few minutes to warm ointment and facilitate flow.
- Tilt head backward or lie down and gaze upward.
- Gently pull down the lower eyelid to form a pouch. Place 0.25 to 0.5 inch of ointment with a sweeping motion inside the lower eyelid by squeezing the tube gently and slowly releasing the eyelid.
- Close eye for 1 to 2 minutes, and roll eyeball in all directions. Temporary blurring of vision may occur; use at night.
- Remove excessive ointment around the eye with a tissue.

ANTIBIOTICS
- Bacterial conjunctivitis is contagious, usually transmitted through direct contact via fingers, towels, handkerchiefs, and similar items moved to the other eye or to other individuals.
- Warm compresses applied to affected eye(s) can aid in the removal of crusting.
- Do not exceed recommended dose or length of treatment; doing so may result in secondary infection.
- Infection can be spread if more than one person uses the medication container.

SPECIFIC DRUGS

See Table 12-2 for characteristics of eye medications.

Antiinfectives

See Chapters 56 to 64 for details on particular antiinfective medications.

Antivirals

See Chapter 68 for details on antiviral agents.

Nonsteroidal Antiinflammatory Agents
ketorolac tromethamine (Acular solution)
INDICATIONS
- Relief of ocular itching caused by seasonal allergic conjunctivitis
- The drug has no significant effect on IOP and does not appear to potentiate the spread of infection.
- The mechanism of its action is thought to be due in part to its ability to inhibit prostaglandin biosynthesis. Ocular administration reduces prostaglandin F_2 levels in aqueous humor.

Mast Cell Stabilizers
nedocromil (Alocril)

Mast cell stabilizers inhibit Type 1 immediate hypersensitivity reactions. Therefore, they inhibit the increased cutaneous vascular permeability that is associated with reagin or immunoglobulin (Ig)E and antigen-mediated reactions. This prevents antigen-stimulated release of histamine and other mast cell inflammatory mediators and inhibits eosinophil chemotaxis. The exact mechanism of action is unknown, but the drug has been reported to prevent calcium influx into the mast cell upon antigen stimulation. The drug has no intrinsic vasoconstrictor or other antiinflammatory activity.

Glaucoma Medications

See Table 12-2.

Other Ophthalmic Medications
Sympathomimetics
phenylephrine hydrochloride (Neo-Synephrine)
- The 0.12% solution is available as an OTC preparation for relief of minor eye irritation.

- Ophthalmologists use 10% and 12% solutions for vaso-constriction and pupil dilation. These higher percentage solutions can cause significant cardiovascular adverse reactions.
- In the eye, phenylephrine acts locally as a potent vasoconstrictor and a mydriatic by constricting ophthalmic blood vessels and the radial muscle of the iris.
- Little rebound vasodilation occurs, and systemic side effects are uncommon.
- Ophthalmic solutions composed of phenylephrine hydrochloride are contraindicated in persons with narrow-angle glaucoma.

Lubricants

artificial tears (Tears Naturale II, Tears Naturale Free)

- Can be used as often as the patient wishes
- Insert systems are indicated in patients with moderate to severe dry eye syndromes such as keratoconjunctivitis sicca, especially those in whom a trial of therapy with artificial tear solutions is unsuccessful.
- Inserts are also indicated for patients with exposure keratitis, decreased corneal sensitivity, and recurrent corneal erosions.

Anesthetics

proparacaine hydrochloride (Alcaine, Percaine)

- Onset of anesthesia after instillation of one drop occurs in approximately 20 seconds. Duration of action is 15 to 20 minutes.

Topical Ear Agents

INDICATIONS

- Superficial infection of the external auditory canal
- Cerumen removal

A large number of otic preparations are available. Some are given by prescription only; others are available OTC. Commonly used prescription topical otic preparations include an antibiotic and an antibiotic plus hydrocortisone. Miscellaneous otic preparations contain a wide variety of combinations of ingredients. Space does not permit a complete listing here, but the components are listed and the most commonly used products are mentioned.

ANATOMY, PHYSIOLOGY, AND PATHOPHYSIOLOGY

The pinna is the visible portion of the ear. The outer ear external auditory canal secretes cerumen to move dirt outward through the canal. The external auditory canal is sealed by the tympanic membrane (TM), which mechanically transmits sound to the middle ear. The middle ear is an air-filled cavity that is connected to the pharynx by the eustachian tube. The eustachian tube opens briefly during swallowing, allowing equalization of pressures on both sides of the TM. The middle ear transmits sound to the inner ear, and the inner ear transduces the sound into nerve impulses.

The two most common problems involving the outer ear are infection and cerumen impaction. Infection often is caused by swimming, or otherwise getting water into the outer ear. Cerumen impaction is associated with hardening of the cerumen, which is associated with old age.

TREATMENT PRINCIPLES
Evidence-Based Recommendations

One study has shown no difference in efficacy between proprietary wax-softening agents and saline/sterile water.

Cardinal Points of Treatment

- These medicines act topically and exhibit minimal systemic absorption. When an ear infection is treated, the other ear also may be treated as a preventative measure. A steroid is usually included with the antibiotic to relieve the symptoms of infection. Use drops for 1 week only.
- To prevent infection in patients at risk (swimmers), use a product that contains 2% acetic acid, boric acid, isopropyl alcohol, or Burow's solution after exposure. These are available OTC or can be made at home.
- To prevent cerumen buildup, use glycerin or an oil such as mineral oil or vegetable oil regularly (usually weekly to monthly). An OTC preparation that contains triethanolamine or carbamide also may be used.
- To treat impacted cerumen, use OTC ear drops nightly for 4 to 7 days. Avoid ear candles because patients may get burned. Excess cerumen may be removed as an office procedure, if necessary.
- For miscellaneous external ear conditions, select an appropriate product from the following list of ingredients:
  - Steroids have antiallergic, antipruritic, and antiinflammatory effects.
  - Antibiotics have antibacterial activity.
  - Phenylephrine is a vasoconstrictor that has a decongestant effect.
  - Acetic acid, boric acid, benzalkonium chloride, and aluminum acetate (Burow's solution) have antibacterial and antifungal activity.
  - Carbamide peroxide and triethanolamine emulsify and disperse earwax.
  - Glycerin is a solvent and vehicle. It has emollient, hygroscopic, and humectant effects.
  - Benzocaine is a local anesthetic.
  - Antipyrine is an analgesic.

How to Monitor

- Monitor for therapeutic effect and hypersensitivity reactions.

Patient Education

- Use only in the ears. Avoid contact with the eyes.
- Notify health care provider if burning or itching occurs, or if the condition persists.
- Use only for a prescribed length of treatment.
- Use ear drops properly:
  1. Wash hands well before instilling eardrops.
  2. Avoid contact of the sterile tip with any part of the ear. For improved accuracy, have another individual instill drops into the ear canal, if possible.

3. Warm bottle to body temperature by holding in hand for 10 minutes before instillation.
4. Shake suspension for 10 seconds to mix well.
5. Patient should lie on side or on back with the affected ear up.
6. For a child, pull ear down and back.
7. For an adult, pull ear up and back.
8. Instill the prescribed number of drops into the ear.
9. Keep the ear tilted for 2 minutes, or insert a cotton plug.
10. Treat for the recommended length of time.

SPECIFIC DRUGS

hydrocortisone 1%, neomycin sulfate 5 mg, polymyxin 10,000 units (Cortisporin Otic Solution) ciprofloxacin 2 mg/ml and hydrocortisone 10 mg/ml (Cipro HC Otic Suspension)

CONTRAINDICATIONS
- Perforated tympanic membrane
- Hypersensitivity to any component

PRECAUTIONS. Prolonged use of antibiotics or steroids may result in the overgrowth of nonsusceptible organisms (e.g., herpes simplex, vaccinia, varicella) and fungus.

ADVERSE EFFECTS
- Rash, itching, and swelling may be signs of hypersensitivity to components of the product.
- Drainage and pain may signify a middle ear infection, and drops are contraindicated.

DOSAGE AND ADMINISTRATION
- The usual adult dosage is four drops instilled three or four times a day. The usual dosage for infants and small children is three drops instilled into the affected ear three or four times a day.

- A wick may be inserted into the canal after the drops have been instilled, and more drops may be applied to saturate the wick. Instruct the patient to instill a few drops to the wick every 4 hours. Remove the wick after 24 hours, and continue to instill the appropriate number of drops three to four times a day.

Topical Mouth and Throat Agents

SPECIFIC DRUGS

ANTIFUNGALS

nystatin (Mycostatin), clotrimazole, other (Mycelex)

INDICATIONS
- Oral candidiasis
- Prophylaxis in immunocompromised patients
- Herpes labialis
- Minor sore throat
- Minor irritation of the throat or mouth
- See Table 12-3 for characteristics of mouth and throat preparations.
- The first group of topical mouth and throat products is antifungals. This section discusses their use only for throat and mouth fungal infections. They usually are associated with antibiotic treatment and immunocompromised patients.
- The antiviral product penciclovir is used (unlabeled) for herpes labialis or cold sores. Carbamide peroxide is indicated for relief of minor oral inflammation such as canker sores, denture irritation, and irritation of inflamed gums.
- Pilocarpine taken as a 5-mg tablet is indicated for dry mouth from salivary gland hypofunction caused by radiotherapy or from Sjögren's syndrome. Because of the risk of serious parasympathomimetic adverse effects, its use should be reserved for patients with a clear indication and significant consequences from dry mouth.
- A wide variety of mouth and throat products with various combinations of ingredients are used for minor irritation of the throat or mouth. These are generally safe and effective

TABLE 12-3 Characteristics of Mouth and Throat Preparations

Preparation	Contraindications, Warnings, Precautions	Adverse Effects	Pregnancy Class	Formulation	Dosage	Administration
nystatin	Hypersensitivity, not for systemic mycoses	Nausea, vomiting, gastrointestinal distress, diarrhea	C	Oral suspension	Adult and child: 400,000-600,000 units Infants: 200,000 units	qid
				Troche (pastilles)	Adults:1 troche	4-5 times/day
clotrimazole	Hypersensitivity, not for systemic mycoses	Increased AST, nausea and vomiting, unpleasant mouth sensations, pruritus	C	Troche	Adult and child >3 yr: 1 troche Prophylaxis: 1 troche during chemotherapy tid	5 times/day
carbamide peroxide	Irritation	Irritation	C	Solution, liquid	>2 yr; swish liquid several drops in mouth for 2-3 minutes and expectorate	qid (after meals and bedtime)
chlorhexidine	Hypersensitivity, not for necrotizing ulcerative gingivitis, increased calculus deposits	May stain teeth, altered taste perception, minor irritation	B	Oral rinse	>18 yr: 15 ml oral rinse for 30 sec after brushing teeth, then expectorate	AM and PM

to various degrees. The most frequently used ingredients include the following:

- Carbamide peroxide (urea peroxide) is used to treat minor oral inflammation because it releases oxygen on contact with mouth tissues to provide cleansing.
- Chlorhexidine gluconate is used for gingivitis because it provides microbicidal activity during oral rinsing.
- Antipyrine is an analgesic.
- Benzocaine and cyclonamine are local anesthetics.
- Hydrocortisone and triamcinolone corticosteroids have antiinflammatory activity.
- Cetylpyridinium chloride, eucalyptus oil, thymol, and hexylresorcinol have antiseptic activity.
- Menthol, camphor, capsicum, dyclonine, and phenol have antipruritic, local anesthetic, and counterirritant activity.
- Saliva substitutes are used for relief of dry mouth and throat.
- Tannic acid is used for temporary relief of pain caused by cold sores because it forms a thin, pliable film over sores within 60 seconds of administration.
- Terpin hydrate is an expectorant.

Patient Education

- To use the suspension form of the drug:
  - Use as directed.
  - Divide dose and place half on each side of the mouth.
- Retain suspension in the mouth for as long as possible before swallowing.
- Continue use for at least 2 days after symptoms disappear.
- To use the troche form, the patient must be competent enough to allow troches to dissolve slowly:
  - Troche should not be chewed or swallowed whole.
  - Troche should be dissolved slowly in the mouth.

OTHER MOUTH AND THROAT PREPARATIONS

carbamide peroxide (Gly-Oxide) and chlorhexidine gluconate (Peridex)

- These agents are not appropriate for treatment of severe or persistent sore throat.
- Do not use these products in children younger than 2 years of age.
- See package labeling for dosage and administration information.

evolve A continually updated list of useful WebLinks may be found in the Evolve Resources at http://evolve.elsevier.com/ Edmunds/NP/

evolve http://evolve.elsevier.com/Edmunds/NP/

Upper Respiratory Agents

BONNIE R. BOCK

DRUG OVERVIEW

Class	Subclass	Generic Name	Trade Name
Decongestants	Oral decongestants	pseudoephedrine HCl	Sudafed (OTC), generic, Entex-PSE (with guaifenesin)
		phenylephrine HCl 🗝	Sudafed PE (OTC)
	Topical nasal decongestants	phenylephrine HCl 🗝	Neo-Synephrine (OTC)
		oxymetazoline	Afrin, Neo-Synephrine 12-hour (OTC)
Antihistamines	Sedating antihistamines		
	Ethanolamine	diphenhydramine HCl	Benadryl (OTC), generic
		clemastine fumarate	Tavist (OTC)
	Alkylamine	chlorpheniramine maleate	Chlor-Trimeton (OTC)
	Low-sedating antihistamines		
	Piperidine	cetirizine HCl	Zyrtec (Rx) ✸ Zyrtec syrup ✸
	Nonsedating antihistamines	fexofenadine HCl ✸	Allegra (Rx) ✸
	Miscellaneous antihistamines	loratadine	Claritin (OTC)
		desloratadine	Clarinex (Rx) ✸
	Intranasal antihistamines	azelastine	Astelin (Rx) ✸
Intranasal Steroids		triamcinolone acetonide	Nasacort AQ (Rx) ✸
		beclomethasone dipropionate	Beconase, Vancenase (Rx)
	Nasal	fluticasone propionate ✸	Flonase (Rx) ✸
Intranasal Mast Cell Stabilizers		cromolyn sodium	NasalCrom (OTC)
Leukotriene Receptor Antagonists		montelukast sodium	Singulair ✸
Antitussives	Narcotic antitussives	codeine phosphate	Generic (Rx)
	Nonnarcotic antitussives	dextromethorphan HBr	Benyin, Delsym, Robitussin Maximum Strength (OTC)
		benzonatate ✸	Tessalon Perles (Rx)
Expectorants		guaifenesin	Robitussin (OTC), Humibid LA (Rx), Mucinex

✸ Top 200 drug; 🗝 Key drug. The antihistamine diphenhydramine is the earliest antihistamine that is commonly used.

INDICATIONS

Decongestants
Oral Decongestants

- Nasal congestion caused by the common cold, hay fever, or other upper respiratory allergies
- Nasal congestion associated with sinusitis and eustachian tube congestion
- *Unlabeled use:* treatment for mild to moderate urinary stress incontinence

Topical Nasal Decongestants

- Symptomatic relief of nasal and nasopharyngeal mucosal congestion caused by the common cold, sinusitis, hay fever, or other upper respiratory allergies
- Adjunctive therapy for middle ear infection by decreasing congestion around the eustachian ostia
- Relief of ear block and pressure pain in air travel

Antihistamines

- Symptomatic relief of symptoms associated with perennial and seasonal allergic rhinitis, vasomotor rhinitis, and allergic conjunctivitis; temporary relief of runny nose and sneezing caused by the common cold
- Skin: allergic and nonallergic pruritic symptoms; mild, uncomplicated urticaria and angioedema
- Amelioration of allergic reactions to blood or plasma, dermatographism, and adjunctive therapy in anaphylactic reactions

Intranasal Steroids

- Vasomotor rhinitis and relief of symptoms of seasonal or perennial rhinitis when effectiveness of antihistamines or tolerance to treatment develops

Intranasal Mast Cell Stabilizers

- Prevention and treatment of allergic rhinitis

Leukotriene receptor antagonists

- Treatment of allergic rhinitis and perennial allergic rhinitis

Antitussives
Narcotic Antitussives

- Codeine for suppression of cough induced by chemical or mechanical respiratory tract irritation

Nonnarcotic Antitussives

- Dextromethorphan HBr (Robitussin) for suppression of nonproductive cough
- Benzonatate (Tessalon Perles) for symptomatic relief of cough

Expectorants

- Guaifenesin may provide some symptomatic relief of respiratory conditions characterized by productive or nonproductive cough.

The seven classes of drugs discussed in this chapter are used to treat a variety of upper respiratory conditions. The two most common conditions in primary care practice that require these medications are upper respiratory viral infection (URI or viral rhinitis) and allergic rhinitis (hay fever). Bacterial infections are covered in the section on antibiotics.

Decongestants and antihistamines are commonly used both OTC and by prescription for treatment of a variety of conditions. Decongestants are used as first-line drugs for URIs. Antihistamines are first-line treatment for allergic rhinitis. Leukotriene receptor antagonists may be used as first-line treatment for allergic rhinitis but are typically prescribed when other treatments fail to relieve symptoms. The antihistamines most commonly seen in primary care practice are discussed here.

Intranasal steroids and cromolyn are generally considered second-line treatment for upper respiratory conditions. Oral formulations of these drugs are used for lower respiratory conditions. These drugs are discussed in detail in Chapter 14; only their intranasal use in upper respiratory conditions is discussed here.

Antitussives and expectorants are used as adjunct therapy in upper respiratory and lower respiratory conditions.

Combination drugs that contain these different categories of medications are available both OTC and by prescription. These combination product ingredients change rapidly, and this may be very confusing to the consumer. Often, OTC combinations purchased by patients contain medications that are not indicated for the condition for which the combination is labeled, and use can be counterproductive to clearing up symptoms. Many nighttime formulations contain alcohol and acetaminophen, which should not be consumed together. Some consumers use products incorrectly, taking an antihistamine for congestion when actually a decongestant is needed. Products with analgesics are often used by patients even in the absence of pain or fever. Many consumers, particularly the elderly, use these products without considering the ingredients and possible drug interactions with medications they are already taking, or preexisting medical conditions that may be adversely affected by certain medications. An example would be patients with hypertension, glaucoma, or urinary retention who take pseudoephedrine for congestion. Many patients self-prescribe OTCs for respiratory problems, so query patients specifically about use of OTC products. (See Chapter 73 for information on OTC use.)

Despite these problems, commonly prescribed combination medications are important in the treatment of respiratory problems and include antihistamine/decongestant combinations (e.g., Allegra-D, Claritin-D, Zyrtec-D), decongestant/expectorant combinations (e.g., Guaifed PD), and antitussive/expectorant combinations (e.g., Robitussin AC, DM), which can be useful in the treatment of multisymptom upper and lower respiratory conditions, if used appropriately. A knowledgeable clinician may suggest special formulations that are available OTC for patients with hypertension (e.g., Coricidin HBP, Coricidin HBP Cough & Cold), and several products are sugar and alcohol free. Despite the multiple combination preparations that are available both OTC and by prescription, many authorities recommend prescribing single-ingredient medications to avoid drug errors and overmedicating.

THERAPEUTIC OVERVIEW OF UPPER RESPIRATORY INFECTION AND ALLERGIC RHINITIS

Anatomy and Physiology

The respiratory system is composed of the upper air passage structure, including the nasal passages, paranasal sinuses, pharynx, and larynx, and the lower air passages, including the trachea, bronchi, and lungs. Air moves through the upper passages (the *conducting portion*) into the lung (*respiratory portion*), where gas exchange occurs through the alveoli of the lung. The respiratory airway is lined with epithelial tissue that contains mucous glands and surface goblet cells that synthesize and secrete thick mucus. Below the larynx to the ends of the bronchi, the airways are lined with columnar epithelial cells that contain hair-like projections or cilia, which continuously beat in an upward motion toward the pharynx. Inhaled irritants stick to the mucus and are moved upward by the cilia to the pharynx, where they are swallowed or expectorated.

Pathophysiology

URIs are often viral in origin, and allergic rhinitis results from an allergic reaction that may have nothing to do with infection. A secondary bacterial infection is common in both URIs and allergic rhinitis that are untreated. Acute sinusitis and otitis media are the most common complications of URI, although pneumonia may develop in susceptible patients. Critical decisions revolve around determining whether the problem is viral or bacterial, and whether the process has an allergic component.

Disease Process

UPPER RESPIRATORY INFECTION. Disease insult to the respiratory tract disturbs the normal physiologic processes: Production of mucus is dramatically increased, but the mucus thickens with dehydration or fever; the mucociliary mechanism is inhibited, and the cilia become sticky and unable to move. Patients cough or swallow enormous amounts of mucus.

URIs are caused by rhinoviruses, adenoviruses, and other viruses. Nasal congestion, watery rhinorrhea, and sneezing are present in 50% to 70% of patients within the first 3 days. Sore throat is reported by 50% of patients in the first 2 days. Other nonspecific symptoms include headache and general malaise. Symptoms are self-limiting, lasting a few days to a few weeks. On physical examination, the nasal mucosa is reddened and edematous with a watery discharge. Diagnosis is based on clinical observation, after absence of signs of bacterial infection is noted—purulent nasal discharge, red tympanic membrane, change in color of discharge, or high fever. URIs should be evaluated by a clinician, particularly if there is any risk of serious disease, including severe acute respiratory syndrome, which is a possible but unlikely differential in the United States.

ALLERGIC RHINITIS. Seasonal allergic rhinitis is caused by a variety of irritations, most commonly allergy to pollen: trees in the spring, grasses in the summer, and ragweed in the fall. Perennial allergic rhinitis usually is caused by allergy to dust, molds, or mites. The symptoms may be similar to URI symptoms, except that they may be more persistent, may fluctuate, and often are related to exposure to allergens. Sneezing, injected conjunctiva, watery itchy eyes, red edematous eyelids, and watery rhinorrhea are often prominent. On physical examination, the turbinates may be pale or violaceous because of venous engorgement rather than red and erythematous as in URI.

MECHANISM OF ACTION

Decongestants

Decongestants are sympathomimetic amines that act to stimulate α-adrenergic receptors of vascular smooth muscle and cause vasoconstriction. This results in nasal decongestion, contraction of gastrointestinal and urinary sphincters, pupil dilation, and decreased pancreatic β-cell secretion. Pseudoephedrine also has β-adrenergic properties that cause relaxation of the bronchi.

In the sympathetic nervous system, adrenergic effector cells contain two distinct receptors, the α- and β-receptors. Sympathomimetic drugs mimic the action of norepinephrine on sympathetic effector organs, thereby affecting the adrenergic receptors. Important α-adrenergic activities include (1) vasoconstriction of arterioles, leading to increased blood pressure; (2) dilation of the pupils; (3) intestinal relaxation; and (4) bladder sphincter contraction. β-Receptors are divided into β$_1$- and β$_2$-receptors because some drugs affect some, but not all, β-receptors. β$_1$-Adrenergic activity includes (1) cardioacceleration and (2) increased myocardial contractility, whereas β$_2$ stimulation leads to (1) vasodilation of skeletal muscle, (2) bronchodilation, (3) uterine relaxation, and (4) bladder relaxation.

Pseudoephedrine HCl is an α-adrenergic receptor agonist (sympathomimetic) that produces vasoconstriction by stimulating α-receptors in the mucosa of the respiratory tract. It also reduces tissue edema and nasal congestion, increases nasal airway patency, promotes drainage of sinus secretions, and opens obstructed eustachian ostia. Pseudoephedrine also is used in the illegal manufacturing of methamphetamine. State and federal regulations now restrict the sale of pseudoephedrine, and it is stored behind the pharmacy counter. In some states, it is available only by prescription. Several manufacturers are using formulations that contain phenylephrine in nonprescription preparations.

Phenylephrine acts directly on α-adrenergic receptors and can be administered orally or topically to relieve nasal congestion in URI, sinusitis, and allergic rhinitis. The efficacy of oral phenylephrine has not been studied extensively.

Nasal sprays or inhaled (topical application of) decongestants to the nasal mucous membranes cause vasoconstriction, resulting in shrinkage, which helps to promote drainage and improve breathing through the nasal passages. These inhaled agents produce reduced systemic effects compared with oral preparations, achieving decongestion without causing sudden or wide changes in blood pressure, cardiac stimulation, or vascular redistribution.

Oxymetazoline is a topical direct-acting sympathomimetic amine that acts on the α-adrenergic receptors of the nasal mucosa, causing vasoconstriction and resulting in decreased blood flow and decreased nasal congestion.

Antihistamines

Antihistamines compete for histamine at the H$_1$-receptor sites and are used to treat immunoglobulin (Ig)E-mediated allergy. Antihistamine therapy is helpful in treating allergic

[handwritten margin notes: Benadryl, Chlor-Trimeton, Nasacort, Flonase, Vancenase, NasalCrom, Singular, Zyrtec, Allegra, Claritin, loratadine]

rhinitis and urticaria in most, but not all, patients. Antihistamines antagonize the pharmacologic effects of histamine. They do not inactivate histamine or block histamine release, antibody production, or antigen–antigen interactions. They also have anticholinergic (drying), antipruritic, and sedative effects to varying degrees. These drugs are classified by the amount of sedation they cause. Azelastine is a topical antihistamine nasal spray with few adverse systemic side effects that is used to treat allergic and vasomotor rhinitis. *[handwritten: Astelin]*

Intranasal Steroids

The steroids used in intranasal products have potent glucocorticoid and weak mineralocorticoid activity. Glucocorticoids inhibit cells, including mast cells, eosinophils, neutrophils, macrophages, lymphocytes, and mediators such as histamine, leukotrienes, and cytokines. They exert direct local antiinflammatory effects with minimal systemic effects. Intranasal corticosteroids effectively control the four major symptoms of allergic rhinitis—rhinorrhea, congestion, sneezing, and nasal itch. They are helpful in managing moderate to severe disease and are used in treating both seasonal and perennial allergic rhinitis. These medications must be used consistently on a daily basis for effectiveness, and maximum effects may not be noted for several days to weeks. For details on the immune system, see Chapter 67.

Intranasal Mast Cell Stabilizers

Cromolyn sodium is an OTC intranasal mast cell stabilizer that is used as a preventative agent that is taken in advance of allergen exposure. It is an antiinflammatory agent that has no intrinsic bronchodilator, antihistaminic, vasoconstrictor, or glucocorticoid activity. Cromolyn inhibits sensitized and mast cell degranulation that occurs after exposure to specific antigens. The drug inhibits the release of mediators, histamine, and slow-reacting substance of anaphylaxis (SRS-A) from the mast cell. It inhibits calcium from entering the mast cell, resulting in the prevention of mediator release. It is effective in reducing rhinorrhea, sneezing, and nasal itch, but it has minimal effect on nasal congestion. Cromolyn acts locally on tissue, inhibiting the release of chemical mediators by preventing mast cell degranulation. It has an excellent safety profile and minimal adverse effects consisting of nasal irritation, stinging, and sneezing. Cromolyn must be taken properly as a nebulized aerosol, inhaled through the mouth, or swallowed orally four to six times a day, and its effect may not be seen for 4 to 6 weeks to months. For details, see Chapter 14.

Leukotriene Receptor Antagonists

Montelukast sodium, a leukotriene receptor antagonist, causes inhibition of airway cysteinyl leukotriene receptors (CysTLs), which are products of arachidonic acid metabolism that are released from mast cells and eosinophils. The CysTL type 1 receptor is found in airway smooth muscle cells, airway macrophages, and proinflammatory cells such as eosinophils and myeloid stem cells. CysTLs are released from the nasal mucosa after allergen exposure and are associated with symptoms of allergic rhinitis.

Antitussives

Codeine and dextromethorphan both act centrally by acting on the cough center of the medulla to suppress cough. Dextromethorphan is the d-isomer of codeine that lacks the analgesic and addictive properties of codeine. However, it is not as effective as codeine in depressing the cough reflex. Benzonatate (dextromethorphan) anesthetizes stretch receptors in the respiratory passages, reducing the cough reflex at its source.

Expectorants

Guaifenesin increases respiratory tract fluid secretions and helps to loosen bronchial secretions by reducing adhesiveness and tissue surface tension. By reducing the viscosity of secretions, guaifenesin increases the efficacy of the mucociliary mechanism in removing accumulated secretions from the upper and lower airways. As a result, nonproductive coughs become more productive, less frequent, and less irritating to the airways. Guaifenesin products that are marketed as sustained or timed release have come under FDA scrutiny. Timed-release OTC drugs require FDA approval because the FDA must ensure that the product releases its active ingredients safely and effectively, sustaining the intended effect over the entire time in which the product is intended to work. Many sustained-release products had been on the market without receiving this approval. Guaifenesin is classed as questionably effective in some studies.

TREATMENT PRINCIPLES

Standardized Guidelines

- A comprehensive algorithm of Treatment Guidelines for Upper Respiratory Illness in Children and Adults from the Institute for Clinical Systems Improvement (ICSI) can be found at http://www.guideline.gov/algorithm/5564/NGC-5564_1.html. Algorithms from previous guidelines for viral upper respiratory infection (VURI), pharyngitis, rhinitis, and sinusitis were incorporated into this algorithm.
- American College of Chest Physicians (ACCP) evidence-based clinical practice guidelines for cough and the common cold provide recommendations and algorithms for care of acute cough due to viral infection (http://www.guideline.gov/summary/summary.aspx?doc_id=8654&nbr=004819).

Evidence-Based Recommendations

- The VURI in adults and children guideline contains an annotated bibliography and discussion of the evidence that supports the recommendations.
- According to randomized controlled trials (RCTs) in allergic rhinitis, oral antihistamines were used first in rhinitis and were found to help control itching, sneezing, rhinorrhea, and stuffiness in most patients; however, they do not alleviate ocular symptoms. Nasal corticosteroids are indicated for patients who do not respond to antihistamines and are considered the most potent medication for the treatment of rhinitis. Nasal cromolyn is less effective than nasal corticosteroids. Intranasal antihistamines are effective in treating nasal symptoms of seasonal, perennial, and vasomotor rhinitis but offer no benefit over conventional treatment. Oral decongestants decrease nasal mucosa swelling, and this reduces nasal congestion.

Cardinal Points of Treatment

UPPER RESPIRATORY ILLNESS

- Hand washing is the most effective way to prevent the spread of VURI. Because this is viewed as mundane and common knowledge, many clinicians fail to reinforce this message and further fail to act as role models by washing their own hands at the beginning of each patient encounter.

- It is important to recognize the signs and symptoms of serious illness in VURI and allergic rhinitis. Symptoms such as upper and lower airway obstruction and severe headache require prompt evaluation and care.
- Do not treat cold symptoms with aspirin-containing products for anyone younger than age 21. Do not use cold or cough medications for children younger than 6 years
- Avoid acetaminophen in patients with liver dysfunction.
- In adults, evidence suggests that zinc gluconate may decrease the duration of a cold if started within 24 hours of onset; however, adverse reactions such as nausea and bad taste may limit its usefulness. No current studies indicate that zinc has effectiveness in treating cold symptoms in children.
- Findings in the medical literature do not support the use of echinacea in preventing VURI.

ALLERGIC RHINITIS

- Allergy testing is rarely helpful in diagnosing allergic rhinitis but may be useful in patients with multiple allergen sensitivities. The goal of therapy is to relieve symptoms, and avoidance of allergens is the first step in this process.
- Controversy is ongoing regarding the use of medication vs. immunotherapy. Risk–cost analyses have not been performed; however, patients with moderate to severe perennial allergies may benefit most from immunotherapy.

COUGH

- Patients with cough associated with viral respiratory infection can be treated with a first-generation antihistamine/decongestant combination preparation. Naproxen can also be used to help to decrease cough. Newer generation, nonsedating antihistamines are ineffective in reducing cough and should not be used.
- Current recommendations have been revised to narrow recommended inhaled anticholinergic agents to a single drug, ipratropium bromide, for cough due to URI or bronchitis. The current guideline supports the use of codeine only in chronic bronchitis and not in cough due to URI. Peripheral and central cough suppressants have limited efficacy in cough due to URI. OTC combination cold medications, other than antihistamine/decongestant combinations, and preparations that contain zinc are not recommended for acute cough due to the common cold.

Nonpharmacologic Treatment

- Nonpharmacologic treatment for URI consists of rest as needed and increased fluids, especially water. Adequate hydration (called *bronchial toilet*) may be more helpful in symptom relief than medication because it helps to decrease cough, thin secretions, and hydrate tissues.
- Use of a teaspoon of honey has been shown to be effective in reducing cough in small children.
- For nonpharmacologic treatment of allergic rhinitis, identify environmental precipitants, which may include time of year, work and home environment, and pets. Implement strategies designed to reduce these factors. Avoid outdoor allergens, use air conditioning in home and car, exercise outdoors in the afternoon when pollen counts are typically low, use high-efficiency particulate air (HEPA) filters in

the home, and use a dryer rather than a clothesline, where clothes can collect airborne pollen.
- For indoor allergens, use strategies for dust, pet, mold, and cockroach avoidance.
- Normal saline nasal sprays or nasal irrigation, twice daily, may help reduce postnasal drip, sneezing, and congestion.

Pharmacologic Treatment

- Patient history reveals which symptoms are most troublesome and can be targeted. Decongestants, antihistamines, or a combination thereof are proven effective. Antitussives or expectorants may be helpful. Because URIs are viral in origin, antibiotics are not indicated. Many patients must have this important fact explained to them.
- Pharmacologic treatment of allergic rhinitis involves identifying and targeting symptoms that are most problematic to the patient; these may include sneezing, runny nose, itching, and nasal congestion.
- Treat mild, intermittent symptoms with an antihistamine, preferably nonsedating, or a decongestant. If the patient is unable to take an oral antihistamine, consider the use of a nasal antihistamine, intranasal cromolyn, or leukotriene receptor antagonist.
- Treat moderate, frequent symptoms with a regular- to high-dose intranasal corticosteroid. Add an oral or a nasal antihistamine and decongestant, if necessary.
- Treat moderate, persistent symptoms with a combination regimen, consisting of intranasal corticosteroids plus a nonsedating or intranasal antihistamine and decongestant, if necessary.
- Treat severe symptoms with a combination regimen consisting of a nonsedating antihistamine with or without a decongestant and intranasal corticosteroid. Consider the use of an oral steroid for 5 days, as well as the use of oxymetazoline as needed for no longer than 3 days.

DECONGESTANTS

- These common drugs, which are widely available without prescription, are very effective in treating nasal congestion. Decongestants are sympathomimetic amines used to relieve nasal congestion caused by colds, allergies, and URIs; they also promote sinus drainage and relieve eustachian tube congestion. Oral forms are often used in combination with antihistamines and expectorants in both OTC and prescription doses (Table 13-1). Topical nasal decongestants provide direct relief to swollen nasal membranes and sometimes are used to decrease congestion of the eustachian tube in middle ear infection and to relieve pressure and blockage of the ear during air travel. Decongestants should be used with caution in patients with hypertension, cardiovascular and peripheral vascular disease, hyperthyroidism, diabetes mellitus, prostatic hypertrophy, urinary retention, and increased intraocular pressure because of their sympathomimetic effects. They are contraindicated in patients with mitral valve prolapse and cardiac palpitations. They also have many side effects that can limit their use, particularly in the elderly.
- Oral decongestants generally do not cause sedation but may cause systemic effects, including nervousness, dizziness, and difficulty sleeping, particularly in infants and the elderly. The clinical problems most often seen with oral decongestants include tachycardia, nervousness, insomnia, palpitations, headache, and irritability, which may be

TABLE 13-1   Commonly Prescribed Respiratory Combination Products

Product Name	Antihistamine	Decongestant	Antitussive	Expectorant
Allegra-D	fexofenadine HCl (60 mg)	pseudoephedrine HCl (120 mg)		
Allegra-D 24 Hour	fexofenadine HCl (180 mg)	pseudoephedrine (240 mg) ER		
Claritin-D	loratadine (5 mg)	pseudoephedrine sulfate (120 mg)		
Claritin-D 24 Hour	loratadine (10 mg)	pseudoephedrine sulfate (240 mg)		
Deconamine SR	chlorpheniramine (8 mg)	pseudoephedrine (120 mg)	hydrocodone (5 mg/5 ml)	guaifenesin (400 mg)
Entex PSE Entex LA Entex HC		pseudoephedrine HCl (120 mg) ER phenylephrine (30 mg) ER phenylephrine (7.5 mg/5 ml)	5 mg hydrocodone	guaifenesin (400 mg) guaifenesin (100 mg/ 5 ml) guaifenesin (10 mg)
Duratuss, Deconsal II		phenylephrine (25 mg) phenylephrine (20 mg) ER		guaifenesin (900 mg) guaifenesin (375 mg)
Decongest II		pseudoephedrine (60 mg)		guaifenesin (600 mg)
Phenergan with codeine	promethazine (6.25 mg/5 ml)		codeine (10 mg/5 ml)	
Semprex-D	acrivastine (8 mg)	pseudoephedrine HCl (60 mg)		
Tussionex Penn Kinetic	chlorpheniramine (8 mg/5 ml)		hydrocodone (10 mg/5 ml)	
Zyrtec-D 12 Hour	cetirizine (5 mg)	pseudoephedrine (120 mg)		

poorly tolerated in the frail elderly; patients with poorly controlled hypertension may experience an increase in blood pressure. The provider should question the patient thoroughly about his history of decongestant use. Patients may voice complaints of their "heart racing," or that the drug keeps them awake. Data suggest that oral decongestants may be used cautiously in patients with controlled hypertension. Sustained-release formulations may have less effect on the cardiovascular system. However, because they may antagonize the effects of antihypertensive medications, alternative agents such as topical decongestants should be used for these patients. The FDA has determined that the combination of pseudoephedrine and caffeine is *not* recognized as safe and effective for OTC use. Cough and cold formulations for children under the age of 6 are not recommended, and most manufacturers have removed these products from the market because of so many cases of accidental overdosing.

- Topical decongestants have little systemic effect, but because of rebound congestion (rhinitis medicamentosa), they should be used only in acute conditions for no longer than 3 consecutive days. Rebound congestion is treated by gradual withdrawal, one nare at a time. Saline nasal spray is often helpful. Overall, topical decongestants are more effective than oral ones, but oral decongestants have longer durations of action and are less irritating.

ANTIHISTAMINES

- Antihistamines are H_1 receptor antagonists that are often used alone or in combination with decongestants and expectorants to relieve symptoms associated with perennial and seasonal allergies with associated rhinitis, vasomotor rhinitis, allergic conjunctivitis, and cold symptoms such as sneezing and runny nose. They also are used to relieve allergic and nonallergic pruritic symptoms, to alleviate mild urticaria and angioedema, for prophylaxis against allergic reactions to blood or plasma products, and as adjunctive therapy in anaphylactic reactions Certain antihistamines also have antiemetic effects and are useful for nausea, vomiting, vertigo, and motion sickness.

- Many OTC cold remedies contain antihistamines; however, their use in the treatment of cold symptoms is controversial. Antihistamines are best used to treat allergic symptoms such as rhinorrhea; watery, itchy eyes; postnasal drainage; and sneezing. Decongestants are preferred for treatment of cold symptoms, such as nasal congestion caused by swollen nasal membranes.

- In general, antihistamines are not recommended to treat lower respiratory tract symptoms, including asthma, because some of their anticholinergic effects may cause thickening of respiratory secretions and may impair expectoration. Several evidence-based reports, however, indicate that antihistamines can be safely used in asthmatic patients with severe perennial allergies without exacerbating the asthma.

- Two generations of antihistamines are available. First-generation agents are usually available OTC and often are used before a health care provider is consulted. Most cause sedation and have sometimes been included in sleep aids. However, they remain highly effective in symptomatic treatment, and some products have been released (by prescription only) that provide new delivery systems that decrease drowsiness.

- Second-generation antihistamines are favored by clinicians for their efficacy/safety ratio and rapid onset of relief from sneezing, pruritus, and watery rhinorrhea. These antihistamines are not very effective against nasal congestion. Local antihistamine nasal sprays and various ocular antihistamines are also effective in less than 30 minutes.

- OTC antihistamines that generally cause sedation may interfere with the patient's activities and contribute to poor adherence. Therefore, an antihistamine and a decongestant often are combined to counteract the side effects of each drug while providing dual treatment. Sedating antihistamines are sometimes preferred if symptoms prevent patients from sleeping. Sedating antihistamines are also used in combination with analgesics as a pain reliever and sleep aid. Prescribed antihistamines are less likely to cause sedation and are generally well tolerated. If a particular antihistamine has lost effectiveness or causes untoward side effects, another antihistamine should be selected from a different class. If the patient requires two antihistamines for severe symptoms, drugs from two different classes should be selected.

INTRANASAL STEROIDS

- Intranasal corticosteroids are *the* most effective agents for the management of allergic rhinitis because of their direct reduction of nasal inflammation and their ability to reduce nasal hyperreactivity. All agents are safe and effective and will improve the patient's quality of life *if* the patient uses them on a daily basis. Many patients do not like the odor or taste associated with specific agents, and one or two different medications may have to be tried before the most tolerable agent can be found for an individual. It is essential for the health care provider to help the patient understand the important role of these agents and to demonstrate how they should be administered correctly.
- Intranasal steroids should be used for at least 1 month before it is decided whether they are effective. Patients should be warned that improvement usually does not begin until 1 to 2 weeks after therapy is started. Intranasal corticosteroids can be used with asthmatic patients and with those who have comorbid nasal polyposis. Intranasal steroids may help to shrink nasal polyps.
- Exceeding the recommended dose may result in systemic effects, including suppression of hypothalamic-pituitary-adrenal (HPA) axis function. Systemic effects are possible with inhaled steroids and are less likely with intranasal corticosteroids when used at conventional recommended doses.
- It should be noted that in some cases, oral corticosteroids may be required for a short time. These powerful drugs reduce nasal inflammation and hyperreactivity but have potentially serious side effects when used over a long period. A short course of tapered corticosteroids is advisable only for moderate to serious exacerbations of allergic rhinitis.

INTRANASAL MAST CELL STABILIZERS (CROMOLYN)

- These agents are particularly effective in patients with intermittent allergies, especially when these are determined to be prevalent during only one season of the year. They are usually available OTC and should be started 3 to 4 weeks before peak allergy season occurs. Their effect on the nose is short-acting and makes compliance more difficult because several doses are needed per day. Intraocular agents are also very effective.

- Continue treatment throughout exposure. In perennial allergic rhinitis, effects of treatment may not appear for 2 to 4 weeks after treatment is first initiated. The need for medication may diminish, and it can be discontinued later.

LEUKOTRIENE RECEPTOR ANTAGONISTS

- Montelukast sodium, a leukotriene receptor antagonist, is used for the relief of symptoms of allergic rhinitis in adults, particularly those with asthma, and pediatric patients, 2 years and older, and for the treatment of perennial allergic rhinitis in adults and pediatric patients 6 months and older. Leuko-trienes are associated with early-phase allergic symptoms such as sneezing, rhinorrhea, and nasal itching, as well as late-phase reactions such as congestion, sneezing, and rhinorrhea. Antileukotriene use is often offered in combination with other therapies, especially when nasal congestion is not ameliorated by other modalities.

ANTITUSSIVES

- Antitussives are used to control or suppress cough caused by respiratory tract irritation, colds, or allergies.

  It is important to determine the underlying disorder that is causing the cough, particularly to rule out serious causes of cough.

- Antitussives should not be given in conditions in which retention of respiratory secretions may be harmful. Antitussives should be used with caution. In general, a cough should not be suppressed. Coughing helps to bring fluid up from the bronchioles and lungs. However, if a patient is having a nonproductive cough that is causing muscle pain or is interfering with sleep, it should be suppressed.
- Antitussive preparations are available in liquid and tablet forms. Patients often expect or prefer a cough syrup for cough suppression. Prescribing cough syrups may provide some psychological benefit. A simple cough syrup that contains guaifenesin but no other drugs, including alcohol, causes no harm, soothes the throat, and makes the patient feel cared for. A cough syrup without sugar is made for diabetic patients. These can also be used in the patient for whom any other medications are unsafe.
- Most effective in suppressing coughs are the narcotic antitussives. Codeine, as a narcotic antitussive, is used to suppress cough induced by chemical or mechanical respiratory tract infection. It also is used as a narcotic agonist analgesic for the relief of mild to moderate pain (see Chapter 42). The antitussive dose of codeine is lower than the required dose for analgesia, and side effects are less frequent at the antitussive dose. Cough suppression with codeine is therefore beneficial at bedtime in patients who have cough-related pain or complications such as costochondritis or sleeplessness caused by deep or persistent cough. Hydrocodone, also a narcotic antitussive and analgesic, has multiple actions similar to those of codeine. Like codeine, it is believed to act directly on the cough center in the brain.
- Nausea, vomiting, sedation, dizziness, and constipation are the most common side effects of narcotic antitussives. Allergic reactions to opiates are infrequent and usually

are manifested by pruritus and urticaria. Narcotic antitussives should be prescribed in small amounts, and patients should be followed closely to determine effectiveness and to prevent excessive use. These drugs can provide good suppression at doses low enough to provoke few side effects.

- Nonnarcotic antitussives lack analgesic properties and are not as effective as codeine in suppressing cough, but they also lack the potential for addiction and other adverse effects associated with narcotic use. Dextromethorphan is a common ingredient in many OTC cold medications and some prescription cough preparations and is frequently used in combination with decongestants, antihistamines, and expectorants (see Table 13-1).
- Benzonatate (in the form of capsules that should be swallowed whole) can cause temporary local anesthesia of the oral mucosa if not taken correctly. It lacks the CNS side effects of codeine or dextromethorphan. However, often it is not as effective. Benzonatate is often used in patients such as the frail elderly; patients who must continue to perform activities that require maximum mental alertness such as driving; and those who are bothered by their cough but cannot tolerate the CNS side effects of other cough suppressants.

EXPECTORANTS

- Guaifenesin (glyceryl guaiacolate) is an expectorant that is used for the symptomatic relief of dry, nonproductive cough associated with respiratory tract infection; it is also used in related conditions such as sinusitis, pharyngitis, bronchitis, and asthma and in the presence of tenacious mucus, mucous plugs, or congestion in the respiratory tract. Guaifenesin is found in many OTC and prescription preparations.
- Expectorants are often used in combination with antitussives to provide relief for dry nonproductive cough and to loosen tenacious mucus or congestion in the respiratory tract. These agents were once believed to stimulate the flow of mucus; however, no evidence supports this view. Expectorants are often used when the patient insists on a cough remedy when cough suppression is not indicated, or when the patient believes the effect to be beneficial.
- Enhancing expectoration by thinning thick secretions helps to promote drainage. This can be accomplished through the use of expectorants, by increasing fluid intake, and by increasing air humidification. Fluid intake—up to a gallon of water a day for those who do not have a fluid restriction—is very important.

How to Monitor

DECONGESTANTS

- Monitor for symptoms of CNS stimulation in oral use (e.g., paradoxical excitation, sleeplessness, ataxia).
- Monitor frequency of topical application, and monitor for symptoms of rebound congestion (rhinitis medicamentosa).

ANTIHISTAMINES

- Monitor for relief of targeted symptoms and for excessive drowsiness and other side effects.

INTRANASAL STEROIDS

- Watch closely for development of infection in the nose or sinus.
- In long-term use, monitor for changes in nasal mucosa such as growth of polyps.

ANTITUSSIVES

- Monitor narcotic antitussives for effectiveness and excessive side effects, especially constipation in the elderly.

Patient Variables

DECONGESTANTS

- Sustained-release products should not be used in nursing mothers or in children younger than 12 years of age.
- Do not give cough or cold products to children under the age of 6. Potential for overdose and death exists and these formulations have been removed from the market. These products, if still available in homes, should be discarded.

ANTIHISTAMES
  Geriatrics

- Antihistamines are more likely to cause excessive sedation, syncope, dizziness, confusion, and hypotension in elderly patients; a decrease in dosage is usually necessary.
- Administer the antitussive codeine with caution in elderly and debilitated patients and in those with severe liver disease or kidney impairment and hypothyroidism, Addison's disease, urethral stricture, or prostatic hypertrophy.
  Pediatrics
- Antihistamines may diminish mental alertness.

> **In young children, antihistamines may produce paradoxical excitation in a syndrome that may include excitement, hallucinations, ataxia, incoordination, muscle twitching, athetosis, hyperthermia, cyanosis, tremor, and hyperreflexia, followed by respiratory depression and cardiorespiratory arrest.**

- Convulsions in children resulting from antihistamine use may be preceded by mild depression and may indicate a poor prognosis. Dry mouth, fever, fixed dilated pupils, and flushing of the face are common. The convulsant dose of antihistamines is close to the lethal dose.
- Use of intranasal corticosteroids in prepubescent children poses a potential risk of growth suppression. Studies with beclomethasone dipropionate used twice daily have shown a significant decrease in growth velocity. This has not been shown in other intranasal steroids (mometasone furoate monohydrate, budesonide, or fluticasone propionate), and it is possible that growth suppression may be associated with certain agents or may be dose related. Children who are currently taking oral inhaled corticosteroids for asthma are at increased risk. When using intranasal steroids in children, use the lowest dosage for a short time, and routinely measure growth.
- Do not use codeine in premature infants; opiates cross the immature blood-brain barrier to a great extent, producing significant respiratory depression. Give to infants and small children with extreme caution, and monitor the dosage carefully.
- Caution is recommended in administering expectorants to children up to 12 years of age with a persistent or

chronic cough or asthma, or if the cough is accompanied by excessive mucus. A medical evaluation should be conducted before treatment with expectorants is provided.

Pregnancy and Lactation

- Decongestant products should not be used in nursing mothers.
- *Category B*: antihistamines (azatadine, cetirizine, chlorpheniramine, clemastine, cyproheptadine, dexchlorpheniramine, diphenhydramine, loratadine) and leukotriene receptor antagonists
- *Category C*: antihistamines (brompheniramine, carbinoxamine, desloratadine, fexofenadine, hydroxyzine, pheniramine, promethazine, triprolidine), intranasal steroids, antitussives (codeine), and expectorants
- Safe use of antihistamines in pregnancy has not been established. Several possible associations with malformations have been found, but the significance is unknown. Use only when clearly needed, and when the potential benefits outweigh the potential risks to the fetus. Do not use during the third trimester of pregnancy; newborn and premature infants may have severe reactions.
- Because of the higher risk of adverse effects for infants in general, particularly for newborns and premature infants, antihistamine therapy is contraindicated in nursing mothers.

INTRANASAL STEROIDS

Pediatrics. Use of intranasal corticosteroids in prepubescent children poses a potential risk of growth suppression. Studies with beclomethasone dipropionate used twice daily have shown a significant decrease in growth velocity. This has not been shown with other intranasal steroids (mometasone furoate monohydrate, budesonide, or fluticasone propionate), and it is possible that growth suppression may be associated with certain agents or may be dose related. Children who are currently taking oral inhaled corticosteroids for asthma are at increased risk. When using intranasal steroids in children, use the lowest dosage for a short time, and routinely measure growth.

Pregnancy and Lactation. *Category C*

LEUKOTRIENE RECEPTOR ANTAGONISTS

Pregnancy and Lactation. *Category B*

ANTITUSSIVES: CODEINE

Geriatrics

- Administer codeine with caution in elderly and debilitated patients and in those with severe liver impairment of kidney function, hypothyroidism, Addison's disease, urethral stricture, or prostatic hypertrophy.

Pediatrics

- Do not use codeine in premature infants; opiates cross the immature blood-brain barrier to a greater extent, producing significant respiratory depression.
- Give to infants and small children with extreme caution, and monitor the dosage carefully.

Pregnancy and Lactation. *Category C*

EXPECTORANTS

Pediatrics. Caution is recommended in children up to 12 years of age with a persistent or chronic cough or asthma, or if the cough is accompanied by excessive mucus. A medical

evaluation should be conducted before treatment with expectorants is provided.

Pregnancy and Lactation. *Category C*

Patient Education

DECONGESTANTS

- Encourage patients to reduce consumption of caffeine-containing beverages (coffee, tea, and cola) because these may increase the restlessness and insomnia caused by pseudoephedrine in sensitive individuals.
- Use medication for only 2 to 3 days, and then stop, to prevent a rebound in symptoms. Treatment–rest cycles may be continued while the patient is symptomatic.

ANTIHISTAMINES

- Antihistamines are used to treat allergy symptoms and should not be used to treat URI, including colds and sinusitis.
- Do not use alcohol, sleeping pills, sedatives, or tranquilizers while taking antihistamines.
- Antihistamines may have a sedative effect, causing dizziness in some patients. Patients should avoid driving a car or performing hazardous tasks until the effects of the medication are known.
- Antihistamines should be stored in a tightly closed container in a cool, dry place away from heat and sunlight, and out of the reach of children.
- Some antihistamines may cause stomach upset; these should be taken with food.
- Antihistamines may cause photosensitivity; the patient should avoid prolonged sunlight exposure.
- Do not crush or chew sustained-release preparations.

INTRANASAL STEROIDS

- Use patient information provided with the product on how to use the nebulizer or inhaler.
- Do not exceed recommended dosage.
- Clear secretions from nasal passages before using; use decongestants if necessary.
- Effects are not immediate; results require regular use and may take up to 7 days.

INTRANASAL MAST CELL STABILIZERS (CROMOLYN)

- Clear the nasal passages before administering the spray, and inhale through the nose during administration.
- Follow the information provided with the product for correct administration of nebulizer, inhaler, or oral ampules of medicine.
- Do not discontinue therapy abruptly without consulting provider.

LEUKOTRIENE RECEPTOR ANTAGONISTS

- Phenylketonuric patients should be aware that the 4-mg and 5-mg tablets contain phenylalanine as an ingredient of aspartame.

ANTITUSSIVES

- Contact health care provider if cough persists for longer than 2 weeks or is accompanied by high fever, rash, or persistent headache.
- Narcotic antitussives such as codeine may impair mental and physical abilities. Patients should be cautioned

to avoid performing potentially hazardous tasks, such as driving or operating heavy machinery.

Expectorants
- Instruct patient to drink plenty of water to help loosen mucus in the lungs.
- Contact health care provider if cough persists for longer than 2 weeks or is accompanied by high fever, rash, shortness of breath (SOB), change in characteristics of cough, increasing fatigue, or persistent headache.

SPECIFIC DRUGS

DECONGESTANTS

Oral Decongestants

pseudoephedrine hydrochloride (Sudafed, Entex-PSE [with guaifenesin])

CONTRAINDICATIONS. Hypersensitivity to sympathomimetics, severe hypertension, or severe coronary artery disease, or use in individuals receiving MAOIs

WARNINGS. Premature infants and newborns are at increased risk for adverse effects.

PRECAUTIONS
- Diabetes, hypertension, cardiovascular disease, prostatic hypertrophy, or hyperreactivity to ephedrine
- Manufacturer's label warns of contraindication in breastfeeding; however, the American Academy of Pediatrics considers pseudoephedrine compatible with breastfeeding.
- Extended-release preparations containing 120 or 240 mg should not be administered to children younger than 12 years of age.

MISUSE AND ABUSE. Because pseudoephedrine is used in the illegal production of methamphetamine, legislation has been enacted on federal and state levels to restrict the sale of OTC products that contain pseudoephedrine. In March 2006, the Combat Methamphetamine Epidemic Act of 2005 (Title VII of the USA PATRIOT Improvement and Reauthorization Act of 2005, P.L. 109-177) was amended and signed into law. Changes on the classification and sale of products containing ephedrine, pseudoephedrine, and phenylpropanolamine have been enacted and include sales limits, "behind the counter" placement, log book recording of sales, and self-certification and training of sellers of these products. The Drug Enforcement Administration (DEA) has issued regulations by which these provisions should be implemented; these can be found online at the DEA Diversion website (http://www.deadiversion.usdoj.gov/meth).

PHARMACOKINETICS
- See Table 13-2.
- Presumed to cross the placenta and to enter the cerebrospinal fluid (CSF); 0.5% of an oral dose is distributed into breast milk over 24 hours.

ADVERSE EFFECTS. See Table 13-3.

DRUG INTERACTIONS
- β-Adrenergic blockers and MAOIs may potentiate the effects of decongestants.
- May reduce the antihypertensive effects of guanethidine, mecamylamine, methyldopa, and reserpine
- Cocaine use with pseudoephedrine may increase the effects of either of these medicines on the heart and may increase the chance of side effects.
- Caffeine use may increase insomnia and restlessness in sensitive individuals.

OVERDOSAGE
- Excessive CNS stimulation, resulting in excitement, tremor, restlessness, insomnia, tachycardia, hypertension, pallor, pupil dilation, hyperglycemia, and urinary retention
- Severe overdose may cause hallucinations, convulsions, CNS depression, cardiovascular collapse, and death.

DOSAGE AND ADMINISTRATION. See Table 13-4.

Topical Nasal Decongestants

phenylephrine hydrochloride (Neo-Synephrine [nasal], Sudafed PE [oral])

CONTRAINDICATIONS
- MAOI use within 14 days
- Topical cocaine and yohimbe

WARNINGS
- Phenylephrtine should be administered with extreme caution to geriatric or hyperthyroid patients or those with bradycardia, partial heart block, myocardial disease, or severe arteriosclerosis.
- After intranasal use of phenylephrine, the possibility of substantial absorption and systemic effects is increased after overdosage or swallowing of excess solution.

PRECAUTIONS
- Severe hypertension or severe coronary artery disease
- Cautious use in thyroid disease, diabetes mellitus, or prostatic hyperplasia
- Topical decongestants should be used in acute states and for not longer than 3 to 5 days.
- Some products may contain sulfites, which can cause allergic reactions in people with sulfite sensitivities.

ADVERSE EFFECTS
- Intranasal use may cause transient burning, stinging, sneezing, and nasal discharge.
- Rebound nasal congestion and rhinitis may occur.
- Systemic sympathomimetic effects include palpitations, tachycardia, ventricular premature contractions, occipital headache, pallor or blanching, trembling or tremors, increased perspiration, and hypertension.
- Nausea, dizziness, CNS stimulation, and nervousness may follow intranasal use of the drug.
- Conduction disorder of the heart, dizziness, headache disorder, hyperhidrosis, insomnia, nervousness, pallor, tachyarrhythmia, and tremors are rare with oral dosages.

TABLE 13-2 Pharmacokinetics of Common Respiratory Medications

Drug	Absorption	Onset of Action	Half-Life	Duration of Action	Metabolism	Excretion
pseudoephedrine	GI; completely absorbed in 30 min	1-2 hr 1.5-2 hr (120 mg) 3-6 hr (ext release) 2.1-2.4 (ped solution)	4-6 hr (30 mg)	4-8 hr (60 mg) 12 hr (extended release)	Liver	55%-96% unchanged in urine
phenylephrine	Nasal mucosa; oral	Immediate	9-16 hr	30 min-4 hr	Liver and intestine, if absorbed	Urine 70%-90%
oxymetazoline	Nasal mucosa	5-10 min	Unknown	5-6 hr with decline over 6 hr	Unknown	Unknown
diphenhydramine	GI	15 min	1-4 hr	4-6 hr	Liver	50%-75% metabolites, 1% unchanged in urine
clemastine	GI	2-5 hr	4-6 hr	5-12 hr	Liver	Urine
chlorpheniramine	GI	30-60 min	12-43 hr	6-24 hr	GI mucosa; liver	Urine 20%-35%, feces 1%
montelukast sodium	GI	3-4 hr (10 mg) 2-2.5 hr (5 mg chew) 2 hr (4 mg chew)	2.7-5.5 hr (adults) 3.4-4.2 hr (children 6-14 yr)	24 hr	Liver CYP450: 2C9 3A4 substrate; potent 2C8 inhibitor	Bile/feces 86%, urine <2%
triamcinolone	Nasal mucosa	10-16 hr	4 hr	Varies	Unknown	Unknown
beclomethasone	Nasal mucosa/GI tract	Several days-2 wk	2.7 hr	Varies	Tissue esterases, liver CYP450 3A substrate	Feces 50%, urine 12%
fluticasone	Nasal mucosa/GI tract	12-48 hr 2-4 days optimum effectiveness	7.8 hr	1-2 wk	Liver, CYP450 3A substrate	Feces
cromolyn	Nasal mucosa	Several days-2 wk	Unknown	Varies	CYP450; <7% systemic absorption	Feces, urine, bile
codeine	GI	1-2 hr	2.5-4 hr	4-6 hr	Liver CYP450 2D6 substrate	Urine
dextromethorphan	GI	15-30 min	11 hr	3-6 hr	Liver; 2D6 substrate, 3A4 substrate (CYP)	Urine
benzonatate	GI	15-20 min	Unknown	3-8 hr	Liver CYP450	Urine
guaifenesin	GI		1 hr		Hydrolysis	Urine

Topical Nasal Decongestants—cont'd

DRUG INTERACTIONS. Anticholinergics, β-blockers, central α$_2$-agonists, linezolid, MAOIs, sortalol, tricyclic antidepressants

DOSAGE AND ADMINISTRATION
- 0.125% and 0.16% are no longer available.
- Prior to initial use of metered sprays, the nasal inhaler must be primed by depressing the pump firmly several times.
- Sprays should be delivered or pumped into each nostril with the patient's head erect, so that excess solution is not released. The nose should be blown thoroughly 3 to 5 minutes later.
- See Table 13-4.

OTHER DRUGS IN CLASS
- Oxymetazoline (Afrin, Neo-Synephrine 12 Hour) is similar to phenylephrine with the following warnings:
  - Do not use for longer than indicated, or rhinitis medicamentosa (RM), also called *rebound rhinitis*, may occur. RM generally is characterized by nasal congestion that begins after use of a nasal spray for longer than 3 days without rhinorrhea, sneezing, or postnasal drip. It occurs equally in men and women and is more common in young and middle-aged adults. Results of studies identifying timing of onset have been inconclusive, in that some studies have shown that rebound congestion does not develop with up to 8 weeks of topical decongestant use, but others show the onset of RM after 3 to 10 days, with symptoms worsening from day 10 to day 30. Several small studies using oxymetazoline showed that rebound

TABLE 13-3   Adverse Effects of Respiratory Medications

Drug	Common Side Effects	Serious Adverse Effects
DECONGESTANTS		
pseudoephedrine	Insomnia, tachycardia, palpitations, headache, dizziness, nausea, nervousness, excitability, agitation, anxiety, weakness, tremor, elevated blood pressure	Arrhythmia, severe hypertension
ANTIHISTAMINES		
diphenhydramine	Somnolence, dry mouth, headache, dizziness, nausea, vomiting, diarrhea, cramps, fever	Dyskinesia, thickening of bronchial secretions
cetirizine	Somnolence, dry mouth, fatigue, pharyngitis, dizziness, abdominal pain, nausea/vomiting, diarrhea	Bronchospasm, hepatitis (rare), hypersensitivity (rare)
loratadine	Headache, somnolence, fatigue, dry mouth, nervousness, abdominal pain	Bronchospasm, hepatitis (rare), hypersensitivity (rare)
desloratadine	Pharyngitis, dry mouth, myalgia, fatigue, somnolence, dysmenorrhea, headache, nausea, dizziness, dyspepsia	Hypersensitivity reaction (rare), hepatotoxicity (rare)
fexofenadine	Headache, dyspepsia, fever, cough, URI, back pain, dizziness, drowsiness, fatigue, myalgia, nausea, sinusitis, skin rash, xerostomia	Hypersensitivity reaction (rare)
azelastine (nasal)	Bitter taste, headache, somnolence, weight increase, myalgia, nasal burning, pharyngitis, dry mouth, paroxysmal sneezing, nausea, rhinitis, fatigue, dizziness	No serious reactions reported
LEUKOTRIENE RECEPTOR ANTAGONISTS		
montelukast sodium	Abnormal hepatic function tests, headache disorder, abdominal pain with cramps, bronchitis, cough, dizziness, fatigue, fever, general weakness, infectious gastroenteritis, myopia, nasal congestion, rhinitis, skin and skin structure infection, skin rash, toothache	Angioedema, anaphylaxis, Churg-Strauss syndrome (rare), hepatic eosinophilic infiltration (rare), hepatotoxicity (rare)
INTRANASAL STEROIDS		
triamcinolone acetonide	Nasal burning, irritation, dryness, rhinorrhea, sneezing, epistaxis, headache, pharyngitis, dry throat, cough, taste changes, light-headedness, dyspepsia, nasal ulcer, urticaria, pruritus	Nasal septal perforation, growth suppression (pediatrics), angioedema (rare), bronchospasm (rare), nasopharyngeal candidiasis, increased IOP
INTRANASAL CROMOLYN		
cromolyn sodium	Sneezing, nasal burning, epistaxis, bad taste	Bronchospasm
ANTITUSSIVES		
codeine	Nausea, vomiting, constipation, hypotension, drowsiness, sedation, palpitations, dizziness, rash, pruritus	Toxic doses—exhilaration, excitement, seizures, delirium, hypotension, miosis, slow pulse, tachycardia, narcosis, flushed face, tinnitus, lassitude, muscular weakness, circulatory collapse, or respiratory paralysis; respiratory depression (at high doses), abuse potential
dextromethorphan	Nausea, sedation, dizziness, abdominal pain, rash	Serotonin syndrome (rare), abuse potential (rare)
benzonatate	Sedation, headache, dizziness, rash, nausea, dyspepsia, pruritus, confusion, nasal congestion, chest numbness, burning eyes	Bronchospasm, laryngospasm, cardiovascular collapse
EXPECTORANTS		
guaifenesin	Drowsiness, headache, rash, nausea/vomiting	None noted

congestion did not begin until after 10 days in healthy volunteers, and that doubling the dose of oxymetazoline in healthy volunteers for 30 days did not increase rebound congestion. The first goal in the treatment of RM is the immediate discontinuation of the topical decongestant. Nasal corticosteroids have been shown in various studies to be beneficial in treating RM by decreasing nasal edema, inflammation, and congestion; however, it is difficult to determine whether rebound congestion is due to the initial nasal condition, RM, or both.

- Clinical evaluation recommended for use in children younger than age 6. Use during pregnancy only when necessary—may constrict uterine vessels, leading to fetal hypoxia

TABLE 13-4   Dosage and Administration Recommendations for Common Respiratory Medications

Drug	Dosage/Administration
pseudoephedrine (Sudafed; generic)	Adults and children >12 yr: 30-60 mg po q4-6h; maximum: 240 mg/day Sustained release: 120 mg po q12h; maximum: 240 mg/day Children 6-12 yr: 30 mg q4-6h; maximum: 120 mg/24 hr Children 2-5 yr: 15 mg q4-6h; maximum: 60 mg/24 hr Children <2 yr: 4 mg/kg/day in divided doses q6h

phenylephrine (Neo-Synephrine; generic)
  Nasal
 	
  Oral
	Adults and children >12 yr: 2-3 drops or sprays (0.25% and 0.5% soln) q4h prn, or 1-3 metered sprays per nostril q4h prn
	0.16% and 0.125% nasal solutions/sprays are no longer available; may dilute 0.25% or 0.5% with saline solution to achieve desired concentration
	Children 6-12 yr: 2-3 drops or sprays (0.25% soln) per nostril q4h prn
	Children 1-5 yr: 2-3 drops or sprays (0.125% soln) per nostril q4h prn
	Infants >6 mo: 1-2 drops (0.16% soln) per nostril q3h prn
	Do not use for longer than 3 days.

oxymetazoline (Afrin; generic)	Adults and children >12 yr: 10-20 mg (as HCl salt) po q4h prn
diphenhydramine (Benadryl; generic)	Adults and children ≥6 yr: 2-3 sprays (0.05% soln) into both nostrils bid; maximum: *3 days* Adults and children >12 yr: 25-50 mg po q4-6h; maximum dose: 300 mg/day Sleep aid: Adults and children >12 yr: 50 mg po qh; children 2-12 yr: 1 mg/kg 30 min before bedtime; maximum: 50 mg Children 6-11 yr: 12.5-25 mg po q4-6h; maximum: 150 mg/day Children 2-5 yr (under direction of provider only): 6.25 mg q4-6h; maximum: 37.5 mg/day
clemastine (Tavist; generic)	Adults and children >12 yr: 1.34-2.68 mg (1-2 mg base) po bid-tid; maximum: 8.04 mg/day (6 mg base). OTC: 1.34 mg po bid; maximum: 2.68 mg/day (2 mg base) Children 6-12 yr: 0.67-1.34 mg po bid; maximum: 4.02 mg/day (3 mg base) Infants and children <6 yr: 0.05 mg/kg/day (clemastine base) or 0.335-0.67 mg/day (clemastine fumarate) (0.25-0.5 mg base/day) divided into 2-3 doses; maximum: 1.34 mg/day (1 mg base)
chlorpheniramine (Chlor-Trimeton [SR]; generic)	Adults and children >12 yr: 4 mg po q4-6h; alternate: 8-12 mg SR q8-12h; maximum: 24 mg/day Children 6-12 yr: 2 mg po q4-6h; maximum: 12 mg/day; alternate: 8 mg SR po qhs Children 2-6 yr: 1 mg po q4-6h; maximum: 6 mg/day
cetirizine (Zyrtec)	Adults and children ≥6 yr: 5-10 mg po once daily; maximum: 10 mg/day Children 2-5 yr: 2.5-5 mg po once daily or in 2 divided doses; maximum: 5 mg/day Children 12-23 mo: 2.5 mg po once daily or bid; maximum: 5 mg/day Children 6-12 mo: 2.5 mg po once daily; maximum: 2.5 mg/day
fexofenadine (Allegra)	Adults and children >12 yr: 180 mg ER po once daily; alternate: 60 mg po bid; renal impairment (<80 ml/min): 60 mg po once daily Children 2-11 yr: 30 mg po bid; renal dose: 30 mg po once daily
loratadine (Claritin)	Adults and children ≥6 yr: 10 mg once daily; renal (Clcr <30 ml/min) and hepatic impairment: 10 mg po every other day Children 2-5 yr: 5 mg po once daily (syrup); renal (Clcr <30 ml/min) and hepatic impairment: 5 mg po every other day
desloratadine (Clarinex)	Adults and children >12 yr: 5 mg po once daily Renal and hepatic impairment (adjust dose frequently): 5 mg po every other day Children 6-11 yr: 2.5 mg po once daily (soln or oral disintegrating tablet) Children 1-5 yr: 1.25 mg po once daily (soln) Children 6-11 mo: 1 mg po once daily (soln)
azelastine (Astelin)	Rhinitis: Adults and children ≥12 yr: 1-2 sprays per nostril bid Children 5-11 yr: 1 spray per nostril bid
montelukast sodium (Singulair)	Rhinitis: Adults ≥15 yr: 10-mg tablet po once daily Children 6-14 yr: 5-mg chewable tablet po once daily Children 2-5 yr: 4-mg chewable tablet or oral granules once daily Children 6-23 mo: 4-mg oral granules once daily

Table continued on following page

TABLE 13-4 Dosage and Administration Recommendations for Common Respiratory Medications (Continued)

Drug	Dosage/Administration	
triamcinolone (Nasacort AQ, Tri-Nasal)	Rhinitis: Adults and children >12 yr: Nasal suspension (Nasacort AQ): 2 sprays (55 mcg/spray) per nostril once daily; may increase to 8 sprays once daily or in 2-4 divided doses, if necessary; maximum: 8 sprays/day. Usual maintenance dose: 1 spray/nostril once daily Nasal spray (Tri-Nasal): 2 sprays (50 mcg/spray) in each nostril once daily Children 6-11 yr: Nasal suspension (Nasacort AQ): 2 sprays (55 mcg/spray) per nostril once daily Nasal spray (Tri-Nasal): 1 spray (50 mcg/spray) in each nostril once daily	
beclomethasone (Beconase AQ)	Adults and children (rhinitis) >12 yr: 1-2 sprays per nostril bid; alternate: 2 sprays per nostril bid Children 6-12 yr: 1 spray per nostril bid. May increase to 2 sprays per nostril bid if necessary; maximum: 2 sprays/nostril bid; decrease to 1 spray/nostril bid when symptoms controlled	
fluticasone (Flonase)	Adults (rhinitis): 2 sprays (50 mcg/spray) per nostril once daily; alternate: 1 spray per nostril bid; may decrease to 1 spray per nostril once daily; maximum: 4 sprays/day Children >4 yr: 1-2 sprays (50 mcg/spray) per nostril daily; start 1 spray/nostril/day; maximum: 4 sprays/day; decrease to 1 spray/nostril/bid once symptoms controlled	
cromolyn	Adults and children >2 yr (allergic rhinitis): 1 spray per nostril tid-qid; maximum: 1 spray per nostril 6 times/day	
codeine	Adults and children >12 yr: 10-20 mg po q4-6h; maximum: 120 mg/day Children 6-12 yr: 5-10 mg po q4-6 h; maximum: 60 mg/day Children 2-5 yr: 2.5-5 mg po q4-6h or 1-1.5 mg/kg/day, codeine divided q4-6 h; maximum: 30 mg/day	
dextromethorphan	Immediate-release (Robitussin CoughGells, others) Suspension, sustained action (Delsym)	Adults and children >12 yr: 10-20 mg po q4h, maximum: 120 mg/day; alternate: 30 mg po q6-8h Children 6-12 yr: 5-10 mg po q4h or 15 mg po q6-8h; maximum: 60 mg/day Children 2-5 yr: 2.5-5 mg po q4h or 7.5 mg po q6-8h; maximum: 30 mg/day Adults and children >12 yr: 60 mg (2 tsp) po q12h; maximum: 120 mg/day (4 tsp) Children 6-12 yr: 30 mg (1 tsp) po q12h; maximum: 60 mg/day (2 tsp) Children 2-5 yr: 15 mg (½ tsp) po q12h; maximum: 30 mg/day (1 tsp)
benzonatate (Tessalon)	Adults and children >10 yr: 100 mg po tid or q4h; maximum: 600 mg/day	
guaifenesin	Immediate-release (Robitussin, generic) Sustained-release (Humibid, Mucinex)	Adults and children >12 yr: 200-400 mg po q4h; maximum: 2400 mg/day Children 6-11 yr: 100-200 mg po q4h; maximum: 1200 mg/day Children 2-5 yr: 50-100 mg po q4h; maximum: 600 mg/day Children <2 yr: 12 mg/kg/day po in 6 divided doses Adults and children >12 yr: 600-1200 mg po q12h; maximum: 2400 mg/day Children 6-11 yr: 600 mg po q12h; maximum: 1200 mg/day

ANTIHISTAMINES

diphenhydramine hydrochloride (Benadryl)

CONTRAINDICATIONS. Newborn or premature infants, nursing mothers, and patients who have exhibited hypersensitivity to antihistamines

WARNINGS

- The FDA warns that oral diphenhydramine should *not* be used concomitantly with any other preparations that contain the drug, including those used topically.
- Use with caution in patients with a history of lower respiratory disease, including asthma, because the anticholinergic (drying) effects may thicken secretions and impair expectoration.
- Avoid sedating antihistamines in patients who have a history of sleep apnea.
- Use with caution in patients with increased intraocular pressure, hyperthyroidism, cardiovascular disease, and hypertension.

PRECAUTIONS

- Use with caution in patients with narrow-angle glaucoma, stenosing peptic ulcer, pyloroduodenal obstruction, symptomatic prostatic hyperplasia, or bladder neck obstruction.

- Commercially available formulations of diphenhydramine may contain sodium bisulfite, which may cause allergic-type reactions, including anaphylaxis and life-threatening or less severe asthmatic episodes, in susceptible individuals.
- Diphenhydramine should be used with caution in infants and young children and should not be used in premature or full-term neonates.

PHARMACOKINETICS
- Diphenhydramine undergoes first-pass metabolism in the liver, and only about 40% to 60% of an oral dose reaches the systemic circulation unchanged.
- See Table 13-5.

ADVERSE EFFECTS
- Diphenhydramine toxicity (e.g., dilated pupils, flushed face, hallucinations, ataxic gait, urinary retention) has been reported in pediatric patients following topical application of diphenhydramine to large areas of the body (often areas with broken skin) or following concomitant use of topical and oral preparations that contain the drug.
- See Table 13-3.

DRUG INTERACTIONS. Additive effects with alcohol and other CNS depressants and sedatives

OVERDOSAGE
- CNS depression to stimulation; stimulation is more common in children, whereas in adults, CNS depression, ranging from drowsiness to coma, is more common
- Coma, cardiovascular collapse, and death may occur.
- Deaths have been reported, particularly in infants and children.

DOSAGE AND ADMINISTRATION. See Table 13-4.

OTHER DRUGS IN CLASS

Other drugs in this class are similar to the key drug, except follows.

clemastine fumarate (Tavist)
WARNINGS
- Safety and efficacy have not been established in children younger than 12 years or in pregnancy.
- Has an additive effect with alcohol and other CNS depressants and is likely to cause dizziness, sedation, and hypotension in the elderly
- Distributed in breast milk

chlorpheniramine maleate (Chlor-Trimeton)
CONTRAINDICATIONS
- Narrow-angle glaucoma, prostatic hyperplasia, stenosing peptic ulcer, pyloroduodenal obstruction, bladder neck obstruction
- MAOIs
- Newborn or premature infants

WARNINGS
- May impair mental alertness; use with caution when performing potentially hazardous tasks or activities

- Safety and efficacy of chlorpheniramine maleate extended-release core tablets in children younger than 12 years of age have not been established.
- Distribution into breast milk is unknown. Decision to discontinue nursing or medication should be made because potential adverse reactions may occur in the nursing infant.
- Do not crush or chew extended-release formulations.
- OTC combination preparations may contain artificial sweeteners that metabolize to phenylalanine.

ADVERSE EFFECTS
- Slight to moderate drowsiness is the most common side effect.
- Other possible side effects are similar to those of diphenhydramine; see Table 13-3.

DRUG INTERACTIONS. Similar to other antihistamines—MAOIs, alcohol, CNS depressants

cetirizine hydrochloride (Zyrtec, Zyrtec syrup)
CONTRAINDICATIONS. Hypersensitivity to hydroxyzine

PRECAUTIONS
- May produce somnolence in some patients and is considered a low-sedating antihistamine
- Caution should be exercised when driving or operating dangerous machinery.
- Use caution with concurrent use with alcohol or other CNS depressants.
- Use caution if impaired liver or kidney function is present.

ADVERSE EFFECTS. Most adverse effects reported with use of cetirizine were mild or moderate.

DRUG INTERACTIONS
- A small decrease in the clearance of cetirizine was caused by a 400-mg dose of theophylline. Larger doses of theophylline could have a greater effect. No significant interactions were noted with low doses of theophylline, azithromycin, pseudoephedrine, ketoconazole, or erythromycin.
- MAOIs

DOSAGE AND ADMINISTRATION
- Renal dosing: Adjust dose amount according to creatinine clearance: for less than 30, give 5 mg po.
- Hepatic dosing: 5 mg po daily
- See Table 13-4.

fexofenadine hydrochloride (Allegra)
- Fexofenadine has a similar clinical profile to other nonsedating antihistamines.
- No significant drug interactions are noted, and serious hypersensitivity reactions are rare.
- Renal dosing should be adjusted frequently.
- Absorption and plasma concentrations are decreased by concomitant administration of antacids that contain aluminum and magnesium hydroxides.
- Extended-release combination tablets with pseudoephedrine should be taken on an empty stomach. Do not break, crush, or chew tablets.

TABLE 13-5   Pharmacokinetics of Prescribed Antihistamines

Drug	Absorptions	Onset of Action	Time to Peak Concentration	Half-life	Duration of Action	Protein Bound	Metabolism	Excretion
cetirizine (Zyrtec)	GI	20 min-1 hr	1 hr	8.3 hr	24 hr	93%	Liver, partially	Urine, 70%; feces, 10%
fexofenadine HCl (Allegra)	GI tract	1-3 hr	2.6 hr	14.4 hr	12 hr	60%-70%	Liver CYP450 3A4 (minor); biliary; renal	Urine, 11%; feces, 80%
desloratadine (Clarinex)	NI; unaffected by food	<1 hr	3 hr	27 hr	24 hr	82%-87%	Liver	Urine and feces
azelastine (Astelin)	40% systemic absorption	3 hr	2-3 hr	22 hr	12 hr	88%	Liver CYP450	Feces, 75%

Miscellaneous Antihistamines

loratadine (Claritin)

- Loratadine is a long-acting tricyclic antihistamine with selective peripheral histamine H_1-receptor antagonistic activity.
- Compatible with breastfeeding according to the American Academy of Pediatrics

CONTRAINDICATIONS. Hypersensitivity to this medication or any of its ingredients

PRECAUTIONS

- Patients with liver disease should receive a lower dose (10 mg every other day) because of reduced clearance of loratadine.
- Impaired renal function
- Safety and effectiveness of use in children younger than 6 years of age have not been established.

DOSAGE AND ADMINISTRATION

- Renal dosing: Adjust dose frequently. See package insert for dosage adjustment recommendations.
- Hepatic dosing: Adjust dose frequently. See package insert for dosage adjustment recommendations.
- See Table 13-4.

desloratadine (Clarinex)

- See Tables 13-4 and 13-5 for specific information regarding dosage and administration recommendations and pharmacokinetics.
- Formulated as tablets, oral solution, and orally disintegrating tablets
- Conventional tablets and oral solution are bioequivalent.
- Oral disintegrating tablets contain aspartame, which metabolizes to phenylalanine.

Intranasal Antihistamines

azelastine (Astelin)

- In comparative studies, intranasal azelastine was more effective than placebo and at least as effective as oral antihistamines or intranasal corticosteroids in relieving allergic rhinitis.

- May be used safely in patients with concurrent asthma and seasonal allergic rhinitis

CONTRAINDICATIONS. Known hypersensitivity

PRECAUTIONS. Use cautiously if lactating.

DOSAGE AND ADMINISTRATION. Available in 137 mcg/spray; see Table 13-4

PATIENT EDUCATION

- Patients should be instructed to prime the delivery system before initial use and after storage for 3 days or longer.
- Patients also should be instructed to store the bottle upright at room temperature with the pump tightly closed and out of the reach of children.
- Use instructions with package.

INTRANASAL STEROIDS

triamcinolone acetonide (Nasacort AQ)

See Chapter 15 for additional details.

CONTRAINDICATIONS

- Untreated localized infection
- Hypersensitivity to the drug or a product component
- Ocular herpes simplex virus (HSV) infection

PRECAUTIONS

- Use cautiously in patients with tuberculosis, systemic infection, nasal septal ulcers, or nasal trauma or surgery.
- Localized infection with *Candida albicans* may develop. Treat infection with appropriate antiinfective therapy.

DOSAGE AND ADMINISTRATION

- Triamcinolone acetonide is supplied as a non-aqueous suspension, aerosol nasal inhalation (Nasacort), and aqueous nasal suspension/solution spray (Nasacort AQ)—see Table 13-4 for dosages.
- If the spray pump that contains the aqueous suspension or solution is not used for longer than 2 weeks, it may have to be partially primed (one actuation for the suspension and three actuations or until a fine mist is observed for the solution).

- The nasal aqueous solution spray pump requires priming—See package insert for instructions.
- Discontinue after 3 weeks if no improvement is noted.
- Monitor height in children/adolescents if treatment lasts longer than 2 months.

OTHER DRUGS IN CLASS

- Beclomethasone dipropionate (Beconase AQ, Vancenase) is similar to triamcinolone acetonide, except as follows:
  - Has a significant systemic effect, especially on growth in children, as a result of the pharmacokinetics of this older agent
  - Undergoes a low degree of first-pass inactivation (40% to 50%), resulting in greater posthepatic bioavailability
- Fluticasone propionate (Flonase) is similar to triamcinolone acetonide, except as follows:
  - Fluticasone is a very potent nasal corticosteroid. Some studies have compared various intranasal corticosteroids, and results suggest that fluticasone has the potential for a greater number of dosage-related systemic effects than do other intranasal corticosteroids. It has been shown to suppress systemic markers such as serum and urinary cortisol and serum osteocalcin in adults. Fluticasone suppresses urinary cortisol in children. Compared with triamcinolone, budesonide, and mometasone, fluticasone shows significant adrenal suppression
  - Used successfully as prophylaxis treatment for seasonal allergic rhinitis when initiated at least 1 week prior to the anticipated start of the grass pollen season

INTRANASAL MAST CELL STABILIZERS

cromolyn sodium (Nasalcrom)

- To prevent nasal allergy symptoms, starting up to 1 week before contact with cause of allergy
- See Chapter 15 for additional information.

CONTRAINDICATIONS. Hypersensitivity to drug or product components

WARNINGS/PRECAUTIONS. Intranasal cromolyn is not to be used for the treatment of acute symptoms.

ADVERSE EFFECTS

- Nasal stinging or sneezing may be experienced. This is rarely a significant problem.
- See Table 13-3.

LEUKOTRIENE RECEPTOR ANTAGONISTS

montelukast sodium (Singulair)

- Montelukast sodium is a prescription medication that has been approved to control the symptoms of seasonal allergic rhinitis in adults and pediatric patients 2 years and older, and perennial allergic rhinitis in adults and children 6 months of age and older.

CONTRAINDICATIONS. Hypersensitivity to any component of the product

PRECAUTIONS

- Phenylalanine is contained in the 4- and 5-mg chewable tablets.
- Use cautiously in nursing mothers because it is not known whether montelukast is excreted in human milk.

ADVERSE EFFECTS

- Adults 15 years and older: headache, influenza, abdominal pain, cough, increased serum alanine aminotransferase (ALT) and aspartate aminotransferase (AST) concentrations, dyspepsia, dizziness, asthenia/fatigue, dental pain, nasal congestion, rash, fever, infectious gastroenteritis, trauma, and pyuria
- Children 6 to 14 years: diarrhea, laryngitis, pharyngitis, nausea, otitis, sinusitis, and viral infection
- Children 2 to 5 years: fever, cough, abdominal pain, diarrhea, headache, rhinorrhea, sinusitis, otitis, otic pain, influenza, rash, dermatitis, urticaria, eczema, gastroenteritis, varicella, pneumonia, and conjunctivitis
- Children 12 to 23 months of age: upper respiratory tract infection, wheezing, otitis media, pharyngitis, tonsillitis, cough, and rhinitis

ANTITUSSIVES

Narcotic Antitussives

codeine phosphate or codeine sulfate

- Codeine is a narcotic that is used for suppression of cough caused by chemical or respiratory tract irritation. Codeine acts on the cough center in the medulla to elevate the threshold for cough, and codeine often is combined with other medications (e.g., guaifenesin) in a syrup or elixir.
- See Chapter 43 for details.

CONTRAINDICATIONS

- Hypersensitivity
- Use in children younger than age 2
- Respiratory depression
- Coma

WARNINGS

- Codeine may be habit forming; psychological and physical dependence and tolerance may occur.
- Codeine may impair the individual's mental and/or physical ability to perform potentially hazardous tasks. Use caution when driving or performing tasks requiring alertness, coordination, or physical dexterity.
- In some ambulatory patients, codeine may produce orthostatic hypotension, dry mouth, and constipation and may cause stomach upset. Take with food or milk.

PRECAUTIONS

- Use with caution in patients with the following:
  - Head trauma and increased intracranial pressure—The respiratory depressant effects of narcotics and their capacity to elevate CSF pressure may be exaggerated in these conditions.
  - Seizure disorders
  - Asthma or pulmonary emphysema
  - Acute abdominal pain

- Use with caution in elderly and debilitated patients and those with severe liver or kidney impairment, hypothyroidism, Addison's disease, and prostatic hyperplasia or urethral stricture.
- Codeine may have a prolonged cumulative effect in patients with liver or kidney dysfunction.

DRUG INTERACTIONS

- Additive depressant effects occur when used in combination with other narcotic analgesics, phenothiazines, tranquilizers, sedative-hypnotics, antidepressants, alcohol, or other CNS depressants. When used in combination, the dosage of one or both agents should be reduced.
- Caution is advised in using with sedating antihistamines because these may increase the risk of CNS depression and may potentiate opiate analgesic efficacy.

OVERDOSAGE. Serious overdose with codeine is characterized by respiratory depression, extreme somnolence progressing to stupor or coma, skeletal muscle flaccidity, bradycardia, hypotension, and cool, clammy skin. In cases of severe overdose, apnea, circulatory collapse, cardiac arrest, and death may occur.

HOW TO MONITOR. Monitor for effectiveness and excessive side effects, especially constipation in the elderly.

PATIENT EDUCATION

- Narcotic antitussives such as codeine may impair mental and physical abilities.
- Patients should be cautioned to avoid performing potentially hazardous tasks, such as driving or operating heavy machinery.

DOSAGE AND ADMINISTRATION

- Codeine is combined with guaifenesin as antitussive syrup, with 10 mg codeine/100 mg guaifenesin/5 ml.
- See Table 13-4.

Nonnarcotic Antitussives

dextromethorphan hydrobromide (Benylin, Delsym, Robitussin maximum strength)

CONTRAINDICATIONS

- Hypersensitivity to any component
- MAOI or MAOI use within 14 days

MISUSE AND ABUSE. In 2005, the FDA issued a talk paper to warn of the abuse of dextromethorphan (DXM), following the deaths of five teenagers who had consumed a powdered encapsulated form. DXM is generally a safe and effective cough suppressant when taken at recommended doses. When taken in very large doses in caplet or liquid form to achieve euphoria, DXM can cause loss of coordination, impaired mental functioning, dizziness, nausea, hot flashes, hallucinations, brain damage, seizures, and death.

WARNINGS

- Administration of dextromethorphan may be accompanied by histamine release, and the drug should be used cautiously in atopic children.
- According to the World Health Organization (WHO) Expert Committee on Drug Dependence, dextromethorphan

can produce very slight psychological dependence but no physical dependence.
- Do not use for persistent or chronic cough, or in cases in which excessive secretions accompany cough. Persons with a high fever, rash, persistent headache, nausea, or vomiting should use the drug only under medical supervision.

PRECAUTIONS

- Use with caution in sedated or debilitated patients and in those confined to the supine position.
- Lozenges containing dextromethorphan hydrobromide should not be used in children younger than 6 years of age.

DRUG INTERACTIONS

- The drug may interact with serotonergic antidepressants—combination may increase risk of serotonin syndrome.
- Avoid use with furazolidone, meperidine, and sibutramine.
- MAOI use within 14 days

OVERDOSAGE

- Acute overdosage: dizziness, drowsiness, blurred vision, nystagmus, shallow respiration, urinary retention, stupor, toxic psychosis, seizures, and coma
- Presentation of intoxication is dose dependent.

DOSAGE AND ADMINISTRATION. Dextromethorphan 15 to 30 mg is equal to 8 to 15 mg of codeine as an antitussive.

benzonatate (Tessalon Perles)

CONTRAINDICATIONS. Hypersensitivity to benzonatate or related compounds (e.g., tetracaine, procaine)

WARNINGS

- Do not chew or break capsules; swallow whole.
- Severe hypersensitivity reactions (including bronchospasm, laryngospasm, and cardiovascular collapse) have been reported that are possibly related to local anesthesia effects caused by chewing or sucking the perle.
- Severe reactions have required intervention with vasopressor agents and supportive measures.

PRECAUTIONS. Release of benzonatate in the mouth can produce temporary local anesthesia of the oral mucosa that could cause choking.

OVERDOSAGE. CNS stimulation may cause restlessness and tremors that may proceed to clonic convulsions, followed by profound CNS depression. Overdose may result in death.

PATIENT EDUCATION. Do not chew or break capsules; swallow whole.

EXPECTORANTS

guaifenesin (Robitussin, Humibid Pediatric, Mucinex)

CONTRAINDICATIONS. Hypersensitivity

WARNINGS. Not for use with persistent cough that occurs with smoking, asthma, or emphysema, or with cough with excessive secretions, unless directed by provider

DRUG INTERACTIONS
- Guaifenesin may affect laboratory results in the following ways:
  - May increase renal clearance of urate, thereby lowering serum uric acid levels
  - May produce an increase in urinary 5-hydroxyindoleacetic acid and therefore may interfere with the interpretation of this test for the diagnosis of carcinoid syndrome
  - May falsely elevate the vanillylmandelic acid (VMA) test for catechols
- Administration of these products should be discontinued 48 hours before urine specimens are collected for such tests.

evolve A continually updated list of useful WebLinks may be found in the Evolve Resources at http://evolve.elsevier.com/Edmunds/NP/

14 Asthma and COPD Medications

SANDRA M. NETTINA

DRUG OVERVIEW

Class	Subclass	Generic Name	Trade Name
Short-acting relatively selective β_2-adrenergic agonist bronchodilators	Aerosol	albuterol 🔑 ✳	Proventil, Ventolin
		levalbuterol	Xopenex ✳
	Oral	pirbuterol	Maxair
		albuterol ✳	Proventil Repetabs, Volmax
Long-acting relatively selective β_2-adrenergic agonist bronchodilators		salmeterol xinafoate 🔑	Serevent Diskus
		formoterol fumarate arformoterol	Foradil Brovana
Methylxanthines		theophylline 🔑	Theo-Dur, Theolair, Slo-bid, Slo-Phyllin, Quibron, Uniphyl
Anticholinergics		ipratropium bromide 🔑 tiotropium bromide	Atrovent Spiriva ✳
Mast cell stabilizers		cromolyn sodium 🔑	Intal
		nedocromil sodium	Tilade
Corticosteroids	Aerosols	beclomethasone dipropionate 🔑	Beclovent, Vanceril, Qvar
		flunisolide	AeroBid
		fluticasone	Flovent ✳
		budesonide	Pulmicort ✳
		triamcinolone acetate mometasone furoate	Azmacort Asmanex
	Oral solutions/tablets (see Chapter 51 for details)	prednisone 🔑	Liquid Pred, Deltasone
		prednisolone ✳	Delta-Cortef, Prelone
		methylprednisolone ✳	Medrol
Leukotriene modifiers	Leukotriene receptor antagonists	montelukast 🔑	Singulair ✳
		zafirlukast	Accolate
	5-lipoxygenase inhibitor	zileuton	Zyflo
Combination products		albuterol/ipratropium	Combivent ✳
		fluticasone/salmeterol budesonide/formoterol	Advair Diskus ✳ Symbicort

✳ Top 200 drug; 🔑 key drug.

INDICATIONS

See Table 14-1.
- Asthma
- COPD
- Other episodes of acute bronchospasm

Six classes of medications that work via different mechanisms of action are used in the treatment of patients with asthma and COPD. Each of these six groups is discussed in detail as part of the treatment of asthma or COPD. These drugs are also used in the treatment of other respiratory disorders that cause inflammation and bronchospasm. These drugs are largely delivered via inhalation and are designated as long-term controller medications (inhaled corticosteroids, long-acting inhaled β_2-agonists, leukotriene modifiers, theophylline, mast cell stabilizers) and quick relief and other medications (rapid-acting inhaled β_2-agonists, oral corticosteroids, anticholinergics). The nurse practitioner should help design a treatment plan for the patient that includes the components of therapy and provides direction for the treatment of symptom exacerbations. Detailed and ongoing patient education is required for adequate management of these diseases.

The standards of care for patients with asthma were developed by the National Asthma Education and Prevention Program (NAEPP) and were most recently updated in the Expert Panel Report 3 (EPR3). Additional guidelines have been put forth by the Global Initiative for Asthma, Global Strategy for Asthma Management and Prevention, revised in 2006. Both sets of recommendations are based on a step approach that is bidirectional. Guidelines for standard of care management of COPD can be found in the National Heart, Lung, and Blood Institute (NHLBI)–World Health Organization (WHO) GOLD, Global Strategies for the Diagnosis, Management, and Prevention of Chronic Obstructive Pulmonary Disease (2006).

Asthma and COPD are similar in their chronicity and in terms of their obstructive component. However, asthma differs from COPD in that asthma is largely an inflammatory condition, and it has a greater degree of reversibility than COPD. Drug therapy has not been shown to alter the long-term decline in lung function that occurs in COPD but should be used to control symptoms. Therapy in COPD is also based on a step approach but is unidirectional and cumulative. Although the same drugs are used in treatment for these disorders, asthma and COPD are discussed separately because responses to pharmacotherapy differ.

THERAPEUTIC OVERVIEW OF ASTHMA
Anatomy and Physiology

The respiratory bronchiole is surrounded by smooth muscle and is lined by pseudostratified columnar epithelium containing mucus-secreting goblet cells and cilia. The smooth muscle is innervated by the autonomic nervous system. Parasympathetic stimulation through the vagus nerve and cholinergic receptors in smooth muscle promotes bronchial constriction. Sympathetic stimulation through the action of catecholamines such as epinephrine on β_2-adrenergic receptors causes bronchodilation. When the need for airflow is increased, such as with exercise, sympathetic stimulation causes bronchodilation, and opposing parasympathetic bronchoconstrictor tone is inhibited.

The lungs also contain α-adrenergic receptors, and their stimulation results in mild bronchoconstriction. No β_1-adrenergic receptors are present in the lungs. β_1-Adrenergic receptors are the predominant adrenergic receptors of the heart, and their stimulation promotes myocardial contractility and conduction, resulting in an increased heart rate (Table 14-2).

Pathophysiology

The key pathophysiologic features of asthma include (1) airway hyperresponsiveness, (2) airway inflammation, and (3) airway obstruction that is largely but not always completely reversible.

TABLE 14-1 Indications for Asthma and COPD Medications

Drug	Indication
β-AGONISTS	
	Relief and prevention of bronchospasm in patients with reversible obstructive airway disease in both asthma and COPD
Short-acting: albuterol, levalbuterol	Acute bronchospasm; prevention of exercise-induced bronchospasm
Long-acting: salmeterol, formoterol	Maintenance treatment of asthma- and COPD-associated bronchospasm; prevention of bronchospasm in nocturnal asthma and exercise-induced bronchospasm
Methylxanthines	Symptomatic relief or prevention of asthma, especially nocturnal symptoms, and reversible bronchospasm associated with COPD. Not a first-line treatment.
Anticholinergics: ipratropium, tiotropium	Maintenance treatment of bronchospasm associated with COPD
Mast cell stabilizers: cromolyn sodium, nedocromil	Prophylaxis of asthma, prevention of exercise-induced bronchospasm Maintenance therapy in mild to moderate asthma
Inhaled corticosteroids	Maintenance therapy for the prophylaxis of asthma
Oral corticosteroids	Short-term management of various inflammatory and allergic disorders such as asthma
Leukotriene modifiers	Prophylaxis and long-term treatment of asthma

TABLE 14-2   Location and Response of Adrenoreceptors

Location	Type	Example of Stimulus Response
Lung (smooth muscle)	α	Mild bronchoconstriction
	β₂	Bronchodilation; dilates arteries; relaxes alveolar walls
Mast cells	α	Augments release of histamine and other inflammatory mediators
	β₂	Inhibits release of inflammatory mediators
Heart	β₁	Increases myocardial contraction, force, and velocity; stimulates glycogenolysis
Blood vessels	α	Vasoconstriction
	β₂	Vasodilation
Skeletal muscle	β₂	Tremor; stimulates glycogenolysis
Multiple	α	Stimulates glycogenolysis; inhibits norepinephrine and acetylcholine release
	β₁	Stimulates lipolysis
	β₂	Stimulates norepinephrine release; inhibits acetylcholine release; moves potassium into cells; stimulates insulin release
Eyes (smooth muscle)	α	Mydriasis

Modified from Lees GM: A hitchhiker's guide to the galaxy of adrenoreceptors, *BMJ* 283:173-178, 1981.

- *Airway hyperresponsiveness:* The airways react abnormally to some triggers such as inhaled allergens, food or recreational drugs, aspirin and related NSAIDs, cold air, exercise, airway irritants (e.g., cigarette smoke, air pollution), respiratory infection, and emotional stress. Conditions such as GERD, chronic sinusitis, and rhinitis also can exacerbate asthma.
- *Airway inflammation:* On exposure to an inhaled antigen, mast cells, eosinophils, epithelial cells, macrophages, and activated T-cells are released. The chemical mediators that they release consist of cytokines, chemokines, histamine, prostaglandins, and leukotrienes (LTs). Their

response in the airways occurs as bronchospasm and inflammation (Figure 14-1); see Chapter 69 on the immune system for additional details.
- *Airway obstruction:* Bronchoconstriction results in a decline in the forced expiratory volume in 1 second (FEV₁). Inflammatory processes occur within the bronchiole, causing epithelial injury. Chronic inflammation can lead to airway remodeling, thickening of goblet cells, mucous hypersecretion, thickening of the basement membrane by collagen deposition, and hypertrophy of smooth muscle, all of which contribute to airway obstruction. In the case of longstanding asthma, symptoms may not be reversible.

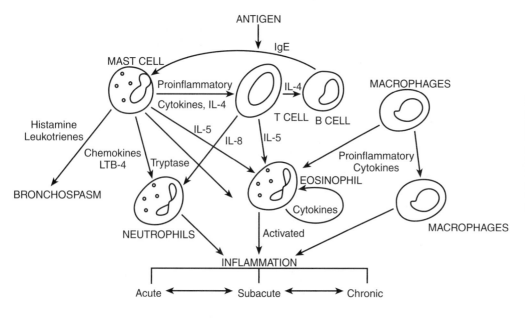

FIGURE 14-1 Cellular mechanisms involved in airway inflammation. (From National Asthma Education and Prevention Program Expert Panel Report 2: *Guidelines for the diagnosis and management of asthma,* Washington, DC, 1997, U.S. Government Printing Office.)

Disease Process

Asthma is the result of complex interactions among inflammatory cells, chemical mediators, and associated changes in the airways. Asthma is classified based on symptomatology, function, risk for exacerbation, and pulmonary function; this classification forms a basis for step therapy. Pulmonary function is determined by comparison of the patient's FEV_1 and forced vital capacity (FVC) vs. predicted averages for the patient's age, height, and gender. Airflow during exhalation is decreased when the airways are narrowed or blocked. Peak expiratory flow (PEF) monitoring can be used by many patients to monitor their lung function at home. This allows them to anticipate when their breathing will become worse and to take appropriate medications or call their health care provider before symptoms become too severe. (*Note: Slight variations in the following classification criteria have been defined for children younger than 12; see website for additional information.*)

1. *Intermittent:* Symptoms ≤2 days per week, symptoms that cause nighttime awakenings ≤2 nights per month, no interference with normal activity, FEV_1 >80% of predicted, and FEV_1/FVC normal.
2. *Mild persistent:* Symptoms >2 days per week but not daily, symptoms that cause nighttime awakenings 3 to 4 times a month, minor limitation of function, FEV_1 >80% of predicted, and FEV_1/FVC normal.
3. *Moderate persistent:* Daily daytime symptoms, symptoms that cause nighttime awakenings >1 time per week but not nightly, some limitation in function, FEV_1 >60% but <80% of predicted, and FEV_1/FVC reduced by 5%.
4. *Severe persistent:* Continuous daytime symptoms, symptoms that occur nightly, extremely limited activity, FEV_1 <60% of predicted, and FEV_1/FVC reduced by >5%.

A patient need only meet one criterion to move into a new severity rating; thus, patients should be reevaluated frequently to determine whether the severity has increased or decreased. Signs of worsening asthma may include increased cough, a greater degree of breathlessness, the occurrence of wheezing, particularly at night, and increased chest tightness. Use of accessory muscles of respiration and suprasternal retractions indicate severe exacerbation. Patients may also complain of chest tightness and productive or nonproductive cough. The chest should be assessed for use of accessory muscles, wheezing, and prolonged forced expiration. Wheezing may be absent between episodes of asthma, as well as during severe airflow limitation.

Asthma is difficult to diagnose in infants and children younger than 5. Viral respiratory infection is the most common cause of asthma symptoms in this age group.

THERAPEUTIC OVERVIEW OF CHRONIC OBSTRUCTIVE PULMONARY DISEASE

Anatomy and Physiology

Inspired air moves through conducting airways as it moves from the environment to the lungs for gas exchange. Conducting airways warm and humidify air and remove foreign material through mucus-secreting goblet cells and ciliary projections in the columnar epithelium. Mucociliary clearance is enhanced by optimal oxygenation, humidification, and coughing. Airway clearance is impaired by low or high oxygen levels, dryness, and cigarette smoking. Alveoli are thin-walled sacs separated by septa and surrounded by a network of capillaries to facilitate gas exchange. Diffusion of gases across the alveolar capillary membrane can be affected by concentration of inspired oxygen; condition of the lung tissue, which affects the surface area available for diffusion; and thickness of the alveolar capillary membrane.

Pathophysiology

Several mechanisms are involved in the pathogenesis of COPD, including airway inflammation, edema, fibrosis of the bronchial wall, hypertrophy of the submucosal glands, hypersecretion of mucus, loss of elastic lung recoil, and destruction of alveolar tissue. Tobacco smoking and other noxious stimuli produce an inflammatory response throughout the lungs, including the parenchyma and vasculature. Inflammatory cells invade the damaged lung tissue and secrete numerous mediators, including tumor necrosis factor (TNF), interleukin-8, and leukotriene B_4 (LTB_4). The larger airways (trachea, bronchi, and bronchioles >2 mm) respond by increasing the number of mucus-secreting glands and reducing mucociliary function. The smaller airways (bronchioles <2 mm) go through repeated cycles of injury and repair, resulting in remodeling, scarring, thickening, and consolidation. This results in increased airflow resistance, as evidenced by decreased FEV_1 and FEV_1/FVC measurements.

As lung parenchyma is destroyed, elastic recoil is lost, thus reducing the force of expiratory airflow and resulting in hyperinflation. Hyperinflation leads to flattening of the diaphragm, an increase in the anteroposterior diameter of the chest ("barrel chest"), and reduced respiratory muscle strength. The loss of alveoli decreases the surface area available for gas exchange. Changes in the vasculature of the lungs caused by the remodeling process can eventually lead to pulmonary hypertension, cor pulmonale, and severe hypoxia and hypercapnia.

Disease Process

COPD is a disease state characterized by airflow limitation that is not fully reversible. Airflow limitation usually is progressive and is associated with an abnormal inflammatory response of the lungs to noxious particles or gases. Although symptoms of COPD vary throughout the illness, they are not a good predictor of degree of airflow limitation. Therefore, COPD has been reclassified by some authors according to spirometry. Predicted values are calculated for each individual patient. The four stages of severity of COPD are as follows:

- Stage I (mild COPD): FEV_1/FVC <0.70, FEV_1 ≥80% of predicted
- Stage II (moderate COPD): FEV_1/FVC < 0.70, FEV_1 50% to 79% of predicted
- Stage III (severe COPD): FEV_1/FVC <0.70, FEV_1 30% to 49% of predicted
- Stage IV (very severe COPD): FEV_1/FVC <0.70, FEV_1 ≤30% of predicted or <50% of predicted plus chronic respiratory failure

Any stage of COPD may be marked by exacerbation of varying severity, but exacerbation is more common in those patients with FEV_1 <50% of predicted value. Many exacerbations are due to respiratory infection or exposure to air pollution, but in about one half of cases, the cause of exacerbation cannot be identified.

The earliest symptom of COPD is often morning cough with sputum that is clear to yellow. Frequent respiratory infections increase cough, often turn the sputum yellow or green, and result in periods of wheezing. Later, shortness of breath develops with exertion and becomes progressively more severe. On auscultation, expiration may be prolonged, expiratory wheezing is often present, and crackles may be audible.

Spirometry is the gold standard by which the diagnosis of COPD should be established and disease severity determined. FEV_1 and FEV_1/FVC are determined before and after bronchodilator therapy to make the diagnosis and determine severity. COPD causes a progressive decline in FEV_1, FVC, and FEV_1/FVC measurements that is greater than would be expected with an age-related decline in lung function.

An arterial blood gas measurement is recommended if FEV_1 is <50% of predicted value. Pulse oximetry is more easily carried out to measure oxygen (O_2) saturation in the blood and can be used for monitoring during rest, activity, and sleep. A chest x-ray film will show hyperinflation of the lungs and flattening of the diaphragm in advanced COPD. These tests are necessary to confirm the correct diagnosis and to rule out other types of respiratory disease.

MECHANISM OF ACTION

β-Adrenergic Agonist Bronchodilators

β-Adrenergic agonists are sympathomimetics. The basic action of β-agonists is to activate the enzyme adenyl cyclase, which increases the production of cyclic adenosine monophosphate (cAMP). Intracellular cAMP inhibits phosphorylation of myosin and lowers intracellular concentrations of calcium. The result is smooth muscle relaxation. Bronchodilation reduces airway resistance as shown by increased FEV_1, mid-expiratory flow rate, and vital capacity. Increased cAMP also inhibits the release of mediators from mast cells in the airways, thereby producing a mild antiinflammatory effect.

Nonselective $β_2$-adrenergic receptor agonists and, to a lesser extent, selective $β_2$-adrenergic agonists cause reflex tachycardia. This produces arterial dilation that results from $β_2$-receptor stimulation of the heart. Albuterol and the other bronchodilators that are relatively $β_2$ selective have their greatest effect on β-adrenergic receptors in the bronchial, uterine, and vascular smooth muscles. Bronchodilators developed to date are only relatively selective in stimulating $β_2$-receptors, and all have varying incidences of cardiac side effects and muscle tremor. At higher doses, the selective drugs may lose their receptor selectivity and cause $β_1$ stimulation.

The role of rapid-acting inhaled $β_2$-agonists (RABAs; also known as short-acting $β_2$-agonists [SABA]) in asthma therapy is to provide relief of bronchospasm during exacerbation or pretreatment before exercise. RABAs and long-acting $β_2$-agonists (LABAs) are considered first-line drugs in the treatment of both asthma and COPD. Increased use of RABAs may signal the need for additional drug therapy. Inability to achieve an adequate response with a $β_2$-agonist during an exacerbation may indicate the need for the addition of a short-term corticosteroid (inhaled or oral).

Methylxanthines

Methylxanthines promote bronchodilation by competitively inhibiting phosphodiesterase, the enzyme that degrades cAMP, which in turn increases intracellular cAMP. (See β-Adrenergic Agonist Bronchodilators [above] for the action of increased cAMP.) Methylxanthines also act as direct central nervous system stimulants that produce vasoconstriction and stimulation of the vagal center, which causes bradycardia.

Methylxanthines in large doses have a positive inotropic effect on the myocardium and a positive chronotropic effect on the sinoatrial node, causing transient increases in heart rate, force of contraction, cardiac output, and myocardial oxygen demand. At high concentrations, vagal stimulation is masked by increased sinus rate and may result in hypotension, extrasystole, and arrhythmia. Additional effects of methylxanthines include diuresis through dilation of renal arterioles, increased cardiac output, and inhibition of reabsorption of sodium and potassium in the proximal renal tubules. The gastrointestinal system is affected by relaxation of smooth muscle, causing reduced lower esophageal sphincter pressure and relaxed biliary contraction, along with stimulation of gastric secretions. The role of theophylline in the control of asthma and COPD is not a primary one because studies have shown that it is not as effective as inhaled LABAs or corticosteroids. It may be beneficial in some cases when given as add-on therapy.

Anticholinergics

Similar to atropine, anticholinergics are nonselective competitive antagonists of muscarinic receptors present in the airways and other organs. The anticholinergic drug blocks acetylcholine-induced stimulation of cyclic guanyl cyclase, thereby reducing production of cyclic guanosine monophosphate (cGMP), a mediator of bronchoconstriction. Airway secretions are reduced by these drugs. Airway resistance also is reduced, as measured by increases in FEV_1 and the middle portion of forced expiratory flow (FEF_{25-75}). Ipratropium and tiotropium when inhaled may be more effective in COPD than in asthma because it is believed that cholinergic tone of the airways is increased in COPD.

Ipratropium exhibits greater antimuscarinic effect on bronchial smooth muscle than on secretory glands, especially with oral inhalation of the drug. Additional antimuscarinic effects may include mydriasis, inhibition of salivary and gastric secretions, tachycardia, and spasmolysis; however, clinical trials have shown these effects to be insignificant in healthy individuals and in those with COPD. Anticholinergics often are used first line as an adjunct or alternative to $β_2$-agonist therapy to avoid $β_2$ side effects, and because they have a longer duration of effect.

Mast Cell Stabilizers

Mast cell stabilizers prevent and reduce the inflammatory response in bronchial walls by inhibiting the secretion of mediators from mast cells.

The exact mechanism of action of these drugs on mast cells remains to be established. Medications in this class act locally to inhibit the release of mediators of type 1 allergic reactions, including histamine and leukotrienes, from sensitized mast cells following exposure to an antigen. They inhibit type III (late) inflammatory reactions to a lesser extent. These drugs are antiasthmatic and antiallergic, and they also may act as bronchodilators.

Corticosteroids

Corticosteroids are hormonal agents that have a profound antiinflammatory effect. Corticosteroids reduce airflow obstruction by reducing airway inflammation in the bronchioles.

Corticosteroids modify the body's immune responses to various stimuli. They suppress cytokine production, airway eosinophil recruitment, and the release of inflammatory mediators. Inhaled corticosteroids (ICSs) provide local therapeutic action with minimal systemic effects. (See Chapter 51 for a detailed discussion of mechanism of action.) ICSs have been shown to reduce asthma symptoms, improve quality of life, improve lung function, decrease airway hyperresponsiveness, control airway inflammation, reduce frequency and severity of exacerbations, and reduce asthma mortality. Oral corticosteroid treatment often is indicated for exacerbation of asthma and some cases of COPD. ICS therapy in COPD does not alter the course of the disease but does control symptoms and has been shown to reduce the frequency of exacerbations.

Leukotriene Modifiers

Leukotriene modifiers act on inflammatory mediators of asthma, the LTs (also known as slow-reacting substance of anaphylaxis [SRS-A]), which contributes to airway obstruction.

Cysteinyl LTs (cysLTs) are more potent and longer-acting bronchoconstrictors than histamine. They are produced in a variety of cells (eosinophils, mast cells, basophils, macrophages, and monocytes) from arachidonic acid through several enzyme pathways (Figure 14-2). Arachidonic acid is released from cell membranes in response to antigen–antibody reactions, immunoglobulin (Ig)E receptor activation, microorganisms, and physical stimuli. LTs enhance responsiveness of the airways to a variety of stimuli and stimulate secretion of mucus in the airways. Zafirlukast and montelukast are potent competitive leukotriene receptor antagonists (LTRAs). They block the action of cysLTs at receptor sites on smooth muscle cells throughout the bronchioles. A single type of receptor is able to mediate profound contractions brought about by the cysLTs. LTRAs prevent the binding of LTs to their receptors in the airways, thereby blocking bronchospasm. Zileuton is a 5-lipoxygenase (5-LO) pathway inhibitor. 5-LO is one of the pathways through which arachidonic acid can be metabolized to form LTs. The effect of both types of drugs is inhibition of the acute bronchoconstriction phase and inhibition of the delayed inflammatory phase of asthma. Bronchodilation with improved FEV_1 and reduced markers of airway inflammation (particularly eosinophils) is the result. Leukotriene modifiers (LMs) may be used as an alternative to ICSs in patients with mild persistent or aspirin-sensitive asthma, but their effect is weaker than that of low-dose ICSs; therefore, they usually are used as add-on therapy in asthma.

TREATMENT PRINCIPLES OF ASTHMA

Standardized Guidelines

Several current guidelines have been recommended for asthma management. The first came from the NAEPP out of the NHLBI in 1991. These guidelines were updated in 1997, 2002, and, most recently, in 2007, in the NAEPP EPR3. The NAEPP guidelines present a step therapy approach to asthma management. An additional guideline came from the Global Initiative for Asthma (GINA), revised in 2006. GINA is a result of collaboration of NHLBI and WHO for the purpose of setting up a network to disseminate information on asthma management around the

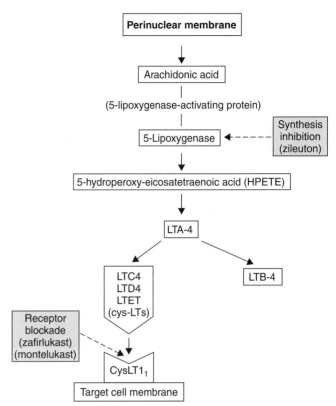

FIGURE 14-2   **The action of 5-lipoxygense (5-LO) inhibitors and leukotriene receptor antagonists on the production of leukotrienes through the 5-LO pathway.** (From Altinger JA: Leukotriene receptor antagonists, *Lippincott's Primary Care Practice* 2:634-642, 1998.)

world and incorporating results of scientific trials pertaining to asthma management. Both guidelines contain detailed information on diagnosis, assessment, pharmacologic management, and patient education for implementation of individual asthma treatment plans. The recommendations of both guidelines are presented in this chapter. Additional guidelines that specifically address optimal asthma control by focusing on assessment and presenting a modified step approach come from the Joint Task Force on Practice Parameters, 2005; however, because they do not outline medication treatment in detail, these guidelines are not discussed in this chapter.

Evidence-Based Recommendations

Meta-analyses and systematic reviews of clinical trials seek to clarify and prioritize drug treatment for optimal control of asthma. Many clinical trials have sought to clarify the use of ICSs in asthma management in terms of dose, systemic side effects, combination therapy, and possible alternative antiinflammatory drugs. It has been found that corticosteroids exhibit a dose-response relationship for efficacy but at the expense of increasing side effects in the high-dose range. People with mild to moderate asthma gained the most benefit from low to moderate doses of beclomethasone, budesonide, and fluticasone. A small decrease has been found in the initial structural growth of bones in children receiving ICSs at high doses, but no difference was noted in adult height, bone mineral density, or urinary or plasma cortisol levels among children treated with long-term corticosteroids. A review of studies in which ICSs were used vs. the combination of ICSs and LABAs showed the combination of ICSs and LABAs to be more efficacious and cost-effective in terms of direct medical costs, episode-free days, and symptom-free days. The addition of the LABA (salmeterol or formoterol) has been found to be more efficacious in terms of preventing exacerbations and in influencing a number of other outcomes, such as rescue-free days, symptom-free days, quality of life, and symptom scores. Nedocromil showed a good safety profile with no significant short- or long-term side effects, but results regarding its efficacy were conflicting. The combination of the bronchodilators albuterol and ipratropium vs. albuterol alone was studied for efficacy and cost in terms of emergency situations associated with asthma exacerbations. Nebulized albuterol vs. the combination product of albuterol and ipratropium was used in the emergency department. Although the cost of the combination product was greater, it was not more efficacious in terms of PEF rate or rate of admission to the hospital.

Cardinal Points of Treatment

- Asthma is a chronic inflammatory disease of the airways that requires daily use of controller medication in most cases, even in young children. Only those with mild, intermittent asthma (symptoms ≤2 days per week or ≤2 nights per month) require no daily medication. They can be treated with as needed use of RABAs.
- The preferred controller medication in adults and children with persistent asthma is low-dose ICS. An LM or a mast cell stabilizer may be considered as an alternative for long-term control.
- The addition of a LABA for patients with moderate persistent asthma improves lung function and symptom control and reduces the need for quick relief medications.
- Alternately, an LM, theophylline, or doubling the dose of ICS may be considered for add-on therapy in those 5 years of age and older.
- For children younger than 5 with moderate persistent asthma, an increase to a medium-dose ICS given as monotherapy is followed by the addition of a LABA or LM. Treatment of severe persistent asthma requires high-dose ICS and a LABA or LM.
- A course of oral corticosteroids may be used in severe asthma, but long-term steroid use should be avoided if possible. Omalizumab (see Chapter 51) may be considered for severe asthma in those 12 years and older.
- Quick relief medication (SABA is preferred) may be used at all stages of asthma for breakthrough symptoms or exacerbations. Ipratropium may be added for severe exacerbations.
- Urgent medical care for exacerbations should include inhaled oxygen; adjunct therapy in refractory cases may include mechanical ventilation and heliox (inhaled helium and oxygen mixture).

Pharmacologic Treatment

- Long-term control
  - Corticosteroids (inhaled, occasionally systemic)
  - Mast cell stabilizers
  - Leukotriene modifiers
  - Long-acting β_2-agonists
  - Methylxanthines
- Quick relief
  - Short-acting β_2-agonists
  - Anticholinergics
  - Systemic corticosteroids

The NAEPP EPR3 guidelines (Figures 14-3 and 14-4) present a stepwise pharmacologic approach that corresponds to the severity of asthma in patients of all ages. Six steps replace a four-step approach from the EPR2 Guidelines. Therapy now varies slightly in the 0 to 4 age group, the 5 to 11 age group, and the 12 and older age group. Information is provided here for ages 5 and older. For stepwise therapy in the 0 to 4 age group, see the EPR2 Guideline website. The goals of therapy are to gain and maintain long-term control of asthma and to quickly and successfully treat asthma exacerbations. *Control of asthma* is defined as prevention of chronic and troublesome symptoms, maintenance of normal or near-normal pulmonary function, maintenance of normal exercise and activity levels, prevention of recurrent exacerbations, avoidance of adverse effects from drug therapy, and satisfaction of patient and family expectations for asthma care.

Referral to or consultation with an asthma specialist is indicated if there is difficulty maintaining control, if step 4 therapy is needed by the adult or child older than 5 years, or if step 3 or 4 therapy is needed by the infant or young child. Referral or consultation also may be considered if the adult or child older than 5 years of age requires step 4 therapy, or the infant or young child requires step 3 therapy.

- *Step 1* therapy for adults and children 5 years and older with mild intermittent asthma involves a quick relief bronchodilator used intermittently with no long-term medication. Inhaled relatively selective β_2-adrenergic agonist bronchodilators are preferred for all severities of asthma because of their minimal side effect profile.
- *Step 2* therapy requires a long-term antiinflammatory medication, in addition to a quick relief bronchodilator. Choices of long-term control medication include an ICS in low dose (preferred), a mast cell stabilizer, an LM, or possibly an oral theophylline.
- *Step 3* therapy distinguishes between the 5 to 11 and 12 and older age groups. For those 12 years and older, an ICS at medium dose as monotherapy or an ICS at low dose with the addition of a LABA is preferred therapy; alternative therapy is a low-dose ICS, given along with one of the following: a LABA, oral theophylline, or an LM. For those in the 5 to 11 age group, any of the therapies may be used without preference.
- *Step 4* therapy uses an ICS at medium dose along with a LABA (preferred); alternatively, medium-dose ICS plus LM or theophylline is given.
- *Step 5* therapy calls for high-dose ICS plus a LABA (preferred); alternatively, in the 5 to 11 age group, a high-dose ICS plus an LM or theophylline may be used. In the 12 and older age group, omalizumab may be added on for those who have allergies.
- *Step 6* therapy calls for high-dose ICS plus LABA plus an oral corticosteroid. Omalizumab may be added on in the 12 and older age group; an LM or theophylline may be substituted for a LABA in the 5 to 11 age group.

Education and use of nonpharmacologic management accompany every step of therapy. Nonpharmacologic management involves controlling environmental triggers and using simple breathing techniques to help control airflow. Patients

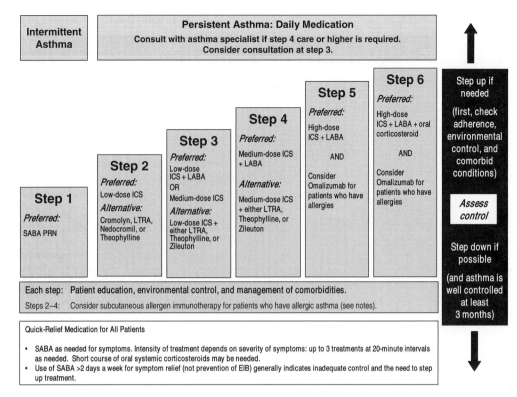

Intermittent Asthma

Persistent Asthma: Daily Medication
Consult with asthma specialist if step 4 care or higher is required.
Consider consultation at step 3.

Step 1
Preferred:
SABA PRN

Step 2
Preferred:
Low-dose ICS
Alternative:
Cromolyn, LTRA, Nedocromil, or Theophylline

Step 3
Preferred:
Low-dose ICS + LABA
OR
Medium-dose ICS
Alternative:
Low-dose ICS + either LTRA, Theophylline, or Zileuton

Step 4
Preferred:
Medium-dose ICS + LABA
Alternative:
Medium-dose ICS + either LTRA, Theophylline, or Zileuton

Step 5
Preferred:
High-dose ICS + LABA
AND
Consider Omalizumab for patients who have allergies

Step 6
Preferred:
High-dose ICS + LABA + oral corticosteroid
AND
Consider Omalizumab for patients who have allergies

Step up if needed
(first, check adherence, environmental control, and comorbid conditions)

Assess control

Step down if possible
(and asthma is well controlled at least 3 months)

Each step: Patient education, environmental control, and management of comorbidities.
Steps 2–4: Consider subcutaneous allergen immunotherapy for patients who have allergic asthma (see notes).

Quick-Relief Medication for All Patients

- SABA as needed for symptoms. Intensity of treatment depends on severity of symptoms: up to 3 treatments at 20-minute intervals as needed. Short course of oral systemic corticosteroids may be needed.
- Use of SABA >2 days a week for symptom relief (not prevention of EIB) generally indicates inadequate control and the need to step up treatment.

Key: **Alphabetical order is used when more than one treatment option is listed within either preferred or alternative therapy.** EIB, exercise-induced bronchospasm; ICS, inhaled corticosteroid; LABA, long-acting inhaled beta$_2$-agonist; LTRA, leukotriene receptor antagonist; SABA, inhaled short-acting beta$_2$-agonist

Notes:

- The stepwise approach is meant to assist, not replace, the clinical decision making required to meet individual patient needs.
- If alternative treatment is used and response is inadequate, discontinue it and use the preferred treatment before stepping up.
- Zileuton is a less desirable alternative due to limited studies as adjunctive therapy and the need to monitor liver function. Theophylline requires monitoring of serum concentration levels.
- In step 6, before oral systemic corticosteroids are introduced, a trial of high-dose ICS + LABA + either LTRA, theophylline, or zileuton may be considered, although this approach has not been studied in clinical trials.
- Step 1, 2, and 3 preferred therapies are based on Evidence A; step 3 alternative therapy is based on Evidence A for LTRA, Evidence B for theophylline, and Evidence D for zileuton. Step 4 preferred therapy is based on Evidence B, and alternative therapy is based on Evidence B for LTRA and theophylline and Evidence D for zileuton. Step 5 preferred therapy is based on Evidence B. Step 6 preferred therapy is based on (EPR—2 1997) and Evidence B for omalizumab.
- Immunotherapy for steps 2–4 is based on Evidence B for house-dust mites, animal danders, and pollens; evidence is weak or lacking for molds and cockroaches. Evidence is strongest for immunotherapy with single allergens. The role of allergy in asthma is greater in children than in adults.
- Clinicians who administer immunotherapy or omalizumab should be prepared and equipped to identify and treat anaphylaxis that may occur.

FIGURE 14-3 Stepwise approach for managing asthma in youths ≥12 years of age and adults. (From National Asthma Education and Prevention Program Expert Panel Report 3: *Guidelines for the diagnosis and management of asthma,* NIH Publication No. 08-4051, Washington, DC, 2007, U.S. Government Printing Office.)

must identify and avoid the factors that trigger their asthma attacks. Allergy skin testing is recommended to identify any outdoor or indoor perennial allergens. Sinusitis, rhinitis, and GERD should be optimally managed and influenza should be prevented through the use of yearly influenza immunization.

Early recognition and treatment of exacerbations of asthma are important in reducing the risk of death and helping to regain control of asthma. Asthma exacerbations are acute or subacute episodes of worsening shortness of breath, cough, wheezing, and chest tightness. Exacerbation can be determined objectively by measurement of a decrease in PEF or FEV$_1$. Ultimate treatment of exacerbation may involve

SABAs, systemic corticosteroids for those with moderate to severe asthma or those who do not respond to inhaled corticosteroids, oxygen to relieve severe hypoxemia, and close monitoring of response through lung function measurements.

Home treatment guidelines for asthma exacerbation are based on monitoring of symptoms or PEF measurements compared with personal best or predicted PEF. Asthma exacerbation should be treated with SABAs as needed based on severity of symptoms; up to three treatments should be used at 20-minute intervals. A written asthma action plan should instruct patients to initiate quick relief medications if PEF drops to below 80%. If PEF is 50% to 79% of

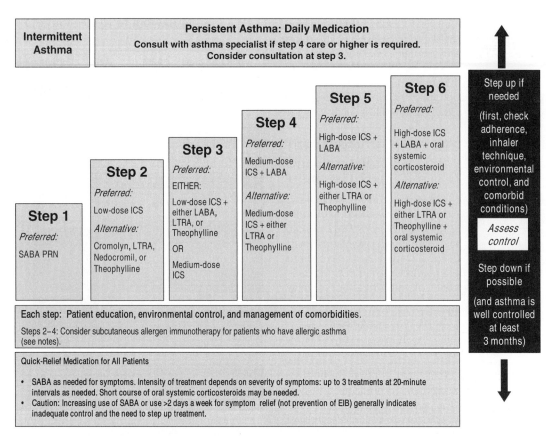

Intermittent Asthma	Persistent Asthma: Daily Medication Consult with asthma specialist if step 4 care or higher is required. Consider consultation at step 3.

Step 1

Preferred:

SABA PRN

Step 2

Preferred:

Low-dose ICS

Alternative:

Cromolyn, LTRA, Nedocromil, or Theophylline

Step 3

Preferred:

EITHER:

Low-dose ICS + either LABA, LTRA, or Theophylline

OR

Medium-dose ICS

Step 4

Preferred:

Medium-dose ICS + LABA

Alternative:

Medium-dose ICS + either LTRA or Theophylline

Step 5

Preferred:

High-dose ICS + LABA

Alternative:

High-dose ICS + either LTRA or Theophylline

Step 6

Preferred:

High-dose ICS + LABA + oral systemic corticosteroid

Alternative:

High-dose ICS + either LTRA or Theophylline + oral systemic corticosteroid

Step up if needed

(first, check adherence, inhaler technique, environmental control, and comorbid conditions)

Assess control

Step down if possible

(and asthma is well controlled at least 3 months)

Each step: Patient education, environmental control, and management of comorbidities.

Steps 2–4: Consider subcutaneous allergen immunotherapy for patients who have allergic asthma (see notes).

Quick-Relief Medication for All Patients

- SABA as needed for symptoms. Intensity of treatment depends on severity of symptoms: up to 3 treatments at 20-minute intervals as needed. Short course of oral systemic corticosteroids may be needed.
- Caution: Increasing use of SABA or use >2 days a week for symptom relief (not prevention of EIB) generally indicates inadequate control and the need to step up treatment.

Key: **Alphabetical order is used when more than one treatment option is listed within either preferred or alternative therapy.** ICS, inhaled corticosteroid; LABA, inhaled long-acting beta₂-agonist, LTRA, leukotriene receptor antagonist; SABA, inhaled short-acting beta₂-agonist

Notes:

■ The stepwise approach is meant to assist, not replace, the clinical decision making required to meet individual patient needs.

■ If alternative treatment is used and response is inadequate, discontinue it and use the preferred treatment before stepping up.

■ Theophylline is a less desirable alternative due to the need to monitor serum concentration levels.

■ Step 1 and step 2 medications are based on Evidence A. Step 3 ICS + adjunctive therapy and ICS are based on Evidence B for efficacy of each treatment and extrapolation from comparator trials in older children and adults— comparator trials are not available for this age group; steps 4–6 are based on expert opinion and extrapolation from studies in older children and adults.

■ Immunotherapy for steps 2–4 is based on Evidence B for house-dust mites, animal danders, and pollens; evidence is weak or lacking for molds and cockroaches. Evidence is strongest for immunotherapy with single allergens. The role of allergy in asthma is greater in children than in adults. Clinicians who administer immunotherapy should be prepared and equipped to identify and treat anaphylaxis that may occur.

FIGURE 14-4   Stepwise approach for managing asthma in children 5 to 11 years of age. (From National Asthma Education and Prevention Program Expert Panel Report 3: *Guidelines for the diagnosis and management of asthma,* NIH Publication No. 08-4051, Washington, DC, 2007, U.S. Government Printing Office.)

predicted or personal best, the patient should consider notifying a clinician. If PEF is 50% or below, immediate medical care is required.

TREATMENT PRINCIPLES OF COPD

Standardized Guidelines

The primary guidelines for COPD management come from GOLD (2006). The GOLD report represents a comprehensive analysis of guidelines from NHLBI, WHO, and the National Institute of Clinical Excellence (NICE) in the

United Kingdom. Recommendations from the GOLD guidelines are presented in this chapter.

Evidence-Based Recommendations

Meta-analyses and systematic reviews seek to clarify the use of corticosteroid therapy and optimal combination therapy in COPD. Oral corticosteroid therapy in COPD provides significant benefit in both stable and acute exacerbations of COPD, but at increased risk of side effects. The benefits are greater in acute exacerbations. The anticholinergics (tiotropium and ipratropium) significantly reduced severe exacerbations and respiratory deaths, and ICSs significantly reduced severe exacerbations and decline in lung function over time, whereas β_2-agonists increased respiratory deaths, probably as the result of tolerance. The use of mucolytic agents (see Chapter 13) has been proposed as a way to reduce exacerbations in patients with COPD. Research has suggested a small reduction in acute exacerbations and number of days of disability with use of a mucolytic agent and has proposed their use throughout the winter months, at least in patients with moderate to severe COPD in whom ICSs are not prescribed.

Additional research suggests that spirometry used for early detection of COPD along with smoking cessation can alter disease progression. Other changes that promote better quality of life for patients with moderate to severe COPD include stopping smoking, allowing breathless patients time to express themselves, encouraging exercise, and providing timely palliative care. Pulmonary rehabilitation relieves dyspnea, improves emotional function, and enhances patients' sense of control.

Cardinal Points of Treatments

1. Bronchodilators are primary to symptom management for as needed or scheduled use; the choice between SABA/RABA, LABA, short-acting anticholinergic, and long-acting anticholinergic is based on individual response, side effects, and access/ease of use.

2. For COPD stage I, prn use of a short-acting bronchodilator is indicated.

3. For COPD stage II to IV, a long-acting bronchodilator should be added if dyspnea persists during daily activities; regular use may be more effective and convenient than as needed use.

4. As needed use of a short-acting bronchodilator may be prescribed, along with regular use of a long-acting or short-acting bronchodilator.

5. Use of a long-acting theophylline preparation is not well tolerated because of common side effects such as cardiac arrhythmia, headache, insomnia, nausea, and toxicity (which may be induced by changes in metabolism caused by food and other drugs).

6. Although past COPD guidelines have recommended a 2-week trial of oral corticosteroids to predict whether there will be long-term benefit, the GOLD 2006 guidelines state that there is insufficient evidence to recommend this, even in severe cases of COPD.

7. Regular use of ICSs is recommended for COPD stages III and IV (<50% of predicted FEV_1) to reduce frequent exacerbations.

8. Influenza and pneumococcal immunizations are recommended to help reduce comorbidity that will affect respiratory status (see Chapter 70). Mucolytic agents may be considered as adjunct therapy.

9. Exacerbations of COPD should be treated with increased dose and frequency of short-acting bronchodilators, systemic corticosteroids (if FEV_1 falls to <50% of predicted), and antibiotics if purulent sputum develops (most exacerbations are caused by infection, although infection may be viral and about one third of exacerbations have no cause).

10. Assessment in the emergency department and possible hospitalization are required for severe exacerbations with respiratory acidosis, significant comorbidity, and the potential need for ventilatory support. The above treatment should be supplemented with oxygen, an anticholinergic bronchodilator (if not already used), inhalation via a spacer or nebulizer, an IV methylxanthine (if insufficient response to short-acting bronchodilators), oral or IV corticosteroid, and possibly mechanical ventilation (noninvasive preferred). Fluid balance, nutritional support, and deep vein thrombosis prophylaxis with heparin are supportive therapies.

Pharmacologic Treatment

- Maintenance
  - Anticholinergics
  - β_2-Adrenergic agonists
  - Methylxanthines
  - Corticosteroids (inhaled, occasionally oral)
  - Expectorants
- Severe exacerbation
  - Anticholinergics
  - β_2-Agonists
  - Methylxanthines
  - Corticosteroids (oral)

The GOLD guidelines treatment of patients with stable COPD is based on severity and is provided in a stepwise approach, starting with one drug and adding drugs as severity increases. Treatment with medications alone often does not effectively manage COPD; therefore, nonpharmacologic treatment strategies are also important.

The goals of COPD treatment are to alleviate symptoms, enhance lung function, improve physical activity, and reduce complications. Pharmacologic treatment does not change the overall long-term decline in lung function; only smoking cessation can slow that progression to the rate of normal age-related decline.

Nonpharmacologic strategies include smoking cessation, patient education, improved nutrition, and exercise. Pulmonary rehabilitation programs are typically multidisciplinary and include individualized, carefully monitored exercise programs, as well as patient education and support. Removal and avoidance of toxins (cigarette smoke and air pollution) are important goals of therapy. Pharmacologic therapy of an adjunct nature includes immunization yearly for influenza, pneumococcal immunization, and possible mucolytic therapy. Every effort should be made to avoid exposing these individuals to upper respiratory infections, which often are carried by children.

- *Step 1* therapy for stage I severity COPD begins with a short-acting bronchodilator as needed to control symptoms.
- *Step 2* therapy for stage II COPD involves the regular use of a long-acting bronchodilator in addition to the as needed use of a short-acting bronchodilator. Pulmonary rehabilitation should be added at this step. For those patients who need additional symptom control, a long-acting theophylline may provide additional benefit.
- *Step 3* therapy for stage III COPD adds an ICS if exacerbations are repeated.
- *Step 4* therapy for stage IV COPD adds long-term oxygen therapy for those with chronic respiratory failure. Surgical options of bullectomy, lung volume reduction, and lung transplantation may be considered.

Treatment for acute exacerbation of COPD includes increased dose and frequency of a short-acting bronchodilator, along with the addition of an anticholinergic bronchodilator if one is not already in use. Inhalation via a spacer or nebulizer may be preferred. Oral corticosteroids should be considered if baseline FEV$_1$ is ≤50% of predicted and should be given to shorten recovery time, improve FEV$_1$, improve hypoxemia, and possibly reduce the risk of relapse, treatment failure, and length of stay. Dosing of 30 to 40 mg per day for 7 to 10 days is considered effective and safe. An antibiotic that covers the most common causative agents (*Haemophilus influenzae*, *Streptococcus pneumoniae*, *Moraxella catarrhalis*, and possibly *Mycoplasma pneumoniae* and *Chlamydia pneumoniae*) should be added if purulent sputum is present. If the patient is not in respiratory acidosis and is not in need of ventilatory support, home management with frequent follow-up and monitoring may be appropriate. If improvement is noted on reassessment, this regimen can be continued and stepped down when possible. If hospital management is necessary, oxygen therapy, IV methylxanthines, IV corticosteroids, and ventilatory support may be necessary.

How to Monitor

β-ADRENERGIC AGONIST BRONCHODILATORS

- Increasing frequency of use of a short-acting bronchodilator, or use beyond the manufacturer's recommended dosing, indicates the need to increase step therapy.
- In general, use of a canister per month indicates inadequate control of asthma and the need for stepped-up therapy.
- Tremor, tachycardia, cardiac arrhythmia (rare), and hypokalemia (when used with thiazide diuretics) limit the dose that can be used.

THEOPHYLLINE

- Serum concentration should be measured at peak steady state, which occurs 8 hours after administration of extended-release formulations and 1 hour after administration of immediate-release formulations, with no dosage change within 3 days.
- Recommended therapeutic serum concentration is 5 to 15 mcg/ml.
- Many drugs and physiologic variables, including tobacco smoking, phenobarbital, and alcohol (all increase metabolism), as well as aging, hypoxemia, respiratory acidosis, heart failure, liver failure, macrolides, quinolones, cimetidine, St. John's wort, and viral infection (all decrease metabolism), affect theophylline metabolism and require adjustment in dosage.
- Serum concentration monitoring should take place whenever signs of toxicity are suspected; on initiation of drug and dosage titration until steady state therapeutic concentration is reached; and routinely every 6 months in children and yearly in adults.

CORTICOSTEROIDS. Some studies have shown a controversial effect on growth; therefore, monitoring the growth of children and adolescents is prudent.

Patient Variables

GERIATRICS

- Bronchodilators may cause increased adverse reactions. Some older adults may not tolerate side effects such as tachycardia.
- Theophylline clearance is reduced in the older adult, causing increased risk of drug toxicity and interaction (see Table 14-8).

- The total daily dosage of theophylline should not exceed 400 mg.
- High-dose ICSs and oral corticosteroids that are often used in COPD may cause or worsen osteoporosis in the older adult.
- Nebulization treatment may be useful when older adults are unable to use inhalers correctly.

PEDIATRICS

- Special delivery devices are available for infants and young children. Caregivers must be taught their proper use. Nebulizer treatments are preferred for children aged 2 years and younger. Children aged 3 to 5 years may use an inhaler with a spacer or a nebulizer.
- The rate of theophylline clearance is highly variable in children from infancy to adolescence and so must be closely monitored.
- Ipratropium safety has not been determined in children younger than 12 years of age.
- The safety and efficacy of montelukast at the 4-mg dose have been established in children 2 to 5 years of age.

PREGNANCY AND LACTATION

- Poorly controlled asthma can result in increased perinatal mortality. In general, little evidence suggests increased risk to the fetus with the use of medications recommended to treat asthma. ICSs do not increase the risk of major malformations, preterm delivery, low birth weight, and pregnancy-induced hypertension. Because of limited research, however, many asthma drugs are categorized as potentially harmful.
- *Category C:* β-Adrenergic agonists (except terbutaline), theophylline, tiotropium, corticosteroids (except budesonide), zileuton
- *Category B:* Ipratropium, mast cell stabilizers, budesonide, montelukast and zafirlukast, and terbutaline
- Most of these medications are excreted in breast milk.
- Theophylline: Patient may need to discontinue breastfeeding because the drug can cause serious toxicity in nursing infants.

Patient Education

- Teach basic facts about asthma.
- Teach inhaler/spacer/holding chamber technique; see Table 14-3 for a summary of inhalation systems.
- Discuss the roles of medications.
- Develop a written self-management plan for both children and adults.
- Develop a written action plan for when and how to take rescue actions, especially for patients with a history of severe exacerbations.
- Discuss appropriate environmental control measures that can be used to avoid exposure to known allergens and irritants.

PROPER USE OF A METERED-DOSE INHALER

1. Remove the cap. (Research studies show that 1% of users fail to remove the cap before using the metered-dose inhaler [MDI]!)
2. Hold the inhaler upright and shake it thoroughly.
3. Tilt head back slightly and breathe out. (Most people take in a large breath before exhaling. This is counterproductive in patients with outflow obstruction and should be specifically noted to patients as a practice to avoid.)
4. The MDI may be placed in the mouth with the lips sealed around it, placed 1 to 2 inches away from the

TABLE 14-3 Inhalation Delivery Devices

Device/Drugs	Advantages	Disadvantages
Metered-dose inhaler (MDI) β_2-Adrenergic agonists Corticosteroids Mast cell stabilizers Anticholinergics	Small and compact Can be used with open or closed mouth technique; open mouth technique may enhance delivery of drug	Requires slow inhalation Requires coordination of inhalation and actuation Up to 80% of dose deposited in oropharynx
Breath-actuated MDI β_2-Adrenergic agonists	Does not require coordination of inhalation and actuation	Requires slow inhalation for optimal deposition, but not so slow as to prevent actuation
Dry powder inhaler (DPI) β_2-Adrenergic agonists Corticosteroids	Requires rapid, deep inhalation May be easier for children 4 yr old and older	Dose lost if patient exhales through device Delivery may be less efficient than with proper use of MDI
Spacer/holding chamber Can be used with standard inhalers (not breath-actuated) and some DPIs	Easier for children 4 yr old and older, or younger than 4 yr with a face mask Decreases oropharyngeal deposition and systemic absorption of drug	Simple tube devices still require coordination of inhalation and actuation; valved holding chambers are preferred. May be bulky and less convenient to carry Requires more extensive cleaning
Nebulizer β_2-Adrenergic agonists Corticosteroids Mast cell stabilizers Anticholinergics	Effective in all age groups and ability levels Slow tidal breathing with occasional deep breaths; most effective	Tightly fitting face mask is needed if unable to use mouthpiece Expensive and less portable than other devices

Adapted from National Asthma Education and Prevention Program Expert Panel Report 3: *Guidelines for the diagnosis and management of asthma,* NIH Publication No. 08-4051, Washington, DC, 2007, U.S. Government Printing Office.

opened mouth, or attached to a spacer or holding chamber with the end of the device placed in the mouth and the lips sealed around it. In infants and young children (or anyone unable to self-administer the device), the spacer can be attached to a face mask and the face mask sealed around the patient's face before the MDI is activated.

5. Press down on the inhaler to release the medication as the patient starts to breathe in slowly.
6. Breathe in slowly for 3 to 5 seconds.
7. Hold breath for 10 seconds to allow deposition of medication deeply into the lungs.
8. Wait 1 minute and repeat inhalation if additional puffs are prescribed.

For inhaled dry powder medications, it is important to close the mouth tightly around the inhaler and breathe in rapidly after activating the dose.

LONG-ACTING β-ADRENERGIC AGONIST BRONCHODILATORS

- The FDA posted an advisory warning to state that although LABAs decrease the frequency of asthma episodes, they also may increase the chance that an asthma episode will be severe. The following recommendations have been put forth by the FDA:
  - LABAs are not first-line asthma agents; they should be added on only if other medications (including low- to medium-dose ICSs) do not control asthma.
  - Do not stop using LABAs and other asthma medications without discussing with your health care provider.
  - Do not use a LABA to treat worsening wheezing; call your health care provider if wheezing worsens while you are using a LABA.
  - A LABA should not be used in place of a SABA to treat sudden wheezing.

THEOPHYLLINE

- Extended-release capsules should be taken 1 hour before or 2 hours after meals; immediate-release forms can be taken with food if gastrointestinal upset occurs.
- Do not change the brand of theophylline without consulting provider.
- Notify physician if nausea, vomiting, insomnia, jitteriness, headache, rash, severe gastrointestinal pain, restlessness, convulsions, or irregular heartbeat occurs.
- Avoid caffeine-containing beverages and other stimulants.

IPRATROPIUM. Avoid contact with eyes; may cause temporary blurring of vision.

CROMOLYN. Do not immerse canister in water.

CORTICOSTEROIDS

- "Swish, gargle, and spit" from mouth after use to reduce systemic absorption and local throat infection.
- Do not abruptly stop medication administration.
- Discard canister when number of doses should have been used; canister cannot be accurately checked.

LEUKOTRIENE MODIFIERS

- Take regularly, even during symptom-free periods.
- Zafirlukast: Take 1 hour before or 2 hours after meals.
- Zafirlukast and zileuton: Report hepatic dysfunction symptoms (e.g., right upper quadrant abdominal pain, nausea, fatigue, lethargy, pruritus, jaundice, flulike symptoms, anorexia).
- Zileuton: Monitor hepatic function tests before and during therapy.

SPECIFIC DRUGS

SHORT-ACTING RELATIVELY SELECTIVE β-ADRENERGIC AGONIST BRONCHODILATORS

albuterol (Proventil, Ventolin) 🔑

CONTRAINDICATIONS. Hypersensitivity to albuterol or any component

WARNINGS
- Discontinue drug if paradoxical bronchospasm occurs.
- Asthma deterioration may be indicated by excessive use of inhalations.
- Consider use of an antiinflammatory agent along with albuterol for treatment of asthma.
- May cause adverse cardiovascular effects in some patients, especially those with coronary insufficiency, cardiac arrhythmia, and hypertension.
- Do not exceed recommended dose because this may lead to death.

PRECAUTIONS. Administer with caution to patients with cardiovascular disorders, diabetes mellitus, hyperthyroidism, or seizure disorder and the elderly.

PHARMACOKINETICS. See Table 14-4. This is a quick-onset, short-acting drug.

ADVERSE EFFECTS. See Tables 14-5 and 14-6.

DRUG INTERACTIONS
- Increased sympathomimetic effects with other sympathomimetic agents
- Enhanced toxicity in patients taking methylxanthines
- Decreased bronchodilating effectiveness with patients taking β-adrenergic–blocking agents
- Decreased effectiveness of insulin and oral hypoglycemic agents

OVERDOSAGE
- Signs and symptoms are those of excessive β-adrenergic stimulation: seizures, hypertension, hypotension, angina, tachycardia, arrhythmias, nervousness, dizziness, etc.
- Cardiac arrest and death may occur.

DOSAGE AND ADMINISTRATION. See Table 14-7.

OTHER DRUGS IN CLASS

Other drugs in this class are similar to the key, except as follows.
- Pirbuterol comes in a breath-actuated inhaler that may be easier for some patients to use.
- Levalbuterol has a longer duration than other drugs in this class.
- Terbutaline is no longer widely available in inhaled form. Subcutaneous injection is used in the hospital setting. It should be used cautiously in labor and delivery because it can inhibit labor.
- Less selective β₂-adrenergic agonists such as epinephrine, isoproterenol, and metaproterenol are not recommended because of their potential for cardiac stimulation, especially at high doses.

LONG-ACTING RELATIVELY SELECTIVE β₂-ADRENERGIC AGONIST BRONCHODILATORS

salmeterol (Serevent) 🔑

CONTRAINDICATIONS. Hypersensitivity to salmeterol or any of its components; acute treatment of bronchospasm

WARNINGS

💣 Warning: Data from a large, placebo-controlled U.S. study that compared the safety of salmeterol (Serevent inhalation aerosol) or placebo added to the usual therapy showed a small but significant increase in asthma-related death in patients receiving salmeterol (13 deaths among 13,176 patients treated for 28 weeks) vs. those on placebo (3 of 13,179) (see WARNINGS and CLINICAL TRIALS).

- Should not be initiated in patients with significant worsening or acutely deteriorating asthma
- Should not be used to treat acute symptoms
- Is not a substitute for ICSs
- Do not exceed recommended dosage.
- May cause paradoxical bronchospasm and immediate hypersensitivity reactions

PRECAUTIONS. Use with caution in patients with coronary insufficiency, hypertension, arrhythmias, thyrotoxicosis, and convulsive disorders.

PHARMACOKINETICS. See Table 14-4. Onset of action is 10 to 20 minutes, so it should not be used for acute bronchospasm. Duration of effect is about 12 hours.

DRUG INTERACTIONS
- Action on the vascular system may be potentiated by concomitant administration of tricyclic antidepressants or MAOIs.
- Decreased effectiveness of bronchodilation with SABA
- Potential for worsened hypokalemia when used with diuretics

DOSAGE AND ADMINISTRATION
- See Table 14-5.
- When using to prevent exercise-induced bronchospasm, use 30 to 60 minutes before exercise.
- Inhalation powder should not be used with a spacer.

OTHER DRUGS IN CLASS

Other drugs in this class are similar to salmeterol, except as follows.

formoterol (Foradil)

- Has a similar black box warning, based on the study of salmeterol showing small but significant increase in asthma-related death among patients receiving the drug.
- Formoterol is administered by capsules inserted into an aerosolized inhaler; store capsules in blister pack until ready for use.
- Formoterol has a quicker onset of action (5 minutes) and a longer duration of action (24 hours), which may increase compliance.
- It should not be used for acute bronchospasm.

TABLE 14-4 Pharmacokinetics of Major Asthma and Chronic Obstructive Pulmonary Disease Medications

Drug	Absorption	Drug Availability (After First Pass)	Onset of Action	Time to Peak Concentration	Half-life	Duration of Action	Protein Bound	Metabolism	Excretion	Therapeutic Serum Level, ng/ml*
RELATIVELY RAPID/SHORT ACTING										
albuterol (inhalation)	Through respiratory and GI tracts	—	10 min (CFC propelled); 25 min (HFA)	0.5-2 hr (therapeutic effect); 2-4 hr (serum conc)	3.8 hr	3-4 hr; up to 6 hr in some	—		Urine	—
albuterol (oral—various forms)	Through GI tract	80%	30 min	2-3 hr	3.8-5 hr	4-8 hr; 12 hr for extended-release tablets	—		Urine	—
levalbuterol	Through respiratory and GI tracts	—	10-17 min	60-90 min	3.3 hr	5-6 hr	—		Urine	—
pirbuterol	Through respiratory and GI tracts	—	5 min	30-60 min (therapeutic effect)	2 hr	5 hr	—		Urine	—
ipratropium	Through respiratory tract; swallowed drug is not significantly absorbed	—	14-30 min	1-2 hr (therapeutic effect)	1.6 hr	4-5 hr	0%-9%	Partially metabolized to inactive ester hydrolysis products		—
RELATIVELY LONG ACTING										
theophylline (extended-release preparations)	Rapidly and completely absorbed through GI tract	Nearly 100%		1-2 hr (immediate release); 8 hr (sustained release)	8 hr (varies with age, comorbid illness, and other conditions)	6 hr (immediate release); 8-24 hr (sustained release)	40%	Hepatic: demethylation	Urine	5-15 mcg/ml (NAEPP EPR2); 10-20 mcg/ml (manufacturer information)
formoterol	Through respiratory and GI tracts	—	5 min		10 hr	12 hr	61%-64%	Hepatic: direct glucuronidation	Urine, feces	—
salmeterol	Through respiratory and GI tracts	—	10-20 min		5.5 hr	12 hr	96%	Hepatic: hydroxylation	Urine, feces	—
arformoterol	Through the respiratory tract	—	6-20 min	1-3 hr	26 hr	12 hr	52%-65%	Hepatic: glucuronidation	Urine, feces	—
tiotropium	Poorly absorbed through GI tract; respiratory tract	—	5 min	5 min	5-6 days	24 hr	72%	Small amount through hepatic cytochrome P450	Unchanged in urine, rest in feces	—
cromolyn sodium	Limited GI and respiratory tracts			15 min; approximately 2-4 wk for therapeutic effect	80 min	6-8 hr		Excreted unchanged	Urine, feces	
nedocromil	Through respiratory tract			28 min; 2 wk for therapeutic effect	3.3 hr	10-12 hr	89%	Excreted unchanged	Urine	—

Table continued on following page

TABLE 14-4 Pharmacokinetics of Major Asthma and Chronic Obstructive Pulmonary Disease Medications (Continued)

Drug	Absorption	Drug Availability (After First Pass)	Onset of Action	Time to Peak Concentration	Half-life	Duration of Action	Protein Bound	Metabolism	Excretion	Therapeutic Serum Level, ng/ml*
beclomethasone dipropionate	Rapidly absorbed through respiratory and GI tracts	Low systemic absorption; about 20% bioavailability from lungs	1-2 wk for therapeutic effect		3 hr		87%	Metabolized in the lung and liver (CYP 3A)	Feces, urine (small amount)	—
budesonide	Rapidly absorbed through respiratory and GI tracts	25% bioavailability from lungs; 5%-15% bioavailability from systemic absorption	Improvement in as little as 24 hr	Maximal therapeutic effect in as little as 1-2 wk	2.8 hr	8-12 hr	85%-90%	Liver (CYP 3A)	Urine, feces	—
flunisolide	Rapid absorption through respiratory and GI tracts	Low systemic absorption and rapid conversion of systemic drug to inactive metabolite			1.8 hr	4-6 hr	—	Liver	Urine, feces	—
fluticasone propionate	Most of the drug is systemically absorbed from the lungs.	13%-30%	Improvement in as little as 24 hr	Maximal therapeutic effect in as little as 1-2 wk	3.1 hr		91%	Liver	Feces, urine	—
triamcinolone acetonide	Rapidly absorbed from the lungs	21.5%			1.5 hr		68%	Liver, kidneys	Feces	—
montelukast	Rapidly absorbed through the GI tract	64%	Rapid	2-4 hr	2.7-5.5 hr		99%	Extensively metabolized through the liver (CYP 3A4 and CYP 2C9)	Feces	—
zafirlukast	Rapidly absorbed through GI tract	Unknown	Rapid	3 hr	10 hr		99%	Extensively metabolized through the liver (CYP 2C9)	Feces	—
zileuton	Rapidly absorbed through GI tract	Unknown	Rapid	1.7 hr	2.5 hr		93%	Metabolized by the liver (CYP 1A2, 2C0, 3A4)	Urine	—

NAEPP EPR2, National Asthma Education and Prevention Program Expert Panel Report 2.

TABLE 14-5 **Common and Serious Adverse Effects of Asthma and COPD Medications**

Drug Class	Drug Name	Common Side Effects	Serious Adverse Effects
Short-acting β-agonists	All	Palpitations, tachycardia, increased BP, cough, dry throat, chest tightness, nausea and vomiting, GI distress, headache, insomnia, tremor, dizziness, vertigo, nervousness, hyperactivity	Arrhythmias, dyspnea, hypokalemia
	albuterol	Heartburn, nasal congestion	Angioedema, bronchospasm, hypertension, angina, rash
	bitolterol		Bronchospasm, elevated LFTs
	levalbuterol	Flu-like syndrome, pain, rhinitis, sinusitis, viral infection	
	pirbuterol		Bronchospasm
Long-acting β-agonists	All	Tremor, nervousness, tachycardia	Bronchospasm
	salmeterol	Palpitations, headache, nasal congestion, joint and muscle pain	Immediate hypersensitivity reactions, rash, angioedema
	formoterol	Dizziness, insomnia	Arrhythmias, angina, hypokalemia, metabolic acidosis
theophylline		Tachycardia, palpitations, tachypnea, nausea, vomiting, diarrhea, GI reflux, headache, insomnia, irritability	Arrhythmias, hypotension, seizures, SIADH, hematemesis, proteinuria, circulatory failure, death
Anticholinergics	All	Headache, dizziness, fatigue, pain, rash, cough, respiratory infection, palpitations, hypertension, dry mouth, GI distress, constipation, urinary retention, eye pain	Anaphylaxis, worsening of narrow-angle glaucoma, bronchospasm, worsening of COPD, tachycardia, urticaria, chest pain
Mast cell stabilizers	All	Headache, nausea, cough, rhinitis	Eosinophilic pneumonitis
	cromolyn	Dizziness, irritation of oropharynx, wheezing, sneezing	Angioedema
	nedocromil	Bad taste, pharyngitis, rash, arthritis, elevated LFTs	Bronchospasm
Inhaled corticosteroids	All	Oral candidiasis; oral, laryngeal, pharyngeal irritation; headache, dyspepsia, cough, respiratory infection	Suppression of HPA axis, cushingoid features, growth velocity reduction, bronchospasm
Leukotriene receptor agonists	All	Headache, fever, rash, dyspepsia, anaphylaxis	
	montelukast	Asthenia, fever	Hepatic eosinophilic infiltrations
	zafirlukast	Dizziness, respiratory infections, elevated LFTs	Systemic eosinophilia, agranulocytosis, bleeding
	zileuton	Dyspepsia, nausea, abdominal pain, asthenia, elevated LFTs, myalgia	Low WBC

METHYLXANTHINES

theophylline (Theo-Dur, Theolair, Slo-Bid, Slo-Phyllin, Quibron, Uniphyl, etc.) 🔑

CONTRAINDICATIONS. Hypersensitivity to xanthines

WARNINGS

💣 **Serious side effects such as ventricular arrhythmias, convulsions, or death may appear without warning as the first signs of toxicity.**

- Active peptic ulcer disease, gastritis, angina, acute ST elevation, myocardial infarction, and a seizure disorder not controlled by medication
- Theophylline has a very narrow therapeutic window; toxicity can cause initially mild signs of toxicity such as nausea and restlessness.
- Reduced theophylline clearance and increased risk for toxicity have been documented, requiring more intensive monitoring of therapeutic level, in those with the following risk factors: age >60 or <1 year old; comorbid conditions such as impaired liver function, acute pulmonary edema, congestive heart failure, cor pulmonale, hypothyroidism, reduced renal function in infants <3 months old; sepsis with multi-organ failure, and shock; fever; administration of certain drugs; and cessation of smoking.

- If theophylline toxicity is suspected because of the presence of nausea and vomiting, particularly repetitive vomiting, additional doses of theophylline should be withheld and the serum concentration of theophylline measured immediately.
- Dosage of theophylline should not be increased in response to acute exacerbation of symptoms.

PRECAUTIONS
- Use cautiously in patients with seizure disorders and cardiac arrhythmias (except bradyarrhythmias).
- Use cautiously and reduce dosage with hepatic insufficiency.

DRUG INTERACTIONS
- Many drugs decrease or increase theophylline levels (Table 14-8, p. 208). Theophylline is a major substrate of cytochrome P450 3A4, 1A2, and 2E1. Food–drug interactions include the following:
  - A high-protein/low-carbohydrate diet increases elimination.
  - A high-carbohydrate/low-protein diet decreases elimination.
- Food may alter bioavailability and absorption. Consistent administration while fasting improves consistency of effects.

OVERDOSAGE
- Symptoms of overdosage may begin with serum concentrations >20 mcg/ml with nausea, tachycardia, vomiting, headache, and insomnia.

Continued

theophylline (Theo-Dur, Theolair, Slo-Bid, Slo-Phyllin, Quibron, Uniphyl, etc.) 🔑—cont'd

- Higher concentrations may cause intractable seizures, hypokalemia, ventricular arrhythmias, and death.

DOSAGE AND ADMINISTRATION
- Theophylline anhydrous and theophylline monohydrate have slightly varying equivalent doses; theophylline anhydrous is 100% theophylline. Dosing intervals vary for immediate-release and extended-release products. Extended-release theophylline products are preferred because of convenience; see Table 14-5.
- Dosage should be individualized based on serum concentration measurements to achieve maximum potential benefit with minimum risk of adverse effects (see Table 14-7). Therapeutic concentration is 10 to 20 mcg/ml; however, the NAEPP recommends 5 to 15 mcg/ml for treatment of asthmatic patients. With risk factors for reduced theophylline clearance, give only 16 mg/kg or 400 mg/day.

Anticholinergics

ipratropium bromide (Atrovent) 🔑

CONTRAINDICATIONS. Hypersensitivity to ipratropium, atropine, or soya lecithin products such as soybean or peanut (inhalation only)

WARNINGS. Do not use as single agent for acute bronchospasm; combine with drug with a faster onset of action.

PRECAUTIONS
- Immediate hypersensitivity may occur.
- Use with caution in patients with narrow-angle glaucoma, prostatic hypertrophy, or bladder neck obstruction.

PHARMACOKINETICS. See Table 14-4. Onset of action is 1 to 3 minutes; duration is about 4 hours.

ADVERSE REACTIONS. Better tolerated by many individuals than β_2-adrenergic agonist bronchodilators; see Tables 14-5 and 14-6.

OTHER DRUGS IN CLASS

tiotropium (Spiriva)
- Tiotropium is a longer-acting anticholinergic for inhalation; however, onset of action is rapid.
- It is indicated for prevention of bronchospasm in COPD.
- Once-daily administration may enhance adherence and thus effectiveness of control in COPD.

MAST CELL STABILIZERS

cromolyn sodium (Intal) 🔑

CONTRAINDICATIONS. Hypersensitivity to cromolyn; acute treatment of bronchospasm

WARNINGS
- Not for use in the treatment of acute asthma attack
- Taper drug slowly if medication withdrawal is desired.

- Severe anaphylactic reaction may occur.
- Should be discontinued if drug causes eosinophilic pneumonia

PHARMACOKINETICS. See Table 14-4. Has a very slow onset with therapeutic effects occurring in about a week; 2 to 4 weeks to maximum therapeutic effect

ADVERSE EFFECTS. Side effects include dizziness, headache, cough, sore throat, and rhinitis. Serious side effects and allergic reactions are very rare.

DRUG INTERACTIONS. No significant drug interactions have been noted.

OTHER DRUGS IN CLASS

Other drugs in this class are similar to the key, except as follows.

nedocromil Sodium (Tilade)
- Although this drug is chemically dissimilar to cromolyn, it is comparable in terms of therapeutic effects.

AEROSOL CORTICOSTEROIDS

beclomethasone dipropionate (Beclovent, Vanceril, QVar) 🔑

CONTRAINDICATIONS
- Initial treatment for severe, acute asthma attack
- Hypersensitivity to any ingredients

WARNINGS
- In patients switched from systemic corticosteroids to inhalation, adrenal insufficiency may occur in times of stress; patient may need to resume systemic delivery.
- Severe infection may occur more readily in patients on corticosteroids; therefore, immune globulin may be indicated for those exposed to chickenpox or measles.
- Combined use of ICS and alternate-day systemic therapy leads to hypothalamic-pituitary-adrenal (HPA) axis suppression more readily than occurs with either treatment used singly.
- Local fungal infections may occur in the mouth, pharynx, or larynx and may require treatment or discontinuation of the aerosol steroid.
- These products are not indicated for rapid relief of bronchospasm.
- Patients may require calcium supplementation while using the product.

PRECAUTIONS
- Use with caution in patients with active or quiescent tuberculosis; untreated systematic fungal, bacterial, parasitic, or viral infection; or ocular herpes simplex.
- Rare pulmonary infiltrates with eosinophilia may occur.

💣 Monitor for hypercorticism and HPA axis suppression. If these occur, discontinue drug gradually. Monitor for growth suppression in children.

PHARMACOKINETICS. See Table 14-3. Beclomethasone is a long-acting drug whose peak therapeutic effects are reached in days rather than hours.

ADVERSE EFFECTS. Adverse reactions of inhaled beclomethasone include oral candidiasis, irritation of the throat, cough, possible bronchospasm, and rare suppression of the HPA axis at high doses.

DOSAGE AND ADMINISTRATION. See Table 14-7.

OTHER DRUGS IN CLASS

Other drugs in this class are similar to the key, except as follows.

flunisolide (AeroBid)

- Mint-flavored, contains menthol
- Absorbed into systemic circulation more readily than other ICSs

fluticasone (Flovent)

- Delivered in a traditional MDI device
- Potent drug and available in a variety of dosages
- Lasts a long time, making it desirable for some individuals

budesonide (Pulmicort)

- Patient inhalation driven, so may be easier to actuate than most MDIs
- However, drug delivery may be dependent on force of inhalation.
- Onset of action may be faster than with other drugs—within 24 hours.

mometasone Furoate (Asmanex)

- Contraindicated in milk protein allergy
- Has unique delivery device; read directions carefully

TABLE 14-6 Adverse Reactions to Asthma and COPD Medications

Body System	β-Adrenergic Agonists	theophylline	ipratropium	Mast Cell Stabilizers	Leukotriene Receptor Antagonists
Body, general		Fever, flushing	Fatigue, pain		Fever
Skin		Rash, alopecia	Rash, alopecia		Rash
Hypersensitivity	albuterol and salmeterol: rash, angioedema		Urticaria, angioedema, rash, bronchospasm, pharyngeal edema	Rash, urticaria, angioedema	Anaphylaxis
Respiratory	Cough, bronchospasm, dry throat; dyspnea; albuterol, salmeterol: nasal congestion	Tachypnea, respiratory arrest	Cough, dyspnea, bronchitis, bronchospasm, upper respiratory infection	Bronchospasm, cough, laryngeal edema, nasal congestion, pharyngitis, wheezing, nasal irritation	zafirlukast: infections
Cardiovascular	Palpitations, tachycardia, increased blood pressure, chest tightness, arrhythmias; levalbuterol: hypotension, syncope	Palpitations, tachycardia, hypotension, circulatory failure, life-threatening ventricular arrhythmias	Palpitations, tachycardia, chest pain		
GI	Nausea/vomiting, GI distress	Nausea, vomiting, diarrhea, epigastric pain, hematemesis, GI reflux	Dry mouth, GI distress, nausea, constipation	Nausea	zileuton: abdominal pain, nausea; dyspepsia zafirlukast: nausea, diarrhea
Metabolic and nutritional		Hyperglycemia, inappropriate antidiuretic hormone syndrome			
Musculoskeletal	salmeterol: joint, muscle pain		Back pain	Joint swelling and pain	
Nervous system	Tremor, dizziness/vertigo, nervousness, hyperactivity, headache, insomnia	Headache, insomnia, irritability, seizures, restlessness, reflex hyperexcitability, muscle twitching	Nervousness, headache, insomnia, paresthesia, drowsiness, coordination difficulty, tremor, dizziness	Headache, dizziness	zafirlukast: headache, dizziness zileuton: myalgia
Special senses			Blurred vision		
Hepatic	bitolterol: increased LFTs				zileuton and zafirlukast: increased LFTs
Genitourinary		Proteinuria, potentiation of diuresis	Urinary retention	Dysuria, urinary frequency	

TABLE 14-7   Dosage and Administration Recommendations for Asthma and COPD Medications

Drug Name	Age Group	Dosage	Administration	Maximum Dose
albuterol (metered-dose aerosol)	Adults and children ≥4 yr	2 inh (90 mcg each) *or* 2 inh 15 min before exercise *or* one 200-mcg capsule for inh to 2 inh qid	q4-6h	
albuterol solution for nebulization (0.5% vial for dilution and 0.083% unit dose)	Adults and children	2.5 mg (unit dose or dilute 0.5 ml of 0.5% solution with 2.5 ml of sterile saline)	tid-qid	
	Children ≥4 yr	0.1-0.15 mg/kg/dose (for 1.25 mg, dilute 0.25 ml of 0.5% solution with 2.75 ml sterile saline)	tid-qid	
albuterol solution for nebulization (0.083% unit dose)	Adults and children 2-12 yr	2.5 mg (3 ml unit dose vial)	tid-qid	
albuterol tablets (extended and immediate release)	Adults and children >12 yr	4-8 mg ER (1-2 tab, 4 or 8 mg each) *or* 2-4 mg IR (1-2 tab, 2 or 4 mg each) Cautiously increase.	q12h tid-qid	32 mg/day
	Children 6-12 yr	4 mg ER (one 4-mg tab) *or* 2 mg IR (one 2-mg tab) Cautiously increase.	q12h tid-qid	24 mg/day
albuterol syrup (2 mg/5 ml)	Adults and children >14 yr	2-4 mg (1-2 tsp) Cautiously increase.	tid-qid	32 mg/day
	Children 6-14 yr	4 mg ER (one 4-mg tab) *or* 2 mg IR (one 2-mg tab) Cautiously increase.	tid-qid	24 mg/day
	Children 2-6 yr	0.1 mg/kg (should not exceed 2 mg) Cautiously increase to 0.2 mg/kg.	tid	4 mg tid
bitolterol (solution for nebulization)	Adults and children >12 yr	2.5 mg 0.2% solution with continuous flow neb; 1 mg with intermittent flow neb	tid-qid with at least 4 hr between treatments	14 mg (continuous); 8 mg (intermittent)
levalbuterol (metered-dose aerosol)	Adults and children ≥ 4 yr	1-2 inh (90 mcg)	q4-6h	
tiotropium	Adults	Inh of contents of 1 capsule with supplied device	qd	
levalbuterol (solution for nebulization)	Adult and children ≥12 yr	0.63 mg (unit dose 0.63 mg/3 ml) If needed, increase to 1.25 mg tid (unit dose 1.25 mg in 3 ml)	tid q6-8h	3.75 mg/day
	Children 6-11 yr	0.31 mg (unit dose 0.31 mg/3 ml)	tid	0.63 mg tid
pirbuterol (metered-dose aerosol)	Adults and children ≥12 yr	2 inh (0.2 mg each)	q4-6h	12 inh daily
salmeterol (dry powder for inhalation)	Adults and children ≥4 yr	1 inh (50 mcg blister)	q12h	Two doses daily
formoterol (dry powder for inhalation)	Adults and children ≥5 yr	1 inh (12-mcg capsule) 1 inh 15 min before exercise Do not use extra doses if already on regular daily dosing.	q12h	Two doses daily
theophylline—immediate-release form	Adults and children >45 kg	300 mg/day po; if tolerated, increase to 400 mg/day after 3 days; if tolerated, increase dose to 600 mg/day after 3 days	Divided q6-8h	Concentration not to exceed 20 mcg/ml or 900 mg/day
	Children 1-15 yr; <45 kg	Dosage based on peak concentration levels 12-14 mg/kg/day; if tolerated, increase to 16 mg/kg/day after 3 days; if tolerated, increase to 20 mg/kg/day after 3 days Dosage based on peak concentration levels	Divided q6-8h	600 mg/day
theophylline—sustained-release form	Adults and children >12 yr	10 mg/kg/day po up to 300 mg; may increase by 25% increments every 3 days, if tolerated, and until optimal clinical response is reached	qd or in 2-3 doses spaced 8-12 hr apart	800 mg/day

TABLE 14-7   Dosage and Administration Recommendations for Asthma and COPD Medications (Continued)

Drug Name	Age Group	Dosage	Administration	Maximum Dose
ipratropium (metered-dose aerosol)	Adults and children >12	2-3 inh (17 mcg each)	q6-8h	12 inh/24 hr
ipratropium (solution for nebulization)	Adults and children >12	250-500 mcg (unit dose vial) via neb	q6-8h	
cromolyn sodium (metered-dose aerosol)	Adults and children ≥5 yr	2 inh (800 mcg each)	qid	
cromolyn sodium (solution for nebulization)	Adults and children ≥2 yr	20 mg (one 2-ml ampule) via neb	qid	
nedocromil (metered-dose aerosol)	Adults and children ≥12 yr	2 inh (1.75 mg each) If good response, can be reduced to tid and then bid	qid	
beclomethasone (metered-dose aerosol) 40 mcg and 80 mcg (CFC free)	Adults	40-80 mcg if previously on bronchodilator (1-2 inh 40-mcg strength); 40-160 mcg if previously on inhaled corticosteroid (1-2 inh 40-mcg strength to 1-2 inh 80-mcg strength)	bid	640 mcg/day
	Children 5-11 yr	40 mcg	bid	160 mcg/day
budesonide (inhalation-driven dry powder)	Adults	200-400 mcg (200 mcg/inh) 400-800 mcg if previously on oral corticosteroid	bid	800 mcg/day bronchodilator therapy alone; 1600 mcg/day if on corticosteroid
	Children ≥6 yr	200 mcg (1 inh)	bid	800 mcg/day
budesonide (inhalation suspension for nebulization)	Children 12 mo to 8 yr	0.5-mg respules via neb (0.25 mg/2 ml or 0.5 mg/2 ml); 1 mg if previously on oral corticosteroid	Daily or can be divided into two equal doses	0.5 mcg/day if on bronchodilator; 1 mg/day if on corticosteroid
flunisolide (metered-dose aerosol)	Adults	2 inh (250 mcg/inh)	bid	8 inh (2 mg/day)
	Children 6-15 yr	2 inh	bid	4 inh (1 mg/day)
fluticasone (metered-dose aerosol)	Adults and children ≥12 yr	88 mcg (2 inh of 44 mcg strength) if previously on bronchodilator; 88-220 mcg if previously on inhaled corticosteroid (2 inh of 44 mcg strength to 1 or 2 inh of 110 mcg strength); 880 mcg if previously on oral corticosteroid (4 inh of 220 mcg strength)	bid	880 mcg/day if on bronchodilator or inhaled corticosteroid; 1760 mcg if on oral corticosteroid
fluticasone (dry powder inhalation)	Adults and adolescents	100-mcg if previously on bronchodilator (one 100-mcg Rotadisk); 100-250 mcg if previously on inhaled corticosteroid (one 100 mcg or 250-mcg Rotadisk); 1 mg if previously on oral corticosteroid (four 250-mcg Rotadisk)	bid	1 mg/day if on bronchodilator or inhaled corticosteroid; 2 mg/day if on oral corticosteroid
	Children 4-11 yr	50 mcg (one 50-mcg Rotadisk)	bid	200 mcg/day
triamcinolone (metered-dose aerosol)	Adults	2 inh (100 mcg each) Alternatively, 4 inh bid	tid-qid	16 inh/day (1600 mcg)
	Children 6-12 yr	1-2 inh (100 mcg each) Alternatively, 2-4 inh bid	tid-qid	12 inh/day (1200 mcg)
mometasone (metered-dose aerosol)	Adults and children > 12 yr	2 inh (220 mcg) if on bronchodilators only or inhaled corticosteroids 2 inh (220 mcg) if on oral corticosteroids	qd in the evening bid	
	Children 4-12 yr	1 inh (110 mcg)	qd in the evening	
montelukast (oral tablets)	Adult and adolescents ≥15 yr Children 6-14 yr Children 2-5 yr	10 mg 5 mg chewable tab 4 mg chewable tab	Daily (evening) Daily (evening) Daily (evening)	
zafirlukast (oral tablets)	Adults and children ≥12 yr Children 7-11 yr	20 mg 10 mg	bid bid	

Table continued on following page

TABLE 14-7   Dosage and Administration Recommendations for Asthma and COPD Medications (Continued)

Drug Name	Age Group	Dosage	Administration	Maximum Dose
zileuton	Adults and children ≥12 yr	600 mg	qid	
albuterol/ipratropium (metered-dose aerosol)	Adults	2 inh (103 mcg albuterol and 18 mcg ipratropium each inh)	qid	12 inh/day
fluticasone/salmeterol (dry powder inhalation)	Adults and children ≥12 yr	1 inh Previously on no corticosteroid therapy, use 100/50 mcg strength; previously on inhaled corticosteroid, strength based on dosage of previous corticosteroid	bid	1 inh bid of 500/50 strength

triamcinolone (Azmacort)

- Has a built-in spacer

Leukotriene Receptor Antagonists

montelukast (Singulair) 🔑

CONTRAINDICATIONS. Hypersensitivity to drug or any of its components

WARNINGS. Not indicated for acute asthma attacks or as monotherapy in exercise-induced asthma; short-term control medications should be available

PRECAUTIONS

- Should not be abruptly substituted for inhaled or oral corticosteroids
- Chewable tablets 4 and 5 mg contain phenylalanine, to which some people are allergic or have contraindications.
- Systemic eosinophilia has rarely occurred.

PHARMACOKINETICS. See Table 14-4. Drug is rapidly absorbed through the gastrointestinal tract and has a long duration of action.

ADVERSE EFFECTS. Rare; may include headache, dizziness, nausea, and diarrhea

DRUG INTERACTIONS. May cause decreased effectiveness when cytochrome P450 (CYP450) inducers such as phenobarbital and rifampin are coadministered.

OTHER DRUGS IN CLASS

Other drugs in this class are similar to the key, except as follows.

zafirlukast (Accolate)

- Take zafirlukast 1 hour before or 2 hours after meals.
- Zafirlukast increases effects of warfarin, cyclosporine, and calcium channel blockers; theophylline and erythromycin decrease levels of zafirlukast.
- Use zafirlukast cautiously in those with liver disease and the elderly; safety in children younger than 5 years has not been established.
- If signs of liver dysfunction become evident (e.g., right upper quadrant pain, nausea, anorexia, pruritus, jaundice, fatigue), discontinue zafirlukast, perform liver function tests (LFTs), and manage accordingly.

zileuton (Zyflo)

- Take 1 hour before or 2 hours after meals.
- Not indicated for children younger than 12 years
- Contraindicated in those with active liver disease; must monitor LFTs and discontinue if enzymes are present at more than three times upper limits of normal.
- Zileuton increases the effects of propranolol, theophylline, and warfarin.

evolve A continually updated list of useful WebLinks may be found in the Evolve Resources at http://evolve.elsevier.com/Edmunds/NP/

TABLE 14-8   Drug Interactions With Theophylline

Action	Drugs
Agents that increase theophylline concentration	Alcohol, allopurinol, β-blockers (nonselective), calcium channel blockers, cimetidine, corticosteroids, disulfiram, ephedrine, estrogen, influenzavirus vaccine, interferon, macrolides, mexiletine, methotrexate, quinolones, tacrine, thiabendazole, thyroid hormones, contraceptives
Agents that decrease theophylline concentration	aminoglutethimide, barbiturates, charcoal, cigarette smoking, ketoconazole, phenytoin, rifampin, sulfinpyrazone, β-blockers
Agents that may increase or decrease theophylline concentration and adverse effects	carbamazepine, isoniazid, loop diuretics, zileuton, ticlopidine, ibuprofen
Agents that are affected by theophylline	adenosine, benzodiazepines, erythromycin, halothane, ketamine, lithium pancuronium, phenytoin

evolve   http://evolve.elsevier.com/Edmunds/NP/

Hypertension and Miscellaneous Antihypertensive Medications

DRUG OVERVIEW

Class	Generic Name	Trade Name
α₁-Receptor blockers (adrenergic agonists)	doxazosin 🔑 ☀	Cardura
	prazosin	Minipress
	terazosin ☀	Hytrin
Centrally acting α₂-agonists (antiadrenergics)	clonidine 🔑 ☀	Catapres ☀
	methyldopa	Aldomet
Peripheral vasodilators	hydralazine ☀	Apresoline
	minoxidil	Loniten
Renin inhibitors	aliskiren	Tekturna

☀ Top 200 drug; 🔑 key drug.

INDICATIONS

Hypertension (HTN)

Other indications and unlabeled uses include the following:
- α₁-Receptor blockers: indicated or unlabeled use for the signs and symptoms of benign prostatic hyperplasia (BPH); prazosin has been used for posttraumatic stress disorder and Raynaud's phenomenon
- Clonidine: many unlabeled uses, including alcohol and opiate withdrawal, smoking cessation, atrial fibrillation, attention-deficit/hyperactivity disorder, menopausal flushing, constitutional growth delay in children, diabetic diarrhea, restless leg syndrome, ulcerative colitis, and the diagnosis of pheochromocytoma
- Methyldopa (unlabeled): hypertension in pregnancy
- Hydralazine (unlabeled): (CHF), pulmonary hypertension
- Minoxidil (indication): topical treatment for baldness

The management of hypertension in general is discussed, with emphasis on the Seventh Report of the Joint National Committee on the Prevention, Detection, Evaluation, and Treatment of High Blood Pressure (JNC 7) guidelines. The drugs most commonly used for hypertension are diuretics, β-blockers, calcium channel blockers, ACE inhibitors, and angiotensin II receptor blockers (ARBs). How these drugs are used to treat hypertension is discussed in this chapter. Detailed information on these antihypertensives is given in the specific drug chapters (Table 15-1). This chapter provides detailed information on other antihypertensive medications used in primary care.

THERAPEUTIC OVERVIEW OF HYPERTENSION

Anatomy and Physiology

Blood pressure (BP) must be kept at a level that is adequate to maintain tissue perfusion as the blood moves into the capillaries. Peripheral resistance, heart rate, and stroke volume interact to determine the mean arterial pressure and capillary flow. Peripheral resistance is determined by the diameter of the arterioles; constriction of the arterioles raises BP. Other factors that influence BP include changes in body position, muscular activity (which causes local warmth, thus dilating vessels), and circulating blood volume. Baroreceptors respond to local changes in BP by constricting or relaxing local smooth muscle to change blood flow. Many hormones also cause contraction or relaxation of arteriolar smooth muscle to bring blood flow to a specific organ. The renin-angiotensin system is an important regulatory feedback loop component of this system. A drop in BP to the renal arteries stimulates the secretion of renin. Renin activates the renin-angiotensin system by cleaving angiotensinogen produced in the liver to yield angiotensin I, which is further converted into angiotensin II by ACE, the angiotensin-converting enzyme. Angiotensin II then constricts blood cells, increases the secretion of antidiuretic hormone (ADH) and aldosterone, and causes reabsorption of sodium in the kidneys, thus leading to water retention, increased blood volume, and increased BP.

TABLE 15-1   Drugs Commonly Used for Hypertension (listed in order of use)

Additional information related to these drugs can be found in the chapters below.

Drug	Abbreviation	Chapter
Thiazide diuretics	THIAZ	30
β-Blockers	BBs	18
Angiotensin-converting enzyme	ACE	20
Angiotensin II receptor blockers	ARBs	20
Calcium channel blockers	CCBs	19
Aldosterone antagonist	ALDO ANT	30

Pathophysiology

Some conditions produce secondary hypertension as a consequence of other disease. The hypertension that results from these conditions is often treatable (see Table 15-3). The cause of primary hypertension (which accounts for approximately 95% of cases of hypertension) remains unknown. Although these are not completely understood, many factors have been linked to primary hypertension, including some that are genetically determined. Involved mechanisms include elevated peripheral resistance, alteration in the cell membrane related to elevated lipids, endothelial dysfunction, changes in sodium or calcium levels, and hyperinsulinemia. Sympathetic nervous system hyperactivity caused by insensitivity of the baroreflexes may contribute to hypertension accompanied by tachycardia and elevated cardiac output in younger patients.

Dysregulation of the renin-angiotensin system leads to hypertension, although this does not appear to be a major factor in the origin of hypertension. African Americans with hypertension and older adult patients tend to have lower plasma renin activity. Approximately 10% of hypertensive individuals have high levels, 60% have normal, and 30% have low renin levels.

Some patients have a decreased ability to excrete sodium, which leads to increased blood volume and increased BP. Sodium restriction may be necessary in these individuals. Abnormalities in sodium transport mechanisms lead to an increased level of intracellular sodium in blood cells. This may result in the increased vascular smooth muscle tone characteristic of hypertension.

Environmental, lifestyle, and dietary factors also play important, and modifiable, roles. Obesity leads to increased intravascular volume and increased cardiac output. Alcohol increases BP by increasing plasma catecholamines. Cigarette smoking raises BP by increasing plasma norepinephrine.

NSAIDs cause fluid retention, which can lead to hypertension. Excessive intake of sodium (salt) or low levels of potassium can contribute to hypertension by increasing blood volume. Physical inactivity is a recently recognized risk factor.

Hypertension is a powerful risk factor for cardiac disease. The higher the BP, the greater is the risk for ischemic heart disease, heart attack, heart failure, stroke, and kidney disease. In adults, each increase of 20 mm Hg in systolic blood pressure (SBP) or 10 mm Hg in diastolic blood pressure (DBP) doubles the patient's risk of cardiovascular disease (CVD). This knowledge has led to an emphasis on the lower spectrum of BP, resulting in the classification of "prehypertension," which is new to JNC 7.

A "metabolic syndrome" has recently been identified as a major cardiac risk factor. This constellation of symptoms is also referred to as syndrome X, the insulin resistance syndrome, or the obesity dyslipidemia syndrome. A patient who has abdominal obesity, hypertension, insulin resistance, and a lipid disorder has a greatly elevated risk of CVD. Instead of serving as separate risk factors, they work together to increase risk. Table 15-2 lists the major cardiovascular risk factors. The WHO diabetes group proposed a set of criteria for diagnosing the metabolic syndrome in 1998 and later updated these (Grundy et al, 2004). This definition is as follows:

Hyperinsulinemia (defined as the upper quartile of a measure of insulin resistance in the nondiabetic population) OR a fasting plasma glucose (FPG) greater than or equal to 110 mg/dl (6.1 mmol/L) or a plasma glucose two hours after an oral glucose tolerance test greater than or equal to 200 mg/dl (11.1 mmol/L)

PLUS at least two of the following:
1. Abdominal obesity, defined as a waist-to-hip ratio greater than 0.90, a body mass index (BMI) ≥30 kg/m², or a waist-to-girth ratio ≥0.9 in men and 0.85 in women
2. Dyslipidemia, defined as serum triglycerides 150 mg/dl (1.7 mmol/L)
3. HDL cholesterol <35 mg/dl (0.9 mmol/L) in men or <39 mg/dl (1.0 mmol/L) in women

TABLE 15-2   Major Cardiovascular Risk Factors for Hypertension

Metabolic syndrome
Hypertension
Dyslipidemia
Obesity (body mass index [BMI] ≥30)*
Diabetes mellitus
Cigarette smoking
Physical inactivity
Microalbuminuria or estimated glomerular filtration rate (GFR) <60 ml/min
Family history of premature cardiovascular disease (men younger than age 55 or women younger than 65 years)

From Joint National Committee on the Prevention, Detection, Evaluation, and Treatment of High Blood Pressure Education Program: *The seventh report of the Joint National Committee on Prevention, Detection, Evaluation, and Treatment of High Blood Pressure,* NIH publication No. 03-5233, Bethesda, MD, May 2003, National Institutes of Health, National Heart, Lung, and Blood Institute.

*Body mass index is calculated as: $\dfrac{\text{Weight (in kg)}}{\text{Height (in m}^2)}$

4. BP ≥140/90 mm Hg or the administration of antihypertensive drugs
5. Urinary albumin excretion rate >20 mcg/min or albumin-to-creatinine ratio >30 mg/g

Disease Process

Fifty million Americans have hypertension, and the prevalence increases with age. Only about 34% of these people are adequately treated. Hypertension is a risk factor for CVD, stroke, CHF, renal failure, and peripheral vascular disease (ALLHAT, 2002). CVD and stroke are the most common causes of death in the United States. Current levels of cardiovascular morbidity and mortality show that much greater effort is required to control hypertension (ALLHAT, 2002).

The pendulum continues to swing regarding which factor is the most important to control: systolic or diastolic BP. Systolic BP was first considered to be most important; subsequently, focus shifted to diastolic BP. Some researchers are exploring the significance of pulse pressure (difference between systolic and diastolic BP). However, ongoing research suggests that management scenarios must address both systolic and diastolic BP levels.

Assessment

The diagnosis of hypertension is based on the average of readings taken at an initial screening and two or more readings taken at each of two or more subsequent visits. The readings on these three separate occasions should not be influenced by any other known mechanism, such as recent exercise, anxiety, or an acute illness. Initial evaluation includes a thorough history, physical examination, and laboratory screening (Box 15-1).

Once the diagnosis of hypertension is made, further evaluation of three factors that are affecting the patient's risk is necessary. Severity should be determined according to the classification in Table 15-3. Next, target organ damage (Table 15-4), which is the damage the hypertension has already caused, should be evaluated. Finally, assessment should be completed for compelling indications (Table 15-5), which include conditions managed in parallel with HTN. These three factors will affect management.

Although primary hypertension is very common, it is essential for the clinician to rule out secondary causes of hypertension. Certain laboratory findings are suggestive of secondary causes, and secondary causes should be suspected if the patient's hypertension does not respond to therapy, the hypertension is of sudden onset (especially before age 20 or after age 50), a patient with well-controlled hypertension demonstrates a sudden increase in BP, or stage 3 hypertension develops.

MECHANISM OF ACTION

α_1-Receptor Blockers (Adrenergics)

α_1-Receptor blockers act by blocking postsynaptic α_1-adrenergic receptors. (Some agents are more selective as blockers than others.) This causes dilation of arterioles and veins and reduces peripheral vascular resistance, as well as supine and standing BP. These drugs tend to affect the diastolic more than the systolic BP. They also relax smooth muscles in the bladder neck and prostate, reducing bladder outlet obstruction without affecting bladder contractility.

Centrally Acting α_2-Agonists (Antiadrenergics)

Centrally acting agonist agents, such as clonidine and methyldopa, act through stimulation of central inhibitory α-adrenergic receptors. They inhibit sympathetic cardioaccelerator and vasoconstrictor centers. Stimulation of α-adrenergic receptors in the brainstem results in reduced sympathetic outflow from the central nervous system (CNS), causing a decrease in peripheral resistance, renal vascular resistance, heart rate, and BP. Renal blood flow and glomerular filtration rate remain essentially unchanged.

Direct Vasodilators

Direct vasodilators relax arteriolar smooth muscle and decrease peripheral vascular resistance. This stimulates the carotid sinus baroreceptors, producing reflex increases in heart rate, renin release, and, consequently, sodium and water retention. Hydralazine and minoxidil decrease arterial BP by reducing peripheral vascular resistance. Reflex sympathetic action results in increased heart rate and cardiac output. Neither agent promotes orthostatic hypotension because of the preferential dilation of arterioles as compared with veins. However, reflex renin release leads to production of angiotensin II, which promotes aldosterone release and sodium reabsorption. Hydralazine increases heart rate and sympathetic discharge, so it is frequently used in combination with β-blockers, clonidine, or methyldopa. Minoxidil triggers cardiac and renal homeostatic mechanisms; therefore, β-blockers and diuretics are included as part of the treatment regimen.

Renin Inhibitors

Aliskiren, the first drug in this new class of drugs, acts to block the action of renin at the top of the renin-angiotensin-system cascade. Thus, it is characterized as providing triple blockage of the renin-angiotensin system (RAS). Aliskiren acts by targeting the RAS at the first and rate-limiting step. Although aliskiren increases renin production, the renin produced is inhibited and its capacity to form angiotensin I, as measured by assessment of plasma renin activity (PRA), is reduced. (By contrast, ACE inhibitors, ARBs, and thiazide diuretics all increase plasma renin concentration and PRA, thereby producing angiotensin I, which is then available for conversion to angiotensin II.) In addition, renin inhibitors do not affect kinin metabolism and hence would not be expected to cause dry cough or angioneurotic edema, both of which are characteristic side effects of ACE inhibitors.

TREATMENT PRINCIPLES

Standardized Guidelines

- Rosendorff C et al: Treatment of hypertension in the prevention and management of ischemic heart disease: a scientific statement from the American Heart Association Council for High Blood Pressure Research and the Councils on Clinical Cardiology and Epidemiology and Prevention. *Circulation* 115:2761-2788, 2007.
- National Institutes of Health, National Heart, Lung, and Blood Institute (NHLBI): The seventh report of the Joint National Committee on the Prevention, Detection, Evaluation and Treatment of High Blood Pressure. *Hypertension* 42(6):1206-1252, 2003.

BOX 15-1   Clinical and Diagnostic Evaluation for Patients with Documented Hypertension

THREE MAIN PURPOSES

- Identify known causes of hypertension.
- Assess presence/absence of TOD and CVD, extent of disease, and response to therapy.
- Identify other cardiovascular risk factors and comorbid conditions; continue/modify treatment as indicated.

HISTORY

- BP history, including duration
- Age of onset (<20 or >50 years, think secondary hypertension)
- Levels of hypertension (>180/110 mm Hg, think secondary hypertension)
- Laboratory or diagnostic testing
- All previous treatments and responses to therapy, including adverse events (resistance to therapy, think secondary hypertension)
- Personal or family history or patient symptoms of coronary heart disease (CHD; especially premature in family), heart failure, cerebrovascular disease, peripheral vascular disease, renal disease, diabetes mellitus, dyslipidemia, or other comorbidity, such as gout or sexual dysfunction
- Listen for symptoms that suggest causes of hypertension (secondary hypertension), such as headache, daytime somnolence, fatigue, tachycardia, claudication, cold feet, sweating, thinning of skin, flank pain, muscle weakness, and tremor.
- Lifestyle assessment, including recent weight changes, physical activity profile, cigarette smoking, dietary intake of sodium, alcohol, saturated fat, and caffeine
- Medication history, including over-the-counter drugs, herbal remedies, and illicit drugs
- Psychosocial and environmental factors that may influence hypertension control

PHYSICAL EXAMINATION

- In particular, look for signs of secondary hypertension, such as variable pressures with tachycardia, sweating or tremors, hyperdynamic apical pulse, murmurs at anterior or posterior thorax, abnormal pulsations in neck, abdominal bruit, abdominal or flank masses, truncal obesity with purple striae, weak femoral pulses, or absent pedal pulses.
- Two or more BP measurements, 2 minutes apart, patient either supine or seated and after standing for at least 2 minutes
- Verification in contralateral arm (higher value should be used)
- Height, weight, and waist circumference
- Funduscopic examination
- Examination of neck (assess for carotid bruits, jugular venous distention, or thyroid enlargement)
- Examination of heart (assess for precordial heaves, enlargement, abnormal rate or rhythm, extra sounds, including murmurs, clicks, S3, S4)
- Examination of lungs (assess for evidence of congestion or bronchospasm)
- Examination of abdomen (assess for abnormal aortic pulsations, bruits, enlarged kidneys, masses)
- Examination of extremities (assess for arterial pulses, bruits, or edema)

NEUROLOGIC ASSESSMENT

Initial Diagnostic Screening

- Before initiation of therapy, focus on determining TOD or other risk factors
- Urinalysis
- CBC
- Blood chemistries (sodium, potassium, creatinine, fasting glucose, and total and HDL cholesterol)
- Twelve-lead electrocardiogram

Optional Laboratory Tests

- 24-Hour urine for microalbuminuria, creatinine clearance, or urinary protein
- Serum calcium
- Uric acid
- Fasting triglycerides and LDL cholesterol
- Glycosylated hemoglobin
- Sensitive TSH
- Limited echocardiography to determine presence of LVH

From Joint National Committee on the Prevention, Detection, Evaluation, and Treatment of High Blood Pressure Education Program: *The seventh report of the Joint National Committee on Prevention, Detection, Evaluation, and Treatment of High Blood Pressure,* NIH Publication No. 03-5233, Bethesda, MD, May 2003, National Institutes of Health, National Heart, Lung, and Blood Institute.

Material on secondary causes modified from Kaplan NM: *Clinical hypertension,* Baltimore, 1998, Williams & Wilkins.

- National Heart, Lung, and Blood Institute: The fourth report on the diagnosis, evaluation, and treatment of high blood pressure in children and adolescents, Bethesda, MD, August 2004, NHLBI.

Evidence-Based Recommendations

In clinical trials:
- Antihypertensive therapy has been associated with 35% to 40% mean reduction in the incidence of stroke; 20% to 25% reduction in MI; and >50% in heart failure.
- It is estimated that control of hypertension to at or below 140/90 mm Hg could, in men and women, prevent 19% and 31% of coronary heart disease events, respectively, whereas optimal control to below 130/80 mm Hg could prevent 37% and 56% of coronary heart disease events, respectively.
- All antihypertensive agents equally reduced total mortality, cardiovascular mortality, and MI.
- α-Blockers were less effective than other antihypertensive agents in reducing rates of stroke and combined cardiovascular events.
- Calcium channel blockers and α-blockers were less effective in reducing heart failure.
- Hypertension during pregnancy: methyldopa and labetalol were preferred. Long-acting nifedipine was also acceptable.

TABLE 15-3   Secondary Causes of Hypertension

Pathology	Signs and Symptoms	Diagnostic Studies
Coarctation of the aorta	Delayed or absent femoral arterial pulses, decreased BP in lower extremities	ECG, chest x-ray studies, echocardiography, Doppler ultrasonography
Cushing's syndrome	Long-term steroid use: truncal obesity with purple striae, moon facies	Morning plasma cortisol after 1 mg hour of sleep dexamethasone
Pheochromocytoma	Labile HTN, tachycardia, headache, palpitations, pallor, sweating, or tremors	Spot urine for metanephrine
Primary aldosteronism	Muscle weakness, polydipsia, polyuria	Hypokalemia, excessive urinary potassium excretion, suppressed levels of plasma renin activity, elevated sodium level
Chronic kidney disease	Abdominal or flank masses (polycystic kidneys)	Urinalysis, creatinine, renal ultrasound
Renovascular disease	Epigastric or renal artery bruits, atherosclerotic disease of aorta or peripheral arteries	Renal duplex ultrasound, renal arteriography
Sleep apnea	Fatigue, loud cyclic snoring	Polysomnography
Hyperthyroidism	Weight loss, fatigue, tachycardia	TSH, T_4, free T_4, free T_4 index
Hypothyroidism	Weight gain, fatigue	May be due to decreased tissue metabolism leading to low production of vasodilating metabolites
Hyperparathyroidism	Renal stones, polyuria, constipation	Serum and urine calcium, urine phosphate, serum parathyroid hormone

Cardinal Points of Treatment

BP targets in men and women with established coronary artery disease (CAD), or who are at high risk of developing CAD, should be 130/80 mm Hg. The BP target of 140/90 remains appropriate for general CAD prevention.
- Initial drug choices:
  - In patients without compelling indications: Thiazide-type diuretics (THIAZs) are used for most. Cardioselective β-blockers (BBs), ACE inhibitors, ARBs, and calcium channel blockers (CCBs), or a combination, may be considered.
  - In patients with compelling indications:

Heart failure—THIAZs, BBs (heart failure [HF] due to diastolic dysfunction only), ACEIs, ARBs, ALDO ANT
Post MI—cardioselective BBs, ACEIs, ALDO ANT
High CVD risk—THIAZs, BBs, ACEIs, CCBs
Diabetes—THIAZs, BBs, ACEIs, ARBs, CCBs
Chronic kidney disease—ACEIs, ARBs
Recurrent stroke prevention—THIAZs, ACEIs
Chronic obstructive pulmonary disease (COPD), asthma—CCBs
African American patients—CCBs + THIAZs, THIAZs (Disease-specific contraindications to these guidelines have been identified.)

TABLE 15-4   JNC 7 Classification and Management of Blood Pressure for Adults

BP Classification	SBP, mm Hg	DBP, mm Hg	INITIAL DRUG THERAPY	
			Without Compelling Indication	With Compelling Indication (see Table 15-5)
Normal	<120	and <80	None indicated	Drugs for compelling indications
Prehypertension	120-139	or 80-89	None indicated	
Stage 1 HTN	140-159	or 90-99	Thiazide-type diuretics for most	Drug(s) for compelling indications
			May consider ACEI, ARB, BB, CCB, or combination	Other antihypertensive drugs (diuretics, ACEIs, ARBs, BBs, CCBs) as needed
Stage 2 HTN	≥160	or ≥100	Two-drug combination for most (usually, thiazide-type diuretic and ACE or ARB or BB or CCB)	Same as above

From Joint National Committee on the Prevention, Detection, Evaluation, and Treatment of High Blood Pressure Education Program: *The seventh report of the Joint National Committee on Prevention, Detection, Evaluation, and Treatment of High Blood Pressure,* NIH Publication No. 03-5233, Bethesda, MD, May 2003, National Institutes of Health, National Heart, Lung, and Blood Institute.

TABLE 15-5   Target Organ Damage Occurring With Hypertension

HEART
Left ventricular hypertrophy
Angina or prior myocardial infarction
Prior coronary revascularization
Heart failure
BRAIN
Stroke or transient ischemic attack
Chronic kidney disease
Peripheral arterial disease
Retinopathy

From Joint National Committee on the Prevention, Detection, Evaluation, and Treatment of High Blood Pressure Education Program: *The seventh report of the Joint National Committee on Prevention, Detection, Evaluation, and Treatment of High Blood Pressure*, NIH publication No. 03-5233, Bethesda, MD, May 2003, National Institutes of Health, National Heart, Lung, and Blood Institute.

Nonpharmacologic Treatment

Lifestyle modification is an important part of treatment for all patients with hypertension (Box 15-2). Those at lower risk may undergo a longer trial of lifestyle modification only. Individuals at higher risk should have treatment initiated with both lifestyle modification and drug therapy.

The importance of lifestyle modification in the management of hypertension cannot be overstated. Lifestyle modifications are not easy to adopt or maintain. However, these changes in behavior are inexpensive and present minimal risk. They may prevent hypertension in some individuals, decrease BP or the need for additional therapeutic agents in others, and ultimately reduce other known risk factors for CVD. Health care providers should be prepared to establish long-term therapeutic relationships with patients and to participate as motivators, educators, and role models in community-based programs as an essential part of the team approach needed to sustain these lifestyle changes.

Pharmacologic Treatment

Table 15-5 summarizes hypertension management based on BP stage and compelling indications. Treatment of hypertension is a complex and multifaceted task. Systematic treatment and monitoring such as that illustrated in Figure 15-1 are essential.

The JNC 7 guidelines should be used to determine drug choice.

- Start lifestyle modifications.
- Start drug treatment as indicated in Table 15-5.
- Make the initial drug choice based on stage and compelling indications.
- Titrate dose: If the clinical goal is not achieved after maximum dose or intolerance of side effects, then substitute another drug from a different class or add a second agent (usually a diuretic).

The JNC 7 places new emphasis on the use of diuretics as the first choice of drug therapy for uncomplicated hypertension. If there are specific indications for a certain drug, it should be used (see Table 15-5). If there are compelling indications, specific drugs should be used.

BOX 15-2   Lifestyle Modifications for Patients with Hypertension

- Lose weight if overweight.
- Limit alcohol intake (≤1 oz ethanol/day for men and ≤0.5 oz ethanol/day for women or lighter-weight persons).
- Increase aerobic activity (30 to 45 min/day most days of the week).
- Reduce sodium intake (≤100 mmol/day, 2.4 g sodium or 6 g sodium chloride).
- Maintain adequate intake of dietary potassium (↑ 90 mmol/day).
- Maintain adequate intake of dietary calcium and magnesium.
- Stop smoking.
- Reduce intake of dietary saturated fat and cholesterol.

From Joint National Committee on the Prevention, Detection, Evaluation, and Treatment of High Blood Pressure Education Program: *The seventh report of the Joint National Committee on Prevention, Detection, Evaluation, and Treatment of High Blood Pressure*, NIH Publication No. 03-5233, Bethesda, MD, May 2003, National Institutes of Health, National Heart, Lung, and Blood Institute.

Commonly used drugs include diuretics, β-blockers, ACEIs, CCBs, and ARBs. The most commonly used diuretic is hydrochlorothiazide. Loop diuretics are used in patients who have renal insufficiency. Potassium-sparing diuretics such as triamterene are used in combination, usually with hydrochlorothiazide, if the patient has low levels of potassium; they should be administered with caution. Aldosterone antagonists such as spironolactone (also a potassium-sparing diuretic) and eplerenone, often are used in patients with CHF and after MI, but the potassium level should be monitored closely.

β-Blockers are effective and have well-demonstrated cardioprotective effects after an MI. However, these effects have not been validated for the treatment of hypertension. The cardioselective β-blockers have a greater effect on the β₁-cardiac receptors than on the β₂-receptors in the bronchi and blood vessels. However, they become less selective as the dosage is increased. Previous JNC recommendations called for use of β-blockers as first-line therapy; many continue to consider them a good first-line treatment for young patients. β-Blockers, however, are not recommended for elderly patients unless the patient has a compelling indication for a β-blocker. β-Blockers with intrinsic sympathomimetic activity (ISA) may be useful for patients who develop symptomatic bradycardia or postural hypotension when taking other β-blockers. Cardioselective β-blockers without ISA are preferred for patients with angina or a history of MI.

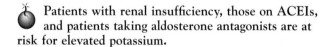 **Patients with renal insufficiency, those on ACEIs, and patients taking aldosterone antagonists are at risk for elevated potassium.**

ACEIs are very effective and safe for the treatment of patients with hypertension. They are cardioprotective. They are useful in preserving renal function but must be used with

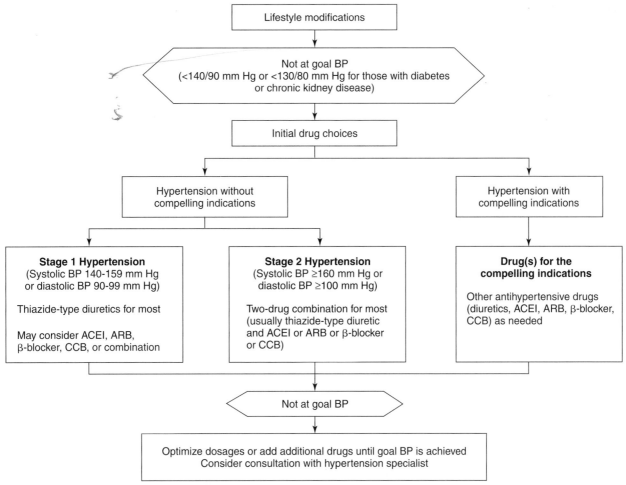

FIGURE 15-1   Hypertension treatment algorithm. (From Joint National Committee on the Prevention, Detection, Evaluation, and Treatment of High Blood Pressure Education Program: *The seventh report of the Joint National Committee on Prevention, Detection, Evaluation, and Treatment of High Blood Pressure,* National Institutes of Health, National Heart, Lung, and Blood Institute, NIH Publication No. 03-5233, Bethesda, MD, NHLBI, May 2003.)

caution in patients with preexisting renal failure because of the risk of hyperkalemia. The first ACEI, captopril, was associated with a dry cough. However, newer ACEIs have a low incidence of cough. ACEIs should be used with caution in women of childbearing age because of the potential for damage to a fetus. ARBs are as effective as ACEIs, and they do not cause cough.

CCBs do not have the cardioprotective characteristics of ACEIs, ARBs, and β-blockers. Short-acting CCBs should not be used for the treatment of patients with hypertension. Verapamil and diltiazem can affect atrioventricular conduction and should be used with caution in patients on β-blockers. Verapamil and diltiazem have numerous drug interactions.

Cost can be an important issue in drug choice. Certain antihypertensive agents are available in generic form and can be much less expensive than drugs that are available only under a trade name. The drug lists in each chapter identify those with generic equivalents, for the provider's review. Practitioners should have a good idea of the relative costs of the medications that they prescribe.

OTHER ANTIHYPERTENSIVE AGENTS. All of the drugs in this chapter can be added to the treatment regimen when initial monotherapy fails.

The α₁-receptor blockers may be used as first-line therapy in patients with BPH. Prazosin is given less frequently than terazosin or doxazosin because of the increased frequency of first-dose syncope. α₁-Receptor blockers cause fewer incidences of reflex tachycardia than are caused by the direct vasodilators, but they more frequently cause postural hypotension. They may cause stress incontinence in women and postural hypotension in older adults.

Clonidine is the only centrally acting antiadrenergic drug in common use. Antiadrenergic agents frequently cause fluid accumulation. Diuretics usually are needed to provide synergistic effects and to prevent fluid accumulation. The centrally acting agents produce an increased incidence of adverse CNS effects such as sedation, depression, dry mouth, and impotence.

Direct vasodilators usually are used in a three-drug regimen. They frequently produce reflex tachycardia but rarely cause orthostatic hypotension. A β-blocker prevents reflex tachycardia caused by decreased peripheral resistance, and a diuretic prevents secondary fluid accumulation. Hydralazine and minoxidil have direct vasodilating actions, but they are reserved for use in those individuals who do not respond to maximal dosages of other medications. Hydralazine is used more often in patients who have CHF, usually as a fourth-line drug. Minoxidil rarely fails to lower BP; it should be reserved for patients who have the most severe hypertension refractory to other drugs because it can cause serious adverse reactions such as fluid retention. ACEIs have largely eliminated the need for minoxidil.

HYPERTENSIVE EMERGENCIES, URGENCIES, AND SEVERE HYPERTENSION.

Hypertensive emergencies and urgencies occur as acute rises in blood pressure. Emergencies are accompanied by end organ damage; urgencies occur without end organ damage. *Hypertensive emergency* is defined as SBP >180 or DBP >120, and patients should be referred to the emergency department for treatment. In hypertensive urgencies, patients should be treated with oral medication over 24 to 48 hours, usually on an inpatient basis. Those with severe hypertension may be treated in the outpatient setting with the goal of long-term control with the use of drugs as directed by JNC 7. Lowering BP too rapidly may cause stroke, symptomatic hypotension, MI, and death.

How to Monitor

α_1-RECEPTOR BLOCKERS.
Monitor BP on a regular basis.

CENTRALLY ACTING α_2-ANTIADRENERGICS: METHYLDOPA
- Monitor BP on a regular basis.
- Obtain baseline and periodic CBC.
- Monitor liver function over the first 12 weeks of therapy.
- Perform periodic liver function tests (LFTs), especially during the first 6 to 12 weeks of therapy, or when unexplained fever occurs.
- Consider direct Coombs' test at baseline and at 6 and 12 months.
- Renal function should be monitored because dosing guidelines are changed by renal impairment.

DIRECT VASODILATORS
- Monitor BP on a regular basis.
- Obtain baseline ECG.
- Monitor for blood dyscrasias.
- Monitor renal function studies, weight gain, and signs of edema.
- Obtain baseline antinuclear antibodies (ANAs) before hydralazine therapy is initiated because lupus-type symptoms may occur.
- Measure serum creatinine/BUN periodically.

Patient Variables

GERIATRICS
- Older adults are more likely than younger patients to have systolic hypertension and are more likely to experience adverse reactions, such as orthostatic hypotension, that can cause falls.
- α_1-Adrenergic blockers: Use is limited because of the side effects of syncope and tachycardia.
- Centrally acting α_2-antiadrenergics:
  - Be vigilant in monitoring for orthostatic hypotension, which may cause falls.
  - Use with caution in renal failure.
  - Clonidine may cause cognitive dysfunction and sedation and may increase the risk of falls.

- Direct vasodilators
  - May precipitate angina in patients with CAD
  - May cause or aggravate pericardial and pleural effusions
  - May increase cerebral and renal blood flow, which may affect dosing

PEDIATRICS.
None of these drugs is indicated in pediatric patients.

Hypertension in children is defined as BP above the 95th percentile for age, gender, and height. Indications for treatment include symptomatic hypertension, secondary hypertension, hypertensive target organ damage, diabetes types 1 and 2, persistent hypertension despite nonpharmacologic measures, and compelling reasons. (See guidelines for tables and additional information. See the National Heart, Lung, and Blood Institute's fourth report for specific recommendations for children.) Acceptable classes for use in children include ACEIs, ARBs, β-blockers, CCBs, and diuretics.

PREGNANCY AND LACTATION.
JNC 7 recommends methyldopa for women when hypertension is first diagnosed during pregnancy.
- The American Academy of Pediatrics considers most β-blockers (refer to specific drugs in database) and CCBs to be "compatible" with breastfeeding. Labetalol and propranolol are preferred because these drugs are not concentrated in breast milk, in contrast to other β-blockers. Methyldopa is classified as category B.

RACE
- Incidence of hypertension in whites is 10% to 15%.
- Incidence of hypertension in blacks is 20% to 30%; African Americans also have higher BP, which is more difficult to treat.
- African Americans tend to respond better than whites to diuretic monotherapy.
- ACEIs, ARBs, and β-blockers are less effective than other agents unless used with a diuretic.
- African Americans are more likely than whites to develop angioedema with ACEIs.
- CCBs and ARBs are preferred for use in African Americans.

GENDER
- α_1-Receptor blockers tend to be used in older men because of their positive effects on BPH.
- Use minoxidil with caution in women because of hirsutism.

Patient Education

ALL ANTIHYPERTENSIVES
- Do not discontinue taking medication unless directed to do so by the health care provider because rebound hypertension may occur.
- Avoid taking cough, cold, or allergy medications that contain sympathomimetics that may cause blood pressure elevations.
- May cause orthostatic hypotension. If dizziness occurs, avoid sudden changes in position. Use caution when rising from a sitting or lying position. A hot bath or shower may aggravate the dizziness. Dehydration may increase the risk of orthostatic hypotension.

α₁-RECEPTOR BLOCKERS

- Warn of the potential for syncope. Make sure the patient takes the first few doses when supine because of the possibility of first-dose syncope.
- Avoid driving and other hazardous tasks.
- Warn men of the possibility of priapism.

CENTRALLY ACTING α₂-ANTIADRENERGICS

- Drowsiness is a common adverse reaction. Take at bedtime.
- Use caution when operating machinery or driving.
- Do not use with alcohol or other CNS depressants; tolerance to these products may be decreased.
- Use hard candy or frequent mouth care to relieve symptoms of dry mouth.

DIRECT VASODILATORS

- Urine exposed to the air may darken.
- Take hydralazine with meals.
- Notify provider if unexplained prolonged fatigue or fever, muscle or joint aches, or chest pain is experienced.

SPECIFIC DRUGS

α₁-RECEPTOR BLOCKERS

doxazosin (Cardura)

CONTRAINDICATIONS. Hypersensitivity to doxazosin, prazosin, terazosin, or tamsulosin

WARNINGS
- Syncope and first-dose effect
- May worsen angina

> ☢ Watch for "first-dose" effect. These drugs can cause marked hypotension, especially postural, and syncope. Hypotension with syncope may occur during the first 30 to 90 minutes after the first several doses.

- Priapism occurs rarely. Administer doxazosin with caution to patients with evidence of hepatic impairment and to patients on other medications metabolized by the liver.

PRECAUTIONS
- Orthostatic hypotension may occur.
- Leukopenia/neutropenia has occasionally occurred.
- Rule out prostate cancer before starting therapy.
- Cardiotoxicity: Rats and mice have had an increased incidence of myocardial necrosis or fibrosis. There is no evidence that similar lesions occur in humans.

PHARMACOKINETICS. See Table 15-6 for pharmacokinetics.

ADVERSE EFFECTS. See Table 15-7. The most common problem is orthostatic hypotension.

DRUG INTERACTIONS. Alcohol, β-blockers, cimetidine, and verapamil may increase effects of α-adrenergic blockers.

DOSAGE AND ADMINISTRATION. See Table 15-8. Extended-release form of doxazosin is not indicated for hypertension.

OTHER DRUGS IN CLASS

Other drugs in this class are similar to the prototype, except as follows:
- Terazosin (Hytrin) has the additional side effects of peripheral edema and weight gain.
- Prazosin (Minipress) has a higher incidence of first-dose syncope and hypotension than doxazosin or terazosin.

CENTRALLY ACTING α₂-ANTIADRENERGICS

clonidine (Catapres)

CONTRAINDICATIONS. Hypersensitivity to clonidine or the components of the transdermal system

WARNINGS
- Use with caution in patients with severe coronary insufficiency, conduction disturbances, recent MI, CVD, or chronic renal failure.
- Tolerance may develop.

PRECAUTIONS

> ☢ Rebound hypertension may occur with abrupt withdrawal.

- Discontinue the drug gradually.
- Symptoms of rebound hypertension include rapid rise in blood pressure, tachycardia, nervousness, agitation, and headache.
- In addition, tremors and confusion may occur with abrupt withdrawal.
- Sedation or drowsiness is a very common adverse effect.
- Stop drug within 4 hours of surgery and resume as soon as possible during immediate postoperative course.
- Clonidine patches are applied every 7 days. Sensitization to transdermal clonidine may produce a generalized rash.

ADVERSE EFFECTS. See Table 15-7. Dry mouth (40%), drowsiness (33%), dizziness (16%) and sedation (10%) are very common. Orthostatic hypotension is also commonly seen.

DRUG INTERACTIONS
- Tricyclic antidepressants (TCAs) decrease the effects of clonidine.
- Clonidine may enhance the CNS depressive effects of alcohol or other sedatives.
- Clonidine can cause bradycardia and so should be used cautiously with β-blockers.

OTHER DRUGS IN CLASS

Other drugs in this class are similar to the key drug, except as follows.

methyldopa (Aldomet)

CONTRAINDICATIONS
- Active liver disease
- Coadministration with MAOIs and sulfite sensitivity if oral suspension is used

TABLE 15-6   Compelling Indications and Recommended Treatment for Hypertension

Compelling Indication	Diuretic	BB	ACEI	ARB	CCB	Aldosterone Antagonist
Chronic kidney disease			X	X		
Diabetes			X	X	X	
Heart failure	X	X	X	X		X
High risk for CAD			X	X	X	
Post MI		X	X	X		
Recurrent stroke prevention	X		X			

From Joint National Committee on the Prevention, Detection, Evaluation, and Treatment of High Blood Pressure Education Program: *The seventh report of the Joint National Committee on Prevention, Detection, Evaluation, and Treatment of High Blood Pressure,* NIH publication No. 03-5233, Bethesda, MD, May 2003, National Institutes of Health, National Heart, Lung, and Blood Institute.

WARNING

 Positive Coombs' test (10%-20% of patients), hemolytic anemia, and liver disorders may occur.

- Hepatic toxicity (elevated liver enzymes, fever, and jaundice) has occurred during the first 3 weeks of therapy. If fever occurs, a workup for adverse reaction is indicated.
- Fatal hepatic necrosis has been reported. This may be a hypersensitivity reaction.

PRECAUTIONS

- Use with caution in patients who have renal insufficiency.
- Transient sedation may occur during initial drug therapy.

DRUG INTERACTIONS

- Coadministration of methyldopa and lithium may cause lithium toxicity (i.e., GI distress, tremor, weakness, and lethargy).
- Use of MAOIs leads to excess sympathetic discharge; concomitant use is contraindicated.
- Coadministration of iron salts may lead to decreased methyldopa absorption.
- COMT inhibitors (tolcapone, entacapone) also decrease methyldopa metabolism.

Peripheral Vasodilators

Hydralazine is discussed; minoxidil is seldom used.

TABLE 15-7   Pharmacokinetics of Other Antihypertensive Medications

Drug	Absorption	Drug Availability	Onset of Action	Time to Peak Concentration	Half-Life	Duration of Action	Protein Bound	Metabolism	Excretion
prazosin (Minipress)	—	43%-82%	2 hr	1-3 hr	2-3 hr	10-24 hr	92%-97%	Extensive; active metabolites	Bile/feces, 90%; urine, 10%
terazosin (Hytrin)	Complete	90%	1-2 hr	1-2 hr	9-12 hr	12-24 hr	90%-94%	70% metabolized	Bile/feces, 60%; urine, 40%
doxazosin (Cardura) (extended-release)	—	65%	—	2-3 hr (8-9 hr)	15-22 hr	>24 hr	98%	Extensive; several active metabolites	Bile/feces, 63%; urine, 9%
clonidine (Catapres)	GI or transdermal	75%-95%	30-60 min	3-5 hr; 2-3 days transdermal	6-20 hr (18-41 hr impaired renal function)	6-10 hr	20%-40%	Extensive hepatic	Kidney, 65%; feces 22%
methyldopa (Aldomet)	Variable	8%-62%	3-6 hr	2-4 hr	2 hr (6-16 hr end-stage renal)	12-24 hr	<15%	Complex liver	Kidney, 70% drug and conjugates
aliskiren (Tekturna)	Poorly absorbed (2.5%)			1-3 hr	24 hr			Liver (CYP 3A4)	25% drug excreted in urine
minoxidil (Loniten)	Rapid	90%	30 min	2-3 hr	4 hr	24-75 hr	0	90% conjugation	Kidney

TABLE 15-8 **Common and Serious Adverse Effects of Antihypertensive Medications**

Drug	Common Side Effects	Serious Adverse Effects
α_1-Adrenergic blockers	Palpitation, nervousness, asthenia, mild GI distress, urinary frequency, nasal congestion, headache, edema, fatigue	Postural hypotension, syncope, CNS depression, dizziness (10%), dyspnea, blurred vision
clonidine	Dry mouth (40%), drowsiness (33%), dizziness (16%), sedation, constipation (10%), GI distress, headache, nervousness, impotence	Syncope, CHF, orthostatic hypotension, tachycardia, bradycardia, Raynaud's disease, conduction disturbances; insomnia, hallucinations, thrombocytopenia, weakness, fatigue, MS pain
methyldopa	Headache, asthenia, dizziness, gynecomastia, GI distress	Bradycardia, angina, CHF, orthostatic hypotension, edema, sedation, parkinsonism; toxic epidermal necrolysis, hemolytic anemia, abnormal LFTs, drug fever, arthralgia, myalgia
hydralazine	Palpitations, headache, constipation, nausea, vomiting, diarrhea	Tachycardia, angina, paresthesia, dizziness, paralytic ileus, blood dyscrasias, hypersensitivity, edema, dyspnea
minoxidil	Hypertrichosis (commonly occurs within 1-2 months of therapy)	Pericardial effusion, angina, cardiac lesions, ECG changes, fluid and electrolyte imbalance, tachycardia, hypersensitivity, hypertrichosis, Stevens-Johnson syndrome

hydralazine (Apresoline)

CONTRAINDICATIONS
- Hypersensitivity
- Mitral valve rheumatic heart disease

WARNINGS
- May cause a drug-induced lupus-like syndrome (more likely on larger doses, longer duration)
- May produce a clinical picture simulating systemic lupus erythematosus (arthralgia, dermatoses, fever, splenomegaly), including glomerulonephritis. Obtain baseline and periodic blood counts and ANA titers.

PRECAUTIONS
- Renal function impairment: may increase renal blood flow; use with caution in patients with advanced renal damage
- Hyperdynamic cardiac status may exaggerate cardiac deficits (pulmonary artery pressure in mitral valve disease; myocardial ischemia or infarction in CAD).
- CAD: myocardial stimulation can cause anginal attacks and ECG changes of ischemia; use with caution in patients with suspected CAD.
- Peripheral neuritis as evidenced by paresthesias, numbness, and tingling has been observed.
- Hematologic effects: bone marrow depression and blood dyscrasias consisting of low CBC, leukopenia, agranulocytosis, and purpura

DRUG INTERACTIONS
- Use MAOIs with caution.
- Cumulative effects are seen with other BP-lowering agents.

RENIN INHIBITORS

aliskiren (Tekturna)
- This is the first of a new class of drugs and little information is currently available. Aliskiren 150- and 300-mg tablets are indicated alone or in combination with other agents for the treatment of patients with hypertension. It has been demonstrated to reduce BP for a 24-hour dosing interval and adds to the therapeutic efficacy of hydrochlorothiazide and valsartan.
- In blocking the RAS, aliskiren produced a dose-response relationship with reasonable effects observed at 300 mg and no clear further increase at 600 mg; 85% to 90% of the BP-lowering effect occurred within the first 2 weeks of therapy.

DRUG INTERACTIONS. Concomitant use of aliskiren has been shown to significantly reduce furosemide exposure and potentially its efficacy.

PATIENT VARIABLES
- Although decreased BP was demonstrated in all subgroups, African American patients tended to have smaller reductions in BP compared with whites and Asian Americans, as has been noted with ACEIs and ARBs.
- No initial dose adjustments are required for the elderly or for patients with mild to severe renal impairment or hepatic insufficiency.

ADVERSE EFFECTS
- The most commonly reported adverse events were diarrhea (dose related), headache, and nasopharyngitis.
- Women and the elderly appeared more susceptible to diarrhea, with incidence rates at the 150 mg/day dose matching those for 300 mg/day therapy in men and younger patients (2.0%-2.3% vs. placebo, 1%). Diarrhea and other GI symptoms were generally mild and brief.
- Rare cases of angioedema were reported in clinical trials. As with all drugs that act on the RAS, aliskiren should not be used in pregnant women because of the risk for fetal and neonatal morbidity and mortality.

PHARMACOKINETICS AND DRUG ADMINISTRATION
- High-fat meals reduce the drug's absorption rate.
- The recommended starting dose of aliskiren is 150 mg given once daily.
- Studies with ambulatory BP monitoring showed reasonable control throughout the 24-hour dosing interval, with the ratio of mean daytime to mean nighttime ambulatory blood pressure ranging from 0.6 to 0.9.

TABLE 15-9 Dosage and Administration Recommendations for Antihypertensive Medications

Drug	Initial Dosage, mg	Administration	Titration	Usual JNC 7 Range	Maximum Daily Dose
prazosin	1	Hour of sleep, then bid or tid	3-15 mg/day 1 mg/dose 2-3 times/day; usual maintenance dose: 3-15 mg/day in divided doses; 2-4 times/day	—	20 mg
terazosin	1	Hour of sleep, then daily	1 mg/day every 1-2 weeks	1-20 mg once daily	20 mg
doxazosin	1	Once daily in morning or evening	2-4 mg/day titrate over several weeks, balancing therapeutic benefit with postural hypotension	—	16 mg
clonidine	0.1 (transdermal)	Once weekly	↑100 mcg weekly ↑ every 1-2 weeks as needed	0.1-0.3 mg once weekly	2400 mg; two 300-mg patches
clonidine	0.1	bid	1 mg once weekly	0.1-0.8 mg/day	2.4 mg
methyldopa	250	bid or tid	Every 2 days	250-1000 mg/day	3 g
hydralazine	10	bid to qid	10-25 mg after 2-5 days, then 50 mg qid	25-100 mg/day in two divided doses	300 mg

- Additional studies showed that the addition of aliskiren (75, 150, or 300 mg) to the diuretic hydrochlorothiazide (6.25, 12.5, or 25 mg) further reduced hypertension vs. monotherapy alone; similar results were obtained when aliskiren (150 or 300 mg) was added to the ARB valsartan (160 or 320 mg).
- Most (85%-90%) of the therapeutic effect is attained by 2 weeks, and up titration to a 300-mg dose may be required for additional response. Doses greater than 300 mg have been observed to increase the risk for diarrhea without increasing BP response and are therefore not recommended.
- Patients with severe renal impairment should be treated with caution because of the paucity of related safety information.

evolve A continually updated list of useful WebLinks may be found in the Evolve Resources at http://evolve.elsevier.com/Edmunds/NP/

Coronary Artery Disease and Antianginal Medications

16

DRUG OVERVIEW

Class	Subclass	Generic Name	Trade Name
Antianginals	Nitroglycerin	nitroglycerin sublingual tablet 🔑 ✺	Nitrostat
		nitroglycerin topical ointment	Nitro-Bid, Minitran
		nitroglycerin translingual spray	Nitrolingual
		nitroglycerin transdermal patch	Nitro-Dur, Transderm-Nitro
	Isosorbide	isosorbide dinitrate sublingual tablet	Isordil
		nitroglycerin oral	Nitro-Time
		isosorbide dinitrate oral	Isordil Dilatrate-SR
		isosorbide mononitrate oral ✺	ISMO, Monoket, Imdur
	Piperazine derivative	ranolazine	Ranexa ER

✺ Top 200 drug; 🔑 key drug. Sublingual nitroglycerin is selected as the key drug because it is the simplest form of the drug.

INDICATIONS

Labeled uses include the following:
- Acute angina: sublingual, translingual spray, and ointment
- Angina prophylaxis: transdermal, sublingual (for activities known to exacerbate angina) transmucosal, and oral sustained-release forms
- Ranexa: reserved for use in treating patients with chronic angina who have not responded to other medications

Unlabeled uses include the following:
- CHF, acute MI: sublingual, topical, and oral forms
- Raynaud's phenomenon, peripheral vascular disease (PVD): ointment

Patients with a history of angina should have sublingual nitroglycerin (NTG) available, and they should know how to use it. Medications other than nitrates used to treat coronary artery disease (CAD) include β-blockers (BBs), calcium channel blockers (CCBs), angiotensin-converting enzyme inhibitors (ACEIs), ACE II inhibitors (ARBs), and antihyperlipidemics. Ranolazine is used in combination with some of these agents for patients with chronic angina. Use of these agents in the treatment of CAD is discussed here. Details on individual drugs are discussed in their respective chapters (Table 16-1).

Angina persisting longer than 20 minutes or continuing after three doses of NTG given 5 minutes apart may indicate progressing infarction, and the patient should go to the nearest emergency department.

THERAPEUTIC OVERVIEW OF CORONARY ARTERY DISEASE

Anatomy and Physiology

The myocardium receives its blood supply from the coronary arteries, a system of small arteries that branch from the aorta (Figure 16-1). The right coronary artery lies in a groove between the right atrium and the right ventricle and supplies the right ventricle. The left main coronary artery is divided shortly after its origin into two branches—the left anterior descending branch and the circumflex branch. The left anterior descending branch supplies blood to the anterior myocardium, apex, and anterior septum and is located on the surface of the anterior myocardium. The circumflex branch lies in a groove between the left atrium and the left ventricle and supplies blood to the left ventricle. Smaller branches arise from the large coronary vessels. In 90% of the population, a posterior descending artery arises from the right coronary artery, and in 10%, it arises from the circumflex branch of the left anterior descending artery.

TABLE 16-1   Drugs Used for Coronary Artery Disease Discussed in Other Chapters

Class	Chapter
β-Blockers	18
Calcium channel blockers	19
ACE inhibitors	20
ACE II inhibitors	20
Antihyperlipidemics	22

Pathophysiology

Determinants in the pathogenesis of MI include the following: atheromatous lesions, increased myocardial oxygen demand, and catecholamine release.

ATHEROMATOUS LESIONS. The atherosclerotic process is the buildup of plaque in blood vessels. This process occurs throughout the body. The arteries most often affected are the coronary arteries (CAD), the cerebral vascular arteries (stroke), and the peripheral arteries (PVD). The first step in the process of atherosclerosis is deposition of the fatty streak. Lipid-laden foam cells derived from macrophages or smooth muscle cells accumulate on the subendothelial lining. The most important lipids in this step are the low-density lipoproteins (LDLs). Smooth muscle cells migrate into the lesion. At this step, the plaque does not affect circulation. Progression of these fatty streaks leads to the development of a collagen cap. The lesion becomes calcified, and the vessel lumen slowly becomes narrowed.

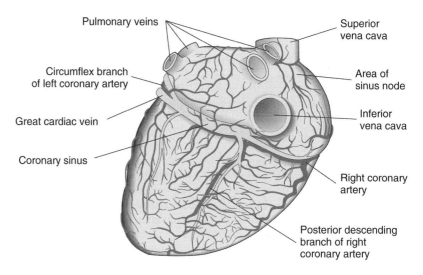

POSTERIOR VIEW

FIGURE 16-1   Anterior and posterior surfaces of the heart, illustrating the location and distribution of the peripheral coronary vessels. (From Berne RM, Levy MW: *Cardiovascular physiology,* ed 7, St Louis, 1997, Mosby.)

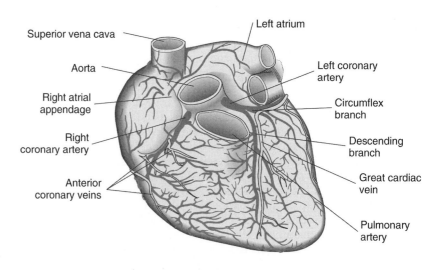

ANTERIOR VIEW

As the plaque grows, it may develop an internal hemorrhage, which then leaks to the surface. The body reacts by formation of a thrombus. Infarction occurs as the result of total occlusion of the artery by the thrombus (Figure 16-2).

INCREASED MYOCARDIAL OXYGEN DEMAND. Myocardial ischemia can be brought on by increased myocardial oxygen requirements such as exercise, mental stress, or spontaneous fluctuations in heart rate and blood pressure. It also can be caused by decreased oxygen supply such as occurs with vasospasm, platelet plugging, or partial thrombosis. Oxygen supply to the myocardium depends on filling of the coronary

arteries during diastole. Filling depends on coronary perfusion pressure and coronary vascular resistance. Coronary vascular resistance depends on the degree of collateralization and the patency of the coronary blood vessels. With exercise, the coronary blood flow may have to increase to as much as four to five times above resting level.

CATECHOLAMINE RELEASE. Catecholamines are released in response to exertional and emotional stress or other activity. Catecholamines cause increased heart rate, blood velocity, and force of myocardial contraction, producing increased oxygen demand and ischemia. Increased heart rate decreases the length of diastole, which occurs when the coronary arteries perfuse the myocardium. Ischemia then stimulates further catecholamine release. If the myocardium does not receive enough oxygen, ischemia may result in pain (angina), arrhythmia, or left ventricular dysfunction (CHF). Ischemia can be either painful or pain free. Silent ischemia is as dangerous as painful ischemia.

Disease Process

RISK FACTORS. Several large epidemiologic studies have identified certain habits and predisposing conditions that correlate with the development of CAD (Box 16-1). One can determine the 10-year coronary heart disease risk based on the Framingham study, as described by the National Cholesterol Education Program (NCEP) Expert Panel (see Chapter 22).

Added to the traditional risk factors is a new group of markers. C-reactive protein (CRP) and homocysteine are markers of inflammation. CRP is a highly sensitive marker for inflammation, but it lacks specificity. Data from more than 30 epidemiologic studies have shown a significant association between an elevated CRP level and the prevalence of underlying atherosclerosis, the risk of recurrent cardiovascular events among patients with established disease, and the incidence of first cardiovascular events among individuals at risk for atherosclerosis. Elevated levels are also found in patients with metabolic syndrome, cigarette smoking, type 2 diabetes, and dyslipidemia. CRP can be decreased through the use of statins, fibrates, and cholesterol absorption inhibitors, as well as by weight loss, increased physical activity, smoking cessation, and the use of thiazolidinediones and β-blockers but not aspirin.

Homocysteine produces a proinflammatory response and is associated with poor dietary folate, vitamin B_6 and B_{12} deficiency, and renal insufficiency. Screening tests for these markers are readily available. Although early data on the relationship between elevated blood homocysteine concentrations and coronary heart disease (CHD) and stroke have been somewhat inconsistent, high homocysteine levels appear to be clearly associated with an increased risk of cardiovascular and cerebrovascular disease. However, homocysteine does not appear to be as important as other risk factors such as hypercholesterolemia, smoking, diabetes mellitus, and hypertension. Recommendations on the use of tests for homocysteine and CRP have not been established; these tests are not recommended for routine screening. They probably are best used with patients at elevated risk for CAD from other risk factors. Elevations in these test results may indicate the need for an aggressive preventative approach.

Additional risk factors include lipoprotein (a) [Lp(a)] and fibrinogen. Lp(a) possesses an atherogenic effect. Most

Coronary syndromes: clinicopathologic correlates

Syndrome	Coronary pathology
a Stable angina	Stenotic endothelialized atheromatous plaque
b Unstable angina	Ruptured atheromatous plaque with subocclusive thrombus
c Variant angina	Coronary spasm with or without atheromatous plaque
d Myocardial infarction	Ruptured atheromatous plaque with occlusive thrombus

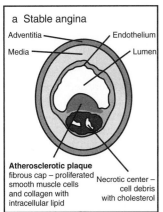

a Stable angina

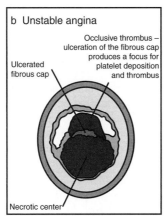

b Unstable angina

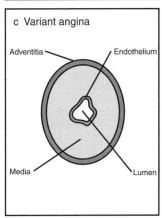

c Variant angina

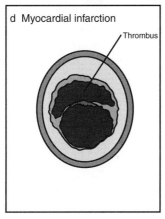

d Myocardial infarction

FIGURE 16-2 Plaque formation in coronary syndromes. (From Timmis AD: *Cardiology,* ed 3, London, 1991, Mosby-Wolfe.)

BOX 16-1   Risk Factors for Coronary Artery Disease

NONMODIFIABLE

Premature family CAD (before age 50 years)
Advanced age
Male gender

POTENTIALLY MODIFIABLE

Diabetes mellitus
Hypertension
Left ventricular hypertrophy
Metabolic syndrome
Chronic kidney disease
C-reactive protein (CRP)

Homocysteine
Lipoprotein Lp(a)
Hyperfibrinogenemia

MODIFIABLE

Physical inactivity
Cigarette smoking
Obesity
Diet
Psychosocial factors—type A personality, anger, hostility, depression, job strain, lack of social support, and isolation

---

patients with an elevated Lp(a) have diabetes or elevated LDL. Lipoprotein may be measured accurately, but a test is not commonly available. Fibrinogen is a plasma protein that plays an important role in thrombosis. Drugs known to lower fibrinogen include tamoxifen, anabolic steroids, ticlopidine, pentoxifylline, and fenofibrate. Measurement is not reliable. It is possible that these tests will be useful in patients with premature atherosclerosis or family history of premature CAD.

Collagen vascular disease is a recently identified risk factor. Patients with rheumatoid and systemic lupus erythematosus have increased risk of cardiovascular disease; this may be related to chronic inflammation or treatment of the disease with steroids and nonsteroidal antiinflammatory drugs (NSAIDs). Coronary artery calcification, as measured by electron beam computed tomography (EBCT), quantifies the amount of calcium in the coronary arteries and correlates well with angiographically defined CAD.

Other possible risk factors are now being explored. These include brain natriuretic peptide (BNP) and endothelial dysfunction, as well as infection (acute or chronic). BNP is a natriuretic hormone that was initially identified in the brain but is also present in the heart, particularly the ventricles. In heart failure, BNP is released in response to high ventricular filling pressures. The plasma concentrations of BNP in patients with asymptomatic and symptomatic left ventricular dysfunction permit their use in diagnosis. The usefulness of BNP in differentiating cardiac from noncardiac causes of dyspnea in difficult-to-assess patients remains uncertain. Levels of generalized and coronary endothelial dysfunction are important prognostic indicators of progression of coronary atherosclerosis and clinical cardiovascular events. Brachial reactivity is a noninvasive measure of endothelial dysfunction that can be obtained relatively cheaply, but its reliability and validity have not been tested. Erectile dysfunction may be related and may be a clinical marker.

Infection, both acute and chronic, may be implicated. Acute infections are associated with a transient higher incidence of CHD. Some theorize that chronic infections such as pneumonia, cytomegalovirus, and *Helicobacter pylori* may stimulate low-grade chronic inflammation and thus atherosclerosis. Trials with long-acting macrolides have not demonstrated benefit. BNP is released from myocardial cells in response to volume expansion and myocardial wall tension, and elevations are associated with the presence of heart failure. The Framingham Heart Study found BNP to be a predictor of cardiovascular disease (CVD) and death in subjects without heart failure. The significance of this remains to be elucidated.

ANGINA. Anginal ischemic myocardial pain has two major causes. By far the most common is arteriosclerotic heart disease, which was described previously. The other cause seen in primary care is coronary vasospasm with or without atherosclerotic CAD.

DEFINITION OF DISEASE. Myocardial ischemia occurs when myocardial oxygen demand exceeds oxygen supply. Increased demand usually occurs as the result of tachyarrhythmias, hypertension, and exercise, all of which increase cardiac workload. Decreased supply usually results from coronary artery stenosis. Angina pectoris is defined as chest pain, pressure, or discomfort caused by myocardial ischemia.

CLASSIFICATION

- *Stable or chronic angina* is defined as no change in the past 2 months in terms of frequency, duration (<15 min), or precipitating causes. The symptom pattern is also reproducible.
- *Unstable angina* is a change in pattern of pain such as an increase in frequency, severity, and/or duration of pain and fewer precipitating factors. Patients with unstable angina should be admitted to a coronary care unit. Treatment for unstable angina is beyond the scope of this text. Immediate care of the patient while hospitalization is awaited is discussed in the section on treatment guidelines.
- *Variant (Prinzmetal's) angina* refers to coronary artery spasm. This is very rare. Pain often occurs at rest and develops because of spasm rather than as the result of increased myocardial oxygen demand.
- *Silent ischemia* is classified as asymptomatic episodes of myocardial ischemia that can be detected with the use of ECG and other diagnostic techniques.

Assessment

The history is crucial to the diagnosis of CAD. Myocardial ischemia causes angina, a symptom of CAD. The sensation of angina is usually described as heavy substernal pressure or pain that may radiate to the left arm. It is brought on by exertion and is relieved by rest. The sensation may be described as tightness, squeezing, gas, indigestion, or a vague discomfort instead of as pain. The pain may occur anywhere from the lower jaw to the epigastrium. It may radiate to the right arm in addition to the left. If the patient identifies the site of pain by pointing to the area of the apical impulse with one finger, angina is unlikely. The episode may last 15 to 30 minutes, but substantial variation has been noted. Patients usually are most comfortable in a sitting position. They may feel short of breath. Occasionally, a patient may have myocardial ischemia with no other symptoms; silent ischemia will show up on ECG.

On physical examination, blood pressure may be elevated or lowered. An occasional extra sound or systolic murmur may be heard. ECG shows characteristic changes of ischemia in about 75% of patients with angina. The other 25% exhibit other abnormalities on ECG. The characteristic change is a horizontal or downsloping ST-segment depression that resolves as the angina resolves. T-wave flattening or inversion also may occur. Occasionally, ST-segment elevation occurs. Examination of the patient between episodes of angina may reveal normal findings, including those obtained via ECG.

Basic diagnostic studies include serum lipid levels, CBC, electrolytes, ECG, and exercise testing. Myocardial perfusion scintigraphy uses radionuclide uptake to identify areas of hypoperfusion. An echocardiogram is useful for assessing left ventricular function. Coronary angiography is the definitive diagnostic procedure for coronary disease. Newer imaging techniques include CT scanning and MRI, but their usefulness remains to be determined.

MECHANISM OF ACTION

Currently, three major classes of antianginal drugs are used in the medical management of angina pectoris: nitrates (short- and long-acting), β-blockers, and calcium channel blockers. (β-Blockers and calcium channel blockers are discussed in later chapters.)

A fourth option, ranolazine, is a new drug that should be used in conjunction with other agents, and whose mechanism of action is unknown. Evidence suggests that ranolazine is an inhibitor of the late sodium current and that its use results in reduction of the intracellular sodium and calcium overload in ischemic cardiac myocytes. This agent does not demonstrate negative chronotropic or inotropic effects, and minimal effects on heart rate and blood pressure have been noted during clinical trials. Most commonly, a combination of these antianginal agents is used for management. In combination with β-blockers or calcium channel blockers, nitrates and ranolazine produce greater antianginal and antiischemic effects.

Nitrates relax vascular smooth muscle via stimulation of intracellular cyclic guanosine monophosphate production. The major effect of nitrates is to reduce myocardial oxygen demand, primarily by decreasing preload and to a lesser extent by decreasing afterload. Nitrates cause major dilation of the venous bed. Vasodilation results in venous pooling of blood, thereby decreasing venous return. Decreased venous return reduces ventricular end-diastolic volume. This reduction in preload results in reduced filling pressure (decreased pressure of blood against the wall of the heart). Reduced wall tension decreases myocardial oxygen demand.

A relatively minor effect of nitrates is the reduction in afterload achieved by arterial relaxation. Reduced afterload decreases myocardial work, which reduces oxygen consumption.

Another relatively minor effect of nitrates is that they improve myocardial oxygen supply by optimizing blood delivery via dilation of coronary arteries. This may be an important mechanism in the prevention and treatment of patients with coronary vasospasm. Nitrates also increase the use of coronary collaterals so that perfusion of the inner layers of the myocardium is improved.

TREATMENT PRINCIPLES

Standardized Guidelines

Fraker TD Jr et al: 2007 chronic angina focused update of the ACC/AHA 2002 Guidelines for the management of patients with chronic stable angina: a report of the American College of Cardiology/American Heart Association Task Force on Practice Guidelines Writing Group to develop the focused update of the 2002 Guidelines for the management of patients with chronic stable angina, Circulation 116(23):2762-2772, 2007.

Canadian Cardiovascular Society; American Academy of Family Physicians; American College of Cardiology; American Heart Association; Antman EM et al: 2007 focused update of the ACC/AHA 2004 guidelines for the management of patients with ST-elevation myocardial infarction: a report of the American College of Cardiology/American Heart Association Task Force on Practice Guidelines, J Am Coll Cardiol 51(2):210-247, 2008.

Evidence-Based Recommendations

Stable angina, effective long-term single drug treatment regimens: β-blockers, calcium channel blockers, nitrates, potassium channel openers

Unstable angina, beneficial or likely to be beneficial: aspirin, clopidogrel/ticlopidine

Cardinal Points of Treatment

1. Control acute attack of angina—use nitrates
2. Long-term management may require the following:
   a. Long-acting nitrate
   b. β-blocker therapy
   c. ACEI
   d. Calcium channel blocker
   e. Ranolazine
   f. Aspirin
   g. Possible revascularization

Patients with symptoms suggestive of CAD should be referred to a cardiologist for evaluation and treatment. The primary care provider usually is responsible for follow-up of patients with stable angina. The provider should be prepared to handle acute angina in the office setting. He should have a protocol to be followed for management of unstable angina and acute MI prior to the arrival of emergency personnel.

RISK REDUCTION. All adults should be educated regarding the efficacy of risk reduction in preventing CAD. Risk reduction is a key component of the treatment of CAD. The three risk factors for which the greatest effort should be made are hypertension, cigarette smoking, and blood lipid abnormalities. Control of these can significantly reduce a person's risk for

CAD. Each of these is important enough to merit a separate chapter in this book. In addition, the control of diabetes mellitus is extremely important. Obesity and physical inactivity should be approached, along with lipid reduction. Exercise is important for weight reduction and for regulation of lipids. Dyslipidemia is positively influenced by exercise.

Pharmacologic Treatment

ACUTE ATTACK

1. Give NTG sublingually at 3- to 5-minute intervals for three doses. If angina is worse or is unimproved 5 minutes after the first dose, then call emergency medical services (EMS) (AHA/ACC guidelines recommendation).
2. Give oxygen, usually at 2 L/min, via nasal cannula.
3. Have the patient chew a regular aspirin (325 mg) while waiting for the ambulance to arrive.
4. Rest and reassurance are helpful.
5. It is important the patient receive thrombolytic therapy as soon as possible, preferably within the first 1 to 3 hours of the MI.
6. Pain management should be administered. Use morphine or other agents to achieve pain relief as required.

USE OF NITRATES IN ACUTE ATTACK

 Nitrates are taken at the time of an anginal attack. Select a fast-acting nitrate.

The most common form used is a sublingual (SL) tablet of NTG. Translingual spray is also acceptable. The usual dose of NTG tablets is 0.3 mg (1/200 gr) to 0.4 mg (1/150 gr) given SL. Use a smaller dose (0.3 mg) for a small, frail, and/or elderly patient. Increase the dose to 0.4 to 0.6 mg if not completely effective. Sublingual NTG is rapid acting, convenient, relatively safe, and inexpensive. NTG spray is equally as effective as the SL tablets but is more expensive. NTG translingual spray may be more convenient for patients who have difficulty handling the small tablets in a stressful situation. It is also more stable, and its effects will last longer than those of the pills. The translingual spray should be sprayed onto or under the tongue, *not inhaled.*

Have the patient take the medicine as soon as pain is experienced. Have the patient lie down and rest. The drug should be effective in 1 to 2 minutes. If the pain is worse or is not relieved after 5 minutes, call EMS and administer a second tablet. If the pain is not relieved within another 3 to 5 minutes, a third pill may be taken. If the patient is having an anginal episode at the time of the office visit, an ECG will document the angina. The effectiveness of the nitrate should be evident on a subsequent ECG.

Fast-acting nitrates can be given before a stressful episode, such as exercise or sex, to prevent angina.

CHRONIC STABLE ANGINA/PREVENTION/POST–MYOCARDIAL INFARCTION MANAGEMENT. Following is a list of general steps that cannot be applied to every variable a patient may have. Use these principles with caution (Table 16-2). The previous protocol assumes that the patient does not have a concomitant illness. However, patients with angina often have other problems, which affect how their angina is treated (Table 16-3).

1. Start with nonpharmacologic lifestyle modifications AFTER the angina is controlled.

2. Manage aggravating factors. Treat other problems and risk factors aggressively as follows:
   - All patients should be given a rapid-acting nitrate and should be instructed in its use for treatment of acute angina. See later discussion for specific details.
   - Long-acting nitrates should be considered. The main limitation is tolerance, which can be limited by providing a nitrate-free period of 6 to 10 hours each day. See later discussion for specific details.
   - β-Blocker therapy should be considered in all patients with angina. These are the only antianginal agents shown to prevent death in patients with angina. A careful evaluation of the patient's risks and indications for β-blockers should be conducted. Allow 1 to 2 months for a drug trial with β-blockers to adjust dose and monitor for therapeutic response and adverse reactions. See Chapter 18 for additional information.
   - ACEIs should be used for all patients with CAD without contraindications, in addition to standard therapy. They decrease the risk of cardiovascular death.
   - Calcium channel blockers are the medications of choice in coronary vasospasm. They may also be useful in stable angina if nitrates and β-blockers have failed. Short-acting nifedipine in moderate to large doses causes an increase in mortality in patients with unstable angina or who are recently post-MI.
   - Recommend aspirin, unless contraindicated. Every patient with CAD should take aspirin 81 to 325 mg daily.
3. Revascularization procedures include coronary artery bypass grafting, percutaneous transluminal coronary angioplasty, and stenting.

USE OF NITRATES IN CHRONIC STABLE ANGINA/PREVENTION/POST–MYOCARDIAL INFARCTION MANAGEMENT. Nitrates are given on a routine basis to prevent anginal episodes. Angina prophylaxis requires a long-acting transdermal patch, an oral sustained-release tablet, or a topical ointment. A transdermal patch is often used because of its ease of administration. Dosage is measured as release rate in milligrams per hour. The usual starting dosage is 0.2 to 0.4 mg/hr, which is increased or decreased depending on the patient's therapeutic response and the adverse effects. Transdermal patches are more convenient but more expensive than oral nitrates. Oral nitrates are effective, safe, and economical. The oral nitrate most commonly used is isosorbide mononitrate. Isosorbide dinitrate is also available. Oral nitrates experience the first-pass phenomenon, in which large amounts of the drug are immediately metabolized by the liver. This means that large doses are required to obtain therapeutic effect. Alternative routes of administration, such as transdermal patches and buccal tablets, were developed to avoid this phenomenon.

Tolerance to nitrates is an issue. To prevent tolerance, it is necessary to interrupt therapy for 8 to 12 hours a day. The usual method is to take off the patch or stop the oral medication in the evening and then restart it in the morning. The problem with this is that early morning is a dangerous time for ischemia and MI. To avoid this risk, nitrates should be omitted for a quiet period during the day. Another antianginal agent may be necessary during the nitrate-free interval.

CHRONIC ANGINA. In patients who continue to experience angina despite adequate treatment with nitrates, ranolazine

TABLE 16-2 Guide to Comprehensive Risk Reduction for Patients With Coronary and Other Vascular Disease

Risk Intervention	Recommendations
Smoking: *Goal* Complete cessation	Strongly encourage patient and family to stop smoking. Provide counseling, nicotine replacement, and formal cessation programs as appropriate.
Lipid management: *Primary goal* LDL <100 mg/dl *Secondary goals* HDL >40 mg/dl males; >50 mg/dl females TG <150 mg/dl	Start AHA Step II diet in all patients: ≤30% fat, <7% saturated cholesterol. Assess fasting lipid profile. In post-MI patients, lipid profile may take 4 to 6 wk to stabilize. Add drug therapy according to the following guide: (see table below)

LDL <100 mg/dl	LDL 100 to 130 mg/dl	LDL >130 mg/dl	HDL <35 mg/dl
No drug therapy	Consider adding drug therapy to diet, as follows:	Add drug therapy to diet, as follows:	Emphasize weight management and physical activity. Advise smoking cessation. If needed to achieve LDL goals, consider niacin, statin, fibrates.
	↘ Suggested drug therapy ↙		
	TG <200 mg/dl	TG 200 to 400 mg/dl	TG >400 mg/dl	
	Statin Resin Niacin	Statin Niacin	Consider combined drug therapy (niacin, fibrates, statin).	
	If LDL goal not achieved, consider combination therapy.		

Risk Intervention	Recommendations
Physical activity: *Minimum goal* 30 min 3 or 4 times per week; Ideal is exercise most days.	Assess risk, preferably with exercise test, to guide prescription. Encourage minimum of 30 to 60 min of moderate-intensity activity three or four times weekly (walking, jogging, cycling, or other aerobic activity) supplemented by an increase in daily lifestyle activities (e.g., walking breaks at work, using stairs, gardening, household work). Maximum benefit 5 to 6 hours a week. Advise medically supervised program for moderate- to high-risk patients.
Weight management	Start intensive diet and appropriate physical activity intervention, as outlined previously, in patients >120% of ideal weight for height. Particularly emphasize the need for weight loss in patients with hypertension, elevated triglycerides, or elevated glucose levels.
Antiplatelet agents/anticoagulants	Start aspirin 81 to 325 mg/day if not contraindicated. Manage warfarin to International Normalized Ratio = 2 to 3.5 for post-MI patients not able to take aspirin.
ACE inhibitors post-MI	Start early post-MI in stable high-risk patients (anterior MI, previous MI, Killip class II [S3 gallop, rales, radiographic CHF]). Continue indefinitely for all with LV dysfunction (ejection fraction ≤40%) or symptoms of failure. Use as needed to manage blood pressure or symptoms in all other patients.
β-Blockers	Start in high-risk post-MI patients (arrhythmia, LV dysfunction, inducible ischemia) at 5 to 28 days. Continue 6 months minimum. Observe usual contraindications. Use as needed to manage angina, rhythm, or blood pressure in all other patients. Individualize recommendations consistent with other health risks.
Blood pressure control: *Goal* ≤140/90 mm Hg	Initiate lifestyle modification weight control, physical activity, alcohol moderation, and moderate sodium restriction in all patients with blood pressure >140 mm Hg systolic or 90 mm Hg diastolic. Add blood pressure medication, individualized to other patient requirements and characteristics (i.e., age, race, need for drugs with specific benefits) if blood pressure is not less than 140 mm Hg systolic or 90 mm Hg diastolic in 3 months, or if *initial* blood pressure is >160 mm Hg systolic or 100 mm Hg diastolic.

From American Heart Association Consensus Panel Statement: *Preventing heart attack and death,* Dallas, TX, 1995, American Heart Association.

may be used in combination with amlodipine, β-blockers, or nitrates, under the direction of a cardiologist.

How to Monitor

Encourage patients to keep a record of prn medication use. This record should be brought to appointments and reviewed by the clinician. Evaluate the record for patterns of increased frequency, multiple dosing to eliminate symptoms, or changes in activity that produce angina and point to worsening anginal status. Decreased frequency of anginal episodes will document the efficacy of NTG. Patients whose episodes of angina do not decrease in number should notify the provider.

Patients who use several drugs to control angina should have cardiac enzymes and electrolytes monitored at least every 3 months.

Patient Variables

GERIATRICS

- Older patients are at increased risk for syncope with administration of NTG.

TABLE 16-3   Treatment of Patients With Conditions Comorbid to Coronary Artery Disease

Clinical Diagnosis	Therapy to Consider
Aortic stenosis	Nitrates (with caution); avoid vasodilators, β-blockers
Asthma, COPD	Calcium channel blockers; avoid β-blockers
Atrial fibrillation	verapamil; if not effective, digoxin plus β-blocker
Congestive heart failure	digoxin, ACEIs, nitrates, diuretics
Diabetes mellitus	Use α_1-selective β-blocker or calcium blocker, ACEI, ARB
Hypercholesterolemia	Low-cholesterol diet, exercise; remove stress
Hypertension	Control blood pressure with β-blocker, calcium channel blocker, ACEI
Second- or third-degree atrioventricular block	Thiazide diuretics; nitrates; avoid β-blockers, verapamil, and diltiazem
Severe peripheral vascular disease	Avoid β-blockers; consider calcium channel blockers
Sick sinus syndrome	Nitrates; avoid β-blockers, verapamil, and diltiazem

- Make sure the patient is seated or lying down before NTG is administered.
- Geriatric patients usually require a lower dose of nitrates.

PEDIATRICS. Safety and efficacy have not been established.

PREGNANCY AND LACTATION. *Category C:* Safety of use in pregnancy has not been established.

GENDER. The effects of ranolazine on angina frequency and exercise tolerance are considerably less in women than in men.

Patient Education

FOR ALL TYPES OF NITROGLYCERIN

NTG is a very unstable medication, and great care must be taken in handling and storing medication, or it may not be effective.

- NTG breaks down rapidly and loses its potency. Sunlight speeds up this process.
- Even under the best storage conditions, all types of NTG lose their strength about 3 months after the bottle has been opened. A new prescription should be obtained every 3 months and the old medication discarded. Patients are reluctant to throw away medication that they have had to purchase, but most NTG costs only pennies, and patients will eventually learn to discard it.
- Medication should be stored in the original dark glass container. Remove all cotton wadding and keep the container tightly capped and out of sunlight. Storage in a plastic or cardboard box allows the nitrate to be absorbed into the container material. If cotton plugs remain in the top of the medicine container, or other drugs are stored with NTG, the nitrate will be absorbed. Refrigeration helps to preserve medication and slow deterioration.
- Natural and predictable side effects of taking NTG include flushing of the face, brief throbbing headache, increased heart rate, dizziness, and lightheadedness when one changes position rapidly. Headache usually lasts no longer than 20 minutes and may be relieved by analgesics such as acetaminophen.
- Patients should rest for 10 to 15 minutes after pain is relieved.
- Notify health care provider if blurring of vision, persistent headache, or dry mouth occurs.
- There is no therapeutic value in not taking NTG for anginal pain. It may prevent damage to the myocardium.
- If medication seems to be less effective after it has been taken for a while, the patient may be developing a tolerance to the drug. The provider should be notified.
- Patients should keep a record of the frequency of their anginal attacks, the number of pills taken, and any side effects and should bring the record to each appointment.
- Patients should use NTG in anticipation of situations in which they can predict that anginal attacks will occur. Taking medication before the activity may prevent or reduce the degree of pain.
- Patients should not change NTG products without notifying the health care provider.
- Combined with this drug, alcohol may lower blood pressure; its use should be avoided.
- Do not stop taking this medicine abruptly.

SUBLINGUAL TABLETS

- For acute anginal attacks, take 1 tablet sublingually as soon as pain is experienced. Do not chew or swallow medication; let it dissolve under your tongue. Lie down and rest. If pain is not relieved within another 3 to 5 minutes, take a second tablet. A third pill may be taken if chest pain is not relieved after the second dose. If pain is worse or unimproved after 5 minutes, call EMS.
- Burning under the tongue after SL medication is taken is not always a reliable indicator that the drug is still potent. Because some NTG products are provided in a much purer form than others, they do not always produce the characteristic throbbing headache.

TRANSLINGUAL SPRAY

- A less popular but equally effective means of administering SL NTG is by metered-dose spray. The spray dispenses approximately 200 doses of 0.4 mg of NTG. It has a shelf life of 2 to 3 years and does not require refrigeration.
- Take spray only when lying or sitting down. Because this is a highly flammable product, put out cigarettes and avoid using spray around fire or sparks.

TRANSDERMAL PATCH

- For transdermal application, select a hairless spot (or clip hair) and apply adhesive pad to skin. Washing, bathing, or swimming does not affect this system. Do not cut or tear patch. If pad should come off, discard it and place a new patch on a different site.

- Discard used NTG patches in a safe place out of reach of children.

TOPICAL OINTMENT

- For topical ointment, spread thin layer on the skin, using applicator and ruler. Do not rub or massage the ointment into the skin. Wash off any medication that may have gotten onto the hands.
- Keep tube tightly closed.
- Discard used paste in a safe place out of reach of children.

ORAL MEDICATION

- Take medication on an empty stomach when possible; follow with a glass of water. Take isosorbide dinitrate 30 minutes to 1 hour before meals; allow a 12-hour nitrate-free period to prevent tolerance.
- Take isosorbide mononitrate tablets on awakening and again 7 hours later. For sustained-release products, do not crush or chew; swallow with a half-glassful of water.
- A dosing schedule of 8 AM, 1 PM, and 6 PM has been recommended; this results in a 14-hour nitrate dose–free interval.

RANOLAZINE EXTENDED-RELEASE

1. This drug may cause changes on ECG; therefore, frequent ECGs are necessary. The patient should not take any drugs without the knowledge of his provider.
2. Grapefruit juice should be avoided while taking this product.
3. Do not use this drug during an acute anginal attack.
4. If a dose is missed, take the regular dose at the next scheduled time and do not double the dose.
5. Medication may be taken with or without food.
6. Swallow medication whole, and do not crush, chew, or break.

SPECIFIC DRUGS

sublingual nitroglycerin (Nitrostat) 🗝

CONTRAINDICATIONS. Hypersensitivity or idiosyncrasy to nitrates, severe anemia, closed-angle glaucoma, postural hypotension, early MI, head trauma, and cerebral hemorrhage.

WARNINGS/PRECAUTIONS

- Use with caution in acute MI; avoid use of long-acting nitrates.
- Postural hypotension may occur accompanied by dizziness, weakness, syncope, or other signs of cerebral ischemia. This is accentuated if the patient is standing or has consumed alcohol. Fatalities have occurred.
- Nitrates may aggravate angina caused by idiopathic hypertrophic cardiomyopathy.
- Tolerance to the effects of nitrates frequently occurs. Nitrate-free periods may decrease this tendency. For discussion of tolerance, see the section on treatment principles.
- Caution is required when treatment is administered to patients with open-angle glaucoma because intraocular pressure may be increased. However, nitrates are not contraindicated with glaucoma.

- Excessive dosage may produce severe headaches.
- Discontinue the drug if blurred vision or dry mouth occurs.
- Severe hypotension may occur in a patient who is volume depleted or hypotensive for any reason.
- Gradually reduce the dosage to prevent withdrawal reactions.

PHARMACOKINETICS

- Isosorbide mononitrate is metabolized primarily by the liver. In contrast to isosorbide dinitrate, isosorbide mononitrate is not subject to the first-pass effect and therefore has nearly 100% bioavailability; see Table 16-4.
- Isosorbide dinitrate is subject to the first-pass effect; therefore, there is only 40% to 50% bioavailability after first pass; see Table 16-4.

ADVERSE EFFECTS

- CNS: headache, light-headedness, syncope, anxiety, nervousness, weakness.
- GI: nausea, vomiting, diarrhea, dyspepsia, abdominal pain.
- Cardiovascular: tachycardia, hypotension, syncope, crescendo angina, rebound hypertension, arrhythmia, premature ventricular contraction, postural hypotension.
- Dermatologic: drug rash, exfoliative dermatitis, cutaneous vasodilation with flushing.
- Miscellaneous: perspiration, blurred vision, diplopia, edema.

Specific dosage formulations cause the following adverse effects:

- Transdermal patch may cause skin irritation. Contact dermatitis may be caused by the transdermal NTG system itself rather than by the NTG molecule.
- A defibrillator must not be used over an NTG patch; arcing may occur and may burn the patient.
- NTG ointment may cause topical skin reactions and anaphylactoid swelling of oral mucosa and edema of conjunctiva.

DRUG INTERACTIONS. Table 16-5 lists common drug interactions with nitrates.

DOSAGE AND ADMINISTRATION. Table 16-6 contains a summary of dosage recommendations.

1. NTG sublingual tablets, 0.3 mg (1/200 gr), 0.4 mg (1/150 gr), and 0.6 mg (1/100 gr); 0.4 mg is most commonly used. To administer, dissolve one tablet under the tongue. Repeat every 5 minutes until pain is relieved, or until three tablets have been taken in 15 minutes.
2. NTG translingual spray, 0.4 mg per metered dose. To use spray, spray onto or under the tongue. Use is the same as for sublingual tablets.
3. NTG transdermal patch, 0.1 to 0.8 mg/hr release rates. Generic patches are available in 0.2, 0.4, and 0.6 mg release rates. Tolerance limits efficacy when patches are used for longer than 12 hr/day.
4. Topical NTG 2% ointment (15 mg/inch): Spread a thin layer on skin using applicator or measuring papers and occlude. Do not use fingers; do not rub or massage ointment into the skin. Keep tube tightly closed. The

Continued

sublingual nitroglycerin (Nitrostat) 🔑—cont'd

dosage is 0.5 to 2 in. Apply first dose upon awakening, and give second dose 6 hours later.

5. Isosorbide dinitrate, oral: 5, 10, 20, 30, and 40 mg scored oral tablets; 40 mg sustained-release tablets.
6. Isosorbide dinitrate, sublingual: For prophylaxis, take 2.5 to 5 mg 2 to 3 hours before anticipated angina. Do not crush chewable tables before administering.
7. Isosorbide dinitrate, extended release: Take on empty stomach.
8. Isosorbide mononitrate, oral: 10- and 20-mg tablets, 60 mg extended-release tablets, 20 mg tablets twice daily, given on awakening and 7 hours later. Extended-release tablets, 30 mg (½ tablet) to 60 mg in the morning; may be increased to 120 to 240 mg
9. Isordil mononitrate, extended release: Do not crush or chew. Take with fluid.

evolve For additional information on antianginal product drug formulations, see the Bonus Reference Tables on the Evolve Resources website at http://evolve.elsevier.com/Edmunds/NP/

Ranolazine Extended Release

Ranolazine is unrelated to other available antianginal agents. The CARISA (Combination Assessment of Ranolazine In Stable Angina) trial showed a significant improvement in exercise duration and angina symptoms when ranolazine was added to therapy for patients already taking antianginal agents. The addition of this drug to standard treatment for acute coronary syndrome does not reduce the risk of major cardiovascular events (e.g., mortality, myocardial infarction) but may provide antianginal and antiarrhythmic benefits. Heart rate and arterial pressure at rest and at peak exercise are unchanged after a single 240-mg dose. Thus, this drug can be added safely to traditional antianginal therapy if no other significant drug interactions occur.

TABLE 16-4 Pharmacokinetics of Common Antianginal Agents

Drug	Availability (After First Pass)	Onset of Action	Time to Peak Concentration	Half-life	Duration of Action	Protein Bound	Metabolism
nitroglycerin, sublingual tablet	Poor	1-3 min	4-8 min	1-4 min	30-60 min	60%	Rapidly metabolizes to dinitrates and mononitrates
nitroglycerin, translingual spray	—	2 min	4 -10 min		30-60 min		
nitroglycerin, transdermal patch	NA	40-60 min	1-3 hr		18-24 hr		
nitroglycerin, topical ointment	NA	15-60 min	1-2 hr		2-12 hr		
nitroglycerin, oral sustained-release tablet	Extensive first-pass effect	20-45 min	1-2 hr		4-8 hr		
isosorbide dinitrate, chewable tablet	Highly variable	3 min	—	1-4 hr (parent drug); 4 hr (metabolite)	0.5-2 hr	2-2.5 hr	Extensively hepatic to conjugated metabolites, including isosorbide 5-mononitrate (active) and 2-mononitrate (active)
isosorbide dinitrate, sublingual tablet	22%	2-10 min	60 min	5 hr	1-3 hr	<4%	Metabolizes to mononitrate and sorbitol
isosorbide mononitrate	Not subject to first pass; nearly 100% bioavailable	30-60 min	30-60 min	4 hr	7 hr	<4%	Metabolizes to sorbitol and isosorbide
isosorbide mononitrate, extended release	Nearly 100%	30-60 min	3-4 hr	4 hr	12 hr after AM dose	5%	Multiple pharmacologically inactive metabolites; metabolized by the liver
ranolazine extended release	76% available as parent or metabolites; with or without food	Variable	2-5 hr	7 hr	Variable	62% bound to plasma proteins	Liver and intestine by CYP 3A isoenzymes and to a lesser extent by CYP 2D6 isoenzymes

TABLE 16-5 Common Drug Interactions With Nitrate Products

Precipitant Drug	Adverse Interaction
Alcohol	Severe hypotension, cardiovascular collapse
aspirin	May increase nitrate serum concentrations or actions
Calcium channel blockers	Marked orthostatic hypotension may occur.
dihydroergotamine	Bioavailability of the ergot may increase, causing an increase in mean standing systolic blood pressure or a functional antagonism between the two agents and a decrease in antianginal effects
heparin	May decrease heparin pharmacologic effects
sildenafil (Viagra)	May precipitate severe hypotension and death

PRECAUTIONS. Ranolazine has been associated with a significant dose- and concentration-related prolongation of the QT interval. These effects are believed to be caused by ranolazine and not by its metabolites. This action places restrictions on wider use of the drug.

CONTRAINDICATIONS
- Patients with mild, moderate, or severe hepatic impairment have about a threefold increase in QTc prolongation.
- Because the QTc prolonging effect is increased approximately threefold in patients with hepatic disease, ranolazine is contraindicated in patients with mild, moderate, or severe hepatic impairment.
- Ranolazine is contraindicated in patients with preexisting QT prolongation, history of torsade de pointes, or congenital long QT syndrome.
- Avoid use in uncorrected hypokalemia or in patients with a history of ventricular tachycardia (ventricular arrhythmia).
- Ranolazine is contraindicated in patients receiving drugs known to prolong the QT interval or drugs known to be moderate or potent cytochrome P (CYP) 3A4 inhibitors (including diltiazem and verapamil). In addition, inhibitors of P-glycoprotein (e.g., cyclosporine) may increase drug absorption.
- Ranolazine should be avoided in patients with severe renal impairment and renal failure, and it should be used with caution in patients with mild to moderate renal impairment.

PATIENT VARIABLES
- The effects of ranolazine on angina frequency and exercise tolerance are considerably smaller in women than in men. The mechanism for reduced antianginal benefit in women is not known.
- In addition to comparable antianginal efficacy for diabetic vs. nondiabetic patients, preliminary data suggest that ranolazine may have a slight benefit for glycosylated hemoglobin (HbA_{1c}) values in diabetic patients.
- No overall differences in ranolazine efficacy have been observed between older and younger patients. However, a higher frequency of adverse events during ranolazine therapy has been reported in patients aged $\geq$75 years but not for patients aged $\geq$65 years. In general, dose selection for

TABLE 16-6 Dosage Recommendations for Antianginal Agents

Drug	Initial Dose	Maintenance Dosage
nitroglycerin sublingual tablet (Nitrostat)	0.3 mg	Usual 0.4 to 0.6 mg sublingual (SL) q 5 min × 3 doses in 15 min. May use 5-10 min prior to activities that may provoke an attack
nitroglycerin translingual spray (Nitrolingual)	0.4 mg/metered dose	1-2 sprays SL q3-5 min × 3 doses in 15 min. May be used 5-10 min prior to activities that may provoke an attack
nitroglycerin transdermal patch (Nitro-Dur, Minitran)	0.2 mg/hr (5 mg patch) to 0.4 mg/hr (10 mg patch)	0.2-0.8 mg/hr patch daily. Remove for 12 of 24 hr to reduce tolerance.
nitroglycerin topical ointment (Nitro-Bid, Nitrol)	0.5-2 inches upon wakening	0.5-2 inches q6h. Include a 10-12 hr nitrate-free interval.
isosorbide dinitrate, chewable tablet (Isordil Titradose)	5-20 mg	5-40 mg q6h
isosorbide dinitrate, sublingual tablet (Isordil SL)	2.5-5 mg	2.5-5 mg q5-10 min for maximum of 3 doses in 15-30 min; may also take 15 min prior to activities that may provoke an attack
isosorbide dinitrate, sustained release (Dilitrate SR)	40 mg	40-80 mg q8-12h
isosorbide mononitrate (ISMO, Monoket [extended release])	5 mg upon awakening	5-20 mg bid given 7 hr apart (e.g., 8 AM and 3 PM) to decrease tolerance development. Titrate to 10 mg twice daily in first 2-3 days.
isosorbide mononitrate, extended release (Isordil, Imdur)	30-60 mg	30-60 mg given in morning as a single dose. Titrate upward as needed, giving at least 3 days between increases; maximum daily single dose: 240 mg
ranolazine extended-release	500-1000 mg po bid	May be taken with or without food. No grapefruit. Monitor adverse effects and possibility of drug interactions.

an elderly patient should be cautious, starting at the low end of the adult dosing range.

- The safety and efficacy of ranolazine have not been established in children.
- Ranolazine is classified as FDA pregnancy risk category C.
- It is not known whether ranolazine is excreted in human milk.

DRUG INTERACTIONS

- Ranolazine is extensively metabolized to numerous metabolites and has the potential for multiple and complex CYP450 drug interactions. Ranolazine also is associated with the potential for drug interactions based on its propensity to prolong the QT interval.
- Ketoconazole, diltiazem, and verapamil increase ranolazine plasma concentrations and should not be given concurrently.
- Cimetidine and paroxetine either do not increase plasma concentrations or do not require dosage adjustments of ranolazine. Digoxin and simvastatin plasma levels are increased by ranolazine, and dosage decreases may be required. No effect on warfarin is apparent.

ADVERSE EFFECTS. Dizziness is common during ranolazine therapy; syncope also may occur infrequently. Patients should use caution when driving or operating machinery.

DOSAGE AND ADMINISTRATION

- Because of extensive and rapid gut and liver metabolism, the systemic availability of ranolazine is highly variable. This is important in that QTc prolongation appears to be dose related.
- The usual dose is 500 mg po twice daily. The maximum recommended dose is 1000 mg po twice daily. It may be taken with or without food. Grapefruit juice should be avoided.

evolve A continually updated list of useful WebLinks may be found in the Evolve Resources at http://evolve.elsevier.com/Edmunds/NP/

Chronic Heart Failure and Digoxin

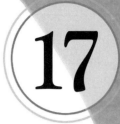

DRUG OVERVIEW

Class	Generic Name	Trade Name
Glycosides	digoxin 🔑 ✹	Lanoxin ✹
		Digitek ✹

 ✹ Top 200 drug; 🔑 key drug.

INDICATIONS

- Chronic heart failure, also called congestive heart failure or heart failure (HF)
- Atrial fibrillation
- Atrial flutter

One of the oldest and most widely prescribed primary care medications in the world is the glycoside digoxin. The principal indication for digoxin is HF. It is used for systolic HF, not diastolic, because of its inotropic properties. It is also used as an antiarrhythmic to control ventricular response to atrial tachyarrhythmia because it is an AV nodal blocker. Digoxin is the only glycoside that is in common use, and it is the only one discussed here. Although digoxin remains only one of the drugs used in the treatment of HF, its wide usage throughout the world, low cost, and narrow therapeutic window dictate that the clinician must understand how and when to use this product. (Additional drugs used in the treatment of HF are discussed in other chapters [Table 17-1].)

Patients with HF commonly take at least two medications: a diuretic and an angiotensin-converting enzyme inhibitor (ACEI).

💣 **The potential for toxicity is the major disadvantage of digoxin use.**

Because of its long half-life and narrow therapeutic window, patients treated with digoxin may easily become toxic. The elderly and those who are renally impaired are at increased risk for cardiac rhythm disturbance, as well as for toxicity from digoxin. Digoxin-induced arrhythmias must be differentiated from digoxin-treated ones, and the dose must be decreased, not increased.

THERAPEUTIC OVERVIEW OF CHRONIC HEART FAILURE

Anatomy and Physiology

- Cardiac output (CO) is the volume of blood ejected from the heart/unit time.
- Stroke volume (SV) is the volume of blood ejected with each beat.

- Heart rate (HR) is the number of beats/minute.
- Calculation of CO: $CO = SV \times HR$
- Left ventricular work and myocardial oxygen consumption depend on HR and blood pressure ($HR \times BP$).
- $BP = CO \times$ systemic vascular resistance (SVR) (afterload)
- Afterload is the force against which the ventricle must contract to eject blood, or the arterial pressure, arterial impedance, or resistance.
- Preload refers to the amount of blood going to the heart and the filling pressure created by systemic vascular resistance.
- The Frank-Starling law of the heart: Within limits, an increase in left ventricular filling increases the ventricular force of contractions, which increases the SV. After optimal filling is attained, increased volume no longer increases the SV. This is when the heart begins to fail. The Frank-Starling law keeps the output of the two ventricles balanced (Figure 17-1).

Pathophysiology

HF usually originates with left-sided ventricular failure (Figure 17-2), which is systolic HF. This side is most affected by hypertension, valvular dysfunction, and coronary artery disease. When the ventricle fails to pump enough blood to meet the metabolic needs of the body, baroreceptors in the circulatory system cause reflex sympathetic

TABLE 17-1 Other Medications Used for Heart Failure

Drug	Chapter
Diuretics	30
ACEIs/ARBs	20
β-Blockers	18
Spironolactone	30
CCBs	19
Hydralazine	15
Nitrates	16

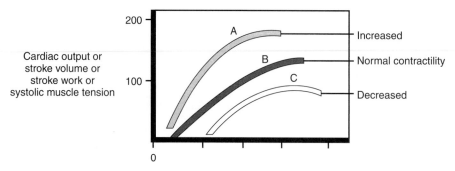

FIGURE 17-1   Frank-Starling law of the heart shows the relationship between length and tension in the heart. End-diastolic volume determines end-diastolic length of ventricular muscle fibers and is proportional to tension generated during systole, as well as to cardiac output, stroke volume, and stroke work. A change in myocardial contractility causes the heart to perform on a different length-tension curve. **A,** Increased contractility. **B,** Normal contractility. **C,** Heart failure or decreased contractility. (From McCance KL, Huether SE: *Pathophysiology,* ed 5, St Louis, 2006, Mosby.)

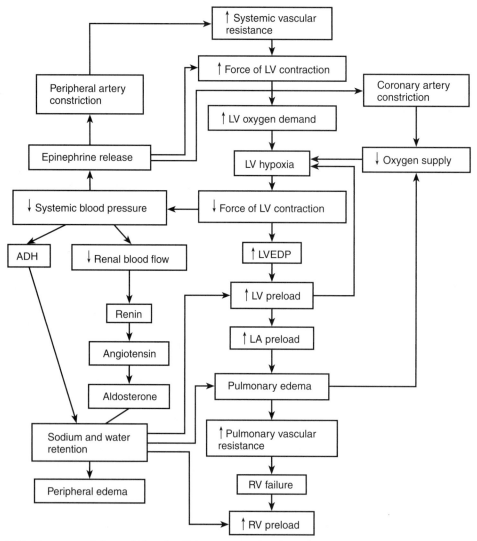

FIGURE 17-2   Left heart failure (CHF) from elevated systemic vascular resistance. Left-sided heart failure leads to right-sided heart failure. Systemic vascular resistance and preload are exacerbated by renal and adrenal mechanisms. (ADH, Antidiuretic hormone; LA, left atrial; LV, left ventricular; LVEDP, left ventricular end-diastolic pressure; RV, right ventricular.) (From McCance KL, Huether SE: *Pathophysiology,* ed 4, St Louis, 2001, Mosby.)

nervous system activation. Veins and arteries constrict to increase critical organ, especially cardiac, perfusion. The Frank-Starling mechanism increases preload to increase myocardial contractile strength. HR increases, also to ensure perfusion. These changes reduce the blood flow to the kidneys, where receptors act to release renin, starting the angiotensin-aldosterone cascade, which leads to further vasoconstriction and sodium and water retention.

As HF progresses, the compensatory mechanisms can no longer maintain homeostasis. Rapid heart rhythm reduces the amount of blood pumped and, consequently, oxygen perfusion. Peripheral vasoconstriction forces the heart to pump harder, and the renin-angiotensin-aldosterone mechanism causes overfilling of the heart. The overall result is left-sided ventricular failure. The pulmonary system experiences increasing capillary pressure and fluid leakage into the interstitial space, resulting in pulmonary edema. As a further result, blood pools in the right ventricle, causing increased pressure in the systemic circulation (right-sided heart failure). This distends visceral veins, the liver and spleen become engorged, and jugular vein distention (JVD) and tissue edema in the extremities become evident, particularly in dependent areas such as the ankles and legs.

Diastolic HF is caused by a stiff left ventricle with decreased compliance and impaired relaxation, causing increased end-diastolic pressure. This leads to decreased ventricular filling. The causes and symptoms are similar to those of systolic failure, but the treatment may be different.

Disease Process

HF is a clinical syndrome characterized by signs and symptoms of volume overload and inadequate tissue perfusion. Common causes of HF are ischemic heart disease, systemic hypertension, valve disease, hypertrophic cardiomyopathy from end-stage hypertension, restrictive cardiomyopathy, hypothyroidism and hyperthyroidism, atrial fibrillation, and COPD.

CLASSIFICATION OF SEVERITY. Severity of HF is rated in accordance with the New York Heart Association (NYHA) functional classification system or its updated 1994 objective assessment system (Table 17-2).

Assessment

Perform a complete history and physical examination that includes measurement of lying, sitting, and standing BP and pulse. In general, left-sided heart failure manifests as pulmonary signs and symptoms; right-sided heart failure causes systemic signs and symptoms. Both left- and right-sided heart failure are present in most patients. The onset is often gradual and subtle. Left-sided symptoms include paroxysmal nocturnal dyspnea (PND), dyspnea on exertion (DOE), S3 (S4 may be present with hypertension) heart sounds, arrhythmias, and pulsus alternans. Right-sided symptoms include fatigue, syncope, decreased exercise tolerance, hepatomegaly, peripheral edema, JVD, ascites, decreased appetite, and early satiety.

Perform diagnostic tests (Table 17-3) to rule out other possible causes for the symptoms, to determine underlying causes of HF, and to establish a baseline from which to monitor the patient. Obtain a complete blood count because anemia can mask heart failure symptoms. Renal function studies are especially important for dosage determination. Potassium levels are crucial because of the risk for arrhythmia. Obtain blood glucose testing because the risk of heart failure was found to be 2.4- and 5-fold increased in men and women, respectively, in the Framingham study. Order thyroid function tests, especially if atrial fibrillation is detected. Brain natriuretic peptide (BNP) is an FDA-approved diagnostic tool that is a reliable measure of cardiac function in both systolic and diastolic failure. A low BNP rules out HF; BNP may have a role in monitoring of patients with HF.

Classify HF according to systolic or diastolic heart failure to determine appropriate treatment.

Examine results from ECG and chest x-ray to identify any treatable causes of HF. The chest x-ray may show pulmonary congestion and cardiomegaly, which are consistent with HF. The ECG is usually abnormal in symptomatic patients with systolic HF. Echocardiograms also help in assessment of left ventricular function and in measurement of ejection fraction. In a person with HF, an ejection fraction less than 40% means left ventricular dysfunction or systolic heart failure; a normal ejection fraction >50% indicates diastolic heart failure. Systolic dysfunction is associated with reduced contractility and increased left ventricular end-diastolic volume. Diastolic dysfunction is associated with reduced ventricular filling. Table 17-4 lists factors that may precipitate an episode.

TABLE 17-2 New York Heart Association Classification of Severity of Heart Failure*

Functional Capacity	Objective Assessment
Class I: Patients with cardiac disease but without resultant limitation in physical activity. Ordinary physical activity does not cause undue fatigue, palpitation, dyspnea, or anginal pain.	A. No objective evidence of cardiovascular disease
Class II: Patients with cardiac disease resulting in slight limitation in physical activity. They are comfortable at rest. Ordinary physical activity results in fatigue, palpitation, dyspnea, or anginal pain.	B. Objective evidence of minimal cardiovascular disease
Class III: Patients with cardiac disease resulting in marked limitation of physical activity. They are comfortable at rest. Less than ordinary activity causes fatigue, palpitation, dyspnea, or anginal pain.	C. Objective evidence of moderately severe cardiovascular disease
Class IV: Patients with cardiac disease resulting in inability to carry on any physical activity without discomfort. Symptoms of heart failure or the anginal syndrome may be present even at rest. If any physical activity is undertaken, discomfort is increased.	D. Objective evidence of severe cardiovascular disease

*When there is reasonable uncertainty that the patient's symptoms are due to cardiac disease, the diagnosis should be no heart disease.
The Criteria Committee of the New York Heart Association: *Nomenclature and criteria for diagnosis of diseases of the heart and great vessels,* ed 9, Boston, MA, 1994, Little, Brown & Co.

TABLE 17-3   Recommended Tests for Patients With Signs and Symptoms of Chronic Heart Failure

Test Recommended	Findings	Suspected Diagnosis
CBC	Anemia	Heart failure caused or aggravated by decreased oxygen-carrying capacity
ECG	Acute ST-T wave changes Atrial fibrillation-tachyarrhythmia Bradyarrhythmia Left ventricular hypertrophy Low voltage Previous MI	MI Thyroid disease, rapid ventricular rate Sick heart Diastolic dysfunction Pericardial effusion Reduced left ventricular performance
Serum albumin	Decreased	Increased extravascular volume caused by hypoalbuminemia
Serum creatinine	Elevated	Volume overload caused by renal failure
Thyroid studies: T_4 and TSH	Abnormal T_4 Abnormal TSH	Hypothyroidism Hyperthyroidism
Urinalysis	Red blood cells and cellular casts Proteinuria	Glomerulonephritis Nephrotic syndrome

Modified from AHCPR: *Quick reference guide for clinicians,* Publication No. 94-0613, Washington DC, 1994, U.S. Government Printing Office.

MECHANISM OF ACTION

Digoxin has an inotropic effect on cardiac cells caused by enhancement of excitation-contraction coupling triggered by membrane depolarization. It acts at the cellular membrane by inhibiting the sodium-potassium pump, thus causing an increase in intracellular sodium. This increases sodium/calcium exchange and subsequent calcium accumulation in the sarcoplasmic reticulum. Activation of cardiac contractile proteins, actin, and myosin follows. The overall result is increased force of contraction of the cardiac muscle.

Cardiac glycosides (1) increase the force of myocardial contraction; (2) depress the sinoatrial node by stimulating vagal activity; (3) prolong conduction to the AV node via vagal stimulation; (4) increase the refractory period of the AV node; and (5) increase peripheral resistance. HR is slowed both vagally and extravagally.

In HF, digoxin increases CO and produces mild diuresis, helping to relieve symptoms. It is most effective in failure caused by decreased left ventricular function and other low-output syndromes. Digoxin is less effective in the high-output syndromes of heart failure such as bronchopulmonary insufficiency, anemia, infection, and hyperthyroidism.

Rapid arrhythmias such as atrial fibrillation, atrial flutter, and paroxysmal atrial tachycardia may provoke pulmonary edema. Oral digoxin maintains tachyarrhythmia suppression.

TREATMENT PRINCIPLES

Standardized Guidelines

- The 2005 American College of Cardiology/American Heart Association published guidelines for the evaluation and management of heart failure. This is an update of the 2001 guidelines. New are the subsets of HF, that is, acute decompensation and diastolic dysfunction. Also discussed are prevention, special populations, and device therapy.
- The Heart Failure Association of America (www.hfsa.org) issued new comprehensive evidence-based guidelines in 2006. This represents a comprehensive sifting of the evidence pertaining to diagnosis, treatment, and management of patients with HF.

Evidence-Based Recommendations

- Improvement in symptoms: ACEIs; angiotensin receptor blockers (ARBs); β-blockers (BBs) such as metoprolol, bisoprolol, and carvedilol; digoxin (in patients already receiving diuretics and ACEIs); and diuretics.
- Prolongation of patient survival: ACEIs, ARBs, BB hydralazine/nitrates (African Americans only). The aldosterone antagonists spironolactone and eplerenone have also been shown to improve survival in selected patients

Cardinal Points of Treatment

1. Loop diuretics for fluid retention
2. ACEI unless contraindicated, or ARB if ACEI is not tolerated

TABLE 17-4   Common Precipitating Factors for Chronic Heart Failure

General Factors	Specific Factors
Patient factors	Alcohol intake Excessive fluid intake Excessive salt intake Increased physical or mental stress Noncompliance with medication regimen Obesity, weight gain
Progression of basic cause	Increasing hypertension, coronary artery disease
Increased cardiac workload	Arrhythmia (possibly caused by digoxin) Electrolyte and acid-base abnormalities Increased or decreased blood volume, anemia Infection (cardiovascular or other, such as urinary tract infection) Pulmonary embolism Renal insufficiency
Medications that impair cardiac performance	Cardiovascular drugs 　Antiarrhythmics 　β-Blockers 　Calcium channel blockers 　Digoxin Corticosteroids Drugs that cause fluid retention 　NSAIDs

3. β-Blockers, especially for diastolic HF; begin when patient is stable on an ACEI
4. Digoxin for systolic HF and atrial fibrillation
5. Spironolactone if drugs listed above are not effective; eplerenone if spironolactone is not tolerated
6. Nitrates and hydralazine in African American patients only, if unable to tolerate the above regimen
7. Calcium channel blocker (CCB) (felodipine or amlodipine) only if needed for angina or hypertension, and if ejection fraction is preserved
8. Salt restriction

Pharmacologic Treatment

Treatment goals include normalizing blood pressure, promoting regression of left ventricular hypertrophy, preventing tachycardia, treating symptoms of congestion, and maintaining atrial contraction (Figure 17-3).

The following drugs are administered to most patients with HF. Figure 17-4 identifies the various medications and their site of action for the treatment of patients with HF.

Drug treatment of mild to moderate heart failure proceeds in the following order:

1. *Diuretics in patients with fluid retention:* Furosemide is more effective than a thiazide diuretic, especially in patients with renal insufficiency. Start at 40 mg po daily or 20 mg for a small, frail, and/or elderly person. The dosage then is gradually increased until excess fluid retention is relieved. The dosage of furosemide needed to maintain a patient is often less than that needed during an acute exacerbation of HF; therefore, consider decreasing the dosage after the acute episode, and always monitor for dehydration and hypokalemia when a patient is on furosemide. Metolazone may be added if the patient is furosemide resistant.
2. *ACEIs or ARBs in all patients unless contraindicated:* Add an ACEI after the diuretic has been taken. These drugs should be used in Stage I HF, before structural abnormalities develop. It is important to make sure that the patient is not overly diuresed before the ACEI is started. If the patient is dehydrated when started on an ACEI, acute renal failure may result. The limiting factor for the dose is often hypotension. If the patient develops a cough from the ACEI, change to an ARB. Start with a very low dose and titrate up, especially slowly every 1 to 2 weeks if the patient is elderly, small, or hypotensive. No difference has been noted between ACEIs. ACEIs cause regression of left ventricular hypertrophy, decrease blood pressure, and prevent or modify cardiac remodeling and are useful in both systolic and diastolic failure. African American patients are less responsive than other patients to ACEIs.
3. *β-Blockers in all stable (minimal fluid retention) patients unless contraindicated:* β-Blockers decrease heart rate, increase diastolic filling time, decrease oxygen consumption, lower blood pressure, and cause regression of left ventricular hypertrophy. They are effective for both systolic and diastolic failure but are of increased importance if diastolic failure is caused by increased diastolic filling time. Bisoprolol, carvedilol, and sustained-release metoprolol have demonstrated effectiveness in treating patients with HF. Metoprolol and carvedilol are most commonly used.
4. *Digoxin:* Add if needed for treatment of patients with systolic failure. Additional medical conditions in which digoxin may be useful include atrial fibrillation and diuretic failure.

If these medications are not sufficient to control heart failure, additional drugs may be given.

1. *Spironolactone, an aldosterone antagonist:* Spironolactone is an effective diuretic that helps to minimize the risk of hypokalemia associated with the use of furosemide. Spironolactone is effective in severe systolic failure. Spironolactone may cause hyperkalemia. Avoid in patients with renal insufficiency.
2. *Nitrates and hydralazine:* Use if the patient is unable to tolerate ACEIs. The combination of nitrates and hydralazine has been approved for use in African American patients only.
3. *CCBs:* May be useful in diastolic HF related to hypertension but can worsen systolic HF. Use a long-acting dihydropyridine such as amlodipine or felodipine only.

Salt restriction is important. Excess salt leads to fluid retention and worsening of symptoms. Patients are at higher risk of hypokalemia when on a high-salt diet. This can be a problem with the frail elderly because easily prepared foods such as canned soup and frozen dinners have a very high salt content.

Certain drugs can exacerbate HF and should be avoided if possible: CCBs, especially verapamil and diltiazem, have a negative inotropic effect on the heart. Other CCBs can cause edema. The exception is use of CCBs for those with diastolic failure not responsive to other therapy. NSAIDs cause sodium retention and peripheral vasoconstriction, thereby decreasing the efficacy of diuretics and ACEIs. Antiarrhythmic agents, except amiodarone and dofetilide, depress cardiac function. Thiazolidinediones used for diabetes, such as rosiglitazone and pioglitazone, may cause fluid retention and are contraindicated for Stage III and IV HF.

> 💣 Patients in diastolic failure are sensitive to fluid depletion, which can cause decreased preload and stroke volume. They should **NOT** receive digoxin.

End-stage HF requires careful control of fluid retention without causing dehydration. The patient should be referred for implantable defibrillators or cardiac transplantation as appropriate. End of life care should be discussed with the patient and family.

DIGOXIN. The administration and dosage of digoxin have changed dramatically over the past few years. In primary care settings, slow digitalization rather than a loading dose is generally recommended because of the risk of toxicity. Digitalization may be achieved within 1 week with the use of small daily maintenance doses. If renal function is poor, modification of dose is required. Digoxin is excreted essentially unchanged, so levels can quickly reach toxic proportions. See Table 17-5 for a summary of dosing regimens.

> 💣 Clinicians should be aware that generic digoxin marketed by different companies may not be bioequivalent to the branded digoxin (Lanoxin). Write the prescription for the trade or generic medication you desire, and then write on the prescription "No substitutions" or "Brand medically necessary."

The clinician may have to contact the pharmacy directly to ensure that the medication dispensed each time is the same. Patients also should be instructed to make certain that they receive the same product, whether brand or generic, each time the prescription is refilled.

Digoxin has a half-life of 36 hours, so it takes 5 to 6 days to achieve steady state. Start with a low dose and increase in 2 to 4 weeks if therapeutic effect is not achieved and the patient is not toxic. Measure digoxin levels monthly until stable, then at least every 6 months.

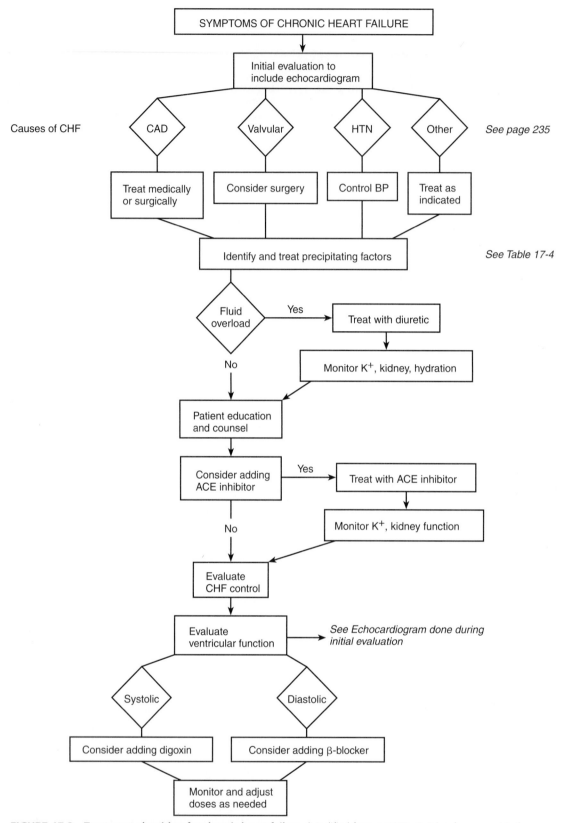

FIGURE 17-3   Treatment algorithm for chronic heart failure. (Modified from AHCPR: *Quick reference guide for clinicians,* Publication No. 94-0613, Washington, DC, 1994, U.S. Government Printing Office.)

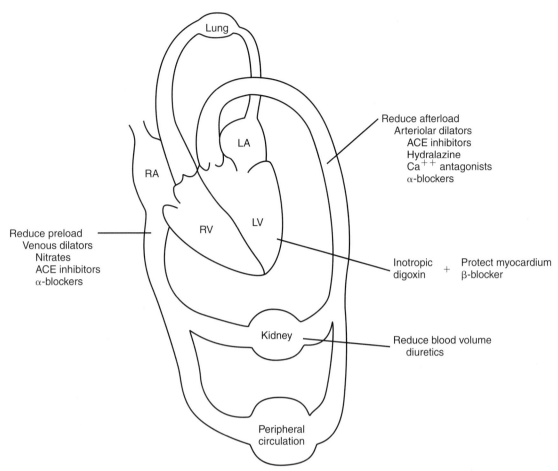

FIGURE 17-4   Sites of action of drugs used in the treatment of patients with chronic heart failure. (Data from Burton L et al, eds: *Goodman & Gilman's the pharmacological basis of therapeutics,* ed 11, New York, 2005, McGraw-Hill; Katzung BG: *Basic and clinical pharmacology,* ed 10, Norwalk, CT, 2006, McGraw-Hill; *Drug facts and comparisons,* Philadelphia, PA, 2008, Kluwer Publishing.)

Digoxin, once initiated, is often a lifetime drug. Occasionally, a patient with HF or arrhythmia may stop taking digoxin if the precipitating factors for the heart problem can be eliminated. The drug may be stopped abruptly without adverse effects. The long half-life allows the drug to be excreted over approximately 6 days.

TABLE 17-5   Digoxin Dosing Schedule

Dosing Regimen	To Maintain Therapeutic Level
Oral loading dose: for adults without increased risk for toxicity	Capsules: 0.4-0.6 mg po, then 0.1-0.3 mg po q6-8h (total of 0.6-1 mg in 24 hr) *or* Tablets: 0.5-0.75 mg po, then 0.125-0.375 mg po q6-8h (total of 0.75-1.25 mg in 24 hr)
Maintenance dose	Capsules: 0.1-0.4 mg po once daily Tablets: 0.125-0.5 mg po once daily
Maintenance dose for patients with renal insufficiency	Clcr 10-50 ml/min: 25% to 75% of dose Clcr <10 ml/min: 10% to 25% of dose or regular dose q48h

How to Monitor

MONITOR FOR THERAPEUTIC EFFECT

- Monitor the patient's clinical response to digoxin, not just serum drug levels. A therapeutic response may be achieved at a "subtherapeutic" drug level (0.5-0.8 ng/ml).
- To monitor for therapeutic effect when digoxin is given for HF, evaluate both signs and symptoms of heart failure. Patients with HF should have a gradual disappearance of subjective symptoms. In the physical examination, monitor weight, pulse rate, heart sounds, JVD, breath sounds, and pedal edema.
- To monitor for therapeutic effect when given for arrhythmia, monitor the ventricular rate. The patient may also be aware of rapid or irregular heartbeat, light-headedness, and dizziness.

MONITOR FOR TOXICITY

- To monitor for toxicity, the health care provider must be alert to early signs of toxicity and must obtain a serum level. A digoxin level >2 ng/ml indicates toxicity, although some patients become toxic at lower doses. Serum levels should be drawn at least 6 to 8 hours after the last dose and, ideally, just before the next dose.

- Hypokalemia is a risk factor for the development of arrhythmia even in patients within the therapeutic range.
- The earliest signs of digoxin toxicity are subtle and are easy to ignore: increased fatigue, visual disturbances, sinus bradycardia, anorexia, weakness, and nausea.
- ECG may show digoxin effect, a nonspecific ST-segment depression, or T-wave flattening.

Patient Variables

GERIATRICS. Use caution in the elderly and in those with renal impairment. Small body mass requires reduced dosage because of the wide distribution of digoxin in the tissue. Dose is based on lean body weight. HF is different in patients older than 75 years in that the incidence of diastolic failure is higher, and almost all patients have significant comorbidity.

PEDIATRICS

- Use of digoxin in children requires extra caution, lower doses, and closer monitoring.
- Newborns exhibit a variable tolerance to digoxin.

PREGNANCY AND LACTATION

- *Category C:* Safe use in pregnancy has not been documented.
- Digoxin does appear in breast milk, a possible contraindication to use.

GENDER. Women on digitalis with HF seem to be at somewhat greater risk of death from all causes.

Patient Education

- Take this drug exactly as directed by the health care provider. If a dose is forgotten, it should be taken as soon as it is remembered. If it is close to the scheduled time for the next dose, do *not* take the missed dose or double the next dose.
- It is important not to switch from trade to different generic products. They may not be the same. Make certain when getting a prescription filled that the same product is received each time.
- For safety, periodic blood tests must be performed to ensure that the drug level is kept within specified limits.
- Because digoxin slows the HR as it strengthens contractions, do not take the medication if HR is very slow. (The health care provider should teach patient and family members how to take a pulse.) Do not take digoxin, without consulting the health care provider, if pulse rate is lower than 60 beats/min.
- Do not take OTC medications, especially antacids or cough, cold, allergy, or diet drugs, without first talking with the health care provider.
- Report new or unusual symptoms to the health care provider. Loss of appetite and increased fatigue are two key symptoms that should be reported.
- Digoxin will kill pets and children. Keep it out of the reach of children and others for whom it is not prescribed.
- Patients should carry an identifying bracelet or card stating that they are taking digoxin.
- Reduce overall salt intake. Avoid high-sodium foods, including salted snacks, pork, luncheon meats, and processed cheese. Do not add salt when cooking; do not use extra salt at the table.
- Do not use salt substitutes because these are potassium chloride and may cause hyperkalemia.

SPECIFIC DRUGS

digoxin (Lanoxin)

CONTRAINDICATIONS. Ventricular fibrillation, ventricular tachycardia, digoxin toxicity, and hypersensitivity to digoxin (allergy is rare)

WARNINGS

- Sinus node disease and AV block: Because digoxin slows sinoatrial and AV conduction, the drug commonly prolongs the PR interval and may cause severe sinus bradycardia and sinoatrial block.

> **Patients with digoxin toxicity may present with arrhythmias identical to the arrhythmias for which digoxin is indicated. Make sure the patient is not digoxin toxic before giving the next dose.**

- A serum digoxin level may be necessary. An ECG may also be helpful.
- Determine the causes of anorexia, nausea, and vomiting before giving the next dose of digoxin because these are frequent symptoms of toxicity.
- Atrial fibrillation may not be controlled with digoxin. Avoid increasing the digoxin dose to toxic levels.
- Acute MI and other severe pulmonary disease or severe cardiac disease may predispose the patient to digoxin toxicity.
- In patients with idiopathic hypertrophic subaortic stenosis (IHSS), use digoxin with extreme caution.
- In Wolff-Parkinson-White syndrome and atrial fibrillation, digoxin may facilitate transmission through accessory pathways, thus increasing the HR.
- In sick sinus syndrome, digoxin may worsen bradycardia or heart block.
- Amyloid heart disease and constrictive cardiomyopathies do not respond to digoxin.
- Renal function impairment delays excretion of digoxin; adjust dosage accordingly. Dialysis has little effect on digoxin.
- Combined renal and hepatic failure may prolong digoxin elimination.

PRECAUTIONS

- Electrolyte imbalance
  - *Potassium:* Hypokalemia makes the myocardium more sensitive to digoxin. It also may reduce the positive inotropic effect of digoxin.
  - *Calcium:* Hypercalcemia predisposes the patient to digoxin toxicity. Hypocalcemia may make digoxin ineffective.
  - *Magnesium:* Hypomagnesemia may predispose to digoxin toxicity.
- *Thyroid dysfunction:* Hypothyroid patients require less digoxin because of decreased excretion rate. Hyperthyroid patients with heart failure may require larger doses. Arrhythmias caused by hypermetabolic states are particularly resistant to digoxin treatment; it is important to avoid toxicity.
- Digoxin may produce false-positive ST-T changes on ECG during exercise testing.

digoxin (Lanoxin) 🖋 —cont'd

PHARMACOKINETICS

- *Absorption:* Digoxin tablets are 60% to 80% absorbed, the elixir is 70% to 85% absorbed, and the Lanoxi-caps, which are solution-filled capsules, are 90% to 100% absorbed. Because of variation in the bioavail-ability of some preparations, absorption may vary between different brands of digoxin. Patients who have changed brand names of digoxin have had significantly altered serum levels of digoxin. Unless a meal is very high in fiber, food does not affect the amount of digoxin absorbed.
- *Distribution:* Digoxin is widely distributed in the tissues. The highest concentrations are found in the myocardium, skeletal muscle, liver, brain, and kidneys. It is not widely distributed in fatty tissue. Digoxin crosses the blood-brain barrier and the placenta. The volume of distribution of digoxin corresponds to the patient's ideal body weight.
- *Metabolism:* Most of the digoxin is not metabolized.
- *Excretion:* From 50% to 75% of digoxin is excreted unchanged by the kidneys. In patients with impaired renal function, significant accumulation may occur. This is especially dangerous because of the 36-hour half-life. Approximately 5 to 6 days is required to achieve steady state or elimination. Digoxin is not removed by dialysis because it is distributed in tissue, not blood.

ADVERSE EFFECTS

- Incidence of adverse effects is 5% to 50%; serious effects, 1% to 4%; toxicity, 0.5%; GI disturbances, up to 50%; CNS and other toxicity, 3% to 5%. The most common adverse effects are as follows:
  - *GI (most common):* anorexia, nausea, vomiting and diarrhea, abdominal discomfort
  - *CNS:* headache, weakness, apathy, drowsiness, visual disturbances (blurring, halo effect, and rarely, yellow or green vision), depression, restlessness, seizures, delirium, hallucinations, neuralgia, psychosis
  - *Cardiac:* Digoxin toxicity may present as almost any known type of arrhythmia. Ventricular tachycardia and unifocal or multifocal premature ventricular con-tractions (especially bigeminy or trigeminy) are the most common toxic arrhythmias. Also common are paroxysmal and nonparoxysmal nodal rhythms, AV dissociation, accelerated junctional (nodal) rhythm, and paroxysmal atrial tachycardia with block. AV block, complete heart block, and atrial fibrillation may also occur. The most common cause of death from digoxin toxicity is ventricular fibrillation.
  - Toxicity in children usually presents as an arrhyth-mia; fewer GI and neurologic disturbances are seen in children than in adults.

DRUG INTERACTIONS.
Many drugs affect digoxin levels (minor substrate of CYP 3A4). However, digoxin does not affect the levels of other drugs (Table 17-6). In addition, when β-blockers are added to digoxin in patients with AV conduction abnormalities, complete heart block can result. Erythromycin and clarithromycin

and tetracycline may increase digitalis absorption and toxicity. Thyroid replacement therapy increases dose requirements of digoxin.

OVERDOSAGE. It is important to monitor closely for digoxin toxicity. Symptoms of acute toxicity include vomiting, hyperkalemia, sinus bradycardia, sinoatrial arrest and AV block, ventricular tachycardia, and fibrillation.

TREATMENT OF TOXICITY

- Hold all digoxin until it is certain the patient is not digoxin toxic.
- Treatment of arrhythmias usually requires hospitalization.
- Digitalis-immune fragments of antibodies (FAB) is a treatment for digoxin intoxication. It is given intrave-nously and binds free digoxin. Improvement in symp-toms usually begins within a half-hour of administration.

DOSAGE AND ADMINISTRATION

- Can be given with or without food; absorption is not affected. Starting dose: 0.125 to 0.25 mg po daily, depending on size, renal function, and age of patient
- Adjust dose according to serum digoxin levels.

TABLE 17-6 **Drug Interactions With Digoxin**

DRUGS THAT MAY INCREASE DIGOXIN LEVELS
amiodarone
alprazolam, diazepam
bepridil
cyclosporine
diphenoxylate
indomethacin
itraconazole
clarithromycin, erythromycin
propafenone
propantheline
quinidine
spironolactone
tetracycline
verapamil

DRUGS THAT MAY DECREASE DIGOXIN LEVELS
Aminoglycosides
Antacids (aluminium and magnesium containing)
Antineoplastics (many)
charcoal, activated
cholestyramine
colestipol
kaolin/pectin
metoclopramide
neomycin
penicillamine
rifampin
St. John's wort
sulfasalazine

evolve A continually updated list of useful WebLinks may be found in the Evolve Resources at http://evolve.elsevier.com/Edmunds/NP/

18 β-Blockers

DRUG OVERVIEW

Class	Subclass	Generic Name	Trade Name
β-Adrenergic blockers	Nonselective	propranolol 🔑 ✴	Inderal ✴, InnoPran XL, generic
		carteolol	
		nadolol ✴	Corgard, generic
		penbutolol	Levatol
		pindolol	Generic
		sotalol ✴	Betapace, Sotalol
		timolol	Betimol, Blocadren, generic
	β_1-Selective	atenolol ✴	Tenormin, generic
		metoprolol ✴	Lopressor, Toprol XL ✴, generic
		acebutolol	Sectral, generic
		betaxolol	Kerlone, Betoptic, generic
		bisoprolol	Zebeta, generic
		esmolol	Brevibloc
	α-β-Blocker	labetalol ✴	Trandate, generic
		carvedilol	Coreg ✴

✴ Top 200 drug; 🔑 key drug. Propranolol was the first β-adrenergic blocker on the market and continues as a popular drug today.

INDICATIONS

- Hypertension: all except sotalol; esmolol is available only in an IV formulation for intraoperative hypertension and arrhythmia. Sotalol is used only for arrhythmia and is not discussed further.
- Angina, long-term management: atenolol, metoprolol, nadolol, propranolol
- CHF: metoprolol, carvedilol, bisoprolol
- Selected arrhythmias: acebutolol, esmolol, propranolol, sotalol
- Prophylaxis of migraine: propranolol, timolol
- Propranolol: hypertrophic subaortic stenosis, pheochromocytoma, essential tremor
- Carteolol is used only for glaucoma as an eye drop.
- MI prophylaxis, acute MI: atenolol, metoprolol, carvedilol

Unlabeled uses include the following:
- Mitral valve prolapse syndrome
- Alcohol withdrawal
- Nadolol, atrial fibrillation, paroxysmal supraventricular tachycardia (PSVT), and ventricular tachycardia prophylaxis

(See Table 18-1 for other indications.)

Since the original introduction of propranolol in the early 1960s, β-blockers have proliferated to include a multitude of drugs. Although the drugs have basic similarities, important differences among them are notable. β-Blockers are used in a wide variety of cardiac and noncardiac conditions. It is important for the provider to pick several β-blockers and know them well, rather than trying to use all of them.

MECHANISM OF ACTION

β_1-Receptors are found mainly in the heart, and stimulation from catecholamines causes an increase in heart rate, blood pressure, myocardial contractility, and AV conduction and a decrease in AV node refractoriness. β_2-Receptors are also present in heart muscle but are more prominent in the lungs and in peripheral vascular smooth muscle. Activation of β_1-receptors causes vasodilation and bronchodilation.

All β-blockers have a similar mechanism of action—competitive blockade of the β-adrenergic receptor. This results in decreased heart rate, myocardial contractility, blood pressure, and myocardial oxygen demand. β-Blockers also reduce the metabolic (glycogenolytic, lipolytic), myocardial

TABLE 18-1   Indications for the β-Blockers

Category	Drug	Hypertension	Angina	CHF	Arrhythmias	ISA	Other uses
NONSELECTIVE	propranolol (Inderal)	√	√		√		Migraine prophylaxis, tremor, hypertrophic subaortic stenosis, pheochromocytoma, Graves' disease
	nadolol (Corgard)	√	√				
	penbutolol (Levatol)	√				√	
	pindolol (Visken)	√				√	
	sotalol (Betapace, Betapace AF)				√		
	timolol (Blocadren)	√					Glaucoma, migraine prophylaxis, MI prophylaxis
β₁-SELECTIVE	atenolol (Tenormin)	√	√				Acute MI, MI prophylaxis
	metoprolol (Lopressor, (Toprol XL)	√	√	√ (extended-release only)	√		Acute MI, MI prophylaxis
	acebutolol (Sectral)	√			√	√	
	betaxolol (Kerlone)	√					Glaucoma
	bisoprolol, (Zebeta)	√					
	esmolol (Brevibloc) (IV only)	√			√		
α-β-BLOCKER	labetalol (Normodyne, Trandate)	√					
	carvedilol (Coreg)	√		√			MI prophylaxis, acute MI

stimulant, vasodilator, and bronchodilator actions of catecholamines, and they suppress renin release (Table 18-2).

As a result of β-blockade, cardiac output and heart rate are decreased. Slowing of the AV conduction system prevents an increase in cardiac automaticity and prolongs the refractory period. Decreased sympathetic peripheral outflow blocks the release of renin (carteolol, labetalol, and pindolol do not consistently inhibit renin release). BP is lowered by the action of β-blockers in decreasing cardiac output, peripheral vascular resistance, venous return, plasma volume, and renin release. The intrinsic sympathomimetic activity (ISA)-active β-blockers do not reduce renin release.

β-Blockers relieve the symptoms of angina by competitively inhibiting sympathetic stimulation of the heart, thereby reducing both heart rate and contractility. Because β-blockers reduce the heart rate–blood pressure product during exercise, symptoms of angina or the ischemic threshold during exercise is delayed or avoided.

CHF is perpetuated by an active renin-angiotensin system coupled with increased tone of the sympathetic nervous system;

thus, decreasing catecholamine levels reduce cardiac congestion and left ventricular hypertrophy (LVH). β-Blockers may increase β₁-receptor sensitivity and restore inotropic response. β₂-receptors promote peripheral vasodilation.

β-Blockers prevent arrhythmia by blocking abnormal cardiac pacemaker potentials, decreasing myocardial oxygen demand, prolonging ventricular filling time, and decreasing microvascular damage of the myocardium.

Clinically significant differences between β-blockers have been noted. These agents are classified by their β-blocking selectivity (β₁- or β₂- α [β-blocking ability]), membrane-stabilizing activity (MSA), ISA, and pharmacokinetics. See Table 18-3 for characteristics of individual agents.

Selectivity (or cardioselectivity) refers to the ability of the drug to preferentially block the β₁-receptors. Cardioselective β-blockers will inhibit β₁-receptors while producing less inhibition of the β₂-receptors that mediate bronchodilation or peripheral vasodilation. However, cardioselectivity is dose dependent, and substantial β₂-blockade occurs in patients with angina for whom higher doses are used. Thus, the advantage of using β₁-selectivity to reduce bronchospasm and decrease peripheral resistance may be diminished with a high-dose regimen. Most providers use selective β-blockers. Cardioselectivity is a clinically important feature of β-blockers.

Intrinsic sympathomimetic activity, or ISA, is another characteristic of β-blockers. Also known as partial agonist activity (PAA), ISA simultaneously blocks natural catecholamine while only partially activating β-receptors. Therefore, side effects such as bradycardia, bronchoconstriction, and resting peripheral vascular resistance may be minimized. ISA is not beneficial in alleviating arrhythmias and may eliminate the effectiveness of the β-blocker in the secondary prevention of MI.

Membrane-stabilizing activity, or MSA, another feature of this drug class, is described as a quinidine-like or local anesthetic effect on cardiac action potentials. High concentrations of the β-blocker are needed to reduce arrhythmias, and these often produce side effects. Thus, the significance of MSA seems to be negligible.

α-Adrenergic blocking activity is another characteristic of two drugs in this class. Labetalol and carvedilol both are

TABLE 18-2   Comparison of Adrenergic Receptors

Receptor	Site	Effect of Stimulation
α₁	Smooth muscle in blood vessels	Vasoconstriction
	Stomach, intestine	Decreased motility and tone
	Kidney	Increased renin secretion
	Liver	Gluconeogenesis
α₂	Smooth muscle in blood vessels	Vasodilation
β₁	Cardiac	Increased rate and force of contraction
	Kidney	Increased renin secretion
β₂	Bronchial, vascular, coronary arteriole, uterine smooth muscle, skeletal muscle	Vasodilation
	Pancreas	Decreased secretion
	Liver	Gluconeogenesis

TABLE 18-3   Characteristics of Individual β-Blockers

Drug	Selectivity	ISA	MSA	Lipid Solubility
propranolol	β_1 and β_2	0	0	High
carteolol	β_1 and β_2	+	0	Low
nadolol	β_1 and β_2	0	0	Low
penbutolol	β_1 and β_2	+	0	High
pindolol	β_1 and β_2	+	0	Low
sotalol	β_1 and β_2	0	0	Low
timolol	β_1 and β_2	0	0	Moderate
atenolol	β_1	0	0	Low
metoprolol	β_1	0	0	Moderate
acebutolol	β_1	+	+	Low
betaxolol	β_1	0	+	Low
bisoprolol	β_1	0	0	Low
carvedilol	α_1, β_1, and β_2	0	+	Moderate
labetalol	α_1, β_1, and β_2	0	0	High

ISA, Intrinsic sympathomimetic activity; MSA, membrane-stabilizing activity.

nonselective β-blockers without ISA. These drugs block β- and α-receptors with a potency ratio of 4:1. The result is a reduction in heart rate and cardiac contractility (as occurs with other β-blockers), and, because of the α-blocking effects of these agents, peripheral and coronary vascular resistance is reduced. Carvedilol is used to treat patients with heart failure; however, the benefit appears to be unrelated to peripheral α-blockade.

Pharmacokinetics is a clinically important characteristic of the β-blockers that may influence their clinical usefulness and side effects. β-Blockers can be classified into two categories: those excreted by the liver and those excreted by the kidney. Propranolol and metoprolol are lipid soluble, are almost completely absorbed by the small intestine, and are largely metabolized by the liver. Because these agents are highly lipophilic, they readily enter the CNS and are responsible for side effects such as lethargy, confusion, sleep disturbance, and probably depression (this matter is under investigation). Lipid solubility of the β-blocker is a clinical necessity when migraine headache or tremor is treated. These drugs also tend to have highly variable bioavailability and relatively short plasma half-lives.

In contrast, drugs such as atenolol and sotalol are more water soluble, are poorly absorbed, are eliminated unchanged by the kidney, and generally do not cross the blood-brain barrier. They show less variance in bioavailability and have longer plasma half-lives.

β-Blockers have adverse metabolic effects; this limits their usefulness in patients with hypercholesterolemia and diabetes mellitus. β-Blockers cause moderate elevation of blood sugar, increased insulin resistance, reduced HDL cholesterol, and elevated triglycerides. They also may blunt the signs and symptoms of hypoglycemia. It has been proposed that inhibition of sympathetic activity may lead to reduction in the patient's quality of life from fatigue, depression, or decreased exercise capacity when compared with ACE inhibitor therapy. However, this quality-of-life disadvantage with β-blockers has not been confirmed in clinical trials.

TREATMENT PRINCIPLES (Guidelines, Evidence-based Findings, and Cardinal Treatment Points are in Chapter 15.)

β-Blockers are important drugs that are known to decrease mortality. However, the choice of a β-blocker must be patient specific because of the many potential side effects that may limit compliance. Selection of agents should be limited to drugs with documented indications and known efficacy. Choose only a few β-blockers and become familiar with their use. Propranolol, atenolol, metoprolol, carvedilol, and labetalol are commonly used.

> β-Blockers must be used with caution in patients with certain heart conditions such as heart block, sinus bradycardia, cardiogenic shock, or heart failure.

Bradyarrhythmia, AV block, heart failure, and exacerbation of peripheral vascular disease (PVD) have occurred. In diabetic patients, β-blockers may intensify hypoglycemia and prolong gluconeogenesis through inhibited release of insulin. Clinical signs and symptoms of hypoglycemia may be blocked. Clinical signs and symptoms of thyrotoxicosis may be masked, and abrupt withdrawal may precipitate thyroid storm. Symptoms of depression may be aggravated in individuals with a history of depression. Asthma and COPD may be exacerbated through the use of β-blockers.

HYPERTENSION. β-Blockers and diuretics generally have been preferred as initial agents because they have been documented to reduce cardiovascular morbidity and mortality in long-term, controlled clinical trials. Newer studies reveal that β-blockers should not be considered as first-line drug therapy for hypertension any longer because the risk for development of diabetes mellitus is high. However, many still consider β-blockers a good first-line medication in select patients only. β-Blockers may serve as an ideal initial agent in patients with angina, arrhythmia, compensated heart failure, post-MI status, tremors, glaucoma, and vascular headache. The Seventh Report of the Joint National Committee on Prevention, Detection, Evaluation, and Treatment of High Blood Pressure (JNC 7) recommends use of a diuretic as first-line therapy for stage 1 hypertension.

Patients who should not be prescribed a β-blocker are African American patients and those with asthma or COPD, severe peripheral vascular disease, Raynaud's phenomenon, depression, bradycardia, or second- or third-degree heart block, as well as hypoglycemia-prone diabetic patients in whom the early warning symptoms of hypoglycemia may be masked. These agents also should not be used for hypertension in the elderly unless a compelling reason such as CAD, MI, or CHF is evident. β-Blockers have not been shown to reduce the risk of stroke that accompanies the use of antihypertensive medications.

See Chapter 15 for information on the management of hypertension.

ANGINA. β-Blockers are the treatment of choice for chronic stable and unstable angina. The goals of therapy are to reduce the frequency and severity of symptoms and to improve exercise capacity without producing significant side effects. The therapeutic effect of β-blockers in relieving angina is dose dependent. Therefore, attainment of adequate β-blockade is important.

The provider can choose among nitrates and β-blockers when selecting a first-line treatment. Although many patients will be taking nitrates, β-blockers will be needed during the necessary nitrate-free time. For simplicity of regimen, many providers simply prescribe β-blockers.

Resting heart rate and drug levels are variable and are poor predictors of control. A more precise approach to treatment involves drug titration that is based on frequency of anginal symptoms and nitrate use (see Chapter 16).

β-Blocker withdrawal may exacerbate angina in patients with CAD.

SECONDARY PREVENTION POST–MYOCARDIAL INFARCTION. The 2004 American College of Cardiology (ACC)/American Heart Association (AHA) Task Force on the management of ST elevation in MI recommended that all patients should receive β-blocker therapy, except those at low risk. Low-risk patients are those with normal or near-normal left ventricular function, successful reperfusion, and absence of significant ventricular arrhythmias, as well as those with contraindications. β-Blockers have been shown to improve survival in patients who have had an MI, primarily by reducing the incidence of sudden death in high-risk patients.

Early treatment of patients with MI with β-blockers occurs during the hospital stay. This approach has shown a small benefit in selected patients. Pooled data from controlled trials in more than 29,000 patients who under-

TABLE 18-4   Pharmacokinetics of Common β-Blockers

Drug	Bioavailability	Onset of Action	Half-life	Duration of Action	Protein Binding	Metabolism	Excretion
propranolol	30%	1-1.5 hr	3-5 hr; 8-11 hr long acting	11 hr	93%	Hepatic 2D6 substrate	Hepatic
nadolol	30%	1-4 hr	10-24 hr	21-39 hr	30%	Negligible	Renal
penbutolol	90%-100%	1.5-3 hr	5 hr	20-24 hr	80%-98%	Hepatic conjugation and oxidation	Renal
pindolol	50%-90%	1 hr	2-4 hr	24 hr	50%	Hepatic	Renal
sotalol	90%-100%	2-4 hr	12 hr	8-16 hr	0%	Not metabolized	Renal
timolol	50%-75%	0.5-2.5 hr	2-3 hr	4 hr	10%	Hepatic 2D6 substrate	Renal
atenolol	40%-50%	2-4 hr	6-9 hr	24 hr	6%-16%	Hepatic, minimal	Renal
metoprolol	40%-50%; long acting, 77%	0.5-2 hr	3-7 hr	14-24 hr	12%	Hepatic 2D6 substrate	Renal
acebutolol	40%	2.5-4 hr	3-4 hr active metabolite 8-13 hr	24 hr	26%	Hepatic	Renal and hepatic
betaxolol	89%-90%	1.5-6 hr	14-22 hr	24 hr	50%	Hepatic	Renal
bisoprolol	80%	2-4 hr	9-12 hr	24 hr	30%	Hepatic 2D6 substrate	Renal and hepatic
labetalol	25%	Oral, 2-4 hr	Oral, 5.5-8 hr	8-24 hr	50%	Hepatic, mainly through conjugation to glucuronide metabolites	Hepatic
carvedilol	25%-35%	1-2 hr	7-10 hr	24 hr	98%	Hepatic 2D6, 2C9; lesser extent 3A4, 2C9, 1A2	Hepatic

TABLE 18-5   Adverse Effects of β-Blockers

Body System	Common Side Effects	Serious Adverse Effects
Body, general	Weight gain, weight loss, decreased exercise tolerance	Lupus-like syndrome, Raynaud's phenomenon, death
Cardiovascular	Bradycardia	Torsades de pointes, cardiac arrest, cardiogenic shock, hypotension, peripheral ischemia, worsening angina, shortness of breath, heart failure, SA block, abnormal ECG, arrhythmias, thrombophlebitis
Circulatory and hematologic		Agranulocytosis, thrombocytopenic purpura, bleeding, thrombocytopenia, eosinophilia, leukopenia, pulmonary emboli, anemia, leukocytosis
Gastrointestinal	Flatulence, gastritis, constipation, nausea, diarrhea, dry mouth, vomiting, heartburn, anorexia, abdominal pain	Ischemia, colitis, dysphagia
Genitourinary	Sexual dysfunction, impotence or decreased libido, dysuria, nocturia, urinary retention or frequency	Renal failure, abnormal renal function
Hepatic		Elevated level of liver enzymes, bilirubin; hepatomegaly, acute hepatitis with jaundice
Hypersensitivity	Pharyngitis, erythematous rash	Photosensitivity, fever with aching and sore throat, laryngospasm, respiratory distress, angioedema, anaphylaxis
Metabolic and nutritional		Hyperglycemia, hypoglycemia, unstable diabetes mellitus
Musculoskeletal	Joint pain, arthralgia, muscle cramps/pain, arthritis	Myalgia, joint disorder, tendinitis, gout
Nervous system	Dizziness, vertigo, tiredness, fatigue, headache, mental depression, confusion	Peripheral neuropathy, paralysis, paresthesias, lethargy, somnolence, restlessness, sleep disturbances, nightmares, incoordination, emotional lability, ataxia, seizures, stroke
Respiratory	Cough, nasal stuffiness	Bronchospasm, dyspnea, bronchial obstruction, wheeziness, laryngospasm with respiratory distress, asthma
Skin, appendages	Rash, pruritus, increased pigmentation, sweating, alopecia, dry skin, psoriasis, acne, eczema	Exfoliative dermatitis, peripheral skin necrosis
Special senses	Taste perversion, eye irritation, visual disturbances	Iritis, cataract, diplopia

went early, short-term IV administration of a β-blocker show a 13% reduction in acute mortality.

Immediate β-blocker therapy may provide an additional benefit in reducing the incidence of intracerebral hemorrhage after thrombolytic therapy. A review of 60,329 patients treated with alteplase in the National Registry of Myocardial Infarction revealed that immediate administration of a β-blocker was associated with a reduction in the incidence of intracerebral hemorrhage of 67% vs. 1% for no immediate β-blocker. This benefit was seen in all age groups and in both men and women.

CHRONIC HEART FAILURE. Patients with symptomatic heart failure have elevated levels of norepinephrine. This increase in sympathetic activity may have harmful effects, and clinical trials have shown that blockade of β-adrenergic receptors leads to symptomatic improvement and enhanced survival in heart failure. β-Blockers produce increased ejection fraction and reduction in left ventricular size and mass. Patients have fewer hospitalizations and less mortality with a reduction in sudden death and death from CHF.

Guidelines from the 2005 ACC/AHA task force recommended that β-blockers should be used in patients with asymptomatic or symptomatic left ventricular dysfunction unless they are contraindicated. Patients who should not receive a β-blocker include those with a heart rate of <60 beats

per minute, a systolic arterial pressure of <100 mm Hg, signs of peripheral hypoperfusion, a PR interval >0.24 second, second- or third-degree AV block, severe COPD, a history of asthma, or severe peripheral vascular disease. β-Blockers with ISA should be avoided.

Carvedilol, metoprolol (extended-release only), and bisoprolol are administered for heart failure. The starting doses of these drugs are significantly lower than those used for hypertension (daily doses of carvedilol 3.125 mg bid, metoprolol 6.25 mg bid, or bisoprolol 1.25 mg). Be aware of the edema caused by carvedilol, although this drug is considered an effective antioxidant.

ARRHYTHMIAS. The role of β-blockers in the treatment of atrial fibrillation (AF) is unclear. Propranolol has not been shown to be effective in maintaining normal sinus rhythm (NSR) after direct current (DC) electroversion. However, other β-blockers such as metoprolol may provide some benefit.

Sotalol is a unique β-blocker because it is classified as a class II and III antiarrhythmic. Sotalol is a 1:1 mixture of the d- and l-isomers and is referred to as dl-sotalol. It has both β-blocking (class II) and cardiac action potential duration prolongation (class III) properties. In clinical studies, sotalol has been shown to be as effective as and less toxic than quinidine and as effective as propafenone, but less effective

TABLE 18-6   Drug Interactions With β-Blockers

β-Blocker(s)	Action on Other Drugs
All β-blockers	Increase flecainide, clonidine, epinephrine, ergot alkaloids, lidocaine, prazosin
propranolol	Increases phenothiazines, haloperidol, anticoagulants, gabapentin
metoprolol, propranolol (lipid soluble)	Increase benzodiazepines, hydralazine
All β-blockers	Alter disopyramide
Other Drug(s)	**Action on β-Blockers**
Calcium channel blockers, oral contraceptives, quinidine, diphenhydramine, flecainide, hydroxychloroquine, ciprofloxacin	Increase β-blockers
Aluminum salts, barbiturates, calcium salts, cholestyramine, colestipol, ampicillin, rifampin, nonsteroidal antiinflammatories, salicylates, sulfinpyrazone	Decrease β-blockers
cimetidine, hydralazine, monoamine oxidase inhibitors, propafenone, selective serotonin reuptake inhibitors, thioamines	Increase metoprolol, propranolol
Thyroid hormones	Decrease metoprolol, propranolol

than amiodarone. Sotalol is a preferred agent in patients with a history of coronary heart disease.

Thus, antiarrhythmic drugs are mainly used as primary therapy in patients who do not want or are not candidates for an internal cardiac defibrillator (ICD) (e.g., because of marked comorbidities or end-stage heart failure that makes death likely). It is far more common to use antiarrhythmic drugs in conjunction with an ICD to reduce the frequency of appropriate shocks or of inappropriate shocks due to atrial arrhythmias. Although it reduces recurrent arrhythmia and the frequency of ICD shocks, sotalol is considered second-line therapy to amiodarone.

Sotalol is also indicated for ventricular arrhythmia. It has been shown to prevent recurrence of sustained VT or VF. However, sotalol is generally less effective than an ICD. This difference is seen largely in patients with an ejection fraction ≤35%.

Bradycardic and proarrhythmic events can occur after initiation of sotolol treatment. Therefore, sotalol should be initiated and doses increased in a hospital in which cardiac rhythm can be monitored.

OTHER USES. Prophylactic treatment of patients with migraine headache with β-blockers helps to reduce the frequency and intensity of headaches. The relative effectiveness is probably influenced by lipid solubility, with more lipid-soluble drugs crossing the blood-brain barrier more easily. Several randomized, placebo-controlled studies

TABLE 18-7   Dosage and Administration Recommendations of β-Blockers

Drug	Indication	Initial Dosage	Titration	Usual JNC 7 Dose Range (for HTN)	Adjustment for Renal Impairment	Maximum Daily Dose
propranolol	HTN	40 mg bid	Every 3-7 days	40-160 mg/day in two divided doses; SR 60-180 mg once daily	None necessary	640 mg
	Angina	SR 80 mg daily 80-320 mg bid-qid SR 80 mg daily				320 mg
	Essential tremor	20-40 mg bid	120 mg/day			320 mg
nadolol	HTN Angina	40 mg daily; 20 mg once daily (elderly)	40-80 mg every 3-7 days; 20 mg every 3-7 days (elderly)	40-120 mg once daily	CrCl 31-40 ml/min: every 24-36 hr, or administer 50% of normal dose CrCl 10-30 ml/min: every 24-48 hr or administer 50% of normal dose CrCl <10 ml/min: q40-60h or administer 25% of normal dose	240-320 mg 160-240 mg
penbutolol	HTN	20 mg once daily	10 mg every 2 weeks	10-40 mg once daily	None necessary	80 mg
pindolol	HTN	10-40 mg/day in two divided doses	10 mg/day q3-4wk		Initially: 5 mg once daily, then increase by 5 mg/day q3-4wk	60 mg
timolol	HTN	10 mg bid	Every week to 20-60 mg/day	20-40 mg/day in two divided doses	None necessary	60 mg
	Migraine		Every week to 20-30 mg/day			30 mg

Table continued on following page

TABLE 18-7   Dosage and Administration Recommendations of β-Blockers (Continued)

Drug	Indication	Initial Dosage	Titration	Usual JNC 7 Dose Range (for HTN)	Adjustment for Renal Impairment	Maximum Daily Dose
metoprolol	HTN	50 mg bid; 25-100 mg/day (extended-release)	Every week	50-100 mg/day in one or two divided doses	None necessary	450 mg in two or three divided doses; 400 mg (extended-release) 200 mg/day
	Angina, SVT, CHF	SR: 25 mg once daily (reduce to 12.5 mg once daily in NYHA class higher than class II)	Double dose every 2 weeks as tolerated			
	Post-MI	50 mg q6h 15 min after last IV dose, then continue for 48 hr; then administer a maintenance dose of 100 mg twice daily				
acebutolol	HTN	400-800 mg/day in divided doses (200-400 mg/day elderly)	Every 4-7 days	200-800 mg/day in two divided doses	CrCl 25-49 ml/min: reduce dose by 50% CrCl <25 ml/min: reduce dose by 75%	1200 mg/day (800 mg/day elderly)
	Angina, ventricular arrhythmia	400 mg/day in divided doses (200-400 mg/day elderly)	600-1200 mg/day in divided doses			
betaxolol	HTN	5-10 mg once daily	Every 1-2 weeks	5-20 mg/day	5 mg/day; increase q2wk up to a maximum of 20 mg/day CrCl <10 ml/min: 50% of usual dose	20 mg
bisoprolol	HTN	2.5-5 mg once daily	Every 1-2 weeks	2.5-10 mg/day	CrCl <40 ml/min: 2.5 mg/day	20 mg
labetalol	HTN	100 mg bid	100 mg every 2-3 days	200-800 mg/day in divided doses	None necessary	2400 mg/day
carvedilol	HTN	6.25 mg bid × 1-2 weeks	Increase to 12.5 mg in 1-2 weeks		None necessary	25-50 mg/day
	CHF	3.125 mg bid × 2 weeks	Increase to 6.25 mg twice daily; double dose every 2 weeks until highest dose tolerated			Mild to moderate CHF: <85 kg: 25 mg bid >85 kg: 50 mg twice daily Severe CHF: 25 mg twice daily

have found that long-term therapy with propranolol reduces the frequency and severity of migraine in as many as 80% of patients. Other β-blockers such as metoprolol, nadolol, and atenolol are commonly used for migraine prophylaxis. Only propranolol and timolol have been approved by the FDA for prophylaxis of migraine headache. The provider should inform the patient that it may take several weeks for therapy to be effective. The dose should be titrated and maintained for a minimum of 3 months before treatment is deemed a failure.

Essential tremor (ET) shows marked improvement with propranolol. Anxiety, with associated tachycardia and tremor, abates with β-blockade of circulating catecholamines. In 2005, the American Academy of Neurology (AAN) concluded that propranolol 60 to 320 mg/day is safe and effective for the treatment of limb tremor associated with ET. Data from 12 prospective, randomized, controlled clinical trials demonstrated that tremor magnitude was reduced by approximately 50% as measured by accelerometry. Clinical rating scales also improved tremor magnitude by 50%. The mean dose of propranolol was 185.2 mg/day in nine of these studies. Side effects of propranolol, including light-headedness, fatigue, impotence, and bradycardia, occurred in 12% to 66% of patients in clinical trials.

Long-acting propranolol has proved effective for the treatment of patients with ET and appears to produce the same therapeutic response as immediate-release propranolol. One study found that long-acting propranolol was preferred to immediate-release propranolol by 87% of patients because of its ease of administration.

Single doses of propranolol taken in anticipation of social situations such as public speaking are useful in some patients.

The AAN recommends following the consensus recommendations of the *American Journal of Cardiology* or consulting with a cardiologist prior to starting propranolol in patients with cardiac disease. Atenolol, metoprolol, nadolol, and timolol have also been used to treat tremor, but this is an off-label use for these agents.

Hyperthyroidism is associated with an increased number of β-adrenergic receptors. Stimulation of these receptors by circulating catecholamines is responsible for the palpitations, tremor, increased heart rate, and anxiety associated with this disorder. β-Blockers are rapidly effective in reducing these symptoms. β-Blockers should be given to most patients with hyperthyroidism who do not have a contraindication for their use. Most often, they are prescribed with drugs that block thyroxine (T_4)-to-triiodothyronine (T_3) conversion. Patients with relative contraindications may better tolerate the cardioselective β-blockers atenolol and metoprolol.

How to Monitor

- Evaluate blood pressure and pulse weekly until stable and then at least every 3 to 4 months.
- Obtain a baseline ECG before initiating drug therapy as needed and on an annual basis thereafter. An ECG provides serial evaluation of electrophysiologic changes that occur during the course of drug therapy and identifies any significant ECG changes such as bradycardia or LVH.
- Based on the specific patient population's appropriate evaluation of blood glucose concentrations, electrolytes, lipid values, and renal and hepatic function tests may be warranted.
- Monitor for toxicity manifested by bradycardia and hypotension. In specific patient subsets, observe for progression of cardiac failure and PVD, exacerbation of bronchospasm, hypoglycemia, hyperthyroidism, and depression.

Patient Variables

GERIATRICS

Recognize the potential for hepatic and renal failure. Drug concentration levels accumulate quickly in the elderly with compromised systems. Thus, therapeutic doses must be small (half the normal dosage) and titrated slowly in the elderly.

- Elderly patients have described sedation and sleep disturbances associated with β-blocker use.
- Confusion, fatigue

PEDIATRICS. The safety and effectiveness of β-blockers, with the exception of propranolol, have not been established in children. However, atenolol, metoprolol, and labetalol have been used to treat children with hypertension.

PREGNANCY AND LACTATION

- The benefits of β-blockers in pregnancy should clearly outweigh any risks. Low birth weight infants have been reported in mothers who used β-blockers during pregnancy.
- Pregnancy categories vary among the different β-blockers:
  - *Category B:* acebutolol
  - *Category C:* betaxolol, bisoprolol (second and third trimester), metoprolol, nadolol, propranolol
  - *Category D:* atenolol

- β-Blockers appear in breast milk. Either breastfeeding or the drug should be discontinued.

RACE

- African Americans should not be treated with β-blockers as first-line therapy. Reduced effectiveness in this population is likely the result of lower plasma renin levels coupled with greater circulating volume. Diuretics and calcium channel blockers are preferred agents.

Patient Education

- Report shortness of breath, nocturnal cough, or lower extremity edema.
- Do not discontinue medication abruptly.
- Report use of β-blockers to ophthalmologist.
- Monitor pulse and contact health care provider if rate is lower than 50.
- Diabetic patients: possibility of masked signs of hypoglycemia
- Use caution when performing hazardous tasks because of CNS side effects.
- Exercise-induced fatigue may develop. Although patients should eat healthy food and should increase exercise, these medications do not always allow them to increase their level of exercise.

SPECIFIC DRUGS

NONSELECTIVE β-BLOCKERS

> **propranolol (Inderal, Inderal-LA, InnoPran XL, generic)** 🔑
>
> **CONTRAINDICATIONS.** Uncompensated heart failure (unless the failure is due to treatment of tachyarrhythmia with propranolol), cardiogenic shock, bradycardia or heart block (second or third degree), pulmonary edema, severe asthma or COPD, Raynaud's disease; pregnancy (second and third trimesters), and hypersensitivity to the product
>
> **WARNINGS**
>
> Administer with caution to patients who have compensated heart failure; β-blockade may further depress myocardial contractility. β-Blockers do not abolish the inotropic action of digoxin; however, both β-blockers and digoxin slow AV conduction.
> Abrupt withdrawal may result in withdrawal symptoms (tremulousness, sweating, palpitations, headache, malaise), exacerbation of angina, MI, ventricular arrhythmia, and death.
>
> - In Wolff-Parkinson-White syndrome, tachycardia may be replaced by severe bradycardia.
> - In patients who have PVD, β-blockers may precipitate or aggravate the symptoms of arterial insufficiency.
> - In general, do not administer β-blockers to patients who have bronchospastic disease. Cardioselective β-blockers are preferred at the lowest dose and are titrated slowly to the desired effect or the development of bronchospastic symptoms.
> - Bradycardia may be caused by a β-blocker and may be symptomatic.

Continued

propranolol (Inderal, Inderal-LA, InnoPran XL, generic) 🖋—cont'd

- Hypotension may occur.
- Anaphylaxis has occurred, with deaths.
- Withdrawal of β-blockers before major surgery and anesthesia is controversial.
- Concomitant use of verapamil or diltiazem may cause heart block.
- Use β-blockers with caution in patients with renal or hepatic function impairment.

PRECAUTIONS

- May mask the signs and symptoms of hypoglycemia
- May mask clinical signs of hyperthyroidism; abrupt withdrawal may exacerbate symptoms
- May alter serum lipid values, including a nonsignificant increase in triglycerides, total cholesterol, and low- and very low-density lipoprotein cholesterol, along with a decrease in HDL
- May potentiate muscle weakness
- May worsen variant angina

PHARMACOKINETICS. See Table 18-4. Duration of action is important when symptoms of cardiovascular disease are controlled. Non–sustained-release metoprolol must be given twice daily because of the 12-hour duration of action. Carteolol is excreted renally and a dosing schedule of every 72 hours is used for patients with creatinine clearance of <20 ml/min.

ADVERSE EFFECTS. The most frequent adverse effects are bradycardia, depression, impotence, diarrhea, dizziness, drowsiness, fatigue and weakness, nausea and vomiting, and insomnia. Table 18-5 lists important adverse effects.

DRUG INTERACTIONS

- Many β-blockers are involved in cytochrome P450 enzyme metabolism; see Table 18-3 for specifics.
- Food may enhance bioavailability.
- See Table 18-6 for drug interactions.

DOSAGE AND ADMINISTRATION

- See Table 18-7 for dosing information.
- Ethanol: slows the rate of absorption
- Propranolol and metoprolol: Food may enhance bioavailability; take at the same time each day.
- Nadolol, pindolol, acebutolol, atenolol, carteolol, bisoprolol, betaxolol, and penbutolol: Take without regard for meals.

OTHER DRUGS IN CLASS

Other drugs in this class are similar to the prototype, except as follows:

- Labetalol (Normodyne, Trandate) is a selective β_1- and nonselective β-adrenergic receptor blocker. Labetalol produces only minimal reduction in heart rate without reflex tachycardia. Hemodynamically, little change in cardiac output is noted, along with a slight drop in peripheral resistance.
- With carvedilol (Coreg), nonselective β-blockade and β_1-blockade counteract increased sympathetic activity that causes progressive myocardial damage. β_1-blockade reduces systemic vascular resistance and helps to compensate for the initial negative inotropic effects of β-blockade. Acebutolol should be used cautiously in the elderly. A twofold increase in bioavailability is noted in the elderly.

evolve A continually updated list of useful WebLinks may be found in the Evolve Resources at http://evolve.elsevier.com/Edmunds/NP/

Calcium Channel Blockers

DRUG OVERVIEW

Class	Subclass	Generic Name	Trade Name
Calcium channel blockers	Dihydropyridine	nifedipine, ✹ nifedipine ER 🗝 ✹	Procardia, Procardia XL, Adalat CC
		amlodipine	Norvasc ✹
		felodipine ✹	Plendil
		isradipine	DynaCirc
		nicardipine	Cardene
		nicardipine SR	Cardene SR
		nisoldipine	Sular ✹
	Phenylalkylamine	verapamil hydrochloride, verapamil SR ✹	Calan, Isoptin SR, Verelan, Verelan PM, Covera-HS
	Benzothiazepine	diltiazem SR ✹, ER, CD ✹	Cardizem ✹, Tiazac, Cartia-XT
	Diarylaminopropylamine	bepridil	Vascor

✹ Top 200 drug; 🗝 key drug.

INDICATIONS

- Hypertension
- Vasospastic angina
- Arrhythmias
- Used off label for treatment of stable angina and Raynaud's syndrome (Table 19-1)

Calcium channel blockers (CCBs) are indicated for a variety of cardiovascular conditions and are categorized into four subclasses. Only one class, the dihydropyridines, includes more than one commercially available drug. The main difference between the dihydropyridines and the other classes is that the dihydropyridines do not affect the cardiac conduction system. Diltiazem is generally considered to have effects that are more similar to those of verapamil than to those of nifedipine. The new CCB bepridil is used only for patients with angina that is not responding to other drugs. About 1% of patients develop a new serious ventricular arrhythmia. Bepridil is not discussed in detail because it is not in common use on an outpatient basis.

💣 **Short-acting nifedipine should not be used for the acute reduction of blood pressure, the control of essential hypertension, immediately after MI, or in acute coronary artery syndrome.**

The warning applies *only* to short-acting nifedipine. Recent studies have shown that CCBs are safe for the long-term treatment of stable symptomatic angina. However, nifedipine did not provide additional protection against new cardiovascular events in patients who were already being treated for angina, hypertension, or hyperlipidemia with effective medications. CCBs are recommended for use when they are necessary to control angina or hypertension in patients who already are receiving proven cardioprotective medications.

THERAPEUTIC OVERVIEW

For an overview of hypertension, angina, and arrhythmias see Chapters 15, 16, and 21, respectively.

MECHANISM OF ACTION

Although these compounds have diverse chemical structures, they all share a basic electrophysiologic property—they block the inward movement of calcium through the slow channels of the cell membranes of cardiac and smooth muscle cells. The drugs differ in their location of action (Tables 19-2 and 19-3). The three types of tissue cells acted on are as follows:
1. Cardiac muscle (myocardium)
2. Cardiac conduction system: SA and AV nodes
3. Vascular smooth muscle: coronary arteries and arterioles, peripheral arterioles

Cardiac Muscle

CCBs decrease the force of myocardial contraction by blocking the inward flow of calcium ions through the slow channels of the cell membrane during phase 2 (plateau phase) of the

TABLE 19-1   Indications for and Unlabeled Uses of Calcium Channel Blockers

	INDICATIONS			UNLABELED USES	
	Stable Angina	Vasospastic Angina	Hypertension	Stable Angina	Raynaud's Disease
nifedipine		√			√
nifedipine SR	√	√	√		√
amlodipine	√	√	√		
felodipine			√	√	
isradipine			√		
nicardipine	√		√		
nicardipine SR			√		
nisoldipine			√		
diltiazem	√		√		√
diltiazem SR			√		√
verapamil	√	√	√		
verapamil SR	√		√		

action potential. The diminished entry of calcium ions into the cells thereby fails to trigger the release of large amounts of calcium from the sarcoplasmic reticulum within the cell. This free calcium is needed for excitation-contraction coupling, an event that activates contraction by allowing cross-bridges to form between the actin and myosin filaments of muscle. The number of actin and myosin cross-bridges formed within the sarcomere determines the force of the heart's contraction. Decreasing the amount of calcium ions released from the sarcoplasmic reticulum causes fewer actin and myosin cross-bridges to be formed, thus decreasing the force of contraction and resulting in a negative inotropic effect. This decreases cardiac output.

Cardiac Conduction System (SA and AV Nodes)

In these tissues, CCBs decrease automaticity in the SA node and decrease conduction in the AV node. *Automaticity* means that a cell depolarizes spontaneously and initiates an action potential without an external stimulus. Automaticity is a normal characteristic of SA nodal cells. *Depolarization* (Phase 0) of the action potential is normally generated by the inward calcium ion current through slow channels. Thus, agents that can block the inward calcium ion current across the cell membrane of SA nodal tissue decrease the rate of depolarization and depress automaticity. The result is a variable decrease in heart rate (a negative chronotropic effect) (Figure 19-1). Similarly, an agent that decreases calcium ion influx across the cell membrane of the AV node slows AV nodal conduction (negative chronotropic effect) and prolongs AV refractory time. When AV conduction is prolonged, fewer atrial impulses reach the ventricles, thus slowing the rate of ventricular contractions.

Vascular Smooth Muscle

The smooth muscle of the coronary and peripheral vessels has a significant influence on afterload and the hemodynamics of circulation. The decreased force of smooth muscle contraction results in coronary artery dilation, which lowers coronary resistance and improves blood flow through collateral vessels, as well as oxygen delivery to ischemic areas of the heart. CCBs dilate the main coronary arteries and arterioles in both normal and ischemic regions. Therefore, drugs with these actions are helpful in the treatment of angina pectoris.

CCBs reduce arterial pressure at rest and at given levels of exercise by dilating peripheral arterioles and reducing the

TABLE 19-2   Major Differences Between the Subclasses of Calcium Channel Blockers

Subclass	Cardiac Muscle	Cardiac Conduction	Vascular Smooth Muscle
Dihydropyridines (nifedipine)	Small decrease	Little or no effect	Strong effect
Phenylalkylamine (verapamil)	Large decrease	Large effect	Moderate effect
Benzothiazepine (diltiazem)	Moderate decrease	Large effect	Moderate effect

TABLE 19-3 Effect of Calcium Channel Blockers on Myocardium

| Medication | CARDIAC MUSCLE | | CARDIAC CONDUCTION SYSTEM | | | | VASCULAR SMOOTH MUSCLE |
	Myocardial Contractility	Cardiac Output	SA Automaticity	AV Refractivity	AV Conduction	Heart Rate	Afterload
nifedipine	0	+−	+−	+	0	−	−−−
amlodipine	0	+	0	+−	0	−	−−
felodipine	0	0	0	−	−	−	−−−
isradipine	−	0	0	+−	+−	0	−−
nicardipine	+−	+−	0	0	0	0	
nisoldipine	0	0	0	+−	0	0	−−−
verapamil	−−	++	−−−	+−	+−	−−	−−
diltiazem	−	+	−−−	+−	+−	−	−−

+++, Pronounced increase; ++, moderate increase; +, some increase; +−, little increase; 0, no effect; −, some decrease; −−, moderate decrease; −−−, pronounced decrease.

total peripheral resistance (afterload) against which the heart works, resulting in reduced blood pressure. This unloading of the heart reduces myocardial energy consumption and oxygen requirements and probably accounts for the effectiveness of CCBs in chronic stable angina and causes a decrease in blood pressure.

CCBs are potent inhibitors of coronary artery spasm. This property increases myocardial oxygen delivery in patients with coronary artery spasm and is responsible for the effectiveness of CCBs in vasospastic angina.

Specific Calcium Channel Blockers

For an overview of the differences between the subclasses of CCBs, see Table 19-2.

Nifedipine is a potent dilator of vascular smooth muscle that causes decreased peripheral vascular resistance in both

Ca^{++} Movements

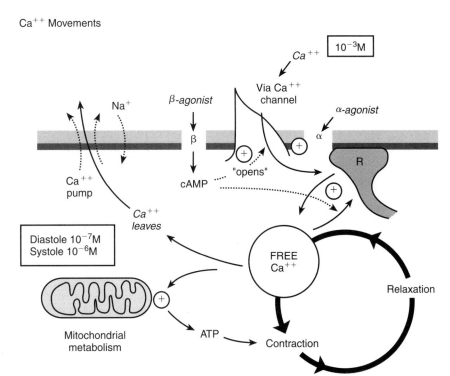

FIGURE 19-1 Physiologic activity of calcium channel blockers. (Data from Burton L et al, eds: *Goodman & Gilman's the pharmacological basis of therapeutics,* ed 11, New York, 2005, McGraw-Hill; National Institutes of Health: *The seventh report of the Joint National Committee on Prevention, Detection, Evaluation and Treatment of High Blood Pressure,* NIH Publication No. 03-5233, Washington, DC, 2003, U.S. Government Printing Office.)

coronary arteries and peripheral arterioles. Nifedipine has a mild negative inotropic effect—less than that of verapamil. Usually, a small increase in heart rate occurs, along with a reflex response to vasodilation. Nifedipine has no tendency to prolong AV conduction, prolong SA node recovery time, or slow sinus rate.

Verapamil also dilates vascular smooth muscle, although it is less potent than nifedipine. Verapamil has a significant negative inotropic effect that prevents and blocks reflex tachycardia and relieves coronary artery spasm. This negative inotropic effect decreases myocardial oxygen demand and thus helps to relieve angina-related ischemia and pain. Verapamil also slows conduction in the SA and AV nodes, although it has a greater effect on the AV node.

Diltiazem has a less negative inotropic effect than verapamil and causes less peripheral vasodilation than nifedipine. Diltiazem selectively has more effect on cardiac muscle than on peripheral vascular smooth muscle. It slows conduction through the SA/AV nodes, but not to the extent that verapamil does.

Bepridil inhibits fast sodium channels in addition to slow calcium channels and has class I antiarrhythmic properties based on the Vaughan Williams classification system.

TREATMENT PRINCIPLES

For information on standardized treatment guidelines, for evidence supporting these guidelines, and for information on nonpharmacologic treatment for hypertension, angina, and arrhythmia, see the related chapters—Chapters 15, 16, and 21. In this chapter, only pharmacologic treatment with CCBs is discussed.

ARRHYTHMIAS. The dihydropyridines—nifedipine and its relatives—are used differently from verapamil and diltiazem, which are similar to each other.

- *Nifedipine and related drugs* cause potent peripheral vasodilation. This often makes them more effective for hypertension than verapamil and diltiazem but more likely to cause peripheral edema. Peripheral edema, namely pedal edema, results from a selective dilution of resistance vessels without concurrent venodilation. An overall increase in proximal capillary pressure drives the increased formation of extravascular fluid. Nifedipine and related drugs are seen to have no effect on cardiac conduction and therefore do not cause arrhythmias nor treat them.
- *Verapamil* and *diltiazem* have a significant effect on cardiac conduction and are used to treat arrhythmia, in addition to hypertension. They are less likely to cause hypotension than nifedipine and related drugs when used to treat angina in a patient who does not have hypertension. However, they are more likely to cause conduction problems than nifedipine and related drugs when used to treat hypertension. They should be used cautiously with β- blockers, if at all, because β-blockers also affect conduction. CCBs are not recommended in heart failure syndrome. These agents have not been shown to improve exercise tolerance, quality of life, or survival. The ACC/AHA 2005 update on the manage-

ment of chronic heart failure did not recommend these drugs in HF.

evolve For a summary of the major actions and uses of CCBs, see the supplemental tables on the Resources website (http://evolve.elsevier.com/Edmunds/NP/).

VASOSPASTIC ANGINA. CCBs are the treatment of choice in variant, or Prinzmetal's, angina. The dihydropyridines, verapamil, diltiazem, and nitrates all are effective as first-line therapy choices. Both classes of drugs reduce vasoconstriction and promote vasodilation in the coronary arteries. Dosing is generally patient specific.

CHRONIC STABLE ANGINA. In chronic stable angina, CCBs are effective in relieving symptoms and increasing exercise tolerance in formal exercise testing. These drugs reduce coronary vascular resistance, increase coronary blood flow, and decrease myocardial oxygen demand. They also reduce ST-segment changes on ambulatory electrocardiographic monitoring. The 2002 ACC/AHA guideline update for the management of patients with chronic stable angina recommended that nitrates and β-blockers should remain first-line therapy. CCBs are reserved for patients with contraindications or adverse reactions to β-blockers or nitrates, and for those whose symptoms are not well controlled with a combination of these agents. Among the available agents, long-acting diltiazem or verapamil or a dihydropyridine (amlodipine or felodipine) should be used.

HYPERTENSION. In the Seventh Report of the Joint National Commission on the Prevention, Detection, Evaluation, and Treatment of High Blood Pressure, thiazide-type diuretics are recommended as the first-line consideration for most patients with stage 1 hypertension without compelling indications. CCBs, along with ACE inhibitors, angiotensin receptor blockers (ARBs), β-blockers (BBs), or combinations of these products, are mentioned as appropriate early considerations. CCBs do not produce hyperlipidemia or insulin resistance as diuretics do, and they do not cause sedation, drowsiness, or sexual dysfunction as β-blockers do. CCBs reduce peripheral vascular resistance without stimulating reactive renal and hormonal responses. CCBs also increase sodium excretion moderately, and, in contrast to most other antihypertensive agents, their effectiveness is not significantly improved by dietary salt restriction.

CCBs are safe and effective for a wide variety of hypertensive patients. African Americans, the elderly, and patients with hyperlipidemia are considered good candidates for CCBs. Treatment with CCBs or diuretics given as monotherapy to African American patients has proved to be more effective vs. some other classes of antihypertensives in terms of degree of blood pressure reduction. These drugs may be preferred in patients taking NSAIDs because they can increase blood pressure moderately by reducing the production of prostaglandins, which are vasodilating substances. The efficacy of CCBs is not blunted by the use of NSAIDs. Overall, CCBs are met with good patient acceptance because of their low incidence of adverse reactions.

How to Monitor

- Follow weekly or biweekly while dosages are being titrated upward.
- Once stable, monitor patient periodically—every 3 to 6 months—for adverse responses and control of the disease process.
- Obtain and monitor serum digoxin levels if CCBs are initiated in patients receiving digoxin.
- Kidney and liver function tests should be performed periodically.

Patient Variables

GERIATRICS. Lower dosages of CCBs should be used because older patients are more susceptible to their side effects such as dizziness, weakness, orthostatic hypotension, syncopal episodes, and falls. However, CCBs generally are well tolerated and are often the drug of choice for elderly patients.

PEDIATRICS. The safety and effectiveness of CCBs in children have not been established. However, increasing experience with long-acting CCBs (such as nifedipine and amlodipine) in children with essential hypertension has been shown to be safe and effective.

PREGNANCY AND LACTATION

- *Category C:* Teratogenic and embryotoxic effects have been demonstrated in small animals.
- Verapamil, diltiazem, and nifedipine are excreted in breast milk.
- It is not known whether the other drugs are excreted in breast milk.

RACE. More effective in African American patients

Patient Education

- Advise patients that they may experience hypotensive effects during dose titration.
- Urge patients to report signs of CHF (e.g., swelling of feet, shortness of breath), irregular heartbeat, nausea, constipation, dizziness, or hypotension.
- Nitrate therapy while patients are on CCBs may cause some dizziness. Consider staggering the times medications are taken to minimize this effect.
- If taking extended-release tablets, patients may pass inert shells in feces (Procardia XL).
- Do not take with grapefruit juice, which is known to affect the liver cytochrome P450 enzyme system and to interfere with drug metabolism. This interaction is most common with the dihydropyridine CCBs, specifically, nisoldipine, nifedipine, and felodipine. The CCBs that exhibit the greatest interactions in this group are the ones that are poorly absorbed (i.e., low bioavailability). Grapefruit juice inhibits CYP450 metabolism of CCBs in the intestinal wall. Therefore, absorption is greatly enhanced and results in a greater pharmacologic effect. For example, nisoldipine and amlodipine are dihydropyridines with very low and very high bioavailability, respectively. Absorption of nisoldipine was increased more than fourfold vs. only slightly increased in patients taking amlodipine. The magnitude of the interaction is highly variable between individuals but reproducible within individuals. Therefore, the implications for patients involve significant blood pressure reduction or minimal blood pressure reduction.

TABLE 19-4 Pharmacokinetics of Selected Calcium Channel Blockers

Drug	Onset of Action	Time to Peak Concentration	Half-life	Duration of Action	Metabolism	Excretion
nifedipine (Procardia)	20 min	0.5-1 hr	2-5 hr	4-8 hr	Liver, 3A4 substrate	Renal, 80%; feces, 20%
amlodipine (Norvasc)	30-50 min	6-12 hr	30-50 hr	24 hr	Liver, extensive 3A4 substrate	Renal
felodipine (Plendil)	3-5 hr	2.5-5 hr	11-16 hr	24 hr	Liver, 3A4 substrate	Renal
isradipine (DynaCirc)	2 hr	1.5 hr	8 hr	12 hr	Liver, 3A4 substrate	Renal
nicardipine (Cardene)	0.5-2 hr	2 hr	2-4 hr	8 hr	Liver, 3A4 substrate	Renal
nisoldipine (Sular)	1-3 hr	6-12 hr	7-12 hr	24 hr	Liver, extensive	Renal
verapamil (Calan, Isoptin) immediate release	1-2 hr	1-2 hr	4-12 hr	6-8 hr	Liver, extensive	Renal and feces
verapamil (Covera-HS, Verelan PM), controlled onset, extended release	4-5 hr	11 hr		24 hr		
verapamil (Calan-SR, Isoptin SR, Verelan), extended release	4-6 hr	7-9 hr		24 hr		
diltiazem (Cardizem)	30 min	2-3 hr	3-4.5 hr	48 hr	Liver, has active metabolite	Renal and bile
diltiazem SR (Cardizem SR)	30-60 min	6-11 hr	3.5-7 hr	12 hr		
diltiazem SR (once-daily dosing) (Cardizem CD, Cartia XT, Dilacor XR Tiazac)		4-6 hr (Dilacor XR); 10-18 hr	5-8 hr	24 hr		

SPECIFIC DRUGS

DIHYDROPYRIDINES

nifedipine (Adalat CC, Adalat capsules, Procardia, Procardia XL) 🗝

CONTRAINDICATIONS. Hypersensitivity

WARNINGS
- Hypotension may occur and may be more common in patients taking concomitant β-blockers. Monitor blood pressure closely.

💣 Patients who took nifedipine and a β-blocker and who underwent coronary artery bypass surgery with high-dose fentanyl anesthesia developed severe hypotension and/or increased fluid volume requirements. Current recommendations are to avoid giving nifedipine for 36 hours prior to surgery.

- Heart failure syndrome may develop rarely when a patient is treated with a CCB, usually when used in combination with a β-blocker.
- Antiplatelet effects have caused inhibition of platelet function. Episodes of bruising, petechiae, and bleeding have occurred.

💣 Withdrawal syndrome: Abrupt withdrawal of CCBs may cause increased frequency and duration of chest pain. To stop drug, gradually taper dosage.

- CCBs do not prevent β-blocker withdrawal symptoms. Be sure to taper any β-blocker, even if the patient is started on a CCB.
- Hepatic function impairment causes a longer half-life of nifedipine. Amlodipine, felodipine, nisoldipine, and nimodipine are extensively metabolized by the liver. Half-life is increased; use these medications with caution or with reduced dosages in patients with impaired liver function.
- Rarely, patients, particularly those who have severe obstructive coronary disease, have developed increased frequency, duration, and/or severity of angina or acute MI on starting or increasing nifedipine or nicardipine.

PRECAUTIONS
- Acute hepatic injury with elevations in liver function tests (LFTs) has occurred rarely with nifedipine and nimodipine.
- Mild to moderate peripheral edema occurs in the lower extremities in about 10% of patients. This is caused by arterial dilation and not by left ventricular dysfunction.

PHARMACOKINETICS. See Table 19-4 for pharmacokinetic information.

ADVERSE EFFECTS. See Table 19-5 for adverse reactions. For additional information on common side effects of various CCBs, see the supplemental tables on the Evolve Learning Resources website.

Table 19-6 compares the adverse reactions among different types of dihydropyridines.

DRUG INTERACTIONS
- Many CCBs are CYP450 3A4 substrates.
- Drug interactions vary in terms of the individual drugs (Table 19-7).

DOSAGE AND ADMINISTRATION
- nifedipine: Avoid administration with grapefruit.
- See Table 19-8 for specific dosage and administration information.

TABLE 19-5 Adverse Effects of Calcium Channel Blockers

Body System	diltiazem	nifedipine	verapamil
Skin, appendages	Rash, erythema multiforme, Stevens-Johnson syndrome	Edema, flushing	Rash, Stevens-Johnson syndrome, erythema multiforme
Respiratory	Dyspnea	Cough, dyspnea	Dyspnea
Cardiovascular	Angina, hypertension, hypotension, AV block, bradycardia, angina, atrial fibrillation, MI, palpitations, syncope	Palpitations, angina, bradycardia, hypotension, syncope, tachycardia	ECG, abnormal bradycardia, AV block, CHF, hypotension, angina, syncope, palpitations, MI, tachycardia
Gastrointestinal	Constipation, diarrhea, nausea	Constipation, nausea	**Constipation** (5%-10%), diarrhea, nausea
Circulatory and lymphatic	Ecchymosis, **pedal edema** (5%-10%)	Leukopenia, thrombocytopenia	Ecchymosis
Musculoskeletal	Arthralgia, muscle cramps	Arthralgia, muscle cramps, **pedal edema** (5%-10%)	Muscle cramps, myalgia
Nervous system	**Headache** (5%-10%), paresthesia, insomnia	**Headache** (10%-15%), tremor, weakness, fatigue, asthenia, **flushing** (5%-10%), **dizziness** (5%-10%), anxiety, ataxia, confusion, depression	Headache, dizziness, fatigue, ataxia, paresthesia, confusion
Genitourinary	Impotence	Impotence	Impotence

Bold, Most common side effect.

TABLE 19-6   Comparison of Adverse Effects (in Percentages) Among Dihydropyridines

Drug	Edema	Flushing	SOB	Dizziness	Headache
nifedipine	20	25	6	10	15
amlodipine	8	2	1	3	7
felodipine	8	5	2	3	12
isradipine	4-30	3	3	5	15
nisoldipine	12	0	1	6	22

Adapted from *Drug Facts and Comparisons,* St Louis, 2008, Kluwer.

OTHER DRUGS IN CLASS

Nicardipine is contraindicated with advanced aortic stenosis because it causes decreased afterload. Additionally, the immediate-release form of nicardipine has prominent peak effects, and this increases the risk of adverse reactions.

Avoid administering nisoldipine with a high-fat meal. It is available in an extended-release tablet.

The combination of dihydropropyridine and β-blockers usually is well tolerated but may increase the likelihood of CHF, severe hypotension, or exacerbation of angina.

PHENYLALKYLAMINE

verapamil hydrochloride (Calan, Calan SR, Isoptin, Isoptin SR, Verelan)

CONTRAINDICATIONS
- Hypersensitivity
- Sick sinus syndrome or second- or third-degree block, except in patients with functioning artificial pacemaker
- Hypotension less than 90 mm Hg
- Patients with atrial flutter/fibrillation and an accessory AV pathway may develop rapid ventricular response or ventricular fibrillation.

WARNINGS
- Hypotension may occur during initial dosing or dosage increases and may be more common in patients taking concomitant β-blockers. Monitor blood pressure.
- Use with caution in patients with heart failure because the negative inotropic effect may precipitate CHF.
- Cardiac conduction: may cause first-degree AV block and transient bradycardia
- Elevated liver enzymes, including elevated transaminases, alkaline phosphatase, and bilirubin, have been reported. Periodic monitoring is prudent. Verapamil is highly metabolized by the liver and should be administered with caution to patients with hepatic insufficiency.
- Renal function impairment: 70% is excreted as metabolites in the urine. Administer with caution to patients with impaired renal function.
- Antiplatelet effects: Bruising, petechiae, and bleeding have occurred.
- Patients with idiopathic hypertrophic subaortic stenosis (cardiomyopathy) (IHSS) may experience a variety of serious side effects, including pulmonary edema and severe hypotension, with verapamil.

TABLE 19-7   Common Drug Interactions With Calcium Channel Blockers

Calcium Channel Blocker	Action on Other Drugs
DIHYDROPYRIDINES	
Dihydropyridines	Increased anesthetics
nifedipine	Increased digoxin, quinidine, tacrolimus, vincristine
nifedipine, isradipine, nicardipine	Increased β-blockers
felodipine, nicardipine	Increased cyclosporine
isradipine	Decreased lovastatin
VERAPAMIL AND DILTIAZEM	
verapamil and diltiazem	Increased midazolam, triazolam, buspirone, carbamazepine, digoxin, statins, imipramine, quinidine, sirolimus, tacrolimus, theophylline, β-blockers, anesthetics
verapamil*	Increased disopyramide, flecainide, doxorubicin, ethanol, nondepolarizing muscle relaxants, prazosin, cyclosporine
diltiazem	Increased nifedipine, methylprednisolone, moricizine

Other Drugs	Action on Calcium Channel Blockers
cimetidine, ranitidine, β-blockers	Increased dihydropyridine
cisapride, diltiazem, quinidine	Increased nifedipine
melatonin, nafcillin, St John's wort	Decreased nifedipine
erythromycin	Increased felodipine
carbamazepine, oxcarbazepine	Decreased felodipine
Azole antifungals	Increased nisoldipine
itraconazole, rifampin	Increased felodipine, isradipine, nifedipine
cyclosporine	Increased nifedipine, felodipine
Barbiturates	Decreased nifedipine, felodipine
phenytoin	Decreased felodipine, nisoldipine
valproic acid	Increased nimodipine
amiodarone, cimetidine, ranitidine, β-blockers	Increased verapamil and diltiazem
rifampin	Decreased verapamil and diltiazem

*Verapamil: many other drug interactions; the most common and clinically important are noted

- Abrupt withdrawal may cause increased frequency and duration of chest pain.

PHARMACOKINETICS. See Table 19-4.

ADVERSE EFFECTS. See Table 19-5.

DRUG INTERACTIONS. Verapamil is a CYP450 3A4 substrate (see Table 19-7 for drug interactions).

TABLE 19-8   Dosage and Administration Recommendations of Calcium Channel Blockers

Drug	Dosage Form	Initial Dose (HTN)	Angina	Titration (HTN)	Usual JNC 7 Dose Range (HTN)	Maximum Daily Dose (HTN)
nifedipine	Capsules	10 mg tid	NA	Increase every 1-2 weeks	Not recommended	120 mg/day
	Tablets, ER	30 mg daily			30-60 mg once daily	120 mg
amlodipine	Tablets	5 mg daily (elderly, 2.5 mg daily)	5-10 mg daily (elderly/hepatic impairment, 5 mg daily)	Increase by 2.5 mg/day every 1-2 weeks	2.5-10 mg once daily	10 mg
felodipine	Tablets, ER	5 mg daily (elderly, 2.5 mg daily)	NA	Increase by 5 mg/day every 2 weeks	2.5-20 mg once daily	20 mg
isradipine	Capsules	2.5 mg bid	NA	Increase by 2.5-5 mg/day every 2-4 weeks	2.5-10 mg/day in two divided doses	20 mg/day (no further benefit and increased side effects >10 mg/day)
	Tablets, CR	5 mg daily		Increase by 5 mg/day every 2-4 weeks		
nicardipine	Capsules	20 mg tid	20 mg tid; usual range: 60-120 mg/day	Increase to 40 mg tid every 3 days		120 mg tid
	Capsules, SR	30 mg bid	NA	Increase to 60 mg bid	60-120 mg/day in two divided doses	120 mg bid
nisoldipine	Tablets, ER	20 mg daily (elderly, 10 mg daily)	NA	Increase by 10 mg/wk to 20-40 mg	10-40 mg once daily	60 mg
verapamil	SR	120 mg bid	NA	Increase to 180-240 mg daily	120-360 mg/day in two divided doses (elderly or small patients, 120 mg/day)	480 mg (no further benefit in doses >360 mg/day)
	Controlled onset, extended release	120-360 mg daily at bedtime (Covera HS); 200-400 mg daily at bedtime (Verelan PM)	180 mg daily at bedtime; maximum dose 540 mg daily		120-360 mg daily (Covera HS); 200-400 mg daily (Verelan PM)	360 mg daily (Covera-HS); 400 mg daily (Verelan PM)
	Tablet (immediate release)		80-120 mg bid (elderly or small stature, 40 mg bid); range: 240-480 mg/day in three or four divided doses		80-320 mg/day in two divided doses	320 mg/day in two divided doses
diltiazem	Tablets (immediate release)	NA	30 mg qid; usual range: 180-360 mg/day	Increase every 1-2 weeks to 180 mg/day	120-540 mg/day	360 mg/day
	Capsules, ER	180-240 mg daily (Cardizem CD, Cartia XT, Dilacor XR, Tiazac) Capsule, SR: 60-120 mg bid; usual range: 240-360 mg/day (Cardizem SR)	Capsule, ER initial: 120-180 mg daily (maximum dose: 480 mg/day) (Cardizem CD, Cartia XT, Dilacor XR, Tiazac)	Increase every 2 weeks	180-420 mg/day	420 mg/day
					Tiazac: 120-540 mg/day	Tiazac: 540 mg/day
	Tablets, extended release	Tablet, ER: 180-240 mg daily. (Cardizem LA)	Tablet, ER: 180 mg daily; maximum dose: 360 mg/day; (Cardizem LA)		120-540 mg/day	540 mg/day

evolve   A continually updated list of useful WebLinks may be found in the Evolve Resources at http://evolve.elsevier.com/Edmunds/NP/

ACE Inhibitors and Angiotensin Receptor Blockers

DRUG OVERVIEW

Class	Subclass	Generic Name	Trade Name
ACEIs	Sulfhydryl-containing	captopril ✹	Capoten
	Dicarboxylic-containing	lisinopril hydrochloride 🔑	Prinivil, Zestril, generic
		benazepril hydrochloride	Lotensin, generic
		enalapril maleate ✹	Vasotec, generic
		quinapril hydrochloride ✹	Accupril
		moexipril hydrochloride	Univasc
		perindopril	Aceon
		ramipril	Altace ✹
		trandolapril	Mavik
	Phosphorus-containing	fosinopril sodium ✹	Monopril, generic
Angiotensin II receptor blockers (ARBs)		losartan	Cozaar ✹
		candesartan	Atacand ✹
		eprosartan	Teveten
		irbesartan	Avapro ✹
		olmesartan	Benicar ✹
		telmisartan	Micardis ✹
		valsartan	Diovan ✹

✹ Top 200 drug; 🔑 key drug.

INDICATIONS

- ACEIs
- Hypertension
- Heart failure
- MI
- Left ventricular dysfunction
- Diabetic nephropathy

Treatment of hypertensive crises is an unlabeled use for captopril.

This chapter discusses the ACEIs and the ARBs as a unit because these drugs are quite similar in terms of their therapeutic uses, mechanisms of action, and adverse effects. Key distinctions are noted.

ACEIs and ARBs are commonly used in the treatment of patients with hypertension. In addition, these drugs have been shown to prolong survival in patients with heart failure, coronary heart disease, and acute MI. They slow the rate of progression of chronic renal failure and, particularly, diabetic nephropathy.

THERAPEUTIC OVERVIEW

For an overview of the disorders indicative of treatment with ACEIs and ARBs, see the respective chapters (Table 20-1).

MECHANISM OF ACTION

Two types of angiotensin receptors have been identified: AT_1 and AT_2. Most of the biologic effects of angiotensin II are mediated by the AT_1 receptor. AT_2 receptors may exert

TABLE 20-1   Disorders Treated With ACEIs and ARBs

Disorder	Chapter
Heart failure syndrome or CHF	17
Left ventricular dysfunction	17
Hypertension	15
Myocardial infarction	16
Diabetic nephropathy	52

antiproliferative and vasodilatory effects. ACEIs block angiotensin-converting enzyme (ACE), which is responsible for the conversion of angiotensin I to angiotensin II. Angiotensin II is a potent vasoconstrictor and is a stimulus for aldosterone release from the adrenal glands (Figure 20-1). Reduction in aldosterone secretion results in less water absorption and sodium/potassium exchange in the distal renal tubule, causing a slight increase in serum potassium.

ACEIs inhibit the breakdown of bradykinin, a potent and naturally occurring vasodilator, by blocking the enzyme kininase II. This is thought to be the cause of the cough commonly experienced by patients who take this class of drugs.

ARBs block the effects of angiotensin II by blocking the binding of angiotensin II to its receptors. They do not affect bradykinin (Figure 20-2). Receptor affinity is highest by candesartan > irbesartan > eprosartan > telmisartan > valsartan > losartan.

ARBs differ from ACEIs in the following four respects:
1. ARBs are more active against AT_1 receptors than are ACEIs.
2. ACE inhibition is not associated with increased levels of angiotensin II, as are ARBs.
3. ACEIs may increase angiotensin levels to a greater degree than ARBs do.
4. ACEIs increase levels of bradykinin, in contrast to ARBs.

Whether these differences translate to significant clinical outcomes is unknown.

The pharmacologic effects of ACE inhibition produce a reduction in systemic vascular resistance, with no effect or a moderate increase in cardiac output. Blood pressure is lowered through decreased systemic vascular resistance. Blood pressure reduction is not accompanied by changes in heart rate. Renal perfusion is increased and renal vascular resistance is decreased, but the glomerular filtration rate is usually unchanged. In patients with heart failure syndrome, ACEIs significantly decrease preload by reducing sodium and water retention (through reduction of aldosterone secretion) and reduce afterload through their effects on angiotensin II (decreasing systemic vascular resistance). This causes a modest increase in ejection fraction and a decrease in ventricular end-diastolic pressure and volume. These in turn improve myocardial energy metabolism. ACEIs also act on the renal vasculature to reduce arteriolar resistance, which improves renal hemodynamics. This may improve the course of patients with diabetic nephropathy and other renal diseases with glomerular hypertension. The ACE escape phenomenon may be seen in some patients when alternate enzyme pathways are used for formation of angiotensin II, thus increasing the benefit of ARBs.

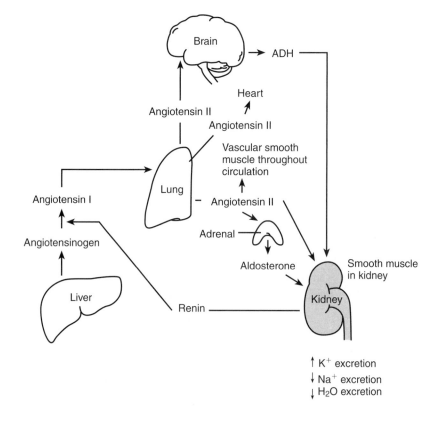

FIGURE 20-1   Essential components of the renin-angiotensin-aldosterone system. (Modified from Levy MN et al: *Physiology*, ed 5, St Louis, 2004, Mosby.)

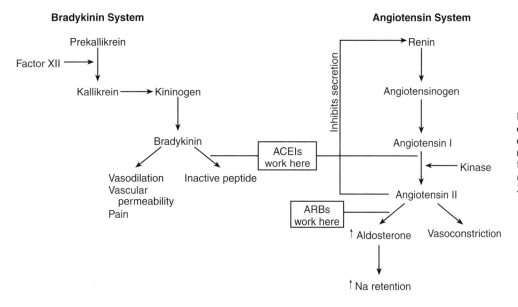

Bradykinin System

Angiotensin System

FIGURE 20-2   **Sites of action of angiotensin-converting enzyme inhibitors (ACEIs) and receptor antagonists.** (Modified from McCance KL, Huether SE: *Pathophysiology,* ed 5, St Louis, 2005, Mosby.)

TREATMENT PRINCIPLES

For information on standardized treatment guidelines, for evidence supporting these guidelines, and for information on nonpharmacologic treatment for patients with hypertension, MI, chronic heart failure, and diabetic nephropathy, see the related chapters—Chapters 15, 16, 17, and 52. In this chapter, only pharmacologic treatment with ACEIs and ARBs is discussed.

ACEIs have similar therapeutic and adverse reactions. They differ basically in terms of pharmacokinetics (Table 20-2). Some are provided as prodrugs that must be metabolized by the liver to the active drug. The duration of hypotensive effects is critical. Many products claim that they provide 24-hour protection, but their effects may wear off within 24 hours. Blood pressure (BP) should be checked shortly before the time of administration to ensure 24-hour BP control. These agents differ in terms of tissue distribution, and this may result in differences in the renin-angiotensin systems affected. Except for fosinopril, these agents are cleared predominantly by the kidney. ACEIs generally are considered safe and effective in patients with mild to moderate renal impairment; however, dosage reduction is required in patients whose renal clearance is diminished. Fosinopril, lisinopril, and ramipril are eliminated by both hepatic and renal mechanisms, and they have the ability to compensate for renal dysfunction by shifting to hepatic elimination. Dehydration and renal insufficiency increase the risk of elevated K when an ACEI is started.

An advantage of ACEIs and ARBs is their relative lack of serious adverse reactions compared with other drugs for hypertension and angina. The most common and often treatment-limiting side effect of the ACEIs is cough. This cough is persistent, dry, and hacking and is seen in up to 20% of patients taking ACEIs. The ARBs were developed, in part, to eliminate this side effect, and clinical trials have demonstrated this benefit. The most serious and potentially life-threatening adverse reaction is angioedema, which occurs in approximately 0.1% to 0.7% of patients. However, because ACEIs are used so often, current clinical practice guidelines suggest that the use of an ACEI should be ruled out for anyone who comes into an emergency department with angioedema.

The main distinguishing clinical features of ACEI-induced angioedema were older age and absence of an allergic history. ARBs are often reserved as alternatives to ACEIs for patients who cannot tolerate an ACEI; in addition, overall costs are reduced because of the availability of generic ACEIs.

Other serious adverse effects of the ACEIs and the ARBs include hyperkalemia, hypotension, and acute renal failure. Abrupt withdrawal of these agents has not resulted in rebound hypertension.

HYPERTENSION. The antihypertensive effects of the ARBs have proved comparable with those of the ACEIs. ACEIs and ARBs are of particular value for the treatment of hypertensive patients who have concomitant illnesses such as diabetes, renal insufficiency, left ventricular dysfunction, and CHF. Fifty to 60 percent of white patients will have a good response to an ACEI; this is comparable with results reported with other first-line antihypertensive drugs. Some African American patients do not appear to respond as well as whites in terms of BP reduction, but cardioprotective or nephroprotective effects can still be seen. The addition of a low-dose thiazide diuretic often allows for efficacy in blood pressure lowering that is comparable with that seen in whites. BP reduction may be progressive, with maximal effects achieved in 2 to 4 weeks.

An additional advantage of ACEIs is regression of left ventricular hypertrophy. However, in ALLHAT (the Antihypertensive and Lipid-Lowering treatment to prevent Heart Attack Trial), an ACEI was shown to be less cardioprotective than a thiazide diuretic. ACEIs have been shown to increase insulin sensitivity and to modestly lower plasma glucose levels. They also minimize or prevent diuretic-induced elevations in cholesterol and uric acid levels.

Another possible benefit of ACEIs may be their ability to reduce the incidence of new-onset diabetes. Multiple clinical trials, such as CHARM (Candesartan in Heart Failure Assessment of Reduction in Mortality and Morbidity), LIFE (Losartan Intervention For Endpoint reduction), HOPE (Heart Outcomes Prevention Evaluation study), ANBP2 (Second Australian National Blood Pressure trial), ALLHAT, and

TABLE 20-2   Pharmacokinetics of ACEI Agents

Drug (Active Metabolite)	Effect of Food on Absorption	Onset of Action	Duration of Action	Time to Peak Concentration	Half-life	Protein Bound	Metabolism	Excreted Unchanged
captopril (Capoten)	Reduced absorption (30%-40%)	0.25 hr	6 hr	1-1.5 hr	2 hr; 20-40 hr (anuria)	25%-30%	50%	Urine, 40%-50%
lisinopril (Zestril)	None	1 hr	24 hr	6 hr	12 hr	25%	—	Urine, 100%
benazepril (Lotensin)	None	1 hr	24 hr	2 hr	10-11 hr	>95%	Liver; metabolized to active drug	Nonrenal (biliary, 12%) and renal (8%)
enalapril (Vasotec)	None	1 hr	12-24 hr	4-6 hr	11 hr	—	Liver; metabolized to active drug	Urine, 60%-80%; some feces
quinapril (Accupril)	Reduced	1 hr	24 hr	2-4 hr	25 hr	97%	Liver; metabolized to active drug	Renal, 96%
moexipril (Univasc)	Reduced	1.5 hr	24 hr	3-6 hr	2-10 hr	50%	Liver; metabolized to active drug	Urine, 52%
ramipril (Altace)	Reduced	1-2 hr	24 hr	1.1-4.5 hr	13-17 hr	56%	Liver; metabolized to active drug	Urine (60%) and feces (40%)
trandolapril (Mavik)	Reduced	4 hr	24 hr	—	5 hr	80%	Liver, 14%	Urine, 33%; feces, 56%
fosinopril (Fosinoprilat)	None	1 hr	24 hr	3 hr	12 hr	95%	Liver; metabolized to active drug	Urine (50%) and feces (50%)
losartan (Cozaar)	Well absorbed	1 hr	12-24 hr	3-4 hr	6-9 hr	99%	CYP450 2C9 substrate and 3A4 substrate active metabolites	Urine, 4%-6%
candesartan	Well absorbed	2-3 hr	>24 hr	6-8 hr	9 hr	99%	Liver	Urine (26%) and feces (67%)
eprosartan	Reduced absorption	1 hr	12-24 hr	1-2 hr	5-9 hr	98%	Liver	Urine (7%) and feces (90%)
irbesartan (Avapro)	Rapidly absorbed	1-2 hr	>24 hr	1.5-2 hr	11-15 hr	90%	Liver	Urine (20%) and feces (80%)
telmisartan	Reduced	1-2 hr	24 hr	0.5-1 hr	24 hr	99.5%	Liver	Feces, 97%
valsartan (Diovan)	Reduced	2 wk	24 hr	2-4 hr	6 hr	95%	Liver, 20%; not CYP450	Urine (13%) and feces (83%)

VALUE (Valsartan Antihypertensive Long-term Use Evaluation], suggest that ACEIs are more likely to prevent diabetes than are other antihypertensive agents. Three major trials are currently under way to determine whether ACEIs and ARBs or combination therapy is more effective than are other antihypertensives in preventing the onset of diabetes.

POST–MYOCARDIAL INFARCTION/HIGH RISK OF CARDIOVASCULAR EVENTS. ACEIs prevent ventricular remodeling and improve endothelial function after MI. They also decrease the action of fibrin, thereby reducing clotting. The 2004 ACC/AHA guidelines on the management of ST-elevated MI (STEMI) recommends that ACEIs should be initiated within 24 hours of presentation in patients who are stable. Those who should not be given an ACEI include patients with the following: ACEI allergy, renal failure, hypotension (systolic blood pressure less than 90 to 100 mm Hg, or systolic pressure 30 mm Hg below baseline), shock, history of bilateral renal artery stenosis, or prior worsening of renal function with ACEIs. Patients with renal insufficiency may be prescribed an ACEI in this setting. ACEIs have been clinically proven to improve survival in patients with serum creatinine concentrations above 3 mg/dl in a study that included more than 20,000 patients 65 years of age who had experienced MI and impaired left ventricular function. Concurrent aspirin therapy attenuated the benefit in these patients.

A landmark trial that supported ACEIs in patients at high risk for cardiac events is the HOPE trial. This trial examined the benefit of an ACEI (ramipril) or placebo for existing therapy in 9541 high-risk patients older than age 55. The trial was halted after 4.5 years because ramipril was shown to significantly reduce the primary end point, cardiovascular mortality, nonfatal MI, stroke, new cases of diabetes. The benefits of ramipril were seen within the first year and were independent of age and gender. These benefits were apparent in patients with significant comorbidities that included impaired left ventricular function, diabetes mellitus, documented coronary heart disease or a prior MI, peripheral vascular disease, or stroke. Results that emerged from the HOPE trial are comparable with those seen in clinical trials of statin drugs.

Although most clinical trial data have been related to the use of ACEIs, ARBs appear to deliver comparable benefits.

CHRONIC HEART FAILURE. ACEIs should be given to all patients with symptomatic or asymptomatic heart failure. Task forces from the 2005 ACC/AHA and the European Society of Cardiology both have given ACEIs a grade 1 recommendation. These agents reduce ventricular dilation, restore the heart to its normal elliptical shape, and reverse ventricular remodeling. They induce a more favorable hemodynamic state by reducing preload, afterload, heart rate, systemic blood pressure, and renovascular resistance. One of the greatest benefits of ACEI therapy is its ability to reduce peripheral vascular resistance and lower BP without compromising cardiac output. These agents also increase renal blood flow, which causes natriuresis. Before therapy is initiated, the patient should be well hydrated to prevent renal failure. A meta-analysis of more than 12,000 patients found that ACEIs have been clinically proven (1) to reduce total mortality (23% vs. 27% for placebo) by preventing deaths from progressive heart failure, (2) to lower the number

of hospital readmissions for heart failure (14% vs. 19%), and (3) to reduce the incidence of MI (9% vs. 11%). The benefit was evident soon after treatment was begun, and this benefit increased over longer than 4 years.

ARBs appear to be as effective or possibly slightly less effective than ACEIs for the treatment of heart failure when compared directly. The 2005 ACC/AHA Task Force recommended administration of an ARB to patients who cannot tolerate an ACEI. A IIa recommendation was given to an ARB as an alternative to an ACEI if the patient is already receiving an ARB for another indication.

The benefits of ACEIs for the African American population have not been as strong as those for other populations. Two major trials (V-HeFT [Vasodilator therapy of Heart Failure Trial] and SOLVD [Studies Of Left Ventricular Dysfunction]) found that African Americans had higher rates of progressive heart failure and of overall mortality. In the SOLVD analysis, hospital admissions and overall mortality rates were higher (13 vs. 8 per 100 patient-years and 12 vs. 10 per 100 patient-years, respectively) than those of whites. These results are somewhat understandable when it is considered that ACEIs have not been shown to be as effective for the treatment of hypertension in this population. In the SOLVD study, both systolic and diastolic blood pressures were reduced (5/3.6) in white patients but not in African Americans.

PREVENTION OF RENAL FAILURE IN DIABETES. ACEIs and ARBs have been proven to dramatically slow the progression of diabetic nephropathy. Although most clinical trials have explored the use of ARBs, the ACEI is believed to confer similar efficacy. With the exception of pregnancy, these drugs should be given to all patients with diabetes who have microalbuminuria or macroalbuminuria. The American Diabetes Association (ADA) 2004 statement on the use of ACEIs and ARBs states the following:

- In patients with type 1 diabetes, with hypertension and any degree of albuminuria, ACEIs have been shown to delay the progression of nephropathy.
- In patients with type 2 diabetes, hypertension, and microalbuminuria, ACEIs and ARBs have been shown to delay the progression to macroalbuminuria.
- In patients with type 2 diabetes, hypertension, macroalbuminuria, and renal insufficiency (serum creatinine >1.5 mg/dl), ARBs have been shown to delay the progression of nephropathy.

How to Monitor

- All patients should have a baseline and a periodic electrolyte panel (serum Na, K, and total CO_2), serum blood urea nitrogen, creatinine, and urinalysis. Once dosage is stable, serum creatinine and potassium should be checked after 2 and 4 weeks. Patients without risk factors for renal deterioration should have these parameters checked every 3 to 6 months during stable maintenance therapy.
- Periodically monitor WBCs for leukopenia.
- Monitor supine BP weekly while titrating dose. Patients with severe hypertension should be monitored more frequently during initial titration.
- Angioedema: This potentially life-threatening complication is common to all ACEIs and develops through the mechanism of action of the drugs. It typically involves the mouth, lips, tongue, larynx, pharynx, and subglottic

tissues. Urticaria is absent. More than 50% of cases occur within 1 week of treatment initiation. Some cases have been reported to occur after several years of therapy. Patients who appear to be at highest risk are those who are older (>65 years), have a history of drug rash, or have seasonal allergies, along with African Americans. Angioedema is not related to ACEI-induced cough.

- Many of these individuals will also be taking diogoxin. Serum digoxin levels should not exceed 1.0 ng/mL (1.3 nmol/mL), particularly in women.
- Because ACE inhibitors and ARBs may cause hyperkalemia in patients with renal failure, these drugs should be avoided or should be used only with great caution when serum creatinine levels are higher than 2.5 mg/dL (220 μmol/L), when glomerular filtration rates (GFRs) are less than 30 mL/minute/1.73 m^2, or when potassium levels are higher than 5.0 mEq/L (5.0 mmol/L).

Patient Variables

GERIATRICS
- Useful in the elderly
- A lower dose may be needed in patients with renal or hepatic insufficiency.
- Evaluate the patient for volume depletion prior to initiating ACEI therapy.

PEDIATRICS
- Safety and effectiveness of ACEIs have not been established in children.
- Irbesartan is indicated in children older than 6 years of age.

PREGNANCY AND LACTATION. The use of ACEIs and almost certainly ARBs in all stages of pregnancy is associated with significant fetal risk. Major congenital malformations, in particular, cardiovascular and central nervous system abnormalities, were seen more often in infants exposed to ACEIs during the first trimester compared with other antihypertensive agents.

These drugs can cause fetal and neonatal morbidity and death. Discontinue as soon as possible after patient becomes pregnant. Several ACEIs have been found in breast milk.

RACE
- Less effective in African Americans than in others when used as monotherapy
- Use of ACEIs in combination with diuretics has been successful for blood pressure reduction in African Americans at rates comparable with those in other populations.

Patient Education

- Take a missed dose as soon as possible. Skip the missed dose if it is almost time for the next dose. Do not take two doses at the same time.
- Common side effects include nonproductive cough, dizziness, and light-headedness.
- The patient should call the practitioner immediately if any of these serious adverse effects occur:
  - Swelling (face, mouth, hands, tongue, or feet), difficulty breathing or swallowing, hives, severe itching,

fainting, cloudy urine, sore throat, fever and sudden onset of abdominal pain, diarrhea, and vomiting (intestinal edema) in an adult
- Signs of excess potassium in the body: irregular heartbeat, leg weakness, numbness or tingling of hands or feet, and extreme nervousness
- Avoid the use of potassium-containing medicines or salt substitutes while receiving this drug.

SPECIFIC DRUGS

lisinopril hydrochloride (Prinivil, Zestril) 🔑

CONTRAINDICATIONS. Hypersensitivity with angioedema with any ACEI, hereditary or idiopathic angioedema; bilateral renal artery stenosis; pregnancy

WARNINGS
- Neutropenia and agranulocytosis have occurred with captopril and occasionally with enalapril, lisinopril, and quinapril. Data are lacking to document whether other ACEIs cause agranulocytosis. Monitor WBCs.
- Anaphylactoid reactions, including angioedema of face, extremities, lips, mucous membranes, tongue, glottis, or larynx, have occurred.
- Proteinuria or nephrotic syndrome has occurred with captopril.

Watch for first-dose effect. Initial dose of ACEI may cause a precipitous, symptomatic fall in blood pressure, particularly in patients receiving diuretics, on sodium-restricted diets, or on dialysis.

- Drug may be associated with oliguria, progressive azotemia, or, rarely, acute renal failure and death. If possible, withhold diuretic for 24 to 72 hours before starting ACEI.
- Renal impairment dose reductions are indicated. The potential for exacerbation of renal insufficiency and hyperkalemia is present.
- Volume-depleted patients (i.e., those who use diuretics or dialysis, or with vomiting, diarrhea, or salt depletion) are at increased risk for symptomatic hypotension.
- Ramipril and fosinopril are primarily metabolized to active drug; increased inactive drug levels may occur with hepatic failure. In severe hepatic dysfunction, dose adjustments may be needed.
- In single renal artery stenosis, the potential exists for increased serum creatinine.
- Hypertensive patients with CHF have increased risk of symptomatic hypotension.

PRECAUTIONS
- Hyperkalemia or use of potassium-sparing diuretics or salt substitutes can induce hyperkalemia.
- Valvular stenosis: Patients with aortic stenosis are theoretically at risk of decreased coronary perfusion.
- Cough has occurred with the use of all ACEIs. The cough is nonproductive and persistent and resolves within 1 to 4 days after therapy is discontinued. It has a higher incidence in women. Incidence ranges from 5% to 25% and can be as high as 39%.
- Photosensitivity may occur.

Continued

lisinopril hydrochloride (Prinivil, Zestril) 🔑—cont'd

PHARMACOKINETICS. See Table 20-2.

ADVERSE EFFECTS. See Table 20-3.

DRUG INTERACTIONS. See Table 20-4.

DOSAGE AND ADMINISTRATION
- See Table 20-5 for dosage and administration directions for all ACEIs and ARBs.
- In general, it takes about 2 weeks for blood pressure reduction to occur and 4 weeks for the full effect to be seen.

- Food affects the rate but not the extent of absorption of fosinopril.
- Take captopril and moexipril 1 hour before meals.
- Ramipril capsules can be opened and mixed with food or water.
- The rate and absorption of quinapril are reduced by approximately 25% when it is taken with a high-fat meal.
- Lisinopril, captopril, enalapril, ramipril: Decrease dose in renal insufficiency.

TABLE 20-3 Adverse Effects of ACEIs and ARBs

Body System	Adverse Effects*
Skin, appendages	Rare: rash, diaphoresis, erythema multiforme, exfoliative dermatitis, flushing, photosensitivity, pruritus
Hypersensitivity	Angioedema (0.1%-0.5%)
Respiratory	Common: cough (ACEIs only); rare: asthma, bronchospasm
Cardiovascular	Orthostatic hypotension; rare: angina, CVA, MI
GI	Rare: abdominal pain, nausea, diarrhea, constipation
Hemic and lymphatic	Leukopenia, agranulocytosis
Musculoskeletal	Myalgia, arthralgia
Nervous system	Headache (<5%), dizziness (3%), fatigue (2%), ataxia, confusion, asthenia
Hepatic	Hepatitis
Genitourinary	Renal insufficiency, hyperkalemia, impotence

*Rare (>1%) unless noted.

TABLE 20-4 Drug Interactions With ACEIs and ARBs

ACEI/ARB	Action on Other Drugs
ACEIs	Increased digoxin, lithium, potassium preparations/potassium-sparing diuretics
captopril	Increased allopurinol
quinapril	Decreased tetracycline
telmisartan	Increased digoxin
telmisartan	Increased and decreased warfarin

Other Drugs	Action on ACEIs and ARBs
Phenothiazines	Increased ACEIs
capsaicin	Increased ACEIs (cough)
Antacids, indomethacin	Decreased ACEIs
probenecid	Increased captopril
rifampin	Decreased enalapril
cimetidine, fluconazole	Increased losartan
indomethacin, phenobarbital, rifampin	Decreased losartan

TABLE 20-5 Dosage and Administration Recommendations of ACEIs and ARBs

Drug	Indication*	Initial Dose	General Titration	Usual Dosage	Maximum Daily Dose
captopril	HTN	12.5-25 mg bid or tid	Increase by 12.5-25 mg/dose every 1-2 weeks.	50 mg tid; 25-100 mg/day in two divided doses (JNC 7)	450 mg
	CHF	6.25-12.5 mg tid; dose dependent upon patient's fluid/electrolyte status		Target dose: 50 mg tid	450 mg
	Diabetic neuropathy	25 mg tid		—	—
lisinopril	HTN	10 mg daily (if presently treated with a diuretic); 5 mg daily (if not treated with a diuretic)	Increase every 2 weeks.	20-40 mg once daily; 10-40 mg once daily (JNC 7)	80 mg
	CHF	2.5-5 mg once daily	Increase by no greater than 10-mg increments every 2 weeks.	20-40 mg once daily (ACC/AHA 2005 Heart Failure Guidelines)	40 mg

Table continued on following page

TABLE 20-5   Dosage and Administration Recommendations of ACEIs and ARBs (Continued)

Drug	Indication*	Initial Dose	General Titration	Usual Dosage	Maximum Daily Dose
benazepril	HTN	10 mg daily (if patient not receiving a diuretic); 5 mg daily (if patient receiving a diuretic)	Increase every 2 weeks.	20-40 mg once daily; 10-40 mg once daily (JNC 7)	40 mg
enalapril	HTN	2.5-5 mg/day	Increase every 1-2 weeks.	10-40 mg in one or two divided doses; 2.5-40 mg/day in one to two divided doses (JNC 7)	40 mg
	CHF	2.5 mg daily (if patient taking a diuretic) 2.5 mg daily or bid		10-20 mg twice daily (ACC/AHA 2005 Heart Failure Guidelines)	40 mg
quinapril	HTN	10-20 mg once daily; 5 mg daily (if patient receiving a diuretic, elderly)	Increase every 1-2 weeks.	20-60 mg daily or divided doses; 10-80 mg once daily (JNC 7)	—
	CHF	5 mg once daily or bid		20-40 mg daily in two divided doses; 20 mg bid (ACC/AHA 2005 Heart Failure Guidelines)	—
moexipril	HTN	7.5 mg once daily (if patient not receiving diuretic); 3.75 mg once daily (with diuretic, elderly, and CrCl <40 ml/min)		7.5-30 mg daily or divided doses; 7.5-30 mg in one or two divided doses (JNC 7)	30 mg
ramipril	HTN	2.5-5 mg once daily	Increase every 1-2 weeks.	2.5-20 daily or divided doses; 2.5-20 mg once daily (JNC 7)	20 mg
	HTN with renal failure	1.25 mg once daily	Increase every 2 weeks.	—	—
	CHF	1.25-2.5 mg bid for 1 wk; initial: 1.25-2.5 mg once daily	Increase every 3 weeks to 5 mg bid as tolerated.	Target dose: 10 mg once daily (ACC/AHA 2005 Heart Failure Guidelines)	10 mg
	CHF with renal failure	1.25 mg once daily	Increase every 3 or more weeks.	1.25 mg bid and up to 2.5 mg bid as tolerated	
	Cerebrovascular risk reduction	2.5 once daily	2.5 mg once daily for 1 week, then 5 mg once daily for the next 3 weeks, then increase as tolerated to 10 mg once daily (may be given as divided dose)	2.5-10 mg once daily	10 mg
fosinopril	HTN	10 mg once daily	Increase every 1-2 weeks.	20-40 mg daily or divided doses	80 mg
	CHF	10 mg once daily	Increase over several weeks.	10-40 mg once daily (JNC 7)	40 mg
	Renal dysfunction	5 mg once daily		20-40 mg daily	
ANGIOTENSIN II RECEPTOR BLOCKERS					
losartan	HTN	25-50 mg once daily	Increase every 2-4 weeks.	25-100 mg in one or two divided doses (JNC 7)	100 mg
	Children (6-16 yrs old)	0.7 mg/kg once daily			
	Diabetic nephropathy	50 mg once daily		50-100 mg in one or two divided doses	50 mg
	Stroke reduction				100 mg
	Hepatic impairment	25 mg daily in two divided doses		—	—

TABLE 20-5   Dosage and Administration Recommendations of ACEIs and ARBs (Continued)

Drug	Indication*	Initial Dose	General Titration	Usual Dosage	Maximum Daily Dose
candesartan	HTN	16 mg once daily	Increase every 2 weeks.	8-32 mg daily in one or two divided doses; 8-32 mg once daily (JNC 7)	32 mg
	CHF	4 mg once daily	Double dose every 2 weeks.	4-32 mg once daily	32 mg
eprosartan	HTN	600 mg once daily	Increase every 2 weeks.	400-800 mg daily or divided doses (JNC 7)	800 mg
valsartan	HTN	80-160 mg once daily	Increase every 4 weeks.	80-320 mg daily in one or two divided doses (JNC 7)	320 mg
	CHF	40 mg bid		80-160 mg bid	
telmisartan	HTN Elderly	40 mg once daily 20 mg once daily	Increase every 2 weeks.	20-80 mg (JNC 7)	80 mg
irbesartan	HTN	150 mg once daily	Increase every 2 weeks.	150-300 mg once daily (JNC 7)	300 mg
	Children (6-12 yr old)	75 mg once daily		75-150 mg once daily	150 mg
	Diabetic nephropathy	75 mg once daily		75-300 mg	320 mg

*HTN dose is when patient IS NOT on a diuretic; CHF dose is when patient IS on a diuretic and digitalis.

evolve A continually updated list of useful WebLinks may be found in the Evolve Resources at http://evolve.elsevier.com/Edmunds/NP/

21 Antiarrhythmic Agents

ELIZABETH MONSON and MAREN STEWART MAYHEW

DRUG OVERVIEW

Class	Subclass	Generic Name	Trade Name
I	IA	quinidine	Quinidex Extentabs, Quinaglute Dura-Tabs
		procainamide	Procan SR
	IB	lidocaine	Xylocaine
		mexiletine	Mexitil
		tocainide	Tonocard
	IC	flecainide	Tambocor
		propafenone	Rythmol
II	β-Adrenergic blockers	propranolol ✹	Inderal ✹
		acebutolol	Sectral
		metoprolol ✹	Lopressor, Toprol XL ✹
III		amiodarone 🔑 ✹	Cordarone, Pacerone
		sotalol ✹	Betapace, Sorine
		ibutilide	Corvert
		dofetilide	Tikosyn
IV	Calcium channel blockers	verapamil ✹	Calan, SR
		diltiazem ✹	Cardizem, SR, CD
Other		digoxin ✹	Lanoxin ✹
		adenosine	Adenocard

✹ Top 200 drug; 🔑 key drug.

INDICATIONS

- Paroxysmal supraventricular tachycardia
- Atrial fibrillation
- Premature ventricular contractions (see Table 21-1 for indications for each medication)

Antiarrhythmics are used for the treatment of fast, slow, or irregular heartbeat. Most drugs used as antiarrhythmics in primary care are used for other indications and are discussed in detail in other chapters. Because amiodarone is the only drug that is used exclusively for arrhythmia, it is the only drug discussed here in detail. The primary care provider who has a patient taking an antiarrhythmic should consult the most recent sources for complete, up-to-date information on the drug and should work closely with a cardiologist, electrophysiologist, or experienced physician. All antiarrhythmic medications have potentially serious adverse effects, including the induction of other serious and even fatal arrhythmias.

THERAPEUTIC OVERVIEW OF ARRHYTHMIAS

Only the three arrhythmias most commonly managed in the outpatient setting are discussed in detail: paroxysmal supraventricular tachycardia (PSVT), atrial fibrillation (AF), and premature ventricular contractions (PVCs).

Anatomy and Physiology

The heart is composed of specialized myocardial muscle cells that have the capacity to generate an electrical potential (automaticity) and spread the electrical current from cell to cell (conductivity) (Figure 21-1). Many cells within the myocardium can serve as a pacemaker of the heart, but the primary pacemaker is found in the sinoatrial node. Electrical

TABLE 21-1   Antiarrhythmic Medication Indications

Class	Drug	Indications
IA	quinidine	Atrial flutter Paroxysmal and chronic atrial fibrillation Paroxysmal ventricular tachycardia without complete heart block
II	propranolol	Paroxysmal atrial tachycardia, especially induced by catecholamines, digitalis, or Wolff-Parkinson-White syndrome Persistent sinus tachycardia Tachycardia and arrhythmia caused by thyrotoxicosis Persistent atrial extrasystoles
III	amiodarone	Documented life-threatening recurrent ventricular arrhythmias not controlled by antiarrhythmic drugs Recurrent ventricular fibrillation Recurrent hemodynamically unstable ventricular tachycardia Suppression of atrial fibrillation
VI	verapamil	Atrial fibrillation, to control ventricular rate with digoxin Paroxysmal supraventricular tachycardia
Other	digoxin	Atrial fibrillation, to control ventricular rate Atrial flutter

waves of depolarization spread through the atrium, the atrioventricular junction, and the bundle of His, and down the left- and right-bundle branches, producing synchronized atrial and ventricular muscular contractions. When the dominant pacemaker slows or does not fire, other cells take over and continue the heartbeat, although at a slower rate. Sometimes aberrant cells take over the pacemaker role, creating irregular rhythms and/or tachyarrhythmias.

Action potential (Figure 21-2) refers to the difference in electrical charge across the myocardial cell membrane that results in polarization and depolarization. *Depolarization* is the electrical impulse that precedes the mechanical contraction of cardiac tissue. *Repolarization* is the recovery stage after muscle contraction.

Pathophysiology

The mechanism of an arrhythmia is theoretically important in determining which drug will be effective. The two basic tachyarrhythmic mechanisms within the heart are (1) increased automaticity, resulting in an ectopic focus, and (2) reentry through abnormal conduction pathways.

However, it is often clinically impossible to determine the mechanism without an electrophysiology mapping study. Arrhythmias that are caused by irritability or increased automaticity are treated with drugs that prolong the action potential, thus decreasing the rate at which impulses can be generated (Figure 21-3). Sustained ventricular tachycardia usually occurs as reentry, and it is treated with a drug that prolongs the effective refractory period.

Disease Process

PSVT is a term that applies to all supraventricular tachycardias except for AF and atrial flutter. In approximately 60% of cases, it is due to reentry within or in close proximity to the AV node known as atrioventricular nodal reentrant tachycardia (AVNRT). It results from atrioventricular reentrant tachycardia (AVRT) in 30% of cases. AVRT refers to accessory pathways that connect the atrium with the ventricle. It is characterized by a heart rate of 130 to 250, 1:1 conduction, and a narrow QRS complex. PSVTs often are seen in patients with no underlying heart disease. Treatment depends on the patient's ability to tolerate the

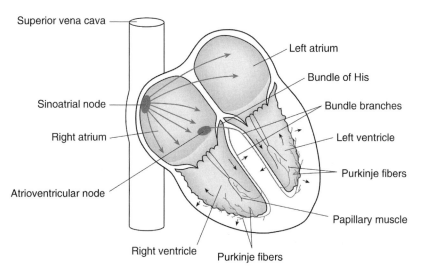

FIGURE 21-1   Conduction system of the heart. (From Berne RM, Levy MN: *Cardiovascular physiology,* ed 7, St Louis, 1997, Mosby.)

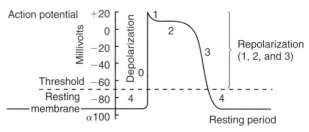

Depolarization
Phase 0—membrane becomes permeable to Na⁺
which rapidly flows into the cell

Repolarization
Phase 1—membrane potential becomes slightly positive
because of the rapid influx of Na⁺
Phase 2—slow inward flow of Ca⁺⁺ and outward flow of K⁺
Phase 3—rapid outward flow of K⁺

Resting period
Phase 4—cell membrane actively transports Na⁺
outside and K⁺ inside, returning cell membrane
to state of polarization

A

FIGURE 21-2   A, Action potential of a single myocardial fiber (cell). B, Ionic exchanges that occur across the cell membrane of a single myocardial fiber during an action potential. (From McKenry LM, Salerno E: *Mosby's pharmacology in nursing,* ed 22, St Louis, 2002, Mosby.)

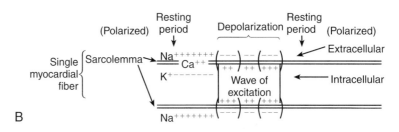

B

tachycardia, the mechanism of the arrhythmia, and how frequently the arrhythmia presents.

AF is a relatively common arrhythmia. Risk factors include male gender, underlying disease, and increasing age. It is due to a total lack of organized electrical activity in the atria. AF is classified according to the duration of the arrhythmia. Paroxysmal AF refers to episodes that self-terminate and last less than 7 days—usually less than 24 hours. Persistent AF lasts longer than 7 days, and episodes fail to terminate on their own. However, they can be terminated by electrical cardioversion after absence of clots in the left atrium has been confirmed by transesophageal echocardiogram and therapeutic warfarin therapy for 3 weeks and initiation of amiodarone. Permanent AF lasts for longer than 1 year, and termination has not been attempted or has failed. Finally, "lone" AF is applied to any form of AF that occurs in patients with no history of structural cardiac disease.

Treatment of patients with AF focuses on rate and rhythm control and anticoagulation to prevent systemic embolization. Rate control with β-blockers, calcium channel blockers, or digoxin and anticoagulation with warfarin is recommended for most patients with AF. Rhythm control is attained through the use of DC or medications. Long-term maintenance of normal sinus rhythm is not usually successful over time if the patient has a history of valvular disease or longstanding hypertension. AF can be classified as paroxysmal, persistent, or chronic and is associated with two problems. The first is rapid ventricular response. The ventricular response usually occurs at a rate of 150 to 220 beats/min. This rapid rate may be

poorly tolerated, precipitating CHF if the patient cannot tolerate loss of atrial kick. The second issue with AF is the risk of thromboembolism. Clots may form in the atria as the result of pooling of blood that occurs with chaotic firing and lack of contractility; they can be released into the systemic circulation, causing arterial occlusion and stroke.

PVCs are caused by increased automaticity. They are classified according to both prevalence and morphologic characteristics. The most important factor in determining whether to treat PVCs is the presence of underlying heart disease. Underlying heart disease (especially myocardial ischemia or recent MI) in the presence of PVCs can be a marker for development of malignant ventricular arrhythmias. Additional factors that place the patient at increased risk are the presence of cardiac scarring, hypertrophy, and/or left ventricular dysfunction. PVCs that are frequent, paired, or sustained are particularly dangerous. PVCs that occur during the QT interval present a risk for initiating ventricular fibrillation. Because of the risks inherent in antiarrhythmic therapy, patients should not be treated unless clearly indicated. Torsades de pointes is a life-threatening ventricular tachycardia that is associated with prolongation of the QT interval. It is most often seen as a drug reaction or an electrolyte imbalance.

Assessment

Take a thorough health history, including history of drug hypersensitivity and review of other medications that may cause drug interactions, other medical comorbidities, and current antiarrhythmic agents that could cause an additive

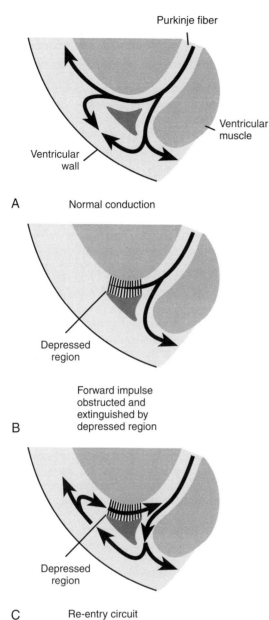

Purkinje fiber

Ventricular muscle

Ventricular wall

A   Normal conduction

Depressed region

Forward impulse obstructed and extinguished by depressed region

B

Depressed region

C   Re-entry circuit

FIGURE 21-3 **Mechanisms of arrhythmias.**

cardiac depressant effect. The patient with an arrhythmia may have no complaints or may complain of chest pain, shortness of breath, fatigue, palpitations, dizziness, weakness, or syncope. The palpitations may be described as fluttering, pounding, skipped beats, or "heart jumping out of the chest." These often are noticed when the patient is sitting quietly or lying in bed.

Auscultation often gives clues as to the rate and rhythm of the heart. AF is recognized by an irregular rhythm and rate, whereas PSVT is a very fast regular rate and rhythm. PVCs are premature ventricular beats with a compensatory pause. Premature atrial contractions (PACs) occur early and cause an occasional skip, with no compensatory pause.

Obtain relevant laboratory studies, such as chest radiograph, graded exercise test, ECG, echocardiogram, and 24-hour Holter monitor results. Obtain baseline laboratory values such as CBC, electrolytes, thyroid panel, and renal and hepatic function tests.

Identify and remove, or correct, any precipitating factors. Treat any underlying factors that may cause arrhythmia, such as hypoxia, acid-base imbalance, increased or decreased potassium or magnesium, thyroid dysfunction, excessive catecholamines, or drug toxicity. Anxiety, caffeine, cigarettes, or stimulants such as decongestants, diet pills, amphetamines, theophylline, nicotinic acid, or alcohol also may precipitate arrhythmia.

MECHANISM OF ACTION

Antiarrhythmic drugs act to reduce electrical irregularity of the heart. They do this by altering the action potential of cardiac cells (Figure 21-4, Table 21-2). All antiarrhythmics have the potential to cause arrhythmia. In 1995, CAST (Cardiac Arrhythmia Suppression Trial) revealed the dangers of aggressive medical treatment of arrhythmias.

Class IA drugs (quinidine, disopyramide, procainamide) depress rapid depolarization (phase 0) of the action potential. These drugs slow conduction by lengthening the effective refractory period of atrial and ventricular myocardium, by depressing the inward sodium current, and by decreasing the automaticity and excitability of ectopic foci of cardiac muscle. Class IB drugs (lidocaine, mexiletine, tocainide) exert less effect on sodium channels at rest but are more prominent during depolarization, so their effect on phase 0 is only slight. Class IC drugs (flecainide, propafenone) depress phase 0 markedly and profoundly slow conduction.

β-Blockers are Class II antiarrhythmics that work by inhibiting sympathetic stimulation. They antagonize the effects of catecholamines released from the adrenergic nerve endings and the adrenal medulla. Blocking sympathetic activity reduces the rate of discharge of the sinus and other foci that act as pacemakers, and it increases the effective refractory period of the AV node.

Class III drugs (amiodarone, ibutilide, dofetilide, sotalol) prolong phase 3 repolarization by blocking potassium channels. The QT interval is thus prolonged on the ECG. This prolongation also increases the risk of torsades de pointes, a ventricular tachycardia. Amiodarone, however, does not appear to have this effect. Amiodarone blocks sodium channels, and this contributes to slowing of conduction and prolongs

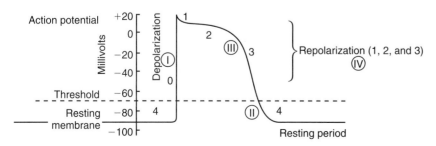

Action potential

Millivolts

+20
0
−20
−40

Depolarization

Threshold −60

Resting membrane −80
−100

Depolarization 0

Repolarization (1, 2, and 3)

Resting period

FIGURE 21-4 **Phases of the action potential and locations of action of the classes of antiarrhythmics.** Circled Roman numerals indicate the major site of action of that category of antiarrhythmic.

TABLE 21-2 Mechanism of Action of Antiarrhythmic Medications

Drug	Heart Rate	Automaticity of Foci	Conduction Velocity		Refractory Period			ECG Changes		
			AV Node	Ventricle	Atrium	Ventricle	Accessory Pathway	PR Interval	QRS	QT Interval
IA										
quinidine	±	↓	±	↓	↑	↑	↑	±	↑	↑
procainamide	±	↓	±	↓	↑	↑	↑	±	↑	↑
IB										
lidocaine	0	↓	0	0	0	±	↑↓	0	0	↓
mexiletine	0	↓	0	0	0	↑	↑	0	0	0
tocainide	0	↓	0	0	↓	↓	↑	0	0	↓
IC										
flecainide	0	↓	↓	↓	0	↑	↑	↑	↑	↑
propafenone	0	↓	↓	↓	0	↑	↑	↑	↑	↑
II (β-Adrenergic Blockers)										
propranolol	↓	↓	↓	↓	±	0	↑	↑	0	↓
metoprolol	↓	↓	↓	0	±	0	↑	↑	0	↓
III										
amiodarone	↓	↓	↓	↓	↑	↑	↑	↑	↑	↑↑
IV (Calcium Channel Blockers)										
verapamil	↓	↓	↓	0	0	0	0	↑	0	0
OTHER										
digoxin	↓	↑	↓	↓	±	↓	↑↓	↑	0	↓
adenosine	↑	↓	↓	0	0	0	0	↑	0	0

refractoriness in the AV node. Its vasodilatory action decreases cardiac workload and therefore decreases myocardial oxygen consumption. Sotalol exhibits β-blocking activity. Ibutilide is available only as an IV formulation and is used for rapid termination of atrial fibrillation and flutter. Dofetilide must be initiated in a hospitalized patient because of its ability to prolong the QT interval.

Class IV drugs are the nondihydropyridine calcium channel blockers (verapamil, diltiazem). These drugs inhibit calcium ion influx through slow channels into conductile and contractile myocardial cells and vascular smooth muscle cells; they also slow AV conduction and prolong the effective refractory period within the AV node.

Digoxin suppresses AV node conduction to increase the effective refractory period and decrease conduction. This results in a decreased heart rate and reduced risk of reentry or supraventricular arrhythmia.

TREATMENT PRINCIPLES

Standardized Guidelines

- ACC/AHA/ESC: 2006 guidelines for the management of patients with atrial fibrillation: a report of the American College of Cardiology/American Heart Association Task Force on Practice Guidelines and the European Society of Cardiology Committee for Practice Guidelines (Writing Committee to revise the 2001 Guidelines for the Management of Patients with Atrial Fibrillation). *J Am Coll Cardiol* 48:e149-e246, 2006.

Evidence-Based Recommendations

Digoxin, diltiazem, and verapamil are effective in controlling heart rate in patients who have recent-onset atrial fibrillation and are hemodynamically stable.

Cardinal Points of Treatment

The primary care provider must work in collaboration with the cardiologist. The cardiologist determines the appropriate medication and begins treatment. The patient, once stable, may be turned over to the primary care provider for long-term monitoring. Table 21-3 outlines specific treatment principles for each type of arrhythmia.

Pharmacologic Treatment

PAROXYSMAL SUPRAVENTRICULAR TACHYCARDIA. Prophylaxis of PSVT usually involves digoxin or β-blockers. Verapamil is a second choice. These medications also may be used in combination. It must be remembered that verapamil increases digoxin serum levels. If the patient has significant heart disease, he or she may require a class IA, IC, or III drug. Radiofrequency ablation is frequently used to eliminate the accessory pathway. This avoids problems with the safety of antiarrhythmic drugs. Digoxin and calcium channel blockers should never be used if an accessory pathway is diagnosed or suspected.

ATRIAL FIBRILLATION. Treatment for patients with chronic AF is threefold: control of rate, rhythm, and thromboembolic events.

1. Control of rapid ventricular response is accomplished with the use of a β-blocker or a nondihydropyridine calcium channel antagonist for patients with persistent or permanent AF.
2. In the absence of preexcitation, intravenous administration of β-blockers (esmolol, metoprolol, propranolol) or nondihydropyridine calcium channel antagonists (verapamil, diltiazem) is recommended to slow the ventricular response to AF in the acute setting; caution is exercised in patients with hypotension or HF.
3. Intravenous administration of digoxin or amiodarone is recommended to control the heart rate in patients with AF and HF who do not have an accessory pathway.
4. Prevention of thromboembolic events is accomplished by anticoagulation. Warfarin is the treatment of choice, particularly in patients who are older than age 70, or who have a history of thromboembolic events, hypertension, coronary artery disease, or left ventricular dysfunction. If the patient is unable to be safely anticoagulated with warfarin, aspirin may be given at 325 mg/day (see Chapter 23).
5. Amiodarone may be used for pharmacologic cardioversion or suppression of AF and maintenance of normal sinus rhythm.

A single oral bolus dose of propafenone or flecainide ("pill-in-the-pocket") can be administered to terminate persistent AF outside the hospital once treatment has proved safe in hospital for selected patients without sinus or AV node dysfunction, bundle-branch block, QT interval prolongation, the Brugada syndrome, or structural heart disease. Before antiarrhythmic medication is initiated, a β-blocker or a nondihydropyridine calcium channel antagonist should be given to prevent rapid AV conduction in the event that atrial flutter occurs.

TABLE 21-3   Suggested Treatment of Common Arrhythmias

Arrhythmia	Treatment Indicated for Acute Problem	Treatment Indicated for Chronic Prophylaxis
Paroxysmal supraventricular tachycardia	Intravenous (IV) adenosine verapamil	digoxin propranolol or other β-blocker therapy verapamil
Premature ventricular contractions	lidocaine IV procainamide	quinidine or procainamide β-Blockers amiodarone
Atrial flutter/atrial fibrillation	IV β-blocker IV calcium channel blocker IV digoxin Cardioversion	digoxin propranolol verapamil Anticoagulants

Nonpharmacologic Treatment

Usually, nonpharmacologic therapy is initiated prior to drug therapy. However, in AF, radiofrequency ablation of foci around the pulmonary veins, the root of the left/right atrium, and the isthmus of the mitral valve may be an appropriate intervention for those with symptomatic AF who are unresponsive to pharmacologic therapy.

PREMATURE VENTRICULAR CONTRACTIONS. In general, PVCs are treated if *any* of the following applies:
- Complex PVCs are present.
- The patient is 1 year or less post-MI.
- The patient has underlying heart disease.
- The patient has angina.
- The patient has other symptoms.
  PVCs are not treated if *all* of the following apply:
- The patient is asymptomatic.
- The patient has a normal heart.
- The PVCs are simple.
- The PVCs disappear with exercise on a graded exercise test.
  Long-term treatment to suppress ventricular arrhythmias is usually selected after provocative testing in an acute care setting. Drugs that may be effective include the class IA drugs and amiodarone. All of the drugs that may be effective are known to cause the arrhythmia that is being treated.

MONITOR FOR THERAPEUTIC EFFECT. A treatment plan specific to the patient is necessary. Total elimination of all irregular beats is not realistic clinically. Usually, the goal is to prevent a potentially fatal arrhythmia or to prevent certain targeted symptoms.

MONITOR FOR TOXICITY. An antiarrhythmic may cause the arrhythmia that one is trying to suppress. Worsening of an arrhythmia after the drug is started may occur as an adverse reaction to the drug. At each visit, ask about specific adverse effects. Monitor drug levels and changes in ECGs as needed. These drugs have significant adverse effects that require close monitoring.

digoxin
- Therapeutic plasma levels should be maintained for the patient. Dosages should be decreased in persons older than 65 years of age. Monitor patient for development of toxicities.

quinidine
- Therapeutic plasma level is 2 to 5 mcg/ml in most laboratories, although patient-dependent therapeutic response has been shown to occur at levels of 3 to 6 mcg/ml. Perform periodic CBC and hepatic and renal function tests. This drug has multiple adverse effects. (See Table 22-5.)

amiodarone
- Plasma concentrations may be helpful in evaluating nonresponsiveness or unexpectedly severe toxicity.
- Perform baseline chest radiographs and pulmonary function tests, including diffusion capacity, before initiation of therapy. Patient history, physical examination, and chest radiograph should be performed every 3 to 6 months.
- Thyroid function is needed at baseline and periodically during therapy.
- Assess liver enzymes at least twice a year.
- Obtain annual ophthalmic examination, including funduscopic and slit-lamp examinations to detect optic neuritis.

Patient Variables

GERIATRICS
- A normal change of aging is loss of conduction fibers in the heart, which predisposes to benign arrhythmia. If treated, the elderly are at increased risk for adverse reactions to the medications. They may require a decreased dosage to avoid possible impaired renal or hepatic function.
- Amiodarone: Healthy subjects older than 65 years show lower clearances of amiodarone than do younger subjects, along with an increased half-life (20-47 days).

PEDIATRICS. Safety and efficacy of these drugs have not been established.

PREGNANCY AND LACTATION
- *Category B:* lidocaine, sotalol
- *Category C:* quinidine, procainamide, mexiletine, tocainide, flecainide, propafenone, propranolol, metoprolol, verapamil, diltiazem, digoxin, and adenosine
- *Category D:* amiodarone; propranolol, metoprolol (second/third trimester [expert opinion]); atenolol
- Drugs are excreted in breast milk.

Patient Education
- Wear a medical alert bracelet and carry a medical identification card specifying that you are taking an antiarrhythmic drug.
- Report any new or uncomfortable symptoms to your health care provider.
  amiodarone
- Photosensitivity and skin discoloration occur in about 10% of those on amiodarone. Advise patients to use sunscreen and protective clothing.
- Advise to call for breakthrough arrhythmia, dyspnea, or cough.
- Advise patients of need for regular visits and testing to monitor for toxic effects.
  digoxin
- Report any occurrence of yellow halo around objects, nausea, decreased appetite, or episodes of extreme fatigue; all symptoms of these may indicate early toxicity.

SPECIFIC DRUGS

amiodarone (Cordarone, Pacerone)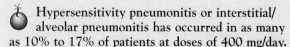

Only the oral form of amiodarone is discussed here. The parenteral form is used only in acute care settings.

CONTRAINDICATIONS
- Hypersensitivity to the drug or its components
- Severe sinus node dysfunction, marked sinus bradycardia, second- and third-degree AV block, syncope caused by bradycardia, cardiogenic shock

WARNINGS/PRECAUTIONS. Amiodarone can exacerbate arrhythmias. Significant heart block or sinus bradycardia has occurred.

Hypersensitivity pneumonitis or interstitial/alveolar pneumonitis has occurred in as many as 10% to 17% of patients at doses of 400 mg/day.

Continued on page 276

TABLE 21-4 Pharmacokinetics of Common Antiarrhythmic Medications

Drug	Absorption	Drug Availability (After First Pass)	Onset of Action	Time to Peak Concentration	Half-life	Duration of Action	Protein Bound	Metabolism	Excretion	Therapeutic Serum Level
IA										
quinidine (as sulfate)	—	80%	—	1-3 hr	6-8 hr	6-8 hr	80%-88%	Hepatic	Urine	2-6 mcg/ml
procainamide	85%	—	30 min	—	3 hr	3 + hr	20%	Hepatic	Renal	3-10 mcg/ml; NAPA 15-25 mcg/ml
IB										
lidocaine	—	—	45-90 sec (IV)	—	1-2 hr	15 min	50%-60%	Hepatic	Renal	1.5-5 mcg/ml
mexiletine	90%	—	—	2-3 hr	10-12 hr	24 hr		Hepatic	Renal	0.5-2 mcg/ml
tocainide	100%	100%	—	0.5-2.5 hr	11-14 hr	5 hr	10%	Hepatic	Renal	5-12 mcg/ml
IC										
flecainide	100%	100%	—	1.5-3 hr	12-27 hr	—	40%	Hepatic	Renal	0.2-1 mcg/ml
propafenone	100%	3%-10%	—	2-3 hr	2-8 hr	—	97%	Hepatic	Hepatic	—
II										
propranolol	100%	30%-40%	1-2 hr	—	4-6 hr	6 hr	90%-95%	Hepatic	Renal	50-100 ng/ml
acebutolol	90%	40%	1-2 hr	2-4 hr	3-4 hr	12-24 hr	5%-15%	Hepatic	Renal	—
III										
amiodarone	35%-65%	50%	2 days-2 wk	3-7 hr	40-55 days	Weeks-months	96%	Hepatic	Hepatic	0.5-2.5 mcg/ml
IV										
verapamil	—	20%-35%	1-2 hr	1-2 hr	5-12 hr	6-8 hr	88%-92%	Hepatic	Renal	50-200 ng/ml
OTHER										
digoxin	—	70%-80%	0.5-2 hr	1 hr	30-40 hr	24 hr	20%-25%	Nonhepatic	Renal	0.5-2 ng/ml
adenosine	—	—	—	—	<10 sec	1-2 min	—	—	—	—

TABLE 21-5   Adverse Effects of Antiarrhythmic Agents

Drug	Common Adverse Effects	Serious Adverse Effects
IA		
quinidine	Light-headedness, diarrhea, nausea, vomiting, heartburn, esophagitis, fatigue, palpitations, weakness, rash, visual problems, tremor	Cinchonism, hepatotoxicity, bronchospasm, lupus erythematosus–like syndrome, convulsions, ventricular tachycardia, ventricular fibrillation, torsades de pointes
procainamide	Myalgias, anorexia, nausea, vomiting, diarrhea, rash	Positive ANA titer, lupus erythematosus–like syndrome, blood dyscrasia, agranulocytosis, neutropenia, hypoplastic anemia, thrombocytopenia, CHF, asystole, ventricular fibrillation, hypotension, hepatic dysfunction
IB		
lidocaine	Light-headedness, nausea, blurred vision, paresthesias, tremors	Respiratory depression/arrest, bradycardia, hypotension, cardiac arrest, allergic reactions
mexiletine	Palpitations, increased PVCs, nausea, vomiting, diarrhea, heartburn, constipation, dizziness, tremor, fatigue, weakness, blurred vision, paresthesias	Hepatic dysfunction, blood dyscrasias, ventricular tachycardia, ventricular fibrillation, angina, hypotension, bradycardia, second- or third-degree heart block, supraventricular arrhythmias, cardiogenic shock
tocainide	Fatigue, palpitations, chest pain, nausea, vomiting, anorexia, diarrhea, dizziness, paresthesias, tremor, headache, anxiety, blurred vision, diaphoresis, increased PVCs	Blood dyscrasias, agranulocytosis, leukopenia, neutropenia, aplastic/hypoplastic anemia, thrombocytopenia, pulmonary fibrosis/edema, interstitial pneumonitis, CHF, hypotension, bradycardia, ventricular tachycardia, ventricular fibrillation
IC		
flecainide	Dizziness, visual disturbances, dyspnea, headache, nausea, fatigue, palpitations, chest pain, asthenia, tremor, constipation, edema	CHF, bradycardia, second- or third-degree heart block, ventricular tachycardia, ventricular fibrillation, supraventricular arrhythmias, hepatic dysfunction, blood dyscrasias, death
propafenone	Unusual taste, nausea, vomiting, headache, fatigue, weakness, palpitations, diarrhea, anorexia, anxiety blurred vision	CHF, bradycardia, second- or third-degree heart block, ventricular tachycardia, ventricular fibrillation, torsades de pointes, bronchospasm
II		
propranolol	Fatigue, light-headedness, depression, short-term memory loss, nausea, vomiting, diarrhea	Bronchospasm, bradycardia, CHF, hypotension, second- or third-degree heart block
acebutolol or metoprolol	Fatigue, dizziness, depression, headache, nightmares, insomnia, peripheral edema, nausea, diarrhea, pruritus, rash	Bronchospasm, bradycardia, CHF, hypotension, second- or third-degree heart block
III		
amiodarone	Photosensitivity, hyperthyroidism, hypothyroidism, malaise, fatigue, tremor, poor coordination, nausea, vomiting, constipation, anorexia	Pulmonary toxicity, hepatic failure, second- or third-degree heart block, blue-gray skin discoloration, bradycardia, ventricular tachycardia, ventricular fibrillation, torsades de pointes, optic neuropathy/neuritis, vision loss, peripheral neuropathy, CHF
IV		
verapamil	Constipation, headache, rash, bleeding, visual problems, upper respiratory infection, dizziness, fatigue, edema, nausea, flushing	Second- or third-degree heart block, bradycardia, CHF, hypotension
OTHER		
digoxin	Palpitations, ventricular extrasystoles, tachycardia, anorexia, nausea, vomiting, diarrhea, headache, dizziness, mental disturbances, rash	Cardiac arrest, second- or third-degree heart block, ventricular tachycardia, ventricular fibrillation
adenosine	Facial flushing, headache, dyspnea, chest pressure, hyperventilation, light-headedness, paresthesias, blurred vision, heaviness in arms, neck/back pain, nausea, metallic taste, tightness in throat	Prolonged asystole, ventricular tachycardia, ventricular fibrillation, bradycardia, atrial fibrillation, bronchospasm

amiodarone (Cordarone, Pacerone) 🔑 —cont'd

Pulmonary toxicity is the main cause of amiodarone-associated death. It most commonly presents as a chronic interstitial pneumonitis; however, an organizing pneumonia, acute respiratory distress syndrome, or a solitary pulmonary mass can be seen. Pulmonary toxicity occurs over months to years of therapy rather than acutely, although a few cases have been reported in as little as 2 weeks. Patients who take more than 400 mg per day are at greatest risk of this problem. Symptoms reported in 50% to 75% of patients include nonproductive cough and dyspnea. Weight loss and fever are seen in one third to one half of patients. Auscultation often reveals bilateral inspiratory crackles. New respiratory symptoms

TABLE 21-6   Dosage and Administration Recommendations of Antiarrhythmic Agents

Drug	Age Group	Initial Dosage	Administration	Maintenance Dosage	Maximum Daily Dose
IA					
quinidine	Pediatric and adult	300 mg q12h	po q8-12h	300 mg q8h	Variable, dependent on serum therapeutic range and presence of ECG changes
procainamide		500 mg bid	po q12h	Dependent on body weight; see prescribing information	5000 mg
IB					
lidocaine	Pediatric and adult	400 mg q8h	IV or injection	Individualize.	Dependent on weight
mexiletine	Adult	200 mg q8h	po q8-12h	200-300 mg q8h	1200 mg
tocainide	Adult	400 mg q8h	po q8-12h	400-600 mg q8h	2400 mg
IC					
flecainide	Adult	50 mg q12h (100 mg q12h for ventricular arrhythmias)	po q12h	100 mg q12h; 150 mg q12h	300 mg; 400 mg (ventricular)
propafenone	Adult	150 mg q8h	po q8-12h	225 mg q8-12h (IR 8 hr; ER 12 hr)	900 mg
II					
propranolol	Pediatric and adult	10-40 mg q6-8h	po q8-12h	80-160 mg bid	640 mg/day
acebutolol	Adult	200 mg q12h	po q12h	600-1200 mg/day in two divided doses	1200 mg
metoprolol	Adult	25 mg bid (Lopressor); 25 mg daily (Toprol XL)	50 mg bid (Lopressor); 100 mg daily (Toprol XL)	200 mg/day	po q12-24h
III					
amiodarone	Adult	800-1600 mg/day (loading dose for 1-3 wk) Requires baseline and periodic PFTs, laboratory tests, ophthalmology examination Monitor ECG closely for prolonged QT interval with initiation or increase in therapy	po once-twice daily (loading doses may require bid scheduling) Reduced creatinine clearance requires longer dosing intervals	200-400 mg/day	400 mg
sotalol	Pediatric Adult and elderly	>2 yr: 180 mg/m² day 320 mg daily Reduced dosage required for impaired creatinine clearance	Give with or without food; use telemetry for titration	320 mg daily	320 mg daily
IV					
verapamil	Adult	80 mg q8h	po q6-8h	240-480 mg/day po daily, if patient not responsive, see product information guide for alternative dosing schedules	480 mg
OTHER					
digoxin	Adult	0.125 mg	po once daily	0.125-0.5 mg once daily	0.5 mg
adenosine	Pediatric and adult	6 mg (adult)	6-mg rapid IV bolus through peripheral line	None	May repeat 12 mg IV if no conversion after 1-2 min

amiodarone (Cordarone, Pacerone) —cont'd

may represent pulmonary toxicity and should be evaluated with a complete history, physical examination, chest radiograph, and pulmonary function tests with diffusion capacity. Preexisting pulmonary disease does not seem to increase the risk of developing pulmonary toxicity, but such patients have a poorer prognosis if pulmonary toxicity occurs.

PHARMACOKINETICS. See Table 21-4 for a comparison of the pharmacokinetics of major antiarrhythmic medications.

ADVERSE EFFECTS. See Table 21-5.

Liver injury is common but is usually mild and manifests only through abnormal liver enzymes. If the increase is greater than two times baseline, consider discontinuing or decreasing the dose. Consult the cardiologist for specific direction. Overt liver disease has occurred and has been fatal in a few cases.

Ocular changes are common and consist of corneal microdeposits and optic neuropathy. Corneal microdeposits are generally benign and occur with long-term therapy. These are visualized as a brownish whorl on the cornea similar to a cat's whiskers, and they are often reversible within 7 months after discontinuation. The patient may report seeing halos around lights at night, blurry vision, and photophobia. Optic neuropathy or optic neuritis resulting in visual impairment has occurred. Some cases have progressed to permanent blindness. Optic neuropathy or neuritis has a prevalence of 1% to 2% after 10 years of therapy. Amiodarone inhibits peripheral conversion of thyroxine (T_4) to triiodothyronine (T_3). It is also a potential source of large amounts of inorganic iodine; therefore, amiodarone can cause hypothyroidism or hyperthyroidism. Altered thyroid function and abnormal thyroid function tests may persist for several weeks or months following discontinuation of amiodarone. Hypothyroidism is managed with dose reduction or a thyroid hormone supplement. Hyperthyroidism may be a greater threat to the patient because of the possibility of aggravation of the arrhythmia. Aggressive medical treatment is needed, including dose reduction or discontinuation of amiodarone treatment. Antithyroid drugs, β-adrenergic blockers, or temporary corticosteroid therapy may be necessary. The action of antithyroid drugs may be delayed in amiodarone-induced thyrotoxicosis because of substantial quantities of pre-formed thyroid hormones that are stored in the gland. Skin reactions that occur as photophobia and a bluish-gray discoloration of the skin are seen with amiodarone therapy. A bluish-gray or slate-gray discoloration of the skin, particularly the face, is seen in approximately 1% to 2% of patients who are on long-term therapy. This has responded to a dose reduction in patients given more than 400 mg per day. Cessation of therapy will reverse this skin discoloration, but results may take up to 1 year.

DRUG INTERACTIONS. Numerous interactions may occur: substrate of 2C8 (major at low concentrations), 3A4 (major); inhibits 2A6 (moderate), 2C9 (moderate), 2D6 (moderate), and 3A4 (moderate). Interactions may occur with drugs administered after amiodarone is discontinued, as a result of the long and variable half-life of 3 to 107 days. Consult a detailed reference for information on specific drug–drug interactions.

- *Anticoagulants:* Potentiation of the anticoagulation response can occur and can result in serious or fatal bleeding. A 30% to 50% reduction in anticoagulant dose is usually required. Onset is 3 to 4 days, and the condition may persist for months after amiodarone has been discontinued.
- *Antiarrhythmics:* Effects of β-blockers, calcium channel blockers, digoxin, flecainide, lidocaine, procainamide, and quinidine are increased in the presence of amiodarone. Concomitant use of antiarrhythmics can increase the risk of hypotension, bradycardia, and potentially fatal arrhythmias.

DOSAGE AND ADMINISTRATION. See Table 21-6 for loading and maintenance dosages.

evolve A continually updated list of useful WebLinks may be found in the Evolve Resources at http://evolve.elsevier.com/Edmunds/NP/

Antihyperlipidemic Agents

JAMES D. HOEHNS and JESSICA L. PURCELL

DRUG OVERVIEW

vastatin (handwritten)

Class	Generic Name	Trade Name
HMG-CoA reductase inhibitors	atorvastatin 🔑	Lipitor ✹
	fluvastatin	Lescol, Lescol XL ✹
	lovastatin ✹	Mevacor, Altocor (extended release), generic
	pravastatin ✹	Pravachol ✹, generic
	rosuvastatin	Crestor ✹
	simvastatin ✹	Zocor ✹, generic
Fibric acid derivatives	gemfibrozil 🔑 ✹	Lopid, generic
	fenofibrate	TriCor ✹
Bile acid sequestrants	cholestyramine	Questran, Questran Light
	colesevelam	WelChol
Other agents	nicotinic acid (niacin)	Niaspan ✹, generic
Combination products	lovastatin/niacin	Advicor
	ezetimibe/simvastatin	Vytorin ✹
Selective cholesterol absorption inhibitors	ezetimibe	Zetia ✹
Fish oil supplements	Omega-3 polyunsaturated fatty acids	Omacor, others

✹ Top 200 drug; 🔑 key drug. Atorvastatin (Lipitor) is the most commonly prescribed antihyperlipidemic drug. Atorvastatin confers robust LDL lowering (30%-50%), has a relatively favorable drug–drug interaction profile, and is well tolerated. It is most important to note that atorvastatin (similar to most other statins) has consistent clinical outcomes data to demonstrate that its use can significantly decrease cardiovascular morbidity and mortality.

INDICATIONS

Hyperlipidemia

Currently, six classes of antihyperlipidemic drugs are available, and each class has its own mechanism for lowering lipid levels and somewhat unique indications. The 3-hydroxy-3-methylglutaryl coenzyme A (HMG-CoA) reductase inhibitors (statins) are indicated for patients with primary hypercholesterolemia, that is, LDL is the primary lipid elevation with minor elevations in triglycerides. Fibric acid derivatives are indicated for reducing the risk that CHD may develop in patients without a history of CHD who have low HDL cholesterol levels and elevated triglyceride levels. They are also indicated for adults with marked hypertriglyceridemia who are at risk of pancreatitis and who have not responded adequately to dietary therapy. Bile acid sequestrants are indicated as adjunctive therapy to diet for reducing LDL cholesterol in patients with primary hypercholesterolemia. Niacin is indicated for patients with hyperlipidemia (all forms of elevated total cholesterol or triglycerides) who respond inadequately to dietary therapy. Selective cholesterol absorption inhibitors are used as monotherapy or in combination with statins for the reduction in elevated total cholesterol, LDL cholesterol, and apolipoprotein B in patients with primary hypercholesterolemia. Omega-3 polyunsaturated fatty acids are indicated as an adjunct to diet to reduce very high (≥500 mg/dl) triglyceride levels in adult patients.

Coronary heart disease is the single largest cause of mortality and cause of disability in both men and women in the United States. Hyperlipidemia is a primary, major risk factor for CHD. The use of statins to treat hyperlipidemia and to lessen the burden of heart disease is one of the greatest advances in therapeutics in recent history. This chapter describes appropriate patient selection, drug selection, and necessary monitoring when one is caring for patients with hyperlipidemia. The National Cholesterol Education Program (NCEP) guidelines are the most widely recognized clinical guidelines for hyperlipidemia, and their application is discussed. Students are encouraged to familiarize themselves with the NCEP guidelines to enhance their ability to provide evidence-based medicine to their patients.

THERAPEUTIC OVERVIEW

Anatomy and Physiology

Cholesterol and triglycerides are classified as lipids, and both are normal and vital constituents of plasma. Because they are hydrophobic and insoluble, they are transported in the plasma via lipoproteins. Five major classes of lipoproteins have been identified: chylomicrons, VLDLs, IDLs, LDLs, and HDLs. Chylomicrons and VLDLs are considered triglyceride-rich lipoproteins, whereas IDLs, LDLs, and HDLs are considered cholesterol-rich lipoproteins. Of the lipoproteins, evaluation of LDLs, which includes IDL and HDL levels, is of primary importance. These two lipoproteins differ in several respects, including their cholesterol transport activities. Simply stated, LDL transports cholesterol from the liver to peripheral tissues; conversely, HDL removes cholesterol from the periphery and transports it to the liver. Chylomicrons are the largest and least dense of the lipoproteins, followed in order of increasing density and decreasing size by VLDLs (or pre-β), intermediate low-density lipoproteins (ILDLs, or broad β), LDLs (or β), and HDLs (or α).

Pathophysiology

A variety of lipid disorders can occur as a primary event or an event that is related to some underlying disease. Dyslipidemia can result from genetic disorders, concomitant disease states, or environmental factors. Alterations in lipoprotein metabolism are complex and often multifactorial. The primary dyslipidemias are associated with overproduction or impaired removal of lipoproteins. Primary dyslipidemias and their associated abnormalities are listed in Table 22-1. Often, the cause of primary dyslipidemia is not identified and plays little or no role in the diagnosis and treatment of most patients.

Table 22-2 provides a list of causes that contribute to secondary hyperlipidemia. If the clinician determines that a patient's hyperlipidemia may be related to another process, correction or modification of this process should be sought before pharmacologic treatment is provided for the hyperlipidemia. Not mentioned in Table 22-2 is obesity, which may also produce lipoprotein alterations. In diabetes, triglyceride levels are related to the degree of glycemic control. In hypothyroidism, lipid abnormalities are corrected with thyroxine replacement. In uremia, an elevated triglyceride and low HDL level is observed. Elevated total cholesterol and triglycerides are seen in patients with nephrotic syndrome. In drug-induced hyperlipidemia, estrogens may increase HDL, whereas β-blockers, progestins, and anabolic steroids may decrease HDL.

evolve For additional information on the classification of hyperlipidemias, see the supplemental tables on the Evolve Resources website.

Disease Process

Overwhelming scientific evidence supports a causal relationship between hyperlipidemia and CHD. Premature coronary atherosclerosis, leading to manifestations of CHD, is the most common and important consequence of hyperlipidemia. Elevated LDL cholesterol is a significant and positive predictor of CHD. Although cholesterol likely contributes to CHD in multiple ways, a major mechanism is LDL oxidation. Oxidation causes the lipoproteins to become "sticky" and facilitates their adhesion to the endothelium of blood vessels, thus causing atherosclerosis. An inverse correlation has been noted between HDL and CHD risk, so that elevated HDL cholesterol is considered protective against the development of CHD. Roughly 50% of Americans have cholesterol levels that place them at increased risk of CHD.

Most data point to an association between elevated triglycerides as an independent risk factor for CHD, although data are conflicting. Obesity, inactivity, cigarette smoking, excess alcohol, high carbohydrate intake, diseases (type 2 diabetes, renal failure, nephrotic syndrome), and drugs (corticosteroids, estrogens, retinoids) are known to be risk factors for elevated triglycerides.

Assessment

As a screening measure, a fasting lipoprotein profile should be obtained every 5 years in adults, beginning at the age of 20 years. Serum cholesterol should be assessed more frequently in patients who have risk factors for CHD. Lipid profiles should be obtained in the fasting state (>12 hours

TABLE 22-1 Primary Dyslipidemia and Associated Abnormalities

Dyslipidemia	Primary Abnormality	Frequency*
Familial hypercholesterolemias	Defective or absent LDL receptors (increased LDL)	0.2%
Familial defective apo-B	LDL receptor binding decreased because of abnormal apo-B (increased LDL)	0.2%
Familial combined hyperlipidemia	Apo-B and VLDL overproduction	0.5%
Familial hypertriglyceridemia	Decreased lipoprotein lipase activity, high VLDL production	1%
Familial hypoalphalipoproteinemia	Decreased apo-A-1 production, increased HDL catabolism	1%

*Percent of general population.

TABLE 22-2   Disorders Associated With Secondary Hyperlipoproteinemia

Underlying Disorder	LDL/Cholesterol	VLDL/Triglycerides
ENDOCRINE/METABOLIC		
Diabetes mellitus		↑↑↑
Cushing's syndrome	↑↑	↑
Hypothyroidism	↑↑↑	
Anorexia nervosa	↑↑	
RENAL		
Uremia		↑↑↑
Nephrotic syndrome	↑↑↑	↑↑
HEPATIC		
Primary biliary cirrhosis	↑	
Acute hepatitis		↑↑↑
IMMUNOLOGIC		
Systemic lupus erythematosus		↑↑
Monoclonal gammopathies		↑↑
STRESS INDUCED		
Acute myocardial infarction		↑↑
Sepsis, excessive burns		↑↑
DRUG INDUCED		
Alcohol		↑↑
Thiazide diuretics	↑	↑↑
β-Blockers		↑↑
Glucocorticoids		↑
Estrogens	↓	↑↑↑
Progestins	↑↑	
Anabolic steroids	↑↑	
Retinoids	↑	↑↑↑

since last meal) for an accurate measurement of triglycerides and LDL. Patients should be evaluated for common secondary causes of hyperlipidemia (diseases and drugs). Assessment of the patient's lifestyle, including diet and exercise, is crucial.

MECHANISM OF ACTION

HMG-CoA Reductase Inhibitors

These drugs (commonly called "statins") are reversible, competitive inhibitors of HMG-CoA reductase, which is the rate-limiting enzyme in cholesterol biosynthesis. HMG-CoA reductase catalyzes the conversion of HMG-CoA to mevalonate, a cholesterol precursor, in the liver. Inhibition of this enzyme decreases cholesterol synthesis, particularly causing a decrease in the serum LDL level. Although the mechanism of action appears straightforward, most LDL lowering observed with these drugs results from secondary, compensatory changes produced by enzyme inhibition. Inhibition of HMG-CoA reductase reduces intracellular cholesterol concentrations, leading to increased synthesis and expression of LDL receptors in the liver. This upregulation of LDL receptors is a compensatory response intended to restore intracellular cholesterol homeostasis. As the concentration of LDL receptors increases, a rise in the catabolic clearance of LDL from the plasma is observed.

In addition to their impressive LDL-lowering effects, HMG-CoA reductase inhibitors increase HDL and decrease triglycerides modestly. New research suggests that these drugs may also decrease levels of C-reactive protein, decreasing inflammatory processes that may be associated with atherosclerosis.

Fibric Acid Derivatives

Despite our lengthy experience with gemfibrozil, several uncertainties surround its precise mechanism of action. Its primary lipoprotein effect is to decrease triglyceride and raise HDL concentrations. The ability of gemfibrozil to lower triglycerides is attributed to an increase in lipoprotein lipase activity, which results in increased catabolism of VLDL. Gemfibrozil also may suppress lipolysis in adipose tissue, decrease free fatty acid flux, and lower the rate of triglyceride synthesis. The increase in HDL observed with gemfibrozil may result from increased synthesis of apolipoprotein A-1, or it may be indirectly related to the drug's ability to lower VLDL. Gemfibrozil exerts a variable and minor effect on LDL levels.

Fenofibrate is a prodrug that is converted to its active metabolite, fenofibric acid. Fenofibric acid inhibits triglyceride synthesis and accelerates the removal of lipoproteins.

Bile Acid Sequestrants

Bile acid sequestrants are unique among the antihyperlipidemics because they are not absorbed systemically, and they are the safest drugs available for the treatment of hypercholesterolemia. Although they differ in their chemical structure, all are large copolymers that function as anion-exchange resins in the intestinal lumen. Here they bind to bile acids, forming an insoluble complex and producing a large increase in the fecal excretion of bile acids. The pathways involved in cholesterol and bile acid metabolism are intertwined and closely related. Although the resin agents are sequestering bile acids and are interrupting their enterohepatic recirculation, a 3- to 10-fold increase has been noted in the diversion of cholesterol into bile acid synthesis. This resultant decline in intracellular cholesterol concentrations leads to two compensatory changes: acceleration of HMG-CoA reductase activity, and upregulation of LDL cell surface receptors. The two homeostatic changes increase intracellular cholesterol concentrations for conversion to bile acids, either by increased cholesterol synthesis or by increased uptake and removal of LDL from plasma. Therefore, bile acid sequestrants increase the diversion of cholesterol to bile acid synthesis, lower intracellular stores of cholesterol, and result in increased catabolism of LDL by the liver.

nicotinic acid (niacin) (Niaspan)

Niacin is believed to act on a hormone-sensitive lipase; this leads to inhibition of release of free fatty acids from adipose tissue (lipolysis). The inhibition of lipolysis leads to reduced free fatty acid transport to the liver and therefore decreased synthesis of VLDL. This decrease in VLDL in turn causes a reduction in LDL. An increase in lipoprotein lipase activity produced by nicotinic acid is believed to increase the rate of chylomicron triglyceride removal from the plasma. The mechanism underlying the increase in HDL is thought to result from reduced lipid transfer of cholesterol from HDL to VLDL and by delayed HDL clearance.

Selective Cholesterol Absorption Inhibitors

Ezetimibe is the first agent in a new class of drugs referred to as *selective cholesterol absorption inhibitors*. Ezetimibe is known to localize in the intestinal wall, where it is converted to its active glucuronide metabolite. It appears to act on the brush border of intestinal epithelial cells, where it selectively inhibits the absorption of cholesterol from dietary and biliary sources. Reduced cholesterol absorption results in a decrease in the delivery of cholesterol to the liver. Less cholesterol is thus available in hepatic stores, allowing more cholesterol to be cleared from the blood. Ezetimibe does not affect the absorption of fat-soluble vitamins or triglycerides—a benefit over bile acid sequestrants. Ezetimibe and/or its glucuronide conjugates circulate enterohepatically, repeatedly delivering the agent back to the intestine and reducing systemic exposure.

Fish Oil Supplements

Omega-3 polyunsaturated fatty acids (PUFAs), mainly eicosapentaenoic acid (EPA) and docosahexaenoic acid (DHA), are essential nutrients. Omacor is a highly concentrated combination of esters of EPA and DHA. The primary mechanism of action for PUFAs is a reduction (approximately 45%) in the hepatic production of triglycerides, which reduces production of VLDL. HDL is largely unaffected and LDL may increase. Adverse events are usually mild and include eructation, dyspepsia, and taste perversion.

TREATMENT PRINCIPLES

Standardized Guidelines

This chapter incorporates the updated Adult Treatment Panel (ATP) III guidelines for the treatment of hyperlipidemia from the National Cholesterol Education Program (NCEP, 2004). (See http://www.nhlbi.nih.gov/guidelines/cholesterol/index.htm.) Other useful hyperlipidemia guidelines from the American Association of Clinical Endocrinologists can be found at http://www.aace.com/pub/guidelines/

Evidence-Based Recommendations

Dyslipidemia is a major treatable risk factor for coronary artery disease. Lowering LDL results in significant decreases in coronary events, including transient ischemic attacks and stroke. As primary prevention, lipid-lowering therapies decrease risk of CHD events and mortality in patients without a history of CHD (1A). In persons with diabetes, LDL reduction produces a more substantial decrease in cardiovascular disease than does blood glucose control (1A). Patients without coronary artery disease should be evaluated with respect to their global cardiac risk to determine whether lipid-lowering therapy is indicated. Statin therapy should be considered as secondary prevention for all patients with coronary heart disease, peripheral vascular disease, or history of stroke. These medications have been shown to decrease coronary heart disease and mortality even if baseline LDL is <100 mg/dl (1A). Statins reduce 5-year overall mortality and cardiovascular morbidity and mortality; the greatest reductions occur in patients at greatest risk (1A).

Cardinal Points of Treatment

- Decreased LDL levels is the primary target of cholesterol-lowering therapy.
- Statins are the preferred initial treatment choice and should be used at a dosage sufficient to lower LDL by 30%-40% in most patients.
- Patients with diabetes (viewed as a CHD equivalent), coronary heart disease, or a 10-year risk of developing coronary heart disease >20% (calculated via Framingham risk scoring) have a goal LDL of <100 mg/dl (with an optional goal of <70 mg/dl if deemed "very high risk").
- If maximal dose statin is unable to achieve goal LDL, then statin+ezetimibe or statin+bile acid sequestrant are useful combinations.
- If triglycerides are 200 to 499 mg/dl after the LDL goal has been reached, consider adding a niacin or fibrate (gemfibrozil or fenofibrate). Of the fibrates, fenofibrate is safer to use concomitantly with a statin.
- If triglycerides are ≥500 mg/dl, the first goal is to lower triglycerides to prevent pancreatitis. Use a fibrate or niacin.
- If HDL is low (<40 mg/dl) after LDL goal is reached, consider adding niacin or a fibrate in patients with CHD or CHD equivalent.

The most widely recognized treatment guidelines for hyperlipidemia, those of the NCEP, were most recently updated in 2004. An important tenet of these guidelines is that the intensity of evaluation and treatment depends on the patient's overall risk status for CHD (Box 22-1), that is, those patients with preexisting CHD or with CHD risk equivalents or those who are at high risk (more than two risk factors) for CHD in the near future are treated more aggressively. Next, patients with two or more risk factors should be further classified into 10-year risk groups based on their Framingham point scores. (See Framingham tables at www.nhlbi.nih.gov/guidelines/cholesterol/risk.) Framingham scores are based on age, total cholesterol level, smoking status, HDL cholesterol, and systolic blood pressure. They are used to assess the individual's 10-year risk of developing CHD. Three levels of 10-year risk are identified: >20%, 10% to 20%, and <10%. Those found to have a risk >20% are categorized as if they had a CHD risk equivalent (for further information, see NCEP guidelines).

A second important feature of the NCEP guidelines is that dietary and drug treatment decisions are based on LDL cholesterol levels (Table 22-3). For example, an individual whose blood pressure is 150/95 mm Hg who currently smokes and has a 10-year risk of 8% would have lifestyle changes initiated at an LDL level 130 mg/dl. According to the recommendations, this individual would initiate drug therapy with an LDL level ≥160 mg/dl. In contrast, an individual with the risk factors listed earlier and a 10-year risk of 12% would initiate therapeutic lifestyle changes and drug therapy at an LDL ≥130 mg/dl. Alternatively, the current guidelines would consider

BOX 22-1   NCEP CHD Risk Equivalents

- Noncoronary vascular disease
- Type 2 diabetes
- 10-year CHD risk >20% (based on Framingham tables)

NCEP RISK FACTORS FOR CORONARY HEART DISEASE OTHER THAN LDL CHOLESTEROL

Positive Risk Factors

- Age
  - Male >45 years
  - Female >55 years
- Family history of premature CHD
  - CHD in male first-degree relative <55 years or female first-degree relative <65 years
- Current cigarette smoking
- Hypertension
- Blood pressure >140/90 mm Hg or presently taking antihypertensive medication
- Low HDL cholesterol (<40 mg/dl)

Negative Risk Factor

- High HDL cholesterol (>60 mg/dl)

drug therapy "optional" for LDL values between 100 and 129 mg/dl in such an individual.

Nonpharmacologic Treatment

The importance of dietary therapy and exercise should not be overlooked. Readers are advised to review the NCEP guidelines for further discussion of dietary strategies. Consider referring the patient to a dietitian for further instruction on low saturated fat and low-cholesterol diets. Try to improve CHD risk factors that can be modified: smoking, hypertension, diabetes, inactivity, and obesity.

Pharmacologic Treatment

Treatment of patients with elevated LDL cholesterol and no prior history of CHD is considered *primary prevention*. Treatment of patients with CHD is called *secondary prevention*. Although therapeutic lifestyle changes are a mainstay of primary prevention, recent evidence shows that lipid-lowering drugs reduce the risk for *developing* CHD. In the case of secondary prevention, it is clear that antihyperlipidemic drugs reduce major coronary artery events, coronary artery procedures, stroke, and coronary and total mortality.

Although achieving the goal LDL value is the first and primary goal, triglycerides and HDL should be considered in drug selection (Table 22-4). If triglycerides are >200 mg/dl after the LDL goal is reached, NCEP recommends setting a goal for non-HDL cholesterol (total cholesterol − HDL cholesterol) that is 30 mg/dl higher than the LDL goal. Once the LDL goal has been reached and triglycerides are <200 mg/dl, the focus should turn to the patient's HDL. The first step in treatment is to increase physical activity and lose weight if overweight. Drug therapy, nicotinic acid, or fibric acid derivatives may be used if the patient's HDL level remains below 40 mg/dl.

HMG-CoA REDUCTASE INHIBITORS. These are among the more expensive drugs used to treat patients with hyperlipidemia, but they are also the best tolerated by patients and are highly efficacious at lowering LDL. Adverse effects are similar for all six of these agents. However, a switch from one drug to another may be advisable if adverse reactions occur. Their onset of activity is evident within 2 weeks, with maximal lipoprotein changes occurring 4 to 6 weeks after initiation. Serum lipoprotein concentrations typically return to baseline values within a similar period after drug discontinuation. In most patients, it is suggested to use a dosage of statin sufficient to achieve at least a 30% to 40% reduction in LDL levels (e.g., atorvastatin 10 mg/day, simvastatin 40-60 mg/day). Hepatotoxicity and muscle toxicity are the two primary adverse effects of greatest concern with statin use. All patients who start statins should be instructed to report immediately episodes of muscle discomfort or weakness or brown urine. Laboratory measurement of AST/ALT and CK-MM levels then should be performed.

At clinically relevant dosages, the LDL-lowering potential of the six drugs in this class can be roughly ranked in the following order: rosuvastatin > atorvastatin > simvastatin = lovastatin > pravastatin > fluvastatin. The comparative potency and efficacy of the HMG-CoA reductase inhibitors are summarized in Table 22-5.

FIBRIC ACID DERIVATIVES. Both fenofibrate and gemfibrozil are highly effective in decreasing triglycerides and increasing HDL. They are not effective for lowering LDL levels, which

TABLE 22-3   Treatment Decisions Based on LDL Cholesterol Levels

Risk Category	LDL Goal, mg/dl	Non-HDL Goal, mg/dl*	Initiate Lifestyle Change, mg/dl	Consider Drug Therapy
High risk: CHD or CHD risk equivalents (10-year risk >20%)	<100 (optional goal, <70)	<130	≥100	≥100 (<100, consider drug options)
Moderately high risk: 2+ risk factors (10 year risk 10%-20%)	<130 (optional goal, <100)	<160	≥130	≥130 (100-129, consider drug options)
Moderate risk: 2+ risk factors (10-year risk <10%)	<130	<160	≥130	≥160
Lower risk: 0-1 risk factor	<160	<190	≥160	≥190 (160-189, LDL-lowering drug optional)

*Non-HDL cholesterol is equal to total cholesterol − HDL cholesterol.

TABLE 22-4   Comparative Percentage Changes in Lipoprotein Concentration Observed With the Antihyperlipidemic Medications

Drug	LDL, %	HDL, %	TG, %
Bile acid sequestrants	↓15-30	↑0-3	No change
niacin	↓10-25	↑15-35	↓25-30
HMG-CoA inhibitors	↓20-60	↑5-10	↓10-30
gemfibrozil	↓10-15	↑15-25	↓35-50
fenofibrate	↓6-20	↑18-33	↓40-50
ezetimibe	↓15-18	↑2-4	↓4-6
Fish oil supplements	↑17-30	↑6-13	↓40-50

may actually increase in some patients. They are generally well tolerated but can cause hepatotoxicity and cholelithiasis. The maximum effect of gemfibrozil is observed within 4 to 5 weeks. Generic gemfibrozil is available and costs less than the HMG-CoA reductase inhibitors.

Fenofibrate causes a decrease in cholesterol and triglyceride levels and elevation of HDL. Uric acid levels also may be decreased in some patients receiving fenofibrate because of uricosuric activity observed with the drug.

Therapy with either a statin or a fibrate protects against the development of nerve damage in patients with type 2 diabetes mellitus. Investigators showed that treatment with statins and fibrates reduced the risk of developing peripheral neuropathy by 35% and 48%, respectively, among diabetic patients during 5-year follow-up.

BILE ACID SEQUESTRANTS. The two bile acid sequestrants are equally efficacious. Patient acceptance is a matter of primary concern because of gastrointestinal adverse effects such as constipation, bloating, and nausea. Selection between agents should be based on cost and palatability. Questran Light (aspartame used for flavoring) should be used before Questran, which contains sucrose and provides unneeded calories for many patients (e.g., diabetic patients, those who are obese). Colesevelam is available in tablet form and may be preferred

by patients who dislike the inconvenience and taste associated with the powder resin.

LDL concentrations begin to decline within a few days with maximum effect observed within 1 month. Triglycerides and VLDL concentrations rise initially in treatment and tend to return to baseline levels after 1 month. Patients who have preexisting elevations in triglycerides may experience a greater and more sustained increase in triglyceride levels. HDL levels are not predictably altered with bile acid sequestrants.

NIACIN. Niacin is one of the most effective antihyperlipidemics in terms of lowering triglycerides and increasing HDL; it is similar to the bile acid sequestrants in lowering LDL. The main limitation of niacin use is the adverse effect of flushing, although tolerance to this phenomenon generally occurs with continued use. Flushing occurs shortly after ingestion and can be blunted with aspirin (30 min before); a slow escalation in niacin dosage over 3 to 4 weeks is encouraged. Extended-release niacin products (e.g., Niaspan) cause less flushing than immediate-release tablets and usually are preferred because of their better tolerability. Niacin impairs glucose tolerance and may cause hyperuricemia.

SELECTIVE CHOLESTEROL ABSORPTION INHIBITORS. Ezetimibe is the only available agent in this novel drug class. When compared with placebo, ezetimibe has been shown to decrease intestinal cholesterol absorption by 50%. As monotherapy, ezetimibe can decrease LDL, increase HDL, and decrease triglycerides. When used in combination with a low-dose statin, an additional 18% reduction in LDL cholesterol has been noted when compared with statin monotherapy. Reduction in LDL cholesterol may be seen as early as 2 weeks following initiation of ezetimibe.

FISH OIL SUPPLEMENTS. Omacor is the only fish oil supplement that has been approved by the FDA. Other brands of fish oil supplements are sold over-the-counter; however, their content or purity is not regulated by the FDA. In studies of patients with a *recent* MI, Omacor significantly reduced total mortality and sudden cardiac death. However, in studies involving patients with *chronic* CHD, the results of using fish oil supplements are equivocal, and some

TABLE 22-5   Comparative Efficacy of Currently Available Statins

HMG-CoA REDUCTASE INHIBITOR, mg						CHANGE IN LIPID AND LIPOPROTEIN LEVELS, %			
atorvastatin	lovastatin	fluvastatin	pravastatin	simvastatin	rosuvastatin	Total	LDL	HDL	Triglycerides
—	20	40	20	10	—	−22	−27	4-8	−10-15
10	40	80	40	20	—	−27	−34	4-8	−10-20
20	80	—	80	40	5 or 10	−32	−41	4-8	−15-25
40	—	—	—	80	—	−37	−48	4-8	−20-30
80	—	—	—	—	20	−42	−55	4-8	−25-35
					40	−47	−60	4-8	−30-35

Data from Maron DJ et al: Current perspectives on statins, *Circulation* 101:207-213, 2000; Oregon Health Resources Commission: *HMG-CoA reductase inhibitors (STATINS) report*—Update 4, October 2006.

concern has arisen about worsened cardiovascular outcomes. No evidence from high-quality trials suggests that fish oil supplements decrease cardiovascular disease in the general population.

COMBINATION THERAPY. Treatment with more than one drug may be required to keep lipoprotein levels within the appropriate range, but combination treatment also contributes to the increased risk of adverse effects. Combining statins with a fibric acid derivative increases the risk of rhabdomyolysis. Statins, fibric acid derivatives, and niacin are known to cause hepatotoxicity. Ezetimibe also may cause hepatotoxicity. The adverse effect risk is additive when these drugs are used together.

How to Monitor

ALL MEDICATIONS. Lipid profiles should be performed to obtain a baseline level and should be repeated at 4 to 6 weeks, and perhaps again at 3 months, to assess response after therapy has been initiated. For long-term monitoring, total cholesterol can be measured at follow-up visits, and a lipoprotein profile (and LDL estimation) can be performed annually.

Liver function tests (LFTs [AST/ALT]) should be performed at baseline, 12 weeks after initiation of therapy or dose escalation, and periodically thereafter (e.g., annually, semiannually). This applies to statins, fibrates, and niacin.

STATINS, FIBRIC ACID, AND NICOTINIC ACID

- Ask the patient about myalgias and check CPK if present. Otherwise, routine monitoring of CPK is probably not necessary.
- If statins, niacin, or fibric acid derivatives are used in any combination, monitor LFTs and CPK more frequently. This is necessary because of concerns about the additive risk of hepatotoxicity and myopathy.

HMG-CoA REDUCTASE INHIBITORS. Although controversy surrounds the necessity of doing so, most clinicians (and drug manufacturers) suggest that LFTs should be performed at baseline, 12 weeks after a statin is begun, and annually/semiannually thereafter. If AST or ALT is three times the upper limit of normal or greater, dosage reduction or discontinuation of therapy is recommended. Some clinicians advocate even less frequent monitoring of LFTs because of the low risk of toxicity of statins. An expert panel recently suggested that there is no need to monitor LFTs in patients receiving long-term statin therapy. The rationale of the experts was that irreversible liver damage is rare and likely idiosyncratic. Less than 1% of patients typically show LFT results greater than three times the upper limit of normal during therapy, although ALT/AST values greater than three times the upper limit of normal have occurred in 2% to 3% of patients on *high*-dose statin therapy (e.g., atorvastatin 80 mg/day). Isolated ALT/AST elevations in the absence of increased bilirubin levels have not been linked with liver injury.

BILE ACID SEQUESTRANTS

- Complete blood counts and liver function tests are recommended at least every 3 months during the first year and periodically thereafter.

- For patients receiving other drugs, monitor for a decreased pharmacologic response and/or drug level of these medications when bile acid resins are initiated. This is especially necessary for patients receiving digoxin, warfarin, levothyroxine, or thiazide diuretics.

nicotinic acid (niacin) (Niaspan)

Repeat the lipid profile 4 to 6 weeks after a dosage of 1500 to 2000 mg/day is reached and perhaps again at 3 months to assess response. For long-term monitoring, total cholesterol can be obtained at most follow-up visits, and a lipoprotein profile (and LDL estimation) can be performed annually.

ezetimibe

- When used in combination with a statin, LFTs (AST/ALT) should be performed at baseline and as indicated for the statin.
- When used as monotherapy, LFTs are not routinely necessary.

Patient Variables

GERIATRICS. In general, the antihyperlipidemics may achieve maximum cholesterol reductions in the elderly at somewhat smaller dosages than those required in younger patients. Significant pharmacokinetic alterations in the elderly do not appear to be a major concern with available antihyperlipidemics.

A common dilemma involves deciding how aggressively one should treat hyperlipidemia in the elderly. Statin therapy does not pose an increased safety risk for older patients with hypercholesterolemia or established cardiovascular disease. Drug therapy is warranted for patients 65 to 75 years of age because of the association between hypercholesterolemia and CHD. Those without CHD but with several risk factors and a markedly elevated LDL also should be strongly considered for drug therapy. No data are available on patients older than age 75, and lipid-lowering therapy is controversial. For patients who are currently on therapy, it should be continued. Before therapy is begun in individuals older than 75 years, a number of factors other than chronologic age must be considered, including quality of life, life span limitations, comorbid conditions, and physiologic age. Although benefits of lipid-lowering therapy in the middle aged are well accepted, the CHD risk reduction associated with treatment in the elderly (>70 years old) is somewhat less certain. When these factors are taken into consideration, elderly patients with established CHD and elevated LDL cholesterol ordinarily should be treated.

PEDIATRICS. Managing hypercholesterolemia in children (10-17 years old) primarily involves dietary and lifestyle changes. Cholestyramine and the statins (lovastatin, fluvastatin, pravastatin, and atorvastatin) are FDA approved for managing hypercholesterolemia in children, yet they are rarely used. If pharmacotherapy is recommended, cholestyramine generally is considered the drug of choice because it is not absorbed systemically and is believed to be safe. Scientific evidence shows a 15% to 20% LDL cholesterol reduction with bile acid sequestrants in pediatrics. It is advised that antihyperlipidemics should be prescribed to children only under the supervision of a lipid specialist.

TABLE 22-6 Pharmacokinetics of Antihyperlipidemic Agents

Drug	Absorption	Drug Availability (After First Pass)	Time to Peak Concentration	Half-life	Protein Bound	Metabolism	Excretion
atorvastatin	14%	14%	1-2 hr	14 hr	≥98%	Hepatic CYP 3A4	Feces, >90%; urine, <5%
lovastatin (prodrug)	—	30%	2 hr	3 hr	>95%	Hepatic CYP 3A4	Feces, 83%; urine, 10%
fluvastatin	—	24%	<1 hr	2.5 hr	98%	Hepatic CYP 2C9 (75%), 2C8 (5%) 3A4 (20%)	Feces, >90%; urine, <10% Urine, 70%;
pravastatin	34%	17%	1-1.5 hr	2 hr	50%	Hepatic	Feces, 60%; urine, 20%
simvastatin (prodrug)	—	5%	2-3 hr	2-3 hr	95%	Hepatic CYP 3A4, 3A5	Feces, 60%; urine, 16%
rosuvastatin	—	20%	3-5 hr	19 hr	90%	CYP 2C9 (10%)	Feces, 90%; urine (unchanged), 10%
gemfibrozil	—	—	1-2 hr	1.5 hr	98%	Hepatic	Feces, 6%
fenofibrate	—	—	6-8 hr	20 hr	99%	Plasma esterases; hepatic conjugation	Urine, 60%; feces, 25%
cholestyramine	—	—	—	—	—	—	Feces, 100%
colestipol	—	—	—	—	—	—	Feces, 100%
colesevelam	—	—	—	—	—	—	Feces, 100%
ezetimibe (prodrug)	—	—	4-12 hr	22 hr	>90	Glucuronidation (hepatic and small intestine)	Feces, 78%; urine, 11%
Niacin	—	—	—	0.75 hr	—	Hepatic	Urine, 88%
Fish oil supplements (Omacor)	—	—	—	—	—	—	—

PREGNANCY AND LACTATION. Triglyceride and cholesterol levels increase during pregnancy, but the increases usually are not considered clinically significant. Drug therapy for hyperlipidemia should be discontinued during pregnancy. The safety of lipid-lowering drugs in pregnant women has not been established. Therapy with HMG-CoA reductase inhibitors is contraindicated during pregnancy and lactation. For patients with severe forms of hyperlipidemia, consultation with a lipid specialist should be considered.

- *Category B:* colesevelam
- *Category C:* fenofibrate, clofibrate, gemfibrozil, niacin, cholestyramine, and ezetimibe
- *Category X:* all statins (atorvastatin, fluvastatin, lovastatin, pravastatin, simvastatin, and rosuvastatin)
- No fetal harm is expected when cholestyramine is given in recommended dosages, although treatment may interfere with absorption of fat-soluble vitamins.

Patient Education

ALL MEDICATIONS. Patients should report any signs and symptoms of liver dysfunction.

STATINS, FIBRIC ACID, AND NICOTINIC ACID. Promptly report any muscle pain, tenderness, or weakness that is unexplained, particularly if malaise or fever is also present.

HMG-CoA REDUCTASE INHIBITORS. May occasionally cause photosensitivity

BILE ACID SEQUESTRANTS. The powders can be blended and stored with any consumable liquid. A mixture of the powders with fruit juice tends to be more palatable than a mixture of them with water. The powders can be mixed with hot food but should not be cooked.

The resins often interfere with absorption of other drugs. Other medications should be taken 1 hour before or 3 to 4 hours after cholestyramine, colestipol, or colesevelam is taken.

nicotinic acid (niacin) (Niaspan)

Facial and upper extremity flushing commonly occurs with niacin use. Pruritus, warm sensations, and tingling also may occur. These adverse effects tend to diminish in severity with continued use. Avoid taking niacin with hot fluids because this may worsen flushing episodes. If episodes are very bothersome, aspirin (81-325 mg) may blunt the effect if given 30 minutes before niacin ingestion.

SPECIFIC DRUGS

HMG-CoA REDUCTASE INHIBITORS

atorvastatin (Lipitor) 🔑

CONTRAINDICATIONS
- Active liver disease or unexplained persistent elevation in transaminases
- Pregnancy and lactation

WARNINGS

💣 Liver dysfunction: HMG-CoA reductase inhibitors have been associated with biochemical abnormalities of liver function. Liver function tests should be monitored. With an increase in transaminase level of three times the upper limit of normal or greater, dose reduction or withdrawal from medication is recommended. Patients who report myalgias should undergo prompt evaluation. With dose reduction, interruption, or discontinuation, transaminase levels usually return to baseline without sequelae.

💣 Skeletal muscle: Rare cases of rhabdomyolysis with acute renal failure related to myoglobinuria have been reported. Patients should be instructed to report immediately unexplained muscle pain, tenderness, or weakness. Therapy should be discontinued if markedly elevated CPK levels occur.

PHARMACOKINETICS. See Table 22-6.

ADVERSE EFFECTS. Statins generally are well tolerated (Table 22-7).

DRUG INTERACTIONS. Administration of atorvastatin with cholestyramine or colestipol decreases atorvastatin area under the curve (AUC) by 25%. However, LDL reduction was greater with the combination than with either drug alone (Table 22-8).

DOSAGE AND ADMINISTRATION. In general, most statins, and particularly atorvastatin, should be taken in the evening (Table 22-9).

OTHER DRUGS IN CLASS

Other drugs in this class are similar to the prototype, except as follows:
- *Lovastatin* should be taken with the evening meal to increase absorption.
- *Altocor*, extended-release lovastatin, provides a slower, prolonged exposure to lovastatin compared with immediate release.
- *Lovastatin*, *pravastatin*, and *simvastatin* are the only HMG-CoA reductase inhibitors available in generic form at this time.
- A combination product, *Advicor*, combines extended-release niacin and lovastatin. The rationale for this combi-

nation involves the potent LDL-lowering effects of lovastatin and the effects of niacin on HDL and triglycerides.
- If the patient requires an 80-mg total daily dose of *fluvastatin (Lescol)*, it should be divided into doses of 40 mg twice daily. Fluvastatin 80 mg is available in an extended-release form, so it may be administered once daily.
- *Pravastatin (Pravachol)* is the most hydrophilic statin on the market; it has yielded favorable efficacy and safety data reported by many large, outcome-based clinical trials.
- After 1 year of therapy with *simvastatin*, LFTs are not required. However, LFTs should be monitored at baseline and every 6 months for the first year.
- Elevated levels of *rosuvastatin* have been found in Asian populations; use lower dosage with caution.

FIBRIC ACID DERIVATIVES

gemfibrozil (Lopid, various generics) 🔑

CONTRAINDICATIONS. Hepatic dysfunction, primary biliary cirrhosis, severe renal dysfunction, preexisting gallbladder disease, hypersensitivity to gemfibrozil

WARNINGS. In some earlier clinical trials, patients who received gemfibrozil (or chemically similar clofibrate) demonstrated increases (or no change) in all-cause mortality compared with groups that were given placebo. This increase in noncardiovascular mortality has been related to increases in cancer and other unknown associations (e.g., accidental and violent deaths). More recent large-scale clinical trials have shown significant decreases in CHD events with gemfibrozil use.

When gemfibrozil is administered concomitantly with HMG-CoA reductase inhibitors, patients may be at increased risk of myositis or rhabdomyolysis. Gemfibrozil monotherapy also may be associated with the development of these conditions. Persistent increases in serum transaminases (e.g., AST, ALT) may be observed; thus, LFTs should be monitored periodically (e.g., at baseline, after 12 weeks, yearly thereafter). Any elevations in serum transaminases are usually reversible with drug discontinuation. Gemfibrozil may increase cholesterol excretion into bile, leading to an increased risk of cholelithiasis. If a patient develops cholelithiasis while receiving gemfibrozil, the drug should be discontinued.

DOSAGE AND ADMINISTvRATION. Gemfibrozil should be taken twice daily 30 minutes before meals. Fenofibrate can be taken once daily (see Table 22-9).

BILE ACID SEQUESTRANTS

cholestyramine (Questran, Questran Light, generic)

CONTRAINDICATIONS
- Complete biliary or bowel obstruction
- Hypersensitivity to cholestyramine or colestipol

WARNINGS. Patients with phenylketonuria (an inborn error of phenylalanine metabolism) should avoid Questran Light

TABLE 22-7   Adverse Effects of Antihyperlipidemic Agents

Body System	Statins	Fibric Acid Derivatives—gemfibrozil	fenofibrate	Bile Acid Sequestrants	Selective Cholesterol Absorption Inhibitor	niacin
Body, general	Fatigue	Fatigue		Fatigue, weight loss/gain, swollen glands, edema, weakness	Fatigue	Flushing
Skin, appendages	Rash, pruritus	Eczema, rash	Rash, pruritus, eczema			Rash, pruritus
Hypersensitivity			Skin rash, Stevens-Johnson syndrome, urticaria, rash	Urticaria, dermatitis, asthma, wheezing, rash		
Respiratory	Cough		Cough, asthma	Shortness of breath	Cough	
Cardiovascular	Chest pain, syncope	Atrial fibrillation	Angina, hypertension, abnormal ECG, peripheral vascular disorder, hypotension, tachycardia, atrial fibrillation	Chest pain, angina, tachycardia (infrequent)		Atrial fibrillation and other cardiac arrhythmias, orthostasis GI
GI	Nausea, vomiting, diarrhea, abdominal pain, constipation, flatulence, dyspepsia, dysgeusia, cholestasis	Dyspepsia, abdominal pain, diarrhea, nausea, vomiting, constipation, acute appendicitis, cholelithiasis	Pancreatitis, cholelithiasis, dyspepsia, flatulence, constipation, diarrhea, nausea, vomiting, increased appetite, rectal disorder, esophagitis, gastritis, colitis, vomiting, anorexia	Common: constipation Less frequent: abdominal pain, distention, cramping, GI bleed, nausea, vomiting, diarrhea, indigestion, flatulence, perianal irritation anorexia, steatorrhea, dental bleeding, sour taste Less common: pancreatitis, diverticulitis, cholecystitis, cholelithiasis, impaction	Diarrhea, abdominal pain	GI upset, activation of peptic ulcer, nausea, vomiting, abdominal pain, diarrhea, dyspepsia, cholestasis
Hemic and lymphatic	Ecchymosis, anemia, lymphadenopathy, thrombocytopenia, petechiae	Anemia, leukopenia, bone marrow hypoplasia, eosinophilia, thrombocytopenia	Anemia, leukopenia, thrombocytopenia, bone marrow hypoplasia	Increased prothrombin time, ecchymosis, anemia		
Metabolic and nutritional		Increased glucose		Malabsorption		Decreased glucose tolerance, hyperglycemia
Musculoskeletal	Rhabdomyolysis, arthralgia, myalgia	Rhabdomyolysis, myopathy, myositis	Rhabdomyolysis, myositis, myalgia, arthritis	Backache, muscle/joint pains, arthritis	Back pain, arthralgia, no rhabdomyolysis seen	Rhabdomyolysis
Nervous system	Headache, dizziness, asthenia, insomnia, paresthesia	Vertigo, headache, paresthesia	Headache, dizziness, insomnia, depression, vertigo, anxiety	Headache, anxiety, vertigo, dizziness, insomnia, fatigue, tinnitus, syncope, drowsiness, femoral nerve pain, paresthesia	Dizziness	Headache
Special senses	Ophthalmoplegia, progression of cataracts	Taste perversion	Conjunctivitis	Uveitis		Toxic amblyopia, vision disturbances
Hepatic	Increased LFTs, hepatitis, jaundice	Hepatotoxicity, increased LFTs	Increased LFTs, hepatitis		Unknown	Increased LFTs, severe hepatic toxicity
Genitourinary	Gynecomastia, loss of libido, erectile dysfunction	Decreased renal function	Decreased renal function	Hematuria, dysuria, burnt odor to urine, diuresis, increased libido		Hyperuricemia

TABLE 22-8 Common Drug Interactions With Antihyperlipidemic Agents

Other Drug	Action on Antihyperlipidemic Agent	Other Drug	Action on Antihyperlipidemic Agent
INTERACTIONS WITH ATORVASTATIN AND:		**INTERACTIONS WITH SIMVASTATIN AND:**	
digoxin	Increased digoxin concentrations 20%	HIV protease inhibitors	
cyclosporine	Increased risk of rhabdomyolysis	erythromycin, clarithromycin, telithromycin	
gemfibrozil/fenofibrate		amiodarone	
niacin		verapamil	
erythromycin		nefazodone	
itraconazole/ketoconazole		Grapefruit juice (avoid >1 quart per day)	
Bile acid sequestrants	Decreased atorvastatin AUC 25%	digoxin	Increased digoxin level (minor)
		warfarin	Increased anticoagulation response
INTERACTIONS WITH LOVASTATIN AND:		**INTERACTIONS WITH ROSUVASTATIN AND:**	
warfarin	Increased anticoagulation response	cyclosporine	Increased risk of rhabdomyolysis
ketoconazole/itraconazole/fluconazole	Increased risk of rhabdomyolysis	warfarin	Increased INR
cyclosporine		gemfibrozil, fenofibrate	Increased risk of rhabdomyolysis
gemfibrozil		Antacids	Decreased rosuvastatin levels
HIV protease inhibitors		Oral contraceptives	Increased hormone levels
nefazodone		**INTERACTIONS WITH FIBRIC ACID DERIVATIVES AND:**	
Grapefruit juice (avoid >1 quart per day)		HMG-CoA reductase inhibitors	Increased risk of rhabdomyolysis
niacin		warfarin	Increased hepatotoxicity
erythromycin		Bile acid sequestrants	Increased anticoagulation response
danazol			Decreased gemfibrozil absorption
INTERACTIONS WITH FLUVASTATIN AND:		**INTERACTIONS WITH BILE ACID SEQUESTRANTS AND:**	
cyclosporine	Increased risk of rhabdomyolysis	warfarin	Decreased absorption; take all medications 1 hr before or 4 hr after ingesting the resin agent
gemfibrozil		levothyroxine	
niacin		digoxin	
erythromycin		thiazides	
Bile acid sequestrants	Decreased fluvastatin AUC 50%	phenobarbital	
ranitidine/cimetidine/omeprazole	Increased fluvastatin AUC	Tricyclic antidepressants	
rifampin	Decreased fluvastatin AUC	**INTERACTIONS WITH NIACIN AND:**	
INTERACTIONS WITH PRAVASTATIN AND:		HMG-CoA reductase inhibitors	Increased risk of rhabdomyolysis
cyclosporine	Increased risk of rhabdomyolysis	gemfibrozil	
gemfibrozil		**INTERACTIONS WITH EZETIMIBE AND:**	
niacin		Fibric acid derivatives	Increased bioavailability of ezetimibe
erythromycin		Bile acid sequestrants	Decreased ezetimibe levels
warfarin	Increased anticoagulation response	cyclosporine	Increased ezetimibe levels
INTERACTIONS WITH SIMVASTATIN AND:			
ketoconazole/itraconazole/fluconazole	Increased risk of rhabdomyolysis		
cyclosporine			
gemfibrozil			
niacin			

(or its generic equivalent), which contains aspartame for flavoring as well as 16.8 mg phenylalanine per 5-g dose.

PRECAUTIONS. Both agents may interfere with normal fat and fat-soluble vitamin (vitamins A, D, E, and K) absorption; thus, long-term use may be associated with increased bleeding potential caused by hypoprothrombinemia associated with vitamin K deficiency. Worsening of constipation, fecal impaction, and aggravation of hemorrhoids have been associated with their use. Earlier animal studies suggested that cholestyramine may be associated with increased gastrointestinal cancers, although this has not been substantiated in humans.

PHARMACOKINETICS. Because these drugs are not absorbed systemically, they are not metabolized and are entirely eliminated by fecal excretion (see Table 22-6).

ADVERSE EFFECTS. Constipation; systemic adverse effects are uncommon with these drugs because they are not absorbed (see Table 22-7).

DRUG INTERACTIONS. Bile acid sequestrants are fraught with numerous drug interactions associated with binding in the gastrointestinal tract. This interaction substantially decreases drug absorption. If patients are taking any other medications, they should be advised to take them 1 hour before or 4 hours after ingesting the resin agent, to minimize this effect (see Table 22-8).

DOSAGE AND ADMINISTRATION. Bile acid sequestrants commonly are titrated upward slowly (over several weeks) to minimize gastrointestinal tract–related adverse effects. They are usually taken before meals. Cholestyramine administration

TABLE 22-9 Dosage and Administration Recommendations of Antihyperlipidemic Agents

Drug	Age Group	Initial Dose	Maintenance Dosage	Administration	Maximum Dosage
atorvastatin	Adults	10 mg	Increase every 4 wk 10-80 mg	daily	80 mg/day
lovastatin	Adults	20 mg	10-80 mg	once daily with evening meal	80 mg/day
fluvastatin	Adults	20-40 mg	20-80 mg	hour of sleep	80 mg/day
pravastatin	Adults	10-20 mg	10-40 mg	hour of sleep	40 mg/day
simvastatin	Adults	5-10 mg	5-40 mg	hour of sleep	40 mg/day
rosuvastatin	Adults	5-20 mg	10 mg	daily	40 mg/day
gemfibrozil	Adults	600 mg	600 mg	q12h	1200 mg/day
fenofibrate	Adults	67 mg	67-201 mg	daily	201 mg/day
cholestyramine	Children Adults	240 mg/kg/day 4 g/day	4-24 g/day	3 divided doses 1-6 divided doses	24 g/day
colestipol	Adults	Granules 5 g Tablets 2 g	5-30 g increase every 4 wk 2-16 g	daily or in divided doses	30 g 16 g
colesevelam	Adults	1.875 g	1.875 g	bid (or 3.75 g once daily)	4.375 g/day
ezetimibe	Adults	10 mg	10 mg	daily	10 mg/day
niacin	Adults	100 mg	500-1000 mg	tid	3-4 g/day
niacin (extended release)	Adults	250 mg	250 mg-2 g	daily	2 g/day
niacin/lovastatin	Adults	500 mg/20 mg	500/20-2000/40 mg	hour of sleep	2000 mg/40 mg
niacin/simvastatin	Adults	500 mg/20 mg	1000/20-2000/40 mg	hour of sleep	2000 mg/40 mg
ezetimibe/simvastatin	Adults	10/20 mg	10/40 mg	hour of sleep	10/80 mg

at mealtime is recommended to decrease gastrointestinal tract–related adverse effects (see Table 22-9).

It is important to explain to patients that they should not ingest the dry resin powders but must first mix each scoopful or packet with 2 to 6 oz of water or another beverage. Mixing the resins with fruit juice has shown improved palatability in comparison with water.

Colesevelam tablets should be swallowed whole. They should not be chewed, cut, or crushed.

OTHER AGENTS

nicotinic acid (Niaspan, various generics)

CONTRAINDICATIONS. Hypersensitivity to niacin, active liver disease, active peptic ulcer, pregnancy, lactation, or arterial hemorrhage

WARNINGS. Use of niacin may lead to persistent increases in serum transaminases, and its use has been associated with jaundice and chronic hepatic toxicity. LFTs should be assessed at baseline, at 6 and 12 weeks after initiation of therapy, and periodically thereafter (e.g., twice yearly). If used in conjunction vwith HMG-CoA reductase inhibitors or gemfibrozil, LFTs should be monitored more frequently (e.g., every 2 months), and measurement of creatine kinase levels should be considered periodically because of concern regarding an increased risk of hepatotoxicity or myopathy with these combinations.

Myopathy and elevations in creatine kinase have been observed in patients receiving niacin alone or with other antihyperlipidemics. Patients with a history of liver or gallbladder disease should use niacin with caution.

Niacin typically worsens glycemic control in diabetic patients and has been shown to increase plasma glucose concentrations by 16% (niacin dosage was 1.5 g three times daily). Close monitoring of blood glucose is recommended if niacin is used in patients with diabetes. Niacin also may worsen peptic ulcer disease and can cause hyperuricemia. Patients with a history of gout or peptic ulcer disease should use niacin with caution.

DOSAGE AND ADMINISTRATION
- Acute adverse effects (flushing, nausea) are lessened with the use of extended-release products, but they may cause somewhat increased hepatotoxicity compared with immediate-release formulations (see Table 22-9).
- Niacin should be taken with meals because it may cause nausea and dyspepsia.
- Patients should not be directly switched from immediate-release to sustained-release preparations at the same dosage per day. A lower dosage (approximately half of the previous immediate-release dosage) of the sustained-release product should be prescribed.
- Most adverse effects associated with niacin are dose related, and this is the rationale for titrating dosages slowly.

SELECTIVE CHOLESTEROL ABSORPTION INHIBITORS

ezetimibe (Zetia)

CONTRAINDICATIONS
- Hypersensitivity
- The combination of ezetimibe and HMG-CoA reductase inhibitors is contraindicated in patients with active liver disease or unexplained persistent elevations in serum transaminase.

PRECAUTIONS
- When administered with HMG-CoA reductase inhibitors, this should be done in accordance with product labeling for that HMG-CoA reductase inhibitor.
- Use is not recommended in hepatic insufficiency.

ADVERSE REACTIONS. Most adverse reactions appear with the same frequency with ezetimibe as with placebo. However, the drug is very new and rare adverse effects may not have been seen (see Table 22-7). No LFT elevation or rhabdomyolysis has been observed in monotherapy.

DRUG INTERACTIONS. The combination of gemfibrozil, fenofibrate, or cholestyramine with ezetimibe is not recommended at this time (see Table 22-8).

DOSAGE AND ADMINISTRATION
- Ezetimibe may be administered with HMG-CoA reductase inhibitors for incremental effect, and for convenience, the two drugs may be administered together (see Table 22-9).
- Ezetimibe may be taken once daily without regard for meals.

FISH OIL SUPPLEMENTS

omega-3-acid ethyl esters (Omacor)

Many of these products are available over-the-counter, and patients purchase them because they are less expensive than prescription products. Care must be taken to ensure that what patients are using consists of acceptable omega-3-acid ethyl esters.

CONTRAINDICATIONS. Hypersensitivity to omega-3-acid ethyl esters or any component of the formulation

PRECAUTIONS. Omacor should be used with caution in patients with known sensitivity or allergy to fish. In some patients, increases in ALT levels have been observed; accordingly, ALT should be monitored periodically during therapy.

DRUG INTERACTIONS. Some studies suggest that omega-3 acids prolong bleeding time. Patients receiving anticoagulants should be monitored.

ADVERSE REACTIONS. Dyspepsia, eructation, and taste perversion (all <5%) have been observed with therapy.

DOSAGE AND ADMINISTRATION. The daily dose of Omacor is 4 g/day. This may be taken as a single 4-g dose or as 2 g twice daily.

evolve A continually updated list of useful WebLinks may be found in the Evolve Resources at http://evolve.elsevier.com/Edmunds/NP/

Don't give 2 drugs from the same. Class at the ~~same time~~ same time

evolve http://evolve.elsevier.com/Edmunds/NP/

23

Agents That Act on Blood

THERESA PLUTH YEO

DRUG OVERVIEW

Class	Subclass	Generic Name	Trade Name
Heparin group *Anticoagulants*	Heparin	heparin sodium 🔑	generic
	Low molecular weight heparin (LMWH)	enoxaparin sodium	Lovenox
		dalteparin	Fragmin
		tinzaparin	Innohep
	Heparinoids	danaparoid	Orgaran
		fondaparinux	AriXtra
	Direct thrombin inhibitors (DTIs)	bivalirudin	Angiomax
		argatroban	Argatroban
		lepirudin	Refludan
Oral anticoagulants		warfarin 🔑 ✷	Coumadin ✷ and generics
		anisindione	Miradon
Platelet aggregation inhibitors *Antiplatelet*	Traditional	acetylsalicylic acid (ASA)	aspirin, generic
		dipyridamole	Persantine, generic
		Extended-release dipyridamole/ASA	Aggrenox ✷
	Adenosine diphosphate (ADP)-induced platelet-fibrinogen binding inhibitors	clopidogrel ✷	Plavix ✷
		ticlopidine	Ticlid, generic
	Platelet glycoprotein IIb/IIIa inhibitors (GPIIb/IIIa)	abciximab	ReoPro
		eptifibatide	Integrelin
		tirofiban	Aggrastat
Platelet-reducing agent	Phosphodiesterase III (PDEIII) inhibitors	anagrelide	Agrylin
		cilostazol ✷	Pletal
Thrombolytic agents		alteplase (tPA)	Activase
		reteplase	Retavase
		streptokinase	Streptase
		tenecteplase	TNKase
		urokinase	Abbokinase
Hemorheologic agent		pentoxifylline	Trental

✷ Top 200 drug; 🔑 key drug.

INDICATIONS

- Prevention or treatment of venous thromboembolism (VTE), which includes deep vein thrombosis (DVT) and pulmonary emboli (PE); arterial ischemic events such as ischemic stroke and TIAs, acute MI, and intermittent atrial fibrillation (AF); and prevention and treatment of peripheral arterial thrombosis. See Table 23-1 for indications for specific drugs.

Anticoagulant drugs prolong the body's ability to form a thrombus (clot) at various points in the coagulation cascade. The goal of therapy is to promote anticoagulation while minimizing hemorrhagic complications through careful monitoring. These medications must be used with great care, and often under the supervision of a specialist.

The list of drugs discussed in this chapter is detailed to give the names the provider may recognize. However, only those drugs used in primary care will be discussed in detail. Unfractionated heparin (UFH) and LMWH are commonly seen in the primary care setting. Warfarin is probably the most important drug in this chapter for the primary care provider. The provider must have a complete understanding of its mechanism of action, dosing, monitoring, and side effects if he is to appropriately prescribe it. The first two groups of platelet inhibitors are seen in primary care. The newer platelet inhibitors remain specialty medications. Thrombolytics and direct thrombin inhibitors (DTIs) are used only in the acute care setting and are included here for those times when the primary provider has contact with patients who are experiencing acute cardiovascular events. Providers need to be aware of the time constraints surrounding initiation of thrombolytic therapy if they are to make timely transfers and referrals to tertiary care centers. The hemorheologic agent is also discussed briefly here.

THERAPEUTIC OVERVIEW
Anatomy and Physiology

A delicate balance must be maintained between the fluidity of the bloodstream and the ability of blood to clot quickly to prevent hemorrhage. In the coagulation system, two pathways

TABLE 23-1 Indications/Uses for Drugs That Act on Blood

Category	Drug	Indications/Uses
Heparin group	Heparin	Prevention of VTE in patients undergoing major abdominothoracic surgery or who for other reasons are at risk of developing thromboembolic disease; prophylaxis and treatment of pulmonary embolism and atrial fibrillation with embolization, for diagnosis and treatment of acute and chronic DIC, for prevention of clotting in arterial and heart surgery, for prophylaxis and treatment of peripheral arterial embolism, and as an anticoagulant in blood transfusions, extracorporeal circulation, and dialysis procedures. Not recommended for treatment of acute ischemic stroke
	LMWH, fondaparinux	Prevention of VTE in patients undergoing major abdominothoracic and orthopedic surgery and in medically ill patients; treatment of pulmonary embolism and acute coronary syndrome; bridge therapy for anticoagulated patients preoperatively and in postpercutaneous intervention; for revascularization therapy; and in patients discharged on recently initiated warfarin with a subtherapeutic INR
Oral anticoagulants	warfarin	Venous thromboembolism, high-risk surgery, prophylaxis (abdominal and orthopedic surgery); short-term treatment of single episode of DVT or PE (3-6 mo); prevention of VTE; indefinite treatment for recurrent DVT or PE; prevention of systemic embolism; post–mechanical prosthetic heart valve replacement, cardiomyopathy, or acute MI (3 mo); and AC cardioversion in atrial fibrillation, tissue cardiac valve replacement (3 mo), atrial fibrillation, valvular heart disease, mechanical prosthetic heart valves
PLATELET INHIBITORS		
Traditional	aspirin	MI (treatment and prophylaxis); stroke, acute ischemic; thromboembolism (prophylaxis in select cases)
	dipyridamole	Adjunctive therapy with warfarin in prevention of postoperative thromboembolic complications in cardiac valve replacement; plays no helpful role when used alone for ischemic stroke or TIA
ADP-induced inhibitors	clopidogrel	Recent MI or stroke; established peripheral arterial disease; to reduce risk of new stroke, acute coronary syndrome, MI
	ticlopidine	Prevention of thrombotic stroke, coronary stenting
GPIIb/IIIa inhibitors	abciximab eptifibatide tirofiban	Angioplasty; patients with unstable angina not responding to conventional medical therapy and for whom percutaneous coronary intervention is planned within 24 hours Angioplasty, adjunct; acute coronary syndrome Acute coronary syndrome
PDEIII inhibitors	anagrelide	Thrombocythemia, thrombocythemia secondary to myeloproliferation
	cilostazol	Intermittent claudication
Thrombolytic agents	Varies with specific drug	MI, acute ischemic stroke, PE, DVT, peripheral arterial occlusion
Hemorheologic agents	pentoxifylline	Intermittent claudication (rarely used)

are necessary for clotting. The *intrinsic clotting pathway* is initiated when the blood is exposed to a negatively charged surface such as the in vitro coagulation activators celite, kaolin, or silica. The intrinsic pathway is triggered when blood comes into contact with damaged endothelium or collagen. The *extrinsic clotting pathway* is triggered by exposure of tissue factor at the site of tissue injury or the addition of thromboplastin to blood. The intrinsic and extrinsic pathways merge on the activation of factor X in what is referred to as the *final common pathway* (Figure 23-1). Factor X then converts factor II (prothrombin) to IIa (thrombin), and factor IIa converts fibrinogen to a fibrin clot (thrombus).

Platelets provide the initial response to tissue injury (bleeding) and are activated by thrombin, ADP, serotonin, and epinephrine. They next adhere to collagen or to the damaged endothelium and then aggregate to form a platelet plug on the damaged cell wall. During this time, platelets also trigger formation of the active clotting factors VII and X, which leads to clot formation. The fibrin-bound clot framework itself stimulates activation of additional platelets. These platelets release thromboxane A$_2$, serotonin, and ADP, which enhance platelet aggregation and reinforce the formed clot.

Studies suggest that flavonoids found in fruits, vegetables, and some beverages such as tea, coffee, beer, and fruit drinks inhibit several measures of platelet activity such as epinephrine- and ADP-induced GPIIb/IIIa and P-selection expression.

Pathophysiology

The normally protective mechanism can become destructive to the body and can serve as the source of further pathology when clots form in certain areas and prevent tissues from receiving blood. Tissue ischemia and necrosis occur distal to the arterial thrombosis and manifest as MI, stroke, and acute peripheral arterial occlusion. Venous thrombi can result in PE.

A number of acquired factors are associated with increased risk for a thromboembolic event (Box 23-1). Most of these factors are linked to decreased circulation, reduced mobility, or obstruction of blood flow. Many are the result of other diseases or disability. One of the critical decisions that a clinician must make is whether it is possible to reduce or control risk factors in order to minimize the chance of thromboembolic events. Clinicians should suspect inherited risk factors, such as deficiency of anticoagulation proteins C and S, antithrombin III deficiency, factor V Leiden mutation, prothrombin G20210A mutation, and factor VIII elevations in patients displaying unusual procoagulable or prothrombotic tendencies. Hyperhomocysteinemia is found in about 5% of the population and is associated with a threefold increase in VTE. Virchow's triad describes inherited and acquired conditions that place patients at increased risk for developing emboli; these include hypercoagulable states, endothelial injury, and circulatory stasis.

Disease Process

Most of these drugs are used to prevent or treat blood clots that cause thromboembolic events such as stroke, MI, DVT, and PE. The most important pathogenic mechanism in angina and MI is an intracoronary, platelet-rich thrombus on a disrupted, ulcerated, or eroded atherosclerotic plaque leading to partial or complete coronary artery occlusion. The same process occurs in the internal carotid artery or the atria of the heart, and this leads to a stroke. Venous stasis frequently gives

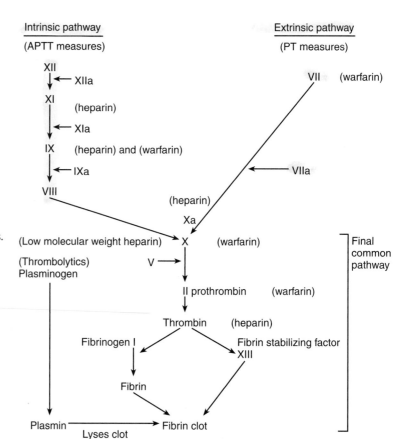

FIGURE 23-1   Coagulation and fibrinogen systems. Site of action of antithrombotic and thrombolytic drugs.

BOX 23-1   Acquired Risk Factors for Thromboembolic Events

- Age >40 years
- General anesthesia >30 minutes
- Cancer
- Oral contraceptive pills
- Prior oral contraceptive therapy
- Polycythemia
- Varicose veins
- Obesity
- Trauma
- Venous stasis
- Bed rest
- Chronic heart failure
- Immobility

rise to clot formation or DVT. If this thrombus dislodges or embolizes, it then causes a PE. PE is the leading cause of preventable hospital death in the United States.

Most cases of chronic peripheral arterial occlusive disease are caused by atherosclerosis. The femoropopliteal, tibioperoneal, aortoiliac, carotid, vertebral, splanchnic, renal, and brachiocephalic arteries are most commonly involved. In chronic arterial occlusive disease, the goals of antithrombotic drug therapy are to relieve symptoms of pain and claudication and to prevent progression of disease that may lead to loss of the limb.

Assessment

- Assess personal and family history of bleeding and vascular disorders, lifestyle, and alterable risk factors such as obesity and immobility.
- Check platelets, INR, aPTT, CBC with platelets, stool Hemoccult, creatinine/blood urea nitrogen, and liver function tests. May wish to test for hyperhomocysteinemia—elevated serum levels of homocysteine have been reported for arterial and venous occlusive disease in relation to low levels of folate, vitamin B_6, and vitamin B_{12}.

MECHANISM OF ACTION

Heparin

Heparin has no effect on existing clots; it prevents or retards formation of new thrombi. Heparin acts at multiple sites in the coagulation system and binds with antithrombin III (AT-III) at two specific sites, resulting in its anticoagulant effect. At the first heparin–AT-III binding site, factor Xa is neutralized, thereby exerting a direct effect on factor X. Factor X is responsible for initiating the final common pathway in the clotting cascade (see Figure 23-1), which ends in clot formation. The second heparin–AT-III binding occurs at the site of conversion of prothrombin to thrombin (factor IIa). With decreased thrombin available, a reduced amount of fibrin is made from fibrinogen. Standard UFH is a mixture of polysaccharide molecules that vary in average molecular weight and composition. Typically, only one third of the molecules in a standard UFH preparation contain the pentasaccharide sequence needed for antithrombin binding and anticoagulation.

LMWH has several advantages over UFH. It has a more predictable anticoagulant effect along with a higher ratio of anti–factor Xa to anti–factor IIa, thus inhibiting the generation of thrombi higher in the clotting cascade. A characteristic of LMWH is that it cannot be monitored with an aPTT as heparin can. Use of LMWH results in a lower incidence of heparin-induced thrombocytopenia and possibly in lower risks of bleeding and osteopenia.

Oral Anticoagulants

Warfarin competitively blocks vitamin K–binding sites and inhibits the synthesis of vitamin K–dependent coagulation factors VII, IX, X, and II (prothrombin) and anticoagulant proteins C and S. At therapeutic levels, warfarin decreases liver synthesis of vitamin K–dependent clotting factors by 30% to 50%. These clotting factors have different half-lives. Factor VII has the shortest half-life (6-9 hr) vs. factors II and X (up to 72 hr). Oral anticoagulants do not reverse ischemic damage or lyse an established thrombus but rather prevent extension of the existing thrombus and the formation of new thrombi by blocking synthesis of clotting factors. Existing clotting factors are not affected; therefore, the onset of action of warfarin is dependent on when existing factors are inactive. This can take several days and should be monitored closely.

It is critical to understand these vitamin K–dependent clotting factors and their half-lives if warfarin is being prescribed. Warfarin is the number one drug causing adverse drug effects in hospitals, sometimes because clinicians do not understand these times. The activity of various clotting proteins (logarithmic scale) is shown in Table 23-2 as a function of time after ingestion of warfarin (10 mg/day po for 4 consecutive days) by a normal subject. Factor VII activity, to which prothrombin time is most sensitive, is the first to decrease. Full anticoagulation, however, does not occur until factors IX and X and prothrombin are sufficiently reduced. Protein C activity falls quickly, and, in some patients, a transient hypercoagulable state may ensue (e.g., coumarin necrosis) (Furie, 2000).

Platelet Inhibitors

Aspirin (ASA) prevents platelet aggregation by inhibiting cyclooxygenase in platelets and endothelial cells, thereby preventing the synthesis of thromboxane A_2 and prostacyclin,

TABLE 23-2   Approximate Half-life of Vitamin K–Dependent Factors and Anticoagulants

Factor or Anticoagulant	Half-life
Factor VII	6 hours
Factor IX	24 hours
Factor X	36 hours
Factor II	50 hours
Protein C	8 hours
Protein S	30 hours

Compiled from Hoffman R et al, eds: *Hematology: basic principles and practice,* ed 3, New York, 2000, Churchill Livingstone.

both of which are potent platelet aggregators and vasoconstrictors.

Dipyridamole increases the body's adenosine levels, producing vasodilation, particularly of the coronary arteries, which improves blood flow. It also inhibits phosphodiesterase, the enzyme responsible for elevating levels of cyclic adenosine monophosphate (cAMP). Low levels of cAMP are associated with reduced platelet adhesiveness.

Clopidogrel inhibits platelet aggregation by inhibiting the binding of ADP to its platelet receptor and the subsequent ADP-mediated activation of the GPIIb/IIIa complex. The effect is irreversible; platelets exposed to clopidogrel are affected for the remainder of their life span (about 10 days). Ticlopidine inhibits platelet aggregation by altering the function of the platelet membrane to inhibit ADP-induced platelet-fibrinogen binding.

Parenteral GPIIb/IIIa inhibitors are used to decrease the rate of ischemic events during balloon angioplasty and to improve coronary patency before stenting. The GPIIb/IIIa receptors are exposed immediately prior to aggregation that allows platelet-to-platelet attachment. This process also requires fibrinogen. The GPIIb/IIIa inhibitor drugs therefore block the binding sites, thereby inhibiting platelet aggregation. These drugs are approved for intravenous use in patients with acute coronary syndrome (ACS) and to prevent restenosis post–percutaneous transluminal coronary angioplasty (PTCA).

The mechanism of action of anagrelide, which reduces platelet counts, is under investigation. Anagrelide inhibits cAMP PDEIII, and PDEIII inhibitors inhibit platelet aggregation. Cilostazol is a quinolinone derivative that inhibits PDEIII.

Thrombolytic Agents

Thrombolytic drugs, also known as fibrinolytics, dissolve blood clots at sites of intravascular injury. They activate tissue plasminogen, which hastens the conversion of plasminogen to plasmin. Enhanced levels of plasmin (a proteolytic enzyme) digest fibrin-bound clots and coagulation factors such as fibrinogen.

Hemorheologic Agents

Pentoxifylline decreases blood viscosity, improves erythrocyte flexibility, increases leukocyte deformability, and inhibits neutrophil adhesion and activation. Although the precise mechanism of action is unknown, these actions improve blood flow through microcirculation and increase tissue oxygenation to the affected area. Because of increased reliance on clopidogrel and ticlopidine clinically, the use of pentoxifylline is currently limited.

TREATMENT PRINCIPLES
Standardized Guidelines

- The Seventh American College of Chest Physicians (ACCP) Conference on Antithrombotic and Thrombolytic Therapy: Evidence-Based Guidelines and the Guidelines for Prevention of Stroke in Patients With Ischemic or Transient Ischemic Attack from the Stroke Council of the American Heart Association statement on primary prevention of stroke have provided important new information on the management and prevention of thromboembolic disorders, acute coronary syndromes, and ischemic stroke.

Evidence-Based Recommendations

Treatments for proximal DVT include the following:
- Beneficial: compression stockings, LMWH
- Likely to be beneficial: oral anticoagulants
  Thrombotic treatment in ischemic heart disease includes the following:
- Beneficial: aspirin, oral anticoagulants in the absence of antiplatelet treatment, thienopyridines
- Likely to be beneficial: combinations of antiplatelets
  Warfarin is superior to ASA for stroke prevention in AF.

Cardinal Points of Treatment

- Identify the drugs to be used in prevention, acute treatment, or maintenance therapy.
- Begin therapy and monitor closely to achieve anticoagulation level desired.
- Provide adequate patient and family education regarding diet, activity, signs for which to monitor, and the need for further laboratory monitoring.

Nonpharmacologic and Pharmacologic Treatment

PREVENTION OF VTE. The use of ASA alone for prophylaxis of VTE is strongly discouraged. Patients undergoing surgery who are considered to be at moderate to high risk for VTE should receive UFH or LMWH. The use of graduated compression stockings or intermittent pneumatic compression devices should be added to the regimen for patients with multiple risk factors for VTE. In addition, all trauma patients with a minimum of one risk factor for VTE, patients admitted to an intensive care unit, those admitted to hospital with CHF or severe respiratory disease, and those who are immobile should receive thromboprophylaxis with either UFH or LMWH. Patients with confirmed, nonmassive PE are treated with intravenous UFH or subcutaneous LMWH. Patients with biosynthetic valves should receive anticoagulation for 3 months (INR goal, 2 to 3). Long-term prophylaxis for these patients should include ASA (75-100 mg daily), unless AF is present. Patients with ball or caged disk prosthetic heart valves require lifelong anticoagulation (INR goal, 2.5 to 3.5) provided in combination with ASA 75 to 100 mg daily.

TREATMENT OF CONFIRMED DVT. Short-term treatment with either UFH or LMWH for at least 5 days with concurrent initiation of warfarin is recommended. UFH is discontinued when the INR reaches a value >2 and has stabilized. For the first occurrence of DVT with at least one known risk factor, anticoagulation is recommended for 6 months. DVT that is idiopathic is treated for 6 to 12 months with anticoagulation, with a target INR of 2 to 3.

TREATMENT OF PE. Patients with stable PE are treated with UFH and warfarin anticoagulation. LMWH is beneficial in submassive PE and DVT but remains controversial for the treatment of massive PE. In those with hemodynamically unstable and life-threatening PE, thrombolytic therapy is the treatment of choice. Intravenous alteplase is the preferred agent.

PREVENTION OF STROKE IN PATIENTS WITH ISCHEMIC OR TRANSIENT ISCHEMIC ATTACK. The American Stroke Association Council on Stroke recognizes that patients with a history of cardiac and/or cerebral vascular disease have an increased risk of recurrent stroke. Those with high-risk sources of cardiogenic embolism such as atrial fibrillation, chronic or paroxysmal, should be anticoagulated. In addition, systemic embolism or stroke occurs in approximately 12% of acute MI patients, particularly when complicated by left ventricular thrombus. ASA and warfarin anticoagulation is recommended for this group.

- The superiority of anticoagulation over ASA for stroke prevention in patients with recent TIA or minor stroke has been demonstrated. An INR of 2 to 3 is necessary to achieve substantial reduction in stroke recurrence and thromboembolic events.

TREATMENT OF ACUTE ISCHEMIC STROKE. For patients experiencing acute ischemic stroke, IV recombinant tissue plasminogen activator (rtPA, alteplase) initiated within 3 hours of symptom onset is recommended. Alteplase is contraindicated if onset of symptoms occurred >3 hours previously. Patients in this group should receive early ASA therapy (160-325 mg daily). The use of streptokinase or full-dose anticoagulation with IV or subQ UFH or heparinoids in acute ischemic stroke is discouraged. In patients who have had a cardioembolic stroke caused by nonvalvular AF, heparin anticoagulation as primary therapy does not reduce the end points of death and disability. Patients with noncardioembolic stroke (atherosclerotic, lacunar, or cryptogenic) are treated with ASA (50-325 mg daily), a combination of ASA and extended-release dipyridamole, or clopidogrel.

TREATMENT OF AF AND PREVENTION OF STROKE IN AF. Patients with persistent or paroxysmal AF who are at highest risk for stroke (prior ischemic stroke, TIA, systemic embolism, or age >75 years) benefit from warfarin anticoagulation, at an INR goal of 2 to 3. For AF patients with more than one moderate risk factor (age >75 years, hypertension, impaired LV function, ejection fraction <35%, or diabetes mellitus), warfarin anticoagulation is recommended. Patients who have persistent, lone AF (no major risk factors) may be treated with ASA (81-325 mg daily). If one or more risk factors are present, either warfarin or aspirin may be used. When mitral stenosis is present or a prosthetic valve is in place, warfarin is indicated, and often ASA is added to the regimen. Warfarin therapy of 3 to 4 weeks' duration is recommended before electrical cardioversion of new onset AF (>48 hours) is attempted. If onset of AF has occurred within 48 hours, cardioversion can be done without anticoagulation. In patients with rheumatic mitral valve disease and AF or a history of systemic embolism, anticoagulation plus ASA (75-100 mg daily) is indicated. If unable to tolerate ASA, clopidogrel or dipyridamole is used. For patients with mitral valve prolapse (MVP), but without a history of systemic embolism or TIA, antithrombotic therapy is not recommended. If these conditions coexist with MVP, ASA (50-162 mg daily) is suggested.

ANTITHROMBOTIC TREATMENT FOR ACS. Patients with non–ST-segment elevation (NSTE) ACS should receive ASA 162 to 325 mg po (chewed) immediately. When patients with ACS continue to exhibit symptoms after 1 hour of conventional therapy, abciximab or eptifibatide should be started. In patients who will not undergo diagnostic cardiac catheterization within 5 days of the event, bolus clopidogrel (300 mg) is recommended, followed by 75 mg daily for 9 to 12 months, in addition to ASA. If angiography is performed immediately, clopidogrel 300 mg should be given 6 hours prior to the procedure if possible. In patients considered at moderate to high risk for future events, eptifibatide or tirofiban therapy is encouraged, in addition to ASA and heparin.

THROMBOLYTIC THERAPY FOR ACS. For patients who are experiencing ischemic symptoms of <12 hours' duration with ST-segment elevation or new left-bundle branch block, a fibrinolytic drug should be given (alteplase, reteplase, or tenecteplase may be used). If symptom duration is <6 hours, the preferred drug is alteplase. In the acute treatment of NSTE ACS, LMWH rather than UFH is considered standard therapy. Contraindications to thrombolytic use include any history of intracranial hemorrhage, closed head trauma, or ischemic stroke within the previous 3 months. All patients without ASA allergy should be given ASA 162 to 325 mg at the time of initial evaluation, regardless of fibrinolytic therapy. Clopidogrel is given if ASA allergy is known.

THERAPY IN PERIPHERAL ARTERIAL OCCLUSIVE DISEASE. Patients with disabling intermittent claudication who are not candidates for surgery or catheter-based intervention should be treated with cilostazol, rather than pentoxifylline. Anticoagulation is not recommended for patients with intermittent claudication. Those with chronic limb ischemia require lifelong ASA therapy. In patients with acute arterial emboli or thrombosis, the use of UFH followed by lifelong warfarin anticoagulation is recommended. Patients with asymptomatic or recurrent carotid stenosis require lifelong ASA therapy.

USE OF ANTITHROMBOTIC DRUGS DURING PREGNANCY. For women requiring long-term anticoagulation with warfarin and considering pregnancy, UFH or LMWH should be substituted for warfarin as soon as pregnancy is achieved. Pregnant women with acute VTE are treated with adjusted-dose LMWH throughout the pregnancy and for at least 6 weeks postpartum. Alternatively, IV UFH may be given for 5 days, followed by LMWH for the duration of the pregnancy.

HEPARIN. UFH is administered as a continuous intravenous infusion on an inpatient basis. For the prevention of VTE, a dose of 5000 units is given every 8 or 12 hours postoperatively. For the treatment of patients with VTE or ACS, a loading dose of ≈80 units/kg is followed by an infusion of 9 to 18 units/kg/hr, depending on the institution. Begin to monitor aPTT ≈ 3 to 4 hours after initiation, so that any necessary adjustments to the dosage can be made. Generally, treatment is discontinued when the patient is past the risk of thromboembolic complications, but this varies with the specific indication. UFH is most often administered intravenously for 5 to 10 days. If indicated, oral anticoagulation with warfarin is given in conjunction (overlapping) with the heparin infusion because the maximal therapeutic effect of warfarin is not fully reached until after 4 to 5 days (Figure 23-2). Heparin resistance is seen in febrile patients and in those with active thrombosis, phlebitis, infection, MI, cancer, or heparin-induced thrombocytopenia (HIT). Concern has arisen about the possibility of increasing the risk of osteoporosis with prolonged standard

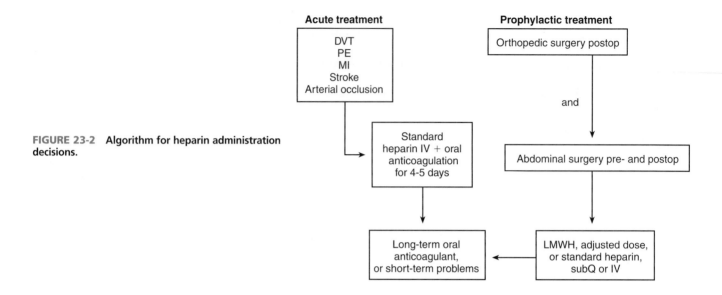

FIGURE 23-2 Algorithm for heparin administration decisions.

heparin administration (> 3 months, at an accumulated dose of 20,000 units).

Low-dose UFH or LMWH is given subcutaneously for prophylaxis of DVT, which may lead to PE in susceptible patients. LMWHs (e.g., enoxaparin) and the anti-Xa inhibitor, fondaparinux, are the preferred treatments for prevention of VTE in patients undergoing major orthopedic surgery such as total hip or knee replacement or hip fracture surgery. UFH, LMWH, or fondaparinux is preferred for major abdominal surgery and for those at risk for DVT or PE because of severely restricted mobility during an acute illness. Use of LMWH as bridge therapy has increased and is indicated for anticoagulated patients removed from warfarin prior to surgery, for AF patients following percutaneous coronary intervention, and for patients discharged on warfarin with a subtherapeutic INR.

A clinically devastating complication of heparin therapy is immune-mediated HIT, which is seen in ≈0.3% to 3% of patients. Although thrombocytopenia is associated with bleeding complications, HIT is uniquely associated with thrombosis. The rate of cross-reactivity between UFH and LMWH is 80% to 100%; therefore, if continued anticoagulation is needed in a situation in which UFH has been used, LMWH cannot be used. DTIs (e.g., argatroban, lepirudin), as well as fondaparinux, may be used in this setting. Warfarin may be prescribed for long-term use in patients with HIT.

ORAL ANTICOAGULANTS. Oral anticoagulation therapy is recommended for long-term use in patients with the following conditions: acute ischemic stroke or TIA, persistent or paroxysmal atrial fibrillation, acute MI and LV thrombus, cardiomyopathy, rheumatic mitral valve disease, mechanical prosthetic heart valves and bioprosthetic heart valves with no other source of thromboembolism, DVT, and PE. In addition, prophylactic anticoagulation therapy is recommended for patients considered at high risk for venous or arterial thromboembolism.

Warfarin therapy often is started concurrently with inpatient heparinization. Warfarin therapy is then continued as short-term adjunct therapy in DVT, post-MI, in PE, and after total joint replacement for up to 3 months. It is used indefinitely for recurrent DVT, PE, chronic AF, and post–embolic stroke, and with cardiomyopathy, left ventricular aneurysm, valvular heart disease, and mechanical cardiac valve replacement. It may be started on an outpatient basis without pretreatment with heparin. No consensus has been reached with regard to perioperative management of patients on warfarin or the INR level that must be reached before surgery can be safely performed.

Loading doses are not necessary and can precipitate thrombotic events in rare cases through rapid depletion of proteins C and S. It is recommended that patients begin with 5 mg once daily (2.5 mg for elderly) for 5 to 7 days and then adjust according to INR. Minor adjustments then can be made because warfarin is available in 1, 2, 2.5, 3, 4, 5, 6, 7.5, and 10 mg dosing strengths. In clinical practice, however, the provider will see patients who are taking warfarin in accordance with unusual dosing schedules (e.g., 5 mg q Tues., Thurs., Sat., and 7.5 mg q Wed., Sun., etc.). This practice arises from prescriber misunderstanding of warfarin pharmacokinetics and dynamics. There is no clinical reason for this, and it adds to poor patient compliance. When a patient is initiated on warfarin therapy, he or she should choose between brand or generic and remain on it. However, choosing a generic can complicate monitoring because many generics are available. Patients who are taking branded warfarin, Coumadin, should not use generic warfarin interchangeably because of differing bioavailability factors and the need to maintain a steady state.

Excessive warfarin anticoagulation is commonly overcorrected. Only in cases of an INR >9, life-threatening bleeding, or emergent surgery does warfarin require high-dose (5-10 mg) vitamin K. Excessive doses of vitamin K can create warfarin resistance and can place the patient at increased risk of thrombosis. In most cases, it is recommended that warfarin be stopped temporarily when INR is >5 and hemoglobin is stable (Table 23-3). Determine the source of excessive anticoagulation; possibilities include medication administration error, dietary indiscretion, alcohol overuse, acute febrile illness, diarrhea, new prescription or OTC medications, new herbal remedies, and vitamin supplements.

Factors that increase sensitivity to warfarin include travel, diet, environment, physical state, prolonged hot weather,

TABLE 23-3   Parameters That Should Be Monitored in Heparin Therapy

Type of Heparin	Parameters That Should Be Monitored
PARENTERAL HEPARIN	
IV or full-dose subcutaneous heparin	Monitor aPTT q6h Daily platelets for HIT Daily hemoglobin for hemorrhage Check stool for occult blood
SUBCUTANEOUS HEPARIN	
All low-dose UFH	CBC with platelets should be obtained if side effects are suspected, or if risk of type II HIT is considered (0.3%-3%). Observe for signs/symptoms of bleeding, including ecchymoses, purpura, hematuria, CNS changes, headache, stool for occult blood. Suspected HIT: serotonin release assay, platelet factor 4 (PF4) immunoassay (heparin-induced antibodies)
Standard UFH: fixed dose, IV	Prolonged aPTT 1.5 to 3× normal; desired therapeutic level varies with disease indication Check platelets every 2 to 3 days from day 4 to day 14, or until UFH is stopped.
LMWH, fondaparinux	No need to monitor aPTT (does not affect aPTT)

increased age, poor nutritional status, vitamin K deficiency, malabsorption, CHF, vascular damage, hepatitis, obstructive jaundice, biliary fistula, febrile states, hyperthyroidism, bowel sterilization for surgery, and recent surgery.

Factors that decrease the response to warfarin include DM, hyperlipidemia, hypothyroidism, edema, hypercholesterolemia, and hereditary or acquired resistance to warfarin.

PLATELET INHIBITORS. Currently, three available antiplatelet agents are effective for secondary prevention of stroke (patients with a history of a stroke or TIA): ASA, clopidogrel, and a dipyridamole-ASA combination.

ASA is the antiplatelet agent of choice for reducing thromboembolic events in patients with atherosclerosis. Used prophylactically, ASA decreases the incidence of MI and/or death in men older than 50 years of age and in patients with unstable angina, non–Q-wave infarction, acute MI, or cerebrovascular disease. The effectiveness of ASA in preventing *arterial* thrombosis is well documented; however, its effectiveness in postoperative prevention of *venous* thromboembolism is controversial. LMWH and warfarin are more effective in decreasing the incidence of venous thromboembolism than is ASA.

ASA is recommended in patients with ischemic CAD (75-162 mg/day), those with mechanical prosthetic heart valves who have had an ischemic stroke despite adequate warfarin therapy, and patients with nonischemic dilated cardiomyopathy. A dose of 75 to 100 mg per day is advised. ASA (81-325 mg/day) is recommended as an alternative to warfarin for AF patients with a low risk of stroke and those with contraindications to warfarin therapy.

Ticlopidine has been evaluated for prevention of stroke, MI, and vascular death in patients with ischemic stroke. Over a 3-year period, the risk of death from recurrent stroke was reduced by 21% compared with a placebo group. The main side effects are diarrhea, neutropenia, and thrombocytopenia.

Clopidogrel is a potent antiplatelet that is useful when a rapid effect is required. It has been shown to be as effective as ASA in reducing stroke in patients with preexisting stroke or MI and persons with diabetes. It is given with ASA to patients undergoing coronary stent implantation angioplasty for prevention of acute and intermediate thrombotic complications. Diarrhea and rash are the most common side effects, but they occur less often than with ticlopidine. "Resistance" to antiplatelet agents has been reported; therefore, an expanded role for the combination of ASA and clopidogrel in high-risk patients should be considered.

The glycoprotein IIb and IIIa receptor antagonists, ReoPro and Integrilin, do not allow binding of fibrinogen, thereby preventing platelet aggregation. Following an acute coronary event, they are used intravenously to stop thrombus formation after plaque rupture.

A combination of ASA and extended-release dipyridamole (Aggrenox) is indicated for secondary prevention of stroke. No excess of adverse cardiac events or increased bleeding has been shown with extended-release dipyridamole. Headache is the most frequently reported side effect.

THROMBOLYTIC AGENTS. Thrombolytics are approved for use in acute ischemic stroke (alteplase only), hemodynamically unstable pulmonary emboli, and acute MI of <12 hours' duration. Numerous treatment eligibility criteria exist. The most important are the absence of brain injury or hemorrhage on computed tomography scan and initiation of intervention within 3 hours from onset of stroke symptoms. Intracerebral hemorrhage is the major complication; its incidence increases when thrombolytic treatment has been delayed, and when the duration of cerebral injury is longer than 3 hours. Absolute contraindications to the use of thrombolytics in all indications include active internal bleeding, pregnancy, recent intracranial or intraspinal surgery, acute bleeding diathesis, uncontrolled HTN, AV malformation or aneurysm, and intracranial neoplasm.

HEMORHEOLOGIC AGENTS. Treatment of occlusive arterial disease includes a regular walking program, control of serum cholesterol, smoking cessation, surgical consideration, and adjunct medical therapy.

Cilostazol has replaced pentoxifylline and is used in patients with chronic occlusive arterial disease to treat intermittent claudication. It is generally considered to be useful only if the disease is of moderate severity. In the treatment of peripheral vascular disease, cilostazol helps to relieve symptoms and improve patient functioning. Improvement may be seen in about 2 to 4 weeks. If improvement is not seen after 8 weeks of therapy, discontinue the medication. If the patient takes the medication and exercises regularly, arterial disease may improve to the extent that the drug is no longer needed. A trial off medication is recommended after 6 months of therapy, to assess benefits.

How to Monitor

Coagulation parameters useful in monitoring the effects of anticoagulant agents include the following:

- aPTT (activated partial thromboplastin time or PTT): reflects the intrinsic pathway, particularly thrombin, factor Xa; most commonly used to monitor heparin therapy
- PT (prothrombin time): measures the extrinsic pathway and reflects depression of vitamin K–dependent clotting factors VII, X, and II; used to monitor warfarin therapy
- INR: mathematical equation used to correct or "normalize" a PT result. The PT value depends on the thromboplastin reagent used by an institution to perform the test. (Laboratories report both determinations [PT/INR] when a PT is ordered.) Used to monitor warfarin therapy

HEPARIN

- IV UFH is monitored via the aPTT, which is most sensitive to factor IIa activity. Platelets should be monitored daily or every other day when UFH is administered IV. Therapeutic aPTT levels vary with the disease state. Low-dose UFH administered SC for prevention of VTE is not monitored.
- See Table 23-3 for parameters to use in monitoring during heparin therapy. The purification process used to develop LMWH renders it incapable of being monitored by the aPTT. The patient should be closely monitored for signs/symptoms of bleeding.

ORAL ANTICOAGULANTS

- According to the Seventh ACCP Guidelines, the initial recommended dose of warfarin is between 5 and 10 mg. In the elderly or in any patient with an increased risk of bleeding, the initial dose may be ≤5 mg (2.5 mg). A minimum of three doses should be given with subsequent INR monitoring before the dose is adjusted.
- Monitor INR every 2 to 3 days until goal is reached, then weekly, decreasing to every 2 weeks, and finally monthly, when stable dose and INR are demonstrated.
- Obtain regular CBC with platelets, liver function tests, stool for occult blood, and urinalysis for albumin and hemoglobin.
- Selected patients manage their warfarin using a home coagulation monitor. The Boehringer-Mannheim CoaguChek Plus Coagulation Monitor is approved by the FDA, but the level of decision-making ability required renders home coagulation monitoring impractical for most patients.
- Query patient at each visit regarding signs and symptoms of bleeding, drug side effects, dietary vitamin K intake/changes, missed doses, alcohol intake, recent illness, new prescription medications, use of OTC medications, vitamin supplements, and herbal remedies. Gingko has been linked to prolonged clotting times.
- The recommended INR goal is 2 to 3 for most indications. In patients with mechanical cardiac valve replacement, the

INR goal is 3 (range, 2.5 to 3.5), which is necessary to prevent clot formation. In patients with acute MI, a higher INR may be beneficial. A lower INR (1.6 to 2.5) may be used for AF patients ≥75 years who are at increased risk of bleeding but do not have frank contraindications to warfarin.

PLATELET INHIBITORS

- Monitor for gastrointestinal (GI) upset and hypersensitivity reactions.
- Routine monitoring of coagulation parameters is not necessary.
- Monitor CBC with platelets, urinalysis, and stool Hemoccult periodically based on coexistent medical conditions.

HEMORHEOLOGIC AGENTS

- Obtain an objective measure of the patient's exercise tolerance, such as the number of blocks the patient can walk before beginning treatment. Monitor ability to walk as a measure of the drug's effectiveness.
- Assess patient's subjective and objective improvement in pain-free walking distance at 4-week intervals.
- Monitor patients for bleeding, including hematocrit or hemoglobin, if the patient is at increased risk for bleeding.

Patient Variables

GERIATRICS

- *Heparin:* Elderly patients may have low levels of AT-III and therefore have increased thrombotic potential. It may be difficult to achieve therapeutic aPTT levels.
- *Warfarin:* Liver function declines with aging, resulting in slower metabolism of warfarin; therefore, a decreased dose is warranted. The elderly exhibit a greater tendency to bleed into the skin while on warfarin because of thinning of the epithelial layer.
- *Thrombolytics:* Use with caution in adults >75 years because of increased risk of bleeding.
- *Clopidogrel:* No dosage adjustment is needed.
- *Pentoxifylline:* Older patients may have renal insufficiency with a decreased ability to excrete this drug. Thus, the geriatric patient may be at higher risk of toxicity.
- *ASA:* Women do not experience the same level of risk reduction from MI and death from daily ASA as do men. This may be due to gender differences in aspirin metabolism.

PEDIATRICS

- Use of oral anticoagulants in children is not well documented.
- *Heparin, thrombolytics, clopidogrel,* and *pentoxifylline:* Safety in children has not been established.
- Children and teenagers should not take ASA without consulting their provider regarding Reye's syndrome. Safety has not been established in children <18 years.

PREGNANCY AND LACTATION

- Heparin (*Category C*): does not cross the placental barrier—Carcinogenic potential and reproductive effects have not been evaluated. If anticoagulation is necessary, heparin is the drug of choice, despite category C classification.
- Warfarin (*Category X*): According to the ACCP, although warfarin may be safe for the fetus after a certain early period (6 to 12 wk), its use is not recommended in

pregnancy because it crosses the placental barrier. Low birth weight, growth retardation, spontaneous abortion, and stillbirth have been seen when the agent is given to pregnant women. Carcinogenicity and mutagenicity have not been determined. If the patient becomes pregnant while on warfarin, she may need to consider termination of the pregnancy. Refer patient to high-risk pregnancy obstetric/gynecology specialist.

- ASA (*Category D*): ASA should not be taken in the last 3 months of pregnancy.
- Dipyridamole (*Category B*)
- Clopidogrel (*Category B*): No adequate studies have been reported.
- Cilostazol (*Category C*)
- Pentoxifylline (*Category C*)
- Heparin: not excreted in human milk
- Warfarin: has not been detected in breast milk; women who are breastfeeding may be given warfarin after careful consideration of available alternatives
- Thrombolytics and clopidogrel: not known if these are excreted in human milk
- Pentoxifylline and its metabolites: excreted in breast milk

Patient Education

FOR ALL PRODUCTS. Emphasize the seriousness of any signs or symptoms of bleeding, what the patient should look for, and especially when to call 911 (e.g., headaches described as the "worst headache of my life," suggesting intracerebral hemorrhage and when to call the health care provider.

Encourage patients to practice safety measures and fall prevention in the home to decrease risk of injury and bleeding and bruising.

HEPARIN. Report any hypersensitivity reactions such as skin rashes, hives, swelling, and itching.

ORAL ANTICOAGULANTS

- Consistency is the key to successful warfarin treatment. Remind patient to take medication at the same time every day.
- For missed doses, caution patient not to "double-up" the next day. Take warfarin as soon as possible on the same day or not at all that day.
- Inform patient of increased risk of bleeding and of signs and symptoms that indicate major or minor bleeding.
- Review relevant safety issues with the patient. Caution in particular about prolonged bleeding associated with falls, abrasions, or cuts.
- Emphasize the importance of laboratory monitoring to keep clotting parameters within the therapeutic range.
- Have patient inform other health care providers, particularly dentists, about anticoagulation medications.
- Diet should be consistent; do not employ rapid weight loss (e.g., Atkins). Beware of foods and their vitamin K content (Box 23-2).
- The effects of alcohol on warfarin can be unpredictable, thereby increasing or decreasing the INR.
- Patient should be aware that many nonprescription multivitamin supplements contain vitamin K. Have patient bring in all OTC preparations, herbs, and vitamins so you can check labels for hidden sources of vitamin K.

BOX 23-2 Vitamin K Content of Common Foods (per Serving)

High vitamin K content (>150 mcg)
- Broccoli, cucumber with peel, endive, kale, red lettuce, raw mint, raw parsley, spinach, Swiss chard, green tea, raw turnip, watercress, brussels sprouts

Moderate vitamin K content (<150 mcg)
- Green beans, raw cabbage, canola oil, coleslaw, green lettuce, salad oil, mayonnaise

Low vitamin K content (<30 mcg)
- Apple, artichoke, dried beans, butter, cauliflower, celery, coffee, cereal, dairy products, eggs, fish, flour, fruit, tomato juice, green pepper, meat, peanut butter, root vegetables, onion, tomato

---

- Vitamin C, vitamin E, selenium, and many herbal remedies can interact with warfarin. Patient should inform provider of all preparations taken.
- Patient should not start new OTC medications or alternative therapies, such as acupuncture or massage, without discussing or informing the provider.
- Address the following safety issues with the patient:
  - The need for a fall-proof home with nonslip rugs, night-lights, and handrails to decrease risk of falls with potential for serious injury and hemorrhage
  - Obtaining medical alert identification (wear bracelet/necklace and carry identification in wallet/purse)
  - The fact that large amounts of cranberry juice may destabilize warfarin therapy, and that excessive consumption should be avoided
- Instruct patient regarding the signs and symptoms of bleeding. Request that patient promptly report any unusual symptoms or unexplained bruising and bleeding.
- Patient should document any missed warfarin doses and any variations in diet or alcohol consumption. These should be brought to office appointments and included in the patient's record.
- Provider should stress the importance of regular laboratory monitoring of PT/INR to maintain therapeutic clotting levels and to avoid complications of warfarin therapy.

ANTIPLATELET AGENTS
- Caution patients that they may bleed longer than usual if they sustain minor cuts.
- Caution about easy bruisability.
- Report bleeding, bruises, and injuries to provider.
- Inform dentist and surgeons of drug use before invasive procedures.

PERIPHERAL VASCULAR DILATORS
- Take this drug with meals to minimize possible GI discomfort.
- Regular leg exercise is important. Daily walking is usually recommended. Patients are to walk until claudication begins, immediately stop and rest for 3 minutes,

then resume walking. This should be done at least eight times a day.
- Cessation of smoking is an extremely important component of treatment.

SPECIFIC DRUGS

HEPARIN GROUP

heparin sodium 🗝

CONTRAINDICATIONS
- Severe thrombocytopenia or previous HIT
- Uncontrolled active bleeding
- Inability to complete coagulation tests

WARNINGS
- Thrombocytopenia has occurred in up to 30% of patients and is classified in two forms:
  - Type I: early, benign, reversible nonimmune thrombocytopenia; rate reported to be as high as 30% of patients; occurs within the first 2 to 3 days of therapy.
  - Type II: a rare, more serious IgG-mediated platelet aggregation seen in 0.3% to 3% of patients. Platelet count generally falls to below 100,000/mm³ or is less than 50% of the baseline value. Alternative anticoagulation is necessary. The FDA has issued a black box warning to inform clinicians of the possibility of this delayed onset of heparin-induced thrombocytopenia (HIT), a serious antibody-mediated reaction that results from irreversible aggregation of platelets. HIT may progress to the development of venous and arterial thromboses, a condition referred to as heparin-induced thrombocytopenia and thrombosis (HITT). Thrombotic events may occur as the initial presentation for HITT, which can have onset up to several weeks after discontinuation of heparin therapy. Patients who present with thrombocytopenia or thrombosis after discontinuation of heparin should be evaluated for HIT and HITT.
- Hypersensitivity to heparin: Use only in clearly life-threatening situations.
- Hemorrhage can occur at any site. Signs and symptoms vary with the location and extent of bleeding. Use with extreme caution in disease states in which danger of hemorrhage is increased:
  - Cardiovascular: subacute bacterial endocarditis, severe hypertension
  - Surgical: during and immediately following spinal tap or spinal anesthesia or major surgery, especially involving the brain, spinal cord, or eye
  - Hematologic: conditions associated with increased bleeding tendencies, such as hemophilia, thrombocytopenia, and some vascular purpuras
  - Gastrointestinal: ulcerative lesions and continuous tube drainage of the stomach or small intestine
  - Other: menstruation, liver disease with impaired hemostasis
- The benzyl alcohol preservative in heparin is reported to be associated with a fatal "gasping syndrome" in premature infants.

- Do not give heparin intramuscularly; it can cause hematoma formation.

PRECAUTIONS
- Thrombi can occur as a result of HIT or "white clot syndrome." This can lead to skin necrosis, gangrene, MI, PE, stroke, and death.
- Heparin resistance is frequently encountered in fever, thrombosis, thrombophlebitis, infections with thrombosing tendencies, MI, and cancer, and in postsurgical patients and those with AT-III deficiency.
- Older women: A higher incidence of bleeding has been reported in women >60 years of age.
- Elevated liver function tests are sometimes seen.

PHARMACOKINETICS. See Table 23-4.

ADVERSE EFFECTS. See Table 23-5.

DRUG INTERACTIONS. Platelet inhibitors, including the NSAIDs such as ibuprofen, ASA, and the GPIIb/IIIa inhibitors, may potentiate the risk of hemorrhage.

DOSAGE AND ADMINISTRATION. See Table 23-6 for heparin dosing schedule, Table 23-7 for administration recommendations, and Table 23-8 for weight-based intravenous heparin dose nomogram.

OVERDOSAGE. Signs of overdosage include the following:
- Minor bleeding: hematoma, ecchymosis, oozing from superficial skin breaks and catheter placement sites, hematuria, mucous membrane bleeding
- Major bleeding: intracranial hemorrhage, sudden unexplained drop in hematocrit, sudden hypotension, sudden change in mental status (suggesting ICH)
  Protamine sulfate (1%) up to 50 mg is given by slow infusion over at least 10 minutes for reversal of heparinization. A dose of 1 mg protamine neutralizes 100 units of heparin. Side effects of protamine include hypotension and anaphylactic reactions.

OTHER DRUGS IN CLASS

LOW MOLECULAR WEIGHT HEPARIN AND HEPARINOID. LMWH has a longer half-life and increased bioavailability compared with UFH because of its reduced binding to plasma proteins and endothelial cells. Therefore, plasma levels of LMWH are very predictable, allowing for fixed schedule dosing once or twice daily. Minor bruising may occur at the subcutaneous injection site. The reported incidence of minor bleeding is less than with UFH, but no difference has been found in the incidence of major bleeding. Thrombocytopenia can result; the incidence is less than with UFH. Hemorrhage is minimally controlled with protamine sulfate. LMWH is more expensive than UFH; however, because regular aPTT monitoring is not required, the overall cost of treatment is lower than with UFH.

💣 Warning: The FDA has issued a black box warning regarding the use of LMWH with neuraxial or spinal anesthesia because of the increased risk of spinal hematoma, which can result in paralysis. This risk is increased when antiplatelet drugs or warfarin is used concurrently with LMWH.

TABLE 23-4   Pharmacokinetics of Drugs Seen in Primary Care

Drug	Absorption	Drug Availability (After First Pass)	Onset of Action	Time to Peak Concentration	Half-life	Duration of Action	Protein Bound	Metabolism	Excretion	Therapeutic Serum Level
heparin sodium	Not absorbed through GI mucosa	Reduced with subQ route	Immediate, IV; 1-2 hr, subQ	3 hr, subQ	Dependent on dose; 30-90 min	Effect gone within hours of discontinuation	Yes	Liver; kidney (partial)	Primarily through the reticuloendothelial system; small amount in urine	Monitor aPTT, 1.5-2.5× normal; narrow therapeutic index; check platelets daily with IV infusion
warfarin	Rapid from GI tract, within 1 hr	Near 100%	24 hr	36-72 hr	25-60 hr, mean 40 hr	2-5 days	99%	Liver: R-1A2 substrate R-3A4; substrate S-2C9; substrate (primary)	Urine and feces	—
aspirin (ASA)	80%-100%	50%-70%	5-30 min	1-2 hr	15-20 min	Dose dependent	50%-80%	Liver	Urine	—
dipyridamole (Persantine)	Incomplete absorption	37%-66%	24 min	2-2.5 hr	10 hr	Unknown	91%-99%	Liver	Feces and urine	—
clopidogrel (Plavix)	Well absorbed; rapid	50%	2 hr	1 hr	8 hr	3 days (single dose); 5-7 days (multiple dose)	98%	Liver	Urine, 50%; feces, 40%	—
cilostazol	Increased by high-fat meal	87%-100%	2-4 wk	2-4 hr	11-13 hr	12 hr (single dose); 2 days (multiple dose)	95%-98%	Liver: 3A4 (primary) and 2C19	Metabolites in urine	—
pentoxifylline	Almost completely absorbed	20%	2-4 wk	2-4 hr	Nonlinear; 30-60 min	Unknown	Unknown	Liver; no CYP450	Urine	—
enoxaparin	90% absorbed		Unknown	3-5 hr	4½ hr	12 hr (40-mg dose)	No	Metabolized by liver and unknown factors	Excreted by kidneys	—
fondaparinux			2-3 hr	1-3 hr	13-21 hr		94%	Minimal	Kidneys	
dalteparin	—	87%	—	4 hr	3-4 hr	—	—	Minimal	Kidney	—

TABLE 23-5   Adverse Effects of Drugs Affecting Blood

Drug	Major Adverse Effects
HEPARIN GROUP	
heparin sodium	Hemorrhage: nosebleeds, hematuria, tarry stools, easy bruising, and petechiae formation
	Local irritation: erythema, mild pain, hematoma, or ulceration may follow deep subcutaneous injection. Do not use intramuscular injection.
	Hypersensitivity reactions may include anaphylaxis, shock, urticaria, rhinitis, asthma, cyanosis, tachypnea, tachycardia, hypertension, fever, chills, headache, and nausea and vomiting.
	Thrombocytopenia: See black box warnings and precautions for delayed and serious thrombocytopenia.
	An association has been noted between long-term heparin therapy and osteoporosis; this occurs when the total heparin dose has exceeded 20,000 units/day for longer than 3 months.
Low molecular weight heparin (LMWH)	Black box warning regarding the use of LMWH with neuraxial or spinal anesthesia because of increased risk of spinal hematoma, which can result in paralysis
ORAL ANTICOAGULANTS	
warfarin (Coumadin)	Hemorrhage: Minor bleeding and hemorrhage are reported in 2% to 20% of patients.
	Hypersensitivity, hepatitis, cholestatic hepatic injury, jaundice, elevated liver enzymes, vasculitis, edema, fever, rash, dermatitis, abdominal pain, fatigue, lethargy, malaise, asthenia, nausea, vomiting, diarrhea, pain, headache, dizziness, taste perversion, pruritus, alopecia, cold intolerance, and paresthesia, including feeling cold and chills
Platelet Inhibitors	
dipyridamole (Persantine)	Epistaxis, purpura, and anemia; thrombocytopenic purpura; dizziness (14%)
clopidogrel (Plavix)	Hemorrhage: Gastrointestinal hemorrhage in 2% of patients; bleeding (major, 4%; minor, 5%), purpura (5%), epistaxis (3%); neutropenia/agranulocytosis GI (27%): abdominal pain, gastritis, constipation, diarrhea; rash; hypersensitivity
cilostazol (Pletal)	Headache, palpitations, tachycardia, diarrhea, abdominal pain, abnormal stools, dyspepsia, nausea, peripheral edema, back pain, myalgia, dizziness, vertigo, cough, pharyngitis, rhinitis, infection
HEMORHEOLOGIC	
pentoxifylline (Trental)	Nausea, vomiting, dyspepsia, belching, bloating, diarrhea, and flatulence (cause 5% of patients to discontinue therapy)
	Dizziness, headache, tremor, nervousness, or agitation
	Angina, edema, hypotension, dyspnea, flushing, and arrhythmia
	Cholecystitis, dry mouth, depression, seizures, epistaxis, laryngitis, nasal congestion, brittle fingernails, pruritus, rash, urticaria, angioedema, blurred vision, conjunctivitis, earache, scotoma, bad taste, excessive salivation, leukopenia, and weight change

ORAL ANTICOAGULANTS

warfarin (Coumadin) 🔑

CONTRAINDICATIONS

- Pregnancy, threatened abortion, eclampsia, and preeclampsia
- Hemorrhagic tendencies or blood dyscrasias
- Recent or contemplated surgery of CNS and eye, and traumatic surgery resulting in large open surfaces
- Bleeding tendencies associated with active ulceration or overt bleeding of GI, GU, or respiratory tract; cerebrovascular hemorrhage; aneurysms—cerebral, dissecting aorta; pericarditis and pericardial effusions; and bacterial endocarditis
- Severe uncontrolled or malignant hypertension
- Severe hepatic disease
- Inadequate laboratory facilities
- Unsupervised patients with senility, alcoholism, psychosis, or lack of patient cooperation for other reasons
- Spinal puncture and other diagnostic or therapeutic procedures with potential for uncontrollable bleeding
- History of warfarin-induced necrosis
- Miscellaneous: major regional or lumbar block anesthesia, malignant hypertension, and known hypersensitivity to warfarin or to any other components of this product

WARNINGS

- Major determinants of warfarin-induced bleeding: intensity of therapy (indicated by INR), patient characteristics, and length of treatment
- Hemorrhage involving any tissue or organ and necrosis and gangrene of the skin and other tissues
- Treatment of each patient is a highly individualized matter. Warfarin has a narrow therapeutic range (index) and may be affected by factors such as other drugs and dietary vitamin K. Dosage should be controlled through periodic determination of PT/INR.
- Caution should be observed when warfarin sodium is administered in any situation, or in the presence of any predisposing condition in which added risk of hemorrhage, necrosis, or gangrene is present.
- Warfarin may enhance the release of atheromatous plaque emboli, thereby increasing the risk of complications from systemic cholesterol microembolization and can present with a variety of signs and symptoms, including sequelae of vascular compromise due to embolic occlusion and the "purple toes syndrome."
- Use with caution in patients with HIT and DVT.
  - Moderate hepatic or renal insufficiency
  - Infectious diseases or disturbances of intestinal flora
  - Trauma that may result in internal bleeding

warfarin (Coumadin) 🔑—cont'd

- Surgery or trauma resulting in large exposed raw surface
- Indwelling catheters
- Moderate to severe hypertension
- Known or suspected deficiency in protein C–mediated anticoagulant response
- Polycythemia vera, vasculitis, and severe diabetes
- Minor and severe allergic/hypersensitivity reactions and anaphylactic reactions have been reported.
  - Warfarin resistance
- Patients with CHF require frequent laboratory monitoring and reduced doses of warfarin.
- Concomitant use of anticoagulants with thrombolytics is not recommended.

PRECAUTIONS
- Periodic determination of PT/INR is essential every 1 to 4 weeks.
- Numerous factors, alone or in combination, including travel and changes in diet, environmental, or physical state, and use of medications, including botanicals, may influence response of the patient to anticoagulants.
- Monitor PT/INR after discharge from the hospital whenever other medications are changed.
- Many important drug interactions may occur with warfarin. See below and Box 23-3.
- For patients with low risk of VTE, warfarin may be stopped 4 days prior to surgery. In patients at high risk for VTE, warfarin should be stopped 4 days prior to surgery to allow the INR to normalize. LMWH should be started as the INR falls. For patients undergoing dental procedures, warfarin does not have to be discontinued if a tranexamic acid mouthwash or an epsilon amino caproic acid mouthwash can be used prior to the procedure to prevent local bleeding.

ADVERSE EFFECTS. The risk of hemorrhage in warfarin therapy is related to the intensity and duration of treatment (Table 23-9).

Acetaminophen is an unrecognized source of excessive anticoagulation in warfarin therapy. Daily use of four regular strength acetaminophen tablets, or 28 tablets per week, greatly increases the risk of a prolonged INR of greater than 6.

DRUG INTERACTIONS. Warfarin reacts with many other drugs, although few reactions are clinically meaningful. Some of these drug interactions are unpredictable, increasing or decreasing warfarin responsiveness in different patients (see Box 23-3). It is advisable to check all medications the patient is taking for possible interactions before starting warfarin and to monitor the INR closely. Also, if the patient is on warfarin, check the INR before and soon after changing any other medications the patient is taking. The categories of drugs in common use that interact with warfarin are listed in Box 23-4.

A strong genetic influence on the patient's response to warfarin has been noted. Individuals with variations in two genes may need lower warfarin doses than those without these genetic polymorphisms. The two genes are *CYP2C9* and *VKORC1*. The *CYP2C9* gene is involved in the breakdown (metabolism) of warfarin, and the *VKORC1* gene helps to regulate the ability of warfarin to prevent blood from clotting. Because routine screening is not done for these genetic polymorphisms, suspect when INR is very responsive to warfarin at low doses, and adjust accordingly.

OVERDOSAGE. Excessive anticoagulation with or without bleeding can be reversed in many instances by discontinuing the drug on a temporary basis. If minor bleeding progresses to major bleeding, parenteral vitamin K may be needed. See Table 23-9 for management of prolonged INR. Vitamin K, especially doses greater than 5 mg, should not be given indiscriminately because its use reduces future response to warfarin. In patients with mildly to moderately elevated INR without evidence of major bleeding, vitamin K may be given orally rather than subcutaneously. In emergency situations of hemorrhage, 200 to 500 ml fresh frozen plasma or whole blood can restore clotting factors to normal.

Signs and symptoms of excessive anticoagulation include the following:
- Minor bleeding (drop in hemoglobin of 3%): ecchymoses and easy bruisability, excessive bleeding from superficial cuts (e.g., shaving), bleeding from oral mucous membranes, nosebleeds, heavy menstrual bleeding, vaginal bleeding, hematuria, hematemesis, joint swelling, and pain
- Major bleeding (drop in hemoglobin >5%): headache, blurred vision, dysarthria, stroke symptoms, weakness, extreme fatigue, and melena

DOSAGE AND ADMINISTRATION. The daily maintenance dose of warfarin is between 2 and 12 mg. The dose is titrated to achieve the INR goal for the specific anticoagulation indication (see Table 23-9).

TABLE 23-6 Heparin Dosing Schedule

Type of Heparin	Dosage Schedule Recommendation
Standard unfractionated heparin IV	5000 unit bolus followed by 800-1000 units/hr infusion
Weight-based IV heparin	Initial dose: 80 units/kg bolus followed by 18 units/kg/hr infusion; then follow Table 23-8
Adjusted-dose IV heparin	Give only amount needed to raise aPTT 1 to 1.5× control.
PROPHYLACTIC subQ HEPARIN	
Unfractionated standard heparin	5000 units subQ q8h or q12h
enoxaparin (LMWH)	40 mg subQ once daily or bid (nonorthopedic use); 30 mg subQ q12h (orthopedic uses); renal dysfunction (<30 ml/min CrCl): 30 mg once daily
dalteparin (LMWH)	2500 units subQ once daily (general surgery; low risk); 5000 units subQ once daily (orthopedic use, general surgery; high risk)
fondaparinux	2.5 mg subQ once daily (all indications)

TABLE 23-7 Dosage and Administration Recommendations

Medication	Dosage	Administration
heparin sodium	5000 units Low-dose prophylaxis preoperative For age >40 yr	subQ 5000 units subQ, 2 hr before surgery 5000 units subQ, q12h postoperatively for 7 days
enoxaparin (Lovenox)	30 mg bid 40 mg daily 1 mg/kg q12 hr	subQ, postoperatively for 7-10 days in total hip and knee replacement subQ, 2 hours prior to abdominal surgery, continuing for 7-10 days subQ, for treatment of DVT and post-ACS for 7-8 days
dalteparin (Fragmin)	2500-5000 units once daily	subQ, 1-2 hr before abdominal surgery and for 5-10 days afterward
aspirin (ASA)	MI: 162-325 mg TIA and stroke: 30-325 mg once daily	po po
dipyridamole (Persantine)	75-100 mg	po qid
clopidogrel (Plavix)	75 mg	po daily, take with or without food
pentoxifylline (Trental)	400 mg	po tid

OTHER DRUGS IN CLASS

Other drugs in this class are similar to the key drug except as follows:

anisindione (Miradon)

Anisindione (Miradon) is a synthetic coagulant indanedione derivative. Its pharmacokinetic properties are similar to those of warfarin. It is reserved for use in cases of warfarin allergy or sensitivity. Managing anisindione and achieving stable, therapeutic PT/INR values is more difficult than with warfarin. It can itself cause a severe hypersensitivity reaction and should be monitored carefully. Do not use in acute stroke patients. See Box 23-3 for drug interaction information.

PLATELET AGGREGATION INHIBITORS

acetylsalicylic acid (ASA) (aspirin)
- The recommended dose of ASA for acute stroke is 160 to 325 mg per day; it should be begun within 48 hours in patients who are not systemically anticoagulated and who are not candidates for alteplase therapy. The dose

for secondary stroke prevention/TIA ranges from 30 to 325 mg/day.
- Routine monitoring of coagulation parameters is not necessary.
- Assess sodium content of ASA preparation for patients with heart failure or edema.
- Individuals with delayed gastric emptying may retain enteric-coated aspirin products. Use with caution in patients who are at increased risk of bleeding from trauma or surgery.

dipyridamole (Persantine)
CONTRAINDICATIONS. Hypersensitivity
PRECAUTIONS.
- *CAD:* Dipyridamole has a vasodilatory effect and should be used with caution in patients with severe CAD. Chest pain may be aggravated.
- *Hepatic insufficiency:* Elevations in hepatic enzymes and hepatic failure have been reported.
- *Hypotension:* Use with caution to avoid peripheral vasodilation.

clopidogrel (Plavix)
CONTRAINDICATIONS
- Hypersensitivity
- Active pathologic bleeding such as peptic ulcer disease or ICH

WARNINGS. Thrombotic thrombocytopenic purpura has been reported rarely and requires prompt treatment.

PRECAUTIONS
- *Bleeding risk:* Use with caution in patients who may be at risk for increased bleeding. Discontinue clopidogrel 5 days before surgery.
- *GI bleeding:* Use with caution in patients with conditions that place them at risk for bleed such as ulcers.
- The combination of clopidogrel and ASA is no more effective than either agent used alone and increases the risk of major bleeding.
- *Hepatic function impairment:* Use with caution.

TABLE 23-8 Weight-Based Intravenous (IV) Heparin Dose Nomogram

aPTT	Dosage
Initial dose	80 units/kg bolus, then 18 units/kg/hr
aPTT <35 sec	80 units/kg/bolus, then 4 units/kg/hr
aPTT 36-45 sec	40 units/kg/bolus, then 2 units/kg/hr
aPTT 46-70 sec	Therapeutic range, no change
aPTT 71-90 sec	Decrease rate by 2 units/kg/hr
aPTT >90 sec	Hold infusion 1 hr, then decrease rate by 3 units/kg/hr

Modified from Hirsh J et al: Heparin: mechanism of action, pharmacokinetics, dosing, considerations, monitoring, efficacy, and safety, *Chest* 108(suppl 4):258S, 1995.

BOX 23-3   Specific Drug Interactions With Warfarin

MEDICATIONS ASSOCIATED WITH AN INCREASE IN INR RESPONSE

acetaminophen
alcohol
allopurinol
aminosalicylic acid
amiodarone
anabolic steroids
aspirin
atorvastatin
azithromycin
cefamandole
cefazolin
cefoperazone
cefotetan, cefoxitin, ceftriaxone
celecoxib
cerivastatin
chenodiol
chloramphenicol
chloral hydrate
chlorpropamide
cholestyramine
cimetidine
ciprofloxacin
cisapride
clarithromycin
clofibrate
co-trimoxazole
cyclophosphamide
danazol
dextran
dextrothyroxine
diazoxide
diclofenac
dicumarol
diflunisal
disulfiram
doxycycline
erythromycin
ethacrynic acid
fenofibrate
fenoprofen
fluconazole
5-fluorouracil
fluoxetine
flutamide
fluvastatin
fluvoxamine
gemfibrozil
glucagon
halothane
heparin
ibuprofen
ifosfamide
indomethacin

influenzavirus vaccine
isoniazid
itraconazole
ketoprofen
ketorolac
levamisole
levofloxacin
levothyroxine
liothyronine
lovastatin
mefenamic acid
methimazole
methyldopa
methylphenidate
methyl salicylate oint (top)
metronidazole miconazole
  (systemic, vag)
moralizing
nalidixic acid
naproxen
neomycin
norfloxacin
ofloxacin
olsalazine
omeprazole
oxaprozin
oxymetholone
paroxetine
penicillin G (IV)
pentoxifylline
phenylbutazone
phenytoin
piperacillin
piroxicam
pravastatin
prednisone
propafenone
propoxyphene
propranolol
propylthiouracil
quinidine
quinine
ranitidine
rofecoxib
sertraline
simvastatin
stanozolol
streptokinase
sulfamethizole
sulfamethoxazole
sulfinpyrazone
sulfisoxazole
sulindac
tamoxifen
tetracycline
thyroid drugs
ticarcillin

ticlopidine
t-PA
tolbutamide
tramadol
trimethoprim-sulfamethoxazole
urokinase
valproate
vitamin E
zafirlukast
zileuton

MEDICATIONS THAT DECREASE INR RESPONSE

alcohol
aminoglutethimide
amobarbital
atorvastatin
azathioprine
butabarbital
butalbital
carbamazepine
chloral hydrate
chlordiazepoxide
chlorthalidone
cholestyramine
clozapine
corticotropin
cortisone
cyclophosphamide
dicloxacillin
ethchlorvynol
glutethimide
griseofulvin
haloperidol
meprobamate
6-mercaptopurine
methimazole
moricizine hydrochloride
nafcillin
paraldehyde
pentobarbital
phenytoin
pravastatin
prednisone
primidone
propylthiouracil
raloxifene
ranitidine
rifampin
secobarbital
spironolactone
sucralfate
trazodone
vitamin C
vitamin K

TABLE 23-9 Management of Prolonged International Normalized Ratio (INR) from Warfarin

INR Value	Signs and Symptoms of Bleeding	Treatment
>therapeutic to 5	None	1. Lower warfarin dose, or 2. Omit a dose and resume warfarin at a lower dose when INR is in therapeutic range, or 3. No dose reduction needed if INR is minimally prolonged.
5-9	None	1. Omit the next one or two doses of warfarin, monitor INR more frequently, and resume treatment at a lower dose when INR is in therapeutic range, or 2. Omit a dose and administer 1 to 2.5 mg oral vitamin K (phytonadione).*
>9	None	Hold warfarin and administer 5 to 10 mg oral vitamin K_1. Monitor INR more frequently and administer more vitamin K as needed. Resume warfarin at a lower dose when INR is in therapeutic range.
≥20	N/A Life-threatening hemorrhage	Hold warfarin and administer 10 mg vitamin K by slow IV infusion; supplement with prothrombin complex concentrate, fresh frozen plasma, or recombinant human factor VIIa, depending on clinical urgency. Monitor and repeat as needed.

*This option is preferred in patients at increased risk for bleeding (e.g., history of bleeding, stroke, renal insufficiency, anemia, hypertension).
Adapted and modified from Ansell, J et al: The pharmacology and management of the vitamin K antagonists: the Seventh ACCP Conference on Antithrombotic and Thrombolytic Therapy, *Chest* 126:204S, 2004.

ADVERSE EFFECTS. See Table 23-5.

DRUG INTERACTIONS
- Coadministration with NSAIDs is associated with increased GI bleed.
- Safety of coadministration with other platelet inhibitors or anticoagulants has not been established.
- Atorvastatin has been shown to increase the effects of bleeding associated with clopidogrel therapy.

DOSAGE AND ADMINISTRATION. No dose adjustments are needed in elderly patients or those with renal disease.

OVERDOSAGE. Reported intentional overdose (1050 mg) of clopidogrel did not result in adverse events or sequelae.

BOX 23-4 Some Categories of Drugs That Interact With Warfarin

Adrenergic stimulants
Analgesics
Antibiotics: aminoglycosides, cephalosporins, macrolides, penicillins quinolones, sulfonamides, and tetracyclines
Anticonvulsants
Antidepressants
Antihistamines
Antihyperlipidemics: bile acid–binding resins, fibric acid derivatives, 3-hydroxy-3-methylglutaryl coenzyme A reductase (HMG-CoA) reductase inhibitors
Gastric acidity agents
Hypnotics
NSAIDs
Oral contraceptives
Steroids
Thyroid medicines
Vaccines
Vitamins

---

ticlopidine (Ticlid)
Ticlopidine can cause life-threatening hematologic adverse reactions, including neutropenia/agranulocytosis and thrombotic thrombocytopenia purpura.

cilostazol (Pletal)
CONTRAINDICATIONS
- CHF of any severity
- Hemostatic disorder or active pathologic bleeding
- Hypersensitivity

PRECAUTIONS. Rare cases of thrombocytopenia or leukopenia progressing to agranulocytosis

DRUG INTERACTIONS. Cilostazol is extensively metabolized by cytochrome P450 (CYP450) 3A4 and 2C19. Significant drug interactions can occur with select drugs.

HEMORHEOLOGIC AGENT
pentoxifylline (Trental)
CONTRAINDICATIONS. Recent cerebral or retinal hemorrhage and sensitivity to pentoxifylline or methylxanthines such as caffeine, theophylline, and theobromine

PRECAUTIONS
- Angina, hypotension, and arrhythmia have been reported occasionally.
- Pentoxifylline is a methylxanthine derivative.
- Caution should be exhibited when prescribing pentoxifylline in patients who have increased risk for hemorrhage such as recent surgery, peptic ulceration, and current warfarin use. These patients must be monitored closely for bleeding with frequent checks of PT and hematocrit/hemoglobin.
- Patients with chronic occlusive arterial disease of the limbs often have other manifestations of arteriosclerotic disease such as angina, hypotension, and arrhythmia. Monitor the patient for signs and symptoms of arteriosclerotic disease.

ADVERSE EFFECTS. See Table 23-5.

DRUG INTERACTIONS
- Concomitant use with theophylline may lead to increased theophylline levels and theophylline toxicity.
- Concomitant use with warfarin may cause bleeding and prolonged PT. Frequently monitor PT in patients taking warfarin.

DOSAGE AND ADMINISTRATION. The usual dose is 400 mg given three times daily with meals. If the patient develops adverse digestive system or CNS side effects, the dose can be lowered to 400 mg twice daily. An extended-release product is now available.

evolve A continually updated list of useful WebLinks may be found in the Evolve Resources at http://evolve.elsevier.com/Edmunds/NP/

24 Antacids and the Management of GERD

DRUG OVERVIEW

Class	Generic Name	Trade Name
Calcium salts	calcium carbonate 🔑	Tums, Rolaids
Sodium bicarbonate		Alka-Seltzer
Aluminum salts	aluminum hydroxide	Amphojel
	aluminum carbonate	Basaljel
Magnesium salts	magnesium hydroxide	Milk of Magnesia
	magnesium oxide	Uro-Mag, Mag-Ox
Combination products	aluminum hydroxide and magnesium hydroxide	Maalox, Mylanta, Gelusil
	alginic acid, magnesium trisilicate, calcium stearate	Gaviscon

🔑 Key drug.

INDICATIONS

- *Hyperacidity:* heartburn, GI reflux, and acid indigestion
- Hyperacidity associated with peptic ulcer, gastric hyperacidity, and sour stomach
- *Calcium carbonate:* gastric hyperacidity, hypocalcemia, hypoparathyroidism, hyperphosphatemia, hypertension, heartburn associated with pregnancy
- *Aluminum hydroxide:* gastric hyperacidity, gastritis, peptic ulcer
- *Magnesium hydroxide:* magnesium deficiencies; magnesium depletion from malnutrition, restricted diet, alcoholism, or magnesium-depleting drugs

Unlabeled Uses

- GERD; not first-line therapy
- *Antacids with aluminum and magnesium or aluminum hydroxide:* prevent stress ulcer bleeding; duodenal ulcer, maybe gastric ulcer
- *Calcium carbonate:* prevention and management of osteoporosis

Antacids are rarely prescribed as first-line treatment. Usually, the patient has been using OTC antacids before coming to the health provider for care. These medications are used commonly for gastroenterologic diseases such as reflux esophagitis and peptic ulcer. The antacids most commonly prescribed have at least one of the following elements as their main ingredient: calcium carbonate, aluminum salts, or magnesium. The ingredient alginate may provide barrier protection and is useful in the management of GERD.

The key antacid is considered to be calcium carbonate because of its widespread popularity, cost-effectiveness, and ease of use. However, combination antacids—in particular, combinations of aluminum hydroxide and magnesium hydroxide—are probably the most commonly used antacids. Antacids vary in sodium content, in magnesium content (a problem in kidney failure), and in the tendency to cause diarrhea or constipation.

THERAPEUTIC OVERVIEW OF GASTROESOPHAGEAL REFLUX DISEASE

Anatomy and Physiology

The pH of saliva is basic, causing the contents of the esophagus to be neutral to basic. Esophageal peristalsis and salivary bicarbonate serve to protect the esophageal mucosa from erosion. The stomach contents are highly acidic, which helps in the digestion of food.

Pathophysiology

The return of stomach contents back up into the esophagus is called gastroesophageal reflux disease (GERD). This reflux frequently causes heartburn, which results from irritation of the esophagus by stomach acid. GERD can lead to scarring and stricture of the esophagus, requiring stretching (dilating) of the esophagus. In all, 10% of patients with GERD develop Barrett's esophagus, which increases the risk of cancer of the esophagus. A total of 80% of patients with GERD also have a hiatal hernia, in which a portion of the stomach protrudes through the diaphragm (where the esophagus normally passes through). Obesity and smoking are considered risk factors.

Many factors may lead to GERD. A very important factor that contributes to GERD is an incompetent lower esophageal sphincter (LES). Reflux of the stomach contents (pH 2) into the esophagus (pH 6) occurs during relaxation of the LES. A decrease in LES pressure allows acidic gastric contents to enter the lower portion of the esophagus. This happens at rest but increases with stress such as that caused by abdominal straining, lifting, or bending. In addition, some people have low basal LES pressure. The highly acidic gastric contents are damaging to the esophageal mucosa, causing inflammation. This mucosal damage may further decrease LES pressure, initiating a self-perpetuating cycle.

Delayed gastric emptying may be caused by gastroparesis or partial gastric outlet obstruction. This can increase GERD because the food stays in the stomach longer. During sleep, peristalsis is decreased, causing an increase in symptoms. Because saliva helps to neutralize stomach contents, anything that decreases salivation such as anticholinergic medications can exacerbate GERD. Hiatal hernias are common and are not a cause of GERD. If the patient with a hiatal hernia has GERD, more reflux will occur.

Disease Process

GERD is one of the most common chronic conditions for which patients in the United States take daily medication. Heartburn and regurgitation associated with GERD were found to occur at least twice a week in 6% and 3% of the adult U.S. population, respectively. GERD involves the movement of stomach contents back into the esophagus. Most patients have very mild disease, although it is possible for the patient to develop complications such as active erosive esophagitis, esophageal adenocarcinoma, and esophageal stricture.

The main symptom of GERD is heartburn that occurs 30 to 60 minutes after meals and when the patient bends over or lies down. Relief is usually reported after antacids are taken. Other symptoms may include nonspecific GI symptoms such as regurgitation of sour or bitter gastric contents, belching, and fullness of the stomach. Atypical symptoms include chronic cough, chronic laryngitis, asthma, sore throat, and noncardiac chest pain. Erosive esophagitis may have more severe symptoms such as pain and dysphagia but also may be relatively asymptomatic. Esophagitis is divided into four grades, which are determined endoscopically. Grade 1 is defined by erythema of the distal esophagus. Grade 2 consists of scattered erosions. Grade 3 involves confluence of erosions involving less than 50% of the diameter of the esophagus; grade 4 involves confluence of erosions involving greater than 50% of the diameter.

Providers must ask specifically about antacids and other OTC remedies when taking a medication history. Many patients will have tried OTC remedies before going to their primary care provider. Most will have tried antacids and OTC histamine blockers (see Chapter 25). Many patients do not consider antacids to be a medication and will not mention taking them when asked about medication use.

An upper endoscopy with biopsy is the standard diagnostic procedure for GERD. It confirms the diagnosis and documents the type and extent of tissue damage. Uncomplicated GERD that is responsive to first-line therapy does not require an endoscopy. For most patients, empiric treatment is initiated based on history and physical examination. Acid suppression therapy with antacids, histamine$_2$ receptor antagonists (H$_2$RAs), or proton pump inhibitors (PPIs) is extremely effective in controlling GERD symptoms but is problematic because of the high associated costs of many of these medications and the need for indefinite therapy duration in most patients. Patients who do not respond and those with suspected complications should undergo an endoscopic examination.

The differential diagnosis includes peptic ulcer, cholelithiasis, nonulcer dyspepsia, and angina pectoris. Patients should be evaluated for *Helicobacter pylori* infection.

MECHANISM OF ACTION

Antacids are weak bases that neutralize gastric hydrochloric acid by combining with it to form salt and water. This process decreases the amount of gastric acid in the stomach, raising the pH. Antacids decrease pepsin activity because pepsin is rendered inactive in alkaline conditions. Antacids also have a number of cytoprotective effects. They may enhance mucosal prostaglandin levels. Aluminum ions inhibit smooth muscle contraction, thereby slowing gastric emptying. This is counterproductive because in GERD, prompt gastric emptying is beneficial. Aluminum binds epidermal growth factor, thus delivering growth factor to the injured mucosa.

Antacids do not protect the stomach by coating the mucosal lining. Alginic acid is not an antacid because in the presence of saliva, it reacts with sodium bicarbonate to form sodium alginate, and it protects the mucosa with its foaming, viscous, and floating properties. This foam may provide a barrier to reflux of stomach contents into the esophagus.

The ability of antacids to neutralize gastric acid has been labeled *acid-neutralizing capacity* (ANC). This ANC is the quantity of 1 M HCl (expressed in milliequivalents) that can be brought to pH 3.5 in 15 minutes (expressed as mEq/ml). Antacids with high ANC usually are more effective than others.

TREATMENT PRINCIPLES
Standardized Guidelines

- American Gastroenterological Association Medical Position Statement: Evaluation of Dyspepsia (http://www.guidelines.gov/)
- DeVault KR, Castell DO: Updated guidelines for the diagnosis and treatment of gastroesophageal reflux disease: the Practice Parameters Committee of the American College of Gastroenterology, *Am J Gastroenterol* 94:1434, 1999

Evidence-Based Recommendations

- H$_2$ inhibitors reduce the risk of persistent esophagitis but are not as strong as PPIs in terms of their ability to neutralize acid.
- Antacids reduce symptoms but do not have a significant effect on healing of erosions or esophagitis.

Cardinal Points of Treatment

- Patients should begin by making lifestyle changes in diet and by managing stress.
- *Diagnostic Guideline 1: Empirical Therapy*—If a patient's history is typical for uncomplicated GERD, an initial trial of empirical therapy is appropriate (with lifestyle modification, particularly weight loss and diet control in obese patients). Lack of response does not rule out GERD. Additional testing should be considered if GERD symptoms are refractory to empirical therapy.
- *Treatment Guideline II: Patient-Directed Therapy*—Antacids, H_2 receptor agonists, and omeprazole are available OTC in the United States. Patients should not self-medicate for longer than 14 days without further evaluation.
- *Treatment Guideline III: Acid Suppression*—The mainstay of treatment for GERD is acid suppression.
- *PPIs*—PPIs are first-line treatment because they are the most effective option. Few data favor one agent over another. Long-term therapy is beneficial in chronic and complicated GERD. Higher than approved dosages may be indicated in certain situations. To achieve optimal benefit, PPIs should be taken 30 to 60 minutes prior to the timing of other medications, breakfast, or the evening meal.
- *H_2 receptor agonists*—H_2 receptor agonists may be used as premedication before meals. Efficacy may outlast that of antacids. Once-a-day dosing is not appropriate as long-term therapy for GERD.
- *Promotility agents (cisapride and metoclopramide)*—These have poor side effect profiles but may be used as adjunctive acid suppression therapy for GERD. Promotility agents may eliminate the root cause of GERD and may make acid suppression unnecessary. Promotility agents are not effective as monotherapy for GERD.
- The goals of treatment include symptomatic relief and prevention of complications. GERD is a lifelong disease that requires lifestyle modifications and medications as indicated.

Nonpharmacologic Treatment

Lifestyle modifications form the foundation of treatment; newer guidelines suggest that lifestyle modifications should be combined with use of an antacid or other medication. Many patients can relieve their symptoms by incorporating lifestyle changes without taking medications. Lifestyle modifications include diet, weight loss if overweight, increased activity, cessation of smoking and alcohol use, and avoidance of drugs that decrease LES pressure (Table 24-1).

Pharmacologic Treatment

- GERD refers to endoscopically determined esophagitis or endoscopy-negative reflux disease. Patients with uninvestigated "reflux-like" symptoms should be treated similarly to patients with uninvestigated dyspepsia. Medical treatment is based on the severity of symptoms.
- Offer patients with GERD a full-dose PPI for 1 or 2 months.
- If symptoms recur following initial treatment, offer a PPI at the lowest dose possible to control symptoms, along with a limited number of repeat prescriptions.
- Discuss with patients using the treatment on an "on demand" basis to manage their own symptoms.
- Offer H_2RA or prokinetic therapy if response to a PPI is inadequate.

MILD, INTERMITTENT SYMPTOMS. Antacids are used for immediate relief of intermittent heartburn. Because their duration of action is only 2 hours, H_2 blockers can be used if symptoms last longer than 2 hours, or if they occur at night. OTC doses are usually sufficient. These drugs require at least 30 minutes to take effect; they also can be taken before a meal that is expected to cause heartburn.

MODERATE SYMPTOMS. Patients who experience symptoms several times a week or daily should be treated with a PPI or a prescription strength H_2 blocker. Twice-a-day dosing of an H_2 blocker or once-daily PPI will provide 24-hour reduction in acidity. PPIs often are used as first-line treatment because they are more effective in reducing acid when compared with H_2 blockers. They provide the advantage of once-a-day dosing, but they are much more expensive. One PPI, omeprazole, is available OTC for 14 days of use in both generic and brand forms. Patients should not self-medicate with omeprazole for longer than 14 days without undergoing further evaluation because of the risks of Barrett's esophagus and other complications. Treatment for moderate symptoms

TABLE 24-1   Lifestyle Modification Treatment for GERD

Lifestyle Area	Modification
Activity	Sit up for at least 1 hr after eating. Elevate head of bed 6-8 in, using blocks. Pillows are less effective and can be counter-effective if they cause bending at the waist. Avoid straining, lifting, bending over, and wearing tight belts, especially on a full stomach.
Avoidance of causative drugs	Avoid drugs that decrease lower esophageal sphincter pressure such as theophylline, nitrates, calcium channel blockers, α-adrenergic antagonists, β-agonists, and benzodiazepines. Avoid anticholinergics and other drugs that decrease salivation; avoid drugs that decrease peristalsis.
Diet	Avoid foods that decrease lower esophageal sphincter pressure such as onions, garlic, mint, and alcohol. Avoid foods that are esophageal irritants such as citrus, vinegar, caffeine, chocolate, peppermint, red sauces, spicy and high-fat foods, and large meals, as well as excessive fluid intake with meals.
Smoking and alcohol intake	Cease smoking and alcohol use to reduce GI and esophageal irritation.
Weight loss	Strive for a gradual, sustained loss of 2 lb per month if overweight.

should continue for 4 to 8 weeks. Intermittent treatment (treatment when symptoms recur) is the usual plan of treatment for mild to moderate disease.

SEVERE SYMPTOMS AND EROSIVE DISEASE. If the patient has severe symptoms, has found treatment for milder symptoms to be ineffective, or has experienced erosion that is documented by endoscopy, he or she should be started on a PPI. Initial dosing is provided at the usual starting dose once a day. If this is not effective, the dose should be increased to twice a day. The usual course of therapy is 8 to 12 weeks, which allows for healing of the erosions. Repeat endoscopy is not required if the patient responds to treatment. Most patients should be allowed a trial off medication, although relapse is frequent, at a rate of about 80%. In cases of relapse (usually within the first 3 months), maintenance therapy should be provided. The dose used for maintenance therapy may not have to be as high as that given for initial treatment. If patients do not respond to therapy, they should be referred for consideration of surgery.

Promotility drugs such as metoclopramide or bethanechol reduce reflux by increasing LES tone and promoting peristalsis and gastric emptying. Because of their potential for serious adverse effects, these agents are not recommended for GERD unless therapy with a PPI or an H_2RA yields no response. Sucralfate enhances mucosal protection. These drugs are frequently added to the standard regimen.

ADDITIONAL CONSIDERATIONS. Antacids with the highest ANC include sodium bicarbonate and calcium carbonate. Sodium bicarbonate is not suitable for long-term use because of side effects. Calcium carbonate requires monitoring for long-term effects.

The clinician must consider drug formulation because it affects efficacy. Suspension and gel formulations have higher ANC than do powders or tablets. Tablets must be chewed thoroughly to be effective; they work best if taken with a full glass of water. Tablets may be more convenient for occasional indigestion.

Timing of antacid administration is important; for the greatest effectiveness, they should be taken 30 minutes after meals. This increases the amount of time that the antacid is in the stomach and is functioning as an antacid. Taking antacids on an empty stomach is not as effective because of the short transit time through the stomach. Taken properly, their duration of action is 2 hours. To avoid drug interactions, it is important to take antacids 1 hour before or 2 hours after taking other medications.

Antacids with calcium may cause constipation. Aluminum may cause constipation; magnesium may cause diarrhea. These second two ingredients usually are given together to balance the effect on the bowels. Antacids with sodium bicarbonate have sufficient sodium to cause problems in patients with hypertension or CHF. Other antacids vary in their sodium content by brand name. If the patient is on a low-salt diet, the sodium content of the antacid should be checked before prescribing. If the patient has any renal insufficiency, magnesium intake should be limited; if given, magnesium levels should be checked periodically. Antacids with calcium may precipitate kidney stones in the predisposed patient.

Antacids were the mainstay of treatment for GERD and peptic ulcer disease for many years, until the antisecretory agents were developed. Antacids are less convenient, less palatable, and less effective than antisecretories in reducing acid, and they have a higher incidence of unpleasant side effects, especially diarrhea and constipation.

How to Monitor

- Monitor electrolytes (magnesium, sodium, or calcium levels as indicated) with long-term use of antacids.
- Evaluate therapeutic effect by following symptom resolution.
- Assess GI and renal status.
- Monitor for adverse effects.

Patient Variables

GERIATRICS
- Avoid using antacids that contain magnesium in elderly patients with renal failure because they may develop hypermagnesemia.
- Avoid sodium-containing antacids because of fluid retention.

PEDIATRICS. Safety has not been established in children.

PREGNANCY. No FDA category has been established, although antacids generally are considered safe for use in pregnancy.

Patient Education

- The patient should notify the health care provider if taking any other medications. Antacids may interact, so they should be taken 1 hour before or 2 hours after other medications are taken.
- If a chewable antacid is prescribed, chew the tablet completely and follow by drinking at least an 8 oz glass of water.
- Shake liquid preparations thoroughly before taking, to ensure accurate dosage.
- Store liquid formulations in a cool place, but do not freeze. Refrigeration may make them taste better.
- Antacids may cause constipation or diarrhea. Either should be reported to the health care provider.
- Notify provider if you see symptoms of bleeding such as black tarry stools or "coffee ground" vomitus.
- The effectiveness of antacids decreases with the age of the medication. Be sure to discard out-of-date antacids.
- Antacids should not be used for longer than 2 weeks without further evaluation by the provider.

SPECIFIC DRUGS

CALCIUM SALTS

calcium carbonate (Tums, Rolaids) 🔑

CONTRAINDICATIONS
- Hypercalcemia, renal calculi, hypophosphatemia
- Patients with suspected digoxin toxicity

WARNINGS
- Sodium content of antacids can be important in patients with hypertension, CHF, or renal failure, and in those on a low-salt diet.

Continued

calcium carbonate (Tums, Rolaids) 🔑 —cont'd

💣 ACID REBOUND

Antacids may cause dose-related rebound hyperacidity within 2 hours after administration. The stomach responds to the higher pH by producing more gastric acid. This is compensated for by the antacids.

It is not clear whether acid rebound is clinically important, except when antacids are discontinued. Monitor for increased symptoms when routinely administered antacids are discontinued.

- *Milk-alkali syndrome:* This may occur as an acute illness with symptoms of headache, nausea, irritability, and weakness, or it may be a chronic illness with alkalosis, hypercalcemia, and possible renal impairment. This syndrome can occur with high doses of calcium carbonate or sodium bicarbonate.
- *Hypophosphatemia:* Prolonged use of aluminum-containing antacids may result in hypophosphatemia, if phosphate intake is not adequate. Hypophosphatemia can cause anorexia, malaise, muscle weakness, and osteomalacia.
- Use with caution in patients with renal function impairment. Hypermagnesemia and toxicity may occur in patients with impaired renal function because of decreased clearance of magnesium ion. Osteomalacia may result; prolonged use of aluminum-containing antacids in patients with renal failure my cause or worsen osteomalacia. Aluminum is deposited in bone, and calcium is relatively safe.

PRECAUTIONS

- *GI hemorrhage:* Use aluminum hydroxide with care in patients with recent massive upper GI hemorrhage.
- *Lipid effects:* Antacids may have an effect on lipid levels, but this effect has not been well studied.
- *Aspirin:* Do not use in combination in chronic pain syndromes. Alkalinization of the urine accelerates aspirin excretion, and systemic alkalosis of increased sodium load may occur.

ADVERSE EFFECTS. Adverse effects depend on the major ingredient(s). Most adverse effects are self-limiting and mild, especially with short-term use (Table 24-2). In long-term use, significant adverse effects can occur.

PHARMACOKINETICS

- Antacids vary in terms of the extent to which they are absorbed. Sodium bicarbonate is absorbed most extensively. About 25% to 35% of the calcium is absorbed. Small amounts of aluminum are absorbed systemically. 💣 Approximately 5% to 20% of the magnesium can be systemically absorbed. It is the systemic absorption that is responsible for many of the adverse reactions.
- Antacids that are not absorbed pass through the intestines and are eliminated in the feces. Aluminum-containing antacids bind with phosphate ions in the intestine to form insoluble aluminum phosphate that is excreted in the feces.
- If ingested 1 hour after meals, antacids reduce gastric acidity for about 2 to 3 hours. However, when ingested during fasting, antacids reduce acidity for only 20 to 40 minutes because of rapid gastric emptying.

DRUG INTERACTIONS

- Antacids inhibit the absorption of many drugs. Take drugs 2 hours before or after an antacid to avoid drug interactions.
- Drug interactions are an important consideration (Table 24-3) and may occur through three different mechanisms. The first involves increasing the gastric pH; disintegration, dissolution, solubility, ionization, and gastric emptying time are altered. This decreases the absorption of weakly acidic drugs (digoxin, phenytoin, chlorpromazine, isoniazid). The absorption of weakly basic drugs is increased, possibly resulting in toxicity or adverse reactions (pseudoephedrine, levodopa).
- The second mechanism of drug interaction occurs when drugs are adsorbed or are bound to the antacid surface, resulting in decreased bioavailability (tetracycline). Magnesium antacids have the greatest adsorption; calcium and aluminum exhibit an intermediate ability to adsorb medications.

TABLE 24-2 Common and Serious Adverse Effects of Antacids

Drug	Common Adverse Effects	Serious Adverse Effects
All antacids		Acid rebound Milk-alkali syndrome (dose dependent)
Calcium	Constipation	Milk-alkali syndrome
Sodium		Sodium retention Milk-alkali syndrome, renal stones
Aluminum	Constipation	Hypophosphatemia; aluminum intoxication; accumulation in serum, bone, central nervous system; encephalopathy Osteomalacia in patients who have renal failure
Magnesium	Diarrhea	Hypermagnesemia in patients who have renal failure

calcium carbonate (Tums, Rolaids) 🗝 —cont'd

- The third mechanism of drug interaction is triggered by increasing urinary pH. This affects the rate of drug elimination; increased urinary pH inhibits the excretion of basic drugs (quinidine, amphetamines) and enhances the excretion of acidic drugs (salicylates).

Sodium antacids have the greatest effect on urinary pH. Have the patient take the antacid 2 hours before or after taking other medications to reduce the likelihood of adverse effects.

DOSAGE AND ADMINISTRATION. See Table 24-4.

TABLE 24-3 Drug Interactions With Antacids

Antacid	Effect
Calcium	Decreased action of fluoroquinolones, hydantoins, iron salts, tetracycline, atenolol
Sodium	Increased action of amphetamines, flecainide, quinidine Decreased action of benzodiazepines, iron salts, ketoconazole, lithium, methotrexate
Aluminum	Increased action of benzodiazepines Decreased action of allopurinol, chloroquine, corticosteroids, diflunisal, digoxin, ethambutol, histamine (H₂) antagonists, iron salts, isoniazid, imidazole, antifungals
Magnesium	Increased action of dicumarol Decreased action of benzodiazepines, chloroquine, corticosteroids, digoxin, H₂ antagonists, hydantoins, iron salts, nitrofurantoin

TABLE 24-4 Dosage and Administration Recommendations for Antacids

Drug	Dosage	Administration
CALCIUM CARBONATE		
Tums	0.5-1.5 g	As needed q2h; maximum 7 g/day
Rolaids chewable		
sodium bicarbonate	325mg-2 g per day dissolved in 6 oz water	1-4 times per day
aluminum hydroxide (Amphojel)	600-1200 mg	tid with meals and q evening
aluminum carbonate (Basaljel)		
MAGNESIUM SALTS		
magnesium hydroxide (Milk of Magnesia)	>12 yr: 5-15 ml liquid or 650 mg-1.3 g	qid (maximum)
magnesium oxide	4-5 capsules (140 mg each)	Once daily with food
	2 tablets (400 mg each)	Once daily with food
COMBINATION PRODUCTS		
alginic acid, sodium bicarbonate, magnesium trisilicate, calcium stearate (Gaviscon)	2-4 tablets (extra-strength tablets); 15-30 ml	qid (20-60 min after meals and at bedtime)
aluminum hydroxide and magnesium hydroxide (Maalox)	2-4 tablets; suspension 10-20 ml	qid (between meals and at bedtime); up to 6× per day
aluminum hydroxide and magnesium hydroxide (Mylanta, Mylanta Double Strength)	5-10 ml	qid (between meals and at bedtime) up to 6× per day

OTHER DRUGS IN CLASS

Other antacids are similar to the key drug, except as follows:
- *Sodium bicarbonate (Alka-Seltzer)* is a well-known antacid that often is used OTC; it has a greater number of adverse effects than other antacids and is not recommended for use. It usually is found in combination with other medications such as aspirin.
- *Aluminum hydroxide (Amphojel)* has a relatively high risk of significant adverse reactions when used on a long-term basis.
- Magnesium hydroxide (Milk of Magnesia) carries the risk of adverse reactions, primarily in patients with renal failure. Avoid in geriatric patients. Do not use in children younger than 12 years.

evolve A continually updated list of useful WebLinks may be found in the Evolve Resources at http://evolve.elsevier.com/Edmunds/NP/

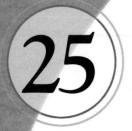

25 Histamine-2 Blockers and Proton Pump Inhibitors

DRUG OVERVIEW

Class	Subclass	Generic Name	Trade Name
Antisecretory agents	H₂ Receptor antagonists/H₂ blockers	ranitidine 🗝 ☀	Zantac ☀, generic, OTC ☀
		cimetidine	Tagamet, generic, OTC
		famotidine ☀	Pepcid, generic, OTC
		nizatidine	Axid, generic
	Proton pump inhibitors	omeprazole 🗝 ☀	Prilosec, generic, OTC
		esomeprazole	Nexium ☀
		lansoprazole	Prevacid ☀
		pantoprazole	Protonix ☀
		rabeprazole	AcipHex ☀

☀ Top 200 drug; 🗝 key drug. Ranitidine is the most commonly used H₂ receptor antagonist. Omeprazole is considered the key PPI because it is available OTC and generic.

INDICATIONS

- Histamine (H₂) blockers/H₂ receptor antagonists
  - Duodenal ulcer treatment and maintenance
  - Gastric ulcer treatment
  - GERD
  - Pathologic hypersecretory conditions
- Proton pump inhibitors (PPIs)
  - Gastric and duodenal ulcers
  - GERD
  - Pathologic hypersecretory conditions
  - *Helicobacter pylori*

H₂ blockers (H₂ receptor antagonists) and PPIs block acid secretion in the stomach but do so via different mechanisms of action. In general, all H₂ blockers, except cimetidine, are considered equally effective and have similar side effect profiles. The indications and off-label uses for each agent are listed in Table 25-1. These distinctions are not always observed in practice.

PPIs generally are considered to be more powerful in terms of action than H₂ blockers because they decrease stomach acidity to a greater extent. Five PPIs are available, and little difference between them has been noted, except for duration of action.

THERAPEUTIC OVERVIEW
Anatomy and Physiology

Several protective factors work together to protect the stomach mucosa from injury. The gastric mucosal barrier resists backward diffusion of hydrogen ions and thus has the ability to contain a high concentration of hydrochloric acid within the gastric lumen, unless an injurious agent breaks the barrier.

Endogenous prostaglandins are thought to provide cytoprotection against injurious agents and are synthesized abundantly in the mucosa of the stomach and duodenum. They are known to stimulate secretion of both mucus and bicarbonate and to maintain mucosal blood flow.

Mucus also mediates mucosal protection. It is secreted by surface epithelial cells and forms a gel that covers the mucosal surface and physically protects the mucosa from abrasion. It also resists the passage of large molecules such as pepsin. Bicarbonate is produced in small amounts by surface epithelial cells and diffuses up from the mucosa to create a thin layer of alkalinity between the mucus and the epithelial surface. Other protective factors include mucosal blood flow, epithelial renewal, and epidermal growth factor that is secreted in saliva and by the duodenal mucosa.

The mucosal surface of the stomach is divided according to type of gland, namely, the oxyntic (parietal) gland area, which secretes acid, and the pyloric gland area, which does not. The most important cell types in these glandular areas are mucous and peptic cells, which are found in both glandular areas;

TABLE 25-1 Indications and Unlabeled Uses for H₂ Blockers and PPIs

	cimetidine	famotidine	nizatidine	ranitidine	esomeprazole	omeprazole	lansoprazole	pantoprazole	rabeprazole
Duodenal ulcer treatment and maintenance	•	•	•	•	•	•	•	X	•
GERD	•	•	•	•	•	•	•	•	•
Gastric ulcer treatment and maintenance	•	•	•	•	•	•	•	X	X
Pathologic hypersecretory conditions	•	•	X	•	•	•	•	•	•
Heartburn/indigestion, sour stomach	•	•		•	X	•	X	X	X
Erosive esophagitis, maintenance	•	•	X		•	•	X	•	•
Prevent upper GI bleeding	•	X	X	X	X	•	X	X	X
NSAID-associated ulcer	X	X	X	X	•	X	•	X	X
H. pylori–associated ulcer	X	X	X	•	•	X	•	X	•

•, Indication; X, unlabeled use.

oxyntic cells, which occur only in the oxyntic gland area; and endocrine cells, which are scattered throughout both glandular areas. The oxyntic gland area occupies most of the mucosal surface of the stomach. The oxyntic cells secrete HCl through an energy-dependent active transport mechanism, along with intrinsic factor, a protein required for the absorption of vitamin B_{12}.

The stomach has three naturally occurring secretagogues that stimulate acid secretion. These include acetylcholine (a neurotransmitter), gastrin (a hormone), and histamine (a paracrine substance). Receptor activation by these secretagogues initiates biochemical steps that lead to active transport of hydrogen by the oxyntic cell. Histamine, released by mast cells, binds to the H_2 receptor that activates intracellular stimulatory protein G and eventually activates membrane-bound adenosine triphosphatase (ATPase). This proton pump provides the energy to extrude hydrogen from the oxyntic cell in exchange for potassium. In this manner, histamine initiates a train of intracellular events that stimulate the continuous secretion of acid.

The rate of secretion varies greatly, depending on the time of day or night and the proximity to the time that a meal was eaten. When the stomach is at rest, the rate of secretion is low. This basal rate contrasts greatly with the high rate of secretion found at mealtime. Basal secretion in the human stomach exhibits a circadian rhythm, characterized by a maximal rate in the evening and a minimal rate in the morning.

The high rates of acid secretion surrounding mealtimes are reduced to the basal rate of secretion through inhibitory processes that begin to occur during a meal. Abatement of hunger suppresses the cephalic phase of gastric secretion. Secretion of HCl by oxyntic cells causes antral mucosal surface pH to fall to below 3.0, prompting the release of the paracrine substance, somatostatin. Somatostatin decreases gastrin release from G-cells and directly inhibits oxyntic cell secretion of acid.

Pathophysiology

Drugs that decrease acid production, or antisecretory agents, are used to prevent the autodigestion of the upper GI tract by the acid–pepsin complex. Drugs or foods that increase acid production may provoke autodigestion. This is often the pathogenesis of PUD. These agents not only cause injury themselves but also augment the injury initiated by other agents.

The mucosa of the upper GI tract is susceptible to injury from a variety of conditions and agents. Endogenous agents include acid, pepsin, bile acids, and other small intestine contents. Exogenous agents include ethanol, aspirin, and NSAIDs.

Acid is essential for the occurrence of peptic injury. A pH of 1 to 2 maximizes the activity of pepsin. In addition, mucosal injury from aspirin, other NSAIDs, and bile acids is augmented in the presence of acid. On the other hand, ethanol causes mucosal injury with or without acid. Corticosteroids, smoking, and physiologic and psychologic stress predispose some people to mucosal injury via mechanisms that are not completely understood. When negative feedback is overwhelmed or is ineffective, erosion (<5 mm lesion) or an ulcer (>5 mm in diameter) may result. Ulcers represent loss of the enteric surface epithelium that extends deeply enough to reach or penetrate the muscularis mucosae. Because pepsin is active only at a pH of 1 to 4,

neutralization of acid or inhibition of acid production eliminates the harmful effects of pepsin.

Disease Process

Peptic ulcer is defined as a break in the gastric or duodenal mucosa that extends through the muscularis mucosae. It arises when the normal mucosal defensive factors are impaired or overwhelmed. Duodenal ulcers are more common between the ages of 30 and 55 years and in males; gastric ulcers are more common between the ages of 55 and 70 years. Ulcers are five times more common in the duodenum than in the stomach. Duodenal ulcers are almost never malignant, whereas 3% to 5% of gastric ulcers are malignant.

Three important causes of PUD have been identified: NSAIDs, *H. pylori,* and acid hypersecretory states such as Zollinger-Ellison syndrome. The provider should confirm the presence of *H. pylori* and NSAID use before determining whether other therapy is warranted.

MECHANISM OF ACTION

Medications that inhibit acid secretion can act in several ways at several locations on or in the oxyntic cell. H_2 receptor antagonist drugs can bind to the H_2 receptor, thereby displacing histamine from receptor binding sites and preventing stimulation of the oxyntic cell by the secretagogue. The four H_2 receptor antagonists have similar chemical structures. They reversibly inhibit basal or histamine-, pentagastrin-, or meal-stimulated acid secretion in a linear, dose-dependent manner by interfering with histamine at the H_2 receptors on the gastric parietal cells. As much as 90% inhibition of vagal and gastrin-stimulated acid secretion occurs with these agents, reflecting the importance of histamine in the mediation of cholinergic and gastrin-stimulated acid secretion. Near-complete inhibition of nocturnal acid secretion may be achieved as well.

PPIs irreversibly inhibit the acid secretory pump embedded within the parietal cell membrane by altering the activity of hydrogen potassium ATPase (H^+/K^+ ATPase). This enzyme affects the secretory pump in the gastric parietal cell by inhibiting hydrogen ion transport into the gastric lumen and by decreasing stimulated acid secretion. It decreases the volume of gastric fluid. An increase in serum gastrin concentrations is observed. Because PPIs act on the basolateral membrane of the parietal cell, they do not affect gastric emptying, basal or stimulated pepsin output, or secretion of intrinsic factor. This type of drug does not seem to affect the ATPase of other organ systems.

TREATMENT PRINCIPLES
Standardized Guidelines

- Talley NJ: American Gastroenterological Association Medical Position Statement: Evaluation of Dyspepsia, *Gastroenterology* 129:1753-1755, 2005.

Evidence-Based Recommendations

- To facilitate healing and to decrease the risk for recurrence of gastric and duodenal ulcers, *H. pylori* should be eradicated in patients with PUD (level of evidence).
- PPIs offer suppression of acid secretion, healing, and symptom relief in patients with peptic ulcers that are superior to those associated with other antisecretory therapies (level of evidence).

- Patients with bleeding peptic ulcers should be treated with a PPI to decrease the need for transfusion or surgery and to reduce the duration of hospital stay. Those with bleeding peptic ulcer and positive *H. pylori* testing should have eradication therapy prescribed (level of evidence).
- Patients with perforated ulcers should undergo eradication of coexisting *H. pylori* infection. Successful eradication should reduce the need for long-term antisecretory therapy and additional surgery (level of evidence).

Cardinal Points of Treatment

- In patients with ulcer symptoms, treat *H. pylori* if present (see Table 25-3). This is cardinal in resolving the problem and not just in treating the symptoms.
- Patients should stop NSAID use if possible.
- Begin PPI therapy along with lifestyle modifications, particularly diet and stress management.

Nonpharmacologic Treatment

Lifestyle modifications are integral to treatment for PUD. Recommendations no longer include bland or restrictive diets. Patients should eat balanced meals at regular times and should avoid foods that exacerbate symptoms. High fiber is encouraged. Caffeine causes increased acid secretion and should be avoided. Alcohol can aggravate an ulcer but usually does not appear to be harmful when taken in moderation. Smoking should be strongly discouraged.

Pharmacologic Treatment

Goals include relief of symptoms and healing of the ulcer. Treatment consists of a course of an H_2 blocker or a PPI. In general, PPIs are used first line because they are more potent and require a shorter course of treatment. H_2 blockers are less expensive and usually are also effective. If the patient does not start to see improvement within a few days, increase the dose of medication or change from an H_2 blocker to a PPI.

H_2 blockers (e.g., ranitidine, famotidine, cimetidine) are associated with 70% to 80% healing of duodenal ulcers after 4 weeks, and with 87% to 94% healing after 8 weeks. PPIs should be given for 4 weeks for a duodenal ulcer and for 8 weeks for a gastric ulcer and are associated with 80% to 100% healing. See Table 25-2 for recommendations on therapy details.

TABLE 25-2 Usual Length of Treatment

Type of Medication	Indication	Length of Time
H_2 blockers	Duodenal ulcer	8 wk
	Eradication of *H. pylori*	Short term
	Erosive esophagitis	Long term
	Gastric ulcer	12 wk
	GERD	12 wk
	Heartburn	Short term
	Hypersecretory conditions	Long term
	Prevention of gastric NSAID damage	Long term
	Upper GI bleeding	Short term
Proton pump inhibitors	Active duodenal ulcer	4-8 wk
	GERD	4-8 wk
	Hypersecretory conditions	Long term

H. PYLORI ULCER. The *H. pylori* organism must be eradicated to prevent recurrence; several treatment regimens are available. In general, an acid suppressant (i.e., an H_2 blocker or a PPI) is combined with an antibiotic. Occasionally, this regimen includes bismuth. After this treatment has been completed, continue treatment of the ulcer with an acid suppressant. See Table 25-3 for dosing regimens for *H. pylori* treatment.

NSAID-INDUCED ULCER. Discontinue the NSAID if possible, and use a standard dosing regimen of an acid suppressant. Sometimes, it is impossible to discontinue the NSAID. Prevention of ulcers is used for high-risk patients on NSAIDs, such as those with a history of ulcer disease, concurrent therapy with corticosteroids or anticoagulants, serious illness, or advanced age. Options include continuous PPI or an H_2 blocker, misoprostol, or a COX-2 selective NSAID.

REFRACTORY ULCERS. Refractory ulcers (nonhealing after 8 to 12 weeks) are uncommon with antisecretory drugs and/or antimicrobial therapy. Consider pathologic hypersecretory conditions, and refer the patient to a gastroenterologist. Patients with a nonhealing gastric ulcer should be evaluated for cancer through repeat endoscopy after 3 to 4 months. Symptomatic response does not preclude the presence of a gastric malignancy.

TABLE 25-3 Treatment of Active *Helicobacter pylori* Ulcer

		Alternate Drug/Comments
STEP 1		
Option 1	PPI before meals bid Clarithromycin 500 mg bid Amoxicillin 1 g bid for 7-14 days	Treatment regimen of choice. If penicillin allergic, metronidazole 500 mg bid
Option 2	PPI before meals bid Bismuth subsalicylate 525 mg qid Tetracycline 500 mg qid Metronidazole 500 mg qid for 7-14 days	Can be used as first-line treatment but generally is reserved for retreatment (14 days)
Option 3	PPI before meals bid Amoxicillin 1 g bid Metronidazole 500 mg bid	First-line treatment in macrolide-allergic patients and retreatment if failed first-line treatment of choice for 14 days
STEP 2	Continue PPI every day for 4-8 weeks longer	H_2 blocker

H₂ BLOCKERS. All H₂ receptor blockers are capable of healing duodenal ulcers, relieving symptoms, and preventing complications. They are well tolerated and have a remarkably low incidence of side effects—less than 3%.

Single dosing at bedtime of H₂ receptor antagonists has been approved for the treatment of acute peptic ulcers. Evening dosing appears to provide optimal 24-hour inhibition. Early evening is the optimal time for once-daily dosing. Because all H₂ blockers have basically the same efficacy, there is no reason to switch from one to another if no symptomatic response is noted. Cimetidine is available OTC but has numerous drug–drug interactions. Ranitidine and famotidine are also available OTC but do not exhibit these interactions.

PROTON PUMP INHIBITORS. The PPIs are the most potent available inhibitors of gastric acid secretion and require a short duration of treatment. Another advantage is their once-daily dosing, which improves patient compliance. Because PPIs affect the actively secreting parietal cells, they should be given at mealtime. H₂ receptor antagonists should not be used concurrently with PPIs. Only omeprazole is available OTC.

How to Monitor

- Check stools and emesis for blood. It takes 72 hours to clear stool from the GI tract from a former bleed. Once the stool is negative for blood, no further hemoccult test is necessary, unless symptoms return or worsen.
- Assess for confusion, especially in elderly or debilitated patients and those with renal or hepatic dysfunction.
- Unusual weakness or tiredness may suggest blood dyscrasias.

H₂ BLOCKERS

- Monitor liver enzymes and platelets.
- Consider monitoring renal function, especially in the elderly.

Patient Variables

GERIATRICS

- Decreased liver and renal function may decrease elimination of drugs; reduce dose by one half.
- No adjustment of dosage is necessary with PPIs.

evolve For additional information, see the supplemental tables on the Evolve Learning Resources website.

PEDIATRICS. Clinical experience in children is limited. Safety and efficacy have not been established. Cimetidine is not recommended for children younger than 16 years of age.

PREGNANCY AND LACTATION

- All H₂ receptor antagonists cross the placenta; although they are believed to be safe, these agents are not recommended for use in the first trimester of pregnancy or by nursing mothers.
- *Category B:* H₂ blockers, lansoprazole, esomeprazole, rabeprazole, pantoprazole
- *Category C:* omeprazole
- H₂ blockers and PPIs are secreted in the milk.

RACE. Higher levels of omeprazole with equivalent doses have been noted in Japanese and Asian subjects. Consider lowering the dose.

Patient Education

H₂ BLOCKERS

- Do not take within 2 hours of antacid ingestion.
- H₂ receptor antagonists should be given after meals and at bedtime. If using once-a-day dosing, give medication before bedtime.
- Report any blood in vomitus or stool or any dark tarry stools, any unusual weakness or tiredness (may suggest blood dyscrasias), or confusion, especially in the elderly.
- Oral suspensions should be shaken vigorously for 5 to 10 seconds before each use.
- Unused constituted oral suspensions should be discarded after 30 days.

PROTON PUMP INHIBITORS

- The capsule should be swallowed whole; instruct patients not to crush or chew capsules.
- PPIs should be taken before meals.
- PPIs and H₂ blockers should not be used concurrently.

SPECIFIC DRUGS

H₂ RECEPTOR ANTAGONISTS

ranitidine (Zantac)

CONTRAINDICATIONS. Hypersensitivity

WARNINGS

- Hypersensitivity reactions: rare cases of anaphylaxis
- Reversible hepatitis and blood dyscrasias occur rarely.
- Because H₂ blockers are excreted by the kidney, dosage should be adjusted in patients with impaired renal function.
- Use with caution in patients with hepatic dysfunction.

PRECAUTIONS

⚫ **Symptomatic response to these agents does not preclude gastric malignancy.**

⚫ **Reversible central nervous system effects have occurred with cimetidine: disorientation, mental confusion, agitation, psychosis, μ depression anxiety, and hallucinations.**

- Use of cimetidine in the elderly is not recommended.
- Hepatocellular injury occurred with nizatidine and ranitidine, as evidence by elevated liver enzymes (AST, ALT, or alkaline phosphatase). All abnormalities reversed on discontinuation of the drug.

PHARMACOKINETICS

- See Table 25-4 for pharmacokinetics of all acid antisecretory drugs.
- All H₂ receptor antagonists are rapidly absorbed from the small intestine but not from the stomach. Absorption is unaffected by food but may be decreased by 30% or more by antacids and/or sucralfate. H₂ receptor antagonists are most often metabolized by the liver, except for nizatidine, which is largely excreted by the kidneys.

ranitidine (Zantac) —cont'd

ADVERSE EFFECTS. H₂ blockers, except for cimetidine, have a very low rate of side effects and are very safe. Because of drug interactions and an increased incidence of side effects, cimetidine is not as safe as the others (see Table 25-5 for adverse effects).

DRUG INTERACTIONS. See Table 25-6 for a summary of the drug interactions of H₂ blockers.

TABLE 25-4 Pharmacokinetics for Medications That Reduce Acidity

Drug	Availability (After First Pass)	Time to Peak Concentration	Half-life	Duration of Action	Protein Bound	Metabolism	Urinary Excretion
ranitidine	48%	2-3 hr	2-3 hr	—	15%	CYP 2D6 substrate; liver	30%-35%, unchanged
cimetidine	60%-70%	1-2 hr	1.5-2 hr	4-8 hr	20%	CYP 1A2, 2C9, and 3A4 inhibitor	48%, unchanged
famotidine	40%-50%	1-3 hr	2.5-3.5 hr	10-12 hr	15%-20%	Liver	30%, unchanged
nizatidine	>70%	1-3 hr	1.1-1.6 hr	—	35%	Liver	>90%, unchanged
omeprazole	45%	0.5-3.5 hr	0.5-1 hr	>2 hr	95%	Liver; CYP 2C19; 3A4	77%, metabolites
esomeprazole	64%	1.5 hr	1.5 hr	—	97%	Liver; CYP 2C19; 3A4	80%, metabolites
lansoprazole	85%	1.7 hr	1.5 hr	24 hr	97%	Liver; CYP 3A4; 2C19	33%, metabolites
pantoprazole	77%	2.4 hr	1 hr	>24 hr	98%	Liver; CYP 2C19; 3A4	71%, metabolites
rabeprazole	52%	2.5 hr	1-2 hr	24 hr	96.3%	Liver; CYP 2C19; 3A4	90%, metabolites

TABLE 25-5 Common and Serious Adverse Effects of Acid Antisecretory Agents

Drug	Common Minor Effects	Serious Adverse Effects
H₂ BLOCKERS	Very low incidence of side effects, most 1%; headache, vertigo, dizziness, diarrhea, constipation, vomiting, rash. May develop B₁₂ deficiency with long-term use	**Very rare: skin reactions, blood dyscrasias, elevated liver function tests (LFTs)**
ranitidine	Muscle aches, malaise, dry mouth	Blurred vision, malaise, reversible leukopenia, anaphylaxis, thrombocytopenia, hepatotoxicity
cimetidine	Arthralgias, myalgia, agitation, gynecomastia, impotence	Neutropenia, thrombocytopenia, agranulocytosis, aplastic anemia, central nervous system (CNS) effects such as confusion, dizziness, somnolence, headache, hallucinations; peripheral neuropathy, galactorrhea, epidermal necrolysis, anaphylaxis, arrhythmia
famotidine	Anorexia, dry mouth, taste changes	Musculoskeletal pain. anaphylaxis, agranulocytosis, thrombocytopenia, leukopenia, seizures, AV block
nizatidine	Fatigue, sweating, rhinitis, abdominal pain, confusion	Tachycardia, hyperuricemia, hepatitis, thrombocytopenia, exfoliative dermatitis, leukopenia
PROTON PUMP INHIBITORS	Headache, diarrhea	Hypertension, tachycardia, blood dyscrasias, hepatic dysfunction, anaphylactoid reactions, pancreatitis, severe skin reactions, interstitial nephritis
omeprazole	Headache, diarrhea, nausea, flatulence, abdominal pain, constipation, dry mouth	Bradycardia, peripheral edema, severe skin reactions, pancreatitis, interstitial nephritis
esomeprazole	Headache, diarrhea, nausea, flatulence, abdominal pain, constipation, dry mouth	Bradycardia, peripheral edema, high blood pressure
lansoprazole	Constipation	Gallbladder disease, esophagitis
pantoprazole		Insomnia, dizziness, somnolence, convulsions, rash
rabeprazole		Migraine, bradycardia, rhabdomyolysis

Bolded categories indicate most common problems.

TABLE 25-6 Drug Interactions With H$_2$ Blockers and Proton Pump Inhibitors

Acid Antisecretory Drug	Effects on Other Drug
HISTAMINE (H$_2$) BLOCKERS	Increased action of ethanol
ranitidine	cefuroxime, cefpodoxime, itraconazole, ketoconazole (decreased absorption); warfarin (increases or decreases prothrombin time)
cimetidine	Increased action of flecainide, fluorouracil, procainamide, succinylcholine, narcotic analgesics
	Decreased action of iron salts, indomethacin, ketoconazole, tetracyclines, digoxin, fluconazole, tocainide
famotidine	cefuroxime, cefpodoxime; delavirdine
nizatidine	itraconazole, ketoconazole
PROTON PUMP INHIBITORS	
omeprazole	Increased action of benzodiazepines, phenytoin, clarithromycin, warfarin
esomeprazole	warfarin, diazepam
lansoprazole	warfarin, indomethacin, ibuprofen, phenytoin, propranolol, prednisone, diazepam, clarithromycin
pantoprazole	warfarin
rabeprazole	warfarin

OTHER DRUGS IN CLASS

Other drugs in this class are similar to the key drug, except as follows:

- *Nizatidine (Axid)* does not inhibit the cytochrome P450 (CYP450)-linked drug-metabolizing enzyme system; therefore, drug interactions mediated by inhibition of hepatic metabolism are not expected to occur.
- *Cimetidine* has extensive drug interactions, many related to its metabolism by the CYP 1A2, 2C9, 2C19, 2D6, and especially 3A4 enzymes. It interacts with numerous medications. Consult a detailed reference for a complete listing. Toxic doses may be associated with respiratory failure and tachycardia that may be controlled by assisted respiration and the use of β-blockers.
- *Famotidine* seems to have similar adverse effects and effectiveness profiles but with fewer drug interactions.
- Calcium carbonate, magnesium hydroxide, and famotidine *(Pepcid Complete)* combines the H$_2$ receptor antagonists with an antacid; this can be very useful for both GERD and PUD.

PROTON PUMP INHIBITORS

omeprazole (Prilosec) 🔑

CONTRAINDICATIONS. Hypersensitivity

WARNINGS/PRECAUTIONS

- Omeprazole should be prescribed only for the conditions, dosages, and durations described.
- This agent crosses the placenta and is distributed in breast milk.
- Patients should be cautioned that capsules should not be opened, chewed, or crushed and should be swallowed whole.
- Safety and effectiveness in children have not been established.

PHARMACOKINETICS. Because the absorption of PPIs is enhanced in an alkaline medium, more is absorbed as they inhibit the secretion of gastric acid.

- The half-life of these drugs is about 60 minutes; however, they have a very long duration of action—at least 72 hours. It takes about 3 to 5 days for gastric acid secretion to return to normal after discontinuation of these drugs because the H$^+$/K$^+$ ATPase enzyme has to be synthesized again.
- Tolerance and rebound hypersecretion after discontinuation do not appear to be issues.
- Protein binding occurs at a rate of 95% to 97%. The drugs are metabolized extensively in the liver and then are excreted in urine.

ADVERSE EFFECTS. PPIs have an even lower incidence of adverse reactions than do H$_2$ blockers.

DRUG INTERACTIONS

- See Tables 25-6 and 25-7 for specific interactions. Omeprazole induces CYP 1A2; inhibits 2C8, 2C9, 2C19, and 3A4 isoenzyme systems; and may interfere with the metabolism of other drugs that use these systems. Lansoprazole uses the CYP 3A4 and 2C19 enzymes without the occurrence of clinically significant drug interactions (does not inhibit these enzymes). Pantoprazole uses the C19 and 3A4 enzymes without significant interactions. Rabeprazole uses 2C19 and 3A4 and inhibits 2C8 and 2C19. Esomeprazole uses 2C19 and inhibits 2C19.
- Because these drugs decrease gastric acid, they may interfere with the absorption of drugs that require absorption in an acid stomach; these include ketoconazole, ampicillin, iron salts, digoxin, and cyanocobalamin.

TABLE 25-7 Other Drug Interactions

Other Drugs	Effect on Antisecretory Drugs
Antacids, anticholinergics, metoclopramide	Decreased action of H$_2$ blockers
clarithromycin, sucralfate	Decreased action of omeprazole
sucralfate	Decreased action of lansoprazole

OTHER DRUGS IN CLASS

Other drugs in this class are similar to the key drug, except as follows:

- *Esomeprazole (Nexium)* is essentially identical to omeprazole, except that it has a longer duration of action, requiring only once-a-day dosing.
- *Rabeprazole (Aciphex)* is less expensive than the others, except for pantoprazole. This drug comes as a small pill and is easy to swallow.

- *Pantoprazole (Protonix)* is the least expensive of the PPIs, except for generic omeprazole.

---

evolve A continually updated list of useful WebLinks may be found in the Evolve Resources at http://evolve.elsevier.com/Edmunds/NP/

26 Laxatives

DRUG OVERVIEW

Class	Subclass	Generic Name	Trade Name
Bulk laxatives		psyllium 🔑	Metamucil, Fiberall
		methylcellulose	Citrucel
		calcium polycarbophil	FiberCon, Fiberall Chewable
Emollients/fecal softeners		docusate sodium, calcium	Colace, Surfak 🔑
		mineral oil	
Osmotic laxatives		lactulose	Chronulac, Cephulac
		sorbitol	
		polyethylene glycol ✴	MiraLax, GoLYTELY
		glycerol (glycerin)	Generic suppositories
		lubiprostone	Amitiza
Saline laxatives	Magnesium	magnesium hydroxide	Milk of Magnesia 🔑
		magnesium sulfate	Epsom salts
		magnesium citrate	Generic
Stimulants	Diphenylmethane derivatives	bisacodyl	Dulcolax 🔑
	Anthraquinone derivatives	cascara sagrada	
		senna	Senokot, X-Prep
		casanthranol	
Enemas		sodium phosphate	Fleet enema
		soap suds	
		tap water	
		oil retention–mineral oil	

✴ Top 200 drug, 🔑 key drug. Drugs marked as key drugs are those most commonly used. Drugs are listed in general order of potency.

INDICATIONS

- All
  - Constipation
  - Prophylaxis of constipation
  - Polyethylene glycol (GoLYTELY), sodium phosphate enema, magnesium citrate: surgical or procedural preparation
  - Saline: expedite cleansing of the body of toxins or parasites

- Psyllium: irritable bowel syndrome and diverticular disease
- Polycarbophil: irritable bowel syndrome, diverticulosis, acute nonspecific diarrhea
- Mineral oil enema: relief of fecal impaction
- Lactulose: hepatic encephalopathy
- Lubriprostone: chronic idiopathic constipation

Laxatives are divided into five primary categories, which vary in terms of mechanism of action, potency, effect, indication, and cost. These five categories consist of bulk, stool softeners, osmotic, stimulants, and enemas.

THERAPEUTIC OVERVIEW

Anatomy and Physiology

The large intestine contains a mixture of the remnants of several meals ingested over 3 to 4 days. The ascending colon holds the contents of the stomach for about an hour. The transverse colon is the primary site for processing feces. The descending colon is a holding tank and conduit for feces for about 24 hours. The sigmoid colon and the rectum act as reservoirs. The nerves responsible for the activation of mass movement are located in the descending colon. Skeletal muscles that maintain continence are located in the surrounding pelvic floor. The integrity of the nervous system is necessary for coordination of the defecation process.

Contractions occur almost continuously in the large intestine and are divided into two basic types. The segmental pattern of motility occurs in the transverse colon, where most of the removal of water and electrolytes occurs and feces are moved forward very slowly. The circular muscles are responsible for segmental contractions. Ring-like contractions divide the colon into chambers called *haustra*. Haustrations mix and compress the feces, facilitating absorption of water while moving the feces backward and slowly forward. The second type of contraction, the mass movement (power propulsion), is a different process that occurs in the transverse and descending colon to promote bowel movements. Evacuation is aided by (1) voluntary muscles of the abdomen that contract to promote propulsion, (2) relaxation of the circular muscles, with disappearance of haustral contractions, and (3) distention of the gut caused by increased contents of the bowel. The increase in mass movements after a meal is called the *gastrocolic reflex*.

Pathophysiology

An abnormality anywhere in the evacuation system can cause constipation. Without enough mass, contractions are not stimulated. Disruption of the nerves that control the process prevents proper stimulation of the muscles. Weakness of the muscles of the abdominal wall, of the circular muscles (segmental contractions), or of the muscles that control mass movement also inhibits a bowel movement. Pain with stretching of the gut inhibits contractions. Any structural defect forms a physical barrier to proper transit.

Disease Process

Constipation is a very common complaint among individuals of all ages, leading to 2.5 million physician visits annually in the United States. Prevalence ranges from 2% to 27%.

Constipation means very different things to different patients. Often it is perceived as infrequent or difficult defecation. Some of these changes normally occur if a patient becomes less active or eats less food. The frequency of bowel movements in normal patients ranges from 3 to 12 a week. Changes in consistency are generally due to changes in the amount of fiber eaten. The objective definition of constipation is two or fewer bowel movements per week, or excessive difficulty and straining at defecation.

Chronic functional constipation (CC) and irritable bowel syndrome with constipation (IBS-C) are both functional GI disorders. The definitions of these conditions, which are diagnosed on the basis of symptom criteria, were updated in 2005 with the use of the Rome III criteria. This framework is particularly helpful for categorizing symptoms in difficult cases. According to Rome III, symptoms must be present over the previous 3 months and must have an onset at least 6 months prior to the time of diagnosis. For CC, symptom criteria include straining, lumpy or hard stool, and a sense of incomplete evacuation. Patients also must have insufficient criteria to be given a diagnosis of IBS.

True clinical constipation includes the diagnostic findings of a large amount of feces in the rectal ampulla on digital examination and/or excessive fecal loading of the colon, rectum, or both on abdominal radiograph. Constipation can be acute or chronic, intermittent or continuous.

Constipation has many causes, ranging from inadequate fiber to colon cancer. Medications are an important cause (Table 26-1). Systemic disease may cause constipation through neurologic gut dysfunction, myopathies, and electrolyte imbalances. Diabetic patients may have autonomic nerve dysfunction. Structural causes can be the result of a congenital defect or the structural obstruction of a mass, which may be cancerous. Any sudden change in bowel habits warrants a thorough investigation. The primary cause is a disturbance in motility; secondary causes include medications, malignancy, and non-GI disease.

Irritable bowel syndrome (IBS) is characterized by a strong relationship between abdominal pain and defecation. Individuals with IBS have visceral hypersensitivity, or increased perception of gut-related events. In IBS, the onset of constipation generally corresponds with an onset of pain at defecation. In patients with functional constipation, some abdominal discomfort or even pain with defecation may occur if a long interval has passed since the last bowel movement, but pain is not a predominant or frequent symptom associated

TABLE 26-1 Medications and Other Agents That Contribute to Constipation

Agents	Example
Analgesics	codeine morphine Prostaglandin inhibitors
Antacids	Aluminum hydroxide Calcium carbonate
Anticholinergics	Antidepressants Antihistamines Antiparkinson drugs Antipsychotics Antispasmodics Anxiolytics
Other	Anticonvulsants Antihypertensives Barium sulfate Iron Lead Monoamine oxidase inhibitors Polystyrene resins verapamil

with defecation. Patients with IBS may report abdominal pain, even if they empty their bowels regularly. By definition, functional GI disorders are diagnosed on the basis of symptoms. For many patients, a complete history and physical examination will allow the clinician to make an accurate diagnosis.

Practitioners should ask specifically about any OTC laxatives that the patient has taken. Evaluate for laxative abuse. Prolonged and habitual use of laxatives can result in cathartic colon, thereby causing reliance on laxatives for a regular bowel movement. Laxative abuse syndrome (LAS) is difficult to diagnose; it often is seen in women with depression, personality disorder, or anorexia nervosa. Clinical features of laxative abuse include factitious diarrhea, electrolyte imbalance, osteomalacia, protein-energy malnutrition, cathartic colon, liver disease, and steatorrhea. Many agents can be detected in urine or stool samples.

MECHANISM OF ACTION

All laxatives work by increasing fluid retention in the colon, resulting in bulkier and softer stools; by decreasing absorption of luminal water through actions on the colonic mucosa; or by increasing intestinal motility. Expected results may take from 5 minutes to several days.

Bulk Laxatives

Bulk laxatives are nondigestible and nonabsorbable. They swell in water to form a viscous solution or gel that absorbs water and expands, increasing both bulk and moisture content of the stool. Increased bulk stimulates peristalsis, and the absorbed water softens the stool. Bulk laxatives also stimulate colonic bacterial growth that increases the weight of the stool and stretches the intestinal wall, further stimulating peristalsis.

Stool Softeners

Stool softeners act to soften stool by lowering surface tension, allowing the fecal mass to be penetrated by intestinal fluids. They also inhibit fluid and electrolyte reabsorption by the intestine.

Docusate sodium is an anionic surfactant that lowers the surface tension of stool to allow mixing of aqueous and fatty substances, which softens the stool and permits easier defecation.

Osmotic Laxatives

Osmotic laxatives are largely nonabsorbable sugars, although small amounts may be absorbed. Bacteria metabolize these agents into lactic acid, formic acid, acetic acid, and carbon dioxide, which act via osmosis. This means that they are present in solution in higher concentration in the bowel, causing water to move from the tissue into the bowel to equalize osmotic pressure. The increased bulk increases colonic peristalsis. Most are disaccharides. Lactulose is a semisynthetic disaccharide of fructose and galactose. Sorbitol is a nonabsorbable sugar. However, glycerin is a naturally occurring trivalent alcohol suppository that acts via hyperosmotic action and through local irritation and lubrication. The American College of Gastroenterology (ACG) Task Force has named osmotic laxatives as among the most effective types.

Stimulants

Stimulant or irritant laxatives increase peristalsis via several mechanisms, depending on the subclass. Stimulants have a direct action on intestinal mucosa or on the nerve plexus. Diphenylmethanes (bisacodyl) stimulate sensory nerves in the intestinal mucosa and increase intestinal chloride secretion. Anthraquinonenone derivatives (i.e., cascara sagrada, senna, and casanthranol) primarily stimulate colonic intramural nerve plexuses.

Senna is protected from small intestinal absorption by its glucose molecules. Colonic bacteria cleave the glucose molecules, releasing active rheinanthrones and producing an action that is specific to the colon.

Saline Laxatives

Saline laxatives attract and retain water in the bowel, thereby increasing intraluminal pressure. Saline laxatives produce an osmotic effect, drawing water into the intestinal lumen of the small intestine and the colon and inducing contractions. Magnesium hydroxide also stimulates the release of cholecystokinin, which increases intestinal secretion and stimulates peristalsis and transit.

Enemas

Enemas work primarily by inducing evacuation as a response to colonic distention and via lavage. They create a barrier between the feces and the colon wall that prevents colonic reabsorption of fecal fluid, thus softening the stool. The lubricant effect also eases the passage of feces through the intestine. Oil retention–mineral enemas also work by lubricating the rectum and the colon. Soap suds enemas provide an irritant action.

TREATMENT PRINCIPLES
Standardized Guidelines

- American College of Gastroenterology guidelines for diagnosis and management of chronic constipation and irritable bowel syndrome: Chronic Constipation Task Force, *Am J Gastroenterol* 100(Suppl 1):S1-S22, 2005.

Evidence-Based Recommendations

Three drugs—polyethylene glycol, lactulose, and tegaserod—are rated as signifying benefit, as demonstrated by two or more randomized controlled trials conducted with appropriate methodology.
- Psyllium is likely to be beneficial.
- Polyethylene glycols are effective.
- Lactulose is likely to be beneficial.
- First-line treatment with unproven benefit: lifestyle changes, paraffin, seed oils, magnesium salts, phosphate enemas, sodium citrate enemas, bisacodyl, docusate, glycerol/glycerin suppositories, and senna

Cardinal Points of Treatment

- Nonpharmacologic treatment fluids and fiber (Table 26-2)
- Treat the underlying cause of constipation first if possible. Start treatment for constipation immediately if it is causing significant discomfort. By understanding the underlying cause of the constipation, the clinician will be better

TABLE 26-2　Drugs of Choice in the Treatment of Constipation

	Short Term	Long Term
First line	Mild: bulk	Bulk
Second line	Severe: enema	Osmotic (saline class)
Third line	Stimulants	Stimulants

TABLE 26-3　Foods High in Fiber

Type of Food	Examples
Fruits (most fruits contain fiber, especially those listed)	Apples Blackberries Peaches Pears Raspberries Strawberries
Grains	Bran cereals Brown rice Popcorn Rye bread Whole wheat bread
Vegetables (most vegetables have fiber; the ones listed are especially high in fiber content)	Beans Broccoli Cabbage Carrots Cauliflower Celery Corn Peas Potatoes Squash

prepared to choose the class of laxative that is most likely to be successful. For example, constipation caused by diseases such as hypothyroidism should be resolved with treatment for hypothyroidism.

Nonpharmacologic Treatment

Nonpharmacologic measures are cost-effective and do not produce the complications associated with laxative use. These measures should be used in all patients with constipation, regardless of whether a medication is prescribed. No medication is an adequate replacement for these measures. Nonpharmacologic management of chronic constipation is encouraged for all ages, especially the young and the old. In the absence of disease, adequate colonic movements can be achieved by a regimen based on four basic components:

- First, adequate fluids are crucial both for laxatives to work and to prevent constipation, with 1500 ml/day minimum essential for maintaining normal bowel activity. Adequate fluids act by keeping fluid in the feces as it passes through the colon. This maintains the bulk of the feces and allows for normal transit. Fluids that are diuretics, such as those that contain caffeine, do not work as well to keep water in the feces. Flavored waters are often an acceptable substitute for plain water. However, data are lacking to support that an increase in fluids to greater than 1500 ml/day is effective in alleviating constipation.
- Second, a high-fiber diet is important. An adult should have a daily intake of 20 to 35 g of fiber; a child should receive 1 g per year of age plus 5 g/day after 2 years of age. This fiber is best obtained from high-roughage foods like bran or vegetables and fruits. See Table 26-3 for a list of foods that are high in fiber. Bran is the outer coating of various grains. The two most commonly found grains are wheat bran and oat bran, which have large amounts of fiber. Other whole grain, unpolished grains, and rice have the outer coating still on, have good amounts of fiber, and may be easier to tolerate than concentrated bran. Sudden increases in fiber in the diet can cause bloating and gas. A high-fiber diet is better tolerated if the change is made gradually. Enough fiber can also be obtained through the regular use of bran slurry (see Box 26-1 for ingredients). Start with 1 tablespoon a day and work up to 3 tablespoons twice a day as needed. It can be mixed with cereal or other foods. Make sure the patient continues to drink enough fluids.
- Third, patients should establish and maintain a regular exercise schedule. Any type of activity is helpful. Simply walking briskly every day facilitates digestion and keeps muscles of the body better toned.

- Fourth, a regular toileting schedule should be established. This includes going to the toilet at the same time each day, 15 to 45 minutes after a meal. Patient should allow for 10 to 15 minutes on the toilet without interruption, stress, or the need to hurry. Patients should not ignore or postpone the urge to defecate.

Pharmacologic Treatment

Pharmacologic treatment may be added if nonpharmacologic treatment is not sufficient, or when immediate or thorough cleansing is indicated. Selection is based on matching the patient characteristics to the effects of the different categories of laxatives. Important factors that should be considered include the cause of constipation, long- or short-term use, severity of constipation, age of the patient, oral food and fluid intake, and prior laxative use (see Table 26-2). Polyethylene glycol, lactulose and tegaserod are recognized as highly effective.

One important decision involves the medication formulation. Remedies are available as oral agents, rectal suppositories, and enemas. Oral formulations may come in tablet, capsule, syrup, powder, or liquid form. Some forms are dissolved in water. Oral treatment is selected for long-term use; it is essential for the clinician to find a formulation that the patient is willing and able to tolerate on a long-term basis. Oral medications also can be used on a

---

BOX 26-1　Bran Slurry Recipe

3 cups applesauce (low sugar)
2 cups wheat or oat bran
1½ cups unsweetened prune juice

short-term basis for severe constipation. Rectal suppositories and enemas should be used only for short-term management because irritation of the rectum can occur with long-term use.

MANAGEMENT
Short Term
- Short-term constipation, whether occasional or caused by external factors, is treated with a short-acting laxative. Another short-term use for laxatives involves preparation for surgery or another procedure.
- Mild short-term constipation can be treated with bulk laxatives or a saline agent such as Milk of Magnesia.
- If the patient is severely constipated or has not responded to increased fiber intake, he or she might need an enema or one of the more potent laxatives. Saline laxatives such as Milk of Magnesia are suggested as second-line treatment by the AGA. Enemas are useful when the patient has stool in the rectum but is unable to push it out. If the patient is impacted, he must be manually disimpacted before any laxative is used. Stimulant laxatives are used for constipation that occurs higher in the colon and should be considered third-line agents.
- If the patient has chronic constipation with a short-term exacerbation, long-term management will be necessary.

Long Term
- Choose a laxative based on the patient's characteristics, and initiate treatment. Table 26-2 provides drug choices.
- If the patient has mild constipation, simple long-term treatment is adequate.
- If the patient has severe constipation, short-term treatment should be instituted while the long-term program is being started. The patient must continue a regimen for at least a week before its effectiveness is evaluated. Increase the dose as necessary.
- If first-line treatment is not effective, consider changing laxatives or adding a second laxative. Change to a more potent category. Use caution if adding a second laxative. Do not use two laxatives from the same category. Bulk and stool softeners can be combined safely with other laxatives. However, this approach will not be needed if the patient is placed on osmotic laxatives, because these also soften stools. Stimulants, saline, and enemas may be given as needed for a short-term problem. Monitor the frequency of their use; if they are needed often, this means that the long-term plan needs adjustment. Stimulant, saline, and osmotic laxatives should not be combined with each other because of increased risk of adverse reactions.
- Biofeedback has been shown to be effective in the management of chronic idiopathic constipation.

Chronic Laxative Abuse
- Many patients already have used pharmacologic treatment and have developed cathartic colon from LAS. These patients should be weaned from their stimulant and saline laxatives and placed on safer long-term laxatives. Long-term management should be initiated with a bulk or stool softener for milder constipation.
- Usually, however, these patients will need a stronger laxative such as an osmotic. Gradually decrease use of the

stimulant or saline laxative as tolerated. Patient education is crucial to success.

BULK LAXATIVES. Bulk laxatives are the most commonly used first-line agents used to treat or prevent mild short-term constipation. They are especially helpful for long-term use because they have a good safety profile. A patient with severe constipation may need a more potent laxative, especially at first. These products are available as powder that is mixed with water. Some form a gritty residue that is unpalatable. Some also are provided as wafers or tablets.

Patients likely to benefit from bulk-forming laxatives include postpartum, elderly, and debilitated patients. Patients who eat a small quantity of food and those who have a low level of mobility are also likely to benefit. However, these agents can be dangerous for patients with poor fluid intake. They can be used to wean patients from long-term stimulant laxatives. Bulk laxatives may reduce the risk of colon cancer. Psyllium lowers serum cholesterol by binding bile salts in the intestine.

STOOL SOFTENERS. Fecal softeners are mild acting and frequently are used for long-term treatment and prevention of constipation produced by a delay in rectal emptying. They are also useful when it is important to reduce straining at stool, as in patients with hernia or cardiovascular disease, during postpartum, or after rectal surgery. Fecal softeners can be helpful in elderly patients who are unable to drink adequate fluids for bulk laxatives to be effective.

Mineral oil now is regarded as not safe for oral ingestion; its use is not recommended. Lipid pneumonitis may result from oral ingestion and aspiration of mineral oil, especially when the patient reclines.

OSMOTIC LAXATIVES. Use of osmotic laxatives has greatly increased in recent years. They are used for short- and long-term constipation and for bowel cleansing. They are especially useful for moderate to severe chronic constipation. These agents are preferred over stimulant and saline laxatives because they have a better safety profile but are not as potent. One drawback is their cost, and different from most other laxatives, they require a prescription.

Sorbitol is used in the short-term treatment of constipation. It also is mixed with activated charcoal in the management of poisoning or drug overdose.

Lactulose is used to treat constipation and also is useful for reducing urea production in the colon, thus lowering blood ammonia levels in patients with portal systemic encephalopathy. It comes as a thick syrup that many patients find unpalatable.

Polyethylene glycol comes in two forms: MiraLax powder for chronic constipation and GoLYTELY for bowel cleansing before a procedure. MiraLax comes as a powder that dissolves in water and is tasteless and nongritty. Because polyethylene glycol is an isotonic solution, dehydration does not occur.

Glycerin suppositories aid rectal evacuation; they are useful in bowel retraining programs and for reestablishing normal function in those who are laxative dependent. They may be used on an occasional basis in the management of chronic constipation. They do not have a powerful osmotic effect.

Lubiprostone is a product that relies on activating the local chloride channels that enhance intestinal fluid secretion without altering sodium and potassium concentrations in the serum. Increased intestinal fluid secretion increases motility in the intestine, thereby promoting the passage of stool and alleviating symptoms associated with chronic idiopathic constipation.

STIMULANTS. Stimulants represent the most potent class of laxatives. They are recommended for short-term treatment but may be used on an occasional basis in a patient with chronic constipation. They should be used only after other methods have failed. Stimulants also are used to cleanse the bowel in preparation for endoscopic examination, x-ray studies, or surgery. Bisacodyl suppositories are used to cleanse the colon in pregnant women before delivery.

SALINE LAXATIVES. Saline laxatives are also potent laxatives. They are used to cleanse the bowel in preparation for endoscopic examination, x-ray studies, or surgery. Saline laxatives are used to hasten evacuation of worms after administration of anthelmintics and to hasten elimination of toxic material after ingestion of poison. They are the laxative of choice for securing a stool specimen.

Milk of Magnesia (MOM) may be used on an occasional basis in patients with chronic constipation. If MOM alone is ineffective, MOM with cascara may be given. MOM is a very popular OTC laxative and is a cause of LAS. The magnesium laxatives have a significant risk for adverse reactions with long-term use; they may cause an accumulation of magnesium, which may be a problem in patients with renal insufficiency.

ENEMAS. Enemas are used for short-term constipation while the patient is being started on a bowel regimen. They also are used to prevent discomfort and tearing or laceration of hemorrhoids or fissures. An enema may be necessary to soften stool after abdominal or rectal surgery. Repeated enemas can cause rectal irritation. Fleet enemas contain only a small amount of liquid to fill the rectum. Oil enemas are very helpful for softening hard stool. Enemas that consist of soap suds or tap water use more liquid and go farther up the colon; these types may be effective in cases of high impaction, but they put the patient at risk for electrolyte imbalance.

Pulsed irrigation enhanced evacuation is used to treat fecal impaction in children and adults that otherwise may require operative disimpaction.

Normal saline or air enemas are used under ultrasound guidance for the nonoperative management of ileocolic intussusception. They may be used for treatment of acute fecal impaction if phosphate-containing enemas are contraindicated.

How to Monitor

SHORT-TERM USE

- Monitor for effectiveness. This includes the ability to pass stool and the resolution of symptoms such as abdominal pain, gastric distention, and excessive straining to stool.

LONG-TERM USE

- All laxatives promote fluid loss; monitor fluid and electrolytes.
- Monitor the effects of laxatives on other medications; reevaluate the use of laxatives according to the status and variability of other comorbid conditions, or whether surgical intervention may alleviate the need for laxative use.

Patient Variables

GERIATRICS

- Constipation increases with age; as many as 30% of healthy older persons regularly use laxatives. Laxatives are second only to analgesics as the OTC drugs most commonly used by the elderly.
- Older adults are more susceptible to dehydration and electrolyte imbalance caused by laxatives than are younger patients.

PEDIATRICS

- Constipation in children may have many causes; contributing factors include emotional, dietary, and environmental changes.
- Dosage adjustments are indicated for specific drugs.
- Magnesium salts and phosphate enemas can cause serious metabolic disturbances in infants and young children. Administer with caution. Do not administer enemas to children younger than 2 years. Infants who receive lactulose may develop hyponatremia and dehydration.

PREGNANCY AND LACTATION. Constipation is common during pregnancy and is thought to be due to an increase in circulatory progesterone. This is compounded by the fact that vitamins, iron, and calcium taken during pregnancy tend to be constipating as well.

- *Category B:* lactulose, psyllium; magnesium salts (*category A/C;* varies by manufacturer)
- *Category C:* methylcellulose, calcium polycarbophil, casanthranol, cascara sagrada, docusate sodium, docusate calcium, mineral oil, senna
- Contraindicated
  - Castor oil during pregnancy; its irritant effect may induce premature labor
  - Improper use of saline cathartics can lead to dangerous electrolyte imbalance; bulk-forming laxatives or stool softeners are preferred.
- Although their absorption is limited, laxatives may be excreted in breast milk.

RACE AND GENDER. Constipation is more frequent among women and nonwhites than among men and whites.

SOCIOCULTURAL. Individuals with a low income and a low level of education are at increased risk for constipation.

Patient Education

- Patients and/or parents may have to be educated about what constitutes a normal bowel movement.
- Nonpharmacologic measures should be reviewed; specific instructions should be written on a prescription pad.

- Information on high-fiber foods should be provided to the patient.

Oral Laxatives

The following information is applicable to all categories of oral laxatives.

CONTRAINDICATIONS. Hypersensitivity, symptoms of appendicitis, fecal impaction, intestinal obstruction, undiagnosed abdominal pain, perforation, or toxic megacolon

WARNINGS
- *Constipation:* Before using laxatives, consider living habits that affect bowel function, including disease state and drug history. Implement nonpharmacologic treatment. Restrict self-medication to short-term therapy for constipation. Long-term use of laxatives (particularly stimulants) may lead to dependence.
- *Fluid and electrolyte balance:* Excessive laxative use may lead to significant fluid and electrolyte imbalance. Monitor patients periodically.
- *Abuse/dependency:* Long-term use of laxatives may result in fluid and electrolyte imbalances, steatorrhea, osteomalacia, diarrhea, cathartic colon, and liver disease (LAS or cathartic colon).

PRECAUTIONS
- Rectal bleeding or failure to respond may indicate a serious condition, which may require further medical attention.
- Some of these products contain tartrazine, to which patients may be allergic.

ADVERSE EFFECTS. Diarrhea, nausea, vomiting, perianal irritation, fainting, bloating, flatulence, cramps

PHARMACOKINETICS. Only lactulose and magnesium are absorbed in appreciable amounts (Table 26-4).

DRUG INTERACTIONS. Laxatives can affect the absorption of drugs in the intestine by decreasing transit time, thus giving the bowel less time to absorb the medication. Important medications in this category are oral anticoagulants, digoxin, aspirin, tetracyclines, and nitrofurantoin. These agents should be taken 2 hours apart to avoid drug interactions (Table 26-5).

DOSAGE AND ADMINISTRATION. See Table 26-6.

TABLE 26-4 Pharmacokinetics of Laxatives

Drug	Onset of Action	Site of Action
BULK LAXATIVES		
psyllium	24-72 hr	Small and large intestines
methylcellulose	24-72 hr	Small and large intestines
calcium polycarbophil	12-24 hr	Small and large intestines
Bran powder	Days	Colon
STOOL SOFTENERS		
docusate sodium	12-72 hr	Small and large intestines
docusate calcium	12-72 hr	Small and large intestines
OSMOTIC LAXATIVES		
lactulose	24-48 hr	Colon
sorbitol	24-48 hr	Colon
polyethylene glycol	1-2 hr	Colon
glycerol (glycerin)	0.25-1 hr (suppository)	Colon
STIMULANT LAXATIVES		
bisacodyl	6-8 hr	Colon
	1 hr (suppository)	Rectum
cascara	6-8 hr	Colon
senna	6-12 hr	Colon
casanthranol	6-12 hr	Colon
SALINE LAXATIVES		
magnesium hydroxide	1-3 hr	Small and large intestines
magnesium sulfate	1-2 hr	Small and large intestines
magnesium citrate	3-6 hr	Small and large intestines
sodium phosphate	1-6 hr	Small and large intestines
ENEMAS		
sodium phosphate	5-15 min	Rectum
Soap suds	2-15 min	Rectum
Tap water	5-15 min	Rectum
Mineral oil	6-8 hr	Rectum

OVERDOSAGE. Diarrhea; discontinue the laxative and monitor fluids

SPECIFIC DRUGS

BULK LAXATIVES

psyllium (Metamucil, Sugar-Free Metamucil, Fiberall) 🔑

CONTRAINDICATIONS. Hypersensitivity to psyllium or any component of the formulation; fecal impaction; GI obstruction

Continued

TABLE 26-5 Drug Interactions With Laxatives

Laxative	Action on Drugs	Drugs	Effect on Laxative
Surfactants	Increased effect of mineral oil	Milk, antacids, H₂- blockers, PPIs	Increased effect of bisacodyl
Mineral oil	Decreased action of lipid-soluble vitamins	Antacids	Decreased action of lactulose
Bulk laxatives	Decreased action of digitalis, salicylates	neomycin and other antiinfectives	lactulose (conflicting reports)
Saline and magnesium	Decreased action of tetracycline		
Magnesium salts	Decreased action of digoxin, chlordiazepoxide, chlorpromazine, dicumarol, isoniazid		

TABLE 26-6 Dosage and Administration Recommendations for Laxatives

Drug	Age Group	Dosage	Administration	Maximum Daily Dose
BULK LAXATIVES				
Psyllium	Adult	Powder: 1 tsp-1 tbsp (varies by product) Capsule: 2-6 Tablet: 1 Wafer: 2	In 8 oz water; tid	
	Child 6-11 yr	Half adult dosage	In 8 oz water; up to tid	
methylcellulose	Adult >12 yr	Powder: 1-2 tbsp (varies by product) Caplet: 2-4 Powder: Half adult dosage	In 8 oz water; 1-3 times/day	
	Child 6-12 yr	Caplet: 1	In 4 oz water; 1-3 times/day In 8 oz water; 1-3 times/day	Up to 6 times/day
calcium polycarbophil	Adult >12 yr	2 tablets (equivalent to 1000 mg polycarbophil)	daily-qid	4 g
	Child 6-12 yr	Half adult dosage	daily-qid	2 g
Bran powder	Adult	6-20 g	daily	
	Child	5 g	daily	
STOOL SOFTENERS				
docusate sodium/calcium	Adult >12 yr	50-500 mg/day	1-4 divided doses	500 mg
	Child 6-12 yr	40-150 mg/day		150 mg
	Child 3-6 yr	20-60 mg/day		60 mg
	Child <3 yr	10-40 mg/day		40 mg
OSMOTIC LAXATIVES				
Lactulose	Adult	10-20 g/day (15-30 ml syrup/day)	Daily; may be mixed with other liquids	40 g (60 ml of syrup)
	Child	5 g/day (7.5 ml syrup/day)	Daily; after breakfast	
sorbitol (70% solution)	Adult	30-150 ml/day	As a single dose	
	Child (2-11 yr)	2 ml/kg		
polyethylene glycol (MiraLax)	Adult	17 g powder (1 heaping teaspoonful)	In 8 oz liquid, once daily	
GoLYTELY	Adult	4 L	Before GI examination; 8 oz (240 ml) q10min	
lubiprostone	Adult	24 mcg po	2 times/day with food	
glycerol (glycerin)	Adult	One adult suppository in rectum	1-2 times/day	
	Child <6 yr	One infant suppository	1-2 times/day	
STIMULANT LAXATIVES				
bisacodyl	Adults	5-15 mg tablet 10 mg suppository	As a single dose	
	Child >6 yr	5-10 mg tablet	Once daily at bedtime or before breakfast	
	Child >2 yr	10 mg suppository	As a single dose	
	Child <2 yr	5 mg suppository		
senna	Adult	Tablet: 8.6 mg Syrup: 10-15 ml	Once daily	4 tablets (34.4-mg)
	Child 6-12 yr	Tablet: 8.6 mg Syrup: 5-7.5 ml	Once daily at bedtime	Two 8.6-mg tablets
	Child 2-6 yr	Tablet: ½ tablet (4.3 mg) Syrup: 2.5-3.75 ml		8.6 mg/day
casanthranol	Adult	One tablet	Daily	
cascara	Adult	5 ml		
	Child 2-11 yr	2.5 ml	As a single dose	

Table continued on following page

TABLE 26-6   Dosage and Administration Recommendations for Laxatives (Continued)

Drug	Age Group	Dosage	Administration	Maximum Daily Dose
SALINE LAXATIVES				
magnesium hydroxide	Adult	Liquid (400 mg/5 ml): 30-60 ml Tablet (311 mg): 6-8	Once daily before bedtime or in divided doses	
	Child 6-12 yr	Liquid: 15-30 ml Tablet: 3-4		
	Child 2-5 yr	Liquid: 5-15 ml Tablet: 1-2		
	Child <2yr	Liquid: 0.5 ml/kg/dose		
magnesium sulfate	Adult	10-30 g/day	In 4 oz of water; in divided doses	
	Child 6-11 yr	5-10 g/day		
	Child 2-5 yr	2.5-5 g/day		
magnesium citrate	Adult	150-300 ml (290 mg/5 ml)	Once daily or in divided doses	
	Child 6-12 yr	100-150 ml		
	Child <6 yr	2-4 ml/kg/dose		
ENEMAS				
sodium phosphate	Adult	4.5 oz (one enema)	As a single dose	
	Child 2-11 yr	2.25 oz (one pediatric enema)		
Mineral oil	Adult	60-150 ml/day (one retention enema)	As a single dose	
	Child 2-11 yr	30-60 ml		
Sorbitol (25%-30% solution)	Adult	120 ml	As a single dose	
	Child 2-11 yr	30-60 ml		
Glycerin	Adult	5-15 ml	As a single dose	

psyllium (Metamucil, Sugar-Free Metamucil, Fiberall) —cont'd

PRECAUTIONS
- Always give with one or more full glasses of water.
- Psyllium products with dextrose should be used cautiously in patients with diabetes.
- Bulk-forming agents may cause impaction, particularly if feces are temporarily arrested in their passage through the alimentary canal (e.g., patients with esophageal stricture). Administer bulk-forming agents with plenty of fluid (8 glasses of water per day), especially in elderly or immobile patients.

ADVERSE EFFECTS
- Abdominal distention and borborygmi are common symptoms, particularly when bulk laxatives are first initiated.
- Bloating appears to be more of a problem with bran.

OTHER DRUGS IN CLASS

Other drugs in this class are similar to the key drug except as follows:
- *Methylcellulose (Citrucel) and calcium polycarbophil (Fiber-Con, Fiberall Chewable):* contraindicated in patients for whom extra calcium is dangerous, and in children younger than 3 years of age. Calcium levels may be monitored in those on calcium polycarbophil. Calcium polycarbophil

releases calcium following ingestion that may impair absorption of tetracycline. This is avoided by spacing the dose of these to 2 or more hours apart.
- *Bran:* See instructions on high-fiber diet and slurry (see Box 26-1).

EMOLLIENTS/FECAL SOFTENERS

docusate sodium (Colace)

WARNINGS. Docusate sodium should be avoided in patients with edema or heart failure and in those on sodium-restricted diets.

ADVERSE EFFECTS. *Docusate:* Intestinal obstruction, diarrhea, abdominal cramping; throat irritation, and a bitter taste have been associated with docusate; rash is uncommon but may occur.

OSMOTIC LAXATIVES
lactulose (Chronulac, Cephulac)

CONTRAINDICATIONS. Patients who require a low-galactose diet

WARNINGS
- To avoid inadequate acidification of stool in treating encephalopathy, other laxatives should not be used concurrently with lactulose.
- *Electrocautery procedures:* A theoretical hazard may exist for patients who are being treated with lactulose.

PRECAUTIONS. *Diabetic patients:* Lactulose syrup contains galactose and lactose; use with caution.

ADVERSE EFFECTS
- Lactulose can cause abdominal distention, epigastric pain, and anorexia; serious events include hypernatremia and lactic acidosis.
- Cramping can occur at an incidence as great as 20%; to avoid, start with a low dose.

OVERDOSAGE. Hypernatremia and lactic acidosis have been seen with high doses of lactulose.

OTHER DRUGS IN CLASS

Drugs that are from the same category or subcategory are similar to lactulose, except in the following ways.
- *sorbitol:* May cause hypernatremia and abdominal bloating
- *polyethylene glycol (MiraLax and GoLYTELY):* MiraLax powder dissolves in water, where it is undetectable. It has become a very popular laxative among the elderly.
- *lubiprostone:* A new product used for chronic idiopathic constipation that stimulates intestinal secretion by acting as a chloride channel activator. It has low systematic availability and is extensively and rapidly metabolized. Pregnancy category C. It may cause nausea or diarrhea. Give with food to decrease the incidence of nausea; does not seem to interact with other drugs

SALINE LAXATIVES

magnesium hydroxide (Milk of Magnesia) ✐

CONTRAINDICATIONS
- Laxatives that contain magnesium are contraindicated in patients with impaired renal function, a colostomy, or an ileostomy.
- Saline laxatives that contain magnesium are contraindicated in children younger than 2 years of age.

WARNINGS
- In pregnancy, sodium salts may promote sodium retention and may result in edema.
- Individuals on a sodium-restricted diet and those with edema, CHF, renal failure, or borderline hypertension should cautiously use preparations that contain sodium.
- *Megacolon, bowel obstruction, imperforate anus, or CHF:* Do not use sodium phosphate and sodium biphosphate in these patients; hypernatremic dehydration may occur.
- *Renal function impairment:* Up to 20% of the magnesium in magnesium salts may be absorbed. In the presence of renal dysfunction, use cautiously products that contain phosphate, sodium, magnesium, or potassium salts. Use sodium phosphate and sodium biphosphate with caution in these patients; hyperphosphatemia, hypernatremia, acidosis, and hypocalcemia may occur.

PRECAUTIONS
- Saline cathartics can produce dehydration if used without adequate fluid replacement.
- Phosphate salts can result in hypocalcemia in children younger than 2 years of age.
- Magnesium levels may have to be monitored.

ADVERSE EFFECTS
- Dizziness, palpitations, weakness, and dehydration have been reported with saline laxatives.
- Excessive bowel activity and cramping may occur.

OVERDOSAGE
- Large doses of magnesium can cause respiratory depression and alterations in neuromuscular activity from hypermagnesemia.
- Other symptoms of hypermagnesemia include muscle weakness, electrocardiographic changes, sedation, and confusion.

OTHER DRUGS IN CLASS

Other drugs in this class are similar to the key drug, except as follows:
- *Magnesium sulfate (Epsom Salts) and magnesium citrate:* Magnesium citrate cherry flavor may produce a red tint in the urine. Use for bowel preparation before surgery or procedures. Refrigerate to improve taste. Take with a full glass of water. Sulfate salts are considered to be the most potent saline laxative.

STIMULANTS

bisacodyl (Dulcolax) ✐

WARNINGS
- Stimulants have a high risk for electrolyte abnormalities and fluid imbalance.
- Daily use of bisacodyl suppositories can cause rectal burning, proctitis, or sloughing of the epithelium.

PRECAUTIONS. All stimulant laxatives have a high abuse potential and can cause cathartic bowel with prolonged use. These laxatives should be used for no longer than 1 week.

ADVERSE EFFECTS. Cramping and nausea and vomiting are more frequent with stimulants.

DRUG INTERACTIONS. Bisacodyl should not be ingested within 1 hour of antacids or foods because the tablets have an enteric coating that interacts with food and can cause severe cramping in the stomach or duodenum. Stimulant laxatives should not be taken within 2 hours of other oral medications.

OTHER DRUGS IN CLASS

Other drugs in this class are similar to the key drug, except as follows:

ANTHRAQUINONE DERIVATIVES

Cascara sagrada may be found in MOM with cascara for added stimulant effect. Both cascara sagrada and senna may discolor acidic urine to yellow-brown or black, and alkaline urine to pink-red, red-violet, or red-brown. Melanosis coli is a darkened pigmentation of the colonic mucosa that results from long-term use of anthraquinone derivatives (casanthranol, cascara sagrada, senna).

Long-term use of senna has been associated with reversible finger clubbing. It is considered to be herbal and hence safe by many patients, but it should not be used on a regular basis. X-Prep (a powdered concentrate of senna) must be used cautiously in diabetic patients because it contains 50 g of glucose per bottle.

ENEMAS

sodium phosphate (Fleet enema, Fleet Phosh-soda)

CONTRAINDICATIONS. Hypersensitivity to phosphate (salts) or any component; hyperphosphatemia, hypocalcemia, hypomagnesemia, hypernatremia, severe renal impairment, severe tissue trauma, heat cramps, heart failure, abdominal pain (rectal forms), fecal impaction (rectal forms). Phosphate enemas are contraindicated in children younger than 2 years of age.

WARNINGS. Phosphate that is absorbed systemically can cause fluid retention and hyperphosphatemia and should be used cautiously in children 2 to 5 years of age and in those with underlying bowel disease or renal dysfunction.

PRECAUTIONS

- Mechanical trauma can occur when sensitive rectal tissues are probed. The lubricated tip should be inserted gently into the adult (3 to 4 inches), the child (2 to 3 inches), and the infant (1½ inches). Use no more than 200 ml of fluid in those with impaired renal function and in those who cannot tolerate large volumes of fluid.
- Enemas should not be relied on to maintain bowel regularity because they disrupt normal defecation reflexes and may result in dependence. Monitor electrolyte losses.

ADVERSE EFFECTS. Cramping, distention, and mucorrhea may result.

OVERDOSAGE. Hypovolemia and potassium depletion may occur when excessive lavage is used. Fatal hyperphosphatemia and hypocalcemia have been associated with excess phosphate doses.

OTHER DRUGS IN CLASS

- *Soap suds, tap water, oil retention, saline enemas:* Soap suds enemas are irritating, can cause proctitis, and should be avoided in the elderly. Hyperkalemia may result when potassium-based soaps are used. Hot water use in enemas can cause acute proctitis. Cold water administration can cause extreme cramping. Repeated tap water enemas can result in water toxicity and/or circulatory overload.

evolve A continually updated list of useful WebLinks may be found in the Evolve Resources at http://evolve.elsevier.com/Edmunds/NP/

Antidiarrheals

27

DRUG OVERVIEW

Class	Subclass	Generic Name	Trade Name
Antidiarrheals	Opiate and opioid derivatives	diphenoxylate hydrochloride and atropine sulfate ☀	Lomotil 🔑
		loperamide hydrochloride	Imodium, Imodium A-D,
		tincture of opium, paregoric	
	Antisecretory	bismuth subsalicylate	Pepto-Bismol, Pink Bismuth
	Adsorbents	attapulgite	Kaopectate, Rheaban
Oral rehydration solution (ORS)		Electrolyte solution	Pedialyte, Gatorade

☀ Top 200 drug; 🔑 key drug chosen based on common usage.

INDICATIONS

- Acute nonspecific diarrhea
- Chronic diarrhea
- Loperamide: for management of acute or traveler's diarrhea
- Attapulgite: mild to moderate diarrhea
- Bismuth: indigestion, nausea, control of traveler's diarrhea, and as an adjunct to treatment of *Helicobacter pylori* peptic ulcer disease
- Oral rehydration solution (ORS): diarrhea in all patients, especially children and pregnant women

Antidiarrheal agents are used as temporary adjunct therapy in the management of acute nonspecific diarrhea and functional chronic diarrhea. Acute episodes of diarrhea are usually benign and self-limiting, by definition lasting less than 2 weeks and usually lasting only 1 to 2 days.

> If diarrhea persists for longer than 72 hours, or if gross blood is present in the stool, the patient should be evaluated further.

Diarrhea should always be evaluated before pharmacologic treatment is begun. Diarrhea is a symptom, so therapy should be targeted at treatment of the underlying cause.

Many antidiarrheal agents are now available OTC and therefore may be overused. Opioid agents may prolong acute infectious diarrhea, leading to potentially serious consequences. Antidiarrheals should never be used for longer than 48 hours without supervision by a health care provider. Short-term use generally is considered safe but should not serve as a substitute for determining the cause of the diarrhea. The American Gastroenterological Association 1999 guidelines form the basis for the recommendations provided in this chapter.

THERAPEUTIC OVERVIEW

Anatomy and Physiology

See Chapter 26 for anatomy and physiology of the bowel.

Pathophysiology

Large-volume diarrhea is caused by excessive quantities of water or secretions in the intestines. Small-volume diarrhea is caused by excessive intestinal motility.

Large-volume diarrhea can be caused by osmosis. A nonabsorbable substance (such as lactose or nonabsorbable sugar) in the gut causes fluid to be drawn into the lumen by osmosis. This condition also may be caused by excessive mucosal secretions. Bacterial toxins and neoplasms that produce hormones also stimulate secretions. Large-volume diarrhea also can be caused by excessive motility of the intestine. Conditions that affect autonomic nervous system control of digestion (e.g., diabetic neuropathy) increase transit time, thereby preventing adequate absorption of water and electrolytes from the feces.

Small-volume diarrhea usually is caused by an inflammatory condition that affects the gut mucosa.

Disease Process

Worldwide, diarrhea is a major cause of morbidity and mortality, especially in children. Diarrhea is the second most common illness among families in the United States, with an annual incidence of up to 63% per year; 4% to 20% of chronic diarrhea results from laxative abuse.

Medically, stools are classified as diarrhea if the patient has increased frequency, which usually is defined as more than two or three bowel movements per day, and the stools are liquid, not just "soft." The emphasis in diagnosis is on consistency, not frequency.

Diarrhea is categorized as acute or chronic. By definition, acute diarrhea persists for less than 2 weeks—usually, a few days to 1 week. It can be subdivided into noninflammatory or inflammatory diarrhea. Noninflammatory diarrhea is watery and nonbloody and usually is caused by a bacterium or a virus that is self-limiting. Inflammatory diarrhea consists of WBCs in the stool; these reflect invasion of the organism or toxin into the wall of the intestine (Table 27-1).

Chronic diarrhea has an extensive number of etiologies. Evaluate the patient carefully for the cause of the diarrhea, and treat the disease—not the symptom. Medications that can cause diarrhea include laxatives, antacids, magnesium-containing products, and antibiotics (Table 27-2).

Acute diarrhea can be of infectious (bacteria, protozoa, or virus) or noninfectious origin (toxons, an inflammatory process, an ischemic process, or a mechanical process). Chronic diarrhea can be classified according to stool type as follows: (1) watery (secretory and osmotic)—no pus, blood, or fat; (2) fatty—fat; or (3) inflammatory—blood and/or pus. Causes of chronic diarrhea include medications, IBS, enteral feedings, malabsorption syndromes (celiac disease, fat malabsorption), and malnutrition.

Assessment

The guidelines put forth by the American Gastroenterological Association emphasize comprehensive evaluation of a patient before treatment is provided. Patient history is important for the diagnosis. Similar illness in contacts points to an infection. Ingestion of improperly prepared or stored food suggests infection or bacterial toxins. Exposure to impure water suggests parasites. Travel abroad exposes patients to infections that are characteristic of the local area. Antibiotic use points to *Clostridium difficile*. The critical laboratory test involves sending the stool for fecal leukocytes, routine stool culture, and *C. difficile*. Obtain ova and parasites if the patient has had diarrhea for longer than 10 days, has traveled to an endemic region, is experiencing a community water-borne outbreak, has human immunodeficiency virus (HIV), or is a homosexual male. If suspicion involves a specific infectious cause, focused stool testing can be ordered (e.g., *Giardia* antigen, Norwalk virus, cryptosporidium).

TABLE 27-1   Causes of Acute Infectious Diarrhea

Cause	Noninflammatory	Inflammatory
VIRAL	Norwalk, rotavirus	Cytomegalovirus
PROTOZOAL	*Giardia, Cryptosporidium*	
BACTERIAL Preformed toxin	*Staphylococcus aureus, Bacillus cereus*	*Escherichia coli, Vibrio parahaemolyticus,*
Enterotoxin production	*E. coli, Vibrio cholerae*	*Clostridium difficile, C. perfringens*
Mucosal innervation		*Shigella, Campylobacter jejuni, Salmonella,* enteroinvasive *E. coli, Chlamydia, Neisseria, Listeria*

TABLE 27-2   Causes of Chronic Diarrhea

Lactose intolerance
Irritable bowel disease
Fecal impaction
Inflammatory bowel disease
Ulcerative colitis
Crohn's disease
Microscopic colitis
Malignancy
Radiation
Malabsorption
Celiac sprue
Pancreatic disease
Neuropathy
Chronic infection
Clostridium difficile
Parasites
Human immunodeficiency virus (HIV)-related enteropathology

MECHANISM OF ACTION

Opioids

Opioid antidiarrheal agents act on the smooth muscle of the intestinal tract to slow GI motility and propulsion. Slowed transit time of intestinal contents allows more fluid to be absorbed from the stool, thereby decreasing fecal volume, as well as fluid and electrolyte loss. Little or no analgesic activity is noted.

The opioids (except loperamide hydrochloride) may be habit forming. Atropine sulfate is added to some formulations to discourage deliberate overdose.

Adsorbents

Adsorbents act by reducing intestinal motility and by adsorbing fluid. In infectious diarrhea, they bind bacteria and toxins in the GI tract.

Antisecretory

Two portions of this salicylate (bismuth and subsalicylates) provide the antisecretory effect; the bismuth portion may exert antimicrobial effects.

TREATMENT PRINCIPLES

Standardized Guidelines

- The CDC has published guidelines on the home management of acute diarrhea in children.
- The WHO has put forth guidelines for ORS and its use (see www. guidelines.gov).

Evidence-Based Recommendations

None found

Cardinal Points of Treatment

- Rehydration
- Opioids are more effective and more palatable than adsorbents but have a greater number of side effects.

Pharmacologic Treatment

This section discusses the empirical treatment of diarrhea as appropriate in the following conditions: initial treatment before diagnostic testing is completed, diarrhea without diagnosis, and diarrhea with diagnosis but no cure.

ACUTE DIARRHEA. Acute diarrhea is usually mild and self-limited. Nonpharmacologic measures, especially bowel rest and adequate hydration, rest, reassurance, and electrolyte replacement, are also helpful. Oral rehydration with electrolyte solution (Gatorade or Pedialyte) is recommended in moderate to severe cases; cola or ginger ale may be sufficient in mild cases. If the patient is not able to replace liquids as fast as they are lost, further treatment is needed to prevent dehydration. Children and frail patients with severe diarrhea may need antidiarrheals or IV rehydration (which can be accomplished in ED without the need for hospitalization). Oral rehydration should be performed rapidly (3 to 4 hours). Continue oral hydration to compensate for ongoing losses. (See WHO guidelines.) An unrestricted diet is recommended as soon as dehydration is corrected. If infants are breastfed, nursing should be continued. Continue present formula; do not dilute or use a special formula.

Treatment of patients with acute diarrhea with the use of antidiarrheals can prolong infection and should be avoided if possible. If patients find the diarrhea significantly inconvenient, they may be given antidiarrheals on a limited basis. Antidiarrheals may be used safely in patients with acute mild to moderate diarrhea. Their main use is to ensure patient comfort. Do not use in patients with bloody diarrhea, high fever, or systemic toxicity because these conditions may worsen the disease. Discontinue if not effective and investigate the origin of the diarrhea. Used on a short-term basis, they are safe and effective for patient relief, allowing patients to function in their usual activities and avoiding distressing episodes of incontinence. Patients with acute inflammatory diarrhea that does not improve within a few days may require antibiotic therapy.

CHRONIC DIARRHEA. Once the source of the chronic diarrhea has been optimally treated, antidiarrheals may be used as needed to control symptoms and prevent dehydration. Opioids are generally safe and effective if used as directed.

OPIATES AND OPIOID DERIVATIVES. Opiates decrease motility, stool number, and liquidity and reduce fecal urgency. They are best used for chronic diarrhea.

ADSORBENTS. Bismuth reduces symptoms through its antiinflammatory and antibacterial properties and decreases nausea and vomiting; it is best used for acute diarrhea.

How to Monitor

- Monitor the number and character of stools, and have the patient keep a record as needed.
- Monitor hydration status, fluid and electrolyte loss, hypotension, and signs of dehydration.
- Observe for signs of toxicity (see specific drug).
- Acute diarrhea should improve within 48 hours of treatment initiation.
- Chronic diarrhea should improve within 10 days.

Patient Variables

GERIATRICS

- Fecal impaction associated with the use of adsorbents is more common in debilitated geriatric patients.
- Diarrhea can be caused by leakage of liquid stool around an impaction.

PEDIATRICS

- Antidiarrheals are not recommended in young children.
- Opioids are contraindicated in children younger than 2 years.
- Bismuth and attapulgite are not recommended for children younger than 3 years of age.

PREGNANCY AND LACTATION

- *Category* B: attapulgite
- *Category* C: loperamide, diphenoxylate/atropine; bismuth (*D* in third trimester).
- Diphenoxylate and atropine are excreted in breast milk.

Patient Education

- Supportive therapy, including rest, hydration, and appropriate diet, is the recommended first-line treatment for acute diarrhea.
- Use safety precautions in driving or operating machinery that requires alertness because the drug may produce drowsiness or dizziness.
- When using opioid agents, avoid alcohol and other CNS depressants; do not exceed the prescribed dose.
- Antidiarrheal agents should not be used for self-medication for longer than 48 hours. If diarrhea is not controlled within 48 hours, or if fever develops, the patient should consult a health care provider.

SPECIFIC DRUGS

OPIATES AND OPIOID DERIVATIVES

diphenoxylate (2.5 mg) and atropine sulfate (0.025 mg) (Lomotil)

CONTRAINDICATIONS. Known enterotoxin-producing bacterium, pseudomembranous enterocolitis, obstructive jaundice, advanced liver disease, known hypersensitivity to diphenoxylate or atropine, enterotoxin-producing bacteria; not for use in children younger than 2 years of age

WARNINGS

- *Diarrhea:* may aggravate diarrhea associated with organisms that penetrate the intestinal mucosa
- *Fluid and electrolyte balance:* must also treat fluid replacement; dehydration increases adverse effects

Continued

diphenoxylate (2.5 mg) and atropine sulfate (0.025 mg) (Lomotil) —cont'd

- Advise safety precautions related to possible drowsiness and dizziness.
- May prolong the half-life of drugs metabolized in the liver
- *Ulcerative colitis:* may induce toxic megacolon
- *Renal and liver disease:* Use with extreme caution in patients with advanced hepatorenal disease and in all patients with abnormal liver function tests because hepatic coma may be precipitated.
- *Atropine:* may cause anticholinergic side effects. Avoid in patients in whom anticholinergic drugs are contraindicated. Although the dose of atropine is subtherapeutic, take precautions related to the use of atropine. Signs of atropinism may occur even at recommended doses, especially in children and patients who have Down syndrome.

PRECAUTIONS

- Schedule V drugs may be habit forming.
- Safety has not been established in children younger than 12 years of age. Only the liquid dosage form is approved for use in children younger than 13 years of age. In treatment of acute enteritis, diphenoxylate (Lomotil) may cause fluid retention in the intestines great enough to mask depletion of extracellular fluid and electrolytes, especially in younger children.

PHARMACOKINETICS. See Table 27-3 for pharmacokinetic information. Diphenoxylate is rapidly metabolized by ester hydrolysis to diphenoxylic acid (diphenoxylate HCl), which is biologically active.

ADVERSE EFFECTS

- *Mild:* drowsiness, dizziness, nervousness, restlessness, headache, depression, dry mouth, difficult urination, blurred vision
- *Severe:* paralytic ileus, urinary retention, respiratory depression

DRUG INTERACTIONS. Effects of medications with anticholinergic activity may be increased.

DOSAGE AND ADMINISTRATION. See Table 27-4.

OVERDOSAGE. Symptoms of overdosage include drowsiness, hypotension, blurred vision, dry mouth, and miosis. Overdosage may cause severe respiratory depression and coma, possibly leading to brain damage or death, especially in children.

OTHER DRUGS IN CLASS

Other drugs in this class are similar to the prototype, except as follows:

- *Loperamide hydrochloride (Imodium):* More specific, longer acting, and two to three times more potent on weight basis than diphenoxylate. Loperamide has no analgesic activity. Some case reports suggest that overdosage may occur at doses around 60 mg. Symptoms of overdosage include CNS and respiratory depression, GI cramping and irritation, nausea, vomiting, and constipation.
- *Camphorated tincture of opium (paregoric):* Hypersensitivity to opium or its other components is also a contraindication. Paregoric is a Schedule III drug and may be habit forming. Do not confuse opium tincture with paregoric. This may lead to a potentially fatal overdose on morphine. Tincture of opium contains 25 times more morphine than paregoric and is a Schedule II drug. Use with caution in patients who have respiratory, hepatic, or renal dysfunction, or a history of narcotic abuse.

Antisecretory

bismuth subsalicylate (Pepto-Bismol)

CONTRAINDICATIONS

- In patient with influenza or chickenpox, it could mask symptoms of Reye's syndrome.
- History of severe GI bleeding

TABLE 27-3   Pharmacokinetics of Selected Antidiarrheal Agents

Drug	Absorption	Onset of Action	Time to Peak Concentration	Half-life	Duration of Action	Metabolism	Excretion
diphenoxylate hydrochloride and atropine sulfate	Well absorbed via oral route; bioavailability 90%	45-60 min	2 hr	12-14 hr	3-4 hr	Liver: diphenoxylic acid is active metabolite.	Feces, 50%; urine, 14%; excreted unchanged in urine, 1%
loperamide hydrochloride	Oral route: <40%; very low levels in breast milk; <50% available after first pass	1-3 hr	2.5 hr (soln) 5 hr (caps)	7-14 hr	41 hr	Liver	Unchanged in feces, 25%; urine, 1%
camphorated tincture of opium (paregoric)			—			Liver	Urine
bismuth subsalicylate	Bismuth minimally absorbed (<1%); salicylate readily absorbed (>90%)		—			Chemical dissociation to bismuth salts and salicylic acid in gastrointestinal tract	Bismuth: feces, 99%; salicylate; urine
attapulgite	Not absorbed after oral administration		—			Liver	—

TABLE 27-4 Dosage and Administration for Antidiarrheal Agents

Drug	Administration and Dosage
diphenoxylate hydrochloride and atropine sulfate	Tablets: 2 tablets (5 mg) qid Liquid: 10 ml (5 mg) qid; maximum dose, 20 mg/day Children: liquid: 0.3-0.4 mg/kg/day in 4 divided doses; maximum: 10 mg/day

loperamide hydrochloride	4 mg initially, then 2 mg after each diarrheal stool; maximum dose: 16 mg/day (8 tablets)
	Acute diarrhea:
	Children: initial doses (in first 24 hours):
	  2-5 yr (13-20 kg): 1 mg three times/day
	  6-8 yr (21-30 kg): 2 mg twice daily
	  9-12 yr (>30 kg): 2 mg three times/day
	After initial dosing, 0.1 mg/kg doses after each loose stool but not exceeding initial dosage
	Chronic diarrhea:
	Children: 0.08-0.24 mg/kg/day divided two to three times/day; maximum: 2 mg/dose

camphorated tincture of opium (paregoric 2 mg/5 ml)	Adults: 5-10 ml; 1 to 4 times daily Children: 0.25-0.5 ml; 1 to 4 times daily
tincture of opium (10 mg/ml)	Adults: 0.6 ml qid
bismuth subsalicylate (262 mg tablets; 262 mg/15 ml)	Take recommended dose every 30 min to 1 hr as needed; chew or dissolve tablets in mouth before swallowing. Adult: 524 mg, maximum 8 doses/24 hr (30 ml, 2 tablets, or 2 caplets) Child 3-5 yr: 1 tsp, 1/3 caplet/tablet Child 6-8 yr: 2 tsp, 2/3 caplet/tablet Child 9 to 12 yr: 1 tablet/caplet or 15 ml; maximum: 8 doses/24 hr
Attapulgite (750 mg caplet; liquid: 600-750 mg/5 ml)	Liquid: Take recommended dose after each loose bowel movement or every 2 hours. Caplets: Swallow whole caplets—1 dose after each loose bowel movement. Adult: 2 tbsp up to six times per day (maximum: 9 g/24 hr) Child 6-12 yr: 600-1500 mg/dose; maximum dose: 4500 mg/day Child 3-6 yr: 300-750 mg/dose; 1 tbsp maximum dose: 2250 mg/day

- History of coagulopathy
- Known allergy to aspirin or nonaspirin salicylates
- Pregnancy (third trimester)

PRECAUTIONS. Use with caution in patients taking medication for anticoagulation, diabetes, and gout.

ADVERSE EFFECTS. These products may cause darkening of stool and tongue discoloration.

DRUG INTERACTIONS. Risk of toxicity is increased with concurrent use of aspirin, warfarin, and hypoglycemics. Decreased effect is often seen with concurrent use of tetracyclines and uricosurics.

OVERDOSAGE. Salicylate toxicity symptoms include tinnitus and fever.

Adsorbents

OTHER DRUGS IN CLASS

- *Attapulgite (Kaopectate):* Do not use this drug if hypersensitivity to any component is present. This agent may impair absorption of oral clindamycin, tetracyclines, penicillamine, and digoxin.

evolve A continually updated list of useful WebLinks may be found in the Evolve Resources at http://evolve.elsevier.com/Edmunds/NP/

28 Antiemetics

DRUG OVERVIEW

Class	Subclass	Generic Name	Trade Name
Antidopaminergic	Phenothiazines	prochlorperazine 🔑 ✸ promethazine ✸	Compazine Phenergan
	Benzamides	metoclopramide 🔑 ✸ trimethobenzamide HCl	Reglan Tigan
Anticholinergics	Antihistamines	meclizine 🔑 ✸ dimenhydrinate	Antivert 🔑 Dramamine
		scopolamine	Transderm-Scop
NK1 Receptor antagonist		aprepitant	Emend
Serotonin 5-HT₃ receptor antagonists		ondansetron HCl dolasetron granisetron HCl palonosetron	Zofran 🔑 Anzemet Kytril Aloxi

✸ Top 200 drug; 🔑 key drug. Other corticosteroids and benzodiazepines may be administered for anticipatory nausea/vomiting associated with chemotherapy. See other relevant chapters.

INDICATIONS

- Nausea and vomiting, particularly that associated with chemotherapy
- Motion sickness
- Vertigo

See Table 28-1.

The mechanisms of action for these drugs are not discussed in detail because drugs with similar mechanisms of action can be found in other chapters. The use of these drugs as antiemetics is discussed in this chapter (see Table 28-1).

The phenothiazine subclass of the antidopaminergic antipsychotics includes prochlorperazine and promethazine, which are used for nausea and vomiting. See Chapter 48 for a detailed discussion of the phenothiazine antipsychotics.

The anticholinergics are divided into two subclasses. The antihistamines commonly used as antiemetics are meclizine and dimenhydrinate. See Chapter 13 for a detailed discussion of antihistamines. The other subclass of anticholinergics includes trimethobenzamide and scopolamine. These are similar to other anticholinergics, which are discussed in detail in Chapter 29.

The serotonin 5-hydroxytryptamine₃ (5-HT₃) receptor antagonists are most useful for the prevention of chemotherapy-induced emesis (CIE) and are discussed in Chapter 29.

The prokinetic agent, metoclopramide, is discussed in Chapter 29.

In all cases of nausea and vomiting or vertigo, the underlying cause should be established because nausea and vomiting are symptoms and are only manifestations of pathophysiologic problems for which further exploration and workup are needed. Severe nausea and vomiting may be the presenting symptoms of underlying conditions such as brain tumor, intestinal obstruction, or appendicitis, and the use of antiemetic medications may slow the diagnosis.

THERAPEUTIC OVERVIEW

Anatomy and Physiology

A "vomiting center" (VC) in the medulla coordinates the respiratory and vasomotor centers and vagus nerve innervation of the GI tract. This center may have four different sources of stimuli. The chemoreceptor trigger zone (CTZ) is located outside the blood-brain barrier near the vomiting center in the medulla (Table 28-2). It communicates with the vomiting center after input is received from drugs and hormones.

Pathophysiology

Normal peristalsis moves the contents of the gut forward. If the forward passage is impeded, reverse peristalsis (retroperistalsis) propels the bolus away from the obstructed segment. During the act of vomiting, retroperistalsis begins in the small intes-

TABLE 28-1 Specific Indications for Antiemetics

Drug	CIE	Nausea and Vomiting	Motion Sickness	Vertigo
Phenothiazines		X	X	
meclizine			X	X
dimenhydrinate			X	
trimethobenzamide		X	X	
scopolamine			X	
NK1 receptor antagonist	X	X		
5-HT$_3$ receptor antagonists	X	X		

CIE, Chemotherapy-induced emesis; 5-HT$_3$, type 3 serotonin; NK, neurokinin.

tine. The gastroduodenal junction, stomach wall, and gastroesophageal junction relax to permit passage of the bolus.

Vertigo is caused by inflammation of the semicircular canals of the inner ear. Motion sickness is caused by repetitive motion, such as angular, linear, or vertical motion.

Disease Process

Nausea is a vague but intensely unpleasant sensation of feeling "sick to the stomach," "queasy," or "about to vomit." This is different from the feelings of discomfort associated with anorexia. Vomiting must be distinguished from the effortless regurgitation that may accompany GERD.

Nausea and vomiting are caused by a wide variety of different factors, ranging from benign fleeting stimuli, such as emotion, to extremely serious disease, such as a brain tumor. Sometimes the cause is obvious, as in motion sickness or reaction to chemotherapy. On other occasions, the diagnosis may be elusive. Accurate diagnosis of the cause also determines which class of antiemetic probably will be most effective.

Motion sickness causes intense nausea and mild vomiting. Patients with vertigo may experience whirling or a feeling of the room spinning around. In true vertigo, the patient can identify the direction in which the room is circling. These patients respond to the sensation with swaying, weakness, and light-headedness. With either of these conditions, the patient may experience sweating, pallor, rapid breathing, and nausea and vomiting.

MECHANISM OF ACTION

Antiemetics act on the VC in the medulla through the four different sources of stimuli input. See Table 28-2.

Antidopaminergics

Phenothiazines block D$_2$-dopamine receptors in the CTZ, as well as other areas of the brain. They also have anticholinergic and antihistamine effects. Examples of antidopaminergic agents include the following.

METOCLOPRAMIDE. Metoclopramide prevents stimulation of the CTZ by antagonizing central and peripheral dopamine receptors and, in higher doses, serotonin receptors. It also accelerates gastric emptying by enhancing the effect of acetylcholine in the upper GI tract.

TRIMETHOBENZAMIDE. The precise mechanism of action of trimethobenzamide is unknown, but it is thought to be mediated through the CTZ. However, direct impulses to the VC are not inhibited.

Anticholinergics

Anticholinergics have antiemetic, anticholinergic, and antihistaminic properties. These antihistamines reduce the sensitivity of the labyrinthine apparatus. This may be mediated through nerve pathways to the VC from the CTZ, peripheral nerve pathways, or other CNS centers. These drugs have a suppressant action on hyperstimulated labyrinthine function. The precise mode of action is not known.

SCOPOLAMINE. Scopolamine is a commonly used anticholinergic that causes inhibition of vestibular input to the CNS, which results in inhibition of the vomiting reflex. Scopolamine also may have a direct action on the VC within the reticular formation of the brainstem.

NK1 Receptor Antagonist

Aprepitant is a selective high-affinity antagonist of human substance P/neurokinin 1 (NK1) receptors and the active ingredient of Emend that recently has been approved by the FDA for the prevention of chemotherapy-induced nausea and vomiting (CINV). Early studies led to the development of a nanoparticle formulation that could be used to enhance exposure and minimize food effects; this improves quality of life without increasing adverse effects.

TABLE 28-2 Sources of Stimuli to the Vomiting Center

Source of Stimuli	Type of Stimulus	Receptors Involved
GI tract: afferent vagal and splanchnic fibers	Distention, irritation, infection, obstruction, dysmotility	Vagal: 5-HT$_3$
Vestibular system	Motion, infection	Histamine$_1$ (H$_1$) and muscarinic, cholinergic
Higher CNS centers	Increased intracranial pressure, infection, tumor, hemorrhage Psychogenic: sights, smells, emotions	Various
Chemoreceptor trigger zone (located outside the blood-brain barrier near the medulla)	Drugs such as opioids, chemotherapy, toxins, hypoxia, uremia, acidosis, and radiation therapy	5-HT$_3$ and dopamine D$_2$

5-HT$_3$, serotonin type 3.

Serotonin 5-HT₃ Receptor Antagonists

These are selective inhibitors of type 3 serotonin ($5\text{-}HT_3$) receptors that exhibit antiemetic activity. They work peripherally in the intestinal wall by blocking $5\text{-}HT_3$ release from enterochromaffin cells and centrally by blocking $5\text{-}HT_3$ receptors in the CTZ. Current data suggest that serotonin receptors play a major role in acute emesis but only a minor role in delayed nausea and vomiting. Examples of $5\text{-}HT_3$ receptor antagonists include ondansetron HCl, dolasetron, granisetron HCl, and palonosetron (which is available only in an IV formulation).

TREATMENT PRINCIPLES

Standardized Guidelines

- The American Society of Clinical Oncology Guidelines for Antiemetics in Oncology were updated in 2006.
- The American Gastroenterological Association has written a position statement on nausea and vomiting.

Evidence-Based Recommendations

None found

Cardinal Points of Treatment

- *Motion sickness:* anticholinergics
- *Chemotherapy-induced vomiting:* $5\text{-}HT_3$ antagonists, metoclopramide, corticosteroids
- *Vomiting from other causes:* antidopaminergic, metoclopramide

  Vomiting can be divided into two types: acute vomiting and anticipated vomiting precipitated by a predicted cause such as motion sickness or chemotherapy.

Nonpharmacologic Treatment for Acute Vomiting

Most causes of acute vomiting are self-limiting and require no specific treatment. The focus of treatment for acute nausea and vomiting is to replace fluids and electrolytes in order to prevent dehydration. General supportive treatment for nausea and vomiting consists of a diet of clear liquids and small quantities of dry foods as tolerated.

Pharmacologic Treatment for Acute Vomiting

If patient intake is disproportionate with fluid loss, antiemetics should be given. Antiemetics also may be given as a comfort measure. If nausea without vomiting is predominant, an oral antiemetic should be adequate. If, however, nausea is accompanied by vomiting, use of a rectal suppository may be necessary. If the patient is experiencing predominantly nausea, an oral antiemetic may be effective. Rectal suppositories are effective for short-term use for acute nausea and vomiting but cause rectal irritation with regular use. Once the vomiting is under control, the patient may be switched to oral antiemetics to prevent recurrence of vomiting until the cause of the vomiting has been resolved.

> 🔹 If vomiting is not controlled, dehydration may occur with associated hypokalemia and metabolic alkalosis. Patients must be treated with IV potassium

and other medications and fluid replacement in a hospital or emergency department setting.

Pharmacologic Treatment for Anticipated Vomiting

In many situations, nausea and vomiting may be anticipated. These situations may involve motion sickness or chemotherapy. Premedicating the patient with an antiemetic may be necessary in order for the patient to receive full therapy; this is the current standard of care. You should also monitor CBC in a patient who is undergoing chemotherapy to ensure that white blood cell count and platelets are adequate.

ANTIDOPAMINERGIC. Commonly used agents include prochlorperazine, promethazine, and metoclopramide. These agents have wide dosing ranges and may be started at the lowest dosage and increased as needed for symptom control. The $5\text{-}HT_3$ receptors are used along with these drugs for CINV.

ANTICHOLINERGICS. Anticholinergic agents seem to be most effective in cases of motion sickness or vertigo. Similar to the antidopaminergic drugs, these agents have wide dosing ranges that allow for dose modification for symptom control. Scopolamine is best used as the transdermal patch for motion sickness. It also can be used in the oncology patient in whom oral and rectal routes are contraindicated.

NK1 RECEPTOR ANTAGONISTS. This drug is highly effective for preventing nausea and vomiting with certain chemotherapeutic agents. It is a relatively new product.

5-HT₃ RECEPTOR ANTAGONISTS. Although most chemotherapeutic agents have emetogenic potential, the use of premedication with $5\text{-}HT_3$ receptor antagonists significantly decreases the nausea and vomiting experienced during and after administration. For CIE, $5\text{-}HT_3$ receptor antagonists used alone or in combination with dexamethasone and other agents are the drugs of choice. They are also effective for postoperative nausea and vomiting (PONV). It has been shown that serotonin, released by the enterochromaffin cells in the GI tract, is the primary neurotransmitter responsible for CIE. They have a favorable toxicity profile but are considerably more expensive than other antiemetics. The most common agent in this class, ondansetron, is now available as a generic.

How to Monitor

Monitor for effectiveness and adverse effects.

Patient Variables

GERIATRICS

- The elderly may require dose reduction and close monitoring because of the increase in adverse effects in this population.
- Resting the bowel by drinking only clear liquids for 8 to 12 hours could be most helpful. It is important to stay hydrated, but water may trigger nausea and more vomiting, so electrolyte drinks would be best.
- Use of relaxation techniques with cancer patients has been effective in decreasing nausea and vomiting.

PEDIATRICS

- The use of antiemetics is discouraged in cases of uncomplicated vomiting.
- *Anticholinergics/antihistamines:* May cause hallucinations, convulsions, or death; mental alertness may be diminished; can produce excitation
- In combination with viral illnesses, the risk of the patient's developing Reye's syndrome may be increased.
- Dopaminergics increase the risk that extrapyramidal symptoms may occur when these drugs are used. Children with acute illnesses such as chickenpox, influenza, and others, are more susceptible than adults to the neuromuscular adverse effects of these drugs.
- Do not give any antiemetic drugs to children younger than 12 years, except for the following:
  - *promethazine, dimenhydrinate:* Do not use in children younger than 2 years of age.
  - *ondansetron:* Approved for use in those older than 4 years of age. Data are not available for use in children younger than 4 years of age.

PREGNANCY AND LACTATION

- None of the antiemetic drugs should be used for nausea and vomiting during pregnancy, unless such usage has been approved by an obstetrician. However, ondansetron has been shown to be safe and effective (off label) for hyperemesis gravidum. Nursing mothers also should not use these products.
- Phenergan and Reglan are commonly used during pregnancy.

Patient Education

- These drugs may have severe sedative effects.
- Patients should not drive or operate dangerous equipment and should use caution while driving or performing other tasks that require concentration.
- Alcohol and other CNS depressants should be avoided.
- Adequate dosing before riding in a vehicle must be ensured for the prevention of motion sickness.
- Antidopaminergic agents may exacerbate preexisting psychiatric conditions.
- Constipation may be severe with the antidopaminergic phenothiazines; patients should be alerted to report problems.
- Males may experience urinary retention.

SPECIFIC DRUGS

ANTIDOPAMINERGICS

Phenothiazines

prochlorperazine (Compazine)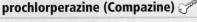

CONTRAINDICATIONS
- Hypersensitivity
- Reye's syndrome
- Pediatric surgery
- Children <2 years or weighing <9 kg

WARNINGS
- Extrapyramidal reactions, such as tardive dyskinesia
- Neuroleptic malignant syndrome (NMS)
- May cause excessive sedation, bone marrow depression, constipation, urinary retention

PRECAUTIONS. Use with caution in patients with cardiac, hepatic, or renal disease, or with glaucoma, prostatic hyperplasia, or decreased GI motility.

PHARMACOKINETICS. *prochlorperazine:* Oral half-life is 3 to 5 hours; metabolized in liver

ADVERSE EFFECTS. Sedation, dry mouth, blurred vision, miosis, mydriasis, constipation, obstipation, atonic colon, urinary retention, decreased sweating, impotence, hyperthermia, hypothermia, hypotension, tachycardia, increased pulse, syncope, dizziness, urticaria, erythema, eczema, photosensitivity

OVERDOSAGE. Symptoms involve extrapyramidal reactions, hypotension, and sedation. CNS depression and coma with areflexia may occur. Early signs of overdose may include restlessness, confusion, and excitement. Treatment generally involves symptomatic and supportive care.

OTHER DRUGS IN CLASS

Other drugs in this class are similar to the key drug, except as follows:
- *promethazine (Phenergan):* Black box warning for respiratory depression: contraindicated in children younger than 2 years old; in children older than 2 years, use the lowest possible dose. Half life: 7-14 hours; metabolized in liver

ANTICHOLINERGICS

meclizine (Antivert) 🔑

Meclizine has an onset of action of 30 to 60 minutes, depending on the dosage. Duration of action is 8 to 24 hours, depending on the dosage.

ADVERSE EFFECTS. See Table 28-3.

DOSAGE AND ADMINISTRATION. See Table 28-4.

OTHER DRUGS IN CLASS

Other drugs in this class are similar to the key drug, except as follows:
- *scopolamine (Transderm Scōp):* The transdermal system allows steady state plasma levels to be reached rapidly and maintained for 3 days. Onset of action is approximately 4 hours.

NK1 RECEPTOR ANTAGONIST

aprepitant (Emend)

Aprepitant is used in the prevention of nausea and vomiting with both highly and moderately emetogenic chemotherapeutic agents and for the prevention of postoperative nausea and vomiting. This medication is given in anticipation of nausea and vomiting and is given at least 3 hours prior to surgery or receipt of emetogenic drugs. Concomitant dexamethasone and methylprednisolone doses should be decreased by 50% and 25%, respectively, when they are given with this drug. It has little affinity for 5-HT₃

TABLE 28-3   Adverse Effects of Antiemetics

| Body System | Antidopaminergic | ANTICHOLINERGICS | | 5-HT$_3$ Receptor Antagonists |
		Antihistamines	Scopolamine	
Skin, appendages	Exfoliative dermatitis	Rash, urticaria	Allergic skin reactions	Pruritus
Hypersensitivity	Hypersensitivity	Hypersensitivity	Hypersensitivity	Hypersensitivity
Respiratory				Hypoxia, bronchospasm
Cardiovascular	Orthostatic hypotension, QT prolongation,	Hypotension, palpitations, tachycardia	Tachycardia	Hypertension, tachycardia
GI	Cholestatic jaundice, dry mouth, constipation, nausea	Dry mouth, anorexia, nausea, vomiting, diarrhea, constipation	Constipation, paralytic ileus	Abdominal pain, constipation, diarrhea, nausea, vomiting
Heme and lymphatic	Blood dyscrasias			Blood dyscrasias
Musculoskeletal	SLE-like syndrome	Muscle cramps		Musculoskeletal pain
Nervous system	EPS: tardive dyskinesia, neuromalignant syndrome, seizures, drowsiness, dizziness, headache	Drowsiness, restlessness, excitation, nervousness, insomnia, euphoria, auditory and visual hallucinations	Drowsiness (15%), restlessness, disorientation, memory disturbances, dizziness, hallucinations, confusion, seizures	Anxiety, dizziness, drowsiness, headache, malaise, fatigue, chills/shivering
Special senses	Blurred vision	Blurred vision, diplopia, vertigo, tinnitus	Blurred vision, dilation of pupils, narrow-angle glaucoma	
Hepatic	Hepatotoxicity			↑ALT, AST
Genitourinary	Urinary retention, impotence	Urinary frequency, difficult urination, urinary retention	Urinary retention	Urinary retention
Other	Menstrual irregularities, weight gain, hyperprolactinemia, hyperglycemia	Dry nose and throat	Dry mouth (67%), toxic psychosis, heat stroke	Fever

receptors, dopamine, or corticosteroid receptors, although it augments their activity. Pregnancy category B. This is a new drug, and little information on adverse effects or use in impaired populations is available. It is highly protein bound.

PHARMACOKINETICS. The drug undergoes extensive metabolism, primarily via cytochrome P (CYP) 3A4–mediated oxidation. It is eliminated primarily via metabolism and is not renally excreted. The apparent terminal half-life in humans ranges from 9 to 13 hours. The drug uses a nanoparticle formulation to enhance exposure and to minimize food effects.

It has been found to be effective with ondansetron and dexamethasone in controlling acute and delayed emesis. No clinically relevant differences in toxicity were noted when aprepitant was added, and improvements in quality of life among patients on chemotherapy were recorded.

ADVERSE EFFECTS. Associated with diarrhea, constipation, headache, and extreme fatigue; some cases of hiccups. Rate of nausea and vomiting with this product in highly emetogenic

substances is roughly equivalent to that seen with other forms of antiemetic therapy.

DRUG INTERACTIONS. Moderate CYP 3A4 inhibitor; care required when used with other drugs that use the P450 enzyme system

SEROTONIN 5-HT$_3$ RECEPTOR ANTAGONISTS

ondansetron hydrochloride (Zofran) 🔑

CONTRAINDICATIONS. Hypersensitivity to the drug (rare but sometimes severe with IV use)

WARNINGS
- Does not stimulate intestinal or gastric peristalsis; not to be used instead of nasogastric suction
- Patients should be informed to stop drug if rash develops.
- Use may mask progressive ileus and/or gastric distention in patients undergoing abdominal surgery.
- In patients with severe hepatic impairment, dosage should be reduced and the drug used with caution.

TABLE 28-4   Dosage and Administration Recommendations for Antiemetics

Drug	Age Group	Dosage	Administration	Maximum Daily Dose
chlorpromazine	Adult	10-25 mg po 50-100 mg pr	q4-6h q6-8h	
	Child	0.5-1 mg/kg po 0.5 mg/kg pr	q4-6h q6-8h	Children <5 yr (<22.7 kg): 40 mg/day Children 5-12 yr (22.7-45.5 kg): 75 mg/day
prochlorperazine	Adult	5-10 mg po	q6-8h	40 mg
	Child	2.5 mg po or pr	10-14 kg: q12-24h as needed; 15-18 kg: q8-12h as needed; 19-39 kg: q8h or 5 mg q12h as needed;	7.5 mg/day 10 mg/day 15 mg/day
promethazine	Adult	25 mg po, IV, IM	bid take 30 min before travel or q6h prn	
	Child ≥2 yr	0.25-1 mg/kg po or pr	q4-6h	25 mg
dimenhydrinate	Adult	50-100 mg po	q4-6h	400 mg
	Child 6-12 yr	25-50 mg po	q6-8h	150 mg
	Child 2-5 yr	12.5-25 mg po	q6-8h	75 mg
trimethobenzamide	Adult	300 mg po 200 mg pr	tid-qid tid-qid	
	Child <13.6 kg (30 lb)	100 mg pr	tid-qid	
	Child 13.6-41 kg (30-90 lb)	100-200 mg pr	tid-qid	
scopolamine	Adult	1.5 mg/patch	Apply patch behind ear, change q3d	

ondansetron	Adult >12 yr	8-24 mg po,
		    8-12 mg IV
			1-2 hr before chemotherapy.
			    May give 8 mg q8-12h
			    post chemotherapy/
			    radiotherapy	

	Hyperemesis gravidum (unlabeled use)	8 mg po, IV	q12h	

	Child 4-11 yr	4 mg po, IV	4 mg 30 minutes before
			    chemotherapy or 1-2 hr
			    prior to radiotherapy and
			    repeated q8h	

granisetron	Adult	2 mg po	Daily or 1 mg q12h, 1 hr before chemotherapy	
dolasetron	Adult	100 mg po, IV	1 hr before chemotherapy or daily	
	Child 2-16 yr	1.8 mg/kg	1 hr before chemotherapy; maximum: 100 mg/dose	
aprepitant	Adult	40 mg po	3 hr before surgery or chemotherapy	

Modified from Minocha A: *Handbook of digestive diseases* (Chapter 3), Thorofare, NJ, 2004, Slack, Inc.

ondansetron hydrochloride (Zofran) 🔑 —cont'd

The manufacturer recommends that the total daily dose should not exceed 8 mg in patients with severe hepatic impairment.

PHARMACOKINETICS. Half-life is 3 to 6 hours.

ADVERSE EFFECTS. See Table 28-3.

DRUG INTERACTIONS. Substrate of CYP 3A4; carbamazepine, nafcillin, phenobarbital, phenytoin, and rifampin will decrease the levels of ondansetron (no dosage change required, however).

OVERDOSAGE. Hypotension, faintness, and short episodes of blindness have been seen.

evolve A continually updated list of useful WebLinks may be found in the Evolve Resources at http://evolve.elsevier.com/Edmunds/NP/

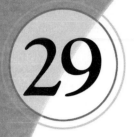

29

Medications for Irritable Bowel Syndrome and Other Gastrointestinal Problems

DRUG OVERVIEW

Class	Subclass	Generic Name	Trade Name
Antispasmodics/anticholinergics		dicyclomine hydrochloride ✱ 🗝 hyoscyamine sulfate	Bentyl Levsin, NuLev
5-HT₃ Receptor antagonist		alosetron	Lotronex
GI stimulants/prokinetic agents		metoclopramide ✱	Reglan
Prostaglandin		misoprostol	Cytotec
Ulcerative colitis treatment		mesalamine sulfasalazine	Asacol ✱ Azulfidine
Locally acting agent		simethicone	Phazyme, Gas-X
Gallstone-solubilizing agent		ursodiol	Actigall

✱ Top 200 drug; 🗝 key drug. Key drug chosen because dicyclomine has a lower incidence of side effects.

INDICATIONS

- See Table 29-1.
- This chapter discusses many diverse classes of medications; the only thing they have in common is their effects on the GI tract. Each class is discussed separately. The disease that is discussed in this chapter is irritable bowel syndrome (IBS).

Irritable Bowel Syndrome

Antispasmodic agents (e.g., dicyclomine hydrochloride [Bentyl], hyoscyamine sulfate [Levsin]) are used primarily to treat patients with IBS and other functional GI disorders. A large number of antispasmodics are available on the market, but they are not used often. Only the two most common antispasmodic drugs are discussed in this chapter. Dicyclomine is used as the prototype.

Alosetron (Lotronex), a type 3 serotonin (5-HT₃) antagonist, is available only through the Prescribing Program for Lotronex because of risk for ischemic colitis; this is not discussed in detail.

THERAPEUTIC OVERVIEW OF IRRITABLE BOWEL SYNDROME

Pathophysiology

The pathophysiology of IBS is not fully understood, but bowel motility is affected. In normal bowel motility, segmenting contractions assist transit through the bowel. When these contractions increase, diarrhea occurs. When they decrease, constipation occurs. External factors include stress, psychologic factors, laxative abuse, food intolerance, and menstruation. Some evidence of inflammation in this process has been obtained.

Disease Process

IBS is a common chronic functional bowel disorder. Other names for IBS include spastic colitis, mucous colitis, nervous colitis, spastic colon, nervous colon, irritated colon, and unstable colon. Functional bowel disorders consist of combinations of chronic or recurrent GI symptoms that cannot be explained by structural or biochemical abnormalities. Generally, the diagnosis is a clinical one that is based on a cluster of symptoms combined with exclusion of a specific organic cause. Diagnostic criteria have been developed to make the diagnosis of IBS more consistent. The history of the patient is critical for diagnosis of IBS. Common symptoms include

TABLE 29-1   Indications for Use of Miscellaneous GI Drugs

Drug Category	Individual Drugs	Indications
Antispasmodics/ anticholinergics	dicyclomine, hyoscyamine	IBS, PUD, hypermotility disorders, ulcerative colitis, diverticulitis
5-HT₃ receptor antagonist	alosetron	IBS with diarrhea
GI stimulants/prokinetic agents	metoclopramide	Diabetic gastroparesis, severe GERD
Prostaglandins	misoprostol	Reduce risk of NSAID PUD
Ulcerative colitis treatment	mesalamine sulfasalazine	Ulcerative colitis Ulcerative colitis, RA, JRA
Locally acting agents	simethicone	Flatulence
Gallstone-solubilizing agents	ursodiol	Gallstones

abdominal pain, altered bowel frequency and stool consistency (often alternating diarrhea and constipation), abdominal distention or bloating, and varying degrees of anxiety or depression. The new Rome III guidelines maintain that IBS of any subtype is characterized by a strong relationship between abdominal pain and defecation. These individuals have visceral hypersensitivity, or increased perception of gut-related events. In IBS with constipation (IBS-C), the onset of constipation generally corresponds with onset of pain at defecation. Patients with IBS-C may report abdominal pain, even if they empty their bowels regularly. The pain is described as sharp, burning, or cramping. The location is usually diffuse. A careful history is necessary to determine what the patient means by such words as "diarrhea," "constipation," and "regular." Nocturnal diarrhea may indicate a serious problem. Patients may be classified into categories based on their predominant symptom: pain, constipation, or diarrhea. Care should be taken to rule out organic causes of symptoms such as celiac disease, lactose or fructose intolerance, and infectious processes.

MECHANISM OF ACTION

- Antispasmodic/anticholinergic agents are also known as antimuscarinic drugs. The muscarinic nervous system is a subcategory of the anticholinergic nervous system. The other subcategory, the nicotinic nervous system, is seldom involved in drug actions. Anticholinergic agents decrease motility, relax smooth muscle tone in the GI tract, and decrease secretions.
- Antispasmodics decrease GI motility by relaxing smooth muscle tone. These medications have anticholinergic properties; thus they compete with acetylcholine for receptors at postganglionic fibers of the parasympathetic nervous system.
- Dicyclomine has indirect and direct effects on the smooth muscle of the GI tract. It indirectly blocks acetylcholine receptor sites and directly antagonizes bradykinin and histamine in GI tract smooth muscle. Both of these actions help to relieve smooth muscle spasm.

- Hyoscyamine, a belladonna alkaloid, inhibits the muscarinic actions of acetylcholine at postganglionic parasympathetic neuroeffector sites, including smooth muscle, secretory glands, and CNS sites. Thus, this drug has an effect on peripheral cholinergic receptors present in the smooth muscle of the GI tract. Specific anticholinergic responses are dose related. Low doses inhibit salivary and bronchial secretions and sweating. Next, pupil dilation and accommodation are affected, and heart rate is increased. Higher doses decrease motility in GI and urinary tracts, and then inhibit gastric acid.
- Antidepressants (particularly the TCAs) and 5-HT₃ (alosetron) and misoprostol have been found to be helpful in some patients. Please see Chapter 46 on antidepressants for a discussion of these products.

TREATMENT PRINCIPLES

Standardized Guidelines for IBS

- The American Gastroenterological Association developed guidelines for the treatment of patients with IBS; these were revised in 2002.

Evidence-Based Recommendations for IBS

Likely to be beneficial are the following:
- *Antidepressants:* Tricyclics have been shown to reduce symptoms; it is not clear whether this is a separate effect from the antidepressant effect.
- Smooth muscle relaxants have been noted to improve symptoms.
- A trade-off occurs between benefits and harms of all medications.
- *5-HT₃ receptor antagonist alosetron (Lotronex):* This agent has improved symptoms in women with diarrhea-predominant IBS and has increased constipation. It may be associated with ischemic colitis.

Cardinal Points of Treatment

- Pharmacotherapy is based on severity and is targeted at specific symptoms.
- All patients with alternating constipation/diarrhea:
  - Increased dietary fiber (25 g/day)
- Pain
  - Antispasmodic (anticholinergic) medication—short term
  - TCAs—long term
- Diarrhea
  - Loperamide—short term; often used for breakthrough diarrhea
  - Antidepressants (TCAs)—long term
  - Alosetron (ordered by GI specialists) if resistant to all other interventions
- Constipation
  - Fiber
  - Laxatives

Nonpharmacologic Treatment

Treatment of patients with IBS begins with patient education. The patient must be reassured that there is no organic cause for the symptoms. Teach that this is a chronic condition and that it will not lead to an organic problem.

Diet with adequate fiber is the cornerstone of treatment. Amounts of fiber and fluid usually have to be increased.

Fiber should be increased gradually to avoid bloating. (See Chapter 26 for a list of high-fiber foods.) The patient should drink 6 to 8 glasses of water a day. The patient should identify and eliminate foods that cause symptoms. Foods that commonly cause problems include raw fruits and vegetables, high-fat foods, beverages such as carbonated beverages, coffee and other forms of caffeine, red wine and beer, and artificial sweeteners such as fructose and sorbitol. Exclude lactose intolerance.

Other important lifestyle changes include good bowel habits and exercise. See Chapter 26 for a discussion of bowel training. The best exercise is usually regular walking.

Pharmacologic Treatment

Treatment of patients with IBS varies with the severity and type of presenting symptoms, which usually occur as diarrhea or constipation. Patients who are experiencing symptoms that become lifestyle limiting should be prescribed a medication on a short-term basis and should be advised to modify diet and behavior and to participate in psychotherapy.
- Cramping abdominal pain—antispasmodic (anticholinergic) medication, as needed, when symptoms are present shortly after a meal
- Abdominal pain, frequent or severe—TCA
- Constipation—increase dietary fiber, laxatives
- Diarrhea—antidiarrheals such as loperamide (Imodium); severe—alosetron (females only) may be considered
- Painful symptoms and diarrhea—TCAs
- Painful symptoms and constipation—SSRIs (conflicting efficacy)
- Simethicone use for problems with gas, including explosive bowel movements, belching, or flatus
- Lubiprostone and polyethylene glycol also used for IBS (see Chapter 26)

Antidepressants often are used over the long term to treat the patient with IBS and associated psychologic symptoms. TCAs have been used extensively. Through their effects on neurotransmitters, they are effective against abdominal pain. A common side effect is constipation, which makes them most useful in patients with diarrhea. SSRIs are used clinically but have shown inconsistent results. Paroxetine (Paxil) has been shown to be effective in improving bowel regularity but not in affecting pain. The other SSRIs do not have the anticholinergic effect that paroxetine has, and they may be more useful in patients with constipation.

How to Monitor

- Monitor for therapeutic response: The patient should be able to report fewer episodes of abdominal cramping and less diarrhea and constipation.
- Monitor for anticholinergic effects: Evaluate for increased heart rate and blood pressure, dry mouth, constipation, blurred vision, or urinary retention.

Patient Variables

GERIATRICS. Lower doses of antispasmodics should be prescribed to geriatric patients because this population may react with increased adverse effects such as agitation, excitement, confusion, or delusions.

PEDIATRICS. Safety and efficacy are not established. Hyoscyamine has been used in infant colic. Dicyclomine is contraindicated in infants younger than 6 months of age.

PREGNANCY AND LACTATION
- *Category B:* dicyclomine, alosetron
- *Category C:* hyoscyamine

Patient Education
ANTISPASMODICS
- Refrain from activities that require mental alertness while taking these medications.
- Stay out of hot and humid environments while taking these medications.
- Take 30 to 60 minutes before a meal.
- Notify physician of side effects, especially eye pain, rash, or flushing.
- Gum or sugarless hard candy may relieve dry mouth.

SPECIFIC DRUGS
ANTISPASMODICS/ANTICHOLINERGICS

dicyclomine hydrochloride (Bentyl)

CONTRAINDICATIONS
- Hypersensitivity
- Glaucoma (narrow angle)
- *Cardiovascular:* tachycardia, unstable cardiovascular status in hemorrhage, MI
- GI tract obstructive disease (pyloroduodenal stenosis, etc.), paralytic ileus, severe ulcerative colitis, and hepatic disease
- Myasthenia gravis
- *Genitourinary (GU):* obstructive uropathy, caused by prostate hyperplasia; renal disease

WARNINGS
Heat prostration potential with extremely high temperatures. These drugs can cause a reduction in sweating, which can predispose a patient to heatstroke and fever.

Use with caution when patients have diarrhea. Diarrhea may be an early sign of incomplete bowel obstruction. Patients who are sensitive to anticholinergic drugs may exhibit signs of psychosis.

PRECAUTIONS. Use with caution in the following:
- *Cardiovascular:* CAD, CHF, arrhythmia, tachycardia, HTN
- *GI:* hepatic disease; early evidence of ileus, hiatal hernia associated with reflux esophagitis (may aggravate)
- *GU:* renal disease; prostatic hyperplasia
- *Ocular:* glaucoma
- *Pulmonary:* COPD reduces bronchial secretions; asthma, allergies
- Myasthenia gravis, hypothyroidism
- Some products may contain tartrazine or sulfites to which many individuals are allergic.

dicyclomine hydrochloride (Bentyl) 🗝—cont'd

PHARMACOKINETICS. Compared with the belladonna alkaloids (hyoscyamine), dicyclomine is poorly and unreliably absorbed orally. It does not cross the blood-brain barrier; therefore, CNS and ophthalmic effects are unlikely. The duration of action is more prolonged than that of the belladonna alkaloids.

ADVERSE EFFECTS. Dry mouth, dizziness, blurred vision, nausea, light-headedness, drowsiness, weakness, nervousness, urinary hesitancy and retention, tachycardia, palpitations, mydriasis, cycloplegia, increased ocular pressure, loss of taste, headache, insomnia, nausea, vomiting, impotence, constipation, and bloated feeling

DRUG INTERACTIONS. The anticholinergics increase the pharmacologic effects of digoxin and atenolol and decrease the effects of phenothiazine. Amantadine, phenothiazines, and TCAs increase the side effects of the anticholinergics.

They may decrease or antagonize the effects of medications used to treat glaucoma. Antacids may decrease absorption of anticholinergics.

DOSAGE AND ADMINISTRATION
- *Adult:* 20 to 40 mg qid ac and daily at bedtime (maximum, 160 mg/day)
- *Geriatric:* Start with 10 mg bid to qid; increase slowly as tolerated (maximum, 160 mg/day).

OTHER DRUGS IN CLASS

Other drugs in this class are similar to the key drug, except as follows:
- *Hyoscyamine* sulfate (Levsin) is a belladonna alkaloid, in contrast to dicyclomine. It is rapidly absorbed and readily crosses the blood-brain barrier, affecting the CNS. Thus, the risk of CNS adverse effects is greater than with dicyclomine.
  - Dosages: *adult, geriatric*—0.125 to 0.25 mg tid to qid or prn before meals or food

5-HT₃ Receptor Partial Agonist

alosetron (Lotronex)

Indicated only for women with severe chronic diarrhea-predominant IBS who have had anatomic or biochemical abnormalities of the GI tract excluded, and who have not responded adequately to conventional therapy. This drug may be prescribed only by providers who enroll in a GlaxoSmithKline prescribing program.

WARNINGS. Black box warning alerts to the potential for serious GI adverse reactions, including ischemic colitis, and serious complications of constipation, including blood transfusion, surgery, and death. Discontinue medication immediately if colitis should develop.

ADVERSE EFFECTS. Constipation, colitis; requires discontinuation of drug

DOSAGE AND ADMINISTRATION. 0.5 mg twice a day is initial adult dosage; after 4 weeks, may be increased to 1 mg twice a day, if required

GI STIMULANTS/PROKINETIC AGENTS

metoclopramide (Reglan)

INDICATIONS. Diabetic gastroparesis; severe GERD unresponsive to standard therapy; prevention of nausea and vomiting in chemotherapy and postoperatively

 Although very effective, this drug has the potential for very serious adverse reactions.

MECHANISM OF ACTION. Metoclopramide stimulates the upper GI tract. Although the exact mode of action is unclear, it appears to increase the responsiveness of tissues in the GI tract to acetylcholine. Metoclopramide increases the tone and amplitude of gastric contractions and relaxes the pyloric sphincter and duodenal bulb. This drug also has been shown to accelerate gastric emptying by increasing peristalsis of the duodenum and jejunum. Its benefit in GERD results from an increased resting tone of the lower esophageal sphincter. Its antiemetic properties are related to metoclopramide antagonism of the central and peripheral dopamine receptors.

HOW TO MONITOR. The patient should be monitored during the first 24 to 48 hours for any adverse reactions. Should extrapyramidal symptoms (EPS) occur, treat with IM diphenhydramine (Benadryl) 50 mg or benztropine (Cogentin) 1 to 2 mg. If parkinsonian symptoms occur (usually within the first 6 months), discontinue use of metoclopramide. Stop the medication if the patient exhibits tardive dyskinesia.

PATIENT VARIABLES

Geriatrics. Older patients may have a slight decrease in elimination of these drugs. Begin with 50% of adult dose and titrate slowly. Geriatric patients are at greater risk of side effects with this drug.

Geriatric patients in particular are at increased risk for adverse effects such as confusion and extrapyramidal symptoms. Use with caution.

Pediatrics. The safety and effectiveness of these drugs have not been established; thus, use of them is not recommended. Metoclopramide has been used in infants and children with symptomatic GERD. Methemoglobinemia has occurred. Infants and children ages 21 days to 3.3 years with GERD have been treated with metoclopramide at dosage of 0.5 mg/kg/day; symptoms improved.

PREGNANCY AND LACTATION. *Category B:* No adequate studies; metoclopramide crosses the placenta and is excreted into breast milk

RENAL DYSFUNCTION
Children and Adults
- *CrCl 40 to 50 ml/min:* Administer 75% of recommended dose.

- *CrCl 10 to 40 ml/min:* Administer 50% of recommended dose.
- *CrCl <10 ml/min:* Administer 25% to 50% of recommended dose.

PATIENT EDUCATION
- Do not consume ANY alcohol-containing food or drink while taking this drug.
- Do not operate heavy equipment or drive a vehicle for at least 2 hours after taking this medication because of the risk of sedation and drowsiness.
- Inform health care provider of the occurrence of any involuntary movements or twitching.

CONTRAINDICATIONS
- Hypersensitivity to the drug
- When stimulation of GI motility might be dangerous, as in GI hemorrhage, obstruction, or perforation
- *Pheochromocytoma:* May cause a hypertensive crisis
- Epilepsy and people receiving drugs that are likely to cause extrapyramidal reactions

WARNINGS
- *Depression:* with suicidal ideation, has occurred in patients with and without prior history of depression

  EPSs manifested as acute dystonic reactions may occur, usually within the first 24 to 48 hours; this is seen more frequently in children and young adults, and in geriatric patients.

- Parkinson-like symptoms occur within the first 6 months of treatment; use with caution in patients with Parkinson's disease.
- Tardive dyskinesia, a syndrome of potentially irreversible, involuntary, dyskinetic movements, may develop. The highest likelihood is among the elderly.
- *Neuroleptic malignant syndrome:* Hyperthermia, muscle rigidity, altered consciousness
- Hypertension has occurred.
- *Anastomosis or closure of the gut:* Metoclopramide theoretically increases pressure on suture lines.
- Elevated prolactin levels persist during long-term administration.

PRECAUTIONS. Use with caution in hazardous tasks.

ADVERSE EFFECTS
- Common mild side effects in 20% to 30% of patients include restlessness, anxiety, drowsiness, fatigue, lassitude, insomnia, headache, dizziness, sedation, nausea, diarrhea, rash, decreased libido, bowel disturbances, and fever.
- Potentially serious adverse reactions include EPS, tardive dyskinesia, dystonic reactions, akathisia, prolactin secretion, hypotension/hypertension, depression with suicidal ideation, seizures, and hallucinations.

DRUG INTERACTIONS. Metoclopramide may decrease the levels of digoxin and cimetidine. It may increase the levels of alcohol, cyclosporine, MAOIs, succinylcholine, and levodopa. Levodopa, anticholinergics, and narcotic analgesics decrease the effects of metoclopramide. The risk of extrapyramidal reactions may be increased when phenothiazine and butyrophenone antipsychotics are given with metoclopramide.

The likelihood of CNS depression may be increased when metoclopramide is given concurrently with antihypertensives, alcohol, sedatives, and TCAs.

DOSAGE AND ADMINISTRATION
- *For gastroesophageal reflux:* 10 to 15 mg po qid, 30 minutes before each meal and at bedtime
- *For diabetic gastroparesis:* 10 mg po qid, 30 minutes before meals and at bedtime

PROSTAGLANDIN
misoprostol (Cytotec)

INDICATION. Reduce risk of NSAID-induced gastric ulcer in patients with high risk of complications from gastric ulcer

MECHANISM OF ACTION. Misoprostol is a synthetic prostaglandin, similar in action to natural substances produced by the body. In contrast to H_2-blockers and acid pump inhibitors, this protective agent does not inhibit the release of acid. Misoprostol shields the stomach's mucous lining from the damage of acid by increasing mucus and bicarbonate production and by enhancing blood flow to the stomach. NSAIDs cause ulceration by blocking prostaglandin synthesis that, in turn, decreases bicarbonate and mucus production. Misoprostol binds with prostaglandin receptor sites, thus causing increased production of bicarbonate and mucus. Prostaglandin receptor sites are saturable, reversible, and stereospecific. These sites have a high affinity for misoprostol.

HOW TO MONITOR
- Ask the patient specifically about diarrhea at follow-up visits.
- Check the stool for occult blood.
- If patient is of childbearing age, administer pregnancy test before starting the drug.

PATIENT VARIABLES
- *Pregnancy Category X:* Do not give to nursing mother.
- *Pediatrics:* Safety and effectiveness have not been established.

PATIENT EDUCATION
- Do not take if pregnant or planning to become pregnant. Make it clear to female patients who are in their childbearing years that pregnant women who take misoprostol may experience a miscarriage. They also may experience life-threatening bleeding as a result of the miscarriage.
- Emphasize the importance of not giving this drug to anyone else.
- Take drug with food to minimize the risk of GI side effects.

CONTRAINDICATIONS. Allergy to any prostaglandins

Category X: To be used only for women who are in their childbearing years if the patient (1) is at high risk of developing gastric ulcers and needs NSAIDs; (2) is capable of complying with effective contraception; (3) has received both oral and written warnings

regarding the hazards of misoprostol therapy, the risk of possible contraception failure, and the hazards this drug poses to other women of childbearing age who might take it by mistake; (4) has had a negative serum pregnancy test within 2 weeks before beginning therapy; and (5) will begin therapy on the second or third day of her next normal menstrual period.

WARNINGS. Must not be taken by women who are pregnant

PRECAUTIONS. Use with caution in patients with preexisting cardiovascular disease.

PHARMACOKINETICS
- Rapidly, extensively absorbed
- *Metabolism:* Liver; rapid deesterification to its free acid, which is the active ingredient
- *Time to maximum concentration:* 10 to 15 minutes; half-life, 20 to 40 minutes
- Availability decreased with food or concomitant antacid
- Serum protein binding: 80% to 90%
- Excreted in urine (65% to 75%)

ADVERSE EFFECTS. The most common adverse effects are diarrhea, abdominal pain, nausea, flatulence, headache, dyspepsia, vomiting, constipation, vaginal spotting, uterine cramps, hypermenorrhea, and dysmenorrhea.

DRUG INTERACTIONS. Concomitant use with antacids may decrease plasma concentration levels of misoprostol.

DOSAGE AND ADMINISTRATION. Usual recommended dose is 200 mcg qid. It is often necessary to start at 100 mcg bid and slowly increase dose to avoid excessive diarrhea.

ULCERATIVE COLITIS DRUGS
sulfasalazine and mesalamine

MECHANISM OF ACTION. Sulfasalazine is split into sulfapyridine and mesalamine (5-aminosalicylic acid, 5-ASA) by bacteria in the colon. Mesalamine is thought to be the active component and is an aminosalicylate. The mechanism of action of sulfasalazine and mesalamine is unknown but is thought to be topical rather than systemic. These agents act by blocking cyclooxygenase and inhibiting prostaglandin production in the colon.

CONTRAINDICATIONS. Hypersensitivity to mesalamine, salicylates, or any component of the formulation

WARNINGS
- *Intolerance/colitis exacerbation:* Acute intolerance syndrome may occur with cramping, acute abdominal pain, and bloody diarrhea.
- *Pancolitis:* Some patients developed pancolitis, although it occurred less often with mesalamine than with placebo.
- Renal function impairment has occurred. Use with caution in patients with renal impairment.
- *Pregnancy Category B:* No adequate studies
- *Lactation:* Low concentrations of mesalamine have been detected.
- Safety and efficacy for use in children have not been established.

PRECAUTIONS
- Pericarditis has occurred rarely with sulfasalazine; investigate chest pain.
- Sulfite sensitivity

PHARMACOKINETICS. Sulfasalazine is not absorbed; it acts locally. Mesalamine is absorbed (20% to 30%).

ADVERSE EFFECTS. Well tolerated. Most effects are mild and transient. Most common are headache, abdominal pain/cramps/discomfort, eructation, diarrhea, constipation, and nausea. Rare are chest pain, anxiety, confusion, and agranulocytosis. Capsules cause fewer adverse reactions than are caused by tablets. Levels of AST, ALT, alk phos creatinine, BUN, amylase, lipase, GGTP, and lactate LDH are elevated. Hepatitis rarely occurs.

DRUG INTERACTIONS
- *Azathioprine, mercaptopurine, thioguanine:* Risk of myelosuppression may be increased by aminosalicylates, warfarin, enoxaparin, and heparin.
- *Digoxin:* mesalamine may decrease digoxin bioavailability.

DOSAGE AND ADMINISTRATION
- 1-g capsules qid for a total dose of 4 g for up to 8 weeks
- Tablets 800 tid for a total dose of 2 to 4 g/day for 6 weeks
- 500-mg or 1000-mg suppositories and suspension for rectal instillation are also available.
- Swallow tablets whole.
- Shake suspension well before inserting into rectum.

LOCALLY ACTING AGENT
simethicone (Phazyme, Gas-X)

The antiflatulent agent simethicone is used to help relieve painful symptoms of trapped air and gas in the GI tract. Overproduction of gas may occur when certain foods are eaten or air is swallowed during the process of eating or chewing. This medication is available OTC.

MECHANISM OF ACTION. Simethicone is a defoaming agent that acts by altering the surface tension of gas bubbles trapped in the GI tract. This action causes the gas bubbles to coalesce and the trapped gas to be expelled through belching or rectal flatus.

PATIENT EDUCATION
- Do not take this medication indiscriminately.
- Patients should report any symptoms that persist to the health care provider.

CONTRAINDICATIONS. Hypersensitivity to simethicone

ADVERSE EFFECTS. Excessive episodes of belching and rectal flatus

DOSAGE AND ADMINISTRATION
- *Ages 12 years and up:* 40 to 125 mg after each meal and daily at bedtime; maximum, 500 mg/day
- *Children (ages 2-12 yr):* 40 mg (0.6 ml) qid after meals and daily at bedtime
- *Infants (<2 yr):* 20 mg (0.3 ml) qid after meals or with formula

GALLSTONE-SOLUBILIZING AGENTS

ursodiol (Ursodeoxycholic Acid) (Actigall)

INDICATIONS. Ursodiol is used to dissolve radiolucent noncalcified gallstones in those patients who either refuse surgery or are poor surgical risks. Ursodiol also is used to prevent stone formation in those who experience rapid weight loss after undergoing gastric bypass surgery or as the result of a low-calorie diet. A functional gallbladder is needed for the drug to be used.

MECHANISM OF ACTION. Ursodiol is a naturally occurring bile acid that suppresses hepatic synthesis and cholesterol secretion and inhibits intestinal absorption of cholesterol. This increases the concentration level at which saturation of cholesterol occurs. The bile changes from cholesterol precipitating to cholesterol solubilizing.

HOW TO MONITOR

- Monitor for fever, pain, and jaundice.
- Monitor for an acute condition in the abdomen that can occur if stones move and block the common bile duct.
- In weight loss patients, monitor for nausea.
- Check baseline LFTs and monitor periodically.

PATIENT VARIABLES

Pediatrics. Safety and usage in children have not been established.

Pregnancy and Lactation. *Category B:* It is not known whether ursodiol is excreted in breast milk; use with caution if administering to a nursing mother.

PATIENT EDUCATION

- Therapy is continued for at least 3 months after apparent dissolution.

- If no dissolution is evident after 12 months, surgery may be necessary. As long as progress toward dissolution is noted, the drug may be continued.

CONTRAINDICATIONS. Patients with stones larger than 2 mm, acute condition in the abdomen, known sensitivity to the drug, acute pancreatic gallstones, or acute cholecystitis are not candidates for the drug.

ADVERSE EFFECTS. Diarrhea, pruritus, rash, dry skin, stomatitis, flatulence, headache, dizziness, fatigue, myalgia, and rhinitis are reported adverse effects.

DRUG INTERACTIONS. Bile-sequestering agents and aluminum-based antacids may reduce absorption. Oral contraceptives, estrogens, and clofibrate increase cholesterol secretion in the liver and may counteract the effectiveness of ursodiol.

PHARMACOKINETICS. Total of 90% absorbed in small bowel; large first-pass effect. Small quantities appear in systemic circulation; metabolized in liver. In all, 80% excreted in feces.

DOSAGE AND ADMINISTRATION

- *Gallstone dissolution:* 8 to 10 mg/kg/day in two or three divided doses
- *Gallstone prevention:* 300 mg bid

evolve A continually updated list of useful WebLinks may be found in the Evolve Resources at http://evolve.elsevier.com/Edmunds/NP/

Diuretics

DRUG OVERVIEW

Class	Subclass	Generic Name	Trade Name
Diuretics	Thiazides and thiazide-like ([NaCl] inhibitors)	hydrochlorothiazide 🗝 ✹ chlorothiazide chlorthalidone indapamide ✹ metolazone ✹	HydroDIURIL Diuril Hygroton Lozol Zaroxolyn
	Loop diuretics (sodium, potassium, chloride inhibitors)	furosemide 🗝 ✹ bumetanide ✹ ethacrynic acid torsemide ✹	Lasix Bumex Edecrin Demadex
	Carbonic anhydrase inhibitors	acetazolamide	Dazamide, Diamox, Diamox Sequels
Potassium-sparing diuretics	Sodium channel blockers	triamterene 🗝 amiloride	Dyrenium Midamor
	Aldosterone antagonists	spironolactone ✹ eplerenone	Aldactone Inspra
Fixed-dose combination therapies		hydrochlorothiazide/ amiloride hydrochlorothiazide/ spironolactone hydrochlorothiazide/ triamterene ✹	Moduretic Aldactazide, Spirozide Dyazide, Maxzide
Potassium supplements		potassium chloride ✹	Kaon-Cl, K-Dur, K-Lor, K-Tab, Micro-K, Slow K

✹ Top 200 drug; 🗝 key drug.

INDICATIONS

- Hypertension
- Chronic heart failure or heart failure syndrome
- Renal failure
- Cirrhosis

Diuretics

The four major subclasses of diuretics—thiazides, loop, carbonic anhydrase inhibitors, and potassium-sparing diuretics (Table 30-1)—act by decreasing sodium reabsorption at different sites along the nephron. The four classes differ in terms of the specific site of action in the nephron. The ability to augment urinary losses of sodium and water is useful in the treatment of hypertension, heart failure, renal failure, and

cirrhosis. A large number of thiazide diuretics are available; only the five most commonly used are discussed here. The use of potassium supplementation is discussed separately at the end of the chapter.

THERAPEUTIC OVERVIEW
Anatomy and Physiology

Sodium and chloride ions and water are freely filtered across the glomerulus. Under normal circumstances, more than 99% of these substances are reabsorbed along the renal tubule. This process requires the renal tubules to reclaim nearly 3 lb of sodium chloride each day. The reabsorption of sodium is, in general, an active transcellular process. By contrast, chloride reabsorption may be passive or active but is most commonly coupled with sodium reabsorption, which explains

TABLE 30-1   Classification of Diuretics

Proximal Tubule	Loop of Henle Inhibitors	Distal Convoluted Tubule	Collecting Tubule
Carbonic Anhydrase Inhibitors		*NaCl Inhibitors*	*Sodium Channel Blockers and Aldosterone Antagonists*
acetazolamide (Diamox)	furosemide (Lasix) bumetanide (Bumex) ethacrynic acid (Edecrin) torsemide (Demadex)	hydrochlorothiazide (Microzide) metolazone (Zaroxolyn) chlorthalidone (Hygroton) indapamide (Lozol)	triamterene (Dyrenium) amiloride (Midamor) spironolactone (Aldactone) eplerenone (Inspra)

the parallel reabsorption of these two ions. Water reabsorption occurs by diffusion, which is driven by solute, particularly sodium, reabsorption.

The first step of sodium and water reabsorption at each site involves the transport of sodium from the tubular lumen into tubular epithelial cells. It is this first step that is inhibited by diuretics. Each segment of the nephron contains different luminal transport proteins or channels that facilitate the entry of filtered sodium into the cell. These transport systems are inhibited predominantly by only certain types of diuretics. It is this specificity that determines the site of action of each diuretic. Once sodium has entered the tubular cells, it is pumped out of the other side of the cell by a sodium-potassium exchanger into the interstitial fluid, from which it may be returned to the circulation.

MECHANISM OF ACTION

The three major classes of diuretics (excluding combination therapy) are thiazide, loop, and potassium sparing. These are generally distinguished at the point where they impair

sodium reabsorption within the renal tubule. Thiazide-type diuretics work in both the distal tubule and the connecting segment (and perhaps in the early cortical collecting tubule). Loop diuretics, the most potent, act in the thick ascending limb of the loop of Henle. Potassium-sparing diuretics work in the aldosterone-sensitive principal cells in the cortical collecting tubule.

The sites of action of the different types of diuretics are outlined in Figure 30-1 and Table 30-1. The ability of each type of diuretic to increase urinary sodium excretion depends on two factors: the amount of sodium reabsorbed at its site of action and the ability of more distal sites to reclaim that sodium. Carbonic anhydrase inhibitors act on the proximal tubule, where up to 65% of sodium is reabsorbed. However, these drugs have limited clinical usefulness as diuretics because sodium lost at this site is effectively reclaimed at more distal sites along the nephron. Loop diuretics act in the ascending limb of the loop of Henle, where 25% of sodium is normally reclaimed. Thiazide diuretics act on the distal tubule, where 3% to 5% of sodium is reclaimed. The collecting

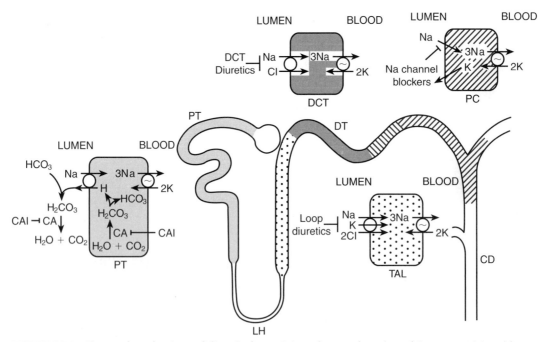

FIGURE 30-1   Sites and mechanisms of diuretic drugs. Spironolactone (not shown) is a competitive aldosterone antagonist that acts primarily in the collecting duct. As the most distal part of the nephron, it exhibits the least amount of reabsorption. *CA,* Carbonic anhydrase; *CAI,* carbonic anhydrase inhibitor; *CD,* collecting duct; *DCT,* distal convoluted tubule; *DT,* distal tubule; *LH,* loop of Henle; *PC,* principal cell; *PT,* proximal tubule; *TAL,* thick ascending limb; ~, indicates primary active transport. (From Ellison DH: The physiologic basis of diuretic synergism: its role in treating diuretic resistance, *Ann Intern Med* 114:887, 1991.)

duct is the site of action of the potassium-sparing diuretics. Normally, only 1% to 2% of the sodium is reabsorbed at this site. These drugs, as their group name implies, limit urinary losses of potassium.

Thiazide Diuretics

In all, 3% to 5% of filtered sodium is reabsorbed in the distal tubule. This reabsorption occurs via an NaCl cotransporter that is inhibited by thiazide diuretics. The therapeutic effect of this class of diuretics is partially blunted by the reabsorption of sodium that takes place distally in the cortical collecting tubule. Thus, the thiazide-type diuretics are less effective in the treatment of edema, where a large amount of fluid loss is the goal of therapy. In the treatment of patients with hypertension, however, these drugs are particularly effective because marked fluid loss is neither necessary nor desirable. The mechanisms that underlie the efficacy of thiazides in the treatment of hypertension are not completely known. Volume loss likely plays an important role. However, during long-term therapy, these drugs may act to decrease peripheral vascular resistance.

The distal renal tubule is also the primary site of calcium reabsorption. The thiazides act to enhance calcium absorption and lessen excretion. This effect is beneficial in the treatment of patients with chronic kidney stones that arise from excessive calcium excretion.

Loop Diuretics   *Lasix Bugc Edecrin oto*

Twenty percent of filtered sodium is reabsorbed in the loop of Henle. A cotransporter in the ascending limb of the loop of Henle and in the macula densa cells of the early distal tubule moves one molecule of sodium and potassium and two molecules of chloride from the tubular lumen into the tubular epithelial cells (see Figure 30-1). Most reabsorbed potassium then moves back out of the cell into the tubular lumen via potassium channels. Loop diuretics inhibit this cotransporter and are able to excrete up to 25% of the filtered sodium. Ototoxicity, caused by intravenous loop diuretic therapy, is thought to be related to inhibition of this cotransporter in the inner ear.

Loop diuretics promote excretion of calcium. This occurs passively as a result of sodium reabsorption inhibition. This is a clinically relevant effect in that loop diuretics and saline hydration are the treatments of choice in cases of hypercalcemia.

Carbonic Anhydrase Inhibitors

Approximately 50% to 75% of filtered sodium is reabsorbed in the proximal tubule. However, the diuretic response is generally weak because most filtered sodium is reclaimed by both the loop of Henle and the distal nephron. An important sodium transport pathway at this site is the sodium/hydrogen (sodium/H) exchanger that is located in the luminal membrane of the proximal tubular cells (see Figure 30-1). An important factor in maintenance of sodium/H exchange is the removal of hydrogen ions from the tubular lumen. If hydrogen ions accumulate, then the activity of the sodium/H exchanger is slowed. Carbonic anhydrase facilitates the removal of luminal hydrogen ions by promoting the dissociation of carbonic acid, H_2CO_3 (formed by the association of filtered bicarbonate with the hydrogen ions secreted into the tubular lumen by the sodium/H exchanger), to yield carbon dioxide and water. This process of carbonic acid formation and dissociation maintains low luminal hydrogen ion levels and thus allows the sodium/H exchanger to continue to reabsorb sodium. If carbonic anhydrase is inhibited, luminal hydrogen ion concentrations rise and the activity of the sodium/H exchanger is inhibited. The carbonic anhydrase inhibitors are relatively weak diuretics because of the ability of more distal sites to increase their reabsorption of sodium.

An important consequence of carbonic anhydrase inhibition is its interference with bicarbonate reabsorption (see Figure 30-1). The distal nephron sites are not able to reclaim all of this additional bicarbonate; as a result, bicarbonate is lost into the urine. This loss of bicarbonate can be an advantage in the treatment of individuals with severe metabolic alkalosis, in whom this bicarbonate loss can limit alkalemia. However, loss of urinary bicarbonate can also lead to severe metabolic acidosis.

Potassium-Sparing Diuretics

SODIUM CHANNEL BLOCKERS. The collecting duct plays a major role in the day-to-day regulation of NaCl and potassium excretion. Sodium reabsorption along this segment, which reabsorbs only 3% to 5% of filtered sodium, occurs via a luminal sodium channel. The reabsorption of sodium generates a voltage gradient that drives potassium from the tubular cell into the tubular lumen and hence into the urine. Blocking of sodium reabsorption at this site slows potassium excretion and leads to the potassium retention for which diuretics that act on this segment are named. The net diuretic effect is approximately 1% to 2% filtered sodium. These diuretics are commonly paired with a loop or a thiazide for refractory edema or to blunt potassium loss.

ALDOSTERONE ANTAGONISTS. Tubular epithelial cells in the collecting duct possess high-affinity receptors for the hormone aldosterone. Occupancy of these receptors by aldosterone initiates a number of events, including activation of previously inactive luminal sodium channels, transport of additional sodium channels from the cytosol to the luminal cell membrane, and stimulation of the production of other sodium channels. Spironolactone and eplerenone competitively inhibit the aldosterone receptor. Eplerenone differs from spironolactone in that it is a more specific inhibitor of aldosterone and produces fewer endocrine side effects. The net diuretic effect of the aldosterone antagonists is approximately 1% to 2% filtered sodium. However, these drugs are particularly useful in the treatment of cirrhosis and ascites and have been shown to improve survival in patients with heart failure.

TREATMENT PRINCIPLES
Standardized Guidelines

- Chobanian AV, et al: The seventh report of the Joint National Committee on Prevention, Detection, Evaluation, and Treatment of High Blood Pressure: the JNC 7 report, JAMA 289:2560, 2003.
- Adams KF, et al: Executive summary: HFSA 2006 comprehensive heart failure practice guideline, *J Cardiac Failure* 12:10-38, 2006 (full 112-page guidelines available online at www.hfsa.org).

Evidence-Based Recommendations

Refer to Chapters 15 and 17 for recommendations in the treatment of hypertension and heart failure.

Cardinal Points of Treatment

- Salt restriction
- First line: thiazide
- Second line: loop diuretic
- Other diuretics as needed for specific conditions

These treatment options may vary if the patient has renal insufficiency.

Pharmacologic Treatment

An important factor in diuretic efficacy is the patient's ability to adhere to a low-sodium diet. As drug concentration falls, a period of positive sodium balance—the period of post-diuretic sodium retention—may follow. If dietary salt intake is high, then the amount of sodium lost in response to the diuretic may be partially or completely offset by postdiuretic sodium retention.

Renal function is another important variable in determination of diuretic response. Patients become less responsive to diuretics as renal function declines. Loop diuretics typically retain efficacy even in the face of moderately severe renal insufficiency; however, patients may require higher diuretic doses to achieve an effect. Most thiazides are relatively ineffective in individuals with a glomerular filtration rate (GFR) <30 ml/min. Exceptions to this are metolazone and indapamide. Potassium-sparing diuretics should be used with great caution or should be avoided in patients with renal insufficiency because of their potential to induce life-threatening hyperkalemia.

In addition, length of time on therapy may contribute significantly to the responsiveness of the kidneys to diuretics. The ability of a diuretic to increase renal NaCl excretion declines over time. This phenomenon, referred to as *diuretic resistance,* is thought to occur in one of every three patients with heart failure (HF). A second drug that is added may act synergistically to mitigate this adaptive process.

For diuretic resistance, evaluate and treat these factors: patient nonadherence (either not taking drug or high NaCl intake), HF, renal failure, increased renal insufficiency, nephrotic syndrome, and cirrhosis. Drugs that may cause diuretic resistance include NSAIDs, captopril, cimetidine, and some antihypertensives. (See Boxes 30-1 and 30-2.)

As with any medication, it is important for the clinician to determine the patient's previous response to treatment and history of any adverse events. Additional considerations include cost, mobility, and toileting concerns that may affect a patient's adherence to prescribed diuretic therapy.

THIAZIDES. Thiazides are the most frequently used and least expensive antihypertensive drugs. Early studies clearly demonstrated blood pressure reduction; however, metabolic effects such as hypokalemia, hyperuricemia, and hyperglycemia were seen. Even more important, demonstration of a significant reduction in coronary events following BP reduction was difficult, and this limited their widespread use. Dosages of hydrochlorothiazide in these early studies were in excess of 50 mg per day. In later studies, doses greater than 25 mg per day were shown to limit the extent of these metabolic effects while reducing blood pressure. These findings led to initiation of the Antihypertensive and Lipid-Lowering treatment to prevent Heart Attack Trial (ALLHAT).

BOX 30-1   Causes of Diuretic Resistance

PATIENT NONADHERENCE

Not taking drug
High NaCl intake

IMPAIRED BIOAVAILABILITY

Chronic heart failure*
Idiopathic edema

IMPAIRED DIURETIC SECRETION BY PROXIMAL TUBULE

Renal failure or worsened renal insufficiency
Old age
Renal transplantation
Chronic heart failure*

Other Medications

NSAIDs—interactions with loop and DCT diuretics; captopril (Capoten)—interaction with furosemide (Lasix); cimetidine (Tagamet)—interaction with amiloride (Midamor) and triamterene (Dyrenium)
Antihypertensives

PROTEIN BINDING IN TUBULE LUMEN

Nephrotic syndrome

HEMODYNAMIC (REDUCED GLOMERULAR FILTRATION RATE [GFR])

Medications

Antihypertensives
NSAIDs
Hypoxemia
Reduced "fullness" of arterial vascular system

ENHANCED NaCl REABSORPTION

Primary

Chronic heart failure*
Nephrotic syndrome
Cirrhosis

Related to Use of Medications

NSAIDs
Adaptation to long-term diuretic therapy

*Chronic heart failure alters primarily the time course of diuretic absorption rather than the percentage of administered dose that is absorbed.

BOX 30-2 Approach to Diuretic Resistance in Patients

ASSESS ADHERENCE WITH TREATMENT REGIMEN (DIET AND MEDICATIONS).

- Measure daily sodium excretion.
  - If >100 mmol/day, reduce intake.
  - If <100 mmol/day, proceed as below.

ASSESS STATUS OF UNDERLYING DISEASE.

- Does patient really need further reduction of extracellular fluid volume?
- Can treatment of underlying disease be improved?

DISCONTINUE NSAIDs AND CONSIDER REDUCING VASODILATORS (ESPECIALLY IF BLOOD PRESSURE IS LOW).

CHANGE TO A LOOP DIURETIC AND INCREASE DOSAGE UNTIL DIURETIC THRESHOLD OR MAXIMUM SAFE DOSE IS ATTAINED.

- Consider constant diuretic infusion.
- May block postdiuretic NaCl retention and may be useful for hospitalized patients

CONSIDER DIURETIC COMBINATIONS.

- Add DCT diuretic (usually the best choice is metolazone or hydrochlorothiazide). Usually avoid combination products in patients with CHF.
- Add distal diuretic (amiloride, triamterene, and spironolactone are primarily effective in cirrhotic edema).
- Add proximal diuretic (carbonic anhydrase inhibitors)

ALLHAT, the largest prospective study on hypertension to date, compared the efficacy of an angiotensin-converting enzyme inhibitor (lisinopril, 10 to 40 mg per day) or a calcium channel blocker (amlodipine, 2.5 to 10 mg per day) or doxazosin (an α-adrenergic blocker) vs. a thiazide diuretic (chlorthalidone, 12.5 to 25 mg per day) in preventing major outcomes in high-risk hypertensive patients. More than 33,000 patients were enrolled in the study from 1994 to 2002 and were followed for a mean of 5 years. Patients were 55 years of age or older with a diagnosis of hypertension and at least one risk factor for coronary heart disease (CHD). The doxazosin arm was prematurely stopped during an interim analysis that showed an increased risk of heart failure (8.1% vs. 4.5% at 4 years) compared with chlorthalidone.

At the end of the study, all three drugs were noted to be effective in reducing blood pressure and providing protection from CHD and nonfatal myocardial infarction. However, chlorthalidone was shown to be superior to the other drugs in terms of the following outcomes.

Compared with chlorthalidone, lisinopril had higher rates of the following:

- Combined cardiovascular disease outcomes (32.3% vs. 30.9%)
- Stroke (6.3% vs. 5.6%)
- Heart failure (8.7% vs. 7.7%; greatest in the first year)

Compared with chlorthalidone, amlodipine had a higher rate of the following:

- Heart failure (10.2% vs. 7.7%; greatest in the first year)

The benefits of chlorthalidone treatment in ALLHAT were evident in men, women, African Americans, non–African Americans, those with and without diabetes, and younger and older patients. Adverse effects, specifically hypokalemia and hyperglycemia, were more frequent in the chlorthalidone group. Hypokalemia occurred in 8.5% vs. 1.9% and 0.8% in the amlodipine and lisinopril groups, respectively. Potassium supplementation, as expected, was more frequent in the chlorthalidone group and was required in 8% of patients. A fasting blood sugar >126 mg/dl was also seen in 11.6% of patients receiving chlorthalidone among those without diabetes.

This was more frequent than in those receiving amlodipine (9.8%) and lisinopril (8.1%).

Based on results from the ALLHAT trial, the seventh Joint National Committee (JNC 7) report recommended that a thiazide diuretic be given as initial treatment of hypertension unless a specific indication for a drug from another class is noted. The authors also believed that the benefits of chlorthalidone would be translated to hydrochlorothiazide at similar doses of 12.5 to 25 mg once daily.

The addition of a thiazide to a loop diuretic and sodium restriction may be useful in the treatment of refractory edema in patients with CHF, cirrhosis, nephrotic syndrome, and renal failure. The rationale for this combination involves inhibition of sodium reabsorption at multiple sites along the nephron and the fact that in CHF, most patients have altered creatinine clearance, so loop diuretics are more effective.

Thiazides are useful in reducing the frequency of new stone formation in patients with idiopathic hypercalciuria because of their ability to decrease renal calcium excretion. This enhanced calcium excretion results in a positive calcium balance that may reduce the number of fractures in older patients. An analysis of 18 observational studies of more than 29,000 patients revealed that the use of a thiazide diuretic on a long-term basis may reduce osteoporotic fractures by up to 20%. The same is not true of loop diuretics because these drugs produce a negative calcium balance and have been shown to increase the risk of hip fracture associated with osteoporosis.

Thiazides also may be used to decrease urine volume in patients with nephrogenic diabetes insipidus. Thiazide diuretics given in combination with a low-salt diet in the management of Ménière's disease may decrease the natural progression of sensorineural hearing loss and may be used to treat vertigo through prevention of flare-ups.

As is the case with most diuretics, major complications of thiazide therapy include fluid and electrolyte abnormalities. Of concern is the increased incidence of sudden death seen in early studies with doses >50 mg per day in patients with hypertension. However, the ALLHAT trial clearly showed that this finding was dose related.

As a general recommendation, thiazides should be started at the lowest dosage, and those with shorter half-lives should be given once or twice daily. Doses no greater than 25 mg daily of hydrochlorothiazide or chlorthalidone should be given for the treatment of hypertension; the adverse effects of hypokalemia, hypomagnesemia, and increased cholesterol, as well as a possible increase in sudden death, among thiazide-treated patients appear to be dose related.

LOOP DIURETICS. The primary use of loop diuretics involves the treatment of states of volume excess that include CHF, nephrotic syndrome, acute and chronic renal insufficiency, and cirrhosis. Furosemide is the most commonly used loop diuretic. Torsemide and bumetanide offer enhanced absorption (90%) over furosemide (50%) and in some cases may provide greater efficacy in patients who do not respond to maximum doses of furosemide. A critical component of loop diuretic dosing is the equivalent dose of each drug. Furosemide 40 mg is equivalent to 1 mg of bumetanide and 20 mg of torsemide. This is important when the change is made from one loop diuretic to another. Diuresis is seen with doses of 10 mg furosemide and at 40 mg in patients with normal renal function. The equivalent doses of bumetanide and torsemide are 1 mg and 20 mg, respectively. Ethacrynic acid is also a loop diuretic; however, its use is limited because of an associated higher incidence of ototoxicity.

In the treatment of patients with HF, loop diuretics relieve the congestive symptoms of pulmonary and peripheral edema. Symptom relief is felt within hours to days, in contrast to other treatments for HF such as ACE inhibitors, β-blockers, and digoxin, which may take weeks to months to provide maximum benefit. A typical starting daily dose of furosemide is 20 to 40 mg; for bumetanide, it is 0.5 to 1 mg, and for torsemide, 10 to 20 mg. Dosing is guided by the diuretic response, and doses should be increased every 1 to 2 weeks because net sodium loss occurs for only 1 to 2 weeks before a new steady state is achieved. A helpful monitoring tool involves asking the patient to record his or her weight each day. If a patient does not respond, the clinician should increase the diuretic dose initially rather than giving the same dose twice daily. Maximum daily doses in patients with normal renal function are 80 mg for furosemide, 3 mg for bumetanide, and 50 mg for torsemide. Higher total doses of up to 200 mg furosemide daily (given as split doses) are necessary in patients with renal insufficiency. It is important to adequately dose the loop diuretics because accuracy of dosing affects the efficacy of other therapies for HF, such as ACE inhibitors, angiotensin receptor blockers (ARBs), and β-blockers.

Except in patients with renal insufficiency (GFR <30 ml/min), thiazide diuretics are more efficacious than loop diuretics for the treatment of hypertension. It is believed that sodium retention is activated by the renin-angiotensin-aldosterone system once the loop diuretic response has dissipated (<6 hours for furosemide and bumetanide). It is not known whether torsemide, which lasts up to 12 hours, would be effective in this setting.

Loop diuretics are also effective for the removal of excess fluid in ascites and chronic kidney disease. In patients with normal kidney function, the maximum effective dose in the treatment of cirrhosis is 40 mg, 1 mg, and 20 mg of furosemide, bumetanide and torsemide, respectively. Doses are higher in the treatment of nephrotic syndrome, where 120 mg, 3 mg, and 50 mg of furosemide, bumetanide, and torsemide, respectively, are used.

The major toxicities related to the loop diuretics result from their ability to induce fluid and electrolyte imbalances, hypersensitivity reaction, and ototoxicity. These fluid and electrolyte imbalances arise from excessive diuresis and occur as hypokalemia, hyponatremia, hypomagnesemia, hypocalcemia, hyperuricemia, metabolic alkalosis, and elevations in BUN and serum creatinine. Excessive sodium and water losses may also lead to volume depletion and hypotension.

The loop diuretics are sulfonamide derivatives, and the provider should pay close attention to the specific reaction of a patient who reports an allergy to a sulfonamide or a "sulfa" drug (e.g., Bactrim, Septra, generic) because individuals with sulfa allergies often have a predisposition to allergic reactions in general, as opposed to cross-reactivity with sulfonamide drugs. The non-sulfonamide loop diuretic ethacrynic acid is reserved for the patient who develops a true allergic reaction to a loop or thiazide diuretic.

Ototoxicity generally manifests as deafness and sometimes is permanent. It has been reported in the treatment of acute renal failure with doses of furosemide >80 to 160 mg per hour (2 to 4 g/day). Concurrent use of aminoglycoside antibiotics and loop diuretics increases the risk of deafness.

CARBONIC ANHYDRASE INHIBITORS. Carbonic anhydrase inhibitors are relatively weak diuretics. They are used primarily in the treatment of patients with open-angle glaucoma and for prophylaxis and treatment of acute mountain sickness. The risk of mountain sickness is directly related to the rate of ascent. Acetazolamide is efficacious above 4000 meters when ascent rates are >500 m/day. Acetazolamide also may be used, usually in combination with other diuretics, to treat edema associated with HF. The ability of carbonic anhydrase inhibitors to increase urinary losses of bicarbonate may be useful in the treatment of individuals with severe metabolic alkalosis.

POTASSIUM-SPARING DIURETICS. Potassium-sparing diuretics are generally used in combination with thiazides. The rationale for this combination is to augment diuresis and blunt the hypokalemia that is seen with use of thiazide and loop diuretics. See later discussion on combination diuretics.

Spironolactone, a nonspecific aldosterone antagonist, has been shown to be of particular benefit in the treatment of severe CHF when added to an ACE inhibitor and a loop diuretic for severe chronic CHF, reducing mortality rates. Hyperkalemia appears to be dose dependent.

Eplerenone is an aldosterone-specific antagonist designed to minimize the unpleasant endocrine side effects of spironolactone. It is effective in the treatment of HF in post–MI patients. It may cause relevant increases in potassium levels >6 mEq/L. The 2005 ACC/AHA guidelines on the management of CHF recommend use of an aldosterone antagonist in patients with moderately severe to severe symptoms of HF (Classes II–IV) and a reduced LVEF. The authors also recommended that a patient's renal function and potassium levels should be followed closely, usually at 1 week and 1 month after dosage adjustments are made.

Patients who should not receive an aldosterone antagonist for the treatment of HF are those with a baseline plasma creatinine concentration >2.5 mg/dl (males) and 2 mg/dl (females), and those with potassium concentration >5 mEq/L.

The authors of the 2004 ACC/AHA guidelines on ST-segment elevation MI also recommend the use of spironolactone or eplerenone in patients who are already receiving an ACE inhibitor, exhibiting an LVEF of 40%, and presenting with symptomatic HF or diabetes.

OSMOTIC DIURETICS. Osmotic diuretics, such as mannitol, act by inhibiting sodium absorption in the proximal tubule and the loop of Henle. Their clinical use is limited primarily to inpatient settings in which they may be used to reduce intracranial pressure or to reduce intraocular pressure in glaucoma. Osmotic diuretics are not used in edematous states or in outpatients because of their potential to induce intravascular volume expansion and pulmonary edema in susceptible patients. These drugs are not discussed further.

COMBINATION DIURETICS. Diuretic combinations are used (1) to minimize the side effects of one diuretic by using lower doses, and (2) to increase urinary sodium losses by blocking sodium reabsorption at two sites along the nephron. Most often, a potassium-sparing diuretic will be used with a thiazide diuretic to minimize the risk of hypokalemia. Another combination consists of a loop diuretic and a thiazide to affect diuresis in individuals with resistance to the effects of loop diuretics used alone. The simultaneous use of two diuretics of the same class (i.e., two loop diuretics or two thiazides) provides no additional therapeutic benefit over that provided by a single agent; thus, these should not be prescribed. Four combinations of diuretics—thiazide and potassium sparing, loop and thiazide, loop and potassium sparing, and loop and carbonic anhydrase inhibitors—may be prescribed. Only thiazide and potassium-sparing agents are available as a fixed dosage. All four combinations of diuretic agents are discussed in the following paragraphs.

THIAZIDE AND POTASSIUM-SPARING COMBINATIONS. Fixed-dose combinations of thiazide and potassium-sparing diuretics are convenient and may enhance patient adherence. The disadvantage of a fixed-dose combination is that it limits flexibility in dose titration. Ideally, the correct doses of individual agents should be determined first, and the patient should be switched to a fixed-dose product if one is found that matches his or her needs. Unfortunately, differences in bioavailability require caution when a change is made from one product to another. Cautions and adverse effects are similar to those associated with the individual agents.

LOOP AND THIAZIDE DIURETICS. Patients may become resistant to the effects of diuretics during treatment. Patients may tolerate these regimens better if the thiazide diuretic is administered every other day or only two or three times per week.

The combination of loop and potassium-sparing diuretics is frequently used to treat patients with decompensated liver disease and ascites. These individuals typically have high aldosterone levels; as a result, they maximally conserve sodium in the collecting duct. The addition of spironolactone is more efficacious than either agent given independently. A typical starting combination of these drugs in patients without hypertension or CHF is 40 mg of furosemide with 100 mg of spironolactone. Amiloride, which also acts in the collecting duct, may be used in lieu of spironolactone. Its onset of action

is faster, and its use does not lead to the complication of gynecomastia, which may be associated with spironolactone.

LOOP AND CARBONIC ANHYDRASE INHIBITORS. During loop diuretic therapy, two factors may make the addition of a carbonic anhydrase inhibitor useful. The first is that loop diuretic–induced volume loss stimulates increased absorption of sodium in the proximal tubule. This increased proximal reabsorption of sodium may blunt the efficacy of the loop diuretic. Second, loop diuretics increase urinary losses of hydrogen ions; this may contribute to the development of a metabolic alkalosis. The addition of a carbonic anhydrase inhibitor may enhance urinary sodium losses and prevent or minimize the development of a metabolic alkalosis.

The combination of a loop diuretic and a carbonic anhydrase inhibitor should be given with caution. Hypovolemia, hypokalemia, and metabolic acidosis are potential complications of this therapy. The health care provider should have a clear understanding of the patient's acid-base status before using a carbonic anhydrase inhibitor. For example, if the patient's serum bicarbonate is elevated as an appropriate response to acute or chronic respiratory acidosis, then the addition of a carbonic anhydrase inhibitor could lead to severe acidemia. A full discussion of acid-base balance is beyond the scope of this chapter.

How to Monitor

Fluid and electrolyte abnormalities are the most common adverse effects of diuretic use. Up to 50% of patients receiving diuretic therapy with loop diuretics experience potassium levels lower than 3.5 mEq/L.

Recent data on the mortality benefits of the aldosterone antagonists in HF have led to an increase in the incidence of hyperkalemia. Following publication of the RALES trial results, significant increases (from 4 to 11 per 1000 patients) occurred during the treatment period in rates of hospital admission for hyperkalemia; rates for hyperkalemia-related death increased from 0.7 to 2 per 1000. Patients who have higher baseline plasma potassium concentrations should not be started on aldosterone antagonists. Studies have identified the following risk factors for the development of spironolactone-induced hyperkalemia:

- Increased age
- More severe HF
- Diabetes
- Preexisting renal dysfunction or altered creatinine clearance
- Volume depletion
- Spironolactone doses >50 mg/day
- Higher-dose ACE inhibitor or ARB
- Combined use of ACE inhibitor and ARB
- β-Blocker use
- Use of potassium supplements or potassium-containing salt substitutes
- Use of NSAIDs

Volume status should be assessed at baseline and periodically during therapy. Patients can be instructed to record their weight and amount of edema on a daily basis at home. Major changes in electrolytes generally occur within the first few weeks of therapy, and, contrary to popular belief, potassium depletion is not progressive with continued treatment. Serum electrolytes should be checked before diuretic therapy is initiated, after 1 week and 1 month of starting therapy, after any dosage changes, and at other times thereafter as warranted by changes in the patient's clinical condition. To prevent significant cardiovascular events such as fatal dysrhythmias, supplementation with magnesium as well as potassium may have to be considered in some patients. See the discussion on monitoring under "Potassium Supplements" later in this chapter.

Patient Variables

GERIATRICS. Older patients are at increased risk for diuretic-induced electrolyte disturbances caused by an age-related decline in renal function. This fall in GFR diminishes the diuretic response, in particular to the thiazides. Despite this fact, isolated systolic hypertension in some conditions may be successfully treated with low-dose diuretic monotherapy in the elderly. The 1991 Systolic Hypertension in the Elderly Program (SHEP) trial demonstrated that chlorthalidone 12.5 to 25 mg daily reduced blood pressure (SHEP, 1991). The incidence of stroke at 4 to 5 years was 5.2%, compared with 8.2% in the placebo group. The incidence of cardiac events was reduced by one quarter to one third, although this reduction was not statistically significant. Benefits were seen in all age groups, including patients older than 80 years, and in both men and women.

PEDIATRICS. Considerable data have supported the safety and efficacy of thiazide diuretics in children. In clinical practice, however, ACE inhibitors, ARBs, and β-blockers are used preferentially over thiazides because of the potential for glucose elevation and lipid and electrolyte abnormalities. The following therapies are used in a variety of clinical situations, including edema, glaucoma, and epilepsy. Acetazolamide is used for glaucoma and epilepsy only. Bumetanide and ethacrynic acid are not recommended in children younger than 18 years of age. Furosemide should be avoided in the premature infant with respiratory distress syndrome because it may increase the risk of persistent patent ductus arteriosus and ototoxicity. Chlorothiazide, hydrochlorothiazide, spironolactone, and hydrochlorothiazide and spironolactone have been safely used in pediatric patients for the treatment of edema and hypertension. Careful monitoring is essential because pediatric patients may be less tolerant of small shifts in fluids and electrolytes.

Subtle changes related to diuretic or potassium replacement therapies may not manifest themselves in pediatric patients as they do in adult patients. Infants especially cannot report symptoms related to weakness, confusion, paresthesias, or muscle cramps. Changes in personality and in eating or sleeping patterns, as well as restlessness, should be reported and investigated promptly.

PREGNANCY AND LACTATION. There is great variability in the safety of diuretics during pregnancy.

> **evolve** Consult the table on Evolve prior to ordering diuretics for pregnant women.

RACE. Race can be a factor when diuretic therapy is considered. In the treatment of hypertension (HTN), African Americans often respond better than whites to monotherapy diuretics.

Patient Education

- Importance of dietary sodium restriction in determining diuretic efficacy
- Symptoms of hypovolemia, including weakness and orthostatic dizziness that might indicate the need for diuretic dose adjustment

- Signs and symptoms of hypokalemia or hyperkalemia, including profound weakness; patients should report these symptoms promptly so that electrolytes may be checked.
- Adherence with intermittent dosing schedules, such as alternate day or weekly dosing, may improve if patients use a calendar to record medication use.
- Patients may wish to avoid taking their diuretics late in the day to minimize disturbance of sleep patterns.
- Urinary volume is expected to increase. Therefore, easy access to a bathroom is essential, especially at initiation of drug therapy. For some patients, this effect does not improve over time.
- May need to monitor daily weight; rapid weight loss (more than 1 to 2 lb/day) might be harmful

SPECIFIC DRUGS

Thiazides and Thiazide-like Diuretics

hydrochlorothiazide (HCTZ) (HydroDIURIL)

CONTRAINDICATIONS
- Hypersensitivity to sulfonamides
- GFR of ≤30 ml/min

WARNINGS. Use with caution in patients with moderate chronic renal insufficiency or hepatic dysfunction because of the potential of both these conditions to deteriorate with volume depletion or electrolyte imbalance.

PRECAUTIONS
- Serum electrolytes should be checked before treatment is initiated and periodically thereafter. Hypokalemia is a common complication of thiazide use (Box 30-3).
- Women may exhibit a greater decrease in serum potassium concentration than men.
- The hyperglycemia seen with thiazide use appears to be a consequence of diuretic-induced hypokalemia.
- Because thiazides interfere with the kidney's ability to completely dilute the urine, patients may retain free water with resultant hyponatremia.

BOX 30-3   Signs and Symptoms of Hypokalemia

Arrhythmias, weak irregular pulse, flattened T waves, presence of U waves
Potentiation of digitalis toxicity
Fatigue
Muscle weakness, cramps
Soft and flabby muscles
Decreased reflexes
Postural hypotension
Rhabdomyolysis
Confusion
Glucose intolerance
Polyuria
Metabolic alkalosis
Nausea and vomiting
Decreased GI motility, ileus

hydrochlorothiazide (HCTZ) (HydroDIURIL) —cont'd

- Thiazides decrease uric acid excretion and may predispose susceptible individuals to episodes of gout.
- The decrease in renal calcium excretion, which may be advantageous in patients with calcium-containing stone disease, may lead to hypercalcemia, particularly in those with hyperparathyroidism.
- Dose-related increases in LDL are seen early in therapy. These increased values tend to return to baseline measurements with long-term therapy.
- Thiazide diuretics have been reported to worsen disease in individuals with systemic lupus erythematosus.
- Potassium supplementation is often required (Box 30-4).

PHARMACOKINETICS. The preparations differ primarily in their duration of action; see Table 30-2.

ADVERSE REACTIONS. A variety of common adverse effects have been described with various thiazides (Table 30-3).

DRUG INTERACTIONS. Thiazides may increase the effects of anesthetics, prolong chemotherapy-induced leukopenia, increase the toxicity of digitalis and lithium, and increase calcium levels in patients also treated with calcium and/or vitamin D supplementation. Decreases in the efficacy of anticoagulants, anti-gout agents, oral hypoglycemics, and insulin may be seen with concomitant thiazide use. Anticholinergics may increase thiazide absorption, whereas bile acid sequestrants decrease it. Methenamines and NSAIDs may decrease the efficacy of thiazide diuretics.

OTHER DRUGS IN CLASS

Other drugs in this class are similar to the prototype except as follows:

- *indapamide (Lozol), metolazone (Mykrox, Zaroxolyn):* Exceptions to avoiding thiazides in patients with GFR ≤30 ml/min are metolazone and indapamide. These two thiazides are effective in patients with diminished GFR. In addition, increases in cholesterol do not occur during treatment with indapamide.

Loop Diuretics

furosemide (Lasix)

CONTRAINDICATIONS
- Volume-depleted patients: These drugs can induce substantial losses of sodium and water.
- Sulfa allergy

WARNINGS. Diuretic-induced hypokalemia is a very common consequence of loop diuretic therapy. The potency of loop diuretics requires careful patient monitoring to assess volume status and to monitor for hypokalemia. Careful

Continued

BOX 30-4   Food Sources Rich in Potassium

HIGH: 5 to 10 mEq/Serving (195-390 mg)

Dairy
Milk, 1%

Meats, Dry Beans, Eggs, and Nuts
Almonds
Beef, lean, ground, broiled/fried
Black bean soup
Chicken, ½ breast
Mussels, cooked
Pork, center loin, broiled
Tuna, canned in water
Turkey, without skin, roasted
Swordfish

Vegetables
Broccoli, boiled
Carrot, raw
Tomato, raw

Fruits
Apple juice
Grapefruit juice
Peaches, canned in water
Pear, raw
Strawberries, raw

VERY HIGH: >10 mEq/Serving (>390 mg)

Dairy
Milk, skim
Yogurt, plain, fat free

Meats, Dry Beans, Eggs, and Nuts
Baked beans, vegetarian or pork, or refried beans
Kidney beans, boiled
Lima beans, boiled

Vegetables
Marinara sauce
Potato, baked with skin
Spinach, boiled

Fruits
Banana
Cantaloupe, raw
Orange juice, canned
Raisins

Condiments
Salt substitutes (1 mEq = 30 mg potassium)

TABLE 30-2 Pharmacokinetics of Diuretics

Drug	Oral Absorption	Onset of Action	Half-life	Duration of Action	Excretion
acetazolamide	NC	Tabs, 1-1.5 hr Caps, 2 hr	6-9 hr	Tabs, 8-12 hr Caps, 18-24 hr	Renal
furosemide	10%-90%	0.3-1 hr	0.5-1 hr	6-8 hr	Renal, 60%; liver, 40%
bumetanide	72%-95%	0.5-1 hr	1-1.5 hr	4-6 hr	Renal, 65%; liver, 35%
ethacrynic acid	NC	<0.5 hr	0.5-1 hr	6-8 hr	Renal, 65%; liver, 35%
torsemide	79%-91%	1 hr	0.8-6 hr	8-12 hr	Renal, 30%; liver, 70%
hydrochlorothiazide	65%-75%	2 hr	15 hr	6-12 hr	Liver, 70%; renal, 30%
chlorothiazide	10%-21%	2 hr	0.75-2 hr	6-12 hr	Renal; liver, 20%-60%
chlorthalidone	60%-70%	2 hr	35-50 hr	24-72 hr	Renal, 65%; liver, 10%; unknown, 25%
indapamide	NC	1-2 hr	10-22 hr	36 hr	Liver
metolazone	65%	1 hr	8 hr	12-24 hr	Renal, 80%; liver, 20%
triamterene	30%-70%	2-4 hr	1.6-2.5 hr	12-16 hr	Liver
amiloride	50%	2 hr	6-9 hr	24 hr	Renal
spironolactone	90%	24-72 hr	1.3-2 hr	48-72 hr	Liver

NC, Nearly complete.

furosemide (Lasix) 🗝 —cont'd

daily monitoring of weight at home can help to reveal patients with too rapid volume loss (>1 to 2 lb/day).

PRECAUTIONS. Loop diuretic–induced hypercalciuria could increase the frequency of stone formation in susceptible individuals. Laboratory abnormalities associated with loop diuretic use include hyperuricemia, which may lead to clinical episodes of gout, impaired glucose tolerance, and increases in LDL cholesterol. Adverse effects on lipid levels may dissipate during long-term therapy.

PHARMACOKINETICS. See Table 30-2. These drugs are highly protein bound and thus are not filtered into the tubular lumen through the glomerulus. Instead, they gain access to the tubular lumen via an organic ion transporter in the proximal tubule.

ADVERSE EFFECTS. See Table 30-3. The most common adverse effects are related to fluid and electrolyte abnormalities.

DRUG INTERACTIONS. Concomitant use of loop diuretics and aminoglycosides or cisplatin can increase ototoxicity. Diuretic-induced volume depletion increases the risk of aminoglycoside-induced acute renal failure. Loop diuretics can increase the activity of anticoagulants and salicylates and may increase blood levels of β-blockers and lithium. Probenecid decreases the efficacy of loop diuretics.

OTHER DRUGS IN CLASS

Other drugs in this class are similar to the prototype except as follows:

- *bumetanide and torsemide:* Metabolized in the liver; better absorbed, more bioavailable; torsemide has a longer duration of action than furosemide and bumetanide. For patients with HF in whom variations in furosemide absorption may be clinically significant, treatment with more completely absorbed loop diuretics may be indicated. Ethacrynic acid is a phenoxyacetic acid derivative; severe diarrhea has been reported.

Carbonic Anhydrase Inhibitors

acetazolamide (Dazamide, Diamox)

CONTRAINDICATIONS

- *Hepatic cirrhosis:* Impaired renal excretion of ammonia caused by these drugs can precipitate hepatic encephalopathy.
- *Advanced renal insufficiency, respiratory acidosis, or metabolic acidosis:* Loss of bicarbonate in the urine as induced by these drugs may cause severe acidemia in these patients.
- *Hyponatremia or hypokalemia:* May be substantially worsened by the use of carbonic anhydrase inhibitors
- Sulfonamide allergy

PRECAUTIONS. Because these drugs may cause hypokalemia and metabolic acidosis, patients' serum electrolyte values should be monitored before and at regular intervals during treatment. A complete blood count before treatment and periodically thereafter will detect hematolytic toxicity, which can occur with sulfonamides such as acetazolamide.

DRUG INTERACTIONS

- Salicylates and diflunisal may increase the activity of carbonic anhydrase inhibitors.
- Acetazolamide can increase cyclosporine levels and decrease levels of primidone.

DOSAGE AND ADMINISTRATION. See Table 30-4 for all dosages and administration.

POTASSIUM-SPARING DIURETICS

triamterene (Dyrenium; Midamor) 🗝

CONTRAINDICATIONS

- Life-threatening hyperkalemia can result if triamterene is used in patients with elevated pretreatment serum potassium (>5.5 mmol/L), patients receiving concomitant potassium supplementation, or patients with moderate or severe renal insufficiency.
- Do not use with other potassium-sparing diuretics.
- Hypersensitivity

Text continued on page 365

TABLE 30-3 Dosage and Administration Recommendations for Diuretics

Drug	Diagnosis	Dose Range	Maximum Daily Dose
acetazolamide	Glaucoma	250 mg one to four times per day 500 mg ER bid	1000 mg
	Mountain sickness prevention	250 mg every 8-12 hours (begin 24-48 hr prior to ascent and 48 hr after arrival) 500 mg every 12-24 hours; (begin 24-48 hr prior to ascent and 48 hr after arrival)	1000 mg
furosemide	HF, Edema HTN	20-80 mg once daily 20-80 mg per day in two divided doses (JNC 7)	600 mg (2005 ACC/AHA guidelines) 80 mg/day in two divided doses (JNC 7)
bumetanide	HF, Edema HTN	0.5-2 mg once daily 0.5-2 mg per day in two divided doses (JNC 7)	10 mg (2005 ACC/AHA guidelines) 2 mg (JNC 7)
torsemide	HF	10-20 mg once daily; double dose until the diuretic response is achieved	200 mg (2005 ACC/AHA guidelines)
	HTN	2.5-5 mg once daily; increase to 10 mg after 4-6 weeks to desired response (JNC 7)	10 mg (JNC 7)
	Chronic renal failure (in patients who produce urine)	20 mg once daily; double dose until the diuretic response is achieved	NA
	Cirrhosis	5-10 mg once daily	10 mg
ethacrynic acid	Edema	50-100 mg per day in one or two divided doses; increase by 25-50 mg every 5-7 days	400 mg
hydrochlorothiazide	HF, Edema HTN	25-100 mg per day in one to two doses 12.5-50 mg once daily (JNC 7) Children <6 months: 2-3 mg/kg/day in two divided doses Children >6 months: 2 mg/kg/day in two divided doses	200 mg (ACC/AHA 2005 guidelines) 50 mg (JNC 7); >50 mg, lose K$^+$ 37.5 mg 200 mg
chlorothiazide *Note:* Chlorothiazide is available as a suspension.	HF, Edema HTN	250-1000 mg in one or two divided doses 125-500 mg per day (JNC 7) Children <6 months: 20-40 mg/kg/day in two divided doses Children >6 months: 10-20 mg/kg/day in two divided doses	1000 mg (ACC/AHA 2005 guidelines) 500 mg (JNC 7) 375 mg 375 mg/day in children <2 years, or 1000 mg/day in children 2-12 years old
chlorthalidone	HF	12.5-25 mg once daily (ACC/AHA 2005 guidelines)	100 mg (ACC/AHA 2005 guidelines)
	HTN Edema	12.5-25 mg once daily (JNC 7) 50-100 mg per day or 100 mg on alternate days	25 mg (JNC 7) 200 mg
indapamide	HF, Edema HTN	2.5-5 mg/day (ACC/AHA 2005 guidelines) 1.25 mg in the morning; increase by 1.25-2.5 mg	5 mg (ACC/AHA 2005 guidelines) 2.5 mg (JNC 7)
metolazone	HF	2.5-20 mg once daily as add-on and only intermittently as needed in patients with CHF (ACC/AHA 2005 guidelines)	20 mg (ACC/AHA 2005 guidelines)
	HTN	2.5-5 mg once daily (JNC 7)	5 mg (JNC 7)
triamterene	HF	50-75 mg per day in two divided doses (ACC/AHA 2005 guidelines)	200 mg (ACC/AHA 2005 guidelines)
	Edema HTN	100-300 mg/day in one or two divided doses 50-100 mg/day (JNC 7)	300 mg/day 100 mg (JNC 7)
amiloride	HF HTN	5 mg once daily (ACC/AHA 2005 guidelines) 5-10 mg per day in one or two divided doses	20 mg (ACC/AHA 2005 guidelines) 10 mg (JNC 7)
spironolactone	HF	12.5-25 mg once daily (ACC/AHA 2005 guidelines)	50 mg (ACC/AHA 2005 guidelines)
	Edema	25-200 mg per day in one or two divided doses	200 mg
	HTN	25-50 mg/day in one or two divided doses (JNC 7)	50 mg (JNC 7)

TABLE 30-4   Adverse Effects of Diuretics

Drug	Common Adverse Effects	Serious Adverse Effects
CARBONIC ANHYDRASE INHIBITORS		
All carbonic anhydrase inhibitors		Metabolic acidosis, hemolytic anemia, erythema multiforme, bone marrow depression
acetazolamide	Drowsiness, paresthesias, confusion, tinnitus, transient myopia, anorexia, altered taste, nausea, vomiting, diarrhea, polyuria, and mild electrolyte imbalances	Severe electrolyte imbalances Gastrointestinal bleeding, aplastic anemia, and sulfonamide-type reactions, including toxic epidermal necrolysis and Stevens-Johnson syndrome
LOOP DIURETICS		
All loop diuretics	Orthostatic hypotension, excessive diuresis leading to dehydration/hypovolemia and hemoconcentration, with subsequent hypotension and severe electrolyte imbalances of potassium (K), chloride (Cl), calcium (Ca), magnesium (Mg), and sodium; ototoxicity Tinnitus Vertigo Hyperuricemia	Cardiovascular collapse Encephalopathy with preexisting liver disease Severe electrolyte imbalances (Ca, Cl, K, Mg, sodium)
furosemide	Photosensitivity	Anemia, neutropenia, and agranulocytosis Hyperglycemia
bumetanide		Reversible azotemia, metabolic alkalosis
ethacrynic acid	Anorexia Diarrhea	Neutropenia Agranulocytosis
Torsemide	Hyperglycemia	Electrocardiographic changes
THIAZIDE DIURETICS		
All thiazide diuretics	Orthostatic hypotension, dizziness, drowsiness, syncope, weakness, nausea, gastrointestinal irritation, hypermotility, electrolyte imbalances, hemoconcentration, transient elevations in blood urea nitrogen (BUN), hypovolemia, depressed respirations and lethargy leading to coma, and elevated glucose levels	
hydrochlorothiazide	Anorexia, nausea, vomiting Abdominal pain, cramping Rash, urticaria	Leukopenia, thrombocytopenia Agranulocytosis
Chlorothiazide	Paresthesias, weakness Photosensitivity	Pancreatitis Leukopenia, agranulocytosis, aplastic anemia, anaphylactic reactions
Chlorthalidone	Vertigo Rash Urticaria Hyperuricemia	Jaundice, pancreatitis Leukopenia, thrombocytopenia
Indapamide	Headache Fatigue Muscle cramps/spasms Hyperglycemia Hyperuricemia	Necrotizing angiitis Vasculitis Cutaneous vasculitis Pruritus
Metolazone	Headache	Lassitude, muscle cramps Joint pain/swelling, chest pain
POTASSIUM-SPARING DIURETICS		
All potassium-sparing diuretics	Dehydration Hypotension Hyperkalemia Nausea Vomiting Gastrointestinal disturbances Weakness	

TABLE 30-4 **Adverse Effects of Diuretics** (Continued)

Drug	Common Adverse Effects	Serious Adverse Effects
Triamterene	Nephrolithiasis Headache Weakness Fatigue	Acute renal failure and megaloblastic anemia Electrolyte imbalance of hyperkalemia or hypokalemia Anaphylactic reactions
Amiloride	Headache	Severe hyperkalemia Encephalopathy
Spironolactone	Headache, lethargy, gastrointestinal irritation Endocrine and androgenic effects (gynecomastia, breast pain, impotence, menstrual irregularities)	Severe hyperkalemia Dehydration and hyponatremia Agranulocytosis, mental confusion Gynecomastia, irregular menses or amenorrhea Postmenopausal bleeding, hirsutism, deepening of the voice

triamterene (Dyrenium; Midamor) 🗝 —cont'd

WARNINGS. Potassium-sparing diuretics can cause life-threatening hyperkalemia. Clinical manifestations of hyperkalemia include profound weakness, paresthesias, flaccid paralysis, bradycardia, hypotension, and ECG abnormalities, including peaked T waves and prolongation of the PR, QRS, and QT intervals. Patients should be advised to avoid large quantities of high-potassium foods, particularly if they were encouraged to eat such foods before therapy with a potassium-sparing diuretic was initiated. Salt substitutes that contain potassium chloride and potassium supplements should be avoided. Electrolytes should be monitored before initiation of therapy and frequently thereafter.

Patients with diabetes-related renal insufficiency are at higher risk of hyperkalemia; these drugs should be used in these patients only with considerable caution and with careful monitoring of electrolytes.

PRECAUTIONS. Hyponatremia may occur with these drugs, particularly when they are used in combination with other diuretics that predispose to the development of hyponatremia. Drugs in this group can also cause a metabolic acidosis:

- Triamterene has been found to be a component of renal stones; use with caution in patients with a history of renal stones.
- Triamterene is a weak folic acid antagonist that can contribute to folate deficiency states.
- Triamterene photosensitivity
- Glucose intolerance or hyperglycemia

DRUG INTERACTIONS. ACE inhibitors commonly raise serum potassium levels and should be used with great caution in combination with potassium-sparing diuretics, although Class III and IV HF patients may receive both under ACC/HFSA guidelines. Spironolactone may decrease the effectiveness of anticoagulants and mitotane. Triamterene increases amantadine levels. Cimetidine may increase the effects of triamterene by increasing its bioavailability and decreasing its clearance.

OTHER DRUGS IN CLASS

Other drugs in this class are similar to the prototype except as follows:

- *spironolactone:* Spironolactone may cause gynecomastia, decreased libido, hirsutism, and menstrual irregularities. Amiloride and spironolactone have complex effects on the elimination of digitalis and may blunt its inotropic activity. NSAIDs lower the therapeutic effects of amiloride and spironolactone and may increase the risk of hyperkalemia.

Potassium Supplements

Most potassium supplements consist of the chloride salt of potassium (KCl). A smaller number are provided as potassium salts of bicarbonate, acetate, citrate, or *l*-lysine. Potassium chloride is the preferred replacement for most patients with diuretic-induced hypokalemia because diuretics induce losses of both potassium and chloride. For this reason, only potassium chloride replacement agents are reviewed here. When metabolic acidosis is present, the use of bicarbonate, citrate, acetate, or gluconate potassium salts may be indicated.

Volume loss associated with diuretic use can stimulate aldosterone production that further increases urinary potassium losses. Guidelines on potassium replacement from the National Council on Potassium in Clinical Practice (released in 2000) underscore the importance of preventing potassium loss and replacing potassium in patients with HTN or CHF; patients with cardiac arrhythmias, stroke, and diabetes; and those with renal impairment. It is recommended that increasing potassium intake should be considered when serum potassium levels are between 3.5 and 4 mmol/L. A goal of ≥4 mmol/L is suggested for patients with asymptomatic hypertension or CHF and for those with cardiac arrhythmias.

Approaches to avoiding hypokalemia in patients treated with diuretics include using the lowest effective diuretic dose, restricting dietary sodium intake to 75 to 100 mEq/day, increasing dietary potassium intake (see Box 30-4), and making concomitant use of potassium-sparing agents (see earlier discussion). Some patients on diuretics are able to obtain enough potassium through diet and do not require medication. Those who require a second agent to control HTN and those who have specific types of cardiac disease could be considered for treatment with medications that tend to increase serum potassium concentration (e.g., ACE inhibitors).

MECHANISM OF ACTION

Potassium, the major intracellular cation, has major regulatory roles in cell metabolism. Many cellular functions may be adversely affected by hypokalemia. For example, hypokalemia may decrease the kidney's ability to respond to antidiuretic hormone, leading to polyuria. Hypokalemia may also impair insulin secretion, leading to worsened glucose control in diabetic patients. Of major importance is the role of potassium in defining resting membrane potential. Because of this role, hypokalemia may predispose to the development of arrhythmias and smooth and skeletal muscle dysfunction. Patients who take digitalis are particularly prone to the arrhythmic potential of hypokalemia. Signs and symptoms associated with hypokalemia are listed in Box 30-3.

TREATMENT PRINCIPLES

How to Monitor

Symptoms of hypokalemia generally are not present until the serum potassium level falls to below 3 mEq/L. Symptoms of hyperkalemia are evident at levels >7 mEq/L. Muscle weakness typically is seen when the potassium level is <2.5 mEq/L or >7 mEq/L. Severe muscle weakness is described as beginning in the lower extremities and progressing upward to the trunk and upper extremities. It is important to note that muscle weakness is a hallmark symptom of hyperkalemia *and* of hypokalemia.

Serum electrolytes should be monitored before diuretic treatment is initiated. Diuretic-induced hypokalemia is dose dependent and severe in approximately 10% to 15% of patients who are receiving high doses. Patients typically develop hypokalemia within the first weeks of therapy; therefore, electrolytes should be checked after 1 to 2 weeks. Hypokalemic patients can increase their potassium intake by augmenting their dietary intake of potassium (see Box 30-4) and/or by using potassium supplements (Table 30-5). Potassium levels should be rechecked approximately 2 weeks after changes are made, to assess the effects of these changes. At that time, a new steady state exists, and potassium levels may then be checked based on clinical concerns or additional changes in therapy.

The amount of potassium replacement required to normalize serum potassium must be determined individually. Relatively low doses (10 to 30 mEq) may be required for the patient on a low-dose thiazide who is adherent with a higher-potassium and sodium-restricted diet, whereas much higher doses are required in the patient who is taking higher doses of a loop diuretic and is unable to maintain a low-sodium and high-potassium diet.

Patient Variables

COMMON CONSIDERATIONS. A normal diet contains approximately 50 to 100 mEq of potassium each day. Individuals whose diet is low in potassium-containing food and those with poor general dietary intake are particularly vulnerable to the development of diuretic-induced hypokalemia.

As indicated above, individuals with underlying cardiac disease and those treated with digitalis are more vulnerable to hypokalemia-induced arrhythmias. Also, patients with preexisting difficulties with any of the symptoms listed in Box 30-3 may be more likely to experience an exacerba-

TABLE 30-5 Potassium Chloride Preparations

Formulation	Brand Name	Concentration (%)*/mEq
Liquid	Generic KCl	10%, 20%
	Kaon-Cl	20%
Powder	Generic	10
	Kay Ciel	20
	Klor-Con	25
Suspension	Micro-K LS	20
Effervescent tablets	Klor-Con	25
Tablets/capsules	Generic	10
	Kaon-Cl	10
	K-Dur	10, 20
	Klor-Con	8
	Klor-Con M	10, 20
	K-Tab	10
	Micro-K	8, 10

*10%: 20 mEq/15 ml; 15%: 30 mEq/15 ml; 20%: 40 mEq/15 ml.

tion of these symptoms should hypokalemia be allowed to develop.

GERIATRICS. Because many elders are on concomitant digitalis therapy, patients should be closely monitored for previously described concerns regarding hypokalemia-related arrhythmias. Because elders are more susceptible to the development of potassium chloride–induced gastrointestinal (GI) lesions, careful monitoring for GI side effects in this population is essential. Because renal function declines with age, monitoring for hyperkalemia caused by impaired potassium excretion is especially important.

PEDIATRICS. Each potassium supplement includes specific guidelines for use in pediatric patients. These should be consulted specifically for each product.

PREGNANCY AND LACTATION. *Category C*

Patient Education

In general, GI upset is a frequent concern in terms of adherence to prescribed potassium replacement therapy. This side effect may be prevented or decreased if the potassium is taken with meals and a full glass of water or other liquid. Because electrolyte imbalances may have severe consequences, educating patients to seek medical care if they develop symptoms of hyperkalemia or hypokalemia (described later in this chapter) is a matter of top priority.

The following should be discussed with patients before they begin oral potassium replacement therapy and periodically should be reinforced as needed:

• Taking potassium with food and a full glass of water or other liquid may prevent nausea or GI upset.
• Do not chew or crush tablets or capsules.
• Mix or dissolve oral liquids, soluble powders, or effervescent tablets completely in 3 to 8 ounces of water, juice, or other liquid.
• Take as prescribed (i.e., frequency and amount), especially if on diuretic or digitalis preparation.
• Report difficulties with swallowing tablets or capsules.

- Because the wax matrix of capsules from which the body has extracted the potassium is not absorbed in the GI tract, patients may observe this in their stool.
- Notify the primary care provider if tarry stools or other signs of GI bleeding develop.
- Do not use potassium-containing salt substitutes while taking potassium supplements.
- Report for potassium monitoring as directed.
- Because potential drug interactions may occur with ACE inhibitors, patients may need closer monitoring of potassium levels to check for hyperkalemia.
- Report to the primary care provider the following signs and symptoms of hyperkalemia or hypokalemia: tingling in hands or feet; unusual tiredness or weakness; leg cramps or muscle weakness; feeling of heaviness in legs; nausea/vomiting; abdominal pain; black or tarry stools; weak, slowed, or irregular pulse; or low blood pressure.

SPECIFIC DRUGS

potassium chloride (Kaon-Cl, K-Dur)

CONTRAINDICATIONS. Sensitivity to tartrazine (found in some potassium preparations, e.g., Kaon-Cl, Kaochlor) may produce some allergic-type reactions. This same sensitivity is frequently seen in patients who are also sensitive to aspirin. The combined use of potassium supplements and potassium-sparing diuretics can lead to life-threatening hyperkalemia. The administration of potassium to patients with chronic renal insufficiency may overwhelm the kidneys' limited ability to excrete potassium and may lead to severe hyperkalemia.

Tablets or capsules can cause GI ulceration in patients with impaired GI transport. Liquid forms of potassium replacement should be used in these patients.

WARNINGS. Life-threatening hyperkalemia may occur in patients whose ability to excrete potassium is impaired by renal insufficiency or the concomitant use of potassium-sparing diuretics. Potassium chloride tablets may cause GI ulceration, bleeding, or strictures, particularly if the tablets are rapidly dissolving.

PHARMACOKINETICS. Absorption of orally administered potassium is nearly complete. In terms of distribution, most potassium is located intracellularly, where potassium concentration is 150 mEq/L. Extracellular potassium concentrations normally range from 3.5 to 5 mEq/L. Biotransformation of potassium does not occur, and the kidney represents the dominant site of excretion; only very small amounts of potassium are lost in the stool (5 to 10 mEq/day) or sweat (0 to 10 mEq/day). Potassium is freely filtered through the glomerulus and then is almost completely reabsorbed in the proximal tubule. Excretion of potassium into the urine occurs as a function of potassium secretion in the collecting tubule. Plasma potassium concentration and aldosterone normally determine the amount of potassium lost in the urine. The normal kidney is capable of regulating potassium excretion to markedly increase excretion in situations of increased potassium intake or to markedly decrease potassium excretion in times of low potassium intake.

ADVERSE EFFECTS. It is important to recognize that hyperkalemia may be entirely asymptomatic, manifesting only as an elevated serum potassium level (5.5 to 8 mEq/L) and as characteristic ECG changes. An elevated serum potassium level predisposes the patient to arrhythmias. Late manifestations include muscle paralysis and subsequent cardiovascular collapse (9 to 12 mEq/L). Unpleasant taste and GI irritation with abdominal discomfort, nausea, vomiting, and diarrhea are the most common adverse effects. More serious complications include hyperkalemia, GI ulceration, bleeding, and, rarely, perforation.

DRUG INTERACTIONS. The combination of potassium supplements with medications that tend to raise serum potassium levels can cause life-threatening hyperkalemia. The concomitant use of potassium supplementation and potassium-sparing diuretics should be completely avoided or should be used only under extreme circumstances with vigilant monitoring. The combination of ACE inhibitors and potassium replacement may also induce hyperkalemia. However, this drug combination may be necessary in patients who are also being treated with diuretics; thus, careful monitoring is required.

DOSAGE AND ADMINISTRATION. Dosage must be individualized based on periodic monitoring of serum potassium levels. Approximately 20 mEq/day is typically required to prevent hyperkalemia; 40 to 100 mEq/day is used to treat patients with hypokalemia. The National Council on Potassium in Clinical Practice recommends administering supplements orally in moderate dosages over a period of several days to weeks to achieve full potassium repletion.

Potassium preparations are available in a number of forms, including liquid, powder, effervescent tablets, capsules, and controlled or extended-release tablets. The potassium concentration of liquid preparations ranges from 20 to 45 mEq/15 ml; values of powders range from 15 to 25 mEq/packet, those of effervescent tablets from 20 to 50 mEq, and those of capsules or tablets from 6.7 to 20 mEq. Liquids, effervescent tablets, and powders may be less likely to cause GI ulceration but frequently are tolerated poorly because of their unpleasant taste (see Table 30-5). The extended-release tablets are large, and many patients have difficulty swallowing them. Smaller tablets are available, but they come in a lower dose, necessitating a larger number of pills.

evolve A continually updated list of useful WebLinks may be found in the Evolve Resources at http://evolve.elsevier.com/Edmunds/NP/

31 Male Genitourinary Agents

DRUG OVERVIEW

Class	Subclass	Generic Name	Trade Name
Benign prostatic hyperplasia (BPH)			
α₁-Adrenergic antagonists	α₁ₐ-Selective	tamsulosin 🔑	Flomax ✴
		alfuzosin	Uroxatral
	Long-acting α₁	doxazosin ✴	Cardura
		terazosin ✴	Hytrin
	Short-acting α₁	prazosin	Minipress
5α-Reductase inhibitors		finasteride	Proscar ✴
		dutasteride	Avodart ✴
Erectile dysfunction (ED)			
PDE5 inhibitors		sildenafil 🔑	Viagra ✴
		tadalafil	Cialis ✴
		vardenafil	Levitra ✴
Other		alprostadil	Caverject
		yohimbine	Yocon

✴ Top 200 drug; 🔑 key drug. Key drug because it was the first on the market and is in common use. Drugs listed in general order of use within class. PDE5, phosphodiesterase type 5.

The drugs used for benign prostatic hyperplasia (BPH) and those given for erectile dysfunction (ED) are discussed in separate sections of this chapter.

Benign Prostatic Hyperplasia

INDICATIONS

- BPH

  Drugs commonly used in the management of BPH are the α₁-adrenergic receptor blockers such as doxazosin and terazosin, which also are indicated for hypertension. Tamsulosin (Flomax) is an α-adrenergic receptor blocker that is specific to the prostate and is indicated only for the treatment of symptoms of BPH. With finasteride, an androgen hormone inhibitor, 6 months of therapy is required to achieve maximum benefit.

THERAPEUTIC OVERVIEW

BPH is a benign neoplasm of the prostate gland that, if large enough, causes voiding dysfunction. BPH, which is extremely common in the aging male, occurs in less than 10% of men aged 31 to 40 years. However, by age 60, nearly half of men will develop BPH, and by age 85, more than 80% will have it. Prostatism has three components: histologic prostatic hyperplasia, an increase in outflow resistance, and response of the bladder (detrusor) muscle to obstruction. The prostate depends on the androgen 5α-dihydrotestosterone (DHT) for growth. The enzyme 5α-reductase metabolizes testosterone to DHT in the prostate gland, liver, and skin. DHT induces androgenic effects by binding to androgen receptors in the cell nuclei of these organs.

The medical history focuses on the urinary tract and on overall health problems that could affect the urinary system such as diabetes, Parkinson's disease, and stroke. It is important to rule out the possibility of prostatic cancer. Medications that can affect bladder function include anticholinergics and sympathomimetics. The American Urological Association (AUA) symptom score for BPH is commonly used to assess symptom severity but not for diagnosis. A patient's symptom score is calculated from the answers to seven questions on a scale of 0 (not present) to 5 (almost always present). These questions address urinary frequency, nocturia, weak urinary stream, hesitancy, intermittence, incomplete bladder emptying, and urgency. A symptom score of 0 to 7 (mild), 8 to 19 (moderate), or 20 to 35 (severe) is given. The AUA symptom score has also been shown to be effective in visually impaired and illiterate patients.

Physical examination emphasizes the digital rectal examination (DRE) and the neurologic system. The DRE is used to estimate the size of the prostate gland, to evaluate anal sphincter tone, and to raise suspicion of prostate or rectal malignancy.

Laboratory tests required to assess renal function include urinalysis, serum creatinine, and BUN. PSA is considered optional under some guidelines. Other tests that may be performed are uroflowmetry, postvoid residual, and pressure flow studies. Tests that are not recommended are filling cystometry, urethrocystoscopy, and imaging of the urinary tract, unless these are indicated by prostatism complicated by additional disease or symptoms.

MECHANISM OF ACTION

The nonspecific α_1-adrenergic receptor blockers (terazosin, doxazosin, and prazosin) reduce sympathetic tone and relax urethral stricture that causes BPH symptoms. Prazosin has a shorter duration of action than the others and generally is not used first line. These drugs also lower blood pressure by blocking α_1-adrenergic receptors on arterioles, causing vasodilation. Newer agents such as tamsulosin and alfuzosin are specific for the α_{1A}-adrenoceptor in the prostate and have little effect on blood pressure.

Finasteride reduces the size of the prostate gland, but 6 to 12 months may be required for improvement of symptoms. It is a 5α-reductase enzyme inhibitor that blocks the conversion of testosterone to dihydrotestosterone, the potent androgen upon which the development of the prostate gland is dependent. Dutasteride is a second-generation 5α-reductase inhibitor. It inhibits both type I and II 5α-reductase.

TREATMENT PRINCIPLES

Standardized Guidelines

- The Agency for Healthcare Research and Quality (AHRQ) Guideline on Benign Prostate Hyperplasia: Diagnosis and Treatment was developed in 1994 and continues as the seminal resource in this area.
- The AUA has developed an algorithm for evaluation and treatment of patients with BPH.

Evidence-Based Recommendations

- α-Blockers and 5α-reductase inhibitors are beneficial.
- *Surgery:* Transurethral microwave thermotherapy and transurethral resection are beneficial.
- *Herbal treatments:* β-Sitosterol plant extract and saw palmetto plant extracts are likely to be beneficial; *Pygeum africanum* and rye grass pollen extract have unknown effectiveness.

Cardinal Points of Treatment

- First line: α_{1A}-Selective antagonist for patients without HTN; long-acting α_1-antagonist for patients with HTN given to reduce symptoms
- 5α-Reductase inhibitor given to shrink the size of the prostate
- Combination therapy with α_1-antagonist plus a 5α-reductase inhibitor

The goals of treatment are to alleviate symptoms and to maintain kidney function. Surgery is the primary treatment for BPH. Watchful waiting is a common plan; symptoms are monitored and treatment is initiated when symptoms become problematic. One review found that 38% of symptoms actually improved and 16% stabilized over a period of 2.6 to 5 years. Surgery is indicated when the patient has refractory urinary retention, recurrent UTIs, hematuria, bladder stones, or renal insufficiency. Medical treatment for BPH is designed to address the impact these symptoms have on the patient's quality of life, or to provide treatment when the patient is reluctant or unable to have surgery, or when the symptoms are mild enough that surgery is not warranted. Treatment decisions generally are made when the patient discusses his options with a urologist. Primary care providers often provide prescriptions and watchful waiting.

All α-blockers used in the treatment of BPH are considered equally efficacious. This was the conclusion of a meta-analysis in which 6333 patients reported that symptom scores improved by an average of 30% to 40%. Selection of one agent over another was based largely on their side effect profiles. The selective α-blockers, tamsulosin and alfuzosin, were found to be better tolerated than their nonselective counterparts in that rates of discontinuation due to side effects were comparable with those of placebo. In contrast, 8% to 20% of patients discontinued treatment with nonspecific α-blockers because of orthostatic hypotension and headache. In elderly patients, tamsulosin was found to have less effect on blood pressure than alfuzosin. Nonspecific α-blockers should be considered in patients with concomitant BPH and hypertension. If the patient does not have hypertension, tamsulosin is probably the first choice. These drugs have an onset of action of approximately 2 to 4 weeks.

Although α-blockers are best for quick symptom relief, finasteride can prevent growth of the prostate over the long term. Treatment for 1 year led to a reduction in AUA symptom scores of 23% and has been shown to reduce the need for surgery by 55% in men treated for 5 years. In general, patients with larger prostates (>40 g) at presentation have been found to derive greatest benefit from treatment with a 5α-reductase inhibitor. Dutasteride has shown to be efficacious and safe for the treatment of BPH and to have side effects comparable with those of finasteride.

Combination therapy with finasteride and doxazosin was shown to lower the risk of clinical progression of BPH by 66%. This was evident in patients treated for longer than 4 years.

Herbal treatment with saw palmetto is popular. It acts as a 5α-reductase inhibitor and should not be used in combination with other β-α-reductase inhibitors. The longest and most clinically useful trial to date failed to demonstrate after 1 year any improvement in AUA symptom scores vs. placebo in 225 men. Saw palmetto appears to be well tolerated and safe.

How to Monitor

- Monitor for symptom relief using the AUA symptom score.
- Monitor closely for complications of BPH, such as obstructive uropathy.

Patient Variables

GERIATRICS. BPH is very common in elderly men.

PREGNANCY AND LACTATION
- *Category C:* Other α_1-adrenergic blockers
- *Category X:* finasteride, dutasteride

💣 Finasteride/dutasteride is teratogenic. Finasteride tablets must not be touched by a woman who may be pregnant because the product may be absorbed through the skin. A pregnant woman should not come in contact with the semen of a man who is taking finasteride.

GENDER. Tamsulosin, alfuzosin, and dutasteride are not indicated for females.

Patient Education
- Report immediately any signs and symptoms of obstructive uropathy.

SPECIFIC DRUGS

α_1-ADRENERGIC ANTAGONISTS

tamsulosin (Flomax) 🔑

CONTRAINDICATIONS. Hypersensitivity; concurrent use with PDE5 inhibitors such as sildenafil (>25 mg), tadalafil (if tamsulosin dose exceeds 0.4 mg/day), or vardenafil

WARNINGS. Orthostatic hypotension with syncope, priapism, patients with *severe* sulfonamide allergies; may affect pupils of the eyes during cataract surgery

PRECAUTIONS. Cancer of prostate and BPH have similar symptoms.

PHARMACOKINETICS. See Table 31-1.
The short-acting drugs have an increased incidence of adverse effects because of the rapid increase in drug levels.

ADVERSE EFFECTS. See Table 31-2.

DRUG INTERACTIONS
- Potentiates other α-adrenergic-blocking agents
- Alcohol, α-blockers, and cimetidine increase the risk of hypotension.

DOSAGE AND ADMINISTRATION. See Table 31-3.

OTHER DRUGS IN CLASS

Drugs that are from the same category or subcategory are similar to the key drug except in the following ways:
- *alfuzosin (Uroxatral) contraindications:* Moderate to severe hepatic impairment, concomitant use with potent 3A4 inhibitors (e.g., itraconazole, ketoconazole, ritonavir) or ED drugs
- *Drug interactions:* Inhibitors of cytochrome P (CYP) 3A4; can increase serum levels; inducers of CYP 3A4 (e.g., carbamazepine, phenobarbital, phenytoin, rifamycin); can decrease serum levels and efficacy of alfuzosin
- *prazosin:* Because of first dose syncope, high incidence of hypotension, and shorter duration of action, it is seldom used for BPH.
- *doxazosin:* Use with caution in severe gastrointestinal narrowing, mild to moderate hepatic impairment (not

recommended in severe hepatic impairment), CHF, and CAD; use with PDE5 inhibitors (e.g., sildenafil).

ANDROGEN HORMONE INHIBITOR

finasteride (Proscar)

CONTRAINDICATIONS
- Hypersensitivity
- Pregnancy

WARNINGS
- A woman who may become pregnant should not handle crushed tablets or come in contact with semen of men taking drug because birth defects may occur.
- Treatment with drug will decrease serum levels of PSA.

PRECAUTIONS. *Obstructive uropathy:* Not all patients have a response to finasteride; monitor carefully for obstructive uropathy.

DRUG INTERACTIONS. None noted at this time

DOSAGE AND ADMINISTRATION. This product is marketed as Propecia to treat male pattern hair loss at 1 mg daily.

Erectile Dysfunction

INDICATIONS

- PDE5 inhibitors
  - ED
  - Unlabeled uses include treatment of ED resulting from vascular or diabetic origins, or from the use of serotonin reuptake inhibitors; also used for orthostatic hypotension and as an aphrodisiac, and for pulmonary hypertension (sildenafil [Revatio] 20 mg)
- *Alprostadil (Caverject):* treatment of ED resulting from neurogenic, vasculogenic, or psychogenic causes, or ED of mixed origin
- *Yohimbine (Yocon):* No indications have been approved by the FDA.

THERAPEUTIC OVERVIEW

ED is defined as the consistent inability to maintain an erect penis with sufficient rigidity to allow sexual intercourse. It is common and frequency increases with age.

Erection and ejaculation involve complex interactions with psychologic, hormonal, neural, and vascular functions. Both sympathetic and parasympathetic pathways are used. Parasympathetic (cholinergic) stimulation controls erection of the penis. Sympathetic (adrenergic) pathways produce ejaculation by causing contraction of the prostate and seminal vesicles, as well as effects on the bulbocavernous and ischiocavernous muscles.

ED may result from malfunction in one or more areas. Causes are categorized into psychologic and organic categories. Psychologic causes are usually abrupt in onset, and incidence varies with partner, position, or situation. This type occurs more commonly in younger men. Organic causes usually have a gradual onset and are consistent.

TABLE 31-1   Pharmacokinetics of Male Genitourinary Agents

Drug	Absorption and Availability	Onset of Action	Peak Effect	Duration of Action	Protein Bound	Metabolism	Excretion
tamsulosin (Flomax)	90% available after first pass; decreased by food	4-8 hr	2-4 wk	24 hr	94%-99%	Hepatic CYP450 pathway not known	Urine, 76% metabolized; urine, 10% unchanged; feces, 21%
alfuzosin (Uroxatal)	49%; increased by food; take following meal	8 hr	4-6 wk	>24 hr	80%-90%	Extensive, some by CYP 3A4	69% feces; urine 24%-30%
doxazosin, extended release	62%-69%; not affected by food	2 wk	4-6 wk	>24 hr	98%	3A4, 2D6, 2C9	63% feces
terazosin	Completely absorbed, minimal effect from food	2 wk	4-6 wk	>24 hr	90%-94%	Liver, extensive	Feces, 55%-60%
finasteride (Proscar)	63% available after first pass	3 months	6 months	2 wk	90%	Hepatic 2D6 3A4	Urine, 40% as metabolites; feces, 60%
dutasteride (Avodart)	60%	3 months	6-12 months	5 wk	99%	3A4, 3A5	Feces, 45%
sildenafil (Viagra)	Rapid, 40% ↓ with high-fat meal	60 min	Peak 2 hr	4 hr	96%	CYP 3A4 2C9	Feces, 80%
tadalafil (Cialis)	Not affected by food	30-45 min	2 hr	36 hr	94%	CYP 3A4	Feces, 61%
vardenafil (Levitra)	15% bioavailable, ↓ with high-fat meal	60 min	2 hr	4 hr	95%	CYP 3A4	Feces, 91%
alprostadil pellets	Absorbed from urethra	30 min	30-60 min	1 hr	81%	—	Metabolized in lungs; 90% kidney as metabolites

TABLE 31-2   Adverse Effects of Drugs That Affect the Urinary Tract

Drug	Adverse Effects
tamsulosin	Orthostasis (7%-16%), dizziness (15%-17%), somnolence, rhinitis (13%-18%), diarrhea, abnormal ejaculation (8%-18%), fatigue, headache (19%-21%)
alfuzosin	Dizziness (6%), syncope (rare), hypotension (rare), abnormal ejaculation has not occurred; QT interval increase (dose higher than 40 mg), fatigue (3%), headache (3%)
doxazosin, terazosin	Orthostatic hypotension (0.3%-2%), syncope, arrhythmias, priapism (rare), dizziness (5%-19%), headache (5%-14%), fatigue (8%-12%), edema, rhinitis, diarrhea
finasteride, dutasteride	Impotence (19%), decreased libido (10%), orthostasis (9%); decreased volume of ejaculate (7%); breast tenderness and enlargement; hypersensitivity reactions, including lip swelling and skin rash, testicular pain
sildenafil, tadalafil, vardenafil	Headaches (16%-46%), flushing (10%), dyspepsia (7%-17%), rhinitis, myalgia, abnormal vision, dyspepsia, diarrhea, dizziness, rash, hypotension, arrhythmia, hypotension, cerebrovascular hemorrhage, photosensitivity, blood dyscrasias, priapism, seizures
alprostadil injection	Penile pain (>10%), urethral burning (>10%); headache (2%-10%), dizziness (2%-10%), vaginal pain (partner; 2%-10%), increased heart rate (<2%)

Workup for ED should include a complete history, including information about sexual history, emotional upheavals, and any drug use. Testing may include measurement of nocturnal penile tumescence with mechanical and elective devices. Injections of papaverine have been used as a screening measure. If the patient fails to have an erection after injection, he may have vasculogenic impotency, and further workup may be necessary. Vascular angiography and hormone levels (e.g., testosterone and prolactin levels) may be obtained to assist with evaluation.

Neurologic causes for ED include diabetes, multiple sclerosis, spinal cord damage, nerve damage after a prostatectomy, decreased blood flow to the penis because of atherosclerosis, and vascular damage resulting from injury, for example, renal transplant, bypass procedures, hyperprolactinemia, and structural abnormalities. Numerous drugs may also be responsible (e.g., antihypertensives, opioids, antidepressants, antianxiety agents, antipsychotic agents, ethyl alcohol, chemotherapeutic agents, cimetidine, estrogenic agents).

TABLE 31-3 Dosage and Administration of Male Genitourinary Agents

Drug	Dosage	Elderly (>65 yr)	Renal/Hepatic Impairment	Dosage and other Considerations	Max Dose
tamsulosin	0.4 mg	None	None	0.4 mg once daily ≈30 min after same meal; titrate q2-4wk; if treatment stopped for 3 to 4 days, resume at 0.4 mg. Do not crush, chew, or open capsule.	0.8 mg
alfuzosin	10 mg		R: Clearance decreased; no recommendations on dosing H: Moderate to severe: contraindicated	10 mg once daily	10 mg
doxazosin	4 mg ER 1 mg	None 0.5 mg once daily	H: Mild to moderate: Use with caution. Severe: Do not use.	4 mg once daily with breakfast; titrate q3-4wk; if treatment stopped for 5 to 7 days, resume at 4 mg 1 mg once daily in morning or evening; may be increased to 2 mg once daily. Titrate q1-2wk.	8 mg
terazosin	1 mg	None	None	1 mg at bedtime; titrate q6wk. Most patients require 10 mg per day. Take with full glass of water.	20 mg
finasteride	5 mg	None	H: Use with caution in hepatic impairment; no specific dosing adjustments recommended	5 mg once daily. Take with a full glass of water.	5 mg
dutasteride	0.5 mg	None	H: Use with caution in hepatic impairment; no specific dosing adjustments recommended	0.5 mg once daily; not to be handled by pregnant women	0.5 mg
sildenafil	50 mg; 30 min to 4 hours before; one dose/24 hr	25 mg	R: 25 mg H: 25 mg	Concurrent use of the following: • α-Blockers: Doses of 50 or 100 mg; should not be taken within 4 hours of an α-blocker; doses of 25 mg may be given at any time. • CYP 3A4 inhibitors: 25 mg if receiving erythromycin, itraconazole, ketoconazole, saquinavir; ritonavir: Max: 25 mg q48hr	100 mg
tadalafil	10 mg; 30-45 minutes prior to sexual activity	Dose based on renal function	R: CrCl 31-50 ml/min: Initial dose 5 mg once daily; maximum dose 10 mg not to be given more frequently than q48h CrCl <30 ml/min or hemodialysis: Maximum dose 5 mg H: Mild to moderate hepatic impairment: Dose should not exceed 10 mg once daily. Severe: Not recommended	Concurrent use of the following: • α₁-Blockers: Use lowest effective dose. • CYP 3A4 inhibitors: Max dose 10 mg; should not be taken more frequently than once every 72 hours with strong CYP 3A4 inhibitors (e.g., amprenavir, atazanavir, clarithromycin, conivaptan, delavirdine, diclofenac, fosamprenavir, imatinib, indinavir, isoniazid, itraconazole, ketoconazole, miconazole, nefazodone, nelfinavir, nicardipine, propofol, quinidine, ritonavir, telithromycin).	20 mg
vardenafil	10 mg; 60 minutes before; one dose/24 hours	5 mg	R: None H: 5 mg (max 10 mg)	Concurrent use of the following: • α-Blocker: 5 mg/24 hr • Erythromycin: Max: 5 mg/24 hr • Indinavir: Max: 2.5 mg/24 hr • Itraconazole: 200 mg/day: Max: 5 mg/24 hr; 400 mg/day: Max.: 2.5 mg/24 hr • Ketoconazole: 200 mg/day: Max: 5 mg/24 hr; 400 mg/day: Max: 2.5 mg/24 hr • Ritonavir: Max: 2.5 mg/72 hr	20 mg

ED in men with diabetes often is associated with diabetic neuropathy and peripheral vascular disease. It occurs at an earlier age in men with diabetes than in men in the general population, and several studies have demonstrated that ED affects 35% to 75% of men with diabetes.

MECHANISM OF ACTION

Erection involves release of nitric oxide (NO) in the corpus cavernosum in response to stimulation. NO increases levels of cyclic guanosine monophosphate (cGMP), producing smooth muscle relaxation in the corpus cavernosum and allowing inflow of blood. PDE5 is the enzyme that breaks down cGMP in the corpus cavernosum. PDE5 inhibitors (e.g., sildenafil) inhibit cGMP and thus allow for increased blood flow into the penis, resulting in an erection.

The PDE5 enzyme is very specific to receptors in the corpus cavernosum smooth muscle. It is also found in much lower concentrations in platelets, vascular and visceral smooth muscle, and skeletal muscle. PDE3 is found in cardiac contractility; therefore, these drugs are not active in this condition. They are closely related to PDE6, which may explain the abnormalities in color vision seen with PDE5 inhibitors. Tadalafil has a different chemical structure than sildenafil and vardenafil. It has less affinity for PDE6 (retina) but greater affinity for PDE11. PDE11 is found in skeletal muscle, testes, heart, prostate, kidney, liver, and pituitary. The clinical significance of these differences is not known.

Alprostadil is a prostaglandin that has many physiologic actions. Vasodilation and inhibition of platelet aggregation are the most important of these. It induces erection via relaxation of trabecular smooth muscle and by dilation of cavernosal arteries. This causes expansion of lacunar spaces and entrapment of blood caused by compression of the venules against the tunica albuginea. This is called *the corporal veno-occlusive mechanism*.

Yohimbine is an alkaloid derived naturally from the West African tree *Corynanthe yohimbine*. Yohimbine is similar to reserpine and has both sympatholytic and mydriatic properties. It is an α_2-adrenergic antagonist that affects erectile function by stimulating presynaptic norepinephrine release in the lower nerve centers. Antidiuresis results from the release of antidiuretic hormone.

TREATMENT PRINCIPLES

Standardized Guidelines

- Montague DK et al: *The management of erectile dysfunction: an update*, Linthicum, MD, 2006, American Urologic Association Education and Research, Inc.

Evidence-Based Recommendations

- Alprostadil increased the chances of a satisfactory erection compared with placebo.
- Some research suggests that vacuum devices were as effective as intracavernosal alprostadil injections for rigidity but not for orgasm.
- Some evidence suggests that intraurethral alprostadil increased the chances of successful sexual intercourse and of at least one orgasm over 3 months compared with placebo. About a third of men suffered penile ache.

- Sildenafil improved erections and increased rates of successful intercourse compared with placebo. Adverse effects, including headaches, flushing, and dyspepsia, have been reported in up to a quarter of men. Deaths have been reported in men on concomitant treatment with oral nitrates.
- Yohimbine improves self-reported sexual function and penile rigidity at 2 to 10 weeks. Transient adverse effects are reported in up to a third of men; not recommended in the latest treatment guidelines

Cardinal Points of Treatment

- Oral PDE5 inhibitors, unless contraindicated, should be offered as first-line therapy for erectile dysfunction.
- Patients who have failed a trial with PDE5 inhibitor therapy should be informed of the benefits and risks of other therapies, including the use of a different PDE5 inhibitor, alprostadil intraurethral suppositories, intracavernous drug injection, vacuum constriction devices, and penile prostheses.
- The initial trial dose of alprostadil intraurethral suppositories and intracavernous injection therapy should be administered under health care provider supervision because of the risk of syncope.

Nonpharmacologic Treatment

Many nonpharmacologic treatments are available for ED. Vascular reconstruction may be appropriate in patients with decreased blood flow. Vacuum constriction devices are safe and effective. A wide variety of implanted penile prostheses have been devised.

Pharmacologic Treatment

Hormonal replacement with testosterone injections or topical patches can be used for men with documented androgen deficiency and no contraindications. This requires a thorough endocrine evaluation.

PDE5 inhibitors have been shown to be safe and effective if used properly and are given as first-line therapy. The major risks associated with their use involve patients with cardiac conditions; these agents are contraindicated in patients who are taking nitrates because of excessive hypotension. Treatment with these drugs in controlled studies has shown that erectile function is improved regardless of patient age, duration of ED, or duration of diabetes. PDE5 inhibitors are effective 50% to 80% of the time. Much controversy has arisen about the possible cardiovascular effects of PDE5 inhibitors. They do not appear to have any direct adverse effects on the heart. Two consensus panels (Second Princeton and the ACC/AHA) have concluded that the use of PDE5 inhibitors is safe and effective in men with stable coronary artery disease who are not receiving nitrates. However, the ACC/AHA consensus statement does identify the following groups of patients as being at increased risk:

- Patients with active coronary ischemia, even those who are not taking nitrates
- Patients with heart failure and borderline low blood pressure and/or low volume status
- Patients on a complicated multidrug antihypertensive drug regimen
- Patients taking drugs that prolong the half-life of PDE5 inhibitors by blocking CYP 3A4

All three PDE5 inhibitors have been shown to be equally effective in the treatment of ED. Tadalafil has a considerably longer period of effectiveness and is better absorbed in the presence of food. Men who are taking tadalafil are able to have an erection for a period of 36 hours vs. 4 hours with sildenafil and vardenafil. Absorption of tadalafil is less affected by high-fat meals and alcohol.

Intraurethral placement of the prostaglandin, alprostadil, is another treatment alternative. This method of administration has largely replaced penile injection as a form of prostaglandin administration in ED. A small pellet is placed into the urethra of the penis prior to anticipated sexual intercourse. In clinical trials, two thirds of men were able to sustain an erection and engage in sexual intercourse vs. 19% in the placebo group.

Yohimbine has a long history of use in ED. However, clinical effectiveness is lacking and treatment is not without risk. In the treatment of men who have ED for psychological reasons, yohimbine may have a role in therapy. Two clinical trials of 101 men found that yohimbine (5.4 mg tid) was shown to allow resumed sexual intercourse in 3 days to 3 weeks. Fifteen percent of men treated with placebo had a similar response. Side effects such as tachycardia and hypertension are possible because of its α_2-blocking effects; caution is advised in patients with heart disease.

How to Monitor

- Monitor for effectiveness.
- Monitor for adverse reactions, especially priapism.

Patient Variables

GERIATRICS

- *sildenafil, vardenafil:* Reduce dosage.
- *tadalafil:* No adjustment necessary
- *alprostadil, yohimbine:* Not indicated

PEDIATRICS

- *PDE5 inhibitors, yohimbine:* Not indicated
- *alprostadil:* Generally not indicated; however, may be used in newborns with congenital heart defects

PREGNANCY

- *PDE5 inhibitors:* Category B: Safety has not been established.
- *alprostadil:* Do not use for sexual intercourse with a pregnant woman unless a condom is used.
- *yohimbine:* Do not use.

GENDER. *PDE5 inhibitors, alprostadil, yohimbine:* Not indicated for use in women

Patient Education

See individual drug.

SPECIFIC DRUGS

PDE5 INHIBITORS

sildenafil (Viagra)

CONTRAINDICATIONS

- Hypersensitivity
- Patients taking nitrates

WARNINGS

- *Renal and hepatic function impairment:* Clearance is reduced; consider lower dose.
- Do not use in patients who have severe hepatic impairment.

PRECAUTIONS

- *Cardiovascular status:* A small potential for cardiac risk is associated with sexual activity. Risk stratification and management recommendations concerning sexual activity and cardiac risk are available to providers through the Second Princeton Consensus Panel.

> **Serious cardiovascular events, including MI, sudden cardiac death, ventricular arrhythmia, cerebrovascular hemorrhage, transient ischemic attack, and hypertension, have been reported in temporal association with sildenafil.**

- *Deformation of penis/priapism:* Use with caution in patients with anatomic deformation of the penis or with risk factors for priapism.
- *Bleeding disorders:* Sildenafil has an effect on platelets but has shown no effect on bleeding time when taken alone or with aspirin. Administer with caution in patients with bleeding disorders or active peptic ulceration.
- *Visual disturbances:* Mild, transient, dose-related impairment of blue or green color discrimination has been noted. Transient loss of vision has been reported, but no proof of cause and effect has been found.
- May be associated with retinitis pigmentosa

PHARMACOKINETICS. See Table 31-1.

DRUG INTERACTIONS. Sildenafil is a 3A4 and 2C9 substrate; inhibitors of these enzymes may reduce sildenafil clearance, causing an increase in plasma concentrations. Inducers will decrease sildenafil concentration.

- Use lower dose of sildenafil when using with ritonavir, ketoconazole, itraconazole, and erythromycin. Do not use with nitrates or α-blockers.
- May add to hypotensive effect of other antihypertensive drugs, especially α-adrenergic blocking agents

PATIENT EDUCATION

- Discuss with patients the potential cardiac risk of sexual activity with preexisting cardiovascular disease.
- Advise patients who experience symptoms (e.g., angina pectoris, dizziness, nausea) upon initiation of sexual activity to refrain from further activity and discuss the episode with their provider.
- Priapism is an emergency. For any erections that last longer than 4 hours, patients should seek immediate medical assistance.
- Take 1 hour before expected use; lasts for 4 hours; take only one per day
- May alter color vision temporarily, producing blue-green hazy vision

DOSAGE AND ADMINISTRATION. See Table 31-3.

OTHER DRUGS IN CLASS

Drugs that belong to the same category or subcategory are similar to the key drug except in the following ways:

- *vardenafil (Levitra):* Manufacturer states that it has a shorter onset of action than sildenafil, but studies have not substantiated this claim. Vardenafil (Levitra) is about ten times as potent as sildenafil.

WARNING. Vardenafil can cause slight prolongation of the QT interval. Do not use with antiarrhythmic drugs or in patients with hepatic insufficiency. Concomitant use with potent 3A4 inhibitors could increase serum levels of vardenafil.

- Tadalafil (Cialis) has a longer duration of action than sildenafil or vardenafil; the period of effectiveness may last up to 36 hours. Visual changes have not been reported. Potent CYP 3A4 inhibitors increase the serum level of tadalafil. This agent does not interact with hypertensive drugs.

OTHER ED DRUGS

alprostadil (Muse)

CONTRAINDICATIONS
- Hypersensitivity
- Conditions that might dispose the patient to priapism
- Anatomic deformation of the penis
- Patients with penile implants

WARNINGS
- Priapism has occurred; to avoid, use lowest dose possible.
- Penile fibrosis may occur.
- Hematoma/ecchymosis may occur because of faulty injection technique.
- Hemodynamic changes such as decreased blood pressure and increased heart rate have been observed.

DRUG INTERACTIONS. Alprostadil increases the effect of anticoagulants and decreases cyclosporine blood concentration. Use with vasoactive agents is not recommended.

OVERDOSAGE. Systemic effects may occur.

PATIENT EDUCATION
- The patient requires an explanation on how to use that is beyond the scope of this text.
- Instructions for injection are included in the package.

- Do not change dose.
- Use condom if partner is pregnant.

DOSAGE AND ADMINISTRATION. Place pellet into urethra of penis and massage for up to 1 minute to ensure adequate distribution.

yohimbine (Yocon)

CONTRAINDICATIONS
- Hypersensitivity
- Renal disease

WARNINGS
- *Special risk patients:* Do not use in patients with cardiorenal problems or psychiatric disorders or those with a history of gastric or duodenal ulcer.
- Cardiovascular side effects include tachycardia and hypertension.

PHARMACOKINETICS. Information is not available.

ADVERSE EFFECTS. Yohimbine penetrates the CNS to cause central excitation, including elevated blood pressure and heart rate, increased motor activity, nervousness, irritability, and tremor. Dizziness, headache, and skin flushing also have occurred.

DRUG INTERACTIONS. Do not use with antidepressants.

OVERDOSAGE. Symptoms include increased heart rate and blood pressure, piloerection, and rhinorrhea. Other symptoms include paresthesias, incoordination, tremulousness, and a dissociative state. Death can occur via respiratory paralysis.

DOSAGE AND ADMINISTRATION. One 5.4-mg tablet three times a day. If side effects occur, the dose may be cut in half.

evolve A continually updated list of useful WebLinks may be found in the Evolve Resources at http://evolve.elsevier.com/Edmunds/NP/

32 Agents for Urinary Incontinence and Urinary Analgesia

MAREN MAYHEW

DRUG OVERVIEW

Class	Generic Name	Trade Name
Anticholinergics	oxybutynin chloride 🔑 ☀	Ditropan XL ☀ Oxytrol patch generic
	tolterodine	Detrol LA ☀
	trospium	Sanctura
Bladder-targeted anticholinergics	darifenacin solifenacin	Enablex VESIcare
Antispasmodics	flavoxate propantheline	Urispas Pro-Banthine
Cholinergic agonist	bethanechol chloride	Urecholine
Posterior pituitary hormone	desmopressin	DDAVP
Urinary tract analgesia	phenazopyridine ☀	Pyridium

☀ Top 200 drug; 🔑 key drug. Key drug because was first marketed for urinary incontinence and remains in popular use.
DDAVP, 1-Deamino-8-D-arginine vasopressin.

INDICATIONS

- *oxybutynin XL:* dysuria, neurogenic bladder, overactive bladder, urge incontinence, frequency, urgency
- *tolterodine LA:* overactive bladder, urge incontinence, frequency, urgency
- *trospium:* treatment of overactive bladder with symptoms of urge urinary incontinence, urgency, and urinary frequency
- *darifenacin:* overactive bladder
- *solifenacin:* overactive bladder
- *flavoxate:* dysuria adjunct in urinary tract infection
- *propantheline:* adjunctive therapy for peptic ulcer
- *desmopressin:* primary nocturnal enuresis (intranasal)
- *bethanechol:* urinary retention
- *phenazopyridine (Pyridium):* dysuria

Unlabeled Uses

- *propantheline:* urinary urge incontinence; similar to dicyclomine (Bentyl) (discussed in Chapter 29)
- *desmopressin:* treatment of overactive bladder in adults
- *phenazopyridine:* interstitial cystitis

This chapter discusses genitourinary drugs used to treat urinary incontinence (UI), urinary retention, nocturnal enuresis in children, and urinary tract pain/discomfort. The condition discussed is UI, which occurs primarily in women and is not really a disease but a geriatric syndrome. Some of the drugs that are used to treat symptoms of UI have not been approved by the FDA for UI. For example, dual SNRIs are being studied for use in stress incontinence. The anticholinergics/antispasmodics, which are FDA approved for UI, are discussed in detail in this chapter. α-Adrenergic agonists, α-adrenergic antagonists, tricyclic antidepressants, sympathomimetics, and estrogens also are used, and information about those drugs may be found in the relevant chapters.

Desmopressin is a medication that is used in children with primary nocturnal enuresis. Phenazopyridine is used on a short-term basis for urinary analgesia, usually resulting from an acute UTI.

THERAPEUTIC OVERVIEW

Urinary incontinence is the unintentional leakage of urine. Four basic types of established incontinence are known: stress, urge, mixed, and overflow.

Stress incontinence is leakage of urine that results from a reduction in urethral resistance and increased abdominal pressure associated with physical exertion (e.g., exercise, coughing, and sneezing). Causative factors include weak pelvic floor muscles, prostatectomy, and obesity. It is the most common type of incontinence in women younger than 60 years and also occurs in men who have had prostate surgery.

Urge incontinence, or overactive bladder, is caused by a hyperactive detrusor muscle and is associated with an intense urge to void before the bladder is full. Urge incontinence is associated with localized conditions (e.g., infection, atrophic vaginitis, stones, calculi or other obstruction), neurologic disorders (e.g., CVA, Parkinson's, Alzheimer's), and metabolic conditions (e.g., diabetes, dehydration, vitamin B_{12} deficiency).

Overflow incontinence results from detrusor muscle underactivity and/or bladder outlet obstruction. Leakage of urine is small in volume and continual. Overflow incontinence is found in women with pelvic organ prolapse and in men with benign prostatic hyperplasia.

Urinary incontinence is a complex syndrome with multiple causes; it is not uncommon for individuals to experience more than one type.

Assessment

A focused history with a careful physical examination is essential for determining the cause of incontinence. Transient or reversible causes should be ruled out (Table 32-1). A bladder diary is a helpful diagnostic tool that reveals toileting habits, fluid intake, and leakage episodes. Urinalysis and postvoid residual are essential laboratory tests. Further evaluation by specialists may involve urodynamic and imaging tests.

MECHANISM OF ACTION

Anticholinergics

Anticholinergic drugs have many actions. They block muscarinic actions (a subset of the parasympathetic nervous system). Primary associated adverse effects are blurred vision, urinary retention, constipation, dry mouth, tachycardia, and confusion.

Anticholinergic medications used for urge incontinence include those in this chapter, TCAs, and dicyclomine (Bentyl) (discussed in Chapter 29).

Anticholinergic drugs inhibit the action of acetylcholine on bladder smooth muscle. This blocks contraction of the bladder and decreases the urodynamic response of detrusor overactivity—the problem in urge incontinence. These actions result in increased bladder capacity, delayed desire to void, and diminished frequency of involuntary bladder contractions. Oxybutynin has both direct antispasmodic effects and anticholinergic effects on smooth muscle. Its direct relaxant effect on smooth muscle is produced by way of phosphodiesterase inhibition. The two newest drugs, darifenacin and solifenacin, have greater affinity for bladder smooth muscle cells than for salivary gland tissue. Darifenacin may have less affinity for the CNS receptors.

Antispasmodics

Flavoxate acts as a direct smooth muscle relaxant. This effect causes relief of bladder spasticity and thereby produces increased bladder capacity. Flavoxate also exhibits local anesthetic and analgesic actions.

Propantheline effectiveness in UI is based on its anticholinergic properties.

Cholinergic Agonist

Bethanechol has an effect that is opposite that of the anticholinergics. It stimulates the parasympathetic nervous system, causing release of acetylcholine at parasympathetic nerve endings. This increases detrusor muscle tone. Increased tone causes a contraction that initiates voiding and bladder emptying, which is useful in some cases of overflow incontinence from urinary retention.

desmopressin (DDAVP)

Desmopressin (1-deamino-8-D-arginine vasopressin; DDAVP) is a synthetic analog of vasopressin that acts as an antidiuretic. Vasopressin is a naturally occurring antidiuretic hormone. Desmopressin is stronger as an antidiuretic than as a vasopressor in smooth muscle. It decreases urine output for approximately 6 hours.

Urinary Tract Analgesia

Phenazopyridine is an azo dye that is excreted in the urine, where it exerts a topical analgesic effect on the urinary tract mucosa. It is useful only for the relief of pain. Phenazopyridine is compatible with antibacterial therapy. It should be

TABLE 32-1 Common Contributors to Transient Urinary Incontinence

Cause	Comment
Delirium	Mental status changes; treat underlying medical condition.
Infection	Irritated detrusor muscle
Atrophic urethritis or vaginitis	May present as dysuria, dyspareunia, burning on urination, urgency, and incontinence; requires a pelvic examination. Treat with estrogen.
Pharmaceuticals	Side effect of numerous agents (e.g., diuretics, NSAIDs, antihypertensives)
Excessive urine output	Peripheral edema, hyperglycemia
Restricted mobility	Cognitive decline, physical weakness
Stool impaction	Requires rectal examination

used short term (2 days) for treatment of UTI until antibiotic action reduces the pain.

DRUG TREATMENT PRINCIPLES

Standardized Guidelines

- Brigham and Women's Hospital: *Urinary incontinence: guide to diagnosis and management* (Available at www.guidelines.gov)

Evidence-Based Recommendations

- Stress incontinence
  - *Beneficial:* Serotonin reuptake inhibitors (SRI) (duloxetine)
  - *Likely to be beneficial:* Pelvic floor electrical stimulation, pelvic floor muscle exercises, vaginal cones
  - *Trade-off between benefit and harm:* Estrogen supplements
- No evidence regarding UI has been reported.

Cardinal Points of Treatment

URGE INCONTINENCE

- *First line:* oxybutynin, darifenacin, solifenacin, tolterodine, trospium
- *Second line:* TCA
- *Third line:* flavoxate, propantheline, dicyclomine

STRESS INCONTINENCE

- Estrogen cream, ring, imipramine, pseudoephedrine, duloxetine

Treatment for UI depends on the type of incontinence. Treatment may include nonpharmacologic therapies, biofeedback, electrical stimulation, and surgical options.

Nonpharmacologic Treatment

Nonpharmacologic approaches constitute the mainstay of treatment for UI. These minimally invasive management techniques include fluid management, bladder training, bladder retaining, and pelvic floor muscle rehabilitation.

Pharmacologic Treatment

In female stress incontinence, α-adrenergic agonists are used. Some research supports the use of estrogen (topically) as first-line therapy in elderly women with atrophic vaginitis that contributes to incontinence. Pseudoephedrine 30 to 60 mg orally up to four times a day (off label) can also be used, although high blood pressure is a risk for some individuals. TCAs increase bladder outlet resistance, which allows for better storage of urine. However, TCAs are not recommended for use in older persons because of orthostasis and anticholinergic side effects. Imipramine is the most commonly used agent (25 mg orally at bedtime). Onset of effect may take several weeks.

In urge incontinence, first-line pharmacotherapy consists of oxybutynin, darifenacin, solifenacin, tolterodine, or trospium. Second-line medications are the TCAs. Propantheline and flavoxate are older drugs that are not often used. Propantheline has strong anticholinergic side effects and is now considered a third-line choice. The theoretical advantage of flavoxate with its direct action on smooth muscle has not been effective in trials. Hyoscyamine or dicyclomine also can be considered.

Bethanechol, a urinary cholinergic, is used for the short-term treatment of urinary retention. The cause of the retention must be diagnosed and treated first.

Phenazopyridine is used in interstitial cystitis.

How to Monitor

- Clinical effectiveness may be monitored through the use of a bladder diary that documents voiding pattern, incontinent episodes, urge symptoms, and urine volumes.
- Monitor for anticholinergic side effects.
- Monitor cardiovascular status in patients with cardiac disease.

Patient Variables

GERIATRICS. Elderly patients are extremely sensitive to anticholinergic effects; both confusion and extreme cardiac effects are commonly seen.

PEDIATRICS

- *Anticholinergics:* Oxybutynin is not indicated in children younger than 5 years of age; safety and efficacy of other products in children younger than 12 years have not been not established.
- Cholinergics are not indicated in children.
- Primary nocturnal enuresis is common in children; desmopressin may be used in children 6 years of age or older.

PREGNANCY AND LACTATION

- *Category B:* oxybutynin, flavoxate, lactation not known; desmopressin, lactation is probably safe
- *Category C:* tolterodine, lactation possibly unsafe; with darifenacin, solifenacin, trospium, propantheline, and bethanechol, safety in lactation is unknown

GENDER. Causes of incontinence vary by gender.

Patient Education

- Careful patient teaching regarding response and side effects is necessary.
- Avoid driving or participating in other hazardous activities until the reaction to the drug is known.
- A dry mouth may be relieved by sugar-free gum or hard candy. Patients should be cautioned to maintain adequate fluid and fiber intake to prevent constipation.
- Avoid hot environments to prevent suppression of sweat gland activity and increased risk for heatstroke. This is a particular problem for the elderly because of age-related reduction in sweat gland activity.
- Alcoholic beverages should be avoided.
- Elderly or debilitated patients should be warned that they may experience agitation, confusion, excitement, or drowsiness with a usual dose. If this happens, they should stop taking the drug and notify the practitioner.
- Postural hypotension and tachycardia may occur during early therapy.
- *Bethanechol:* Take on an empty stomach to avoid the side effects of nausea and vomiting.
- Because orthostatic hypotension may occur, patients should be taught how to change positions slowly.

SPECIFIC DRUGS

ANTICHOLINERGICS

oxybutynin chloride (Ditropan, Ditropan XL, Oxytrol transdermal patch)

CONTRAINDICATIONS

- Hypersensitivity to oxybutynin or to any other anticholinergic drug
- Untreated narrow-angle glaucoma, partial or complete GI obstruction, paralytic ileus, intestinal atony in the elderly or debilitated, megacolon, ulcerative colitis, obstructive uropathy, myasthenia gravis, unstable cardiovascular status, and acute hemorrhage

WARNINGS

> When taken by patients who live in areas of high environmental temperature, risk for heatstroke is increased because of suppression of sweat gland activity.

- Diarrhea may be an early sign of intestinal obstruction in patients with a colostomy or ileostomy. In this situation, the use of oxybutynin chloride would be harmful.
- Use with caution in patients who have GERD or who are taking drugs (such as bisphosphonates) that may cause or exacerbate esophagitis.
- May induce drowsiness or blurred vision. Concomitant use of alcohol or other sedating drugs may enhance the drowsiness caused by oxybutynin.
- Use with caution in patients with clinically significant bladder outflow obstruction because of the risk of urinary retention.
- *Renal/hepatic function impairment:* Use with caution in patients with hepatic or renal impairment.

PRECAUTIONS. All drugs that have anticholinergic and smooth muscle relaxant properties have troublesome systemic anticholinergic side effects. The elderly are particularly sensitive to these effects and frequently experience dry mouth, constipation, and increased confusion. Careful dosing and close monitoring of clinical response and of tolerance of side effects are essential. The medication may aggravate symptoms of heart disease (including angina, CHF, arrhythmias, tachycardia, hypertension), hyperthyroidism, reflux esophagitis, hiatal hernia, and prostatic hyperplasia.

PHARMACOKINETICS. See Table 32-2.

ADVERSE REACTIONS. See Table 32-3.

DRUG INTERACTIONS. Concurrent use of other anticholinergics or drugs with anticholinergic activity may enhance the anticholinergic effects of oxybutynin chloride.

Oxybutynin may increase serum concentrations of digoxin, decrease serum concentrations of haloperidol, and enhance the development of tardive dyskinesia.

DOSAGE AND ADMINISTRATION. See Table 32-4.

The usual dosage for adults is 5 mg given two or three times per day. This may be increased to 5 mg four times per day. The recommended geriatric dosage is 2.5 to 5 mg two or three times daily. This may be increased to 5 mg three times per day every 1 or 2 days. The dosage for the XL formulation is 5 to 10 mg once daily. This dosage should be increased gradually in 5-mg increments to a maximum of 30 mg per day. Oxytrol is available as a transdermal patch that delivers 3.9 mg/day when applied twice weekly (every 3 to 4 days).

The usual pediatric dosage for children 5 years of age and older is 5 mg given twice per day. This may be increased to 5 mg three times a day. In children 6 years of age, the extended-release formulation is initiated at 5 mg once daily and is increased to a maximum of 20 mg daily.

OTHER DRUGS IN CLASS

Research findings are mixed and show no clear advantage of one drug over another. Other drugs in this class are similar to the key except as follows:

- *trospium:* Does not cross the blood-brain barrier; excreted unchanged in urine; can be used in patients with liver insufficiency; must be taken twice a day
- *darifenacin:* May cause less dry mouth, increased drug interactions, and fewer CNS effects; do not chew or crush tablets
- *solifenacin:* May result in less dry mouth; long half-life may or may not be beneficial for older adults, who will have the drugs in their system for a long time

ANTISPASMODICS

propantheline (Pro-Banthine)

CONTRAINDICATIONS. Hypersensitivity to propantheline; ulcerative colitis, toxic megacolon, obstructive disease of the GI or urinary tract, narrow-angle glaucoma, myasthenia gravis

DRUG INTERACTIONS. An increased effect will occur with narcotic analgesics, type I antiarrhythmics, antihistamines, phenothiazine, TCAs, corticosteroids, CNS depressants, amiodarone, β-blockers, and amoxapine. A decreased effect has been observed with antacids.

DOSAGE AND ADMINISTRATION. The usual adult dosage is 15 mg given three times a day 30 minutes before meals and 30 mg at bedtime. The dosage will have to be adjusted as needed and tolerated, with a maximum dosage not to exceed 120 mg daily. The recommended geriatric dosage is 7.5 mg given two or three times a day, with a maximum dosage not to exceed 30 mg three times a day. The usual pediatric dose is 2 to 3 mg/kg/day given in four to six divided doses (pediatric administration is limited because of availability of dosage forms).

If the patient is also receiving antacids, propantheline should be taken at least 1 hour before or after the other drug.

CHOLINERGIC AGONIST

bethanechol chloride (Urecholine)

CONTRAINDICATIONS. Hypersensitivity, hyperthyroidism, asthma, PUD, bradycardia, AV conduction defects, recent urinary or GI surgery, CAD, hypotension, hypertension, parkinsonism, epilepsy, and vasomotor instability

TABLE 32-2   Pharmacokinetics of Medications Used in Urinary Incontinence/Genitourinary Problems

Drug	Absorption	Onset of Action	Half-life	Duration of Action	Protein Bound	Metabolism	Excretion
oxybutynin XL	6%-10%	Onset 30-60 min	6-10 hr	24 hr	0	Hepatic, 3A4	Renal, 1%
tolterodine	77%	Onset 30-60 min	2-10 hr	5 hr	>96%	Hepatic 2D6	Renal, 1%
trospium	10%, decreased with food	—	20 hr	3 hr	50%-85%	Unknown	Urine unchanged, <10%
darifenacin	15%-25%	2 wk	13-19 hr	—	98%	3A4, 2D6	Urine metabolites, 60%
solifenacin	90%	2 wk	45-68 hr	2 wk	98%	3A4	Urine (3%-6%)
propantheline	<50%	30-45 min	1.-3 hr	4 hr	—	Hepatic, gastrointestinal tract	Renal, 70% as metabolites
flavoxate	—	60 min	—	—	—	—	Renal, 57%
bethanechol	Poor	30-90 min	1-6 hr	6 hr	—	Unknown	Unknown
desmopressin	Intranasal, 3.3%-4.1%	60 min	1.5-3 hr	6 hr	—	—	Unknown
phenazopyridine	3%	1 hr	2-4 hr	4 hr	—	2D6 and 3A4	Renal, 65% unchanged

TABLE 32-3   Common and Serious Adverse Effects of Medications Used in the Treatment of Urinary Tract Conditions

Drug	Common Side Effects	Serious Adverse Effects
Anticholinergics	Dry mouth, constipation, diarrhea, ↓ sweating, headache, dizziness, anxiety, vision changes, fatigue, sinusitis, dysuria, somnolence	Urinary retention, ↑ IOP, drowsiness, confusion and delirium, heatstroke, hallucinations, seizures, tachycardia, arrhythmias, HTN, anaphylaxis, angioedema
propantheline	Anticholinergic effects	Anaphylaxis
flavoxate	Anticholinergic effects Antispasmodic effects: nausea, vomiting, nervousness, vertigo	Tachycardia, leukopenia, confusion, respiratory distress
bethanechol	Flushing, sweating, abdominal cramps, colicky pain, nausea, belching, diarrhea, borborygmi, salivation, lacrimation, malaise, urinary urgency, headache	Bronchial constriction, asthma, miosis, orthostatic hypotension, tachycardia, seizures, fecal incontinence
desmopressin	Flushing, headache, rhinitis, nausea, abdominal pain, dizziness; nasal irritation, nosebleed when given intranasally	Severe fluid overload and hyponatremia, seizures, anaphylaxis, thrombosis
phenazopyridine	Headache, rash, pruritus, nausea, vertigo, GI disturbances, staining of contact lenses	Anaphylaxis, anaphylactoid reaction, renal and hepatic toxicity, anemia

WARNINGS/PRECAUTIONS

- *Reflux infection:* In urinary retention, if the sphincter fails to relax as bethanechol contracts the bladder, urine may be forced up the ureter into the kidney pelvis. If bacteriuria is present, this may cause reflux infection.
- Some products that contain tartrazine may cause allergies.

DRUG INTERACTIONS

- When bethanechol chloride is given concomitantly with other cholinergics, additive cholinergic effects and toxicity may occur.
- Ganglionic-blocking compounds may raise the level of bethanechol, causing severe abdominal symptoms and a critical fall in blood pressure.
- Quinidine and procainamide can raise the level of bethanechol and antagonize the cholinergic effects of bethanechol.

DOSAGE AND ADMINISTRATION. Dosage is highly individualized. The minimally effective dosage should be determined by beginning the adult patient on 5 to 10 mg, then repeating hourly to a maximum of 50 mg until a satisfactory response occurs. Take the medication on an empty stomach.

POSTERIOR PITUITARY HORMONES
desmopressin

Primary nocturnal enuresis should be used as an adjunct to behavioral conditioning or other nonpharmacologic intervention. Desmopressin is effective in some cases that are refractory

TABLE 32-4   Dosage and Administration Recommendations for Urinary Incontinence/Genitourinary Agents

Drug	Starting Dosage, mg	Administration	Titration	Maximum Daily Dose, mg
oxybutynin (Ditropan XL)	5-10	Daily	Increase by 5 mg in 1 week.	30
tolterodine (Detrol LA)	2-4	Daily		4
trospium	20	bid		40
darifenacin	7.5	Once daily	Increase to 15 mg once daily in 2 weeks.	15
solifenacin	5	Once daily	10 mg	10
flavoxate	100-200	tid-qid		800
propantheline	15-30	Before meals, 30 mg at bedtime		240
bethanechol	5-10	q1h until response; usual dose, 10-50 mg two to four times per day		400
desmopressin	0.2 (oral)	At bedtime		0.6
phenazopyridine	100-200	tid after meals for 2 days		

to conventional therapies. Desmopressin rapidly reduces the number of wet nights per week. However, the tendency is that this effect is not maintained after cessation of therapy. Desmopressin is more expensive than TCAs but is safer. Alarm interventions are intermediate in cost and are more disruptive but do not have the potential for adverse effects.

CONTRAINDICATIONS
- *Hypersensitivity:* Severe allergic reactions; anaphylaxis has not been reported with intranasal administration
- Intranasal delivery may be inappropriate when level of consciousness is impaired; moderate to severe renal impairment (CrCl <50 ml/min)

WARNINGS
- *Water intoxication:* Fluid overload and hyponatremia may result from excessive fluid intake. Severe hyponatremia may induce seizures and coma. Serum electrolyte monitoring is a reasonable precaution with initiation of the medication. Patients with electrolyte or fluid balance abnormalities, such as CHF and cystic fibrosis, should be monitored carefully. Particular attention should be paid to the possibility of the rare occurrence of an extreme decrease in plasma osmolality that may result in seizures, leading to coma. Very young or elderly patients should be cautioned to drink only enough fluid to satisfy thirst so as to decrease the potential for water intoxication and hyponatremia.
- *Desmopressin:* Children and infants require careful fluid intake restriction to prevent possible hyponatremia and water intoxication.

PRECAUTIONS
- *Cardiovascular effects:* High intranasal dosage has infrequently produced a slight elevation of blood pressure that disappears with dosage reduction. Use with caution in coronary artery insufficiency or hypertensive cardiovascular disease.

- Nasal mucosa changes (e.g., scarring, edema, discharge, blockage, congestion, severe atrophic rhinitis)
- Decreased response with time (longer than 6 months) has been reported.

DRUG INTERACTIONS
- Desmopressin may enhance the effects of pressor agents.
- Carbamazepine and chlorpropamide may potentiate the effects of desmopressin.

ADMINISTRATION AND DOSAGE. Individualize dosage. Initial dose is 20 mcg given intranasally at bedtime. This may be increased up to 40 mcg or may be decreased to 10 mcg, depending on the response. Give one half dose in each nostril. Duration of treatment is usually 4 to 8 weeks. The bottle accurately delivers 25 or 50 doses. Discard any solution remaining after 25 or 50 doses because the amount delivered may be less than that prescribed.

URINARY TRACT ANALGESIA
phenazopyridine (Pyridium)
CONTRAINDICATIONS
- Hypersensitivity, kidney or liver disease
- Patients with a CrCl <50 ml/min
- Glomerulonephritis

PRECAUTIONS
- Use with caution in GI disturbance and glucose-6-phosphate dehydrogenase deficiency.
- Do not delay definitive diagnosis and treatment of the causative condition.
- Discontinue when symptoms of infection are controlled, usually within 2 days.

ADVERSE EFFECTS. Stains urine (and underwear) orange; may cause headache, dizziness, and stomach cramps

PATIENT EDUCATION

- Stains the urine orange or red and may stain fabrics
- Notify provider if patient develops a yellowish tinge to the skin and/or sclera.
- Do not use long term.
- Does not treat infection, just reduces the pain associated with infection
- May stain contact lenses
- Should be taken after a meal

DOSAGE AND ADMINISTRATION. The usual dosage for adults is 200 mg given three times a day after meals. Continued use after 2 days when given with an antibiotic for the treatment of UTI is not recommended. It is available as an OTC product at 100 mg and by prescription at 200 mg.

evolve A continually updated list of useful WebLinks may be found in the Evolve Resources at http://evolve.elsevier.com/Edmunds/NP/

evolve http://evolve.elsevier.com/Edmunds/NP/

Acetaminophen

33

DRUG OVERVIEW

Drug Class	Generic Name	Trade Name
Antipyretic/analgesic	acetaminophen	Tylenol

INDICATIONS

- Antipyretic
- *Analgesic:* acute mild to moderate pain and chronic pain in conditions like osteoarthritis and rheumatoid arthritis
- Weak antiinflammatory effects

Unlabeled Use

- To decrease fever and pain in children receiving DPT vaccination

Acetaminophen (N-acetyl-p-aminophenol, or APAP) is an OTC medication that is commonly used to alleviate fever and mild pain. It can be used in patients who have experienced gastric irritation with aspirin or NSAIDs. Acetaminophen is similar to aspirin in terms of its effectiveness in decreasing fever and pain. It is the drug of choice for relief of minor pain in children, adults, and the elderly. APAP is different from aspirin in that it has a weak antiinflammatory effect, little GI adverse effect, and no impact on platelet aggregation. It is very well tolerated at recommended dosages. Maximum adult total daily dose is 4 g/day.

Acetaminophen is a metabolite of phenacetin. Phenacetin was introduced in 1887, was used extensively for many years, and then was taken off the market because its use led to nephropathy. APAP has been in use since 1893 but has become very popular since 1949. APAP has the effectiveness of phenacetin without the adverse reactions. However, acetaminophen overdosage may still cause nephropathy.

The problem most frequently noted with APAP involves difficulty in determining proper dosing in children. The FDA continues to issue safety alerts on various preparations to state that the dosing is confusing. All cough and cold medications that contain acetaminophen and are marketed for children younger than 2 years have been withdrawn from the market. Current guidelines recommend avoiding use of these products in children younger than 2 years because of the risk of toxicity associated with improper dosing.

The use of acetaminophen in the management of fever is discussed in this chapter. For additional information on the use of APAP in the treatment of pain, see Chapter 42.

THERAPEUTIC OVERVIEW

Pathophysiology

Fever is an elevation of the setpoint of body temperature. The hypothalamus is the site of the heat-regulating center. The setpoint is elevated through several mechanisms. The most common of these involves the monocyte-macrophages, which, when stimulated, release pyrogenic cytokines such as interleukin-1. These stimulate the heat-regulating center to raise the setpoint. This prompts increased heat production via shivering or decreased heat loss through peripheral vasoconstriction.

Disease Process

It is essential for the clinician to identify and treat the cause of fever and not just the symptoms. Fever is a symptom with many causes, the most common of which is infection. The danger in treating a fever involves the risk that symptoms of a worsening infection may be masked. A fever may be an important indication of antibiotic resistance. Fever of unknown origin is defined as an unexplained case of fever exceeding 38.3° C on several occasions for at least 3 weeks in patients without neutropenia or immunosuppression. Causes of fever and hyperthermia are listed in Table 33-1.

MECHANISM OF ACTION

Antipyretic

Acetaminophen reduces fever through direct action on the hypothalamic heat-regulating center, thereby lowering the setpoint to normal. It does this by inhibiting the action of pyrogenic cytokines on heat-regulating centers. This action increases dissipation of body heat via vasodilation and sweating.

Analgesic

Acetaminophen is a centrally acting analgesic. Its site and mechanism of analgesic action are not clear but may result from inhibition of prostaglandin synthetase in the CNS. APAP differs from ASA in that it does not inhibit peripheral prostaglandin synthesis. This may account for the absence of antiinflammatory and platelet-inhibiting effects.

TABLE 33-1 Causes of Fever and Hyperthermia

Common Causes of Fever	Less Common Causes of Fever	Causes of Hyperthermia
Infections: bacteria, virus, rickettsia, fungus, parasites	Cardiovascular disease: myocardial infarction, thrombophlebitis, pulmonary embolism	Heatstroke
Autoimmune disease	GI disease: inflammatory bowel disease, alcoholic hepatitis, granulomatous hepatitis	Malignant hyperthermia of anesthesia
CNS disease, including head trauma and mass lesions	Medication: drug fever	Malignant neuroleptic syndrome
Malignant disease, especially renal cell, liver, leukemia, and lymphoma	Other: sarcoidosis, tissue injury, hematoma, and factitious causes	

TREATMENT PRINCIPLES

Standardized Guidelines

- Simon LS, et al: *Pain in osteoarthritis, rheumatoid arthritis and juvenile chronic arthritis*, ed 2, Glenview, IL, 2002, American Pain Society.

Evidence-Based Recommendations

For the person with osteoarthritis (OA), acetaminophen is the medication of first choice for mild pain. Little evidence suggests that acetaminophen provides any benefit when peripheral inflammation is a causative factor for the pain.

Cardinal Points of Treatment

- Acetaminophen is an OTC medication; many patients self-administer this product for both pain relief and fever reduction.
- APAP use appears relatively straightforward in adults. However, in all individuals, particularly in children, its use becomes more complicated and presents many opportunities for overdosage. Different dosages are used for different age and weight groups, and many formulations with different strengths are available. APAP is a frequent constituent of other OTC combination products. These formulations change frequently. See Table 33-2 for a list of formulations and strengths. Note the broad array of products with different strengths.
- Evidence from past studies suggests that acetaminophen is the drug of choice for reduction of fever. Treatment of minor fever is not generally indicated. Symptomatic relief of a fever greater than 40°C is usually required. A temperature greater than 41.5°C (hyperpyrexia) constitutes a medical emergency.
- The decision to treat a fever is based on the circumstances. All fevers do not have to be treated with an antipyretic. Fever may serve as a protective physiologic mechanism. Treating the fever may prolong the course of the infection, obscure symptoms, or make it difficult for the clinician to assess the patient's response to the infection.
- Fever should be treated if it is deleterious to the patient, or if the patient is in significant discomfort as a result of the fever. For example, the elderly can have tachycardia from fever that may decompensate their CHF. Children may experience seizures if their temperature is high. The patient may experience fluid and electrolyte imbalance because of perspiration.

TABLE 33-2 Strengths of Various Formulations of Acetaminophen

Formulation	Strength
Drops, infant	80 mg/0.8 ml
Elixir, liquid, child suspension/syrup	160 mg/5 ml
Caplets, geltabs, extra strength	500 mg
Tablets	325 mg
Tablets, extra strength	500 mg
Adult liquid, extra strength	500 mg/15 ml
Extended-release geltabs	650 mg
Suppositories	80, 120, 125, 300, 325, 650 mg

These formulations vary in terms of flavors and ingredients: saccharin, alcohol, phenylalanine, aspartame, sucrose, corn syrup, and others.

Nonpharmacologic Treatment

Nonpharmacologic treatment of fever consists of heat removal measures such as cold water or alcohol sponge baths or the use of ice bags. Untreated fever may cause fluid and electrolyte losses through perspiration; these fluids and electrolytes must be replaced.

Pharmacologic Treatment

FEVER. Pharmacologic treatment of fever may consist of aspirin, NSAIDs, or APAP. APAP generally is preferred in children to avoid Reye's syndrome, which is associated with some other antipyretic agents. Some adults may find aspirin or ibuprofen more effective. Acetaminophen is given every 4 to 6 hours, depending on its strength. If the patient has an illness that causes a fever, it is often advisable to give the medication routinely rather than as needed to prevent uncomfortable swings in temperature; however, the maximum dose per day must not be exceeded.

ACUTE MILD TO MODERATE PAIN. Acetaminophen is useful in the treatment of mild to moderate noninflammatory acute pain such as headache, muscle ache, and the malaise that accompanies minor viral infection. It is commonly used in children to relieve the pain of teething. It is not effective in the treatment of acute inflammation. The effectiveness of pain relief is better if APAP is given routinely and not on a prn basis.

CHRONIC PAIN. Acetaminophen is a very effective pain medication for chronic pain of malignant or nonmalignant origin. It is useful for the pain of OA in the elderly, who often cannot tolerate NSAIDs. It often is used in combination with other medications to enhance their effectiveness. It frequently is combined with codeine and similar opioids as an adjunct medication. See Chapter 42 for a discussion of analgesics.

When acetaminophen is given in combination products, such as acetaminophen with codeine, it is important for the clinician to monitor the daily intake of acetaminophen to avoid an overdose.

DPT VACCINATION USE. A dose of acetaminophen should be given immediately following vaccination and every 4 to 6 hours for 48 to 72 hours. This decreases the incidence of fever and reduces injection site pain.

How to Monitor

- Monitor temperature and track reduction of fever.
- Monitor relief of pain and the presence of adverse effects.
- Acetaminophen may be found in many combination OTC products (cold and sinus). Ask specifically about acetaminophen when taking a medication history, to avoid potential overdosing.

Patient Variables

GERIATRICS. Geriatric patients often have subclinical hepatic insufficiency and are at risk for APAP toxicity. All patients, but particularly those who are older, who are taking hepatic toxic drugs, who are alcoholics, or who have cirrhosis, should use this product with great care.

Use APAP with caution in geriatric patients, especially when given in combination with alcohol, and in patients with known impaired hepatic function. Use lower doses and increased dosage intervals. This agent is safer than other drugs for the treatment of chronic pain.

PEDIATRICS. Acetaminophen is used commonly for pain and fever in children and generally is well tolerated. Use caution to avoid overdosage (see "Dosage and Administration" section). In contrast to aspirin, acetaminophen may be given to children with viral infection because it is not associated with Reye's syndrome. Because of the risk of Reye's syndrome, children should *never* receive aspirin.

Most overdosage occurs with conscientious parents who inadvertently overdose sick children.

> **Failure to give APAP in proper concentration and dosage may lead to serious acetaminophen toxicity. Infant drops (80 mg/0.8 ml) are three times more concentrated than the elixir/solution (160 mg/5 ml).**

PREGNANCY AND LACTATION. Acetaminophen crosses the placenta. It is used routinely in pregnancy (category B) and appears safe for short-term use. No evidence has been found of a relationship between APAP ingestion and congenital malformations.

Acetaminophen is excreted in breast milk. No adverse effects have been reported in nursing infants.

Patient Education

- Keep medication away from children.
- Severe pain or high fever may indicate serious illness. If fever or high fever persists, consult a health care provider.
- Avoid consumption of large amounts of alcohol while taking acetaminophen because of the increased risk of liver damage or nephropathy.
- Generic acetaminophen is as effective as and less expensive than brand name products.
- Discuss mild cyclic elevations in temperature vs. true fever that requires treatment.

SPECIFIC DRUGS

acetaminophen (Tylenol)

CONTRAINDICATIONS. Hypersensitivity to acetaminophen

WARNINGS/PRECAUTIONS

- Do not exceed recommended maximum dosage (4 g/day) for an adult.
- Use with caution in patients with hepatic function impairment.
- Use with caution in patients with chronic alcoholism and in those who consume ≥3 alcoholic drinks/day.
- Known glucose-6-phosphate dehydrogenase deficiency (G6PD) problems

PHARMACOKINETICS. Acetaminophen is rapidly and almost completely absorbed from the GI tract. Peak plasma concentration occurs in 30 minutes to 2 hours. Liquid preparations are absorbed faster than tablets. The rate and amount of absorption from rectal suppositories are variable, and the half-life is 1 to 3 hours. Acetaminophen is metabolized in the liver. About 4% is metabolized via the cytochrome P450 oxidase system, and the toxic metabolite is detoxified with hepatic glutathione. Hepatic necrosis can occur if glutathione stores have been depleted by long-term or toxic doses of acetaminophen. Approximately 95% of this drug is metabolized and excreted in the urine.

ADVERSE EFFECTS. When acetaminophen is used as directed, adverse effects are rare. Hypersensitivity presents as skin eruptions, urticarial and erythematous skin reactions, and fever. Extremely rare hematologic reactions include hemolytic anemia, leukopenia, neutropenia, and pancytopenia. Other reactions are hypoglycemia and jaundice. Adverse effects are usually dose dependent. Hepatic toxicity may occur following intake of >7.5 g within 8 hours. Alcoholics and patients on hepatic metabolizing medications are more susceptible to hepatic toxicity. This is very important because hepatic toxicity can be caused by binge drinking.

DRUG INTERACTIONS. Concurrent use with the following drugs may increase the risk of hepatotoxicity: barbiturates, hydantoins, carbamazepine, rifampin, sulfinpyrazone, and ethanol.

OVERDOSAGE. Acute overdosage of acetaminophen can result in hepatotoxicity and is life threatening. Toxicity is likely to occur if a patient takes more than 250 mg/kg in a single dose or greater than 12 grams within a 24-hour period. However, nearly all patients who ingest more than 350 mg/kg develop severe liver toxicity (AST/ALT levels greater than 1000 international units/L) unless they are treated quickly. Children must be monitored carefully for signs of toxicity. APAP is metabolized to a highly toxic intermediate product, which normally is detoxified by glutathione. When glutathione is depleted, the toxic intermediate attacks other cells, causing necrosis. Symptoms that appear in the first 24 hours are nausea, vomiting, drowsiness, lethargy, malaise, and confusion.

After 24 hours up until 72 hours, symptoms abate and liver toxicity (AST/ALT elevation) normally occurs. An increase in liver enzymes within 24 hours is a sign of permanent injury. Liver enzyme elevation usually peaks at between 72 and 96 hours after ingestion, along with other markers of liver function such as the INR and a total bilirubin concentration above 4. The last stage, which consists of recovery, lasts anywhere from 4 days to 2 weeks; recovery is complete in many cases.

TREATMENT OF OVERDOSAGE. The patient should immediately receive activated charcoal. Further treatment should take place in a hospital setting with the patient receiving N-acetylcysteine (NAC), the specific antidote for acetaminophen poisoning. The dose is based on the serum level of APAP. NAC increases glutathione stores; this allows further metabolism of acetaminophen and thus prevents accumulation of the toxic metabolite. NAC also possesses potent antiinflammatory and antioxidant effects.

DOSAGE AND ADMINISTRATION. The dosage for adults is 325 to 650 mg for fever and 325 to 1000 mg for pain (Table 33-3). Acetaminophen should be administered every 4 to 6 hours. It can be given prn or routinely. The maximum dose over a 24-hour period for adults and children ≥12 years old is 4 g. Elderly patients frequently do well on 1000 mg every 6 hours because they metabolize the drug more slowly.

Dosage for children is based on the formula of 10 to 15 mg/kg/dose (oral) and 10 to 20 mg/kg/dose (rectal); the maximum daily dose should not exceed 2.6 g/day. Administer every 4 to 6 hours. See Table 33-3 for a list of dosages by age and weight. Weight is the preferred dosing method over age.

TABLE 33-3   Dosage of Acetaminophen by Age and Weight*

Age Group	Weight, lb	Dosage, mg
0-3 mo	6-11	40
4-11 mo	12-17	80
1-< 2 yr	18-23	120
2-3 yr	24-35	160
4-5 yr	36-47	240
6-8 yr	48-59	320
9-10 yr	60-71	400
11 yr	72-95	480

*Follow manufacturer's guidelines. Weight recommendations should be followed in preference to age recommendations. Children may repeat dose every 4 to 6 hours; do not exceed 5 doses in 24 hours. Not to exceed 2.6 g/day. Adults: 325 to 650 mg every 4 to 6 hours, or 1 g 3 or 4 times/day. Not to exceed 4 g/day.

Formulation is an issue for children. Many confusing formulations are based on the age and the weight of the child. Conscientious parents may easily overdose their children if they do not use the proper formulation for age of the child.

Infant formulations (drops; 80 mg/0.8 ml) are three times more concentrated than child formulations (suspensions; 160 mg/5 ml). Chewable tablets are available in two strengths (80 mg and 160 mg) and are easily confused. Suppositories (80 mg, 120 mg, 325 mg, and 650 mg) are needed if the child is vomiting or refuses the medication. Give specific instructions on the type of formulation recommended. Instruct the parent to read the label carefully to avoid overdosage.

evolve A continually updated list of useful WebLinks may be found in the Evolve Resources at http://evolve.elsevier.com/ Edmunds/NP/

Aspirin and Nonsteroidal Antiinflammatory Medications

34

DRUG OVERVIEW

Class	Subclass	Generic Name	Trade Name
Salicylates		acetylsalicylic acid 🔑	aspirin, OTC
NSAIDs	Propionic acids	ibuprofen 🔑 ✹	Motrin, OTC
		fenoprofen	Nalfon
		flurbiprofen	Ansaid
		ketoprofen	Orudis, OTC
		naproxen ✹	Naprosyn, Anaprox OTC
		oxaprozin	Daypro
	Acetic acids		
	Indole and indene acetic acids	indomethacin ✹	Indocin
		etodolac ✹	Lodine
		sulindac	Clinoril
	Heteroaryl acetic acids	diclofenac sodium ✹	Voltaren, Cataflam
		ketorolac	Toradol
		tolmetin sodium	Tolectin
	Alkanones	nabumetone ✹	Relafen
	Fenamates (anthranilic acids)	meclofenamate	Meclomen
		mefenamic acid	Ponstel
	Oxicams	piroxicam ✹	Feldene
		meloxicam ✹	Mobic ✹
	COX-2 inhibitors	celecoxib	Celebrex ✹

✹ Top 200 drug; 🔑 key drug. Ibuprofen was chosen as the key drug because it was the first NSAID and is still in common use.

INDICATIONS

ASPIRIN

- Short- or long-term symptomatic treatment of mild to moderate pain, rheumatoid arthritis, and osteoarthritis
- Reduces risk of recurrent TIAs or stroke in patients who have had TIAs caused by fibrin platelet emboli
- Reduces the risk of death or nonfatal MI with previous infarction or unstable angina pectoris

Unlabeled Uses

- Prevention of cataracts, toxemia in pregnancy
- Reduction of risk for colorectal adenoma

The action of aspirin (ASA) on blood clotting is discussed in Chapter 23.

MOST NONSTEROIDAL ANTIINFLAMMATORY DRUGS (NSAIDs)

- Osteoarthritis (OA)
- Rheumatoid arthritis (RA)
- Mild to moderate pain: dental extractions, minor surgery, soft tissue athletic injury
- Primary dysmenorrhea

Unlabeled Uses

- Tendinitis, bursitis, migraine

This chapter discusses the use of salicylates and NSAIDs in the treatment of osteoarthritis and acute inflammatory/pain conditions. Salicylates and NSAIDs are closely related. They have antiinflammatory, analgesic, and antipyretic effects. ASA is the only salicylate discussed here because it is the only salicylate in common use.

> All of these drugs can cause GI irritation and bleeding, which can be fatal. GI bleeding may occur without any prodromal symptoms.

NSAIDs constitute a large group of drugs that are used to treat a variety of conditions. Official FDA indications vary among the NSAIDs and do not correlate well with their common usage. Table 34-1 lists some indications for the use of aspirin and individual NSAIDs. Recent research suggests that long-term NSAID use may decrease the incidence of Alzheimer's disease. However, these neurologic effects are negated if the individual has been taking ASA for its cardioprotective effects. The different classes are chemically unrelated but share the same therapeutic actions and adverse effects. For the purpose of this chapter, NSAIDs are divided into seven classes: propionic acids, indole and indene acetic acids, heteroaryl acetic acids, alkanones, fenamates, oxicams, and COX-2 inhibitors. Significant differences among the drugs have been noted. Although COX-2 inhibitors may decrease the risk of GI side effects, they are much more expensive than the other classes.

A broad body of literature demonstrates that NSAIDs are associated with an increased risk of serious and potentially fatal thrombotic events, MI and stroke, and adverse cardiovascular events, These adverse effects were once thought to occur only with COX-2 NSAIDs, but additional studies have demonstrated this risk with older NSAIDs as well. Clinicians should follow the findings of continuing study in this area.

THERAPEUTIC OVERVIEW
Anatomy and Physiology

In joints, the ends of the bones are capped by cartilage, and the joint structure is held together by a very tight capsule. A very fine membrane, the synovium, lines that capsule. The synovium normally stops at the point where the cartilage begins. The synovium does not extend across the whole joint; otherwise, trauma to the synovium would occur every time the joint was flexed (Figure 34-1). The tendons attach to the bones, and, when the muscle contracts, the joint opens or closes.

INFLAMMATION. See Chapter 69, Immunizations and Biologicals, for a review of the immune system. Prostaglandins cause increased vascular permeability and neutrophil chemotaxis (movement), and they induce pain. Increased vascular permeability allows diffusion of large molecule inflammatory substances across cell walls into the site of inflammation. Prostaglandins are produced in the mast cell from arachidonic acid by the action of the COX enzyme and are classified into groups according to their structure. Prostaglandins E_1 and E_2 are active in the inflammatory response. Aspirin and NSAIDs act to block the COX enzyme from producing prostaglandins, thereby inhibiting inflammation (Figure 34-2).

Two types of cyclooxygenase have been identified: COX-1 and COX-2. COX-1 is found in the blood vessels, stomach, and kidneys; COX-2 is found in the brain, kidneys, and bone. Inhibition of COX-2 is necessary to prevent inflammatory action.

COX-1 prostaglandins protect the gastric mucosa. They encourage mucosal blood flow and elaboration of bicarbonate to produce a more neutral or less acidic layer next to the gastric mucosa. Prostaglandins also produce a significant layer of mucus that serves as a barrier to the acid. They maintain normal renal function, mental function, and temperature. Although these effects are desirable, it is through COX-1 inhibition that salicylates and NSAIDs are thought to have their direct detrimental effects on the gastric mucosa. Selective COX-2 inhibitor drugs are designed primarily to inhibit COX-2 while sparing COX-1. Because this selectivity is not perfect, these drugs may exert some detrimental effect on the gastric mucosa. COX-1 drugs are widely available, but relatively few COX-2 drugs are currently in use.

When an inflammatory process occurs, the synovium becomes lumpy. The synovium also starts to grow into and across the cartilaginous area, producing pits in the cartilage. At the same time, the tendon sheath that surrounds the tendon becomes inflamed, so that motion of the joint is painful. If this process is not checked, ultimately, the ends of the bones are denuded and bone grates upon bone, with resultant eventual destruction of the joint (Figure 34-3). The inflammatory response is accompanied by symptoms of erythema, edema, tenderness, and pain.

TABLE 34-1   Indications for Specific Drugs

	OA	RA	Mild to Moderate Pain	Primary Dysmenorrhea	Juvenile RA	Acute Gout	Acute Tendinitis/ Acute Bursitis
aspirin	X	X	X				
ibuprofen	X	X	X	X			
fenoprofen	X	X	X				
flurbiprofen	X	X					
ketoprofen	X	X	X	X			
naproxen	X	X	X	X	X	X	X
oxaprozin	X	X			X		
indomethacin	X	X				X	X
etodolac	X	X	X		X	Y	
sulindac	X	X			Y	X	X
diclofenac	X	X	X	X	Y		
ketorolac		X					
tolmetin	X	X					
nabumetone	X	X					
meclofenamate	X	X	X	X			
mefenamic acid			X	X			
piroxicam	X	X			Y		
meloxicam	X	Y					
celecoxib	X	X		X			

X, Indication; Y, unlabeled use.

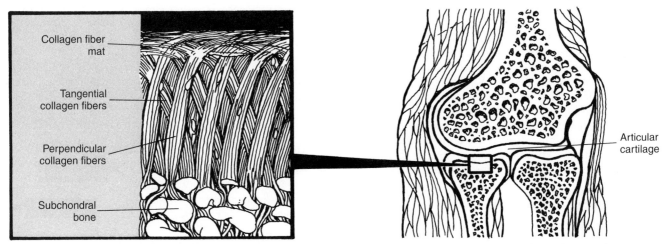

FIGURE 34-1   Organization of collagen fibers in articular cartilage. (From McCance KL, Huether SE: *Pathophysiology,* ed 4, St Louis, 2001, Mosby.)

Pathophysiology: Osteoarthritis

In OA, the articular cartilage degenerates, is roughened, and then is worn away. The body attempts to repair the lost cartilage, but the integrity of the new cartilage is inferior to that of the original, and the integrity of the surface of the cartilage is lost. Bone compensates by hypertrophy at the articular margins, forming spurs and causing lipping at the edge of the joint surface. The synovial membrane thickens, but it does not form adhesions. A low level of inflammation usually is present (see Figure 34-3).

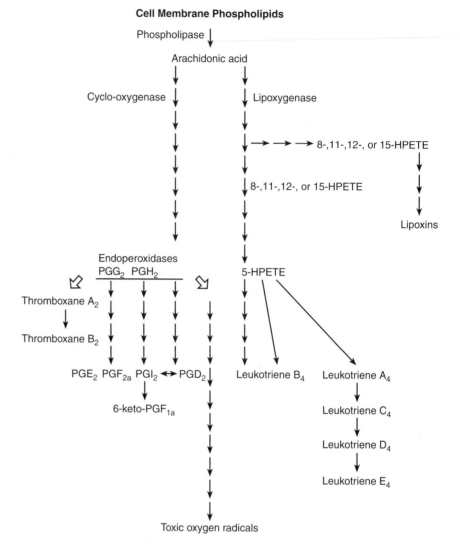

FIGURE 34-2 Arachidonic acid synthesis to prostaglandins. (Modified from Melmon K, Morrelli-Howard F: *Clinical pharmacology: basic principles in therapeutics,* ed 3, New York, 1992, McGraw-Hill.)

Disease Process

More than 100 types of arthritis are known. The one thread that is common to all arthritic conditions is inflammation. Treating the inflammation is only one component of treating arthritis, but it is extremely important.

Characteristic symptoms of OA are pain with movement and weight bearing that is relieved by rest. The patient often has brief morning stiffness (less than 30 minutes) with minimal articular inflammation and no systemic manifestations. Joints commonly affected are terminal joints of the fingers, thumb, hip, knee, and spine. No signs of acute inflammation are seen, and the erythrocyte sedimentation rate is normal.

MECHANISM OF ACTION

Acetaminophen (APAP) is different from salicylates and NSAIDs in that it does not have significant antiinflammatory action. This is because APAP affects COX in the brain but not in peripheral tissue.

Salicylates and NSAIDs reduce inflammation by inhibiting the production of prostaglandins, prostacyclin, and thromboxanes in both CNS and peripheral tissue. They do this by blocking the COX enzyme. This major mechanism is involved in most of the effects achieved by salicylates and NSAIDs (see Figure 34-2) and may be responsible for the fact

that the incidence of colon cancer has been found to be lower in patients who take ASA on a regular basis.

Pain

The mechanism for decreasing pain occurs through the antiinflammatory process. Pain is relieved when inflammation is decreased and when prostaglandins are reduced. Salicylates may cause some pain reduction centrally at subcortical sites.

Antipyretic Effects

ASA blocks the effect of interleukin-1 on the hypothalamus, which is responsible for temperature control. Peripherally, salicylates reduce fever by causing vasodilation of superficial blood vessels. This effect results in dissipation of heat.

Platelet Effects

Platelet activation is stimulated by thromboxane; this results in aggregation, and the clotting cascade ensues. The antiplatelet effects of NSAIDs are caused by blocking of the COX-1 enzyme and production of thromboxane. Any drug that inhibits the COX-1 enzyme reduces the production of thromboxane. This effect is applied in the treatment of patients with cardiovascular disease. Aspirin causes irreversible inactivation of COX, allowing decreased production of

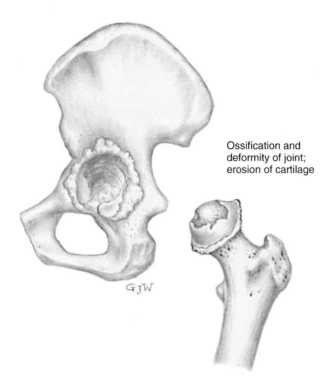

Ossification and deformity of joint; erosion of cartilage

FIGURE 34-3   Osteoarthritis (OA). Cartilage and degeneration of the hip joint from osteoarthritis. (From Mourad L: *Orthopedic disorders,* St Louis, 1991, Mosby.)

thromboxane for the life of the platelet (8 to 10 days). NSAIDs, however, exhibit reversible inactivation of COX, which lasts only for the duration of drug activity, so continuous platelet aggregation is not found. This is why aspirin—not NSAIDs—is used for prevention of stroke and MI.

Ongoing research is examining the use of NSAIDs in the treatment of patients with a variety of problems:

1. The use of NSAIDs to reduce the risk of Alzheimer's is under study at the NIH.
2. A strong inverse link is apparent between breast cancer and NSAID use.
3. NSAIDs may protect against Parkinson's disease.
4. NSAIDs seem to decrease the risk of colon cancer.

Adverse Effects

When prostaglandins are inhibited, more gastric acid is produced and the risk of mucosal damage is increased. ASA and NSAIDs, by inhibiting prostaglandins, increase gastric acid production at the same time that they decrease defenses to that acid. This process serves as the basis for the adverse GI effects of these medications.

Kidneys that are impaired also rely on prostaglandins to cause vasodilation. When prostaglandins are inhibited, vasodilation is lessened and blood flow to the kidneys is decreased.

As with other NSAIDs, long-term use of celecoxib can lead to renal papillary necrosis, renal insufficiency, acute renal failure, and other renal injuries. In patients for whom renal prostaglandins have a compensatory role in the maintenance of renal perfusion, NSAIDs may cause a dose-dependent reduction in prostaglandin formation and, secondarily, renal blood flow that may precipitate overt renal decompensation.

Patients with impaired renal function, heart failure, or liver dysfunction; elderly patients; and those taking diuretics, ACE

inhibitors, and angiotensin II receptor antagonists are at greatest risk for this reaction. Discontinuation of NSAID therapy usually is followed by recovery to the pretreatment state.

TREATMENT PRINCIPLES
Standardized Guidelines

- Brigham and Women's Hospital: *Lower extremity musculoskeletal disorders: a guide to diagnosis and treatment,* Boston, 2003, Brigham and Women's Hospital.
- Many others on specific topics in osteoarthritis

Evidence-Based Recommendations

- A total of 509 clinical studies on osteoporosis are listed in PubMed.
- Patient education and exercise improve a patient's well-being.
- Topical NSAIDs, acupuncture, and tramadol are effective for pain relief in knee OA.
- Glucosamine and chondroitin do not relieve most OA pain, but they may be effective in moderate to severe knee pain resulting from trauma or overuse.

For the person with moderate to severe pain and/or inflammation, a COX-2 selective NSAID is the first choice, unless the person is at significant risk for hypertension or renal disorder.

In persons at increased risk for hypertension and edema, clinicians should use any NSAID cautiously because of the risk of exacerbating hypertension or edema. Nonselective NSAIDs should be considered only if the person is not responsive to or is not able to take COX-2 selective NSAIDs and/or acetaminophen up to 4000 mg per day, and only after a risk analysis has been done to determine the risk for a significant NSAID-induced GI complication. If such risk factors exist, then a prophylactic agent such as a proton pump inhibitor or misoprostol should be given along with the nonselective NSAID.

The person at risk for a cardiovascular event should be given a regular low dose of aspirin (between 75 and 160 mg per day), whether the patient is treated with a nonselective or a COX-2 selective NSAID.

Tramadol may be used alone or in combination with acetaminophen or NSAIDs for therapy at any time during the treatment of a person with OA, when NSAIDs alone produce inadequate pain relief.

Cardinal Points of Treatment

- Begin with nonpharmacologic treatment.
- First line: acetaminophen
- Second line: NSAIDs
- The underlying goals of treatment are to limit the inflammatory process, protect the joint, and relieve pain.
- Nonpharmacologic methods are important in all uses of NSAIDs. If a patient has moderate pain, consider starting NSAIDs at the same time that nonpharmacologic treatment is initiated.

DRUG CHOICE. All NSAIDs differ from one another in terms of a number of drug properties. Evaluation of these properties in relationship to the patient and his or her condition will aid drug choice. Wide variation has been noted in how patients respond to a particular medication. As always, when many drugs are included in the same class, one should select a few and become familiar with them. Clinically, no clear guidelines and no evidence-based decision making are available to assist the provider in selecting the most appropriate NSAID for a particular patient.

Aspirin can be effective and inexpensive. Up to 12 tablets a day are required, so compliance can be difficult. Salicylates are generally less expensive than NSAIDs. Because salicylates almost always cause GI distress or ulceration, their use is significantly limited.

The following drug characteristics must be considered:
- *Degree of COX-1 vs. COX-2 inhibition:* Varying degrees of COX-1 inhibition may occur. Even COX-2 inhibitors exhibit a small amount of COX-1 inhibition at higher doses. These differences cause differences in the frequency of adverse GI effects.
- *Potency of the different therapeutic effects:* For example, one drug may be a relatively weak antiinflammatory but a potent analgesic that may be used for pain rather than for inflammation.
- Pharmacokinetic components that should be considered include duration of action (frequency of dosing), protein binding (drug interactions), and renal excretion (renal function).

- Relative frequency of adverse effects, especially GI, renal, hepatic, and cardiovascular, should be reviewed.
- The specific use that is intended and the specific indications for each drug must be known.
- Whether the drug is an OTC product or is available by prescription only should be considered.

Patient variables that should be considered include the following:
- Medical condition, especially renal and hepatic function and cardiovascular status
- Age
- Ability to comply with dosing schedules
- Reliability of the patient in promptly reporting adverse effects
- Cost—All of these drugs except celecoxib are now available as generics.

See Table 34-2 for other unique properties of antiinflammatory drugs.

A common practice is to use ASA/NSAID for antiinflammatory purposes for a specified period, whereas these agents often are used for acute pain only once or twice.

TABLE 34-2　Individual Characteristics of Aspirin and NSAIDs

	Inflammation	Pain	COX-1*	COX-2†	Renal AR	Hepatic AR	Comments
aspirin			↑	↑			High risk for ARs; cardioprotective
ibuprofen	↑		↑	↑			Key drug
fenoprofen		↑					AR: Headache
flurbiprofen		↑					
naproxen			↑			2C9, ↑	
oxaprozin						2C9	
indomethacin	↑		↑	↑	↑	↑	High risk for ARs, esp CNS, headache, hyperkalemia; aggravates epilepsy and parkinsonism; short-term use only
etodolac			↓	↑		↓ 2C9	
sulindac					↓	↑	AR: Pancreatitis; prodrug, bypasses kidney
hepatic risk							
diclofenac		↑	↑			↑	
ketorolac	↓	↑↑	↑↑			2C9	↑ AR: Headache, black box warning; short-term use, not primary care
tolmetin		↑					
nabumetone			↓	↓	↓	2C9	Prodrug
meclofenamate		↑					Toxicity manifests as diarrhea.
mefenamic acid		↑				2C9	Toxicity manifests as diarrhea, ↑ AR
piroxicam			↑		↑	↓	High risk of AR; daily dosing, largely replaced by COX-2 inhibitors
meloxicam			↓	↑		2C9	↑ GI in dose >30 mg
celecoxib			↓↓	↑			AR: Headache, sulfa allergy, daily dosing

Blank, Average; ↑ increased; ↓ decreased AR, adverse reaction.
*COX-1 action correlates with GI protection, platelet aggregation, and kidney function.
†COX-2 action correlates with inflammation; located in brain, kidney, and bone.

Initiate treatment with the starting dose. The analgesic effect should be noticed within 1 to 4 hours of administration. However, the full antiinflammatory effect will not be apparent until after a few weeks. Increase the dose until therapeutic effects are seen, or the patient experiences adverse effects. Patient response to one NSAID does not predict what the response will be to any other NSAID, even one within the same drug class. If pain cannot be managed adequately with NSAIDs, see Chapter 42 for information on analgesia.

If the patient experiences GI distress or is at high risk for GI bleed, coadministration of misoprostol may be considered. H_2-blockers and proton pump inhibitors may provide some benefit, but only misoprostol is acceptable for preventing both gastric and duodenal ulcers. Misoprostol may be started at the approved dose of 200 mcg qid with food. If the patient experiences severe diarrhea, the dose should be decreased to 100 mcg qid or 200 mcg bid with food.

Women who are of childbearing age should not take misoprostol unless appropriate contraception is being used because it is an abortifacient.

Aspirin products have largely been replaced by NSAIDs. A trend toward increasing use of COX-2 inhibitors has occurred because they offer a reduced risk of GI distress. This has allowed the use of NSAID treatment for many patients who formerly were unable to use these agents. However, NSAIDs still have adverse renal, hepatic, and cardiovascular effects. Cost is also a major limitation. Insurance companies often limit reimbursement or require preauthorization unless the patient has had an adverse reaction to NSAIDs.

Nonpharmacologic Treatment for Osteoarthritis

Nonpharmacologic treatment includes proper exercise with rest periods. A supervised walking program can improve functional status. Recommend weight loss to overweight patients to reduce strain on joints. The patient must be realistic about the limitations of medications and about his own prognosis.

Pharmacologic Treatment for Osteoarthritis

Acetaminophen may be effective in treating the pain of OA because many patients have minimal inflammation. Patients with mild OA should be started on acetaminophen. If this is not effective, NSAIDs can be used. NSAIDs are more effective than acetaminophen for OA of the knee or hip. They are also more effective in moderate to severe disease. Some patients' conditions can be managed via long-term acetaminophen therapy with short-term use of NSAIDs for flareups. Because of the decreased risk of GI toxicity, COX-2 inhibitors are useful for long-term management of OA in elderly patients.

Intraarticular injection of steroids can be provided on a limited basis. Topical creams such as capsaicin can also help with the pain. Surgical measures such as hip or knee replacement may be necessary in joints that are seriously affected.

Pharmacologic Treatment for Rheumatoid Arthritis

NSAIDs are frequently prescribed in RA and other rheumatologic diseases. See Chapter 35.

Nonpharmacologic Treatment for Acute Mild to Moderate Pain

Nonpharmacologic treatment includes rest, ice, compression, and elevation (RICE) for the first 24 to 48 hours, as indicated. These actions are the cornerstones of therapy.

Pharmacologic Treatment for Acute Mild to Moderate Pain

For minor problems, start the patient on NSAIDs immediately. In large muscle injury with the possibility of continued bleeding into the tissue, wait 24 hours because of the NSAID effect on platelets. Usually, short-acting products such as ibuprofen are used. These are given for a limited time, usually for 1 to 2 weeks.

In addition to these indications, NSAIDs are used for a large variety of minor musculoskeletal problems such as low back pain, bursitis, and tendinitis. NSAIDs also are frequently used for chronic pain. See Chapter 42 for more information.

Pharmacologic Treatment for Primary Dysmenorrhea

NSAIDs should be started 24 to 72 hours before the patient starts menstrual bleeding. The medication should be taken on a routine basis for 2 to 3 days. It is important that NSAIDs are not used during pregnancy.

Pharmacologic Treatment for Reduction of Cardiovascular Risk

Aspirin at the dosage of 325 mg taken every other day or 81-mg daily is effective in reducing the incidence of MI and stroke. An 81-mg enteric-coated aspirin is commonly used because of the decreased risk of GI toxicity. Concomitant use of an NSAID with aspirin has been shown to reduce the cardioprotective effects of aspirin.

How to Monitor

ALL DRUGS
- Adverse reactions, especially GI distress
- Monitoring of renal and hepatic function
- Subjective report of relief of pain

SALICYLATES
- Monitor for vertigo, tinnitus, or impaired hearing.
- Serum concentration can be measured.

NSAIDs
- *Short-term:* Acute minor pain should be relieved within 1 hour.
- *Long-term:* Get a baseline CBC and differential, creatinine, UA, K, and liver function tests. Check when product is started and then every 3 months until the patient is stable, then every 3 to 6 months.
- Follow patients weekly after initial prescription to determine pain relief and/or early side effects.
- Relief of pain such as in RA may take up to 2 weeks.
- GI bleeding can occur at any time during therapy. Assess for bleeding tendencies by monitoring CBC, PT, UA, and stool for occult bleeding.

Patient Variables

GERIATRICS. Elderly patients are more susceptible to the adverse effects, especially GI, CNS, and renal effects. NSAIDs can cause confusion, particularly in the elderly patient. Renal clearance may be decreased. Rarely observed increases in serum potassium can occur in the elderly, those with renal disease, and those on potassium-sparing diuretics. Use with antihypertensive agents requires monitoring for increasing hypertension (especially with diclofenac), edema, or other signs of CHF.

PEDIATRICS

A possible association has been noted between the development of Reye's syndrome and the use of salicylates as an antipyretic in children and teenagers who have varicella or an influenzavirus infection. Dehydrated children have increased susceptibility to salicylate toxicity.

The use of NSAIDs in the pediatric population is not common, except in children with a diagnosis of juvenile arthritis. Ibuprofen, naproxen, and indomethacin are available in liquid form. Naproxen may be useful because it does not have to be given as often as ibuprofen and is safer than indomethacin. The elixir or suspension dosage should be watched carefully because the drug concentration may vary. It is very easy to give a small child an overdose if the correct product and dosage are not given.

PREGNANCY AND LACTATION

- Use in pregnant women generally is not recommended; NSAIDs must be discontinued prior to the expected due date to prevent excess bleeding.
- *Category C:* Ibuprofen, naproxen, and celecoxib
- *Category D:* salicylates (aspirin); may be teratogenic or produce hemorrhage; avoid use during pregnancy, especially in the third trimester
- *Category D:* NSAIDs are not recommended in the third trimester or near the time of delivery.
- Salicylates and NSAIDs (e.g., naproxen, ibuprofen, COX-2 inhibitors) are excreted in breast milk.

Patient Education

ALL DRUGS

These drugs can cause serious GI bleeding. Report immediately signs of GI irritation, pain, emesis, diarrhea, or the presence of blood; stop taking the drug.

- Take with meals or with food or milk to avoid GI distress. A full glass of water is also recommended.
- May take with antacids
- Refrain from drinking alcohol.
- Take medication around the clock (e.g., every 6 hours, not just qid) for best serum concentration.
- Do not take more than one drug from these two classes of drugs concurrently.

SALICYLATES

- Discard aspirin if tablets exude a strong vinegar-like odor.
- If necessary or per doctor instructions, stop taking aspirin 5 to 10 days before surgery (depends on procedure and surgeon preference) to avoid any problem with platelets.

NSAIDs

- Patients should notify health care provider if they become aware of shortness of breath (SOB), wheezing, dizziness, GI distress, pruritus, or skin rash.
- If necessary or per doctor instructions, stop taking NSAIDs 3 days before surgery (depends on procedure and surgeon preference) to avoid any problem with platelets.

SPECIFIC DRUGS
SALICYLATES

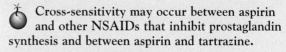

aspirin

CONTRAINDICATIONS. Suspected hypersensitivity to salicylates or NSAIDs because anaphylaxis is not uncommon. Hypersensitivity may be exhibited by acute bronchospasm, generalized urticaria and angioedema, severe rhinitis, and shock within 3 hours of ingestion. Foods that contain salicylates may contribute to a reaction. These include curry powder, paprika, licorice, Benedictine liqueur, prunes, raisins, tea, and gherkins.

Cross-sensitivity may occur between aspirin and other NSAIDs that inhibit prostaglandin synthesis and between aspirin and tartrazine.

- Pregnancy (third trimester)
- Hemophilia, bleeding ulcers, and hemorrhagic states

Use of salicylates in children (<16 years old) with influenza or chickenpox may be associated with Reye's syndrome. Reye's syndrome presents with vomiting, lethargy, and belligerence and progresses to delirium and coma. Reye's syndrome is rare, but the mortality rate is 20% to 30%.

- Asthma; rhinitis; nasal polyps (aspirin hypersensitivity is more prevalent)
- Tinnitus, dizziness, or impaired hearing probably represents high blood salicylic acid levels and can be helpful in dosage titration. Temporary hearing loss disappears gradually when the drug is discontinued.

WARNINGS/PRECAUTIONS

- *Chronic renal insufficiency:* ASA can impair renal function.
- *Hepatic function impairment, hypothrombinemia, and vitamin K deficiencies:* ASA may cause hepatotoxicity and bleeding.
- Gastric ulcer, peptic ulcer, mild diabetes, gout, erosive gastritis, or bleeding tendencies may occur because of GI irritation and bleeding.
- Severe anemia, history of coagulation defects, or use of anticoagulants because aspirin interferes with hemostasis

Aspirin 🔑 —cont'd

- Salicylates are included with many other combination medication products. Patients taking long-term therapy should be careful not to overdose with other nonprescription analgesics.
- Controlled-release aspirin has a long onset of action and is not recommended for fever or short-term pain control or for children younger than 12 years of age. It is also contraindicated in children with fever and dehydration.

PHARMACOKINETICS. Rapid and complete absorption of aspirin occurs after oral administration (Table 34-3). The bioavailability of aspirin depends on the dosage formulation, particle size, presence of food, gastric emptying time, gastric pH, and antacids or buffering agents in the stomach. Food slows the absorption of salicylates. Bioavailability of enteric-coated products may be erratic. Absorption from rectal suppositories is slow with lower salicylate levels. hey are partially hydrolyzed to salicylic acid during absorption. Salicylic acid is distributed to all body tissues and fluids, including the CNS.

ADVERSE EFFECTS. See Table 34-4.

DRUG INTERACTIONS. See Table 34-5.

OVERDOSAGE. An overdosage of salicylates is life threatening and requires intensive supportive treatment in a hospital. Initial symptoms include respiratory alkalosis with hyperpnea and tachypnea, nausea, vomiting, hypokalemia, tinnitus, headache, dizziness, confusion, dehydration, hyperthermia, hyperactivity, and hematologic abnormalities, progressing to coma and respiratory collapse.

DOSAGE AND ADMINISTRATION. See Table 34-6.

TABLE 34-3 Pharmacokinetics of Aspirin and NSAIDs

Drug	Drug Availability, After First Pass	Time to Peak Concentration	Half-life	Protein Bound	Metabolism	Excretion
aspirin	50%-75%	1-2 hr	15-20 min	76%-90%	Liver via conjugation	Renal, depends on urinary pH
ibuprofen	80%	1-2 hr	1.8-2 hr	99%	Liver via oxidation	45%-79%, renal
fenoprofen	—	1-2 hr	2-3 hr	99%	Liver	90%
flurbiprofen	—	1.5 hr	5.7 hr	99%	Liver via 2C9	70%
ketoprofen	90%	0.5-2 hr; 6-7 hr for ER	2-4 hr; 3-8 hr ER	99%	Liver via glucuronidation	80%
naproxen	95%	1 hr	12-17 hr	99%	Liver	95%
oxaprozin	95%	2-4 hr	42-50 hr	99%	Liver via oxidation and glucuronidation	65%; fecal, 35%
indomethacin	98%	2 hr	4.5 hr	90%	Liver; significant enterohepatic recirculation	60%; fecal, 33%
etodolac	80%	1.5 hr; 5-7 hr ER	5-8 hr; 12 hr ER	99%	Liver	72%; fecal, 16%
sulindac	90%	2-4 hr	7.8 hr	93%	Liver, extensive	50%; fecal, 25%
diclofenac	50%-60%	2 hr	2 hr	99%	Liver, several metabolites	65%; fecal, 35%
ketorolac	100%	2-3 hr	2-8 hr	99%	2C9	61%
tolmetin	—	0.5-1 hr	2-7 hr	—	Liver, conjugation or oxidation	100%
nabumetone	80%	4-12 hr	22.5 hr	99%	2C9	80%; fecal, 9%
meclofenamate	100%	0.5-2 hr	1.3 hr	99%	Liver	70%; fecal, 30%
mefenamic acid	—	2-4 hr	2 hr	90%	2C9	52%; fecal, 20%
piroxicam	—	3-5 hr	50 hr	99%	2C9	≈ 60%; fecal, ≈ 30%
meloxicam	89%	5-10 hr	15-20 hr	99%	Liver via 2C9 and 3A4 (minor)	50%; fecal, 50%
celecoxib	—	3 hr	11 hr	97%	2C9	27%; fecal, 57%

NSAIDs

ibuprofen (Motrin, etc.) 🔑

CONTRAINDICATIONS

- Hypersensitivity
- *NSAID:* potential of cross-sensitivity to other NSAIDs or salicylates. If patient has had asthma, rhinitis, urticaria, nasal polyps, angioedema, bronchospasm, or other symptoms of allergic or anaphylactoid reactions, he or she should never receive another NSAID.
- *Ketorolac:* contraindicated in patients with previously documented peptic ulcer and GI bleeding
- *Indomethacin:* Do not give to patients with active GI lesions or a history of recurrent GI lesions unless the high risk is warranted and patients can be monitored closely.
- Pregnancy (third trimester)
- Congenital heart disease in which patency of the PDA is necessary for pulmonary or systemic blood flow
- Bleeding (especially with active intracranial hemorrhage or GI bleed)
- Thrombocytopenia; coagulation defects
- Proven or suspected necrotizing enterocolitis
- Significant renal dysfunction
- Perioperative pain management post–coronary artery bypass graft surgery

WARNINGS

- Black box warning
  - Cardiovascular—May increase risk of serious and potentially fatal cardiovascular thrombotic events, MI, and stroke; risk may increase with duration of use; possible increased risk with cardiovascular disease or cardiovascular disease risk factors
  - GI—Increased risk of serious GI adverse events, including bleeding, ulceration, and stomach or intestinal perforation, which can be fatal; may occur at any time during use and without warning symptoms; elderly patients at greater risk for serious GI events
- *GI effects:* Many minor upper GI problems (e.g., dyspepsia) are common; these usually develop early in therapy.
- *CNS effects:* depression, drowsiness, headache, and dizziness, especially in the elderly
- *Renal function impairment:* NSAID metabolites are eliminated primarily by kidneys; use with caution in those with renal function impairment. Reduce dosage as recommended by drug manufacturer.
- Hepatic function impairment may occur.

PRECAUTIONS

💣 **A patient with a prior history of GI disease should exercise extreme caution. The risk for GI bleeding increases with age.**

- The risk of GI bleeding for a person between the ages of 25 and 49 is almost zero; this risk increases steeply from 60 to 69 years; from 70 to 80 years of age, the risk almost doubles.

- *Corticosteroids:* NSAIDs are not a substitute for corticosteroids. Do not discontinue corticosteroids abruptly. Corticosteroids should not be given concurrently with NSAIDs.
- NSAIDs reversibly inhibit platelet aggregation.
- *Cardiovascular effects:* May cause fluid retention and peripheral edema. Use caution in cases of compromised cardiac function or hypertension, in patients on long-term diuretic therapy, and in those with other conditions that predispose to fluid retention. Agents may be associated with significant deterioration of circulatory hemodynamics in severe heart failure and hyponatremia, presumably because of inhibition of prostaglandin-dependent compensatory mechanisms.
- *Ophthalmic effects:* Perform ophthalmologic studies in patients who develop eye complaints during therapy. Effects include blurred or diminished vision, scotomata, changes in color vision, corneal deposits, and retinal disturbances. Discontinue therapy if ocular changes are noted.
- *Infection:* NSAIDs may mask the signs of infection.
- *Renal effects:* Acute renal insufficiency, interstitial nephritis with hematuria, nephrotic syndrome, proteinuria, hyperkalemia, hyponatremia, renal papillary necrosis, and other renal medullary changes may occur. Administer with caution to dehydrated patients. Hyperkalemia is a potentially serious NSAID-induced renal electrolyte abnormality.
- *Hepatic effects:* Borderline LFT elevations may occur in about 15% of patients and may progress, remain essentially unchanged, or become transient with continued therapy. The alanine aminotransferase test is probably the most sensitive indicator of liver dysfunction.
- Alcoholics are at risk for adverse effects because of the toxic effects of alcohol on the gastric mucosa and liver. Patients commonly underreport their drinking, so all patients should be warned about the risks of bleeding and liver toxicity associated with concurrent use of alcohol and NSAIDs.
- Photosensitivity may occur.

PHARMACOKINETICS. See Table 34-3. Analgesic effect onset generally occurs after 30 to 60 minutes and lasts 4 to 6 hours. Antiinflammatory response onset may take 1 to 3 weeks. Indomethacin has a faster onset of antiinflammatory effect than do other NSAIDs.

ADVERSE EFFECTS. The most important adverse effects have been discussed in the Warnings and Precautions sections. These drugs have a large number of possible side effects. *Drug Facts,* a well-known drug compendium, lists 175 effects. The frequency of the various adverse reactions varies by drug. The most common effects are listed in Table 34-4.

DRUG INTERACTIONS. See Table 34-5.

DOSAGE AND ADMINISTRATION. See Table 34-6.

TABLE 34-4 Common and Serious Adverse Effects of Salicylate and NSAIDs (by Body System)

Body System	Common Side Effects	Serious Adverse Effects
Body, general	Headache, dizziness	—
Skin, appendages	Increased sweating, photosensitivity	Rash, pruritus
Hypersensitivity	Rash, pruritus, fever	Urticaria, Stevens-Johnson syndrome, toxic epidermal necrolysis, anaphylaxis, pulmonary infiltrates, asthma
Respiratory		Asthma, acute bronchospasm
Cardiovascular	Palpitations, tachycardia	Hypertension, MI, CHF, arrhythmia, PE
GI	Diarrhea, nausea, constipation, flatulence, dyspepsia	GI bleeding
Hemic and lymphatic	—	Blood dyscrasias
Nervous system	—	CVA, sedation, confusion
Special senses	Taste disturbances	Blurred vision
Hepatic	↑ LFTs	Hepatic failure, tinnitus, hearing loss, vertigo*
Genitourinary	↑ Creatinine	Fluid and electrolyte changes, sodium and water retention, hyperkalemia, acute renal failure

*Salicylates only.

TABLE 34-5 Drug Interactions of Salicylates and NSAIDs

Salicylate/NSAID	Action on Other Drugs
ASA	↑ Anticoagulants, heparin, carbonic anhydrase inhibitors, nitroglycerin, valproic acid, methotrexate, sulfonylureas, insulin
ASA	↓ NSAIDs, ACE inhibitors, β-blockers, loop diuretics, probenecid, sulfinpyrazone, spironolactone
NSAIDs	↑ Aminoglycosides, anticoagulants (especially celecoxib), cyclosporine, hydantoin, lithium, methotrexate, penicillamine, ASA
NSAIDs	↓ ACE inhibitors, β-blockers, loop diuretics, lithium
ibuprofen, indomethacin	↑ digoxin
indomethacin	↑ dapiprazole
indomethacin, naproxen, sulindac	↓ Thiazides
indomethacin, diclofenac	↓ Potassium-sparing diuretics
Other drugs	**Action on Salicylate/NSAID**
Oral anticoagulants, alcohol, ammonium chloride, ascorbic acid, methionine, carbonic anhydrase inhibitors, nizatidine	↑ ASA
Antacids, urinary alkalinizers, charcoal, corticosteroids	↓ ASA
cyclosporine, bisphosphonates, probenecid	↑ NSAIDs
cholestyramine, colestipol, sucralfate	↓ NSAIDs
diflunisal	↑ indomethacin
fluconazole	↑ celecoxib
cimetidine	↑↓ NSAIDs
ketoconazole	↑ ketorolac
phenobarbital	↓ fenoprofen
Salicylates	↓ NSAIDs, except ↑ ketorolac

TABLE 34-6   Dosage and Administration of Salicylates and NSAIDs

Medication	Formulation	Acute	Chronic	Administration	Maximum Dose
aspirin	Many	325-650 mg q4h	3.2-6 g/day	dd	500 mg q3h
ibuprofen	Liquid, tablet	200 mg q4-6h	300 mg	qid	3.2 g/day (inflammatory disease); 1.2 g/day (pain/fever/dysmenorrhea)
fenoprofen	Caplet	200 mg q4-6h	300-600 mg	tid-qid	3.2 g/day (inflammatory disease); 2.4 g/day (pain)
flurbiprofen	Tablet	100 mg q12h	200-300 mg/day	Two to four dd (no more than 100 mg per dose)	300 mg
ketoprofen	Caplet	25-50 mg q6-8h (12.5-25 mg q4-6h [OTC])		tid-qid	300 mg/day; 75 mg (OTC)
naproxen	Liquid, tablet, ER	500 mg q12h or 250 mg q6-8h			1500 mg/day
naproxen sodium		220 mg q8-12			660 mg/day
naproxen, delayed release		500 mg q12h			1000 mg/day
naproxen, controlled release		500-1000 mg once daily			1500 mg/day
oxaprozin	Tablet	—	600-1200 mg (OA); 1200 mg (RA)	Once daily	1800 mg
indomethacin	Liquid, tablet SR	75-150 mg/day 75 mg bid		In three or four dd One or two times per day	200 mg 150 mg
etodolac	Tablet	200-400 mg q6-8h	300 mg	bid-tid	1000 mg
sulindac	Tablet	200 mg bid	150 mg	bid	400 mg
diclofenac	Tablet	50 mg tid	100-150 mg/day	dd	150 mg
ketorolac	Tablet, injection	20 mg once, then 10 mg q4-6h	—	prn	40 mg/day, 5 days; intended as a continuation of IV/IM dosing only
tolmetin	Tablet	—	400 mg	tid	2000 mg
nabumetone	Tablet	—	1000 mg	One or two times per day	2000 mg
meclofenamate	Caplet	50-100 mg q4-6h	200-400 mg/day in three or four dd		400 mg
mefenamic acid	Caplet	500 mg, then 250 mg q6h	—		1000 mg
piroxicam	Caplet	—	10-20 mg	Once daily	20 mg
meloxicam	Tablet	—	7.5 mg	Once daily	15 mg
celecoxib	Caplet	400 mg, then 200 mg bid	200 mg	Once daily	400 mg

dd, Divided doses.

OTHER DRUGS IN CLASS

All drugs in this category have the same black box warnings as ibuprofen. Other drugs in this class are similar to the key drug except as follows:

- *ibuprofen* and *naproxen* are available as a liquid suspension and can be useful in pediatric arthritis.
- *fenoprofen* (Fenoprofen): Used for pain

- *flurbiprofen* (Ansaid): Used for acute pain associated with musculoskeletal injuries; relatively high risk of GI adverse reactions
- *ketoprofen* (Orudis): Used in osteoarthritis
- *naproxen*: Has longer half-life than ibuprofen. Can be used bid instead of qid ibuprofen; excellent for both musculoskeletal pain and arthritis

- *indomethacin* (see Chapter 36, Gout Medications): Very good with acute inflammation but with very high risk of adverse reaction. Avoid in the elderly.
- *etodolac* (Lodine): Lower risk of GI adverse reactions than most
- *sulindac* (Clinoril): Lower risk of renal adverse reactions; considered safer than other NSAIDs in patients with renal dysfunction
- *diclofenac* (Voltaren): Good for pain; relatively high risk of GI adverse reactions
- *ketorolac* (Toradol): Acute to severe pain only; increased adverse reactions. The FDA has a black box warning reminding patients and clinicians that it is appropriate only for short-term (5 day) treatment of moderately severe acute pain; contraindicated perioperatively; contraindicated in renal impairment; hypersensitivity symptoms range from bronchospasm to anaphylactic shock, in addition to GI black box warning; no cardiovascular black box warning for this product
- *tolmetin* (Tolectin): Was once a popular drug used in arthritis treatment; now used as alternative drug
- *nabumetone* (Relafen): Relatively low risk of GI and renal adverse reactions; commonly used for acute musculoskeletal injuries

- *meclofenamate* (Meclomen): High incidence of adverse reactions; used in patients with chronic arthritis who need alternative medications
- *mefenamic* (Ponstel): Increased adverse reactions
- *piroxicam* (Feldene): Long half-life with daily dosing, but high GI and renal adverse reactions. Infrequently used now. Avoid in elderly.
- *meloxicam* (Mobic): Very low risk of GI adverse reactions and increased COX-2, but not quite as low a risk of GI adverse reactions as the COX-2 inhibitors; higher doses (>15 mg daily) are not COX-2 selective
- *celecoxib* (Celebrex): The remaining COX-2 on the market with probably the fewest adverse reactions, especially GI and renal. May be used every day with chronic pain of arthritis. Cannot be used by people who are allergic to sulfonamides. Drug should be used cautiously in patients with heart disease because of risk for increased cardiovascular mortality in this group. Consider risk vs. benefit.

evolve A continually updated list of useful WebLinks may be found in the Evolve Resources at http://evolve.elsevier.com/Edmunds/NP/

35 Disease-Modifying Antirheumatic Medications and Immune Modulators

DRUG OVERVIEW

Class	Subclass	Generic Name	Trade Name
Conventional DMARDs	Antimalarials	hydroxychloroquine sulfate ✷	Plaquenil
	Sulfonamides	sulfasalazine	Azulfidine
	Antineoplastic	methotrexate sodium ✷	Rheumatrex, Folex
Immunomodulators	Cytokine blockers TNF-α inhibitor	adalimumab	Humira
		etanercept	Enbrel
	Cytokine blockers, IL-1 receptor antagonist	infliximab anakinra	Remicade Kineret
	T-cell modulators	abatacept leflunomide	Orencia Arava
Corticosteroids		prednisone ✷	See Chapter 50

✷ Top 200 drug.

INDICATIONS

See Table 35-1.

The drugs in this section generally are initiated by a rheumatologist. Patients on these medications are seen in the primary care setting. All patients with suspected rheumatoid arthritis (RA) should be referred to a specialist for evaluation and initiation of medication. Primary care providers should work with the specialist in monitoring the course of the disease and identifying possible adverse reactions. Therefore, this chapter emphasizes the principles of drug use and ways to monitor the effects of medications. Methotrexate is discussed in detail because it is by far the most commonly used disease-modifying antirheumatic drug (DMARD). It is also well tolerated and produces beneficial effects within 2 to 6 weeks.

Drug treatment for RA continues to evolve. The conventional DMARDs methotrexate, hydroxychloroquine, and sulfasalazine remain in common use. Previously, gold salts, penicillamine, and azathioprine were used, but their use now is indicated only if all other therapy has failed because of the toxicity of these drugs. The newer immunomodulators are becoming increasingly important in the treatment of RA. The field continues to change rapidly as agents with new mechanisms of action are being developed. Many agents are currently being investigated in clinical trials.

THERAPEUTIC OVERVIEW

Anatomy and Physiology

See Chapter 69, Immunizations and Biologicals, for discussion of the immune system.

Pathophysiology

The pathophysiology of RA is much the same as that of any autoimmune disease. For unknown reasons, the body fails to distinguish between self- and non–self-protein found in the body and proteins carried by foreign invaders. In all

TABLE 35-1 Important Characteristics of DMARDs

Drug	Indication	Formulation	Onset of Action	% Who Respond
hydroxychloroquine	SLE, RA, malaria	Tablets, take with food	2-4 mo	25-50
sulfasalazine	RA, ulcerative colitis, JRA	Tablets	2-3 mo	>30
methotrexate	Severe RA	Tablets, subQ qwk	1-2 mo, some relief in 3-6 wk	>70
adalimumab	RA, psoriasis with arthropathy, ankylosing spondylitis	40 mg subQ q2wk	2-4 wk	50-70
etanercept	RA, psoriasis with arthropathy, ankylosing spondylitis	25 mg twice a wk	1-2 wk generally, by 3 mo in almost all patients	50-70
infliximab	RA, ulcerative colitis, ankylosing spondylitis, psoriatic arthritis, Crohn's disease	3 mg/kg IV at 2 and 6 wk after the first infusion, then every 8 wk thereafter	2-4 wk	50-70
anakinra	RA	100 mg subQ daily	1-3 mo	38
abatacept	RA	IV infusion, given at 2 and 4 wk after first infusion, then every 4 wk	3 mo	50
leflunomide	RA	Loading dose of 100 mg/day for 3 days, then 20 mg po daily	2-3 mo	50

individuals, it is not uncommon for a T– or B–immune cell lymphocyte to react to a self-protein during its development in the thymus or bone marrow. Normally, these self-reactive immune cells are destroyed, but occasionally, they escape destruction. Years later, they are activated to trigger an immune response. Activation is thought to occur after infection with a common bacterium or virus that contains a protein with a stretch of amino acids that match a stretch of amino acids on the tissue protein. The organisms most commonly implicated in this activation include *Streptococcus*, *Mycoplasma*, and *Borrelia* (the agent of Lyme disease), although retroviruses also may be responsible.

In RA, the causative agents first gain access to the joint and cause an inflammatory response. This results in damage to small blood vessels and leads to the accumulation of inflammatory cells (macrophages and lymphocytes). Macrophages process the pathogenic material and transfer the antigen to lymphocytes. Among the lymphocytes, the B-cells produce antibodies, and the T-cells produce cytokines that activate B-cells and cytotoxins that attack tissues directly inside the joint capsule, causing synovitis. As the disease progresses, the inflammatory process spreads from the synovium into the cartilage and bone, with collagen-destroying enzymes causing destruction of the joint. These changes begin within the first 2 years of the disease, making early diagnosis and aggressive treatment very important.

Disease Process

The clinical presentation of RA is extremely variable, but it is chiefly characterized by disfigurement and inflammation of multiple peripheral joints. Articular signs and symptoms include symmetric joint swelling with stiffness, warmth, tenderness, and pain. Stiffness is usually worse in the morning. Duration of stiffness is a measure that can be used to evaluate disease activity. Although any joint may be affected, the joints most often affected are the proximal interphalangeal and metacarpophalangeal joints and the wrists, knees, ankles, and toes. Systemic symptoms include a prodrome of malaise, fatigue, fever, and weight loss.

Physical examination reveals acute inflammation of the joint, seen as tenderness and swelling. Heat and redness are not prominent features of RA, although an involved joint is often warmer on examination. Anemia, high-spiking fever, rash, and other extraarticular features occur in systemic onset juvenile arthritis. Later in the disease, the examination becomes specific for RA. X-rays of the wrists or feet are usually the earliest way to detect changes but are not diagnostic in the early phase of RA. The erythrocyte sedimentation rate is a very nonspecific but sensitive indication of inflammation. It is elevated in active disease and usually is monitored as an indicator of the effectiveness of therapy. RA factor (an immunoglobulin [Ig]M antibody) is positive in 75% to 85% of patients with RA. Antinuclear antibodies are elevated in approximately 20% of patients with RA.

Over time, the disease involves skin and blood vessels, lymph tissues, eyes, chest cavity, lungs, nerves, and blood. Patients with classic RA and the need for aggressive treatment have joint symptoms that persist beyond 2 years, positive rheumatoid factor, poor functional status, a large number of inflamed joints, and extraarticular manifestations of disease.

MECHANISM OF ACTION
Conventional DMARDs

DMARDs have antiinflammatory effects that may slow disease progression and preserve joint function. The exact mechanism of how they work in RA is unclear.

HYDROXYCHLOROQUINE. It has been suggested that hydroxychloroquine sulfate acts by mimicking the action of its parent compound, chloroquine. The antimalarials possess antiinflammatory properties, which possibly are seen as inhibiting the conversion of arachidonic acid to prostaglandin F_2. In vitro, these agents interfere with the chemotaxis of polymorphonuclear leukocytes, macrophages, and eosinophils.

SULFONAMIDES. The mechanism of action of sulfasalazine remains unknown. It has antiinflammatory action and reaches high concentrations in serous fluids in connective tissue.

METHOTREXATE. Methotrexate is used because it possesses both antiinflammatory and immunosuppressive properties. Evidence of clinical efficacy has been shown in numerous studies. This agent acts by inhibiting dihydrofolate reductase and 5-amino-imidazole-4-carboxamide ribonucleotide transferamylase, resulting in impaired DNA synthesis. Furthermore, it exhibits inhibitory effects on cytokines, especially interleukin-1, and may alter arachidonic acid metabolism. Methotrexate also exerts an antiproliferative effect on synovial cells.

Immunomodulators

Agents that regulate the extent and duration of the immune response are known as immunomodulators. Cytokines such as tissue necrosis factor (TNF) and interleukin (IL) are some of the many substances the body releases during the inflammatory response. Through genetic research, these agents have been cloned so that they can be produced outside the body and given to patients who are immunodeficient. Many are indicated for the treatment of RA. Some are indicated for multiple sclerosis.

CYTOKINE BLOCKERS. Cytokines are cellular messengers that initiate and perpetuate the inflammatory response by stimulating the production of cartilage-degrading enzymes and allowing pannus, an inflammatory exudate, to attach to cartilage and bone. The two cytokines targeted by the new immune modulators are TNF and IL-1.

The cytokine blockers–TNF inhibitors adalimumab, etanercept, and infliximab bind to TNF and inhibit its interaction with cell surface receptors. The cytokine blocker–IL-1, anakinra, blocks IL-1 by competitively inhibiting binding to the receptor. IL-1 mediates inflammatory responses and causes cartilage degradation. Abatacept is a T-cell modulator that inhibits T-cells by binding to CD80 and 86, thereby blocking interaction with CD28. Leflunomide blocks the synthesis of pyrimidine, which is required for proliferation of T-cells.

CORTICOSTEROIDS. Corticosteroids inhibit the production of interleukins. This inhibition decreases the immune response through diminished activity of T-cells. Corticosteroids also affect both the type and the number of leukocytes and monocytes in serum. The antiinflammatory effects of corticosteroids overlap with their immunosuppressive actions. They affect carbohydrate, protein, and lipid metabolism and increase hepatic gluconeogenesis. Detailed information regarding corticosteroids can be found in Chapter 50.

TREATMENT PRINCIPLES

Standardized Guidelines

- Simon LS et al: *Pain in osteoarthritis, rheumatoid arthritis and juvenile chronic arthritis*, ed 2, Glenview, IL, 2002, American Pain Society (APS) (179 pp; clinical practice guideline no. 2).

Evidence-Based Recommendations

The DMARD methotrexate is widely used as first-line treatment in individuals with RA because of consensus about its effectiveness in practice.

- Sulfasalazine and combined treatment with methotrexate and sulfasalazine are as effective as methotrexate in improving pain, joint swelling, and function in people with early rheumatoid arthritis who have not previously received DMARDs.
- Antimalarials may improve symptoms and function in DMARD-naive people, and are reasonably well tolerated, but radiologic evidence of erosion is more marked with antimalarials than with sulfasalazine.

A variety of DMARDs are available for second-line treatment of RA, and no clear evidence suggests that either is superior.

- Methotrexate, sulfasalazine, penicillamine, and leflunomide cause similar improvements in symptoms and function when given to individuals as second-line DMARD treatment, although methotrexate causes fewer adverse effects.
- The combination of methotrexate plus sulfasalazine plus hydroxychloroquine is more effective in reducing measures of disease activity in patients given second-line treatment than are any of the drugs used alone. Adding the cytokine inhibitors infliximab or etanercept to methotrexate is more effective than using methotrexate alone.
- Although antimalarials and oral gold seem to improve clinical disease activity when given as second-line treatment, they are not as effective as methotrexate or sulfasalazine. Parenteral gold is more effective than oral gold; however, it leads to higher levels of toxicity when compared with most of the other commonly used DMARDs.
- Cyclosporine offers short-term control of RA when used as second-line treatment, but it is associated with nephrotoxicity.

Cardinal Points of Treatment

- For the patient with active RA, DMARDs are the first choice of pharmacotherapy. For the individual who is receiving any of the five known DMARDs shown by radiograph to slow damage from disease progression (sulfasalazine, methotrexate, leflunomide, etanercept, and infliximab, as of this writing), acetaminophen may be used as concomitant medication for mild pain. However, because RA is an inflammatory disease, many more patients will benefit from concomitant therapy with an antiinflammatory medication.
- A COX-2 selective NSAID should be used as a concomitant medication for the person with moderate to severe pain with or without inflammation, unless clear risk factors for exacerbation of renal disease are present, or the medications are not tolerated because of GI complications.
- If the antiinflammatory medication and the DMARD provide inadequate pain relief, then acetaminophen should be added. (If GI risk factors are present, then a prophylactic proton pump inhibitor or misoprostol should be given along with the nonselective NSAID.) The patient at risk for a cardiovascular event should be given a regular low dose of aspirin (between 75 and 160 mg per day), whether treated with a nonselective or a COX-2 selective NSAID.
- Low-dose oral glucocorticosteroids (<15 mg per day of prednisone or equivalent as a single dose) should be considered for short-term use in patients with RA. These medications have been shown to decrease progression of erosion for the first 2 years. When oral glucocorticoids are used, prophylaxis with a bisphosphonate should be considered, along with calcium supplementation and daily

supplemental vitamin D to lower the risk of glucocorticoid-induced osteoporosis.

- Intra-articular glucocorticoids should be used in patients with intense flares of OA or RA as evidenced by high degrees of inflammation and effusion in the joint; they can be used at any time during the course of the illness.
- Opioids should be used for patients with OA or RA when other medications and nonpharmacologic interventions produce inadequate pain relief and the patient's quality of life is affected by the pain. Morphine, oxycodone, hydrocodone, or other mu agonist opioids, given as a single agent or combined with an NSAID or with acetaminophen, should be used for moderate to severe OA or RA pain that has not responded to other treatments. The use of codeine and propoxyphene should be avoided because of their side effects and limited analgesic effectiveness.
- DMARDs and immunomodulators generally are prescribed by a rheumatologist. Other health care providers are often involved in monitoring the response to medication and adverse reactions.

Nonpharmacologic Treatment

Treatment for RA must include nonpharmacologic measures. These include patient education, addressing the emotional impact of RA, physical and occupational therapy, systemic rest, articular rest, exercise, use of heat and cold applications, assistive devices, splints, and weight loss if overweight.

Pharmacologic Treatment

Analgesic and antiinflammatory medications are important in arthritis pain management but should be used concurrently with nutritional, physical, educational, and cognitive-behavioral interventions. Clinicians should consider efficacy, adverse side effects, dosing frequency, patient preference, and costs when selecting medication for pain management.

Of several monotherapies with DMARDs for adults with RA, research suggests no regimen is clearly superior. Combination therapies improve response rates in some patients who were previously taking monotherapy.

As a diverse group of drugs, DMARDs have in common slowing the disease process in RA. On the negative side, DMARDs produce a high incidence of adverse effects and drug interactions, some of which can lead to death.

The importance of early, aggressive disease-modifying treatment in improving outcomes has been well established. DMARDs are used as first-line treatment as soon as the disease is diagnosed, to prevent joint destruction and deformity. Methotrexate and leflunomide are considered first-line choices in patients with more aggressive rheumatic disease (synovitis plus extraarticular manifestations). If the disease is mild, NSAIDs at full therapeutic doses are recommended for 2 to 3 months. Hydroxychloroquine and sulfasalazine are added if the disease does not remit after a trial of NSAIDs. They generally are chosen for their lower incidence of serious adverse effects when compared with the other DMARDs.

> ☼ Use hydroxychloroquine with caution in patients with renal/hepatic function impairment or history of alcohol use. It can cause irreversible retinal damage. Patients should wear sunglasses in bright sunlight because the eyes may become photosensitive.

The immunomodulators share common untoward effects. Serious infections, sepsis, and fatalities have been observed in treated patients, many of whom were receiving other immunosuppressive agents concomitantly. Rare cases of TB have been reported.

> ☼ All candidates for immunomodulator therapy should be assessed for TB risk; anti-TB therapy should be considered before initiation of the cytokine blocker in those deemed to be at risk. Patients with serious chronic infection and those who require live-virus vaccinations should not be given a cytokine blocker.

Combination therapy generally is used because it is more effective and provides a more sustained response. Immunomodulators often are used with methotrexate. Immunomodulators generally are not used in combination because of the increased rate of adverse effects. Overall, the response rate is about 50%. This means that half of patients with RA do not have a good response to any of these drugs. Treatment regimens for RA are evolving as newer drugs are introduced.

How to Monitor

- The rheumatologist or clinician specialist working in rheumatology who follows these patients should monitor the patient closely.
- Indicators of reduced disease activity include decreased ESR and C-reactive protein. ESR is used over time to monitor disease activity.
- Patients who are taking DMARDs should be monitored closely for adverse effects. The usual parameters that should be monitored include the following:
  - CBC with differential and platelets for blood dyscrasias, metabolic panel for hepatic and renal function, and urinalysis
  - *Hydroxychloroquine:* Periodic blood cell counts during prolonged therapy. Refer to ophthalmologist for baseline and every-3-month examination. Assess patient for muscle strength and knee and ankle reflexes.
  - *Sulfasalazine:* Perform CBC, including differential WBC, and LFTs before starting and at every second week during the first 3 months of therapy. During the second 3 months, perform the same tests once monthly and thereafter once every 3 months and as clinically indicated. Also perform urinalysis and an assessment of renal function periodically during treatment.
  - *Methotrexate:* CBC, albumin, creatinine, and LFT at baseline and then monthly for 6 months and every 1 to 2 months thereafter; baseline alkaline phosphatase, chest radiograph, and hepatitis B and C serology in high-risk patients
- The usual parameters that should be monitored for patients who are taking immunomodulators include the following:
  - Perform TB test before initiation of therapy.
  - Assess risk factors for infection.
  - Monitor for signs and symptoms of infection.
  - Monitor CBC and LFTs.

Patient Variables

Use with caution in patients with hepatic or renal insufficiency because the drug may accumulate and cause toxicity.

GERIATRICS. Geriatric patients are more susceptible than others to adverse effects. The frail elderly do not usually tolerate this very aggressive category of drugs. Use methotrexate with caution; decrease the dose because hepatic and renal functions are diminished in this population.

PEDIATRICS. Use extreme caution when administering these drugs to children. These agents have caused deaths.

PREGNANCY AND LACTATION
- *Category C:* hydroxychloroquine, lactation probably safe
- *Category B:* sulfasalazine, lactation safety unknown
- *Category X:* methotrexate: lactation unsafe
- *Category B:* TNF inhibitors, no studies have been performed in pregnant women; lactation unknown
- *Category B:* IL-1 receptor antagonist, lactation safety unknown
- T-cell modulators: safety unknown
- *Category C:* abatacept, lactation safety unknown
- *Category X:* leflunomide, lactation unsafe

Patient Education

Thorough patient education regarding potential adverse reactions and ways to monitor for them is important because these medications can cause death. See Table 35-2 for the adverse reactions that may occur with each particular drug.

SPECIFIC DRUGS

ANTINEOPLASTICS

methotrexate (MTX) sodium (Rheumatrex, Folex)

CONTRAINDICATIONS
- Hypersensitivity
- Nursing mothers
- Pregnancy

WARNINGS

> **Black box warning: Toxic effects, potentially serious, have been seen at all doses. Deaths have occurred.**

- Marked bone marrow depression may occur with resultant anemia, leukopenia, or thrombocytopenia.
- Coadministration of methotrexate with NSAIDs increases the risk of severe marrow suppression and GI toxicity.
- Close monitoring for toxicity is necessary. See the section "How to Monitor."
- *Liver:* Hepatotoxicity, fibrosis, and cirrhosis, usually after prolonged use. Acutely, liver enzyme elevations are frequent, are usually transient and asymptomatic, and do not appear predictive of subsequent hepatic disease.
- Methotrexate-induced lung disease is a potentially dangerous lesion that may occur acutely at any time.
- *Renal use:* Use methotrexate in patients with impaired renal function with extreme caution and at reduced dosages because renal dysfunction will prolong elimination.
- *GI:* Diarrhea and ulcerative stomatitis require interruption of therapy; hemorrhagic enteritis and death from intestinal perforation may occur.
- *Mutagenesis:* Causes embryotoxicity, abortion, and fetal defects, as well as impairment of fertility

PRECAUTIONS
- Use with extreme caution in the presence of active infection; usually contraindicated in patients with immunodeficiency syndromes
- *Neurologic:* A transient acute neurologic syndrome with behavioral abnormalities; focal sensorimotor signs and abnormal reflexes have been observed in patients treated with high dosages

TABLE 35-2   Adverse Effects of DMARDs and Immunomodulators

Drug	Adverse Reactions
hydroxychloroquine	Irreversible retinal damage, agranulocytosis, skin reaction, GI distress, muscular weakness, CNS toxicity (irritability, psychosis, dizziness, convulsions), alopecia
sulfasalazine	GI intolerance; death from hypersensitivity, agranulocytosis, aplastic anemia, or other dyscrasias; renal and liver damage; irreversible neuromuscular and CNS changes; fibrosing alveolitis; anorexia; headache; reversible oligospermia (33%); infection; bruising; bleeding; swelling
methotrexate	Hepatotoxicity, lung disease, bone marrow depression, GI distress, thrombocytopenia, hypertension, rash/pruritus, diarrhea, alopecia, dizziness, headache, infection, fetal death
adalimumab	Serious infection, TB; neurologic events (MS, confusion), malignancies, arrhythmias, heart failure, respiratory infection, nausea, abdominal pain, headache, injection site reaction
etanercept	Infection (38%), injection site reaction (37%), malignancies, headache (17%), CNS demyelinating disorders, lymphadenopathy, hypersensitivity, heart failure, myocardial ischemia, stroke, paresthesias, GI distress, interstitial lung disease
infliximab	Serious infection, TB; malignancies, demyelinating syndromes, respiratory infection, acute infusion reaction, heart failure, hepatotoxicity
anakinra	Infection (35%), neutropenia, hypersensitivity, injection site reaction (28%), headache, nausea, dizziness
abatacept	Infection, malignancies, headache, respiratory infection, nausea, cough, dizziness
leflunomide	Hypersensitivity, hepatotoxicity, renal function impairment, carcinogenesis, diarrhea, hypertension (10%), headache, alopecia (10%), GI distress, rash, hypertension, infection, and many more

PHARMACOKINETICS. Effects may be seen in 3 to 6 weeks.

ADVERSE EFFECTS. Hepatotoxicity, fibrosis, and cirrhosis have occurred after long-term therapy. Lung disease, marked bone marrow depression, unexpectedly severe bone marrow depression, diarrhea, ulcerative stomatitis, impaired renal function, severe skin reactions, and opportunistic infection also may occur; also, elevated LFTs, nausea/vomiting, and dizziness are possible.

DRUG INTERACTIONS

Methotrexate toxicity may occur when administered with protein-bound agents and with drugs that alter renal elimination, such as NSAIDs, sulfonamides (including trimethoprim/sulfamethoxazole), tetracycline, and chloramphenicol. Phenytoin and cyclosporine may interfere with the elimination of methotrexate and vice versa; thus, concomitant use of these two agents may lead to increased risk of toxicity.

Although concern has arisen that vitamins containing folic acid or its derivatives may decrease the response of methotrexate, concomitant therapy with folic acid may reduce methotrexate toxicity without compromising its therapeutic effect.

PATIENT EDUCATION

- The patient should report immediately to the health care provider signs and symptoms of infection, bleeding, shortness of breath, or dysuria.
- Alcohol should be avoided while the patient is on methotrexate.
- The patient should avoid prolonged exposure to sunlight.
- Methotrexate must be stored at room temperature.

DOSAGE AND ADMINISTRATION. Begin with single oral doses of 7.5 mg/wk or divided doses of 2.5 mg at 12-hour intervals for three doses given as a course once weekly. Optimal duration of therapy is unknown.

evolve A continually updated list of useful WebLinks may be found in the Evolve Resources at http://evolve.elsevier.com/Edmunds/NP/

36 Gout Medications

CHRISTY L. CROWTHER

DRUG OVERVIEW

Class	Generic Name	Trade Name
NSAIDs	indomethacin 	Indocin
	naproxen	Naprosyn
	sulindac	Clinoril
Colchicine	colchicine	Generic
Uricosuric agents	probenecid	Benemid
Xanthine oxidase inhibitors	allopurinol	Zyloprim
Combination product		ColBenemid

Top 200 drug. Drugs are listed in approximate order of use.

INDICATIONS

- Hyperuricemia
- Prophylaxis of gouty arthritis
- Acute gouty arthritis

Pharmacologic management of gout relies on the use of NSAIDs (see Chapter 34), colchicine, uricosuric agents (probenecid and sulfinpyrazone), and xanthine oxidase inhibitors (allopurinol) (Table 36-1).

THERAPEUTIC OVERVIEW

Pathophysiology

Gout is a term that is used to describe a collection of disorders caused by the deposition of monosodium urate crystals in body tissue. Gout can be classified as primary or secondary. Primary gout, which affects males 10 times more often than females, is caused by an inborn error of purine metabolism that results in the overproduction or underexcretion of uric acid. Secondary gout is associated with hyperuricemia that results from other diseases or drugs that interfere with uric acid secretion. Secondary gout arises from a multitude of causes, including endocrine disorders, lead poisoning, high-dose salicylates (more than 3 g/day), myeloproliferative disorders, and chronic renal disease.

The basic pathology of gout generally is classified into one of two categories: overproduction or underexcretion of uric acid. A 24-hour urine collection is used to differentiate overproducers from underexcreters of uric acid.

Disease Process

Four phases generally are recognized in the development of gout. The first is asymptomatic hyperuricemia, which, as the name implies, is not associated with any clinical symptoms. Evidence suggests that the higher an individual's serum uric acid level, the greater is the likelihood that acute gout will develop. Acute gouty arthritis, the next phase, typically presents as a sudden, exquisitely painful monoarthropathy. Although any synovial joint can be affected, the most common site for this painful manifestation is the metatarsophalangeal joint of the great toe. The third phase, the intercritical period, is the period between acute attacks. Most individuals who develop gout have a second episode of gout within 6 months to 2 years of the first attack. Untreated gout tends to result in more frequent, severe attacks of longer duration. However, some patients will never have a second attack. Finally, chronic tophaceous gout can occur. Tophi are sodium urate crystals that are deposited in the soft tissues and can occur in up to 50% of patients with gout. They tend to appear at any time from 2 or 3 years to 10 years after the onset of gout. The most common locations for tophi are synovium, prepatellar and olecranon bursae, the Achilles tendon, and the helix of the ear.

Hyperuricemia, defined as serum urate level >6 mg/dl in men and >7 mg/dl in women, is the strongest risk factor for development of gout. The higher the serum urate level, the greater is the incidence of acute gouty arthritis. Hyperuricemia alone, however, is not diagnostic. Studies involving acute gout attacks have found that uric acid levels have been low to normal in 12% to 43% of patients. Key risk factors for gout include hypertension, thiazide and loop diuretics, obesity, and alcoholism. These risk factors seem to be additive in terms of

TABLE 36-1 **Pharmacologic Management of Different Phases of Gout**

Preferred Class of Drugs	Goal of Therapy	Stage and Duration of Treatment
(1) Colchicine used as initial therapy (2) NSAIDs (3) Glucocorticoids (intraarticularly, orally, or parenterally as needed) (4) Intramuscular corticotropin	Reduce pain; reduce inflammation	*Acute Stage* usually requires treatment 1-2 wk
Colchicine NSAIDs	Prevention of further inflammatory episodes and pain	*Post-Acute Stage:* Drugs used to prevent rebound flare until serum urate <6 mg/dl, if urate-lowering therapy has been started
Uricosuric agents (probenecid) Uricostatic agents: xanthine oxidase inhibitors (e.g., allopurinol)	Prevent disease by reducing hyperuricemia to serum urate level <6 mg/dl	*Chronic Stage:* Usually requires lifelong treatment

Modified from Schlesinger N: Management of acute and chronic gouty arthritis: present state-of-the art, *Drugs;* 64(21):2399-2416, 2004; Morgan L: Colchicine in acute gout, *Aust Fam Physician* 37(3):103, 2008.

risk. Other risk factors for developing gout include age older than 60, family history, lead exposure (patients who consume "moonshine" whiskey have an even greater risk because moonshine tends to have a high lead content), and the use of other medications (e.g., low-dose aspirin [<2 g/day], cyclosporine, tacrolimus, ethambutol, pyrazinamide, nicotinic acid). Dietary intake of meat and seafood has been shown to significantly increase the risk that a gout attack will occur; consumption of dairy products is associated with the lowest risk of attacks. Excessive alcohol consumption, specifically, beer and spirits but not wine, is associated with increased risk of an attack. Conditions such as thyroid problems, kidney disease, anemia, hyperlipidemia, diabetes, vascular disease, trauma, surgery, and radiation treatment also may serve as triggers for gout.

Up to 90% of individuals with gout are underexcreters of uric acid. Normally, the kidneys turn over approximately 700 mg/dl of uric acid per day. Of that amount, about 10% is excreted. Normal serum uric acid in males ranges from 2 to 7 mg/dl; the normal range for females is 2 to 6 mg/dl. Any factor that interferes with the glomerular and renal tubular reabsorption of uric acid can result in elevated serum uric acid levels.

Overproduction of uric acid is much less common. It is often the result of another disease, frequently one associated with excessive rates of cell turnover. Hemolytic anemias, myeloproliferative and lymphoproliferative diseases, and psoriasis are examples of processes that may cause secondary gout resulting from overproduction of uric acid. Some inherited diseases and genetic abnormalities can cause primary gout through overexcretion of uric acid.

The most important differential diagnosis to be made in a patient with gout is the exclusion of a septic joint. Synovial fluid aspiration and examination helps confirm the diagnosis. Fluid is sent for WBC and differential, crystal analysis, and Gram stain with culture. Examination of joint fluid with the use of a polarized microscope will reveal the presence of crystals. The presence of birefringent crystals in the synovial fluid does not exclude the possibility of infection because gout and infection can coexist in a joint.

MECHANISM OF ACTION

Use the following three mechanisms in the treatment of gout (Figure 36-1):
1. Increase the excretion of uric acid (uricosurics).
2. Decrease the synthesis of uric acid (allopurinol).

3. Decrease or stop the inflammatory response (NSAIDs, colchicine).

NSAIDs inhibit prostaglandin synthesis, thereby reducing the intensity of inflammation and pain in injured tissue. See Chapter 34 for a detailed discussion of prostaglandin inhibition.

The exact mechanism of action of colchicine is unknown. Colchicine affects leukocyte function to reduce lactic acid production. This results in decreased deposition of uric acid and reduction of the inflammatory response. Colchicine has no effect on uric acid metabolism and is not an analgesic.

Uricosuric agents (probenecid and sulfinpyrazone) are tubular blocking agents. They decrease serum uric acid levels by increasing urinary excretion of uric acid caused by inhibition of tubular reabsorption of urate. During this process, high concentrations of uric acid develop in the proximal renal tubules. This may predispose the patient to the development of urinary stones. For this reason, increased fluid intake is necessary and alkalinization of the urine is desirable when uricosuric therapy is initiated. Probenecid also inhibits the tubular secretion of most penicillins and cephalosporins. This increases the effectiveness of antibiotics.

Allopurinol inhibits xanthine oxidase, the enzyme that converts xanthine to uric acid. This reduces uric acid production by altering the breakdown of purines to produce xanthines rather than urates. Xanthines are much more soluble than uric acid and therefore have a much greater renal clearance. Different from uricosuric agents, allopurinol does not promote uric acid secretion, so the level of uric acid in the renal tubules is not increased.

TREATMENT PRINCIPLES
Evidence-Based Recommendations

- *Treatment:* colchicine, corticosteroids, and NSAIDs have unknown effectiveness.
- *Prevention of recurrence:* allopurinol, colchicine, sulfinpyrazone

No firm evidence-based guidelines have been put forth regarding when in the course of gout it is most appropriate to start urate-lowering therapy. This is essentially up to the patient and the clinician.

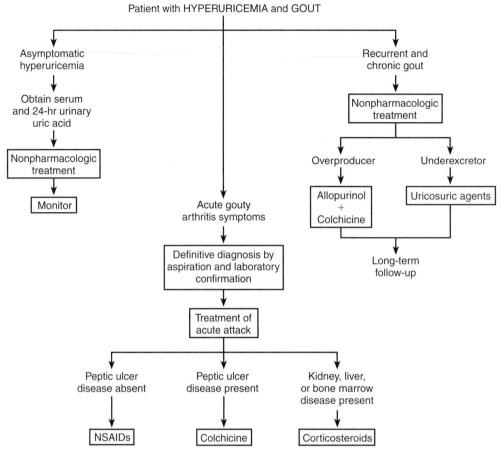

FIGURE 36-1   Suggested treatment algorithm for gout. (Modified from Gall EP: Hyperuricemia and gout. In Greene HL II, et al, editors: *Decision-making in medicine,* ed 4, St Louis, 2007, Mosby.)

Cardinal Points of Treatment

- Gout treatment should be individualized and guided by principles of pharmacology.
- Acute flares can be managed with antiinflammatory agents such as NSAIDs and glucocorticoids.
- *Prevention of acute attacks:* First line—colchicine; second line—uricosuric drug if underexcretor; allopurinol if overproducer
- Urate-lowering drugs are used for long-term treatment.
- Management of gout requires characterization and modification of risk factors and associated disorders.

ASYMPTOMATIC HYPERURICEMIA. Although the treatment of asymptomatic patients is somewhat controversial, a blood uric acid level greater than 7 mg/dl may warrant treatment if the patient has multiple other risk factors. However, most clinicians recommend that asymptomatic hyperuricemia *not* be treated.

Nonpharmacologic management of asymptomatic gout is generally attempted. Adequate fluid intake is necessary. Preventive measures include managed weight loss, primary prevention of hypertension, decreased alcohol consumption, and dietary modifications to reduce purine intake. A low-purine diet restricts the consumption of meat and prohibits alcohol, liver, kidney or sweetbreads, dried beans and peas, mushrooms, lentils, spinach, anchovies, sardines, and whole grain and bran breads and cereals.

ACUTE GOUTY ARTHRITIS. The goal of therapy is to decrease or stop the inflammatory response. Treatment of acute gout usually begins with NSAIDs; pharmacologic treatment of hyperuricemia must be started after the acute attack has subsided. Initiate treatment immediately, and put the patient on bed rest for the first 24 hours.

NSAIDs are the drugs of choice for reducing the inflammation and pain of acute gout. NSAIDs indicated for gout include indomethacin, naproxen, and sulindac, but all NSAIDs are somewhat effective. Indomethacin traditionally has been used most frequently; however, it is associated with a high risk of adverse effects, and the newer NSAIDs are considered equipotent. If the patient is at high risk for GI bleeding, a COX-2 inhibitor may be appropriate.

Colchicine is used for the acute attack, but it is no longer recommended as first-line treatment because of the nausea and vomiting that often occur prior to the relief of pain. Corticosteroids are very effective but should be reserved for patients who are unable to take NSAIDs or colchicine. Corticosteroids are given by intraarticular injection if the gout is monoarticular. Opioids are used to treat severe pain, if required.

PREVENTION OF RECURRENCE. The rationale that underlies therapy is that increasing the excretion of uric acid and/or decreasing the synthesis of uric acid reduces the frequency and severity of acute attacks and minimizes urate deposition in tissues—the cause of chronic tophaceous arthritis. The decision to treat during the intercritical period is based on the likelihood of additional attacks. Patients who are able to make significant lifestyle changes may not need medication. Patients at high risk for recurrence (e.g., on diuretics, elderly, with mild renal failure) probably need treatment.

Colchicine may be sufficient prophylaxis in patients with normal renal function. Because the primary mechanism of pain in an acute gout attack appears to be the inflammation that results when granulocytes phagocytize monosodium urate crystals, interference in this cycle will prevent an attack. It is also used as adjunct therapy, to prevent acute attacks when uricosuric and allopurinol therapies are started. Significantly fewer attacks (0.1 flares) were seen at 6 months in patients receiving colchicine 0.6 mg twice daily vs. those in the placebo group given 1.8 mg. If an acute gout attack occurs while the patient is on colchicine, the drug should be continued or increased and another agent (such as an NSAID) should be added. Colchicine has a fairly narrow therapeutic window and a high risk of adverse effects such as nausea, vomiting, diarrhea, and abdominal pain.

Reduction in serum uric level is accomplished with uricosurics or allopurinol. Uricosurics are used to prevent and treat tophi and, in combination with colchicine, help to prevent acute attacks. Probenecid should not be given within the first 2 to 3 weeks of an acute gout attack because it may intensify and prolong the inflammation. An increased frequency of attacks is fairly common during the first 6 to 12 months of probenecid therapy.

Allopurinol lowers uric acid levels in both underexcreters and overproducers. It is especially useful in overproducers, those with tophaceous gout, unresponsive patients, and patients with uric acid renal stones. Decreases in uric acid in both serum and urine are usually evident within 2 to 3 days after initiation of therapy. Allopurinol should not be started during the acute phase of gout because the drug has no antiinflammatory or analgesic action, and it may prolong the acute phase of gout. It should not be used for the treatment of asymptomatic hyperuricemia. As with probenecid, allopurinol has a tendency to increase the frequency of attacks during the first few months of therapy, so concurrent administration of colchicine is recommended. Allopurinol is very effective in shrinking and eliminating tophi. A serum level of uric acid below 5 mg/dl may be necessary. This can be accomplished through the addition of a uricosuric. Colchicine will not prevent the progression of tophaceous gouty arthritis.

How to Monitor

Perform baseline serum uric acid level, then monitor every 2 to 3 months. Normal serum uric acid levels in men range from 2 to 7 mg/dl. In women, normal serum uric acid levels range between 2 and 6 mg/dl.

NSAIDs
- Obtain baseline kidney and liver function tests, especially in the elderly.
- Short-term use (i.e., until the attack subsides) is recommended.
- Monitor for adverse reactions.
- GI disturbances may occur in up to 60% of patients taking NSAIDs. The incidence of GI side effects increases with age.

COLCHICINE
- *First-time administration of colchicine:* Patient should be monitored weekly for signs of toxicity. These include weakness, nausea, vomiting, diarrhea, and anorexia.
- Periodic liver function tests and blood counts (every 3 to 6 months) should be performed if the patient is on long-term therapy.
- Colchicine can cause reversible malabsorption of vitamin B_{12}; periodic monitoring of B_{12} levels may alert the clinician to the potential deficiency.

URICOSURIC AGENTS
- Obtain baseline CBC and serum levels and repeat every 2 to 3 months for those receiving allopurinol. Serum uric acid is the best test used to evaluate the efficacy of therapy.
- Renal function testing, especially BUN, creatinine, and creatinine clearance, should be monitored in patients with renal disease or any other disease that can affect renal function.
- Allopurinol hypersensitivity syndrome occasionally may develop and may be life threatening. It is apparently a dose-dependent hypersensitivity that presents with fever, eosinophilia, dermatitis, hepatic dysfunction, renal failure, and vasculitis and is associated with a mortality rate of approximately 20%.

Patient Variables

GERIATRICS

Elderly patients frequently have diminished renal function, and the risk of adverse renal effects is increased. Begin at the lowest recommended dosage. Monitor renal function.

- Colchicine adverse reactions have resulted in death. Gastrointestinal toxicity occurs in up to 80% of patients. Bone marrow suppression, blood dyscrasias, hepatic necrosis, and seizures are more common in the elderly.

PEDIATRICS
- Safety and efficacy not established for colchicine, sulfinpyrazone
- Probenecid is contraindicated in children younger than 2 years of age. It is used with penicillins and cephalosporins to prolong duration of action.
- Allopurinol should be used only in children with hyperuricemia related to malignancy or in those with certain rare inborn errors of purine metabolism.

PREGNANCY
- *Category B:* probenecid
- *Category C:* colchicine, allopurinol
- *Category C/D:* sulfinpyrazone

Patient Education

ALL GOUT THERAPIES
- Lack of patient education is probably the most important barrier to optimal management of gout. Education about the disease, triggering factors, lifestyle changes, and rationale of using various drugs may improve patients' adherence with treatment and treatment outcomes.
- Maintain adequate fluid intake.
- Take medication with food to prevent GI upset.

- Report any symptoms of GI distress.
- Lose weight slowly on an approved weight loss diet. Quick weight loss may bring on a gout attack.
- Stress the importance of medication compliance despite the absence of attacks.

NSAIDs
- Notify the health care provider if increased swelling or pain develops.
- NSAIDs can mask symptoms of infection.
- Dizziness may occur when some NSAIDs are initiated. Engaging in tasks that require mental alertness may be hazardous.

COLCHICINE. Notify the practitioner if skin rash, sore throat, fever, unusual bleeding, bruising, tiredness, weakness, numbness, or tingling occurs.

URICOSURIC AGENTS
- Avoid taking aspirin or other salicylates because these may cancel the efficacy of each drug.
- Increased fluid intake is necessary to prevent uric acid kidney stones. Patients should drink at least six to eight 8-oz glasses of water per day. Drinking 10 to 12 glasses of water daily helps to keep urine diluted.
- Notify the practitioner if a rash develops.

ALLOPURINOL
- It has been shown that almost half of patients who are taking allopurinol for gout do not take the dosage as prescribed. Patient education is essential if this statistic is to change.
- Notify the provider of skin rash, painful urination, blood in urine, irritation of the eyes, or swelling of the lips and mouth.
- Large doses of vitamin C may increase the possibility of kidney stone formation.
- Advise the patient that acute attacks of gout may occur during the early stages of allopurinol therapy.
- Allopurinol usually is better tolerated if taken with food or milk. Fluid intake sufficient to produce urine output of at least 2 L per day is necessary to prevent the formation of kidney stones.
- It may take 6 weeks for optimal benefit to be attained with the drug; until then, the patient must continue to take any other anti-gout medications used previously.

SPECIFIC DRUGS

COLCHICINE

colchicine (generic, ColBenemid)

CONTRAINDICATIONS. Serious GI, hepatic, renal, and cardiac disease; blood dyscrasias

WARNINGS/PRECAUTIONS

Nausea, vomiting, abdominal discomfort, and diarrhea are early signs of toxicity. Colchicine should be discontinued if these signs appear, and the drug should not be reinstituted until the symptoms subside (usually within 24 to 48 hours). Death has occurred with ingestion of as little as 7 mg of colchicine, although patients have survived larger doses. Bone marrow suppression can occur with prolonged administration.

- Reduce dosage or discontinue drug if weakness, anorexia, nausea, or vomiting occurs.
- Long-term colchicine therapy has been linked to chromosomal aberrations in some patients.

PHARMACOKINETICS. See Table 36-2.

ADVERSE EFFECTS. See Table 36-3. GI disturbances are the most common manifestations.

DRUG INTERACTIONS. The effects of CNS depressants and sympathomimetic agents may be enhanced by colchicine. Colchicine may interfere with vitamin B_{12} absorption. Increased colchicine toxicity is seen with concurrent use of clarithromycin, erythromycin, and grapefruit juice. Cyclosporine levels are increased and possible toxicity is seen with the use of colchicine. Interferon α-2a efficacy is decreased with concurrent use of colchicine.

DOSAGE AND ADMINISTRATION. Initially, dosage is 0.6 to 1.2 mg followed by 0.6 mg every 1 to 2 hours until the pain is relieved or until GI symptoms occur. Pain usually is much improved within 12 hours and is gone within 24 to 48 hours. Do not repeat therapy in less than 72 hours. For long-term use, the usual dosage is 0.6 mg twice daily.

URICOSURIC AGENTS

probenecid (Benemid, ColBenemid)

Probenecid is frequently the uricosuric agent of choice because it seems to cause fewer GI and hematologic side effects than sulfinpyrazone; the latter is associated with fewer dermatologic and hypersensitivity reactions.

CONTRAINDICATIONS. Hypersensitivity to the product, blood dyscrasias, the presence of uric acid kidney stones, high-dose aspirin therapy, and children younger than 2 years of age

WARNINGS/PRECAUTIONS
- Probenecid may exacerbate or prolong acute gout; concurrent use of colchicine reduces this risk.

TABLE 36-2   Pharmacokinetics of Selected Drugs Used to Treat Gout

Drug	Time to Peak Concentration	Half-life	Duration of Action	Protein Bound	Metabolism	Excretion
colchicine	12-24 hr	4 hr	Not applicable	10%-30%	Liver	Feces primarily; kidney, 10%-20%
probenecid	3 hr	5-8 hr	8 hr	85%-95%	Liver	Kidneys, 75%-88%
allopurinol	1-2 wk	1-3 hr	24 hr	<1%	Liver	Kidney, 70%; feces, 20%

TABLE 36-3 Adverse Effects of Gout Medications

Drug	Common Side Effects	Serious Adverse Effects
NSAIDs (indomethacin, naproxen, sulindac)	More frequent: GI upset, sodium and water retention, dizziness	More frequent: gastric/duodenal ulcers, reversible acute renal failure, hepatotoxicity, renal papillary necrosis, bronchospasm
colchicine	More frequent: nausea, vomiting, diarrhea, abdominal pain	Less frequent: severe diarrhea, hemorrhagic gastroenteritis, hepatocellular damage, bone marrow depression, seizures
probenecid	More frequent: headache, anorexia, nausea, vomiting, precipitation of acute gout	Less frequent: hypersensitivity reactions, development of uric acid renal stones
sulfinpyrazone	More frequent: nausea, dyspepsia, GI pain and blood loss, aggravation of peptic ulcers	Less frequent: blood dyscrasias, development of renal acid stones
allopurinol	More frequent: pruritic maculopapular rash, nausea, vomiting, drowsiness	Less frequent: reversible clinical hepatotoxicity, transient elevations in liver function tests; rare but acute hypersensitivity reaction (fever, eosinophilia, dermatitis, hepatic dysfunction, renal failure, vasculitis), Stevens-Johnson syndrome, fever, chills, acute attacks of gout, granulocytosis, granulocytopenia

- Salicylates antagonize the uricosuric effect of probenecid and should not be used. Probenecid should be discontinued if hypersensitivity reactions occur.
- Alkalinization of urine may prevent formation of uric acid stones, hematuria, and costovertebral pain associated with probenecid therapy.
- This drug must be used with caution in patients with a history of peptic ulcer.
- The false diagnosis of glycosuria may be made on the basis of the presence of a reducing substance in the urine. False reports of elevated theophylline levels also have occurred.

PHARMACOKINETICS. See Table 36-2.

ADVERSE EFFECTS. See Table 36-3. Headache, dizziness, and precipitation of acute gouty arthritis are the most common reactions.

DRUG INTERACTIONS. Plasma concentration of β-lactam antibiotics is increased, thus raising the risk of antibiotic-related side effects. The action or effect of oral sulfonylureas may be enhanced, causing hypoglycemia. Plasma concentrations of indomethacin, acetaminophen, rifampin, naproxen, ketoprofen, methotrexate, meclofenamate, lorazepam, and other drugs may be increased. Sulindac can reduce the uricosuric effect of probenecid, but the clinical significance of this has not been determined. Zalcitabine (Hivid) toxicity (peripheral neuropathy, pancreatitis, lactic acidosis, hepatomegaly, hepatic failure) has been seen with probenecid administration.

DOSAGE AND ADMINISTRATION. Therapy should not begin until after the acute attack has subsided. If an acute attack of gout occurs during probenecid therapy, continue the drug and add therapeutic doses of colchicine or an NSAID.

- Initial dosing is 250 mg twice daily for 1 week, followed by 250 to 500 mg twice daily. A maximum dose of 2 g per day, in four divided doses, may be necessary for some patients. If the patient has not had any attacks in at least 6 months and has a normal serum uric acid level, the daily dosage can be decreased by 500 mg every 6 months.

XANTHINE OXIDASE INHIBITORS
allopurinol (Zyloprim)

CONTRAINDICATIONS. Prior severe reaction to allopurinol

WARNINGS/PRECAUTIONS

Allopurinol has caused hepatotoxicity. Hypersensitivity reactions, including Stevens-Johnson syndrome, have occurred. Skin rash is one of the earliest signs of allergic reaction.

- Patients with impaired renal function require a reduction in dosage and careful monitoring of renal parameters.
- Acute attacks of gout may occur during the early stages of therapy. Colchicine should be given concurrently for the first 3 to 6 months of allopurinol therapy to decrease this risk.
- Bone marrow depression has occurred from 6 weeks to 6 years after initiation of therapy.
- Risk of skin rash may be increased in patients receiving amoxicillin or ampicillin.

PHARMACOKINETICS. See Table 36-2.

ADVERSE EFFECTS. See Table 36-3.

DRUG INTERACTIONS. Potentiates oral anticoagulants, hypoglycemics, and theophylline. Uricosurics reduce the effect of allopurinol. Incidence of rash is increased with ampicillin and amoxicillin. Avoid urinary acidifiers; monitor renal function with thiazides. Mercaptopurine and azathioprine doses should be decreased to reduce risk of side effects.

Concomitant administration of thiazides may induce hypersensitivity reaction in patients with diminished renal function. Dosages of mercaptopurine and azathioprine must be decreased. Use of iron preparations results in increased hepatic iron concentration. Half-life of theophylline is increased.

DOSAGE AND ADMINISTRATION. Allopurinol dosage will vary according to the patient's serum uric acid level and symptoms of gout. Initial therapy should be given at 100 mg per day. The dosage can be increased by 100 mg per week until the patient's serum uric acid is below 6 mg/dl. The usual effective range for allopurinol is 100 to 800 mg daily.

The effective range for patients with mild gout is usually 200 to 300 mg per day. Doses of 400 to 600 mg per day are appropriate for patients with moderately severe tophaceous gout.

Doses up to 300 mg may be given as a single dose; amounts greater than 300 mg should be given in divided doses.

Normal serum urate levels generally are achieved in 1 to 3 weeks.

evolve A continually updated list of useful WebLinks may be found in the Evolve Resources at http://evolve.elsevier.com/ Edmunds/NP/

Osteoporosis Treatment

JAN DiSANTOSTEFANO

37

DRUG OVERVIEW

Class	Subclass	Generic Name	Trade Name
Bisphosphonates		alendronate sodium 🔑	Fosamax 🔑 ✹ Fosamax Plus D ✹
		risedronate	Actonel 🔑 ✹ Actonel Plus Calcium
		ibandronate sodium	Boniva ✹
		zoledronic acid	Reclast
Hormones		calcitonin	Miacalcin Nasal, ✹ Calcimar, Fortical, Osteocalcin
	Parathyroid hormone	teriparatide	Forteo
	Hormone replacement therapy	estrogen/progesterone	Menostar
Selective estrogen receptor modulators (SERMs)		raloxifene	Evista 🔑 ✹

✹ Top 200 drug; 🔑 key drug. Alendronate is a key drug because it was the first in its class and is still commonly used.

INDICATIONS

- Treatment and prevention of osteoporosis in postmenopausal women and osteopenia
- Treatment to increase bone mass in men with osteoporosis
- Treatment of glucocorticoid-induced osteoporosis in men and women
- Treatment of Paget's disease in men and women (teriparatide excluded)
- Treatment of bone pain of severe osteoporosis
  This chapter concentrates on the use of these medications for osteoporosis because this is the condition that is most commonly treated by the primary care provider.

THERAPEUTIC OVERVIEW

Anatomy and Physiology

The bony skeleton is made up of an outer shell of cortical dense bone that surrounds an internal honeycomb-like structure of trabecular bone. Bone is composed of a protein framework that hardens when the minerals calcium and phosphorus are deposited on it. Without enough calcium, bones get weak.

Bone is constantly changing. This occurs in an ongoing cyclic pattern that allows both proper bone health and appropriate use of calcium in the bones for other body functions, such as maintaining normal heart rhythm. Bone remodeling is a process in which old bone is removed and new bone is laid down. The two stages of bone remodeling are resorption and formation. The first stage of remodeling is bone breakdown or resorption, when old bone is removed. The osteoclasts scoop away the bone over a period of about 2 weeks and are replaced by osteoblasts. The calcium in the broken-down bone tissue circulates throughout the body and is used for other key functions. The second stage, bone formation, follows when new bone fills in the spaces from which the old bone was removed. When the bone has been completely replaced, bone strength is maintained.

Pathophysiology

In osteoporosis, too much bone is removed, too little bone is formed, or a combination of both occurs. This leads to a loss in bone amount and strength. During childhood and through early adulthood, new bone is added to the skeleton faster than old bone is removed. As a result, bones become stronger, larger, and denser. Peak bone mass, the maximum amount of bone that a person can have, is reached at between 20 and 30 years of age. After age 30, bone is removed faster than it forms. Osteoporosis also may be linked to long-term glucocorticoid use, including use of inhaled steroids for treatment of chronic obstructive lung disease. Table 37-1 lists risk factors associated with osteoporosis.

Disease Process

Osteoporosis now is widely recognized as a progressive systemic disease, characterized by low bone density (osteopenia) and microarchitectural deterioration of bone that predisposes patients to increased bone fragility and fracture. Because of decreased bone mass, fragility fractures result from trauma that would not cause normal bone to fracture. Osteoporosis of the spine may lead to crowding of internal organs, spinal cord compression, GI disorders, or restrictive lung disease. Increased mortality and morbidity are associated with limited physical activity, back pain, skeletal deformity, height loss, and kyphosis. Osteoporosis of the spine is associated with significant morbidity, reduced quality of life, and soaring medical costs.

Women are more susceptible to osteoporosis because their peak bone mass tends to be 10% to 30% less than that of males. The prevalence of osteoporosis in men increases after age 80. Men have a shorter life span than women, so they account for only 21% of hip fractures. By the age of 90, only 17% of men have had a hip fracture, compared with 32% of women.

Assessment

Bone loss does not show up on conventional radiographic films until one fourth or more of the bone's mineral content is gone. The most commonly used technique is central dual energy x-ray absorptiometry (DXA), which measures the spine, hip, or total body. It is the most sensitive test and provides the most precise T-scores. Peripheral dual energy x-ray absorptiometry (pDXA) measures the wrist, heel, or finger. Quantitative computed tomography (QCT) measures the spine, hip, or total body. Ultrasonometry uses sound waves to measure density at the heel, shinbone, and kneecap. This technique can be performed easily in the office setting but is currently less sensitive than DXA.

Bone density testing is indicated for women and men with an increased risk for osteoporosis. If a woman is at least 5 years postmenopausal or has several risk factors, she should be strongly encouraged to have bone density testing and should be placed on therapy if the testing is indicative of osteoporosis or osteopenia. Box 37-1 lists indications for bone mineral density (BMD) testing.

A T-score represents the number of SDs above or below the mean BMD for the young, healthy female population (women who are younger than 35 years of age). A T-score of -1 signifies a 10% to 12% loss of bone mass, compared with mean values for young normal adults. According to recommendations of the WHO Task Force for Osteoporosis, osteoporosis is defined as a T-score ≤ -2.5 in women without a history of fragility fractures (Table 37-2). Treatment generally is indicated if the patient is two or more standard deviations below the normal premenopausal level.

In addition, researchers recently have developed a mathematical formula for predicting women's risk of osteoporotic fracture. A woman's risk for bone fracture, known as her "FRISK (fracture risk) score," is obtained by using her BMD at the spine and femoral neck, the number of previous fractures sustained, her body weight, and a falls score derived from the number of falls in the past year. On a scale of 0 to 10, a FRISK score of 5.4 or higher is associated with an expectation of fracture. For every one unit increase in a patient's FRISK score, the odds of having a fracture increase by 1.75. In initial trials, the formula has been shown to be as

TABLE 37-1   Risk Factors Associated With Osteoporosis

Potentially Modifiable	Nonmodifiable
Current cigarette smoking Diet low in calcium/vitamin D Use of glucocorticoids, anticonvulsants for ≥3 months Thyroid replacement therapy Alcohol intake >2 per day Sedentary lifestyle Body weight <127 lb or BMI <21 Lack of estrogen Environmental risks (loose rugs, dark stairs, etc.) Poor eyesight (increased risk of falls) History of organ transplant	Personal history of fracture as an adult (other than skull, facial bone, ankle, finger, and toe) First-degree relative with fracture (especially hip fracture) Race (white or Asian) Older age Poor health Dementia Hormonal disorders—gonadal insufficiency Early menopause (45 years either natural or surgical) Neoplastic disorders—lymphoma, leukemia, multiple myeloma Metabolic abnormalities—primary hyperparathyroidism, type 1 diabetes mellitus Connective tissue disorders—rheumatoid arthritis Genetic disorders—thalassemia, hemochromatosis, osteogenesis imperfecta

BOX 37-1   Indications for Measuring Bone Mineral Density

- Postmenopausal women who are 2 years postmenopausal and have two or more risk factors
- Postmenopausal women who are 5 years postmenopausal and have no other risk factors
- Patients with osteopenia on plain radiographs
- Patients being treated for osteoporosis to monitor changes in bone mass
- Patients receiving long-term glucocorticoid therapy
- Patients with hyperparathyroidism or another disease associated with high risk of osteoporosis
- Men with hypogonadism
- Patients with gastrointestinal disease such as malabsorption and hemigastrectomy (10 years after surgery)
- Patients with prolonged immobilization
- Patients with rheumatoid arthritis or ankylosing spondylitis
- Those being treated with methotrexate
- Patients with prolonged use of thyroid replacement
- Those who have used anticonvulsants for 5 years or longer
- Those who sustained previous fracture in adult years with minimal trauma or with classic fracture sites for osteoporosis (vertebra, wrist, hip, pelvis)
- Patients with lifelong low calcium intake

TABLE 37-2   WHO Criteria for Diagnosis of Osteoporosis

T-Score*	Classification
≥ −1	Normal
≤ −1 to −2.5	Osteopenia
≤ −2.5	Osteoporosis
≤ −2.5 fracture	Severe osteoporosis

*T-score indicates the number of standard deviations below the average peak bone mass in young adults.

much as 75% accurate in predicting fracture in women with osteoporosis.

MECHANISM OF ACTION
Bisphosphonates

Bisphosphonates are nonhormonal agents that have an extremely high affinity for bone. Alendronate was the first of the newer bisphosphonates to be approved by the FDA for the treatment and prevention of osteoporosis. Risedronate is the second bisphosphonate to be approved for the treatment of osteoporosis. Ibandronate is the newest bisphosphonate and may be taken on a monthly basis. Bisphosphonates inhibit the activity of osteoclasts to normalize the rate of bone turnover. This results in an indirect increase in bone mineral density. The bisphosphonates are very specific to the skeleton; they reduce risk for both vertebral and nonvertebral fractures without demonstrating other benefits outside of the skeleton. One exception to this is ibandronate, which has not been shown to significantly reduce the incidence of hip fracture. These agents are incorporated into bone matrix but are not pharmacologically active thereafter. It is unknown whether the incorporated bisphosphonates, when released by resorption, could eventually interfere with bone remodeling.

A recent study of women who discontinued alendronate after 5 years showed a moderate decline in BMD and a gradual rise in biochemical markers but no higher fracture risk other than for clinical vertebral fractures compared with those who continued alendronate. These results suggest that for many women, discontinuation of alendronate for up to 5 years does not appear to significantly increase fracture risk. However, women at very high risk of clinical vertebral fracture may benefit by continuing treatment beyond 5 years.

SERMs

Another class of agents used in treating patients with osteoporosis is SERMs. Raloxifene and tamoxifen are both SERMs; however, raloxifene is the only one that is used for osteoporosis. Raloxifene was designed to exert an estrogenic effect in bone but not in reproductive tissue. It reduces resorption of bone and decreases overall bone turnover. Although raloxifene reduces the risk for developing vertebral fracture and increases hip and spine BMD, it has no significant effects on most nonvertebral fractures, including hip fracture. Raloxifene prevents endometrial thickening, reducing the risk of endometrial cancer, but does not relieve the vasomotor symptoms of menopause. It also may reduce the risk of cardiovascular effects by lowering low-density lipoprotein cholesterol. It seems to exert antiestrogenic effects on breast tissue, which theoretically might decrease the risk of breast cancer. Raloxifene does, however, increase the risk of venous thromboembolism, similar to traditional estrogen therapy.

Hormones

Calcitonin is a naturally occurring hormone that is produced by C-cells in the thyroid gland. Although its mechanism of action in osteoporosis has not been fully delineated, calcitonin is known to block bone resorption through its potent inhibitory effects on osteoclasts. Calcitonin is a protein and therefore cannot be taken orally because it would be digested before it could work. Intranasal salmon calcitonin is 50- to 100-fold more potent than human calcitonin.

Calcitonin lowers serum calcium concentration primarily by direct inhibition of bone resorption. Osteoclasts are reduced in number and function, and osteocytic resorption is decreased. Calcitonin also has a direct effect on the kidneys. Through inhibition of tubular reabsorption, calcium, phosphate, and sodium are increased. However, urinary calcium is decreased rather than increased in some patients because calcitonin-induced inhibition of bone resorption has a greater effect on calcium excretion than does the drug's direct renal action. In the Prevent Reoccurrence Of Osteoporosis Fractures (PROOF) study, treatment with nasal calcitonin produced a 1.2% increase in spinal BMD, along with a 36% risk reduction for new vertebral fractures. Calcitonin also has an analgesic effect through mechanisms that may involve increased release of endorphins. It may therefore produce beneficial pain relief after a fracture.

Synthetic human PTH, teriparatide, was approved by the FDA in 2003 and is the first approved agent for the treatment of osteoporosis that stimulates new bone formation. Once-daily injections stimulate new bone formation on trabecular and cortical bone surfaces through preferential stimulation of osteoblastic activity over osteoclastic activity. This effect is manifested as an increase in skeletal mass and an increase in bone turnover markers. By increasing new bone formation, teriparatide improves bone mass and bone strength. PTH also acts on the kidneys by reducing renal clearance of calcium. Patients treated with PTH along with calcium and vitamin D supplementation have statistically significant increases in bone mineral density (10% to 20% after 1½ years) at the spine and hip when compared with patients taking only calcium and vitamin D.

TREATMENT PRINCIPLES
Standardized Guidelines

- Armstrong C: *Practice guidelines: NAMS updates recommendations on diagnosis and management of osteoporosis in postmenopausal women,* American Academy of Family Physicians, 74(9):2006. (Available at http://www.aafp.org/afp/20061101/practice.html#p1)

Evidence-Based Recommendations

A review of 90 randomized controlled trials evaluated the use of alendronate, etidronate, risedronate, raloxifene, or teriparatide to reduce the risk of osteoporotic fracture in postmenopausal women. All five medications were shown to reduce the risk of vertebral fracture in women with severe osteoporosis with adequate calcium intake. Alendronate and raloxifene also have been demonstrated to reduce the risk of vertebral fracture in women with adequate calcium or vitamin D intake who have osteoporosis without fracture. However, only risedronate and teriparatide have also been demonstrated to reduce the risk of nonvertebral fracture in women with severe osteoporosis and adequate calcium intake. Alendronate has been shown to do so in women with osteoporosis with or without fracture and with adequate calcium or vitamin D intake. However, none of these drugs has been demonstrated, by direct comparison, to be significantly more effective than each other, or than the other active interventions reviewed in the report.

Of the five interventions, only raloxifene appeared to reduce the risk of vertebral fracture in postmenopausal women unselected for low BMD. However, because the full data have not been made public, some uncertainty continues regarding this result. None of the five interventions has been shown to reduce the risk of nonvertebral fracture in women unselected for low BMD.

Cardinal Points of Treatment

- The primary goal of osteoporosis management is to reduce fracture risk via nonpharmacologic treatment. Even when medication is initiated, these nonpharmacologic steps must be continued.
- Bisphosphonates and raloxifene are useful in the prevention of osteoporosis.
- Bisphosphonates are first-line treatment and are chosen according to patient choice of dosing. Raloxifene is an alternative therapy for people who cannot tolerate bisphosphonates, for those who are physically unable to comply with special recommendations related to bisphosphonate therapy, for patients in whom bisphosphonates are contraindicated, and for those who do not show satisfactory improvement on bisphosphonates.
- Teriparatide is recommended as a treatment option for the secondary prevention of osteoporosis in patients who do not tolerate bisphosphonates, have an unsatisfactory response to bisphosphonates, have an extremely low BMD of -4 SD or a very low BMD of -3 SD and a history of more than one fracture, and have one or more age-independent risk factors (i.e., low BMI, prolonged immobility, maternal history of hip fracture before the age of 75, and/or untreated premature menopause).

Nonpharmacologic Treatment

- Counsel all women on the risks of osteoporosis and related fractures.
- Advise all patients to consume adequate amounts of calcium ($\geq$1200 mg per day, including supplements if necessary) and vitamin D (400 to 800 IU per day for individuals for risk of deficiency). Table 37-3 lists recommended daily requirements of calcium. Table 37-4 shows the calcium content of common foods.
- Recommend regular weight-bearing and muscle-strengthening exercises to reduce the risks of falls and fractures.
- Advise patients to avoid tobacco smoking and excessive alcohol intake.
- Recommend BMD testing (see Box 37-1).

TABLE 37-3 Recommended Daily Requirements for Calcium

Life Stage	Daily Requirement
Adolescent girls, aged 9-17 yr	1300 mg
Pregnancy, ≤18 yr of age	1300 mg
Pregnancy, 19-50 yr of age	1000-1200 mg
Lactation, ≤18 yr of age	1300 mg
Lactation, 19-50 yr of age	1000 mg
Men, 24-65 yr of age	1000 mg
Men, >65 yr of age	1500 mg
Premenopausal women	1000-1200 mg
Postmenopausal women on HRT	1000 mg
Postmenopausal women not on HRT	1500 mg

- Initiate therapy to reduce fracture risk in postmenopausal women with BMD T-scores by central dual DXA below -2 in the absence of risk factors and in women with T-scores below -1.5 if one or more risk factors are present.
- Consider postmenopausal women with vertebral or hip fractures as candidates for osteoporosis treatment.

Pharmacologic Treatment

The oral bisphosphonates alendronate, ibandronate, and risedronate all are effective for the prevention and treatment of osteoporosis. Side effects and costs are similar, although risedronate may be slightly less expensive. All must be taken on an empty stomach first thing in the morning, and the patient must remain upright and must not eat or drink anything for 30 to 60 minutes. Effectiveness is greatly decreased if these agents are not taken correctly. Low bioavailability, GI upset, and dyspepsia are frequent and may be significant enough to interfere with compliance. Some women are unable to take oral medications and will benefit from IV bisphosphonates. Weekly or monthly bisphosphonates allow for greater ease of dosing.

Raloxifene is as effective as the bisphosphonates in promoting bone density, and it has the added benefit of protecting patients against breast cancer. Side effects include hot flashes, leg cramps, and a threefold increase in relative risk of venous thromboembolism, with the greatest risk occurring during the first 4 months of use. Because immobilization increases the risk of venous thromboembolic events independent of therapy, raloxifene is not indicated for women who are not fully ambulatory, and it should be discontinued for women who undergo prolonged immobilization. It generally is regarded as a second-line treatment option.

Calcitonin is a less potent agent and therefore is reserved as an alternative for women who cannot or choose not to use one of the other therapies. The nasal spray is convenient (but expensive) and causes few side effects except for occasional nasal irritation, but it is not as effective as the bisphosphonates. Calcitonin is not recommended in osteoporotic women during the first 5 years after menopause because few data are available to support its efficacy during this period. It may have a place for use in immobile patients who are unable to sit up for the time required after taking a bisphosphonate.

TABLE 37-4   Calcium Content of Readily Available Foods

Food	Serving Size	Calcium, mg
Yogurt, unflavored	1 cup	415
Mackerel, canned	5 oz	400
Sardines, in oil	4 oz	400
Milk, skim, nonfat	1 cup	302
Milk, 1%, low-fat	1 cup	300
Collard greens, frozen, cooked	1 cup	300
Salmon, baked, broiled	6 oz	300
Milk, 2%, low-fat	1 cup	297
Milk, whole	1 cup	291
Cheese, Swiss	1 oz	272
Cheese, provolone	1 oz	214
Cheese, mozzarella (part skim)	1 oz	207
Frozen yogurt	1 cup	200
Dried figs	10	200
Macaroni and cheese (box mix)	1 cup	199
Ice cream, plain	1 cup	176
Ice milk	1 cup	176
Cheese, American	1 oz	174
Molasses, blackstrap	1 tsp	172
Cheese, mozzarella (whole milk)	1 oz	163
Cottage cheese, 2%	1 cup	155
Bok choy	1 cup	150
Instant oatmeal	1 packet	150
Rhubarb, cooked with sugar	½ cup	150
Cottage cheese, 1%	1 cup	138
Broccoli, cooked	1 cup	136
Cottage cheese, regular	1 cup	130
Almonds	1.5 oz	100
Soybeans, cooked	1 cup	100
Turnip greens, frozen, cooked	½ cup	100

PTH, given as a daily subcutaneous injection, is reserved for patients with severe osteoporosis who cannot tolerate or are unresponsive to other therapies. Patients who are at risk for osteosarcoma should not take teriparatide (see listings under Contraindications section). Safety and efficacy are not approved for use beyond 2 years of treatment.

Because the risk–benefit balance of hormone replacement therapy is generally unfavorable in older postmenopausal women, it is regarded as a second-line treatment option. However, it may be an appropriate option in younger postmenopausal women at high risk of fracture, particularly those with vasomotor symptoms.

How to Monitor

- Creatinine at baseline
- Monitor levels of serum calcium and phosphorus prior to treatment initiation and yearly thereafter.
- Central BMD should be measured by DXA to establish the diagnosis of osteoporosis prior to treatment initiation and every 2 years to monitor therapy.
- The rate of bone loss can be monitored with a urine test called NTx (N-telopeptide cross-links) prior to treatment initiation, 3 months later, and yearly or whenever therapy is changed. This test measures urine levels of a compound linked to bone breakdown, and samples should be collected at the second void of the day. Normal levels are less than 38 (values above normal indicate a faster rate of bone loss). If therapy is effective, then subsequent tests will show decreased levels. A reduction of 30% or more in NTx levels is considered a favorable response. A Clinical Laboratory Improvement Amendments (CLIA)-waived, point-of-care urine test for NTx (Osteomark) is available from Ostex International (Seattle, WA, USA). This rapid, disposable, noninvasive test yields results in 5 minutes and is convenient for use in offices.
- Periodic nasal examinations performed to observe crusts, dryness, erythema, and irritation are recommended for patients receiving calcitonin nasal spray.
- Patients should undergo routine dental monitoring while taking these drugs.

Patient Variables

GERIATRICS. No overall differences in efficacy or safety were observed between patients older than 65 and younger patients who were receiving any of these medications.

Calcitonin nasal spray: Compared with patients younger than 65 years of age, the incidence of nasal adverse events (rhinitis, irritation, erythema, and excoriation) was higher in patients older than age 65, particularly in those over the age of 75.

PEDIATRICS. Safety and effectiveness of these medications in patients younger than the age of 18 have not been evaluated. Teriparatide should not be used in pediatric populations and in young adults with open epiphyses.

PREGNANCY AND LACTATION

- *Category C:* alendronate, risedronate, ibandronate, teriparatide, calcitonin
- *Category D:* zoledronic acid
- *Category X:* raloxifene, estradiol

Raloxifene, teriparatide, and transdermal estrogen are not indicated for premenopausal women. Raloxifene is contraindicated in women who are or may become pregnant. These agents are indicated only for postmenopausal women. Estrogen is known to decrease the quantity and quality of breast milk. It is not known whether alendronate, risedronate, ibandronate, raloxifene, and teriparatide are excreted in human breast milk. The impact of these drugs has not been studied in nursing women, so they are not recommended for nursing mothers.

Calcitonin has been shown to cause a decrease in fetal birth weight in animals. Calcitonin does not cross the placenta and is not indicated for use in pregnancy. Safety of use in lactation is unknown. Calcitonin is distributed in breast milk. In animal studies, it has been shown to inhibit lactation.

RACE. Pharmacokinetic differences due to race have not been studied. Osteoporosis is more common in whites and Asians than in members of other races. Darker-skinned races genetically are found to have denser bones.

GENDER

Bisphosphonates. Bioavailability and pharmacokinetics following oral administration are similar in men and women. Safety and effectiveness of bisphosphonates have been demonstrated in clinical studies in men being treated for glucocorticoid-induced osteoporosis and Paget's disease.

Raloxifene. No significant differences were noted between age-matched men and women with the use of raloxifene; however, safety and efficacy have not been evaluated in men.

Teriparatide. Absorption occurs at a rate that is approximately 20% to 30% lower in men than in women.

Estrogen. Indicated only for postmenopausal women

Patient Education

- Include adequate amounts of calcium (1000 to 1500 mg/day), vitamin D (400 international units), and general good nutrition in the diet (see Tables 37-3 and 37-4).
- Weight-bearing exercise, particularly walking, should be encouraged, along with modification of other risk factors for osteoporosis such as smoking and alcohol consumption.
- Alendronate and risedronate must be taken at least 30 minutes before and ibandronate must be taken 60 minutes before the first food, beverage, or medication is taken. To facilitate absorption, the bisphosphonates should be taken with a full glass (6 to 8 oz) of plain water, and the patient should avoid lying down for 30 to 60 minutes thereafter, to facilitate delivery to the stomach and reduce the potential for esophageal irritation.
- Raloxifene can be taken without regard for food intake.
- *Calcitonin nasal spray:* Advise patient on pump assembly, pump priming, and use of the pump. Any significant nasal irritation should be reported. Once the pump has been activated, the bottle may be maintained at room temperature for 2 weeks until the medication is finished. Explain the action of absorption through the mucosal membranes into the bloodstream to facilitate patient understanding of mechanisms of action and compliance with medication. Calcitonin can be taken without regard for food or beverage intake.
- Teriparatide is administered by subcutaneous injection with a prefilled delivery device; instructions should be given to inject once daily into the thigh or abdomen. This agent can be injected at any time of day. Teriparatide should be refrigerated at 36° F to 46° F both before and after use. It should not be frozen and should be discarded if it has been frozen. Do not use teriparatide that is discolored or cloudy, or that has particles in it. Do not use after the expiration date on the pen has passed. One pen provides 28 days of medication. No foods, beverages, or activities are restricted when teriparatide is taken. Data are not available on safety and efficacy after the drug is taken for longer than 2 years.

- The adhesive side of the Menostar estradiol transdermal system should be placed on a clean, dry area of the lower abdomen. Menostar should not be applied to or near the breasts. The sites of application must be rotated, with an interval of at least 1 week allowed between applications to a particular site. The area selected should not be oily, damaged, or irritated.

SPECIFIC DRUGS
BISPHOSPHONATES

alendronate (Fosamax), risedronate (Actonel), ibandronate (Boniva) 🔑

CONTRAINDICATIONS. Hypocalcemia, renal insufficiency, inability to stand or sit upright for 30 to 60 minutes, abnormalities of the esophagus that delay emptying such as stricture or achalasia

PRECAUTIONS
- Patients must have adequate nutrition, calcium, and vitamin D.
- Hypocalcemia and vitamin D deficiency must be corrected before therapy is initiated. Severe bone, joint, and or muscle pain has been reported in postmenopausal women.
- Osteonecrosis of the jaw with delayed healing has been reported in patients taking bisphosphonates; most cases have occurred in patients with cancer who are treated with IV bisphosphonates, but some have occurred in patients with postmenopausal osteoporosis.
- Renal insufficiency: not recommended for patients with renal insufficiency (CrCl <35 ml/min)

PHARMACOKINETICS. Bisphosphonates have an affinity for hydroxyapatite crystals in bone and act as antiresorptive agents. Their primary mechanism of action involves inhibition of osteoclastic bone resorption.

ADVERSE EFFECTS. Osteonecrosis, primarily in the jaw, is a rare dental condition in which bone in the lower jaw or, less commonly, the upper jaw becomes exposed, and the wound fails to heal within the typical time frame. This is more common in patients on IV bisphosphonates but has been reported in patients taking oral bisphosphonates. See Table 37-5.

DRUG AND FOOD INTERACTIONS. Recent research showed a 44% increase in risk of fracture among patients taking proton pump inhibitors for a year or longer, probably caused by decreased absorption of calcium from reduced stomach acid. A similar but smaller risk was found for patients on H₂-blockers. These are poorly absorbed from the GI tract so should not be taken with any food or drink other than water.

The incidence of adverse GI events is increased with concomitant use of aspirin or NSAIDs. Calcium-, aluminum-, and magnesium-containing medications may interfere with absorption and should not be administered within 2 hours of the dose.

OVERDOSAGE. Hypocalcemia, hypophosphatemia, and upper GI adverse events such as upset stomach, heartburn, esophagitis, gastritis, or ulcer may result from overdosage.

alendronate (Fosamax), risedronate (Actonel), ibandronate (Boniva) —cont'd

Death has occurred with significant overdosage of both alendronate and risedronate in rats.

DOSAGE AND ADMINISTRATION
alendronate (Fosamax)

- Osteoporosis (treatment): 10 mg po once daily or 70 mg once weekly. Fosamax also is available in a preparation to which vitamin D and calcium have been added. Information about vitamin D and calcium may be found in Chapter 72.
- Osteoporosis (prevention): 5 mg po once daily or 35 mg once weekly. Must be taken at least 30 minutes before the first food or drink of the day. Patient should be in upright position and should not lie down for 30 minutes after taking the medication. Should be taken with 8 oz plain water

risedronate (Actonel)

- Osteoporosis (prevention and treatment): 5 mg po once daily or 35 mg po once weekly. Must be taken at least 30 minutes before the first food or drink of the day. Patient should be in upright position and should not lie down for 30 minutes after taking medication. Should be taken with 8 oz plain water
- 35 mg of risedronate is taken once weekly on day 1, then 500 mg calcium is taken once daily with food on days 2 to 7 of each week.

ibandronate (Boniva)

- Osteoporosis (prevention and treatment): 2.5 mg po once daily or 150 mg once monthly. Must be taken at least 60 minutes before the first food or drink of the day. Patient should be in upright position and should not lie down for 30 minutes after taking medication. Should be taken with 8 oz plain water
- Dosage is 3 mg intravenously given every 3 months by the health care provider. 3 mg/3 ml IV bolus injection over 15 to 30 seconds, then 3 mg IV bolus every 3 months. If a dose is missed, give as soon as possible and resume 3 month cycle.

HORMONES

calcitonin (Miacalcin, Calcimar, Osteocalcin)

CONTRAINDICATIONS. Clinical allergy to calcitonin-salmon

PRECAUTIONS. Because calcitonin is a polypeptide, the possibility of a systemic allergic reaction exists. Skin testing should be considered prior to treatment for patients with suspected sensitivity.

PHARMACOKINETICS. See Table 37-6. Calcitonin is destroyed in the GI tract and therefore must be administered parenterally or intranasally. Calcitonin causes inhibition of osteoclast function with loss of the osteoblast border responsible for resorption of bone. It also has been shown to increase spinal bone mass in postmenopausal women with established osteoporosis but not in women in early postmenopause.

Calcitonin is not recommended in osteoporotic women during the first 5 years after menopause because few data are available to support its efficacy during this period

TABLE 37-5   Adverse Effects of Osteoporosis Drugs

Medication	Adverse Effects
alendronate, ibandronate, and risedronate	Abdominal or musculoskeletal pain, nausea, heartburn, irritation of the esophagus, and, rarely, osteonecrosis of jaw
raloxifene	Hot flashes, leg cramps, increased risk of venous thromboembolic events
teriparatide	Nausea, dizziness, cramps; injection site pain, swelling, bruising, erythema
calcitonin nasal spray	Intranasal: rhinitis, epistaxis, sinusitis, mucosal ulcerations
estrogen transdermal, low-dose	Breast cancer, endometrial hyperplasia, myocardial infarction, stroke, ovarian cancer, gallbladder disease, blood clots, dementia, breast pain, headache, irregular bleeding or spotting, abdominal cramping or bloating

ADVERSE EFFECTS. See Table 37-5.

DRUG INTERACTIONS. Formal studies designed to evaluate drug interactions have not been done. No drug interactions have been observed.

DOSAGE AND ADMINISTRATION. Osteoporosis: 200 units/once daily intranasally, alternating nostrils daily. Calcitonin also can be administered IM or subQ and is dosed 100 units every other day.

PARATHYROID HORMONE

teriparatide (Forteo)

CONTRAINDICATIONS. Hypersensitivity to teriparatide

PRECAUTIONS. Avoid use in the treatment of patients with increased risk of osteosarcoma, such as those with Paget's disease of the bone or unexplained high levels of alkaline phosphatase in the blood, patients from a pediatric or young adult population, and anyone who has ever been given a diagnosis of bone cancer or other cancers with metastasis to the bone, has had radiation therapy involving the bone, has a metabolic bone disease other than osteoporosis, or had preexisting hypercalcemia. Transient episodes of orthostatic hypotension have been observed infrequently, but these resolved spontaneously and did not preclude continued treatment. Use with caution in patients with active or recent urolithiasis to avoid exacerbation of the condition. Because of transient increases in serum calcium, use with caution in patients who are taking digitalis. Monitor for teriparatide-induced hypercalcemia.

PHARMACOKINETICS. PTH is the primary regulator of calcium and phosphate metabolism in bone and kidney. Physiologic actions include regulation of bone metabolism, renal tubular reabsorption of calcium and phosphate, and intestinal calcium absorption. Once-daily administration of PTH stimulates new bone formation via preferential stimulation of osteoblastic activity over osteoclastic activity.

ADVERSE EFFECTS. See Table 37-5. Usually mild and did not require discontinuation of therapy.

TABLE 37-6 Pharmacokinetics of Osteoporosis Drugs

Drug	Absorption	Time to Peak Concentration	Half-life	Metabolism	Excretion
alendronate	Oral bioavailability is 0.64% (women) and 0.59% (men). Food decreases bioavailability significantly.	Concentrations of drug in plasma following therapeutic oral doses are too low (<5 ng/ml) for analytical detection.	>10 years—accumulates in bone	Not metabolized	Urine: The portion that is not removed from circulation via absorption is eliminated unchanged by the kidney (approximately 50%-60% of absorbed dose). Unabsorbed alendronate is excreted unchanged in the feces.
calcitonin	Destroyed in GI tract; nasal, 31-39 minutes	Peak concentration plasma attained within first hour of administration	70-90 min	Primarily kidneys, some in blood and peripheral tissues	Urine: minimally unchanged
ibandronate	0.6%—decreased by 90% if taken with food	Concentrations of drug in plasma following therapeutic oral doses are too low (<5 ng/ml) for analytical detection.	37-157 hr (po) 4.6-25.5 hr (IV)	Not metabolized	The portion that is not removed from circulation via absorption is eliminated unchanged by the kidney (approximately 50%-60% of absorbed dose). Unabsorbed ibandronate is excreted unchanged in the feces.
estradiol transdermal patch	Continuously releases estradiol, which is transported across intact skin, leading to sustained circulating levels of 14 mcg/day			Cytochrome P450, although transdermal application avoids first pass of liver	Urine
raloxifene	2%		32.5 hr	Liver extensively	Feces primarily
risedronate	0.62%—food decreases bioavailability significantly	Concentrations of drug in plasma following therapeutic oral doses are too low (<5 ng/ml) for analytical detection.	480 hr	Not metabolized	The portion that is not removed from circulation via absorption is eliminated unchanged by the kidney (approximately 50%-60% of absorbed dose). Unabsorbed risedronate is excreted unchanged in the feces.
teriparatide	95%	30 min	5 min IV 1 hr subQ	Believed to occur by nonspecific enzymatic mechanisms in the liver	Renal

OVERDOSAGE. Not reported in clinical trials. However, no specific antidote is known. Treatment should include discontinuation of therapy, monitoring of serum calcium and phosphorus, and supportive measures such as hydration.

DOSAGE AND ADMINISTRATION

- Osteoporosis: 20 mcg subcutaneously once daily into the thigh or abdominal wall. Has not been evaluated beyond 2 years of treatment, so use of drug is not recommended beyond 2 years. Administer initially under circumstances where the patient can sit or lie down if symptoms of orthostatic hypotension occur. Forteo should be stored under refrigeration (36° F to 46° F) at all times. It should not be used if it has been frozen.

SERMS

raloxifene hydrochloride (Evista) 🗝

CONTRAINDICATIONS. Active or past history of venous thromboembolic events, including deep vein thrombosis, pulmonary embolism, and retinal vein thrombosis. Prolonged immobilization.

PRECAUTIONS. The greatest risk for thromboembolic events occurs during the first 4 months of treatment. Raloxifene should be discontinued at least 72 hours prior to and during prolonged immobilization and should be resumed only after the patient is fully ambulatory. Patients should be advised to avoid prolonged restriction of movement during travel. There is no indication for premenopausal women. Safety and efficacy in women with severe hepatic insufficiency have not been established.

PHARMACOKINETICS. Raloxifene reduces resorption of bone and decreases overall bone turnover.

ADVERSE EFFECTS. See Table 37-5.

DRUG AND FOOD INTERACTIONS. Cholestyramine causes a 60% reduction in the absorption and enterohepatic recycling of raloxifene and should not be coadministered. Coadministration with warfarin has not been observed under chronic conditions; however, 10% decreases in prothrombin time have been observed, and prothrombin time should be monitored. Raloxifene is highly bound to plasma

raloxifene hydrochloride (Evista) 🔑 —cont'd

proteins, and caution should be used when it is administered with other highly protein-bound medications such as clofibrate, indomethacin, naproxen, ibuprofen, diazepam, and diazoxide.

DOSAGE AND ADMINISTRATION

Osteoporosis. 60 mg po once daily; may be administered at any time of day without regard to food.

Hormone Replacement Therapy. Estrogen-progestin therapy is no longer considered first-line treatment for menopause. See Chapter 54 on hormone replacement therapy. Estradiol transdermal therapy (Menostar) is the only estrogen therapy specifically indicated for osteoporosis prevention. It is not indicated for vasomotor symptom relief or osteoporosis.

CONTRAINDICATIONS. Undiagnosed abnormal genital bleeding; known, suspected, or history of cancer of the breast. Known or suspected estrogen-dependent neoplasia. Active deep vein thrombosis, pulmonary embolism, or a history of these conditions. Active or recent (e.g., within the past year) arterial thromboembolic disease (e.g., stroke, myocardial infarction) or liver dysfunction or disease; known hypersensitivity to product ingredients

PRECAUTIONS. Despite the rarity of endometrial hyperplasia in the clinical trial on which FDA approval was based, the manufacturer recommends that patients with an intact uterus take a progestin for 14 days every 6 to 12 months, and that they have an endometrial biopsy at least once a year. This "long-cycle" progestin regimen has been reported to protect against endometrial hyperplasia in women taking a low dose (0.3 mg/day) of oral estrogens. In women who have had a prior hysterectomy, oral conjugated estrogens without a progestin did not increase the risk of coronary disease but did increase the risk of venous thromboembolism and stroke; the incidence of breast cancer, surprisingly, was lower with unopposed estrogen than with placebo.

PHARMACOKINETICS. The new patch releases 14 mcg/day of 17-β-estradiol (E2). Other estrogen patches deliver 25 to 50 mcg/day. The systemic availability of transdermal E2 is 20 times greater than that of oral estrogen because absorption from the skin avoids first-pass metabolism in the liver.

ADVERSE EFFECTS. During the 2-year, double-blind trial, in which no progestin was given, endometrial hyperplasia developed in only one woman in the E2 treatment group and in none in the placebo group (see Table 37-5). Overdosage produces nausea and withdrawal bleeding in females.

DRUG AND FOOD INTERACTIONS. Patients dependent on thyroid replacement therapy may need to increase the dose when taking estrogen. Estrogens are metabolized partially by cytochrome P450 3A4 (CYP 3A4). St. John's wort preparations (*Hypericum perforatum*), phenobarbital, carbamazepine, and rifampin may reduce plasma concentrations of estrogens, possibly resulting in a decrease in therapeutic effects and/or changes in the uterine bleeding profile. Inhibitors of CYP 3A4 such as erythromycin, clarithromycin, ketoconazole, itraconazole, ritonavir, and grapefruit juice may increase plasma concentrations of estrogens, possibly causing side effects.

DOSAGE AND ADMINISTRATION. Each 3.25 cm^2 system contains 1 mg of estradiol USP, thus providing 14 mcg/day. Apply one patch weekly.

Zoledronic Acid

This agent is to be administered annually IV over 15 minutes. Zoledronic acid 5 mg was highly effective in women with postmenopausal osteoporosis in reducing the incidence of bone fracture across the most common fracture sites—hip, spine, and nonspine—with sustained effect over 3 years. Women who received this product had a 70% lower risk of spinal fracture and a 40% lower chance of hip fracture than those given placebo. Side effects include headaches, but these tended to be minor and short-lived.

evolve A continually updated list of useful WebLinks may be found in the Evolve Resources at http://evolve.elsevier.com/Edmunds/NP/

38 Muscle Relaxants

DRUG OVERVIEW

Class	Subclass	Generic Name	Trade Name
Antispasmodics	Centrally acting sedatives/CNS depressants	metaxalone	Skelaxin ✹
		methocarbamol ✹	Robaxin
		chlorzoxazone	Paraflex, Parafon Forte
	TCA relatives	cyclobenzaprine ✹	Flexeril
Agents with both antispasmodic and antispasticity	Benzodiazepines	diazepam ✹	Valium
	β₂-Adrenergic agonists	tizanidine ✹	Zanaflex
Antispasticity agents	GABA receptor stimulants	baclofen ✹	Lioresal

✹ Top 200 drug. Drugs are listed in order of common use. See Chapter 47 for a full discussion of diazepam.

INDICATIONS

- Centrally acting sedatives: musculoskeletal conditions; as an adjunct to rest, physical therapy, and other measures for relief of discomfort associated with acute, painful musculoskeletal conditions
- Cyclobenzaprine: musculoskeletal pain, muscle spasm
  - *Unlabeled use:* fibromyalgia
- Tizanidine: spasticity
  - *Unlabeled use:* muscle spasm
- Benzodiazepines
  - Diazepam: muscle spasm
  - Lorazepam, *unlabeled use:* muscle spasm
- Baclofen: spasticity resulting from multiple sclerosis, spinal cord trauma

- *Unlabeled uses:*
  - Trigeminal neuralgia
  - Hiccoughs
  - Spasticity from cerebral lesions
  - Cerebral palsy
  - Huntington's chorea
  - Rheumatic disorders
  - Rigidity from Parkinson's disease
  - Schizophrenia
  - Stroke
  - Alcohol withdrawal

Muscle relaxant drugs are chemically unrelated. For the purposes of this chapter, they are divided into two types: antispasmodic agents and antispasticity agents. Some drugs have properties of both types. The first group consists of the centrally acting sedatives and the tricyclic antidepressant (TCA) relative cyclobenzaprine. Metaxalone is treated as the key drug for the centrally acting sedatives because it is most commonly used. Cyclobenzaprine is also discussed in detail. The benzodiazepines and the centrally acting α₂-adrenergic agonist tizanidine have antispasmodic and antispasticity actions. The GABA-receptor stimulant baclofen is used only for spasticity.

THERAPEUTIC OVERVIEW

Pathophysiology

Muscle spasms are painful involuntary muscle contractions. They often are seen in skeletal muscle after acute injury (muscle strain) and in many chronic conditions.

Disease Process

Muscle spasms are commonly provoked by low back irritation that follows a motor vehicle accident after musculoskeletal injury has occurred. If a patient with this condition is not treated adequately, the condition can become a chronic, disabling problem. Other causes of chronic skeletal muscle spasm include rheumatic disorders, stroke, cerebral palsy, and Parkinson's disease.

The second common source of muscle spasms is CNS disorders. Examples include multiple sclerosis and injury to and disease of the spinal cord. These are mentioned briefly.

LOW BACK PAIN. Low back pain is the second leading reason, behind upper respiratory infection, for visits to primary care. The lifetime prevalence of at least one episode of back pain is 70% to 85%. It is not possible to determine the exact cause of the pain in about 80% of cases. The differential diagnosis is broad. Most low back pain appears to be due to muscular or ligamentous injuries that usually are self-limited. Acute low back pain may become chronic even if properly treated. Careful evaluation is necessary to rule out a serious cause. Simple acute back pain does not require imaging studies unless trauma has occurred. Box 38-1 summarizes the classification of back pain.

MECHANISM OF ACTION
Centrally Acting Sedatives/CNS Depressants

The centrally acting sedatives are CNS depressants. Their exact mechanism of action is unknown. These agents do not work directly on skeletal muscle, nor do they work at the neuromuscular junction. They achieve their effect on localized muscle spasms by producing sedation in the patient. This sedation causes a decrease in facilitative and inhibitory neuronal activity, which affects the muscle stretch reflex. These agents do not have analgesic or anti-inflammatory properties. They have been found to reduce the involuntary contractions and muscle spasms that result from skeletal muscle injury and are effective against peripherally caused muscle spasms. Centrally acting sedatives are ineffective in treating spasticity of muscles caused by CNS disease.

Methocarbamol causes CNS depression. It has no direct action on the contractile mechanism of striated muscle or on nerve fiber. Chlorzoxazone acts at the spinal cord and subcortical levels, inhibiting multisynaptic reflex arcs. Carisoprodol, which blocks interneuronal activity in the descending reticular formation and spinal cord, is metabolized to meprobamate, which is similar to barbiturates. Therefore, it is not recommended and is not discussed further here.

TCA Relatives

Cyclobenzaprine (Flexeril) is structurally related to TCAs. It acts in the CNS to reduce tonic somatic motor activity. It causes reserpine antagonism, norepinephrine potentiation, potent anticholinergic effects, and sedation. It also is effective in the treatment of non-CNS muscle spasms such as TMJ pain. Cyclobenzaprine works at the brainstem. Orphenadrine is similar to cyclobenzaprine but is not commonly used. Cyclobenzaprine provides an added benefit of aiding sleep, which often presents a problem for patients with back pain.

Benzodiazepines

Diazepam (Valium) is the only benzodiazepine with the indication for muscle spasm. It has direct skeletal muscle relaxant action in the brainstem and at the spinal cord level, enhancing GABA-mediated presynaptic inhibition. Diazepam may be used for both skeletal muscle strain and spasticity caused by upper motor neuron disorders.

α$_2$-Adrenergic Receptor Agonists

Tizanidine is an imidazoline derivative, an α$_2$-adrenergic receptor agonist that is related to clonidine and has centrally mediated myospasmolytic action. It has muscle relaxant, antinociceptive, and gastroprotective properties; lowering gastric acid secretion. Tizanidine is effective for both CNS and non-CNS spasms.

GABA Receptor Stimulants

Baclofen is effective only for muscle spasm caused by CNS disease. It inhibits monosynaptic and polysynaptic reflexes at the spinal level and is a structural analog of γ-aminobutyric acid (GABA), the inhibitory neurotransmitter.

BOX 38-1   Classification of Back Pain

MUSCULOSKELETAL BACK PAIN
Back Pain Without Sciatica

- Simple back pain in those younger than age 50, with no systemic illness or neurologic deficit, may be sacroiliac dysfunction
- Complicated back pain in those older than age 50 or with systemic signs may result from vertebral fracture

Sciatica

- Simple radiculopathy without bladder or bilateral findings from disk herniation, degenerative disease, spondylolisthesis
- Urgent radiculopathy (cauda equina syndrome) with urinary retention, saddle anesthesia, or bilateral neurologic findings

- Back and leg pain relieved by sitting indicates probable spinal stenosis in older adults, often caused by osteoporosis and osteoarthritis
  - Tolerable symptoms without neurologic deficit
  - Intolerable symptoms or neurologic defect

NONMUSCULOSKELETAL BACK PAIN

- Infection, associated with fever, adenopathy, IV drug use, immunosuppression
- Malignancy, associated with weight loss, history of cancer (often prostate), hematuria
- Renal disease
- Vascular disease
- Psychosocial issues

TREATMENT PRINCIPLES

Standardized Guidelines

- U.S. Preventive Services Task Force: Primary care interventions to prevent low back pain in adults: recommendation statement.
- Chou R, Huffman LH; American Pain Society; American College of Physicians: Medications for acute and chronic low back pain: a review of the evidence for an American Pain Society/American College of Physicians clinical practice guideline, *Ann Intern Med* 147(7):505-514, 2007.

Evidence-Based Recommendations

- Medications with good evidence of short-term effectiveness for low back pain include NSAIDs, acetaminophen, skeletal muscle relaxants (for acute low back pain), and TCAs (for chronic low back pain).
- Evidence is insufficient to identify one medication as offering a clear overall net advantage because of complex trade-offs between benefits and harms.
- Individual patients are likely to differ in how they weigh potential benefits, harms, and costs of various medications.

Cardinal Points of Treatment

ANALGESICS
- First line: NSAIDs, acetaminophen
- Second line: tramadol; opioids if severe or debilitating pain

MUSCLE RELAXANTS
- First line: cyclobenzaprine, centrally acting sedatives

This section is limited to discussion of the treatment of peripherally caused muscle spasms. Management of CNS spasms is beyond the scope of this book. Patients often seek OTC medications and complementary and alternative medicine for their back pain before visiting a primary care physician. They frequently do not tell their health care provider about their use of other treatments unless questioned, and they frequently continue to use them, regardless of the therapeutic regimen that is established.

Nonpharmacologic Treatment

Treatment of acute injury consists of rest and ice. Ice is used for the first 24 to 48 hours; heat, or ice alternating with heat, then may be applied. Physical therapy may be indicated as the injury begins to heal. Chronic muscle spasm also should be treated with physical therapy. Special pillows may be used, along with bed rest, office chairs, or car seats, to help take pressure off the low back area and keep the body in good alignment.

Pharmacologic Treatment

Medication for acute muscle injury begins with NSAIDs and acetaminophen. If these used alone are ineffective in relieving pain, or if muscle spasm is a significant component of the patient's complaint, a muscle relaxant may be considered. Skeletal muscle relaxants should not be used for longer than a week because muscle spasm seldom lasts longer than that. When prescribed for acute muscle spasm, these drugs are used as adjunctive therapy.

TREATMENT OF LOW BACK PAIN. Research shows that muscle relaxants are effective in the management of nonspecific low back pain. However, they must be used with caution because of the risk of adverse effects. Chronic muscle spasm may be treated with short-term muscle relaxants to help break the cycle of pain, muscle spasm, and pain.

Treat acute episodes of low back pain with an analgesic for 1 to 2 weeks. Add a skeletal muscle relaxant if spasms are a source of pain. If no improvement is noted, order additional diagnostic tests to look for additional problems. Complicated back pain should be assessed and the specific cause treated.

Simple radiculopathy (sciatica) calls for 6 weeks of the same care that is given for simple back pain. If a neurologic deficit progresses, order a CT scan or MRI. Urgent conditions with bilateral neurologic findings require an immediate consult and CT or MRI to identify disk herniations.

Provide symptom management in cases of possible stenosis with tolerable symptoms. Intolerable symptoms or pronounced neurologic deficits require imaging studies to evaluate the need for laminectomy, insertion of an artificial disk, or another therapeutic regimen.

DRUG SELECTION. Because of similarities among drugs, the provider should become familiar with one or two of the sedative muscle relaxants; metaxalone and methocarbamol are most commonly used, but research suggests that they provide only limited effectiveness. Cyclobenzaprine, which has a different mechanism of action, is an important muscle relaxant.

> Diazepam is the only benzodiazepine indicated for muscle relaxation and is the only drug in this category with direct muscle relaxant effects. It is very effective for short-term relief of severe muscle spasms. However, because of its abuse potential, it should be used only on a short-term basis, and the amount of medication taken should be closely monitored.

Other benzodiazepines have indirect effects as muscle relaxants. They offer the advantage of a shorter half-life with fewer adverse reactions. Lorazepam is used often.

Baclofen is used for CNS disorders with severe muscle spasm.

How to Monitor

- Watch for a reduction in severity and duration of muscle spasms.
- Monitor for sedation or dizziness.
- Perform liver function tests in patients at risk.
- All these drugs have some risk of abuse and addiction. Carefully evaluate patient use of the drug and response to it. Consider giving a limited amount of drug to patients who seem at high risk for abuse.

Patient Variables

GERIATRICS
- Elderly patients may be more susceptible to the sedative effects of muscle relaxants; thus, these medications must be used very cautiously in this patient population.

- Use of these agents put elderly patients at increased risk for falls.
- Patients who engage in driving for long distances are particularly at risk and should use special pillows to support the lower back area.

PEDIATRICS. Safety of use in children younger than age 12 has not been established.

PREGNANCY AND LACTATION
- Safety for use in pregnant women has not been established.
- Lactation: not known whether excreted in breast milk.

Patient Education

- May cause sedation and may decrease mental alertness; patients should use caution when performing hazardous tasks.
- Do not drink alcohol or take any other CNS depressants concomitantly with skeletal muscle relaxants because effects are additive.
- Notify provider if skin rash or jaundice occurs because these may be linked to more significant adverse effects.

SPECIFIC DRUGS

CENTRALLY ACTING SEDATIVES/CNS DEPRESSANTS
metaxalone (Skelaxin)

CONTRAINDICATIONS. Hypersensitivity

WARNINGS
- Hepatic function impairment: Administer with great care to patients with preexisting liver damage, and perform serial liver function studies as required. Discontinue if signs or symptoms of liver dysfunction are observed.
- May impair mental or physical abilities; patients should use caution while driving or performing other tasks that require alertness, coordination, or physical dexterity.
- Do not give to those with a history of drug-induced hemolytic anemia or other anemias.

PHARMACOKINETICS. Table 38-1 outlines the pharmacokinetic activity of selected muscle relaxants.

ADVERSE EFFECTS
- CNS: drowsiness, dizziness, headache, nervousness, irritability
- GI: nausea, vomiting, GI upset
- Miscellaneous: hypersensitivity (light rash with or without pruritus), leukopenia, hemolytic anemia, jaundice

DRUG INTERACTIONS
- May enhance the effects of alcohol, barbiturates, and other CNS depressants
- May produce false-positive Benedict's test results when blood sugars are tested

DOSAGE AND ADMINISTRATION. Table 38-2 outlines dosage and administration recommendations for selected muscle relaxants.

TABLE 38-1 Pharmacokinetics of Selected Muscle Relaxants

Drug	Onset of Action	Half-life	Duration of Action	Metabolism	Excretion
ANTISPASMODIC metaxalone (Skelaxin)	1 hr	9 hr	4-6 hr	Liver	Metabolites in urine
methocarbamol (Robaxin)	1 hr	1-2 hr	—	Liver	Urine, inactive metabolites; small amount in feces
chlorzoxazone (Paraflex, Parafon Forte)	1 hr	1 hr	6-12 hr	Liver, extensive	Urine
carisoprodol (Soma)	30 min	2 hr; meprobamate: 10 hr	4-6 hr	Liver; active metabolite meprobamate	Urine
cyclobenzaprine (Flexeril)	Well absorbed orally but great deal of variance in serum levels	18 hr	12-24 hr	Highly protein bound 1A2 2D6 3A4	Urine
BOTH ANTISPASMODIC AND ANTISPASTICITY diazepam (Valium)	Almost immediately when given IV; 30-60 min po dose	20-80 hr		Highly protein bound	
tizanidine (Zanaflex)	1-2 hr to peak; food increases rate to achieve peak concentration	2 hr	3-6 hr	Extensive first-pass metabolism in liver	Urine, 60%; feces, 20%
ANTISPASTICITY baclofen (Lioresal)	30-60 min following intrathecal bolus	3-4 hr	4-8 hr	Liver (≈15%)	Excreted in urine unchanged

OTHER CENTRALLY ACTING AGENTS

cyclobenzaprine (Flexeril)

CONTRAINDICATIONS
- Hypersensitivity
- Acute recovery phase of MI; patients with arrhythmias, heart block, or conduction disturbances or CHF
- Hyperthyroidism

> ✹ Concomitant use of MAOIs within the past 14 days may cause hyperpyretic crisis, seizure, and death.

WARNINGS
- Not effective in the treatment of cerebral or spinal cord disease spasticity
- Use for short periods, usually 2 to 3 weeks
- TCAs: closely related; may cause the same adverse reactions

PRECAUTIONS
- Use cautiously in patients with urinary retention, angle-closure glaucoma, or increased intraocular pressure, and in those taking anticholinergic medication.
- May impair mental or physical abilities; patients should use caution while driving or performing other tasks that require alertness, coordination, or physical dexterity.

ADVERSE EFFECTS. Cyclobenzaprine may cause all the adverse effects produced by TCAs. The most common of these are drowsiness, dry mouth, dizziness, fatigue, nausea, constipation, asthenia, dyspepsia, unpleasant taste, headache, confusion, nervousness, and blurred vision.

DRUG INTERACTIONS. Cyclobenzaprine may interact with MAOIs and may enhance the effects of alcohol, barbiturates, or other CNS depressants; may exhibit all the drug interactions characteristic of TCAs.

DOSAGE AND ADMINISTRATION. See Table 38-2.

tizanidine (Zanaflex)

CONTRAINDICATIONS
- Hypersensitivity
- Concomitant therapy with ciprofloxacin or fluvoxamine or other potent inhibitors of CYP 1A2

WARNINGS
- Experience with long-term use is limited.
- Orthostatic hypotension
- Hepatocellular injury
- Sedation (50%)
- Hallucinations, delusions

PRECAUTIONS
- Prolongation of QT interval, bradycardia
- Retinal degeneration and corneal opacities in animals
- Renal disease: Clearance is reduced by more than 50%.
- Monitor ophthalmic and liver function at baseline and at 1, 3, and 6 months, then periodically.

ADVERSE EFFECTS.
Serious. Hepatotoxicity, bradycardia
Common. Orthostatic hypotension, dizziness, dry mouth, somnolence, weakness
Other. Asthenia, urinary urgency, blurred vision, flu syndrome, dyskinesia, nervousness, pharyngitis, rhinitis, increased spasticity/tone

DRUG INTERACTIONS
- Oral contraceptives: Use with caution; reduce dose.
- Tizanidine delays the action of acetaminophen.
- Alcohol increases the blood level of tizanidine.
- Potent CYP 1A2 inhibitors may increase the effects of tizanidine. Significant orthostatic hypotension may be

---

TABLE 38-2   Dosage and Administration Recommendations for Selected Muscle Relaxants

Drug	Dosage and Administration
ANTISPASMODIC	
metaxalone (Skelaxin)	800 mg tid or qid daily
methocarbamol (Robaxin)	Give three 500 mg tablets qid or two 750 mg tablets qid; then decrease to two 500 mg tablets qid or two 750 mg tablets tid for maintenance.
chlorzoxazone (Paraflex, Parafon Forte)	250-500 mg tid to qid; maximum 750 mg qid
carisoprodol (Soma)	350 mg tid to qid; take last dose at bedtime
cyclobenzaprine (Flexeril)	5-10 mg tid; limit use to 2-3 wk
BOTH ANTISPASMODIC PROPERTIES AND ANTISPASTICITY	
diazepam (Valium)	*Adults:* 2-10 mg po bid to qid *Geriatrics:* 2-5 mg po bid to qid
tizanidine (Zanaflex)	*Adults:* Begin with 4 mg. Increase dosage gradually by 2-4 mg to maximum of 8 mg. Dose can be repeated q6-8h with maximum dosage 36 mg/day. Little experience with doses >8 mg
ANTISPASTICITY	
baclofen (Lioresal)	Start low; increase dosage gradually until effective. Usually begin with 5 mg tid × 3 days; 10 mg tid × 3 days; 15 mg tid × 3 days; 20 mg tid × 3 days; maintenance dosage is usually 40-80 mg/day, not to exceed 80 mg daily.

seen. Drugs such as ketoconazole, norfloxacin, ofloxacin, and rofecoxib are contraindicated.

- Ciprofloxacin may increase the levels/effects (e.g., hypotension) of tizanidine. Concurrent use is contraindicated.
- Diuretics, other α-adrenergic agonists, and antihypertensives may induce additive hypotensive effects.
- Fluvoxamine may increase levels/effects (e.g., hypotension) of tizanidine; concurrent use is contraindicated.
- Mirtazapine may antagonize the α-agonist effects of tizanidine.

DOSAGE AND ADMINISTRATION. See Table 38-2.

evolve A continually updated list of useful WebLinks may be found in the Evolve Resources at http://evolve.elsevier.com/Edmunds/NP/

39

Overview of the Nervous System

V. INEZ WENDEL and MAREN STEWART MAYHEW

The ability to understand the pharmacotherapy of the nervous system is highly dependent on the clinician's mastery of basic concepts of nervous system anatomy and physiology. This section reviews pertinent information about the CNS for easy review and retrieval.

NERVE CELL (NEURON) AND SYNAPTIC TRANSMISSION

The neurologic system is composed of the central, peripheral, and autonomic nervous systems. The *neuron* is the specialized cell of the nervous system. Neurons, or nerve cells, transmit an impulse from the body of the cell through the axon to the dendrite for the synapse. The axon may be covered with a myelin sheath, which enhances conduction (Figure 39-1). A *Schwann cell* forms the myelin sheath around a single axon in the peripheral nervous system. The *node of Ranvier* is the unmyelinated portion of the axon between nodes. The myelin sheath increases conduction velocity by causing depolarization across one or more nodes. Each nerve cell is separated from the next cell by a space called a *synapse*.

Chemicals that transmit the signal from one neuron to the next are called *neurotransmitters*. They are synthesized in the cell body or nerve terminal of the presynaptic neuron (Figure 39-2). Neurotransmitters are released from the synapse and cross the synaptic cleft. The dendrite on the nerve cell body receives the signal. Various receptors on the postsynaptic membrane of the dendrite accept only certain neurotransmitters. The receptors are discussed in greater detail in the section on the autonomic nervous system.

Modifying levels of neurotransmitters with medication is an important concept in the management of many neurologic diseases and conditions, including depression, dementia, Parkinson's disease, and seizures. In the brain, 30 different neurotransmitters have been classified as amino acids, amines, and neuropeptides. The amino acid neurotransmitters consist of glutamate, γ-aminobutyric acid (GABA), and glycine. Glutamate is an excitatory neurotransmitter. GABA and glycine are inhibitory neurotransmitters. GABA is the target of many anticonvulsants. The amines include the catecholamines—dopamine, norepinephrine, and epinephrine—as well as serotonin, histamine, and acetylcholine. Most neuropeptide neurotransmitters are also hormones; these include vasopressin, oxytocin, insulin, somatostatin, gastrin, substance P, endorphin, and enkephalin. Other neurotransmitters include nitric oxide, carbon monoxide, ATP, and adenosine. Table 39-1 summarizes neurotransmitters and their synthesis, location, function, and receptors.

CENTRAL NERVOUS SYSTEM

The central nervous system consists of the brain and the spinal cord. It coordinates information that makes interaction with the environment possible.

Brain

The brain consists of the cerebrum, cerebellum, pituitary, diencephalon, and brainstem (Figure 39-3). Each part of the brain is responsible for specific functions.

The *cerebrum (cortex and corpus callosum)* is responsible for global function, which is measured by level of consciousness (LOC) and mental status (MS). LOC is the patient's ability to relate to himself or herself and to the environment. MS consists of mental function, intellectual abilities, memory, orientation, and judgment. The dementias are disorders of cerebral function.

Specific areas of the cerebrum are responsible for specific functions. The *frontal lobe* is responsible for complex problem solving, value judgments, language expression, and expression of emotions. The *parietal lobe* allows for voluntary interpretation of touch, pressure, temperature, and position sense. The *temporal lobe* is responsible for interpretation of sounds and comprehension of language. Seizures often originate here. The *occipital lobe* interprets visual images. The *motor cortex* is the posterior portion of the frontal lobe, just anterior to the central fissure, which extends laterally across the brain in an organized pattern. It is responsible for voluntary movements. The *sensory cortex* lies just posterior to the motor cortex and is responsible for conscious interpretation of sensation. The *basal ganglia*, located in the subcortical gray matter surrounding lateral ventricles, are responsible for modulation and integration of voluntary body movements. Parkinson's disease is associated with dysfunction of neurotransmitters in the basal ganglia.

The *diencephalon* consists of the hypothalamus and thalamus. The *hypothalamus* controls the peripheral autonomic nervous system and endocrine processes and regulates body temperature, sleep, appetite, and emotions. The *thalamus* is a relay center for interpretation and integration of sensory impulses and complex reflex movements. The pituitary gland lies at the base of the brain at the sella turcica and is connected to the hypothalamus. The pituitary gland supplies numerous hormones that govern many vital processes.

The cerebellum, located in the posterior fossa, is connected to the brainstem. The cerebellum is responsible for coordination of involuntary muscular activity, balance, timing, posture, and position in space. The *brainstem*, which

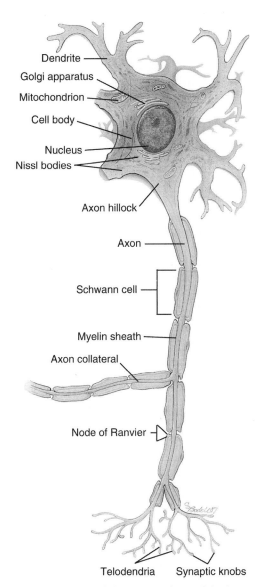

FIGURE 39-1 **Structure of the neuron.** (From Thibodeau FA, Patton KT: *Anatomy and physiology*, ed 6, St Louis, 2007, Mosby.)

Labels in Figure 39-1: Dendrite, Golgi apparatus, Mitochondrion, Cell body, Nucleus, Nissl bodies, Axon hillock, Axon, Schwann cell, Myelin sheath, Axon collateral, Node of Ranvier, Telodendria, Synaptic knobs

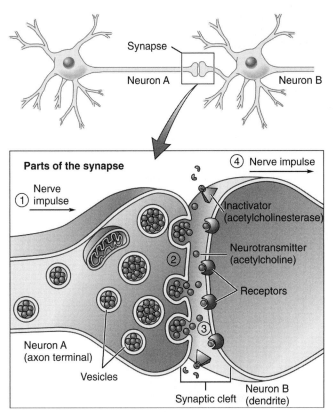

FIGURE 39-2 **Structure of a synapse showing an axon terminal of a presynaptic neuron, a synaptic cleft, and a postsynaptic neuron with receptor sites.** On the arrival of an action potential at a synaptic knob, neurotransmitter molecules are released from vesicles in the knob into the synaptic cleft. The combining of neurotransmitter and receptor molecules in the plasma membrane of the postsynaptic neuron initiates impulse conduction in the postsynaptic neuron. (From Herlihy B, Maebius N: *The human body in health and illness,* ed 3, Philadelphia, 2007, Saunders.)

consists of the midbrain, pons, and medulla, is the point of origin of cranial nerves III to XII. The *midbrain* is responsible for coordination of motor, sensory, and reflex functions. The *pons* coordinates movement and regulates respiratory rate. Heart rate, blood pressure, respiration, and swallowing are regulated in the medulla. The *medulla* is where the motor tracts cross over, a process that accounts for contralateral control. The *reticular activating system (RAS)* controls consciousness, arousal from sleep, wakefulness, alertness or how attention is directed, perceptual association, and direct introspection. It consists of neurons from the brainstem and thalamus to the cerebral cortex and receives stimuli from the sensory system. The *pituitary gland* supplies numerous hormones that govern many vital processes.

Spinal Cord

The spinal cord, which is a continuation of the medulla, connects the brain to the body (Figure 39-4). Nerves are grouped into bundles or tracts, and each tract performs specific functions (Table 39-2). The center *gray matter* contains cell bodies with projections to the periphery. The surrounding *white matter* contains myelinated axons of the ascending and descending tracts. The ascending tracts relay sensory impulses from the periphery to the brain. The descending tracts control voluntary and involuntary movements. The descending pathways are composed of the upper motor neurons, which originate and terminate within the central nervous system and modify spinal reflexes. Lower motor neurons originate in the gray matter of the anterior horn and terminate at the muscle fibers.

PERIPHERAL NERVOUS SYSTEM

The peripheral nervous system consists of cranial nerves and spinal nerves.

Cranial Nerves

Cranial nerves I and II are integrated in the brain, and cranial nerves III to XII are integrated in the brainstem. (Table 39-3 outlines functions of the cranial nerves.)

Spinal Nerves

A total of 31 pairs of spinal nerves run through the intervertebral foramina: 8 cervical, 12 thoracic, 5 lumbar, 5 sacral, and 1 coccygeal. Each spinal nerve receives and supplies

TABLE 39-1　**Neurotransmitters**

Neurotransmitter	Synthesis	Inactivation	Location	Function	Receptors
Glutamate	Krebs cycle metabolite, α-ketoglutarate, and glutamine	Astrocytes	CNS	Excitatory	Ionotropic and metabotropic
GABA	Glutamic acid by glutamic acid decarboxylase	Reuptake into nerve terminals or glial cells	CNS	Inhibitory	GABA$_A$ and GABA$_B$
Glycine	Serine by serine hydroxymethyltransferase	Reuptake		Inhibitory	
Catecholamines Dopamine	L-Tyrosine to L-dihydroxyphenylalanine (DOPA) by tyrosine hydroxylase; DOPA to dopamine by aromatic amino acid decarboxylase; dopamine to L-norepinephrine by dopamine	Uptake into nerve terminal with storage in synaptic vesicles or degradation by monoamine oxidase (MAO) and catechol-O-methyltransferase (COMT)	Substantia nigra Medial mesencephalic tegmentum Hypothalamus	Control movement Controls primitive functions such as emotions and visceral function Inhibits release of prolactin	D$_1$ cause excitation. D$_2$ cause inhibition.
Norepinephrine (noradrenaline)	β-Hydroxylase L-norepinephrine to L-epinephrine by phenylethanolamine-N-methyltransferase	Uptake also occurs in glial cells and smooth muscle that contain MAO or COMT.	Locus ceruleus Ventral brainstem reticular formation	Memory, information processing, emotions, energy, psychomotor function, movement, blood pressure, heart rate, bladder emptying Attention	α-Adrenergic receptors β-Adrenergic receptors
Epinephrine (adrenaline)			Ventral pontine and medullary reticular formation	Blood pressure and heart rate, attention	
Serotonin	L-tryptophan to L-5-hydroxytrytophan (5-HTP) by tryptophan hydroxylase; 5-HTP to L-5-hydroxytryptamine (5-HT or serotonin)	Degradation by glial cells with MAO and aldehyde dehydrogenase to 5-hydroxyindoleacetic acid (5-HIAA)	Pontomedullary caudal raphe nucleus, midbrain rostral raphe nuclei, gastrointestinal neurons	Stimulates release of growth hormone, adrenocorticotropic hormone (ACTH), and prolactin; regulates circadian rhythms; regulates food intake, satiation; controls mood, most often in association with inhibitory responses	Fourteen or more types of receptors, including 5-HT$_1$, 5-HT$_2$, 5-HT$_3$, and 5-HT$_4$; also associated with various effector mechanisms, including G proteins, cAMP, cyclic guanosine monophosphate (cGMP), IP3, and gated channels
Histamine	L-Histidine to histamine by histidine decarboxylase	Inactivated in glial cells by monoamine oxidase and histamine methyltransferase	Tuberal and mammillary regions of the hypothalamus	Arousal, biorhythms, pain control, temperature regulation, and food and water intake	H$_1$, H$_2$, H$_3$
Acetylcholine	Acetyl CoA and choline by choline acetyltransferase	Acetylcholinesterase breaks down to choline and acetic acid; reuptake of choline occurs	Neuromyal junctions; preganglionic sympathetic and parasympathetic axons; most parasympathetic and some sympathetic postganglionic axons in autonomic effect organs; basal nucleus of Meynert, hippocampus, and cerebral cortex	Voluntary movement; regulation of autonomic nervous system target organs (eye, salivary glands, heart, gastrointestinal tract, sweat glands); memory	Nicotinic receptors in the peripheral nervous system; muscarinic in the brain and autonomic target organs

TABLE 39-1   Neurotransmitters (Continued)

Neurotransmitter	Synthesis	Inactivation	Location	Function	Receptors
Neuropeptides (substance P, neurotensin, endorphin, enkephalin, vasopressin, oxytocin, insulin, gastrin, somatostatin, and others)	Processed in the cell body from a large precursor peptide molecule	Removed from the synaptic cleft by peptidase	Stored in vesicles in the nerve terminal	Modulate the release or action of neurotransmitters, or act as growth factors; involved in pain modulation, control of cardiovascular system, and stress responses	
Nitric oxide	Arginine and reduced nicotinamide-adenine dinucleotide phosphate		Hippocampus	Memory	
Adenosine triphosphate	Adenosine	Degraded by 5′-nucleotidases, resulting in ADP, AMP, and adenosine	Synaptic vessels, co-released with classic neurotransmitters	Mediates contraction of urinary bladder, vas deferens, and blood vessels and relaxation of intestines and some blood vessels; involved in nociceptive pain responses	Purinergic

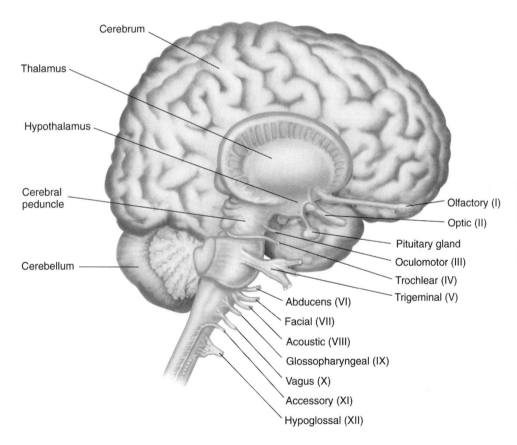

FIGURE 39-3 The brain, including major components of the cerebrum, diencephalons, and brainstem, as well as the cranial nerves. (From Rudy EB: *Advanced neurological and neurosurgical nursing,* St Louis, 1984, Mosby.)

information to a specific region called a *dermatome* (see Figure 39-4).

AUTONOMIC NERVOUS SYSTEM

The autonomic nervous system controls involuntary (smooth) muscle and gland activity. This area is not assessed directly during neurologic examination, although blood pressure, pulse, sweating, bladder, and rectal sphincter tone are regulated by the autonomic nervous system. Function of the heart, eyes, uterus, urinary bladder, and gastrointestinal tract, from the salivary glands to the anal sphincter, is governed and maintained by the autonomic nervous system (Table 39-4).

The autonomic nervous system is a complex set of neurons that originate in the hypothalamus; it is composed of two antagonistic systems, which are described as follows.

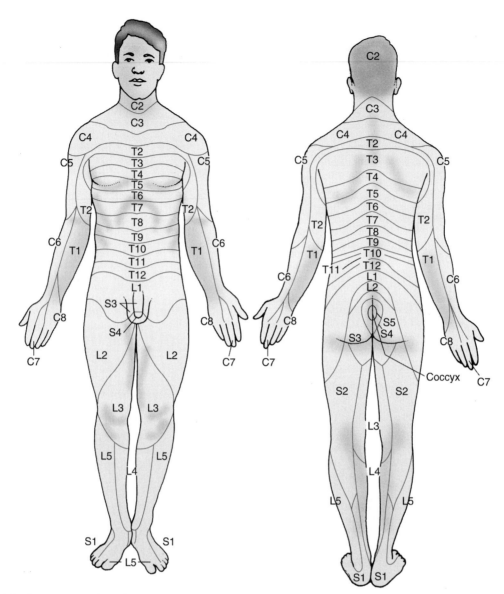

FIGURE 39-4   Spinal nerves. Location of exiting spinal nerves in relation to the vertebrae. (From Shpritz DW: Assessment of the nervous system. In Ignatavicius DD, Workman ML: *Medical-surgical nursing: critical thinking for collaborative care,* ed 5, Philadelphia, 2006, Saunders.)

TABLE 39-2   Major Ascending Tracts of Spinal Cord

Name	Function	Location*	Origin	Termination†
Lateral spinothalamic	Pain, temperature, and crude touch opposite side	Lateral white columns	Posterior gray column opposite side	Thalamus
Anterior spinothalamic	Crude touch and pressure	Anterior white columns	Posterior gray column opposite side	Thalamus
Fasciculi gracilis and cuneatus	Discriminating touch and pressure sensations, including vibration, stereognosis, and two-point discrimination; also conscious kinesthesia	Posterior white columns	Spinal ganglia same side	Medulla
Anterior and posterior spinocerebellar	Unconscious kinesthesia	Lateral white columns	Anterior or posterior gray column	Cerebellum
Spinotectal	Touch related to visual reflexes	Lateral white columns	Posterior gray columns	Superior colliculus (midbrain)

From Thibodeau GA, Patton KT: *Anatomy and physiology,* ed 6, St Louis, 2007, Mosby.
*Location of cell bodies of neurons from which axons of tract arise.
†Structure in which axons of tract terminate.

TABLE 39-3   **The Cranial Nerves and Their Functions**

Cranial Nerves	Function
Olfactory (I)	Sensory: smell reception and interpretation
Optic (II)	Sensory: visual acuity and visual fields
Oculomotor (III)	Motor: raising of eyelids, most extraocular movements Parasympathetic: pupillary constriction, change in lens shape
Trochlear (IV)	Motor: downward, inward eye movement
Trigeminal (V)	Motor: jaw opening and clenching, chewing, and mastication Sensory: sensation to cornea, iris, lacrimal glands, conjunctiva, eyelids, forehead, nose, nasal and mouth mucosae, teeth, tongue, ear, facial skin
Abducens (VI)	Motor: lateral eye movement
Facial (VII)	Motor: movement of facial expression muscles, except jaw; closing of eyes; labial speech sounds (b, m, w, and rounded vowels) Sensory: taste—anterior two thirds of tongue, sensation to pharynx Parasympathetic: secretion of saliva and tears
Acoustic (VIII)	Sensory: hearing and equilibrium
Glossopharyngeal (IX)	Motor: voluntary muscles for swallowing and phonation Sensory: sensation of nasopharynx, gag reflex, taste—posterior one third of tongue Parasympathetic: secretion of salivary glands, carotid reflex
Vagus (X)	Motor: voluntary muscles of phonation (guttural speech sounds) and swallowing Sensory: sensation behind ear and part of external ear canal Parasympathetic: secretion of digestive enzymes; peristalsis; carotid reflex; involuntary action of heart, lungs, and digestive tract
Spinal accessory (XI)	Motor: head turning, shrugging of shoulders, some actions for phonation
Hypoglossal (XII)	Motor: tongue movement for speech sound articulation (l, t, n) and swallowing

Modified from Rudy EB: *Advanced neurological and neurosurgical nursing,* St Louis, 1984, Mosby.

TABLE 39-4   **Actions of Autonomic Nervous System Neuroreceptors**

Effector Organ or Tissue	Receptor	Adrenergic Effect	Cholinergic Effect
EYE, IRIS			
Radial muscle	α_1	Contraction (mydriasis)	—
Sphincter muscle	—	—	Contraction (miosis)
Eye, ciliary muscle	β_2	Relaxation for far vision	Contraction for near vision
Lacrimal glands	—	—	Secretion
Nasopharyngeal glands	—	—	Secretion
Salivary glands	α_1	Secretion of potassium and water	Secretion of potassium and water
	β	Secretion of amylase	—
HEART			
SA node	β_1	Increased heart rate	Decreased heart rate; vagus arrest
Atrial	β_1	Increased contractility and conduction velocity	Decreased contractility; shortened action potential duration
AV junction	β_1	Increased automaticity and propagation velocity	Decreased automaticity and propagation velocity
Purkinje system	β_1	Increased automaticity and propagation velocity	—
Ventricles	β_1	Increased contractility	—
ARTERIOLES			
Coronary	α_1, β_2	Constriction, dilation	Dilation
Skin and mucosa	α_1, α_2	Constriction	Dilation
Skeletal muscle	α, β_2	Constriction, dilation	Dilation
Cerebral	α_1	Constriction (slight)	—
Pulmonary	α_1, β_2	Constriction, dilation	—
Mesenteric	α_1	Constriction	—
Renal	$\alpha_1, \beta_1, \beta_2,$ D	Constriction, dilation	—
Salivary glands	α_1, α_2	Constriction	Dilation
Veins, systemic	α_1, β_2	Constriction, dilation	—
LUNG			
Bronchial muscle	β_2	Relaxation	Contraction
Bronchial glands	α_1, β_2	Decreased secretion; increased secretion	Stimulation

Table continued on following page

TABLE 39-4 **Actions of Autonomic Nervous System Neuroreceptors** (Continued)

Effector Organ or Tissue	Receptor	Adrenergic Effect	Cholinergic Effect
STOMACH			
Motility	α_1, β_2	Decreased (usually)	Increased
Sphincters	α_1	Contraction (usually)	Relaxation (usually)
Secretion	—	Inhibition (?)	Stimulation
Liver	α, β_2	Glycogenolysis and gluconeogenesis	Glycogen synthesis
Gallbladder and ducts	—	Relaxation	Contraction
PANCREAS			
Acini	α	Decreased secretion	Secretion
Islet cells	α_2, β_2	Decreased secretion; increased secretion	—
INTESTINE			
Motility and tone	α_1, β_1, β_2	Decreased	Increased
Sphincters	α_1	Contraction (usually)	Relaxation (usually)
Secretion	α_2	Inhibition (?)	Stimulation
Adrenal medulla	—	—	Secretion of epinephrine and norepinephrine (nicotinic effect)
KIDNEY			
Renin secretion	α_1, β_1	Decreased; increased	—
URETER			
Motility and tone	α_1	Increased	Increased
URINARY BLADDER			
Detrusor	β_2	Relaxation (usually)	Contraction
Trigone and sphincter	α_1	Contraction	Relaxation
Sex organs, male	α_1	Ejaculation	Erection
SKIN			
Pilomotor	α_1	Contraction	—
Sweat glands	α_1	Localized secretion	Generalized secretion
Fat cells	α_2; β_1 (β_3)	Inhibition of lipolysis; stimulation of lipolysis	—
Pineal gland	β	Melatonin synthesis	—

From Sugerman RA: Structure and function of the neurologic system. In McCance KL, Heuther SE, editors: *Pathophysiology: the biologic basis for disease in adults and children,* ed 5, St Louis, 1996, Mosby.

Sympathetic

A primary response of the sympathetic nervous system is to prepare the body to expend energy. The "fight or flight" response is part of this system. The neurotransmitter norepinephrine, also called *adrenaline*, is released at the postganglionic fibers. Therefore, this system is also known as the *adrenergic system*. The two types of adrenergic receptors—α and β—are further subdivided according to their actions.

Parasympathetic

The parasympathetic nervous system prepares the body for energy conservation. The primary neurotransmitter is acetylcholine. Anticholinergic medications block the action of acetylcholine and interfere with the parasympathetic nervous system.

FUNCTION

Reflexes

The reflexes reflect a primitive response mediated by the nervous system and combining sensory and motor functions. A specific motor or efferent response occurs in response to sensory or afferent input. Reflexes, which regulate most bodily functions and homeostasis, are triggered without perception or input from the cerebrum (Figure 39-5).

Sensory System

Cell bodies of the afferent or sensory neurons are located in the dorsal or posterior horn of the gray matter of the spinal cord (Figure 39-6). The ascending spinothalamic tract is re-

sponsible for the primary sensations of crude touch, pressure, temperature, and pain. The spinocerebellar tract is responsible for discriminatory sensation, that is, it perceives details about the stimulus and its location, or proprioception, and the position of the body in space.

Motor System

The motor system controls skeletal muscle, somatic, and voluntary activity with use of the neurotransmitter, acetylcholine. Two different pathways are involved in the motor system, as follows:

- *Corticospinal (also called pyramidal):* Upper motor neurons (CNS) from the motor cortex cross over in the brainstem to the spinal cord to synapse with lower motor neurons (peripheral nervous system) that run from the spinal cord to muscle. This pathway controls voluntary movements, integrates complex movements, and serves as a direct connection between periphery and brain.
- *Extrapyramidal (affected in Parkinson's disease):* This complicated pathway, with its many interrelated neurons, provides background muscle control to allow voluntary movement, maintain muscle tone, and control (especially gross automatic movements such as walking) and coordinate body movement. Two extrapyramidal pathways originate in the basal ganglia. The "direct" pathway facilitates movement through the D_1-dopamine receptors with the use of GABA and substance P neurotransmitters. The "indirect" pathway inhibits movement through the D_2-dopamine receptor with GABA and enkephalin used as neurotransmitters.

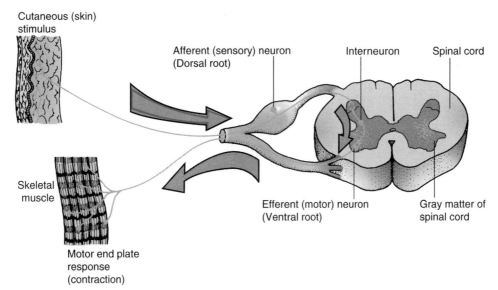

Cutaneous (skin) stimulus

Afferent (sensory) neuron (Dorsal root)

Interneuron

Spinal cord

Skeletal muscle

Motor end plate response (contraction)

Efferent (motor) neuron (Ventral root)

Gray matter of spinal cord

FIGURE 39-5 **Cross section of the spinal cord shows simple reflex arc.** (From Shpritz DW: Assessment of the nervous system. In Ignatavicius DD, Workman ML: *Medical-surgical nursing: critical thinking for collaborative care,* ed 5, Philadelphia, 2006, Saunders.)

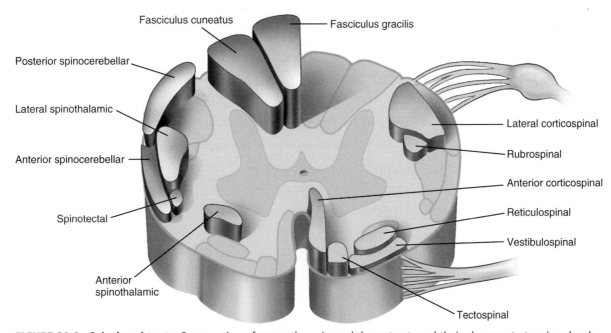

Fasciculus cuneatus

Fasciculus gracilis

Posterior spinocerebellar

Lateral spinothalamic

Anterior spinocerebellar

Spinotectal

Anterior spinothalamic

Lateral corticospinal

Rubrospinal

Anterior corticospinal

Reticulospinal

Vestibulospinal

Tectospinal

FIGURE 39-6 **Spinal cord tracts.** Cross section of upper thoracic cord shows tracts and their placement at various levels of the cord. (Courtesy Barbara Cousins. From Thibodeau FA, Patton KT: *Anatomy and physiology,* ed 6, St Louis, 2007, Mosby.)

• The *cerebellar area of the brain* coordinates muscular activity, maintains equilibrium, and controls posture.

evolve A continually updated list of useful WebLinks may be found in the Evolve Resources at http://evolve.elsevier.com/Edmunds/NP/

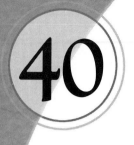
40 Medications for Attention-Deficit/Hyperactivity Disorder

LAURIE SCUDDER

DRUG OVERVIEW

Class	Subclass	Generic Name	Trade Name
Analeptics	—	caffeine	Vivarin
Amphetamine-like drugs	Short-acting	methylphenidate 🔑 ✹	Ritalin
	Intermediate-acting	methylphenidate ✹	Ritalin SR; Metadate SR
	Long-acting	methylphenidate SR	Concerta ✹, Metadate CD, Ritalin LA, Daytrana Transdermal System
		dexmethylphenidate	Focalin
Amphetamines	Short-acting	dextroamphetamine	Dexedrine
		methamphetamine	Desoxyn
	Intermediate-acting	amphetamine/dextroamphetamine	Adderall
	Long-acting	amphetamine/dextroamphetamine	Adderall XR ✹
Analeptic	Short-acting	modafinil	Provigil ✹
Norepinephrine reuptake inhibitors	—	atomoxetine	Strattera ✹
Antidepressants	Tricyclics	imipramine ✹ desipramine	Tofranil Norpramin
	Aminoketone	bupropion, bupropion SR ✹	Wellbutrin, Zyban, Wellbutrin XL ✹

✹ Top 200 drug; 🔑 key drug.

INDICATIONS

See Table 40-1.

Labeled Uses

- Attention-deficit/hyperactivity disorder (AD/HD)
- Narcolepsy
- Obesity
- Sleep apnea

Unlabeled Uses

- Depression in frail elderly, cancer, and poststroke patients
- Improvement in pain control, sedation, or both in patients receiving opiates
- Cognitive impairment following traumatic brain injury
- Chronic fatigue syndrome

This chapter discusses drugs used primarily in the treatment of AD/HD. Both amphetamines and amphetamine-like drugs act to alter levels of neurotransmitters in the brain, thereby modifying behaviors to improve and maintain function in patients with attention deficit disorder with or without hyperactivity and narcolepsy.

Atomoxetine, which is indicated only for the treatment of AD/HD, increases extracellular concentrations of norepinephrine, although the precise mechanism for efficacy in AD/HD is unknown. Antidepressants are used occasionally in children who have failed to respond to other therapy. Modafinil, a CNS analeptic with a unique mechanism of action, is used to treat excessive sleepiness associated with narcolepsy, obstructive sleep apnea, and shift work sleep disorder. Analeptics are not discussed in detail. An *analeptic* is a drug that acts as a stimulant to the CNS. Caffeine is the only

TABLE 40-1 AD/HD Drug Indications and Unlabeled Uses

Class	Drug	Trade Name	Indications	Unlabeled Uses
Analeptics	caffeine	Vivarin	Fatigue, drowsiness, analgesia adjuvant	Atopic dermatitis (topical), obesity, headache (adjunct in migraine)
	modafinil	Provigil	Narcolepsy	AD/HD; depression
Amphetamines	amphetamine salt	Adderall	Narcolepsy, AD/HD	
	dextroamphetamine sulfate	Dexedrine	Narcolepsy, AD/HD, obesity	Cocaine dependence, autism
	methamphetamine	Desoxyn	AD/HD, obesity	
Amphetamine-like drugs	dexmethylphenidate	Focalate	AD/HD	Depression in medically ill, elderly; improvement in pain control, sedation, or both in patients receiving opiates; chronic fatigue syndrome
	methylphenidate	Ritalin, Concerta	ADD, AD/HD, narcolepsy	
Norepinephrine reuptake inhibitors	atomoxetine	Strattera	AD/HD	

See Chapter 46 for antidepressants used for AD/HD.

other analeptic seen in primary care. It is used on an OTC basis to help people stay awake and restore mental alertness, and as an adjunct in analgesic formulations. It is a methylxanthine and is not discussed here in detail. Chapter 14 provides a discussion of the theophyllines, which are related chemically to the methylxanthines.

Amphetamines, which have very high potential for abuse, are category II drugs. They are used primarily in long-acting formulations, which may make dosing easier for AD/HD in primary care. Methylphenidate, a commonly used drug, is similar to the amphetamines but has less abuse potential, although it is a Schedule II drug. New, longer-acting formulations provide dosing options.

THERAPEUTIC OVERVIEW

Pathophysiology

AD/HD is a heterogeneous disorder of unknown cause. Structural and functional neuroimaging studies have not identified a unique origin. Although a positive family history is typical, no specific genetic marker has been identified, and studies that have found a familial association fail to distinguish between the actions of genes and family-specific environmental causes. The neurobiologic processes involved in attention and inhibition necessitate coordination of cortical and subcortical functioning; the most critical structure for maintaining alertness and attention is the reticular activating system, whereas the ability to inhibit distractions is cortically mediated at the prefrontal cortex. Circuits that connect these areas help to control how the brain both sustains and filters attention in response to stimuli. Both dopamine and norepinephrine appear to be important in linking subcortical areas to the frontal lobe. Stimulant drugs probably work by increasing "background" dopamine levels in the synapses. However, diagnostic trials of stimulant medications have failed to distinguish between children with and those without AD/HD.

The key features of AD/HD are inattention and hyperactivity/impulsivity. Although the disorder occurs in individuals of all races and socioeconomic strata, a 6:1 male/female ratio has been noted in childhood, and a positive family history is common. Environmental factors associated with AD/HD include poverty, maternal psychopathology, and family conflict, although none of these has been determined to be causally linked with AD/HD. Substance abuse, school failure, and, later, difficulty in maintaining a job may be associated with AD/HD; however, evidence suggests that patients who are treated properly with medication and who are given support do very well. It is estimated that up to 65% of children with AD/HD have at least one other comorbid condition such as depression, conduct disorder, oppositional defiant disorder, Tourette's syndrome, or a learning disability.

Disease Process

The diagnosis of AD/HD in children is made after observation and history taking. It requires a documented history of inattention and impulsivity, with or without hyperactivity, causing impairment in at least two settings (usually home and school) before the age of 7. Symptoms must have been prominent for at least 6 months. AD/HD is common, affecting 4% to 12% of school-age children and 3% to 4% of adults. Childhood AD/HD is a prerequisite for the diagnosis of AD/HD in adults, but it is increasingly recognized that adults may have the disorder, along with symptoms that were present in childhood, without ever having received a formal diagnosis as a child.

The *Diagnostic and Statistical Manual for Mental Disorders, Fourth Edition (DSM-IV-TR)* defines three subtypes of AD/HD. In children with AD/HD, Predominantly Inattentive Type, inattention is the major problem. The child cannot focus on instructions or tasks, fails to finish schoolwork, often loses things, cannot organize, and is forgetful and easily distracted. Inattentive children may not be noticed in the school setting because they are not disruptive. Thus, their condition often is not diagnosed until they are attending middle or high school.

The second subtype of AD/HD defined by the DSM-IV-TR is AD/HD, Predominantly Hyperactive-Impulsive Type. These children receive more attention in the classroom—often negative attention—because they fidget, cannot wait their turn, interrupt others, act as if "driven by a motor," talk incessantly, have difficulty enjoying quiet leisure activities, and act impulsively. These children often come to the attention of the health care provider because of concerns expressed by parents and teachers as early as preschool or kindergarten.

Finally, children with AD/HD, Combined Type, exhibit both behavior sets.

AD/HD is a dimensional, not a categorical, disorder with varying degrees of severity, some so mild that they may almost appear normal. In children, hyperactivity usually predominates. Although the hyperactive behavior may abate, or may be better controlled, with age, the attentional cluster of symptoms—inattention, lack of concentration, forgetfulness, shift in activities, executive operation dysfunction, and disorganization—tend to persist. Adolescents often display oppositional and restless behavior. Adults have increased problems with attention and executive level functioning and may underperform in their jobs.

Before AD/HD is diagnosed, other causes of impaired concentration and memory should be ruled out through a comprehensive neurologic and behavioral examination. Laboratory studies typically are not necessary but may include comprehensive metabolic panel, thyroid studies, and heavy metal screening, with particular attention to lead and toxicology screens. Absence and simple partial seizures can present with staring spells; an electroencephalogram may be indicated to rule out seizures. Children with sleep disorders that interfere with REM sleep may present with inattention and poor school performance; a comprehensive sleep study may be needed to evaluate this possibility. Other psychiatric diagnoses that should be considered and ruled out include anxiety disorders, affective disorders, adjustment disorders, behavioral disorders, and developmental disorders, including speech and language delays, which may cause a child to appear inattentive as a result of an inability to understand classroom directions.

Even though AD/HD has been recognized in children, awareness is only now increasing about the fact that adolescents and adults may have AD/HD and may not have had treatment. In many of these individuals, the condition is diagnosed when they have problems with employment, or when they seek treatment for depression or another type of medical problem. Much of the information generated by research about children with AD/HD appears to apply to adults also. Adults benefit from behavioral therapy and from the use of medication to keep them focused and functional.

MECHANISM OF ACTION
Analeptics

Caffeine, a methylxanthine, competitively blocks adenosine receptors and is a potent stimulant of the CNS. It also produces cardiac stimulation, dilation of coronary and peripheral blood vessels, constriction of cerebral blood vessels, skeletal muscle stimulation, augmentation of gastric acid secretion, and diuretic activity. It may produce tachycardia or premature ventricular contractions as well. The CNS-stimulating effects and associated constriction of cerebral blood vessels are effective as analgesic adjuncts. It also increases absorption of ergot alkaloids. Tolerance to these effects may develop.

Modafinil is a pharmacologically distinct psychostimulant approved for use in narcolepsy. Although the exact mechanism of action is unknown, studies have demonstrated that it inhibits the reuptake of dopamine and activates glutaminergic circuits while inhibiting GABA. It is thought to have less abuse potential because of the absence of euphoric effects.

Amphetamine-like Drugs

Methylphenidate is a mild cortical stimulant with CNS actions similar to those of the amphetamines. It inhibits the reuptake of both norepinephrine and dopamine in the cerebral cortex. This results in an increase in neurotransmitter in the synaptic cleft and enhanced stimulation of the cerebral cortex and subcortical structures. In normal children, as well as in children with AD/HD, this effect enhances the child's ability to selectively filter stimuli, leading to a decrease in motor activity and an increase in attention and cognition. Dexmethylphenidate contains the more pharmacologically active of the dextro and levo isomers.

Amphetamines

Amphetamines are sympathomimetic amines with CNS stimulant activity. Norepinephrine is released from central noradrenergic neurons. At high doses, dopamine may be released. The site of action for appetite suppression is thought to be the lateral hypothalamic feeding center. Peripheral α and β activity includes elevation of systolic and diastolic blood pressures and weak bronchodilator and respiratory stimulant actions.

Norepinephrine Reuptake Inhibitors

The mechanism of action of atomoxetine is selective reuptake of presynaptic norepinephrine. It does not bind to monoamine receptors in the brain, thereby decreasing the risk of adverse reactions compared with older norepinephrine reuptake inhibitors.

Antidepressants

See Chapter 46 for information on depression and the mechanism of action of antidepressant agents.

TREATMENT PRINCIPLES
Standardized Guidelines

- Clinical practice guideline: Treatment of the school-aged child with attention-deficit/hyperactivity disorder, American Academy of Pediatrics, October 2001 (Available at http://aappolicy.aappublications.org/cgi/content/full/pediatrics;108/4/1033)

Evidence-Based Recommendations

- Likely to be beneficial: atomoxetine, dexamphetamine sulphate, methylphenidate, methylphenidate plus psychological/behavioral treatment
- Methylphenidate improves core symptoms and school performance in children with AD/HD when used alone, and it may be beneficial when added to psychological/behavioral treatment.
- Dexamphetamine and atomoxetine may also reduce symptoms of AD/HD but can cause adverse effects.

Cardinal Points of Treatment

Treatment options are listed in order of preference:
- Counseling for parent(s) or guardian(s)
- First line: All agents are similarly effective. Methylphenidate has the best track record.
- Long-acting methylphenidate if the child has difficulty taking multiple doses during the day

- An amphetamine salt
- A TCA antidepressant (desipramine or nortriptyline) or atomoxetine for patients with a history of substance abuse
- Bupropion for patients with a history of cardiac disease or other medical contraindications to stimulants

Nonpharmacologic Treatment

Drug therapy is not indicated for all children with this syndrome. Stimulants are not intended for use in the child who exhibits symptoms related to environmental factors and/or primary psychiatric disorders, including psychosis. Appropriate educational placement is essential, and psychosocial intervention generally is needed.

Classes or counseling for parents in behavior modification (such as point systems that allow children to earn rewards) is often considered an integral part of the treatment plan for AD/HD. Additionally, social skills training, cognitive-behavioral therapy, support groups, biofeedback, and meditation all have been integrated into comprehensive, multidisciplinary management programs, although empirical evidence for the efficacy of these interventions is lacking.

Pharmacologic Treatment

When nonpharmacologic measures alone are insufficient, the decision to prescribe stimulant medication will depend on the clinician's assessment of the chronicity and severity of the child's symptoms.

All available stimulants appear to be equally effective. Methylphenidate is usually the first-line drug of choice for AD/HD. When giving medications to children, the clinician first must obtain permission from a parent or guardian. Although some families may choose not to inform their child's teacher of the decision to medicate, teachers may be very helpful in evaluating response to therapy. The Connors Teacher's Rating Scale, completed prior to initiation of therapy and 1 to 2 weeks after initiation of therapy, may provide a standardized assessment of response. Additionally, parent rating scales should be completed before and after therapy is begun.

A once-daily formulation of methylphenidate (Concerta) may be used to help children for whom multiple doses per day are difficult. If paradoxical aggravation of symptoms or other adverse effects occur, reduce dosage or, if necessary, discontinue the drug. Duration of therapy is unknown and is highly individualized. Most studies of stimulants have been short-term trials that demonstrated efficacy over weeks to a year. Increasingly, treatment is continuing into adulthood. Although "drug holidays" during school breaks and the summertime are still common, children who exhibit impairment in both home and school settings may require treatment on all days.

If the patient does not respond to methylphenidate, other medications from another class may be considered. Amphetamines usually are used. Adderall contains both amphetamine and dextroamphetamine. In higher doses, its duration of action is prolonged. In clinical practice, many adults with AD/HD do respond to dosing within FDA-approved maximums, which currently are 20 mg daily for *d*-methylphenidate XR (Focalin) and 20 mg daily for mixed amphetamine salts XR (Adderall). Other stimulant preparations approved for child and adolescent AD/HD have not yet been approved for adults. Approved doses reflect the failure of studies submitted to the FDA to demonstrate significantly greater benefit with higher doses. Emerging evidence indicates that some adults with AD/HD may tolerate and benefit from higher doses than those approved by the FDA.

The TCA antidepressants have been used as both primary and adjunctive therapy in children who fail to achieve a positive response to stimulants. The specific agents used are desipramine and nortriptyline, primarily because of their effects on norepinephrine reuptake. They have produced a favorable response in patients with AD/HD and generally are avoided in patients with cardiac disease, specifically, conduction abnormalities.

Bupropion is an atypical antidepressant that has weak effects on norepinephrine and dopamine. It has been shown to be effective for AD/HD in as little as 2 weeks. Studies are limited and this use is off-label.

An alternative choice is atomoxetine. Currently, it is used for patients who cannot tolerate CNS stimulants, although it also may be used for patients who wish to avoid stimulants or in patients with a history of substance abuse.

Alternative therapies include antioxidants; vitamin and mineral preparations, especially copper, zinc, selenium, and B vitamins; and herbal extracts. Valerian root, kava kava, ginkgo biloba, and Pycnogenol (pine bark extract) have been used. The safety and efficacy of the herbal extracts remain unknown.

How to Monitor

- Patients should be seen more frequently during the dosage adjustment period, although some follow-up may be conducted through phone consultation. Once patients are stable, they should be followed about once every 6 to 12 months.
- Monitor blood pressure levels.
- Monitor weight.

> **Children with known seizures or tics should be followed closely, particularly at therapy initiation and following a dose increase, for an escalation in events.**

Patient Variables

GERIATRICS. Methylphenidate has an unlabeled use in the elderly population. It may increase mental alertness and stimulate appetite. Low dosages and careful monitoring are required. Monitor cardiovascular status closely. Many patients will be unable to tolerate the stimulant effects.

PEDIATRICS. Use in children younger than 6 years of age is off-label.

PREGNANCY AND LACTATION. Studies conducted for any of these drugs have not been adequate to determine safety; they are not recommended for women of childbearing age.

GENDER. Women who use modafinil and oral contraceptives should take precautions to avoid pregnancy. See Drug Interactions for more information.

USE AND ABUSE. *Drug dependence:* Use with caution in emotionally unstable patients and in those with a history of alcoholism or other drug dependence. Chronic abuse can cause frank psychotic episodes. Withdrawal from the drug should be monitored because severe depression may occur. Chronic abusive use can lead to marked tolerance and psychic dependence with varying degrees of abnormal behavior. Frank psychotic episodes can occur.

SPECIFIC DRUGS

AMPHETAMINE-LIKE DRUGS

methylphenidate (Ritalin); methylphenidate SR (extended-release tablet) (Concerta); methylphenidate transdermal system (Daytrana); dexmethylphenidate (Focalin) 🔑

CONTRAINDICATIONS
- Hypersensitivity
- Marked anxiety, tension, and agitation
- Glaucoma
- Motor tics or family history or diagnosis of Tourette's syndrome
- Concomitant use of MAOIs
- Preexisting severe GI disease, such as esophageal motility disorders, small bowel inflammatory disease, and others

WARNINGS
- Some evidence suggests that methylphenidate may lower the convulsive threshold in patients with a prior history of seizures, in those with prior EEG abnormalities in the absence of seizures, and, very rarely, in the absence of a history of seizures and no prior EEG evidence of seizures. Safe use concomitant with anticonvulsants has not been established.
- Sudden death has been reported in children with underlying structural cardiac disorders, cardiomyopathy, and rhythm disorders.
- Modest increases in blood pressure have been reported; caution should be exercised in patients whose underlying medical condition may be affected by this increase.
- Exacerbation of behavioral and processing symptoms may occur in patients with preexisting psychosis. Manic episodes have been reported in those with bipolar disorder. Mania and psychotic symptoms, including hallucinations and delusional thinking, can be caused by stimulants, even in the absence of a known psychiatric disorder.
- Blurring of vision occasionally has been reported.
- Temporary slowing in growth rate has been reported in some studies in children, although it is unclear whether this leads to long-term growth suppression. Height and weight should be monitored with long-term use.

PRECAUTIONS
- Agitation and aggressive behavior may be exacerbated.
- Watch for symptoms of abuse.

PHARMACOKINETICS. Methylphenidate is thought to block the reuptake of norepinephrine and dopamine. It is readily absorbed; both the immediate-release formulation and transdermal methylphenidate reach peak concentrations in 2 hours. The once-daily formulations (Metadate CD and Concerta) have a biphasic release system that mimics an immediate-release product and is followed by a second, sustained-release phase.

The fact that the oral medication is drawn so slowly into the brain is a likely explanation for why patients do not experience euphoria. In general, if brain concentrations of a substance peak quickly, the potential for abuse and addiction increases because the individual experiences the drug more dramatically and thus is more likely to try to repeat the experience more frequently. This explanation helps to clarify why use of methylphenidate rarely leads to abuse and addiction when it is taken properly as a treatment for AD/HD.

ADVERSE EFFECTS. Side effects may subside after the first few weeks of treatment. Nervousness and insomnia are the most common adverse effects; they usually are controlled by reducing dosage and omitting the drug in the afternoon or evening. Other common side effects include decreased appetite, abdominal pain, headache, depression, irritability, weight loss, and rebound symptoms (particularly at the end of the day); potential concerns regarding decreased growth velocity have been expressed. Less common side effects include headache, dizziness, tachycardia, psychotic symptoms, and tics, although the drug should be used only with caution in children with known tic disorders. A rare hypersensitivity reaction consists of hives, fever, arthralgia, exfoliative dermatitis, erythema multiforme, and thrombocytopenic purpura. Occasionally, visual disturbances, including difficulty accommodating and blurring, have been reported.

DRUG INTERACTIONS
- Use cautiously with pressor agents.
- May inhibit metabolism of coumarin anticoagulants, anticonvulsants (e.g., phenobarbital, diphenylhydantoin, primidone), and tricyclic drugs (e.g., imipramine, clomipramine, desipramine). Downward dosage adjustments of these drugs may be required when they are given with this product. Serious adverse events have been reported with concomitant use of clonidine, although a causal relationship has not been established.

DOSAGE AND ADMINISTRATION. Immediate-release methylphenidate usually is initiated at 2.5 to 5 mg orally before breakfast and before lunch. Dosage may be increased by 5 to 10 mg at weekly intervals. Maximum dose is 60 mg/day. The drug's short half-life often necessitates a dose during the school day. Many children and parents object to the use of medications that require a daily visit to the school nurse, and, particularly for these children, sustained-release (SR) formulations may be useful. SR products (Concerta) are initiated at 18 mg/day for children who are naïve to the product; children already on short-acting preparations may be converted to longer-acting products at a higher maximum daily dose.

methylphenidate (Ritalin); methylphenidate SR (extended-release tablet) (Concerta); methylphenidate transdermal system (Daytrana); dexmethylphenidate (Focalin) 🔑—cont'd

The dose may be gradually increased to a maximum of 72 mg/day. Some children metabolize the psychostimulants more quickly than do others, and some children experience a "rebound" effect of increased impulsiveness and activity, which requires more frequent dosing. As children grow up, their need for medication changes and should be reevaluated periodically. Individualize the dosage according to the needs and responses of the patient.

Adults. Administer in divided doses two or three times daily, preferably 30 to 45 minutes before meals. The average dosage is 20 to 30 mg daily. Some patients may require 40 to 60 mg daily; in others, 10 to 15 mg is adequate. Patients who are unable to sleep if medication is taken late in the day should take the last dose before 6 PM.

SR tablets: SR tablets have a duration of action of approximately 12 hours. Tablets must be swallowed whole and must never be crushed or chewed.

Children 6 Years and Older. Initiate medication in small doses, increasing weekly in gradual increments. If improvement is not observed after appropriate dosage adjustment, the drug should be discontinued. However, children who fail to respond to one formulation may respond to a different formulation even in the same drug class.

Tablets (short acting): Start with 5 mg twice daily (before breakfast and before lunch), increasing in gradual increments of 5 to 10 mg each week. Give the last dose before 6 PM to avoid insomnia. Because anorexia may be associated with administration, it is recommended but not necessary for the medication to be taken 30 to 45 minutes before meals.

SR tablets: For those who have never taken methylphenidate, start with an 18 mg tablet (Concerta) every morning.

A conversion table included with the prescribing information should be used to determine appropriate dosage for those who are already taking methylphenidate. Children on short-acting methylphenidate 10 mg bid or tid may initiate long-term methylphenidate at a dose of 36 mg qAM; children on 15 mg of the short-acting drug may be started on the 54 mg dose of the long-acting formulation.

- Concerta 18 mg every morning provides an initial dose of 4 mg plus an extended dose of 14 mg.
- Concerta 27 mg every morning provides an initial dose of 6 mg plus an extended dose of 21 mg.
- Tablets must be swallowed whole and must never be crushed or chewed.

Transdermal system: Supplied in patches from 12.5 to 37.5 cm². Doses of 12.5 provide a nominal dose equivalent to 10 mg delivered over 9 hours. The highest dose is equivalent to 30 mg/day. Patches provide a much lower first-pass effect, and a lower dose may produce an equivalent response. The patch should be applied daily to alternating hips and should be removed after 9 hours. The patch is a dermal irritant. Application to inflamed skin leads to an increase in rate and extent of absorption, as does applying an external heat source to the patch. Patches applied to areas other than the hip may result in variance in absorption; this has not been adequately studied.

- Methylphenidate is available in many formulations with different pharmacokinetic profiles. The generic form is significantly less expensive. It should be used first to monitor for adverse reactions. Because half-life is the shortest, adverse effects resolve quickly. Once the dosage has been established, the patient can be switched to a longer-acting methylphenidate. Some formulations are not consistent in their rate of absorption.
- An expanded indication for methylphenidate Hcl extended-release tablets, allowing its once-daily use for the treatment of AD/HD in adults 18 years and older has been approved.

OTHER DRUGS IN CLASS

Other drugs in this class are similar to the key drugs except as follows:

- *Amphetamines* may be useful in patients who do not respond to methylphenidate. The risk of adverse effects is higher.

modafinil (Provigil)

CONTRAINDICATIONS. Known hypersensitivity

WARNINGS. Patients with narcolepsy and sleep disorders should be warned that their level of wakefulness may not return to normal, and that they may need to avoid activities that require alertness, such as driving. Provigil has not been studied in pregnancy and lactation. Safety in children younger than 16 years of age has not been established, and leukopenia has been reported in children.

PRECAUTIONS

- Not recommended for patients with a history of angina, cardiac ischemia, recent MI, or left ventricular hypertrophy
- Not recommended for patients with mitral valve prolapse who have developed mitral valve prolapse syndrome with previous CNS stimulant use
- Caution should be exercised when modafinil is given to patients with a history of psychosis; caution is warranted when one is operating machinery or driving. Although functional impairment has not been demonstrated with modafinil, all CNS-active agents may alter judgment, thinking, and/or motor skills.
- Stimulants may unmask tics in individuals with coexisting Tourette's syndrome.
- Use caution in patients with renal or hepatic impairment.
- Safety and efficacy in children younger than 16 years of age have not been established.

PHARMACOKINETICS. The precise mechanism(s) through which modafinil promotes wakefulness is (are) unknown. Modafinil has wake-promoting actions similar to those of amphetamine and methylphenidate, although the pharmacologic profile is not identical.

ADVERSE EFFECTS. Generally well tolerated. Adverse effects most often are reported to be mild and may include headache, nausea, nervousness, rhinitis, diarrhea, back pain, anxiety, insomnia, dizziness, and dyspepsia.

DRUG INTERACTIONS. Modafinil is a reversible inhibitor of the drug-metabolizing enzyme CYP 2C19. Coadministration with drugs that are metabolized via that pathway, including diazepam, phenytoin, and propranolol, may increase the circulating levels of those compounds. In addition, in individuals deficient in the enzyme CYP 2D6, the levels of CYP 2D6 substrates such as TCAs and SSRIs, which have ancillary routes of elimination through CYP 2C19, may be increased by coadministration of modafinil. It is thought that 7% to 10% of the white population is deficient in this enzyme; the percentage is similar or lower in other populations. Dose adjustments may be necessary for patients who are being treated with these and similar medications (see PRECAUTIONS, Drug Interactions). Coadministration of modafinil with other CNS-active drugs, such as methylphenidate and dextroamphetamine, did not significantly alter the pharmacokinetics of either drug.

Women who are taking modafinil and hormonal contraceptives should be cautioned that excessive metabolism of the latter drug may increase the risk of pregnancy. Selection of an oral contraceptive that contains a higher level of ethinyl estradiol may be necessary; use of a backup method of birth control, including condoms, is advised.

DOSAGE AND ADMINISTRATION. 100 to 300 mg once daily

Norepinephrine Reuptake Inhibitors

atomoxetine (Strattera)

Atomoxetine is thought to be as effective as the stimulants. It is not a controlled substance and it is not a stimulant, so it is useful for patients who cannot tolerate stimulants. It is the only FDA-approved nonstimulant treatment for AD/HD that has been shown to be safe, well tolerated, and efficacious in the treatment of children, adolescents, and adults with AD/HD. It has a relatively low potential for abuse compared with other medications given for AD/HD.

CONTRAINDICATIONS
- Hypersensitivity
- Glaucoma
- Concomitant use of MAOIs or use of an MAOI within the previous 2 weeks

WARNINGS
- Atomoxetine carries a black box warning advising of an increased risk for suicidal ideation.
- Postmarketing reports have described rare instances of severe liver injury.

PRECAUTIONS
- Use with caution in patients with known hypertension, tachycardia, or cardiovascular disease because the drug may increase blood pressure and heart rate.
- Urinary retention may occur.
- Height increase and weight gain have been reported to be slowed, although evidence of rebound growth has been observed.
- Pregnancy category C; use during lactation has not been studied.
- Safety in geriatric patients has not been established.

PHARMACOKINETICS. Atomoxetine is metabolized by the 2D6 enzyme system. Its half-life is 4 hours in most patients, although this may be prolonged to 30 to 40 hours in poor metabolizers (7% of population). An active metabolite is excreted in the urine. Atomoxetine is not a controlled substance, no evidence of abuse potential has been found.

ADVERSE EFFECTS. Atomoxetine causes more vomiting (11% to 15%) and insomnia (16%) than methylphenidate. Adverse effects with a frequency greater than 2% include headache, rhinitis, upper abdominal pain, decreased appetite, constipation, increased cough, flu syndrome, and psychiatric symptoms such as irritability and mood swings. Adults experienced a higher incidence of chest pain, palpitations, insomnia, and urinary retention when compared with those taking placebo. Sexual dysfunction, including erectile dysfunction, impotence, and orgasmic abnormalities, also has been reported, although the exact incidence is unknown.

DRUG INTERACTIONS
- Concomitant use with oral albuterol may exacerbate increases in blood pressure and heart rate.
- Blood pressure should be monitored in patients who are concomitantly using pressor agents.
- Dosage adjustment may be necessary when coadministered with CYP 2D6 inhibitors (e.g., paroxetine, fluoxetine, quinidine).

DOSAGE AND ADMINISTRATION. For children, start with 0.5 mg/kg/day. Titrate at three or more daily intervals to 1.2 mg/kg/day. The maximum dosage regardless of age or weight is 1.4 mg/kg/day or 100 mg/day, whichever is less. It may be administered once a day without regard for meals. Dose should be adjusted in patients with hepatic failure. Patients on CYP 2D6 inhibitors may be started on the usual dose with subsequent increases if well tolerated.

evolve A continually updated list of useful WebLinks may be found in the Evolve Resources at http://evolve.elsevier.com/Edmunds/NP/

Medications for Dementia

V. INEZ WENDEL

DRUG OVERVIEW

Class	Subclass	Generic Name	Trade Name
Cognitive function	Cholinesterase inhibitors	donepezil 🗝	Aricept ✹
		rivastigmine	Exelon
		galantamine	Razadyne Razadyne ER
	Receptor antagonists	memantine	Namenda ✹

✹ Top 200 drug; 🗝 key drug. Donepezil has been designated a key drug because it was the first to be developed and is the most commonly used.

INDICATIONS

Cholinesterase Inhibitors

- Delay the progression of Alzheimer's disease (AD) symptoms
- Donepezil approved for treatment of severe AD

Unlabeled Uses

- Modification of problematic behaviors associated with moderate to severe dementia of Alzheimer's type, vascular dementia, dementia with Lewy bodies, or mixed dementia

NMDA Receptor Antagonists

- Management of moderate to severe dementia of Alzheimer's type

Unlabeled Uses

- Management of catatonic schizophrenia, mild to moderate dementia, neurogenic bladder, parkinsonism, and phantom limb syndrome

Alzheimer's disease (AD) is a chronic neurodegenerative illness characterized by cognitive and functional decline, as well as emergent behavioral disturbances. Currently, cholinesterase (ChE) inhibitors (donepezil, rivastigmine, and galantamine) are the standard therapy for AD. The three cholinesterase inhibitors are medications that are currently available specifically for the treatment of mild to moderate dementia of the Alzheimer's type. These drugs do not cure the disease; however, they may slow the progression of the disease and at best may modestly improve function. These medications often are initiated by primary care practitioners

for patients who meet the criteria for mild to moderate Alzheimer's-type dementia, or they may be initiated after consultation with a provider who specialize in geriatrics or with a neuropsychiatrist.

Memantine hydrochloride is available for moderate to severe dementia. It is the first N-methyl-D-aspartate (NMDA) receptor antagonist, a new subclass of medications that have a different mechanism of action from the cholinesterase inhibitors. Memantine may slightly improve function, reduce care dependency (in one study by as much as 40 minutes a day of provider time), and slow clinical decline in patients with moderate to severe dementia (those who are stage 5 through 7 on the Global Deterioration Scale, or who have a Mini Mental State Exam score <10; see "How to Monitor"). It may be given in addition to the cholinesterase inhibitors.

Medication treatment for AD is a topic of intense research that is limited by our lack of understanding of the cause and pathology of the disease. Drug treatment is sought to increase cerebral metabolism and blood flow, prevent or reverse degeneration of neurons, and facilitate function in the remaining neurons that support memory and cognition. No drugs have been found that prevent or reverse degeneration of neurons.

THERAPEUTIC OVERVIEW

Pathophysiology

In patients with AD, loss of neurons occurs in the nucleus basalis of Meynert, the origin of the cholinergic neurons. A decrease in cholinergic activity results from loss of neurons and from a decrease in the activity of choline acetyl transferase, the enzyme responsible for acetylcholine synthesis.

The brain of a patient with AD often shows marked atrophy, with widened sulci and shrinkage of the gyri. In the great majority of cases, every part of the cerebral cortex is involved; however, the occipital pole often is relatively spared. The cortical ribbon may be thinned and ventricular dilation apparent, especially in the temporal horn, as the result of atrophy of the amygdala and hippocampus. Microscopically, significant loss of neurons is apparent, in addition to shrinkage of large cortical neurons. Many investigators believe that loss of synapses, in association with shrinkage of the dendritic arbor of large neurons, is the critical pathologic substrate. The neuropathologic hallmarks of AD are neuritic plaques and neurofibrillary tangles. Classic neuritic plaques are spherical structures that consist of a central core of fibrous protein known as *amyloid* that is surrounded by degenerating or dystrophic nerve endings (neurites). Two other types of amyloid-related plaques are recognized in the brains of patients with AD: diffuse plaques, which contain poorly defined amyloid but no well-circumscribed amyloid core, and "burnt-out" plaques, which consist of an isolated dense amyloid core.

Disease Process

More than 50 causes of dementia, a syndrome of impaired cognition involving memory, language, and reasoning, have been identified. AD and vascular dementia are the most common causes of dementia. Mixed vascular dementia and AD are other common causes. The incidence of AD varies from 5% in those older than 65 years of age to 30% to 50% in those older than age 85. Some evidence suggests that women who drink more caffeine and people with higher education have some neuroprotection from AD, perhaps because of some cognitive reserve; however, people with higher education seem to have AD in which symptoms progress rapidly. Diagnosis of AD is based on exclusionary and inclusionary data. The criteria for dementia are listed in the *Diagnostic and Statistical Manual of Mental Disorders, Fourth Edition* (DSM-IV). Workup includes CBC, chemistries, B_{12}, folate, thyroid profile, VDRL test, and, if relevant, CT scans or MRIs to rule out treatable causes of impaired cognition.

MECHANISM OF ACTION

Cholinesterase Inhibitors

Cholinesterase inhibitors act by blocking the enzyme that degrades acetylcholine in the brain. This results in more acetylcholine in the synaptic cleft and enhances cholinergic transmission. The intended effect is to diminish signs and symptoms of dementia, thereby improving function and slowing the progression of the disease, which may delay the need for nursing home placement. The effectiveness of the drugs wears off as the disease progresses, as more neurons are destroyed. No evidence suggests that cholinesterase inhibitors alter the disease process or cure the disease. Although these drugs diminish symptoms, when the medications are stopped, symptoms return, and the patient may soon become as symptomatic as if he or she had never taken the drug.

NMDA Receptor Antagonists

Memantine is an NMDA receptor antagonist. The NMDA receptor is linked to learning and memory and is stimulated by glutamic acid, the principal excitatory neurotransmitter.

Excessive stimulation of the NMDA receptor, however, leads to excitotoxicity. Blocking of this receptor is thought to prevent cognitive damage in patients with vascular dementia. Memantine blocks the excitotoxic effects associated with abnormal transmission of glutamate. It improves overall patient function, but no evidence indicates that it prevents or slows down neurodegeneration.

TREATMENT PRINCIPLES

Standardized Guidelines

- Qaseem A et al: Current pharmacologic treatment of dementia: a clinical practice guideline from the American College of Physicians and the American Academy of Family Physicians, *Ann Intern Med* 4;148(5):370-378, 2008.
- Doody RS, Stemves JC, Beck C, et al: Practice parameter: management of dementia (an evidence-based review): report of the quality standards subcommittee of the American Academy of Neurology, *Neurology* 56:1154-1166, 2001.
- U.S. Preventive Services Task Force: Screening for Dementia: recommendation and rationale, *Ann Intern Med* 138:925-926, 2003.

Evidence-Based Recommendations

- The evidence is insufficient to compare the effectiveness of different pharmacologic agents for the treatment of dementia.
- An overview of research suggests that donepezil improves cognitive function and global clinical state for up to 2 years in people with mild to severe AD. Quality of life was improved at 24 weeks. Donepezil given to patients with more severe dementia produced improvement in cognitive function at 24 weeks. Research suggests that donepezil delayed the median time to clinically evident functional decline by 5 months.
- Additional studies suggest that galantamine improves cognitive function and global clinical state over 6 months in people with AD or vascular dementia.
- One study in people with AD found no significant difference between donepezil and galantamine in cognitive function or adverse effects at 1 year.
- Ginkgo biloba and memantine are likely to be beneficial.

Cardinal Points of Treatment

- Evidence from various trials suggests that the cholinesterase inhibitors stabilize cognitive and functional ability for about 1 year.
- Pharmacologic treatment should begin as soon as disease is suspected.
- Clinicians should base the decision to initiate a trial of therapy with a cholinesterase inhibitor or memantine on individualized assessment
- Clinicians should base the choice of pharmacologic agents on tolerability, adverse effect profile, ease of use, and cost of medication.
- Depression and/or delirium should be identified and treated.
- Avoid medications with sedating or anticholinergic side effects because drugs with these side effects contribute to falls in the elderly.
- Avoid polypharmacy; use the least number of medications and the smallest doses of medication, including OTC medications.

- Treat any metabolic disorders, infections, and comorbid illnesses.
- Advise patients with dementia to avoid alcoholic beverages.

Nonpharmacologic Treatment

Educate caregivers regarding behavioral and environmental management, recommend caregiver support groups, and use community resources, including respite care.

Pharmacologic Treatment

Approximately one third of those treated with cholinesterase inhibitors exhibit a modest improvement in cognitive testing scores, function, and behavior; one third show no change; and one third are not able to tolerate the medication because of adverse effects.

- Tacrine was the first drug of this class approved for the treatment of dementia. However, it required dosing four times a day, had adverse hepatic effects, and required frequent monitoring of liver function. Tacrine has not been widely prescribed since the introduction of newer cholinesterase inhibitors. The newer drugs offer two main advantages over tacrine. First, because they do not have adverse hepatic effects, they do not require extremely frequent liver function monitoring, as tacrine does. Second, they can be given once or twice a day.
- Donepezil or galantamine ER is considered first-line therapy because it allows once-a-day dosing; donepezil is easier to titrate. Treatment should be started at 5 mg a day, which, if tolerated after 4 weeks, can be increased to 10 mg daily. Donepezil may be better tolerated than the other cholinesterase inhibitors.
- Although cholinesterase inhibitors have proved effective in stabilizing symptoms, it appears that in clinical practice, many patients receive treatment with only one ChE inhibitor for a short time, relative to the long-term course of AD. For example, in the United States, the average total duration of treatment with a ChE inhibitor is less than 200 days, which is of concern given the fact that the disease course of AD lasts approximately 7 to 10 years.
- A proportion of patients with AD fail to attain sustained clinical benefit from ChE inhibitor treatment, mainly because of lack of initial efficacy, loss of efficacy during long-term treatment, or the occurrence of safety/tolerability issues. In most instances, once a treatment is thought to be ineffective or poorly tolerated, the trial often is considered definitive and treatment is stopped altogether. Thus, many patients with AD are being "given up on" early in the course of their illness because no alternative treatment is offered. Currently, if treatment with a certain ChE inhibitor fails to provide initial or sustained efficacy or is associated with poor tolerability, patients still may benefit from another ChE inhibitor.
- Patients who should be switched include those who (1) show initial lack of efficacy, (2) initially respond to treatment but subsequently fail to benefit, or (3) experience safety/tolerability issues. Every effort to increase dose to maximize efficacy or decrease dose to reduce side effects should be made first.
- Switching should be considered only after a minimum of 6 months of treatment, beginning when the optimal dose of initial medication is reached. Treatment evaluation should be based on realistic objectives.

- Follow specific published guidelines for the medications involved. For some drugs, a drug-free period is necessary to "wash out" the drug before a new drug is introduced .

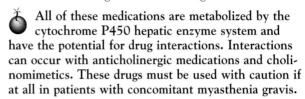 **All of these medications are metabolized by the cytochrome P450 hepatic enzyme system and have the potential for drug interactions. Interactions can occur with anticholinergic medications and cholinomimetics. These drugs must be used with caution if at all in patients with concomitant myasthenia gravis.**

- Patients with moderate to severe dementia (stages 5 through 7 on the Global Deterioration Scale, or a Mini-Mental State Examination score <10; see "How to Monitor") may be started on memantine, which may be given concomitantly with donepezil. Slight improvement in function, reduction in dependence on caregivers, and slowing of clinical decline may result.
- Some controversial studies suggest that patients with long-term ASA or nonsteroidal antiinflammatory use may have some reduction in the incidence of AD. Other evidence suggests that vitamin E slows the progression of Alzheimer's-type dementia by protecting cell membranes from the oxidative damage of free radicals. Still other studies are examining whether diet might have a protective or harmful role in the origin of AD.
- If the patient cannot tolerate a cholinesterase inhibitor because of GI or cardiac effects, NMDA inhibitors can be used alone.

How to Monitor

A variety of cognitive assessment tools are available to monitor therapeutic response to treatment. The most commonly used standardized assessment tool is the Folstein Mini-Mental State Exam (MMSE). The Global Deterioration Scale (GDS) can be used to stage dementia based on functional ability. The Katz assessment of activities of daily living (ADLs) and instrumental activities of daily living (IADLs) is useful in monitoring improvement or decline in function. Clinical evaluation and family observation of behavior and function are also helpful.

Because the liver metabolizes these drugs, periodic monitoring of hepatic function may be justified, particularly in those receiving multiple medications and in those with weight loss, anorexia or nausea, vomiting, and abdominal pain—signs and symptoms that suggest hepatic dysfunction.

- Monitor CBC and routine serum chemistry for toxic adverse events.
- Monitor heart rate and blood pressure, particularly in patients with cardiovascular disease.
- Monitor for signs and symptoms of toxicity, such as vomiting and diarrhea, diaphoresis, urinary incontinence, psychosis (including hallucinations, nervousness, and behavioral changes), and tremor. Changes in these symptoms are important to follow. If exacerbations occur, consider adjusting the medications or looking for other potential causes of delirium. It is important to note that visual hallucinations are a hallmark feature of Lewy body dementia.

Patient Variables

PEDIATRICS. Efficacy has not been established for any dementing conditions that occur in children. These drugs are used in head injuries in children.

GERIATRICS. Age does not influence the metabolism or clearance of the cholinesterase inhibitors.

 However, reduce dose and use galantamine and memantine with caution in patients with severe renal impairment (CrCl, 5-29 ml/min).

PREGNANCY AND LACTATION

- *Category C:* donepezil
- *Category B:* rivastigmine, galantamine, memantine
- No controlled studies of these drugs in pregnancy have been conducted.
- It is unknown whether these drugs are excreted in breast milk.

GENDER. Plasma concentrations are up to 50% higher in women.

Patient Education

- Caution patients not to change their dosage without consulting their health care provider.
- Advise of initial and long-term/delayed side effects. GI side effects are common; sleep disturbances may be addressed by changing the time medication is given.
- Advise of purpose, expectations from treatment, and time frame to note improvement, not cure.
- Counsel regarding behavioral and environmental management of the disease.
- Advise patients regarding long-term care, including in-home services, adult day care, assisted-living facilities, and nursing homes.
- Take donepezil in the evening, just before going to bed. Donepezil or memantine may be taken with food or on an empty stomach. Inform health care provider of medication taken before surgery. Avoid eating grapefruits or drinking grapefruit juice concurrent with medication administration.

evolve Many excellent sources of education and support are available for patients and families. See Resources for Patients and Providers on the Evolve website.

SPECIFIC DRUGS

CHOLINESTERASE INHIBITORS

donepezil (Aricept)

CONTRAINDICATIONS. Known sensitivity to the drug

PRECAUTIONS

- These drugs are cholinesterase inhibitors and, as such, may exaggerate succinylcholine-type muscle relaxation in anesthesia. Synergistic affects may occur with cholinomimetics and other cholinesterase inhibitors, such as bethanechol.
- Vagotonic effects on heart rate may be provoked, causing bradycardia. Use with caution in patients with conduction abnormalities.
- Because of their cholinergic activity, these drugs may increase gastric acid secretion. Use with caution in patients who are at increased risk for developing ulcers or who have a history of ulcer disease, as well as in patients who are taking nonsteroidal antiinflammatory drugs. Nausea, vomiting, and diarrhea may result.

- *Genitourinary effects:* may cause bladder outflow obstruction
- Use caution in patients with a history of asthma.
- These drugs may have some potential to cause generalized convulsions. However, seizure activity may also be a symptom of AD.

PHARMACOKINETICS. Donepezil is absorbed completely and reaches peak levels in 3 to 4 hours with linear pharmacokinetics. Neither food nor time of administration influences the rate or extent of absorption. Half-life is about 70 hours, and steady state is reached within 15 days. Ninety-six percent of the drug is protein bound. Seventeen percent is excreted in urine intact. The drug is extensively metabolized in the liver by the P450 2D6 and 3A4 enzyme systems.

ADVERSE EFFECTS. Donepezil is associated with nausea, vomiting, diarrhea, headache, dizziness, insomnia, fatigue, muscle cramps, and anorexia. It also may contribute to depression, abnormal dreams, and hot flashes. Use cautiously in patients with a history of asthma, COPD, cardiac disease, and seizure.

DRUG INTERACTIONS. Donepezil interacts with other drugs that are highly bound to plasma proteins. It also may interact with other drugs metabolized by P450 3A4 or 2D6 enzyme systems. No effect on the pharmacokinetics of theophylline, cimetidine, warfarin, and digoxin has been found. Donepezil may decrease the effects of anticholinergic medications.

OVERDOSAGE. Cholinergic crisis may occur. Symptoms include severe nausea, vomiting, bradycardia, sweating, convulsions, collapse, and death, if respiratory muscles are involved. Atropine is used as an antidote.

DOSAGE AND ADMINISTRATION. The newer cholinesterase inhibitors—rivastigmine and galantamine—have a similar mechanism of action and a similar adverse reaction profile. See Table 41-1 for specific dosing. Individual patients, however, may respond better to or may tolerate a different agent. At this time, these medications are not approved for combination therapy.

OTHER DRUGS IN CLASS

Other drugs in this class are similar, except that fewer adverse events seem to be associated with donepezil than with rivastigmine. It may true be that dosing and titration of donepezil is easier, and the lowest dose of donepezil is worth considering. In a sample population of nursing home residents, those taking galantamine were more likely to experience diarrhea than those taking rivastigmine or donepezil. Donepezil and galantamine have been demonstrated to be mildly effective in dementia caused by cerebral ischemia.

Rivastigmine has demonstrated a benefit for patients with dementia with Lewy bodies and for those with dementia associated with Parkinson's disease (PD).

Formulations of rivastigmine include 1.5, 3.0, 4.5, and 6.0 mg capsules and a 2 mg/ml oral solution. The recommended maintenance dosage for these oral formulations is 6 to 12 mg/day for Alzheimer's dementia and 3 to 12 mg/day for dementia associated with PD.

Rivastigmine is also available as a transdermal system (Exelon Patch) for the treatment of mild to moderate

TABLE 41-1   Dosage and Administration of Cognitive Function Drugs

Drug	Dosage	Half-life	Onset	Time to Peak Concentration	Duration	Administration
donepezil	5-10 mg po daily	70 hr		Several weeks	6 wk	Administer at bedtime; increase to 10 mg after 4-8 wk at 5 mg; 10-mg dose may have improved effect at expense of increased cholinergic side effects.
rivastigmine	1.5-6 mg po bid

4.6 mg 24 hr patch or 9.5 mg 24 hr patch | 1.5 hr | Within 2 wk | Up to 12 wk | | Administer with morning and evening meals; increase dosage by 1.5 mg bid q2wk; if GI side effects occur, hold dose for several days and restart at lower dosage. Apply patch every 24 hours at the same time daily at a different body site as directed to reduce skin irritation; exposure of the patch to external heat sources (e.g., excess sunlight, saunas, solarium) for long periods should be avoided. |
galantamine	4-12 mg po bid	7 hr		1 hr	12 hr	Administer with morning and evening meals; increase dosage by 4 mg bid q4wk; if treatment is interrupted, restart at lowest dosage and titrate up.
galantamine ER	8-24 mg po daily	7 hr		1 hr	24 hr	Start with 8 mg daily given with morning meal; increase dosage by 8 mg per day q4wk if tolerated for maximum of 24 mg/day.
memantine	10 mg po bid	60-80 hr		3-7 hr	12 hr	Start with 5 mg in AM; increase in 5-mg increments to 5 mg bid—5 in AM, 10 in PM; then 10 mg bid with 1 wk interval between dosage increases. Take with or without food.

Alzheimer's dementia and mild to moderate dementia associated with PD. Rivastigmine patches are available in two sizes: 5 cm^2 (4.6 mg/24 hr dosage) and 10 cm^2 (9.5 mg/24 hr dosage). The patch was designed with compliance in mind and has been well received by caregivers as a method of drug delivery because it helps them follow the treatment schedule, interferes less with their daily lives, and is easier to use overall than the oral medication. Side effects include nausea, vomiting, and diarrhea.

When patients are switched from capsules or oral solution formulations, those receiving a total daily dose of <6 mg of the oral formulation initially should use the 4.6 mg/24 hr patch. Initial use of the 9.5 mg/24 hr patch is advised for patients taking a total daily oral dose ranging from 6 to 12 mg. The first patch should be applied on the day following the last oral dose. No dose adjustments are required for patients with hepatic or renal impairment. However, those with body weight <50 kg may be at increased risk for adverse events. Treatment should be interrupted for several days if significant adverse events occur and then should be resumed at the same or next lower dose level. Treatment that is interrupted for longer than several days should be reinitiated at the lowest daily dose and uptitrated after 1 month as tolerated.

Patients or caregivers should be taught the importance of applying the correct dose to the correct part of the body. Application sites should be rotated to reduce skin irritation; the same site should not be used within 14 days.

NMDA RECEPTOR ANTAGONISTS

memantine (Namenda)

CONTRAINDICATIONS. Hypersensitivity

PRECAUTIONS
- Seizures occur in a small number of patients.
- Reduce dose in patients with severe renal impairment.
- Genitourinary conditions, drugs, and diets that raise urine pH will increase plasma levels of memantine.
- Observe caution with concomitant use of other NMDA antagonists.

PHARMACOKINETICS. Memantine is well absorbed. It has a half-life of 60 to 80 hours and is excreted unchanged in urine. The CYP system plays no significant role.

ADVERSE EFFECTS. Hypertension, tachycardia, dizziness, headache, back pain, gait abnormalities, arthralgia, confusion, somnolence, hallucination, cough, weight gain or loss, sweating, nausea, vomiting, diarrhea, constipation, anorexia, and urinary incontinence. Use cautiously in patients with impairment or a history of seizures.

DRUG INTERACTIONS. Use caution with acetazolamide, cimetidine, dichlorphenamide, hydrochlorothiazide, methazolamide, nicotine, quinidine, ranitidine, and sodium bicarbonate.

DOSAGE AND ADMINISTRATION. May take concurrently with cholinesterase inhibitors for better results. See Table 41-1.

evolve A continually updated list of useful WebLinks may be found in the Evolve Resources at http://evolve.elsevier.com/Edmunds/NP/

42 Analgesia and Pain Management

V. INEZ WENDEL

DRUG OVERVIEW

Class	Subclass	Generic Name	Trade Name
Opioid agonists	Phenanthrenes	morphine sulfate (extended release)	MS Contin, Avinza, Kadian
		morphine 🔑, morphine (short acting)	MS-IR
		codeine with or without acetaminophen ✺	Codeine Tylenol #3
		hydrocodone with acetaminophen ✺	Lortab, Vicodin
		hydrocodone with ibuprofen ✺	Vicoprofen
		oxycodone ✺	OxyContin ✺
		oxycodone with aspirin	Percodan
		oxycodone with acetaminophen ✺	Endocet ✺ Percocet, Roxicet ✺, Tylox
		hydromorphone	Dilaudid
	Phenylpiperidines	meperidine	Demerol
		fentanyl	Sublimaze, Duragesic transdermal, Actiq (transmucosal)
	Diphenylheptanes	methadone	Dolophine
		propoxyphene	Darvon
		propoxyphene-N (with acetaminophen) ✺	Darvocet
Mixed agonist-antagonists	—	pentazocine	Talwin
Partial agonists	—	tramadol ✺	Ultram
		tramadol with acetaminophen ✺	Ultracet

✺ Top 200 drug; 🔑 key drug. Morphine has been designated a key drug because, traditionally, all opioids were compared with morphine.

Information about acetaminophen can be found in Chapter 33.
Information about aspirin and NSAIDs can be found in Chapter 34.

INDICATIONS

- Symptomatic treatment for moderate to severe acute pain
- Used to induce sedation as a form of anesthesia (preoperative medication)
- Postsurgical pain
- Severe diarrhea and cramping
- Dyspnea related to left ventricular failure or pulmonary edema
- Methadone only: detoxification of opioid addiction
- Codeine only: persistent cough

This chapter discusses pain management in the outpatient setting, including the use of drugs other than opioids, but it focuses on the use of opioids in pain management; only the common drugs listed above are discussed in detail.

Natural opioids come from opium, which is obtained from unripe seed capsules of the poppy plant. Opium contains more than 20 distinct alkaloids. The main phenanthrenes are morphine, codeine, and thebaine. The benzylisoquinolines are papaverine (a smooth muscle relaxant) and noscapine. Heroin is diacetylmorphine, which is metabolized to morphine.

Synthetic opioids were developed in the hope of producing a less addictive drug. These attempts failed, but the drugs have proved to be extremely useful for management of both acute and chronic pain. Many semisynthetic derivatives are made through simple modifications of morphine or thebaine. Morphine is the precursor of the synthetic opioid analgesics hydrocodone, hydromorphone, and oxycodone. Thebaine is the precursor of naloxone, an opioid antagonist. The phenylpiperidines and the diphenylheptanes are chemical classes that are structurally distinct yet similar to morphine. These drugs have actions similar to those of morphine.

The opioids are classified as narcotics and thus are considered controlled substances because of their abuse potential, as mandated by the Controlled Substances Act of 1970. Clinicians should be familiar with regulations regarding the use and dispensing of narcotic analgesics. Methadone is prescribed chiefly for the treatment of opiate detoxification and may be dispensed only by pharmacies and maintenance programs approved by the FDA and by state authorities, according to the requirements of the Federal Methadone Regulations. Methadone also is used for pain management; it may be prescribed by any provider with a DEA license to prescribe Schedule II drugs and can be dispensed by any licensed pharmacy (see Chapter 8). Because of the potential for abuse, the health care provider must justify the use of opioid analgesics for ambulatory patients.

Morphine is the standard opioid with which all others are compared. It is used extensively in acute care and hospice settings. Codeine, hydrocodone, and oxycodone are used frequently in combination with acetaminophen in both acute and primary care settings. Hydromorphone is very potent (five times the potency of morphine) and is reserved for severe pain not relieved by morphine; primary care providers generally will not prescribe this drug. Opioid agonist-antagonists also are used and may be preferred over traditional opioids for use in ambulatory patients because their potential for abuse is lower. Pentazocine has limited use because of CNS toxicity. Tramadol is a weak opioid agonist that inhibits the reuptake of norepinephrine and serotonin, thus modifying the patient's perception of pain.

THERAPEUTIC OVERVIEW

Pathophysiology

Melzack and Wall's gate control theory of pain is the most comprehensive pain theory proposed to date. They suggest that four processes are required for pain to occur: transduction, transmission, modulation, and perception. Sensory receptors, or nociceptors, that are sensitive to painful or tissue-damaging (noxious) stimuli are present in the skin, bone; muscle; connective tissue; and thoracic, abdominal, and pelvic viscera.

Transduction occurs when a noxious stimulus depolarizes peripheral nerve endings and sets off electrical activity. The nerve endings that transduce the noxious stimuli conduct electrical signals to the spinal cord through two types of nerve fibers: A delta fibers and C fibers. A delta fibers are myelinated, and their activation is associated with sharp, stinging sensations. C fibers are unmyelinated, and their activation is associated with vaguely localized pain that may be dull or burning.

Next, transmission occurs, whereby electrical impulses are carried throughout the peripheral and CNS. Modulation is the central neural activity that controls the transmission of pain impulses. Finally, during perception, the neural activities involved in transmission and modulation result in a subjective correlate of pain that includes behavioral, psychologic, and emotional factors (Figure 42-1).

Disease Process

Pain is defined by the International Association for the Study of Pain (IASP) as "an unpleasant sensory and emotional experience associated with actual or potential tissue damage, or described in terms of such damage. Pain is always subjective."

OPIOID TOLERANCE, DEPENDENCE, AND ADDICTION. All opioid drugs cause tolerance and dependence. This is not the same as abuse. *Tolerance* is a pharmacologic phenomenon characterized by decreasing drug effect over time. More drug is needed to produce the same effect. *Dependence* is the physiologic development of abstinence syndrome or withdrawal symptoms when a drug is discontinued or an antagonist is given. Slowly tapering the drug can eliminate withdrawal symptoms. Psychologic dependence, or *addiction*, is the overwhelming obsession with obtaining and using a drug for a non–medically approved purpose. Tolerance and dependence

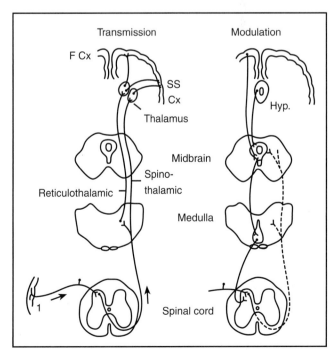

FIGURE 42-1 Pain transmission and modulation. (From Fields HL: *Pain,* New York, 1987, McGraw-Hill.)

are the consequences of regular use of an opioid for a particular length of time and are not a problem. Addiction is a problem; however, a patient in pain should not be deprived of adequate pain relief because of fear of addiction.

Some patients exhibit specific behaviors when pain is undertreated; this has come to be called *pseudoaddiction*. These individuals watch the clock, demand pain medication, and may even resort to illegal means to get drugs. This phenomenon can be distinguished from true addiction in that the behavior ceases when the patient attains adequate pain control.

ORIGIN OF PAIN. Although the trend is to consider pain as a single entity, some authors still distinguish between acute and chronic pain. Acute pain usually is related to an identifiable injury, such as recent surgery, trauma, or infection, and resolves within a predictable and expected time interval. Chronic pain seems to be the result of physiologic changes in the nervous system caused by untreated or undertreated, persistent acute pain. Although injury may initiate chronic pain, factors remote from its cause may perpetuate it, leading to unexplainable persistence. Currently, an estimated 50 million Americans suffer from chronic pain. This number will increase as the population ages and treatment for pain-related chronic health problems, such as back disorders, degenerative joint diseases, rheumatologic conditions, visceral diseases, and cancer, is increased. In the person with cancer-related pain, about 60% to 70% of pain is related to the tumor, 15% to 20% is related to diagnostic procedures or treatment for cancer, and the remaining 0% to 15% is completely unrelated to cancer or its treatment.

CLASSIFICATION OF PAIN. Pain can be classified as nociceptive or neuropathic (Table 42-1). Nociceptive pain is further divided into two categories: somatic and visceral. Nociceptive pain arises from the direct stimulation of afferent nerves in cutaneous or deep musculoskeletal tissues. It occurs in response to tissue injury or disease infiltration of the skin, soft tissue, or viscera. Somatic pain is well localized in skin and subcutaneous tissues but not in bone, muscle, blood vessels, and connective tissue and is often described as dull or aching. Visceral pain is poorly localized and often is described as a continual aching, or a deep, crampy, or sharp, squeezing pain. Visceral pain may be referred to dermatomal or myotomal sites that are distant from the source of pain. Visceral pain occurs in response to stretching, distention, compression, or infiltration of organs such as the liver.

Neuropathic pain, which results from injury to peripheral nerves or to the CNS, is described as episodes of shooting or stabbing pain superimposed over a background of aching and burning. Because it originates from peripheral nerves, spinal cord, or brain, it is poorly localized and often is associated with paresthesias and dysesthesias.

Assessment

It is important for the clinician to determine the cause of pain whenever possible. Even in a patient with terminal cancer, each new pain should be evaluated for a proximate cause that may be specifically treated. For example, bone pain may be ameliorated by radiation. Severe flares of pain are called "breakthrough pain" because they may break through the pain medication. Patients learn what triggers these breakthrough episodes so they can plan with the provider for how to prevent or resolve them.

Initial pain assessment seeks to characterize the pathophysiology of the pain, identify its cause, determine its intensity, and evaluate its impact on the patient's ability to function. Assessment should include a detailed history and physical examination, psychosocial and functional assessment, and diagnostic evaluation as indicated. Associated findings of acute pain can include facial grimacing, tachycardia, hypertension, pallor, diaphoresis, mydriasis, and nausea. Chronic pain may be accompanied by fatigue, depression, sleep disturbance, decreased appetite, increased irritability, and decreased libido. Visible facial expressions of pain usually are lacking, and physiologic signs may be absent. Patients also can have intermittent chronic pain, such as recurrent episodes of neuralgia, headache, or angina.

Because pain is a subjective experience, assessment also must include patient self-report, which includes a description of pain and its onset, duration, and diurnal variation, as well as information on the location and radiation of pain, its intensity or severity, aggravating and relieving factors, and the patient's goal for pain control. A variety of common pain assessment tools can be used with to help grade pain severity in children and adults.

Follow-up assessment of the outcome of pain management is required to assess the effectiveness of the intervention.

TABLE 42-1 Classification of Pain

Category	Characteristics	Examples
NOCICEPTIVE		
Somatic	Well localized Dull, aching, or throbbing	Laceration, fracture, cellulitis, arthritis
Visceral	Poorly localized Continual aching Referred to dermatomal sites that are distant from the source of pain	Subscapular pain arising from diaphragmatic irritation Right upper quadrant pain arising from stretching of the liver capsule
NEUROPATHIC		
	Shooting or stabbing pain superimposed over a background of aching and burning Pain not well localized	Post-herpetic neuralgia, post-thoracotomy neuralgia, poststroke pain, trigeminal neuralgia, diabetic polyneuropathy

Changes in pain pattern or the development of new pain should trigger reassessment, diagnostic evaluation, and modification of the treatment plan. Documentation of a patient's adherence with regard to dosing and duration of prescriptions is essential for all pain management. The provider should assess functioning and barriers to or facilitators of nonprescription treatment, especially sleep, activity, diet, diversion, and so forth.

The Agency for Health Care Policy and Research (AHCPR) clinical practice guidelines, although dated, include the following classic principles of pain assessment (A-A-B-C-D-E-E):
- Ask about pain at every office visit or phone call.
- Assess pain systematically. (Be consistent in using the same pain intensity scales for pain measurement.)
- Believe the patient and family regarding their reports of pain and what relieves it.
- Choose pain control options that are appropriate for the patient, family, and setting.
- Delivery of pharmacologic or nonpharmacologic interventions should be made in a timely, logical, and coordinated fashion.
- Empower patients and their families.
- Enable them to control their course to the greatest extent possible.

MECHANISM OF ACTION

Opioid Agonists

Opioid analgesics are thought to inhibit painful stimuli in the substantia gelatinosa of the spinal cord, brainstem, reticular activating system, thalamus, and limbic system. Opiate receptors in each of these areas interact with neurotransmitters of the autonomic nervous system, producing alterations in reaction to painful stimuli. The opioid action of the drug manifests as analgesia, sedation, euphoria, mental clouding, respiratory depression, miosis, decreased peristaltic motility, depression of the cough reflex, and orthostatic hypotension.

Opiate receptors in the CNS mediate analgesic activity. Opioid agonists occupy the same receptors as endogenous opioid peptides, and both alter the central release of neurotransmitters from afferent nerves sensitive to noxious stimuli.

Actions of opioid analgesics can be defined by their activity at three specific receptor types: mu, kappa, and delta. The mu receptors mediate morphine-like supraspinal analgesia, miosis, respiratory depression, euphoria, physical dependence, and suppression of opiate withdrawal. The kappa receptors mediate spinal analgesia, respiratory depression, and sedation. The delta receptors mediate antagonist activity (Table 42-2). Morphine-like agonists have activity at the mu, kappa, and delta receptors. Mixed agonist-antagonist drugs, such as pentazocine, have agonist activity at some receptors and antagonist activity at other receptors. The opioid antagonist naloxone does not have agonist activity at any opioid receptors.

The mechanism by which opioids produce euphoria is not clear. They alter hypothalamic heat regulation in such a way that body temperature often falls slightly. They also affect the hypothalamus by causing decreased levels of testosterone, cortisol, ACTH, and β-endorphin. With long-term use, this effect diminishes. CNS effects in the limbic system can include dysphoric mood, especially with long-term use, intense and unusual dreams, and hallucinations. Pupillary miosis results from excitatory effects on the parasympathetic nerves that cause constriction of the pupil.

The respiratory depression associated with opioids is caused by a direct effect on the brainstem respiratory centers by which the brainstem becomes less responsive to carbon dioxide. Death from morphine overdose is usually the result of respiratory arrest. The cough reflex is depressed by a direct effect on the cough center in the medulla. This event is separate from respiratory depression.

Opioids produce nausea and vomiting through direct stimulation of the chemoreceptor trigger zone for emesis in the medulla. A vestibular component is part of the effect, in that nausea and vomiting are more common in ambulatory patients than in those on bed rest.

Opioids produce peripheral vasodilation, reduce peripheral vascular resistance, and inhibit baroreceptor reflexes, causing orthostatic hypotension and fainting.

The effects of opioids on the GI system are many. They decrease gastric motility, thereby prolonging gastric emptying time and increasing the likelihood of esophageal reflux. With opioid use, the absorption of other orally administered drugs is retarded. Opioids diminish biliary, pancreatic, and intestinal secretions. The sphincter of Oddi constricts and causes increased pressure in the common bile duct, leading to biliary colic. Opioids delay digestion of food in the small intestine. Propulsive peristaltic waves in the colon are diminished and

TABLE 42-2   Action of Opioids on Pain Receptor Sites

Receptor	Primary Location	Function	Associated With	Opioids Involved
Mu$_1$	Supraspinal, periphery	Mediate somatic primarily, and visceral analgesia	Supraspinal analgesia, peripheral analgesia euphoria, sedation	morphine-like, endorphin
Mu$_2$	Spinal		Spinal analgesia, respiratory depression, dependence, decreased GI motility, miosis, pruritus	
Kappa$_1$	Spinal	Mediate visceral pain	Spinal analgesia, sedation, miosis,	pentazocine, morphine (slight), dynorphin
Kappa$_2$	Spinal		Dysphoria	
Kappa$_3$	>Supraspinal		Supraspinal analgesia	
Delta	Spinal >supraspinal	Antagonist activity	Spinal and supraspinal analgesia, tachycardia, tachypnea, dysphoria, hallucinations, mydriasis, hypertonia	Antagonists, enkephalins

tone is increased to the point of spasm. This delays the passage of stool and leads to constipation.

Opioids inhibit the urinary voiding reflex and may cause urinary retention. They also may prolong labor. Opioids cause dilation of cutaneous blood vessels, resulting in flushing. Some opioids—morphine and meperidine, but not methadone or fentanyl—cause histamine release. This may lead to pruritus, sweating, and urticaria. The opioids affect the immune system in a manner that is poorly understood, but they seem to cause suppression of natural killer cells.

Mixed Agonist-Antagonists

The mixed agonist-antagonists produce potent analgesic effects by stimulating the kappa receptor and blocking the mu receptor. Thus, they may produce withdrawal symptoms in patients with opioid dependency but are also less likely to be abused when compared with pure opioid agonists.

evolve For additional information, see the supplemental tables on the Evolve Learning Resource website.

TREATMENT PRINCIPLES

Standardized Guidelines

- Gruener D, Lande SD, editors: *Pain control in the primary care setting*, Glenview, IL, 2006, American Pain Society. (Available at www.ampainsoc.org)
- American Pain Society: *Principles of analgesic use in the treatment of acute pain and cancer pain*, Glenview, IL, 2003, American Pain Society.
- Chou R, Huffman LH, American Pain Society, American College of Physicians: Medications for acute and chronic low back pain: a review of the evidence for an American Pain Society/American College of Physicians clinical practice guideline, *Ann Intern Med* 147:505-514, 2007.

Evidence-Based Recommendations

- Some evidence suggests that long-term management of chronic pain with opiates may significantly improve functional outcomes and quality of life.
- Morphine is effective in providing relief of moderate to severe pain but is associated with the adverse effects of constipation, nausea, and vomiting.
- Limited evidence suggests that there is very little difference between hydromorphone and other opioids in terms of analgesic efficacy, adverse effects, and patient preference.
- Limited evidence indicates that methadone is effective for relief of cancer pain, and it is available for administration via multiple routes.
- Randomized, controlled trials conducted to support the practice of switching opioids to manage inadequate pain relief and intolerable side effects are lacking.

Cardinal Points of Treatment

- Chronic pain requires routine administration of drugs. Giving medication before pain is severe means that the patient will use less of the drug. The clinician should instruct that medication is to be given regularly without waiting until the patient is in severe pain and is begging for medication. Experts agree that addiction generally is not a concern, especially for patients with chronic pain or terminal illness. Primary care providers should be comfortable about treating patients who have chronic pain. Pain

of greater severity may be relieved by combining therapies. More severe pain may require the addition of an opioid preparation that is useful at higher dosages. Analgesic adjuvants may be useful. Frequent follow-up is needed to assess outcomes and side effects, provide reassurance, and establish goals. It is unrealistic to expect total pain relief in patients with chronic pain. Concurrent problems such as depression, anxiety, and insomnia augment the perception of pain in many patients.

- The variety of patients who present with pain is extensive, and treatment should be individualized to the patient's response. Acute mild to moderate pain, such as that seen with strains and sprains, is commonly managed in the primary care setting. Acute severe pain usually is managed in an acute care setting to address the underlying cause, such as acute myocardial infarction or fracture. Chronic pain, both benign and malignant, is managed in primary care or by referral to specialty pain management clinics. Hospice referral is important for the management of pain and other symptoms associated with terminal disease and dying. Because of reimbursement mechanisms and changes in practice, pain management is being moved increasingly from the purview of the specialist to the primary care setting.

- Patients with chronic pain may have multiple problems, including psychiatric responses to chronic pain and other comorbid conditions. Simply prescribing a pill is not an effective way to manage pain. These patients require a comprehensive pain management program that includes the patient, the family, and caregivers, along with all health care providers, including specialists. The plan must be consistent from one health professional to the next. Primary care clinicians may have to refer patients to pain management clinics for evaluation and specialized treatment, such as nerve block. Hospice referral must be considered for terminal conditions.

Nonpharmacologic Treatment

- For adequate treatment of pain, first, the cause must be identified, then management of the underlying disease must be maximized. Refer the patient to appropriate specialists and members of the interdisciplinary team, such as orthopedists, neurosurgeons, psychiatrists, pain specialists, physical and occupational therapists, or hospice staff, for further evaluation and additional interventions. Provide the patient with education regarding the nature of pain, assessment tools (use of pain scales and pain diaries), and the purposes and expected results of nonpharmacologic and pharmacologic management. To reduce anxiety, allow the patient to have some control over the situation and to make decisions when possible.

- Nonpharmacologic treatment of pain can be used alone or in combination with medications. Nonpharmacologic measures include patient education, management of anxiety and depression, cognitive-behavioral therapy, and appropriate exercise and activity. Common cognitive-behavioral interventions include distraction, meditation, and progressive relaxation therapy. Expressive therapies such as art, music, and movement therapy also have proved effective. Complementary and alternative medicine therapies may be helpful, although little scientific evidence is available to support the use of chiropractic manipulation, homeopathy, and spiritual healing. Heat, ice, massage, topical analgesics, acupuncture, and transcutaneous electrical nerve stimulation (TENS) may provide relief when used alone or in combination with analgesic medications.

Pharmacologic Treatment

- Whenever possible for mild to moderate pain, begin pharmacologic pain management with acetaminophen on an around-the-clock schedule if the patient has not yet tried this regimen. The maximum dose for patients without renal or hepatic dysfunction or alcohol use is 4000 mg/day given in divided doses. If acetaminophen is not effective, an NSAID can be used. The combined use of NSAIDs and acetaminophen is unlikely to improve pain relief. NSAIDs have a side effect of GI bleeding; in addition, they elevate blood pressure, cause fluid retention, and may provoke renal failure, particularly in the elderly.
- If nonopioid medications are not effective or are not tolerated, opiates can be given alone or with acetaminophen for nonmalignant and malignant pain. Dosage may depend on whether the patient is opiate naïve. Fear of drug dependency or addiction does not justify withholding of opiates or inadequate management of pain. Advise patients regarding side effects and driving. Prophylactically treat constipation.
- Adjuvant drugs, which are medications developed for purposes other than analgesia, use different pain pathways in reducing pain. They are particularly useful for neuropathic pain when given alone or in combination with NSAIDs or opioids. Gabapentin and other, newer anticonvulsants are good first-line choices and have fewer side effects than the older tricyclic antidepressants (Table 42-3). Serotonin reuptake inhibitors such as Paxil and serotonin norepinephrine reuptake inhibitors such as Cymbalta have also proved effective.

If opioids are to be used, particularly in the patient who has never been on opiates, the following recommendations apply:
- Start at the lowest possible dose.
- If converting from one opioid to another, use an equianalgesic dose.
- Adjust the dosage to achieve pain relief with acceptable levels of adverse effects.
- Titration rate depends on the half-life of the selected opioid.
- No ceiling effect is seen with analgesia with pure opioid agonists; the ceiling is limited only by side effects.

STEPS TO CHANGING OPIOIDS
- Calculate the 24-hour dose of current opioids, including around-the-clock and rescue doses.
- Use an equianalgesic table to convert the dosage of the current drug to the equivalent dosage of the new drug.
- Adjust the dosage of the new drug to accommodate patient variability and to account for incomplete cross-tolerance.
- Determine the dosing interval according to the duration of action of the new opioid.
- Calculate rescue doses.

GUIDELINES FOR STARTING DOSES OF NEW OPIOIDS.
After the 24-hour dosage of the new opioid has been determined, reduce the dosage by 25% to 50% based on the following:
- Patient age
- Pain intensity
- Renal/hepatic dysfunction
- Incomplete cross-tolerance

The new dosage may have to be reduced by 75% when one is treating frail, elderly patients or those who have the following:
- Moderate pain
- Major organ dysfunction (renal/hepatic disease)
- History of adverse reactions to opioids

Rescue Doses (rarely ordered by primary care clinicians except for hospice care)
- Administer rescue doses to patients to relieve breakthrough pain that occurs despite their regularly scheduled around-the-clock drug regimen:
  - Give 5% to 15% of the 24-hour oral dose.
  - Administer oral rescue doses every 1 to 2 hours as needed.
  - Administer parenteral rescue doses every 15 to 60 minutes.

How to Monitor

- The severity of pain experienced by the patient determines which parameters should be monitored. The initial database should be used to formulate treatment goals and to monitor progress.
- The patient who is taking opioids should be seen at least weekly until pain is controlled, and perhaps more frequently, depending on the nature of the condition. Once stable, the patient should be seen regularly.

TABLE 42-3   Adjuvant Analgesics

Drug Class	Indications	Comments	Examples
Anticonvulsants	Neuropathic pain from diabetic neuropathy, trigeminal neuralgia, post-herpetic neuralgia, glossopharyngeal neuralgia, and neuralgia from nerve trauma or cancer infiltration	Especially useful for episodic lancing or burning pain	clonazepam gabapentin pregabalin
Neuroleptics	Chronic pain syndromes, moderate to severe pain unrelieved by opioids, or the presence of severe side effects with use of opioids	Antiemetic and anxiolytic effects	chlorpromazine
Tricyclic antidepressants	Neuropathic pain, including post-herpetic neuralgia and neuropathy	These drugs have innate analgesic properties and may potentiate the analgesic effects of opioids. Anticholinergic side effects	amitriptyline nortriptyline
Serotonin/norepinephrine reuptake inhibitors	Pain from diabetic neuropathy	Only drug of its class that is FDA approved for the treatment of diabetic neuropathy	duloxetine

- Assess for therapeutic effect. Use a standard pain assessment tool.
- Assess the patient for the occurrence of common side effects, dependency, and interference with activities of daily living or lifestyle patterns.
- Most patients on opioids become constipated.
- Monitor for nausea, especially when the patient is starting to take opioids.

For very fragile patients, specific signs and symptoms that should be assessed at baseline and as necessary while the patient is taking medications include the following:

- Vital signs, including orthostatic blood pressure
- *Respiratory function:* Rate, breath sounds
- Cardiac heart sounds
- *Abdomen:* Abdominal sounds, bowel and urinary functions
- *Psychiatric:* Dysphoria, confusion, disturbing dreams, insomnia, and hallucinations

Patient Variables

GERIATRICS. Elderly patients are more susceptible to CNS side effects of opioids and to constipation. Usually, they should be placed on a bowel regimen when opioids are started. Use a lower dose of opioids. In elderly patients, avoid or use with caution propoxyphene, tramadol, and methadone.

PEDIATRICS. Children experience pain in the same way that adults do. Sometimes, they have greater difficulty communicating their pain, so providers must be alert. A pain scale that uses smiling or frowning faces may facilitate assessment of pain. Use morphine, codeine, or meperidine; do not use oxycodone, propoxyphene, methadone, or pentazocine. The safety of hydromorphone in children has not been established.

PREGNANCY AND LACTATION. Every drug discussed in this chapter except oxycodone belongs to Category C (Category D with prolonged use or high doses at term); oxycodone belongs to Category B (maternal addiction and neonatal withdrawal occur after illicit use). Some association of first-trimester exposure and congenital defects with codeine has been shown. Although significant respiratory depression of the mother may be lacking when morphine is administered before delivery, the neonate may exhibit respiratory depression because of an immature blood-brain barrier. Opioids cross the placental barrier and are excreted in breast milk.

Patient Education

- Take medications exactly as prescribed. It may be important to jot down times when medication was last taken to prevent overdosing.
- Work to taper doses if taken over a long time.
- Although this product has the potential for addiction, used properly, this should not be a problem.
- It is most effective when taken before severe pain is experienced.
- Use other methods of relieving pain whenever possible.
- Do not take any other medications without informing your health provider.
- Do not drink alcoholic beverages.
- Inform your health care provider of all prescribed, over-the-counter, and herbal medications that you are taking.

- Report to your health care provider any new or troublesome symptoms. Common side effects include constipation, suppression of the cough reflex, dizziness, nausea, drowsiness, sweating, and flushing.
- After you have taken this medication, avoid operating heavy machinery, driving, or performing tasks that require alertness.
- Urinate frequently and monitor bowel habits daily. Report to your health care practitioner any problems associated with constipation.
- Rise slowly from a lying or sitting position to minimize feelings of light-headedness. Avoid standing in one position for long periods.
- During initial doses, lie down for short periods to avoid developing nausea.
- Family members should alert the health care practitioner if any of the following are noted in the patient: presence of shallow, slow respirations; shortness of breath; pupil constriction; deep sleep; vomiting; abdominal pain; palpitations; and skin rash.
- Keep this medication out of the reach of children and all others for whom it is not prescribed. Dispose of all extra medication when it is no longer needed. Do not keep it for another time. Do not share this medicine with any other person.

SPECIFIC DRUGS

OPIOID AGONISTS
Phenanthrenes

---

morphine (MS Contin, Avinza, and Kadian) (Schedule II Drug) 🔑

Other opioids are compared with morphine in terms of efficacy (Table 42-4). Morphine is the primary opioid analgesic used for relief of severe pain. It is classified as a Schedule II controlled substance. Morphine is more effective against dull, continuous pain than for sharp, spasmodic pain.

CONTRAINDICATIONS
- Hypersensitivity to opioids
- Acute bronchial asthma and/or upper airway obstruction
- Premature infants or during the delivery of a premature infant
- Epidural or intrathecal morphine should not be given in the presence of infection at the injection site or to a patient on anticoagulation therapy or with any condition or medication therapy that would contraindicate epidural or intrathecal anesthesia
- Respiratory insufficiency, CNS depression, increased intracranial pressure, acute alcohol intoxication, convulsive disorders, heart failure secondary to chronic lung disease, and cardiac arrhythmias
- Patients taking MAOIs or who have received MAOIs within 14 days
- Pregnancy (prolonged use or high doses at term)

WARNINGS

💣 Fatal overdose may result if the extended-release form is chewed, crushed, or diluted.

---

morphine (MS Contin, Avinza, and Kadian) (Schedule II Drug) 🔑 —cont'd

- In cases of head injury and increased intracranial pressure, opioids may obscure the clinical picture.
- In asthma and other respiratory conditions, use with extreme caution because opioids depress the respiratory drive while increasing airway resistance.
- These products may cause severe hypotension, especially in patients at risk for orthostatic hypotension.

PRECAUTIONS

- When given to patients with renal or hepatic dysfunction, these products may have a prolonged duration and a cumulative effect, requiring reduced dosage and longer intervals between doses.
- Opioids may obscure diagnosis in acute abdominal conditions.
- Use with caution in patients who are elderly, debilitated, hypoxic, or sensitive to CNS depressants and in those who have hypercapnic cardiovascular disease, myxedema, convulsive disorder, increased ocular pressure, acute alcoholism, delirium tremens, cerebral arteriosclerosis, ulcerative colitis, fever, decreased respiratory reserve, hypothyroidism, kyphoscoliosis, Addison's disease, prostatic hypertrophy, urethral stricture, CNS depression, coma, gallbladder disease, recent GI or genitourinary tract surgery, or toxic psychosis.
- Use with caution in patients with supraventricular tachycardias; vagolytic action may increase the ventricular response rate.
- Opioids suppress the cough reflex, which may be a problem in elderly or frail patients with pulmonary problems.
- Some products contain sulfites, which produce asthma-like symptoms in sensitive individuals.
- These agents may produce drowsiness or dizziness; advise patients to observe caution while driving or performing other tasks that require alertness or physical activity.
- Monitor for drug abuse and dependence.

PHARMACOKINETICS. Opioids are readily absorbed from the GI tract (Table 42-5). Opioids that are more lipophilic are absorbed through the nasal or buccal mucosa and through the skin. All are readily absorbed after subcutaneous or intramuscular injection. Oral opioids undergo a variable but significant first-pass effect, thus decreasing the bioavailability of oral preparations. Morphine is 17% to 33% bioavailable. The time-effect curve is prolonged by the oral route; this lengthens the duration of action. Approximately 30% to 35% of the drug is protein bound. Opioid analgesics are metabolized in the liver through glucuronidation and to a lesser extent by the cytochrome P450 2D6 enzyme system. They are excreted through the kidney in a conjugated form. Genetic variability produces wide differences in how quickly opioids are metabolized. All opioids are excreted in urine; some are excreted to a small extent in feces.

ADVERSE EFFECTS. The most common adverse effects are constipation, dry mouth, headache, light-headedness, dizziness, sedation, nausea, vomiting, and sweating (Table 42-6).

DRUG INTERACTIONS

- *With P450 2D6:* See Table 42-7.
- *With analgesics.* In general, CNS depressant effects may be potentiated by the concomitant use of other opioid analgesics, alcohol, antianxiety agents, barbiturates, anesthetics, nonbarbiturate sedative-hypnotics, phenothiazines, skeletal muscle relaxants, and tricyclic antidepressants. (Respiratory depression, hypotension, profound sedation, and coma also may result.) Use of opioids with furosemide may aggravate or produce orthostatic hypotension. Concurrent use of opioids with anticholinergics may produce paralytic ileus. The phenothiazines enhance the sedative effects of the opioids. Plasma amylase or lipase levels may be unreliable for 24 hours after administration of opioids. Morphine may potentiate the anticoagulation effects of warfarin.

OVERDOSAGE. Signs and symptoms of overdosage include the following:

- *Acute overdose:* Profound respiratory depression, respiratory rate less than 12 breaths/min; irregular and shallow respirations, deep sleep, stupor or coma, miosis, cyanosis, gradually decreasing blood pressure, oliguria, clammy skin, hypothermia
- *Chronic abuse:* Constricted pupils, skin infection, mood changes, depressed level of consciousness, itching, needle scars, abscesses

DOSAGE AND ADMINISTRATION. The dosage and formulation of opioid analgesic used depends on the severity of pain experienced by the patient, the response to pain and medication, the nature of the illness, and the route of administration. This category may be administered via oral, rectal, sublingual, intramuscular, subcutaneous, and intravenous routes. The oral route is used most often in primary care, except in terminally ill patients. In some patients with chronic pain, long-acting delivery systems may be used more often, along with transmucosal systems for breakthrough pain.

Refer the patient to the hospice for assistance.

Morphine sulfate comes in immediate-release and extended-release formulations. The immediate-release formulation, IR morphine, is given for breakthrough pain. IR morphine comes in tablet and liquid formulations. Morphine oral concentrate at 20 mg/ml can be used sublingually in patients who are unable to swallow.

ER formulations such as MS Contin and Avinza are used for routine administration in chronic pain. MS Contin is commonly used in hospice. Given twice a day, it provides around-the-clock pain control. MS Contin can be given rectally when the patient is unable to swallow.

Morphine sulfate extended-release capsules (Avinza) consist of two components: an immediate-release component that rapidly achieves plateau morphine concentrations, and an extended-release component that maintains plasma concentrations throughout the 24-hour dosing interval. The amount absorbed is similar to that absorbed in other forms of oral morphine.

The extended-release formulation of morphine must be taken correctly: Tablets must be swallowed whole and must not be chewed, crushed, or dissolved. If chewed, crushed, or dissolved, the patient may receive a fatal overdose.

Continued

morphine (MS Contin, Avinza, and Kadian (Schedule II Drug) 🔑 —cont'd

Guidelines for use of long-acting medications have been published to help patients maintain as much of their normal life as possible; use of adjuvants may decrease overall narcotic use. Patients can take one capsule in the morning and go out and function all day long; they do not have to take the medication with them.

Table 42-8 summarizes dosage and administration information for all of these agents.

OTHER DRUGS IN CLASS

Other drugs in this class are similar to the key drug except as follows:

codeine (Schedule II-III)

Codeine has two primary therapeutic effects: analgesic and antitussive. Ten percent of codeine is metabolized to morphine. Codeine is relatively less potent than morphine and does not have the abuse potential of morphine. It is more likely than other opioids to cause constipation and nausea. Codeine often is combined with nonopioid analgesics, centrally acting muscle relaxants, antihistamines, and decongestants. Noncombination forms of codeine are classified as Schedule II controlled substances. Oral codeine is as effective as the parenteral form.

hydrocodone (Lortab, Vicodin) (Schedule III)

Hydrocodone is a semisynthetic opioid with primary actions that affect the CNS and smooth muscle organs. Its principal actions are analgesia and sedation. It is similar to codeine in that at least one half of its analgesic activity is retained in the oral form. It is used to treat moderate to severe pain of an acute nature, or as an antitussive. It is available in combination only with acetaminophen, aspirin, or ibuprofen and with antihistamines, decongestants, and expectorants for cough suppression. Similar to morphine, hydrocodone produces

drug dependence. It should not be used in patients who are hypersensitive to any of the combination tablet ingredients. Hydrocodone preparations may be less constipating than codeine, especially in older adults.

oxycodone (Percocet With acetaminophen, OxyContin) (Schedule II)

Oxycodone is similar to hydrocodone; it is a semisynthetic opioid that is similar to codeine in that in oral form, it retains at least one half of its analgesic activity. The immediate-release form is used to treat moderate to severe pain.

The controlled-release form is indicated only for chronic pain that requires continuous analgesia for an extended period; it is not to be used on an as-needed basis.

💣 Controlled-release tablets are not to be broken, crushed, or chewed because this allows rapid release and absorption of a potentially lethal dose of oxycodone, particularly with the 80 and 160 mg tablets.

These high-dose tablets are to be used only for those with opiate tolerance because they have become popular for drug abuse. Oxycodone is also available in combination with aspirin or acetaminophen. Similar to morphine, it produces drug dependence.

hydromorphone (Dilaudid) (Schedule II)

Hydromorphone is a very potent synthetic compound that maximizes analgesic effects and minimizes some of the common side effects of morphine. Hydromorphone has approximately five times the potency of morphine (i.e., 10 mg morphine is equivalent to 2 mg hydromorphone). Hydromorphone produces less sedation, nausea, vomiting, and constipation than its counterpart. The incidence of associated respiratory depression is marked, requiring close observation. Use the lowest dose possible to prevent this adverse effect. Rectal suppositories are particularly useful for producing a prolonged effect. It is a very desirable drug among intravenous drug abusers and is not usually prescribed by primary care providers.

Phenylpiperidines
meperidine (Demerol) (Schedule II)

Meperidine is a synthetic opioid analgesic with less potency than morphine. It is used for relief of moderate to severe pain, for preoperative sedation, for postoperative analgesia, for obstetric anesthesia, and, when given intravenously, for supportive anesthesia.

CONTRAINDICATIONS. Meperidine should not be used to treat patients with chronic pain because of the high risk of seizure, even in those with normal renal function.

WARNINGS. It should be used with particular caution, if at all, in the elderly. It is a drug of choice among drug abusers and must be used with extreme caution.

PHARMACOKINETICS. The onset of action is more rapid, but the duration of action is shorter, than that of morphine.

ADVERSE EFFECTS. It causes less sedation and pruritus than morphine. The major metabolite, normeperidine, can cause irritability, dysphoria, and seizures.

TABLE 42-4 Equagesic Opioid Analgesic Doses Equivalent to Morphine 10 mg IM

Medication	Oral Dose	Subcutaneous Dose
morphine	30 mg	10 mg
MS Contin	30 mg	ND
hydromorphone	7.5 mg	1.5 mg
fentanyl (Duragesic patch)*	ND	ND
codeine	200 mg	120 mg
hydrocodone	30 mg	ND
oxycodone	20-30 mg	ND
meperidine	300 mg	75-100 mg
methadone	20 mg	10 mg

ND, Not determined.
*100 mcg/hr = morphine 10 mg IM q4h.

TABLE 42-5 Pharmacokinetics of Selected Oral Analgesic Medications

Drug	Availability After First Pass	Onset of Action	Time to Peak Concentration	Half-life	Duration of Action	Metabolism (Primarily in Liver)
OPIOID AGONISTS						
morphine, immediate release	25% (low lipid solubility)	15-60 min	0.5-1 hr	2-4 hr	4-5 hr	Glucuronidation; lesser extent 2D6
MS Contin	40%	—	1.5 hr	2-4 hr	8-12 hr	
Avinza	About 25%	15-60 min	30 min	15 hr	24 hr	
codeine	60%; lipid soluble	10-30 min	0.5-1 hr	2-4 hr	4-6 hr	10% converted to morphine; 2D6
hydrocodone (Vicodin)	—	10-20 min	1 hr	4 hr	4-8 hr	2D6 (minor)
oxycodone (Percodan)	50%-87%	15-30 min	1 hr	3 hr	3-4 hr	2D6 (minor)
oxycodone, time-release formula (OxyContin)	50%-87%	1 hr	1.6 hr	4.5 hr	12 hr	
hydromorphone (Dilaudid)	Very highly lipid soluble; 62%	15-30 min	0.5-1 hr	2-3 hr	4-5 hr	
meperidine (Demerol)	50%	10-15 min	0.5-1 hr	3-4 hr	2-4 hr	2D6
fentanyl (Duragesic transdermal)	Very highly lipid soluble	12-24 hr	24-72 hr	≈17 hr	3 days	Via CYP 3A4 in liver
methadone	About 80% (highly lipid soluble)	30-60 min	3-5 days	8-59 hr	Analgesia: 4-7 hr (increases to 24-48 hr with repeated dosing)	2D6
propoxyphene (Darvon)	—	15-60 min	2-2.5 hr	6-12 hr; 30-36 hr for metabolite	4-6 hr	Liver
MIXED AGONIST-ANTAGONISTS pentazocine (Talwin)	≈20%	15-30 min	1-3 hr	2-3 hr	4-5 hr	
PARTIAL AGONISTS tramadol (Ultram)	75%	60 min	2 hr	6-7 hr	6 hr	20% protein bound; extensive metabolism by 2D6, 3A4

DRUG INTERACTIONS. When administering with phenothiazine and many other tranquilizers, reduce the dosage of meperidine by 25% to 50% because these agents potentiate the action of meperidine.

DOSAGE AND ADMINISTRATION. Each dose of syrup should be taken in one-half glass of water because, if undiluted, it can exert a topical anesthetic effect on mucous membranes.

fentanyl (Sublimaze, Duragesic Transdermal, Actiq Transmucosal) (Schedule II)

Intravenous fentanyl is a very potent short-acting opioid that is used for relief of moderate to severe pain and for preoperative sedation and operative and postoperative analgesia. A 0.1 mg dose of fentanyl is equivalent to 10 mg of morphine (100 times as potent).

Transdermal fentanyl is useful in the outpatient setting for long-term relief of pain, especially for a patient who is unable to take oral medications. It can be useful in tapering opioids and is to be used only in patients with moderate to severe chronic pain in opioid-tolerant patients age 2 years and older who require a total opioid dose at least equivalent to a 25 mcg/hour patch. Because of the risk for potentially fatal respiratory depression, the patch is not indicated for the management of postoperative, mild, or intermittent pain.

Initiate therapy with the 25 mcg patch, particularly in the elderly, who may have decreased fat stores and altered clearance. This agent is very lipid soluble and has enhanced CNS penetration. The patient must have adequate fat stores. The patch strength is roughly equivalent to that of the 12 hour MS Contin dose. It has a depot or holding effect, is deposited in the skin, and will continue to be absorbed for hours after the patch is removed.

The product also is available as a transmucosal "lozenge on a stick" product that is inserted between the buccal area and the teeth. The patient sucks on the lozenge. Doses include 200, 400, 600, 800, 1200, and 1600 mcg.

WARNINGS. The transdermal or transmucosal system is to be used for breakthrough or rescue doses only in hospitalized patients or those in hospice. Use of the patches in opioid-naive patients, concomitant use of more patches than prescribed, too-frequent patch replacement, and patch exposure to heat may create overdosage situations and be life threatening.

TABLE 42-6   Adverse Effects of Opioid Analgesics

Body System	Adverse Effects
Body, general	Interference with thermal regulation, paresthesia, pain at injection site, local tissue irritation and induration after SC injection, particularly when repeated; facial flushing, chills, faintness, pruritus (not an allergic reaction)
Hypersensitivity	Pruritus, urticaria, other skin rashes, diaphoresis, laryngospasm, edema, hemorrhagic urticaria; anaphylactoid reactions after IV administration; morphine thrombocytopenia, flushing
Respiratory	Bronchospasm, depression of cough reflex, laryngospasm, respiratory depression, apnea, and respiratory arrest
Cardiovascular	Peripheral circulatory collapse, tachycardia, bradycardia, arrhythmia, palpitations, chest wall rigidity, hypertension, hypotension, orthostatic hypotension,* syncope, asystole, shock, coma
GI	Nausea,* vomiting, diarrhea, cramps, abdominal pain, taste alterations, dry mouth, anorexia, constipation,* biliary tract spasm; exacerbation of ulcerative colitis
Musculoskeletal	Muscular rigidity
CNS	Euphoria, dysphoria, delirium, insomnia, agitation, anxiety, fear, hallucination, disorientation, drowsiness,* sedation,* lethargy, impairment of mental and physical performance, skeletal or uncoordinated movement, mood changes, weakness, headache, mental cloudiness, tremor, convulsions, psychic dependence, toxic psychoses, depression, increased intracranial pressure, miosis, sweating headache, dizziness, light-headedness, coma
Special senses	Blurred vision, visual disturbances, diplopia, miosis; hydromorphone nystagmus
Hepatic	propoxyphene—reversible jaundice
Genitourinary	Ureteral spasm and spasm of vesical sphincters, urinary retention or hesitancy, oliguria, antidiuretic effect, reduced libido or potency

*Very common.

ADVERSE EFFECTS

The respiratory depressant effects of fentanyl are particularly dangerous and mandate that the provider have resuscitative measures and opioid antagonists available, making it unacceptable for the outpatient setting.

DRUG INTERACTIONS. CYP 3A4 inhibitor

DOSAGE AND ADMINISTRATION (FENTANYL TRANSDERMAL SYSTEM). See Box 42-1.

Diphenylheptanes
methadone (Dolophine) (Schedule II)

Methadone hydrochloride is a synthetic opioid analgesic that is used primarily in the detoxification, treatment, and maintenance of persons with opiate addiction. It may be used orally for management of severe and chronic pain in patients unable to tolerate other narcotics. When it is used for persons with heroin and other opiate addiction for longer than 3 months, methadone use moves from a treatment phase to a maintenance phase.

WARNINGS. Regulations for its use for narcotic detoxification and maintenance are complicated. Refer patients to pain specialists with experience in the use of methadone.

PHARMACOKINETICS. It is long acting (36 to 48 hours) and should be used with caution, if at all, in the elderly.

ADVERSE EFFECTS. Side effects are similar to those seen with other opioids. Methadone is less sedating and euphoric than morphine. Respiratory depression and arrest remain one of its serious adverse effects.

DRUG INTERACTIONS. Methadone is a major substrate for CYP 3A4 and therefore has numerous drug interactions. Consult a detailed reference if prescribing methadone. Methadone can also prolong the QT interval, especially when used in conjunction with other drugs, in patients with hypokalemia, or in those with abnormal liver function tests. Fluoxetine and St. John's wort both increase metabolism, and their use may result in withdrawal symptoms.

DOSAGE AND ADMINISTRATION. See Table 42-8.
- *Opioid detoxification:* Individualize treatment.
- *Adults:* Adjust dose to severity of withdrawal symptoms: 5 mg tid po for 21 days, with the dose gradually reduced every few days
- *Opioid maintenance:* 40 to 120 mg or higher once daily po

propoxyphene (Darvon; Darvocet [with acetaminophen])

Propoxyphene is a centrally acting opioid that is structurally related to methadone. It is a weak analgesic with efficacy similar to that of acetaminophen or aspirin alone, but it has physically and psychologically addictive properties. To improve its overall effect, the drug often is combined with nonopioid analgesics. It is not recommended to be used alone for treatment of chronic pain.

It is classified as a Schedule IV controlled substance.

CONTRAINDICATIONS. Hypersensitivity

TABLE 42-7 Drug Interactions With Selected Analgesics

Drug	Increase Level	Decrease Level	Drug	Increase Level	Decrease Level
OPIOID AGONISTS			meperidine	Barbiturates chlorpromazine thioridazine MAOIs furazolidone cimetidine Hydantoins Protease inhibitors	Agonist-antagonist analgesics
morphine	amitriptyline Antihistamines Barbiturates chloral hydrate chlorpromazine cimetidine clomipramine furazolidone glutethimide MAOIs methocarbamol nortriptyline thioridazine	Agonist-antagonist analgesics	Fentanyl	Barbiturates chlorpromazine thioridazine MAOIs furazolidone diazepam droperidol nitrous oxide Protease inhibitors	Agonist-antagonist analgesics
codeine	Barbiturates chlorpromazine furazolidone MAOIs thioridazine	Agonist-antagonist analgesics	methadone	Barbiturates chlorpromazine thioridazine MAOIs furazolidone cimetidine fluvoxamine Hydantoins Protease inhibitors	Agonist-antagonist analgesics rifampin
hydrocodone	Barbiturates chlorpromazine furazolidone MAOIs Protease inhibitors thioridazine	Agonist-antagonist analgesics	propoxyphene	Barbiturates chlorpromazine thioridazine MAOIs furazolidone Protease inhibitors	Agonist-antagonist analgesics Charcoal Cigarette smoking
oxycodone	Barbiturates chlorpromazine furazolidone MAOIs Protease inhibitors thioridazine	Agonist-antagonist analgesics	**MIXED AGONIST-ANTAGONISTS**		
			pentazocine	Barbiturates	
			PARTIAL AGONISTS		
hydromorphone	Barbiturates chlorpromazine furazolidone MAOIs thioridazine	Agonist-antagonist analgesics	tramadol	MAOIs	carbamazepine

WARNINGS. Norpropoxyphene has cardiac conduction effects and increases PR and QRS intervals. Propoxyphene products in excessive doses, given alone or in combination with other CNS depressants (including alcohol), are a major cause of drug-related death.

> Alternative analgesic therapy may be safer and more effective, especially when narcotic therapy is initiated in patients who have not used propoxyphene.

PHARMACOKINETICS. The active metabolite, norpropoxyphene, has a half-life of up to 36 hours.

ADVERSE EFFECTS. The drug can cause ataxia and dizziness that may contribute to falls, particularly in the elderly.

DRUG INTERACTIONS. Propoxyphene may inhibit the metabolism and increase the serum levels of carbamazepine, phenobarbital, MAOIs, tricyclic antidepressants, and warfarin. See Table 42-7 for drug interactions with narcotics.

DOSAGE AND ADMINISTRATION. See Table 42-8. A dose of 100 mg propoxyphene napsylate is required to equal 65 mg of propoxyphene HCl because of differences in molecular weight.

MIXED AGONIST-ANTAGONISTS
pentazocine (Talwin)

Alternative analgesic therapy may be safer and more effective than pentazocine, especially when narcotic therapy is initiated in patients who have not used propoxyphene.

Pentazocine is a synthetic opioid that is believed to induce analgesia by stimulating the kappa opioid receptors while blocking the mu receptors. It is used primarily for the relief of moderate to severe pain or as a preoperative or preanesthetic medication. It is not recommended for long-term use, nor is it recommended for use in the elderly. It is a category IV narcotic.

CONTRAINDICATIONS. Hypersensitivity

TABLE 42-8   Dosage and Administration of Selected Opioid Analgesics

Drug	Dosage	Administration
OPIOID AGONISTS		
morphine	10-30 mg 10-20 mg 10 mg (5-20 mg)/70 kg 2.5-15 mg/70 kg	po q4h pr q4h subQ or IM q4h IV in 4-5 ml of sterile water over 4-5 min; have opiate antagonist immediately available during IV administration
morphine, controlled release (MS Contin)	15-60 mg; total daily dose of morphine	po q8-12h; total daily dose divided in 2-3 doses
codeine (pain relief)	Adult: 15-60 mg Child >1 yr: 0.5-1 mg/kg/dose	po, IM, subQ, or IV q4-6h po, IM, subQ q4-6h; do not administer IV in children
codeine (antitussive)	Adult: 10-20 mg Child 6-12 yr: 5-10 mg Child 2-5 yr: 2.5-5 mg	po q4-6h; do not exceed 120 mg/24 hr po q4-6h; do not exceed 60 mg/24 hr po q4-6h; do not exceed 30 mg/24 hr
hydrocodone	2.5-10 mg	po q4-6h up to 60 mg/24 hr
oxycodone	2.5-5 mg Immediate release (OxyIR): 5 mg Controlled release (OxyContin) 10-160 mg; *Note:* 80 mg and 160 mg tablets used only in opioid-tolerant patients	po q6h po q6h po q12h
hydromorphone	Adult only: 2-8 mg 3 mg 1-2 mg	po q3-4h pr q4-8h subQ, IM, or slow IV q4-6h
meperidine	Adult: 50-150 mg Child: 1-1.5 mg/kg/dose (maximum 100 mg/dose)	po, IV, IM, or subQ q3-4h po, IV, IM, or subQ q3-4h
fentanyl	25-100 mcg/hr patch (initial dosage may be approximated from the 24 hour morphine dosage)	Change patch every 3 days; see text discussion for details.
methadone (pain relief)	2.5-10 mg	po, subQ, or IM q8-12h
methadone (detoxification)	40-120 mg	po once daily (if possible); see text discussion for details
propoxyphene	65 mg (as HCl); 100 mg (as napsylate)	po q4-6h
MIXED AGONIST-ANTAGONISTS pentazocine	30-60 mg 50 mg	IM q3-4h po q3-4h
PARTIAL AGONISTS tramadol	50-100 mg	po q4-6h, not to exceed 300-400 mg/24 hr; 300 mg/day in elderly

WARNINGS/PRECAUTIONS. See also warnings and precautions for morphine.

- Use with extreme caution in patients who are emotionally unstable and in those with a history of drug abuse. Because both psychologic and physiologic dependence may occur, this drug should be given under careful supervision. It should be prescribed only in limited amounts.
- Because the tablets are popular with drug addicts for intravenous injection, Talwin NX with naloxone was developed. When taken orally, naloxone is not absorbed, allowing the pentazocine to exert its analgesic effects. When the drug is misused by injection, severe effects, such as pulmonary emboli, vascular occlusion, ulceration and abscesses, and withdrawal symptoms in opioid-dependent individuals, may occur.
- If patients who are receiving therapeutic doses demonstrate any evidence of hallucinations, confusion, or disorientation, the medication should be discontinued.

- In patients who have demonstrated dependence on opioids, switching to pentazocine may produce withdrawal symptoms.
- Pentazocine has been known to provoke seizures, especially in those patients with known seizure disorders.

ADVERSE EFFECTS. See adverse effects for morphine. In addition, pentazocine causes the following effects:

- *Cardiovascular:* Circulatory depression, shock
- *CNS:* Agitation, clammy feeling, confusion, crying, dizziness, dysphoria, faintness, floating feeling, hostility, lethargy, light-headedness, nervousness, nystagmus, numbness, paresthesias, syncope, tingling, tinnitus, tremor, unreality, unusual dreams, vertigo
- *Dermatologic:* Burning, edema of face, urticaria, rash, severe sclerosis, soft tissue induration, sting on injection, ulceration

---

BOX 42-1 Dosage and Administration of the Fentanyl Transdermal System

1. *Initial Dose Selection.* Individualize dosage. If the patient is opioid naïve, start with the lowest dose—25 mcg/hr. Generally, however, this is not the first opioid the patient has used. The fentanyl patch should be used only in those with chronic pain whose condition cannot be managed with short-acting narcotics. The usual use of fentanyl transdermal systems is to convert the patient from oral or parenteral opioids to the transdermal system, as follows:
   * Calculate the previous 24 hour analgesic requirement.
   * Convert this amount to the equianalgesic oral morphine dose (see Table 42-8).
   * Convert from 24 hour morphine dose to transdermal fentanyl dose (Janssen Pharmaceutical Company provides a dosage conversion calculator).
2. *Application of Patch.* Apply to nonirritated skin on a flat surface of the upper torso. Clip, but do not shave, the hair. Clean the skin with clear water; do not use soaps, oils, lotions, alcohol, or any other agents that might irritate the skin or alter its characteristics. Allow the skin to dry completely before system application.
   * Apply the patch immediately on removal from the sealed package. Press firmly with palm of hand for 10 to 20 seconds, making sure contact is complete, especially around the edges.
   * Each system works continuously for 72 hours. However, occasionally patients may find that they need to replace the system every 48 hours. Remove the old system, and apply the new system to a different skin site. Dispose of the old system carefully.
3. *Wearing the First System.* Because peak levels are not reached for 24 hours, the patient may need short-acting analgesics. After 24 hours, assess the efficacy of the system by counting the number of times the patient needs a rescue dose of short-acting analgesic.
4. *Titrate Dosage.* Titrate upward if necessary after use of the initial 3 day system. Because the conversion system from morphine to fentanyl is conservative, about half of patients will need upward titration. If the patient is using rescue doses of analgesic equivalent to 90 mg/24 hr of morphine, increase the fentanyl system dose by 25 mcg/hr.
   * After the first titration, titrate upward every 6 days. For delivery rates in excess of 100 mcg/hr, multiple systems may be used.
5. *Discontinue.* If the patient requires more than 300 mcg/hr, change the patient to another method of opioid administration. Remember that it takes about 18 hours for the fentanyl concentration to decrease by 50% after the system has been removed.
   * A fentanyl patch can be used to discontinue opioids by wearing the patch, then simply removing and allowing the concentration to gradually decrease.

---

* *Hematopoietic:* Depression of white blood cells, transient eosinophilia
* *Other:* Speech difficulty

DOSAGE AND ADMINISTRATION. See Table 42-8.

PARTIAL AGONISTS

tramadol (Ultram)

Tramadol is not a scheduled drug.

PHARMACOKINETICS. Tramadol is metabolized by cytochrome P450 2D6 isoenzymes.

WARNINGS
* See warnings for morphine. Seizure risk is present, especially in patients with a history of seizures or in those who are taking a medication that increases the risk of seizures.

* Anaphylactoid reactions have occurred.
* Use great caution in combination with MAOIs.

ADVERSE EFFECTS. See adverse effects for morphine; the most common are dizziness/vertigo, nausea, constipation, headache, and somnolence.

DRUG INTERACTIONS. Inhibitors such as chlorpromazine, fluoxetine, paroxetine, quinidine, quinine, ritonavir, and ropinirole may decrease the effects of tramadol. Use with carbamazepine causes an increase in tramadol metabolism.

DOSAGE AND ADMINISTRATION. See Table 42-8.

evolve A continually updated list of useful WebLinks may be found in the Evolve Resources at http://evolve.elsevier.com/Edmunds/NP/

43 Migraine Medications

DRUG OVERVIEW

Class	Subclass	Generic Name	Trade Name
Abortive agents	Serotonin 5-HT$_{1D}$ receptor agonist	sumatriptan 🗝	Imitrex ☀
		frovatriptan	Frova
		naratriptan	Amerge
		rizatriptan	Maxalt
		almotriptan	Axert
		zolmitriptan	Zomig
	5-HT$_{1B/1D}$	eletriptan	Relpax ☀
	Ergotamine derivatives	ergotamine tartrate 🗝	Cafergot
		dihydroergotamine (DHE)	DHE-45, Migranal
		isometheptene mucate	Midrin
Prophylactic agent		cyproheptadine	Periactin

☀ Top 200 drug; 🗝 key drug. Key drugs chosen because they were first in their class and are still used. See Table 43-1 for discussions in other chapters of drugs commonly used for prophylaxis.

INDICATIONS

- Acute treatment of migraine with or without aura
- *Prophylaxis of migraine:* valproate, topiramate

A wide variety of drugs are used for the treatment of migraines. They are divided into medications that are effective in acute treatment of migraine symptoms and medications used for chronic prophylaxis. The most commonly used migraine medications are the serotonin$_1$ (5-HT$_1$) receptor agonists, commonly known as the "triptans." Migraine-specific products are discussed in detail in this chapter. Abortive medications include acetaminophen, aspirin, and NSAIDs, as well as triptans. Preventative medications approved by the FDA also include β-blockers, calcium channel blockers, TCAs, SSRIs, and anticonvulsants. Only their use in the treatment of migraines is discussed in this chapter.

THERAPEUTIC OVERVIEW

Pathophysiology

Migraine is a primary disorder of the brain that still is poorly understood. Genetics is linked to the incidence of hemiplegic migraines, and because 70% to 80% of migraine sufferers have a family history of migraine, genetic components that have not been identified are probably involved. A single explanation that encompasses all of the phenomena that

occur with migraine has eluded researchers to date. Many neural events can cause dilation of blood vessels, which causes pain and other nerve activation. The underlying physiologic problem appears to be the dysfunction of an ion channel in brainstem neurons that normally modulate sensory input and exert neural influence on cranial vessels. The brain neurotransmitters involved are primarily from the serotonergic system. Serotonin receptor subtypes, including 1B, 1D, and 1F, play a role in cerebral vasodilation and trigeminal nerve activation, which are believed to be the precursors of migraine pain.

Disease Process

Headaches represent a very common complaint in primary care. They have many causes, ranging in seriousness from stress to brain tumor; therefore, the cause must be determined whenever possible for effective therapy to be determined.

Tension headache (THA), the most common type of headache, usually is described as vise-like pressure associated with stress and/or fatigue. The pain of THA usually is generalized but may be worse in the area of the neck and the back of head. These patients are generally treated with analgesics for mild to moderate pain. (See Chapter 42 for more information on pain management.)

Approximately 23 million Americans are afflicted with migraine headaches. Migraine headaches usually begin in the teenage years, peaking between the ages of 25 and 34; they are three times more prevalent among women than men.

462

TABLE 43-1 **Drugs Commonly Used for Prophylaxis Discussed in Other Chapters**

Class	Generic Name	Trade Name	Dosage 24 Hours	Chapter
β-Blockers	atenolol	Tenormin	25-200 mg	18
	metoprolol	Toprol XL, Lopressor	50-200 mg	
	nadolol	Corgard	20-120 mg	
	propranolol	Inderal	20-160 mg	
Calcium channel blockers	verapamil	Calan, Isoptin, Verelan	120-480 mg	19
Antidepressants	fluoxetine	Prozac	10-80 mg	46
	amitriptyline	Elavil	10-150 mg	
Anticonvulsants	divalproex	Depakote	125-200 mg	44
	topiramate	Topamax	50-150 mg	
	gabapentin	Neurontin	300-2400 mg	
Analgesics	NSAIDs	aspirin	1300 mg/day	42
	acetaminophen	Ibuprofen	800 mg/day	
	Combinations of above with caffeine	Tylenol		

These headaches represent a debilitating and costly medical problem. For a variety of reasons, a large group of persons do not seek medical care for their migraines.

Migraine symptoms vary. All migraines are paroxysmal in nature—clearly defined attacks separated by symptom-free intervals. Daily or continuous headaches usually are not migraines but are tension or vascular headaches. Migraines are classified as with aura or without aura and are graded as mild, moderate, or severe in intensity. The duration of migraine is an important variable because the clinician must choose medications whose duration of action is adequate. Classic migraines go through specific phases (Table 43-2).

Complicated migraines, which are less common, are characterized by attacks in which neurologic symptoms last for the entire headache or for several days or weeks or, in some cases, leave a permanent neurologic deficit. Complicated migraines are divided into three subtypes. An *ophthalmoplegic* migraine affects the third, fourth, or sixth cranial nerve; permanent damage to the third nerve has been reported. *Hemiplegic* migraine is characterized by both motor and sensory symptoms that are unilateral and may last longer than the headache itself; this type is very rare. Complete recovery from these symptoms may take weeks, and permanent weakness can occur following multiple attacks. *Basilar-type* migraine is characterized by any combination of vertigo, diplopia, dysarthria, tinnitus, decreased hearing, ataxia, simultaneous bilateral paresthesias, and altered consciousness. It may be difficult sometimes to distinguish between visual symptoms of a classic migraine and basilar artery migraine, although the latter is more likely to affect both visual fields.

A transformed migraine is a long-lasting headache that results from overuse of pain and/or migraine medications. Following a migraine episode, the patient has rebound headache daily or nearly daily. Medications that can cause this include caffeine, acetaminophen, NSAIDs, barbiturates, sedatives, narcotics, ergots, and triptans.

Assessment

Diagnosed migraine must meet specific criteria established by the National Headache Foundation (Box 43-1). A diagnostic workup headache history includes age of onset of headaches; duration of complaint; frequency and duration of each headache; site, quality, and time of onset; associated phenomena; and aggravating and relieving factors. Physical examination, including neurologic examination, is typically normal. Some patients experience substantial burden from their migraines. The Migraine Disability Assessment Scale (MIDAS) is a five-item questionnaire that is used in practice (see Goadsby et al, 2002, for questionnaire) to help the clinician measure how much intervention is required to improve the patient's quality of life.

💣 It is essential that adequate evaluation and diagnostic testing be completed to confirm the diagnosis of migraine. Some headaches that patients may call migraines are actually other pathologic conditions;

TABLE 43-2 **Phases of a Migraine**

Phase	Experienced by	Symptoms	Timing
Prodrome	50%	Increased/decreased perception, irritability or withdrawal, food cravings, yawning, speech difficulties	Starts 24 hr before overt migraine
Aura	20%	Visual disturbances (flashing lights, shimmering zigzag lines), numbness or tingling in hands, dysphagia, olfactory and auditory changes	Starts 30-60 min before headache, lasts 5-60 min
Headache		Severe, pulsating, unilateral; accompanied by nausea and vomiting, photophobia, or phonophobia; all reversible	Lasts 4-72 hr
Postdrome		Fatigue, aching muscles, or euphoria	Lasts up to 24 hr

---

BOX 43-1   Diagnostic Criteria for Migraine

MIGRAINE WITHOUT AURA

A. At least five attacks that fulfill criteria B through D
B. Headache that lasts 4 to 72 hours (untreated or unsuccessfully treated)
C. At least two of the following pain characteristics:
   1. Unilateral location
   2. Pulsating quality
   3. Moderate or severe intensity
   4. Aggravation by walking stairs or similar physical activity
D. During headache, at least one of the following:
   1. Nausea and/or vomiting
   2. Photophobia and phonophobia

MIGRAINE WITH AURA

A. At least two attacks that fulfill criterion B
B. At least three of the following characteristics:
   1. One or more fully reversible aura symptoms indicating focal cerebral, cortical, and/or brainstem dysfunction
   2. At least one aura symptom develops gradually over longer than 4 minutes, or two or more symptoms occur in succession.
   3. No aura symptoms last longer than 60 minutes; if more than one aura symptom is present, accepted duration is proportionally increased.
   4. Headache follows aura, with a free interval of less than 60 minutes (headache may begin before or simultaneously with aura).

Adapted from Headache Classification Committee of the International Headache Society: Classification and diagnostic criteria for headache disorders, cranial neuralgias and facial pain, *Cephalalgia* 8(suppl 7):1-96, 1988.

---

some of these headaches represent significant problems that must not be ignored. Box 43-2 lists headache symptoms that warrant further evaluation.

Migraine headache often is stimulated by visual, olfactory, or other environmental triggers that may be identified. (See Box 43-3.) The patient must be screened for concurrent illnesses, especially cardiovascular problems such as increased blood pressure and CAD. These concurrent illnesses may affect treatment options.

MECHANISM OF ACTION

Abortive Agents

See Table 43-3 for drug effects on serotonin receptors.

All 5-HT$_1$ receptor agonists (triptans) have a similar chemical structure and a comparable mechanism of action. 5-HT$_{1B}$ and 5-HT$_{1D}$ receptors are located on the extracerebral, intracranial blood vessels that become dilated during a migraine attack and on nerve terminals in the trigeminal system. Therapeutic activity is caused by activation of these receptors, which results in cranial vessel constriction, inhibition of neuropeptide release, and reduced transmission in trigeminal pain pathways. Each product varies with regard to onset of action, duration of action, and incidence of recurrent headache.

BOX 43-2   Headache Danger Signals That Warrant Investigation

Sudden onset of new, severe headache
Progressively worsening headache
Onset of headache after exertion, straining, coughing, or sexual activity
Presence of associated neurologic symptoms, nausea/vomiting, physical signs, "worst headache they have ever had"
Onset of first headache after the age of 50 years

Ergotamine derivatives demonstrate partial agonist and/or antagonist activity against dopaminergic, tryptaminergic, and α-adrenergic receptors, depending on their site. Ergotamine derivatives have three primary actions. They (1) depress central vasomotor centers, (2) constrict peripheral and cranial blood vessels, and (3) reduce extracranial blood flow and decrease hyperperfusion of the basilar artery area. In unrelated actions, these drugs also increase the force and frequency of uterine contractions.

Ergotamine tartrate is an α-adrenergic–blocking agent with direct stimulating effects on the smooth muscle of the peripheral and cranial vessels. Ergot drugs also produce an increase in central vasomotor center stimulation. Although dihydroergotamine (DHE) is an ergot, it is also a 5-HT$_{1B/1D}$ receptor agonist that is not as selective as the triptans. DHE binds to norepinephrine (noradrenaline) α$_1$, α$_{2A}$, and α$_{2B}$ and dopamine D$_{2L}$ and D$_3$ receptors. It is a stronger venoconstrictor and a weaker arterial vasoconstrictor than ergotamine.

BOX 43-3   Migraine Triggers

Change in hormone levels in women
Illness
Unaccustomed exercise, activity
Change in sleep pattern
Change in eating pattern
Bright or flickering lights
Noise
Odors, tobacco smoke
Weather changes
High altitude
Stress/stress cessation
Medications
Food: chocolate, wine, certain cheeses

TABLE 43-3 Drug Effects on Serotonin (5-HT) Receptors

Drug	1	1A	1B	1D	1E	1F	2A/2C	5A	7	2 to 4
sumatriptan	High	Weak						Weak	Weak	None
naratriptan				High		Weak				None
rizatriptan		Weak	High	High	Weak	Weak			Weak	
zolmitriptan		Weak	High	High		Weak				
almotriptan		Weak	High	High		High			Weak	
frovatriptan			High	High						
eletriptan		Weak	High	High	Weak	High			Weak	
DHE		High		High			High			

Combination Drugs

Isometheptene mucate is a sympathomimetic agent that acts as a vasoconstrictor of dilated cranial and cerebral arterioles. Midrin is a combination capsule that contains 65 mg of isometheptene mucate, 325 mg of acetaminophen, which exerts an analgesic effect, and 100 mg of dichloralphenazone, a mild sedative that acts centrally to allay anxiety. Caffeine, which is added to many migraine combinations, helps to promote constrictive properties and enhances absorption. ASA, acetaminophen, ibuprofen, and caffeine, all of which are commonly found in combination analgesic products used for the treatment of patients with mild to moderate migraine, have been shown through evidence-based studies to be effective in the prophylaxis and treatment of migraine.

Prophylactic Agents

See Box 43-4 for a list of prophylactic medications.

The β-blockers are postulated to exert antimigraine effects through stabilization of vascular tone. Postulated mechanisms by which this stabilization may occur include (1) inhibition of norepinephrine release by blocking prejunctional β-receptors, (2) reduction in enzyme activity (tyrosine hydroxylase) that is the rate-limiting step in norepinephrine synthesis, and (3) delayed reduction of locus ceruleus neuron firing. Blocking of central β-receptors interferes with vigilance-enhancing adrenergic pathways that are important in headache prevention. Interaction with serotonin receptors by some β-adrenergic blockers may stabilize vascular tone.

Calcium channel blockers regulate cellular functions, including vascular smooth muscle contraction, neurotransmission, and hormone secretion enzyme activity. These products also block intracerebral vasoconstriction caused by vasoactive neurotransmitters such as 5-HT (serotonin) and norepinephrine. In addition, calcium channel blockers may impede neurovascular inflammation and prevent hypoxia of cerebral neurons.

Tricyclic antidepressants act to reduce migraine activity by increasing the availability of synaptic norepinephrine or serotonin "downregulation" of 5-HT receptors and β-receptor density. Thus, they enhance the opiate mechanism and provide inhibition of 5-HT and norepinephrine reuptake, while binding to receptors on platelets and neurons that are blocking 5-HT uptake. The net result is an increased threshold for precipitation of a migraine attack in selected individuals.

SSRIs are potent, specific 5-HT receptor reuptake inhibitors that reduce migraine frequency and intensity. They act to prevent the vasoconstrictive effects of decreased serotonin levels during headache. Such constriction sets up a cascade of neuron inflammatory changes that produce headache pain. Maintaining the serum level of 5-HT with SSRIs prevents initiation of this pathway, thereby preventing migraine.

Anticonvulsants are believed to exert antimigraine activity through their influence on cerebral arteries and circadian rhythms. They also may help to regulate secretion of hormones from the anterior pituitary gland that help to relax vascular structures.

TREATMENT PRINCIPLES
Standardized Guidelines

- Silberstein SD: Practice parameter: evidence-based guidelines for migraine headache (an evidence-based review), *Neurology* 55:754-762, 2000. (Noted as still accurate as of June 2008.)

BOX 43-4 Abortive Medications

MILD TO MODERATE

acetaminophen
aspirin
Caffeine-containing combination products
isometheptene
naproxen, ibuprofen, indomethacin

MODERATE TO SEVERE

Triptans
dihydroergotamine
ergotamine
Opioids
Corticosteroids

From: Silberstein SD: Practice parameters: evidence-based guidelines for migraine headache, *Neurology* 55: 754-762, 2000.

Evidence-Based Recommendations

ACUTE TREATMENT

- *Beneficial:* Salicylates, ibuprofen, almotriptan, eletriptan, frovatriptan, naratriptan, rizatriptan, sumatriptan, zolmitriptan
- *Likely to be beneficial:* diclofenac, ergotamine, naproxen, flufenamic acid
- *Children:* Ibuprofen is effective; acetaminophen is probably effective.
- Sumatriptan nasal spray is effective.
- Combination products, including ASA, acetaminophen, NSAIDs, and caffeine, are effective.

PREVENTIVE TREATMENT

- *Adults:* Propanolol, timolol, divalproex, sodium and topiramate have been found to be helpful.
- *Children:* Evidence is insufficient for any treatment to be recommended.

Cardinal Points of Treatment

- Establish a diagnosis.
- Establish realistic patient expectations through education and counseling.
- Treat attacks rapidly and consistently.
  - *First line:* Triptans
  - *Second line:* DHE
  - *Third line:* Combination analgesics of NSAIDs, ASA, and caffeine
  - Emergency rescue drugs include prochlorpemazine PR/IM, IV; opiates, corticosteroids
- Encourage patient to identify and avoid triggers.

The goals of migraine treatment are to correctly diagnose HA, to decrease pain and associated symptoms, to prevent recurrence, to improve quality of life, and to allow the patient to maintain function. Treatment of migraine headache must be individualized for each patient. Some of the critical decisions that must be made by the clinician in determining appropriate treatment for a patient with migraine are illustrated in Figure 43-1.

Nonpharmacologic Treatment

Although this text focuses on pharmacology, the successful management of migraine headache has a lot to do with the willingness of primary care providers to explore sources of stress and anxiety in their patients, to teach them about migraine headache, and to work with them in using multiple strategies to reduce stresses and triggers in their lives.

Prevention or reduction of episodes of migraine requires healthy regular daily habits pertaining to sleep, meals, and exercise. Patients should avoid peaks of stress and troughs of relaxation because acute stress and the abrupt removal of stress are common triggers. Regularity of habits, rather than just searching for triggers, is essential for enhancing the effectiveness of nonpharmacologic approaches.

The second step in the management of migraine headache involves the identification and avoidance of headache triggers. The patient should try to determine the factors responsible for initiating his or her headaches. Have the patient keep a diary that correlates the patient's activity, food, and stressful events with occurrence of migraine. Common migraine triggers include loud noises, strong smells (e.g., perfumes), flashing lights, changing time zones, weather and altitude changes, smoke, and menstruation. Food triggers include caffeine withdrawal, aged cheese, chocolate, MSG, nitrate/nitrite-preserved foods, glutamate, excessive vitamin A, and alcohol. Psychologic stressors may serve as triggers; drug triggers include oral contraceptives, nitroglycerin, histamine, reserpine, corticosteroid withdrawal, and hydralazine. Frequently, the patient will not be able to identify specific triggers.

Treatment of the acute attack begins with resting in a quiet dark place. This reduces external stimuli and allows the patient to relax. Sleep has been found to reduce the duration of headache. Other effective techniques include local pressure, acupuncture, Botox injections, local application of cold, and sleep. These approaches frequently are not feasible when people are at work or have responsibilities that they must meet.

Relaxation training, thermal biofeedback, and cognitive-behavioral therapy may help to prevent migraine. Alternative therapies that have been described in the evidence-based literature include feverfew, riboflavin, and magnesium.

Pharmacologic Treatment

Factors that the clinician should consider when determining appropriate drug therapy include frequency, duration, and severity of headaches; symptoms other than pain, such as nausea; and therapies that have been tried previously. Complicated and transformed migraines should be managed by a specialist.

ABORTIVE TREATMENT (FOR THOSE WHO ARE HAVING AN ACUTE MIGRAINE). Patients in whom migraine has been diagnosed should have medication on hand in anticipation of an acute migraine attack. Abortive agents are used in the absence of prophylactic management in patients who have less than four attacks each month. It is important that any abortive agent be administered no more often than 2 days per week to avoid the possibility of rebound headache. Usually, patients will have headaches of variable intensity, so they should be given different treatment options to try. No drug works perfectly every time. Patients should be encouraged to try products for at least two or three episodes of migraine before they decide that they are ineffective.

The major initial treatment choice involves selection between ergots and triptans. Triptans have become the first-line treatment for abortive treatment of migraines. In general, triptans cause fewer adverse reactions, but some patients may be unable to tolerate them. Triptans are also expensive. Ergotamine formulations are effective and cost less than the triptans. If the patient is able to take medication at the earliest onset of headache, ergots usually are effective. If a patient wakes up with a headache or has difficulty "catching the headache in time," a triptan will be more effective. All triptan and ergotamine drugs have the same cardiovascular cautions.

Although all triptans are similar, patient responses may vary. One agent might be more effective than another for a particular patient. For example, zolmitriptan and rizatriptan are lipid soluble; this trait facilitates penetration across the blood-brain barrier. Duration of action may become an issue

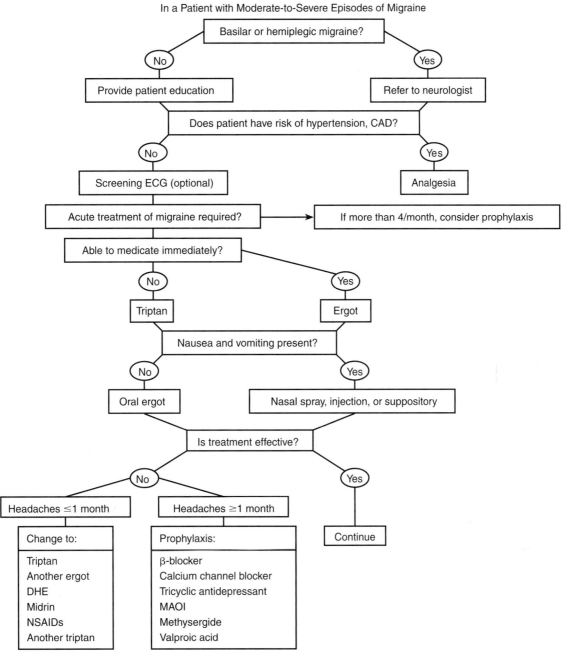

FIGURE 43-1 **Critical decision making in the treatment of migraine.**

for patients with long-lasting or recurring migraine if duration of effect is shorter than they need. Frovatriptan has a half-life of 26 hours and a headache recurrence rate as low as 7%. Often, formulation choice will determine which medication should be prescribed. Imitrex has a formulation that, when swallowed whole, dissolves similarly to Alka-Seltzer and begins to work in 15 minutes.

Isometheptene is a mild ergotamine that is safe and effective for mild migraine. Isometheptene is found in an OTC combination product that contains 65 mg isometheptene, 100 mg dichloralphenazone, and 325 mg acetaminophen (e.g., Midrin). It does not have the adverse effects commonly associated with ergotamines. Ergotamine tartrate is seldom

used any more because of the increased risk of adverse reactions. It has been used for migraines of long duration, but newer triptans have a longer half-life. DHE is being used increasingly for severe migraine. It is safer than other agents because of the decrease in arterial vasoconstriction; it relieves pain reliably and quickly.

Mild to Moderate Migraines. Analgesics such as aspirin, NSAIDs, or a combination product are commonly used. Combination OTC migraine medications that contain aspirin, acetaminophen, and caffeine are approved migraine treatments. Commonly used NSAIDs such as naproxen and ibuprofen are effective; indomethacin is often more effective than other NSAIDs.

Nausea and Vomiting. Administer triptan migraine medication in nasal spray or injection formulation for patients who have severe nausea or vomiting and are unable to take oral products. Nasal spray is easy to use and is effective for mild to moderate migraine. Commonly used antiemetics include prochlorperazine (Compazine) and trimethobenzamide (Tigan). Metoclopramide (Reglan) has the added effect of speeding up absorption of other drugs and is used with aspirin for mild to moderate migraine. Although it appears to be the most effective antiemetic, metoclopramide has potentially serious adverse reactions (see Chapter 28).

Moderate to Severe Migraine. Evidence-based studies suggest that triptans are first-line drugs and are generally very effective. Ergotamine tartrate may be used if triptans are not effective. DHE, which is very effective for severe migraine, is available as nasal spray or intramuscular or subcutaneous injection for the treatment of patients with moderate to severe migraine. It produces a quick response and a low recurrence rate. If triptan drugs have not been adequate, DHE is a good second-line drug to try.

Migraine Recurrence. Migraines may recur within 24 hours after initial response to medication in 30% to 40% of patients. Research meta-analyses suggest that clinicians should consider giving a long-acting triptan such as frovatriptan.

Severe Migraine. Consider injection of a triptan or DHE; these generally are very effective. Corticosteroids or opioids may be required as rescue medications. Corticosteroids should be administered intravenously, intramuscularly, or orally at 2 to 4 mg bid for 2 days and tapered over 3 more days at one event per month. Opioids can be used for patients who have infrequent but severe migraines. If rescue medications are required, reexamine the patient for whether he or she is using other medications correctly, that is, in terms of dosages, timing, and so forth.

PROPHYLACTIC MEDICATIONS. Prophylactic medications typically are used when patients experience more than two or three attacks each month, or when headaches do not respond adequately to abortive medication. Quality of life may be so poor that these products have to be used. These products may not eliminate migraine headaches but do decrease their frequency, intensity, and duration. Best evidence for use is available for propranolol, timolol, amitriptyline, valproate, and topiramate.

Select a medication that has a low adverse effect profile and is compatible with the patient's coexisting conditions. Use once-daily dosage if possible to improve compliance. Start slowly and gradually increase dose until headache is relieved or patient has side effects. Give a medication an adequate trial of at least 2 to 6 months. Consider tapering medication if headaches are well controlled after 6 months.

β-Blockers reduce headache frequency and severity in 60% to 80% of cases. Propranolol is most commonly used. Atenolol, metoprolol, and nadolol also have been shown to be effective. Gradually increase dosage to minimize adverse reactions. Three to four weeks of therapy is required before effectiveness can be evaluated. These agents may aggravate neurologic symptoms associated with hemiplegic or basilar migraine.

Second-line agents include calcium channel blockers. These agents decrease headache frequency, intensity, and duration in 40% to 60% of migraineurs. Verapamil is used most commonly. Clinical improvement may not be noted for 4 to 6 weeks after initiation of therapy. As with many other products, tolerance to calcium channel blockers commonly develops.

TCAs also are used in the prophylactic treatment of patients with migraine. Amitriptyline is considered first line; the others are considered second line. TCAs provide sedation and stabilization of the sleep cycle—disruption of the sleep cycle is a common problem with migraineurs. Amitriptyline, doxepin, nortriptyline, and imipramine are the more sedating TCAs. Less sedating TCAs include protriptyline and desipramine. Tricyclics are rapid acting, providing benefit to 60% of individuals in 10 to 14 days. Dosages required for migraine treatment are lower than those needed for that treatment of mood disorders.

SSRIs are considered second-line treatment. They are less effective than TCAs. Fluvoxamine and paroxetine have been studied most extensively.

The anticonvulsants divalproex, gabapentin, and topiramate have been used for severe migraine. The most in-depth study involved divalproex. See Silberstein, 2007, for details on the strength of evidence available for each of these medications and their uses.

How to Monitor

Patients should develop the habit of keeping a headache diary to document the frequency and severity of their headaches and to help identify triggers. Patient should bring a diary for review by the provider at regular intervals.

When using triptans or ergots, monitor cardiovascular status via periodic ECGs and cardiac enzyme laboratory work.

For those patients who are taking cyproheptadine, liver function studies should be performed at regular intervals. Patient weight should be checked and monitored for abnormal weight gain. Questions regarding anticholinergic side effects such as dry eyes, dry mouth, constipation, urinary retention, and excessive drowsiness should be included in the general follow-up assessment. The effectiveness of cyproheptadine is apparent within 3 weeks of treatment initiation.

Patient Variables

GERIATRICS
- Use all products with caution because the elderly are more susceptible to adverse effects than are younger patients. Begin with a very low dose and increase slowly.
- Although many individuals with a lifelong history of migraine report a decrease in headache during their 50s, migraines are very rare in geriatrics, and an intracranial lesion should be suspected. New headaches in this age group require further evaluation.

PEDIATRICS
- Children's migraines frequently last less than 2 hours.
- The safety and efficacy of most migraine medications have not been established in children.
- Although evidence does not support the recommendation of any prophylaxis medication in children, cyproheptadine

often is used; use in those younger than age 2 is contraindicated.

- Sumatriptan is used by clinicians in children older than 5 years, but this drug does not have the approved FDA indication.

PREGNANCY AND LACTATION
- *Category B:* cyproheptadine
- *Category C:* Triptans; may be secreted in milk
- *Category X:* Ergotamines; should not be used in women who are likely to become pregnant

GENDER
- Three times as many women have migraines.
- The frequency and severity of migraines often decrease or change character in postmenopausal women.

Patient Education

Extensive education regarding diagnosis, disease course, lifestyle modifications, and treatment medications (their uses and side effects) is necessary, so patients can make decisions and manage their headaches when they occur.

Education should include the following:
- Use a product no more than twice a week to avoid rebound headaches.
- Instruct patients on how to use the medication, particularly nasal sprays and injections, at the first sign of pain.
- Avoid alcohol with these medications.
- Report any adverse symptoms at their first occurrence.

PROPHYLACTIC AGENTS. Patients should take the product daily regardless of whether they have headache symptoms. It often takes 3 to 4 weeks to determine the efficacy of specific products.

SPECIFIC DRUGS

ABORTIVE AGENTS

Triptans

---

sumatriptan (Imitrex) 🔑

CONTRAINDICATIONS
- Hypersensitivity
- *Significant cardiovascular disease:* CAD, stroke, transient ischemic attacks, uncontrolled hypertension, peripheral vascular disease, ischemic bowel disease
- Basilar artery, hemiplegic, or complicated migraine
- Concomitant use of monoamine oxidase inhibitors, ergots, or SSRIs
- Individuals younger than 18 years of age
- Pregnancy
- Severe hepatic impairment

WARNINGS

💣 Risk of myocardial ischemia or infarction and other adverse cardiac events; these agents have the potential to cause coronary vasospasm. Do not give to patients with cardiac risk factors unless a cardiovascular evaluation shows no underlying disease. Give first dose in office with adequate

---

medical equipment; consider obtaining an ECG during administration. Ventricular fibrillation/tachycardia and myocardial infarction have occurred.

- *Cerebrovascular events and fatalities:* Cerebral hemorrhage, subarachnoid hemorrhage, stroke, and other cerebrovascular events may be seen.
- Markedly increased blood pressure, including hypertensive crisis, has been reported.
- Nasal spray may cause local irritation.
- Hypersensitivity reactions are rare, but severe anaphylaxis reactions have occurred.
- *Renal function impairment:* Use rizatriptan and sumatriptan with caution.
- *Hepatic function impairment:* Administer with caution; dose may have to be decreased.
- Carcinogenesis and impaired fertility have been observed in animal studies.

PRECAUTIONS
- Chest, jaw, or neck tightness has occurred after administration; monitor for angina.
- Seizures have occurred rarely.
- *Ophthalmic effects:* Binds to melanin; can accumulate over time; causes corneal effects in animals
- Photosensitivity may occur.

PHARMACOKINETICS. Table 43-4 compares all migraine products. Onset of action varies among these agents; sumatriptan, rizatriptan, almotriptan, and Relpax have an onset of action of less than 2 hours; naratriptan, frovatriptan, and zolmitriptan take longer. Duration of action is also a consideration; frovatriptan lasts the longest.

ADVERSE EFFECTS. See Table 43-5.

DRUG INTERACTIONS
- Cimetidine may increase drug levels of zolmitriptan and other potent cyp 3A4 inhibitors.
- Ketoconazole increases levels of almotriptan.
- Oral contraceptives increase levels of frovatriptan.
- Propranolol increases levels of rizatriptan, eletriptan, and frovatriptan.
- Sibutramine increases levels of naratriptan, sumatriptan, zolmitriptan, and rizatriptan.
- Triptans increase levels of SSRIs.

OVERDOSAGE. Symptoms to be expected include hypertension and other more serious cardiovascular symptoms such as pressure in the chest, palpitations, pain, and shortness of breath.

DOSAGE AND ADMINISTRATION. See Table 43-6.

Patients should take the initial dose at the first sign of migraine. If the first dose is not effective, patients may repeat the dosage once, generally after 2 hours. Patients should repeat with the same dosage as the initial dose. With the next migraine, patients may start with a higher dose if the first dose was ineffective. Do not give any more triptan within that 24-hour period.

Patients should administer a triptan no more often than 2 days per week. A 24-hour hiatus should be taken between use of this medicine and use of an ergot.

Continued

sumatriptan (Imitrex) 🔑 —cont'd

The most commonly used formulation is the tablet. A nasal spray will work if the patient has nausea and vomiting that interfere with absorption of a tablet. Orally disintegrating tablets dissolve on the tongue, requiring no water. This makes it a very convenient dosing system. Patients with severe migraine prefer the injection formulation because it has the fastest onset of action. The thigh is the preferred site for injection.

The initial dose, whether oral tablet, nasal spray, or subcutaneous injection, should be administered in the office, so the provider can monitor blood pressure and pulse. In addition, the provider should be present to answer questions about any side effects that may occur.

OTHER DRUGS IN CLASS

Other drugs in this class are similar to the key drug except as follows:

- All drugs in this category are very similar; the main differences lie in their pharmacokinetics.
- The newest drug, *eletriptan (Relpax)*, is a potent CYP 3A4 inhibitor. Concentrations of eletriptan may increase up to fourfold if given with ketoconazole, itraconazole, clarithromycin, erythromycin, or nefazodone. Studies suggest faster headache relief and less headache recurrence with this drug as compared with other triptans.
- *Frovatriptan* has the longest half-life of the triptans but is similar in other respects.

ERGOTAMINE DERIVATIVES

ergotamine tartrate (Cafergot) 🔑

CONTRAINDICATIONS
- Coronary heart disease or coronary artery vasospasm, uncontrolled hypertension, impaired hepatic or renal function, hemiplegic or basilar migraine, and concomitant use with peripheral and central vasoconstrictors
- In pregnancy and in women who may become pregnant, uterine stimulant actions may cause fetal harm.
- Do not use ergots within 24 hours of using triptans.

WARNINGS
- Possible vasospastic reactions may occur with the use of ergots; the clinician and the patient should be aware of the signs and symptoms of such vascular changes.

💣 Overuse of ergot agents may lead to ergotism. Manifestations include symptoms of intense arterial vasoconstriction with evidence of peripheral vascular ischemia, headache, intermittent claudication, muscle pain, numbness, coldness, and pallor of the extremities. If the condition progresses, gangrene may occur.

- Vasospasm-related events include peripheral vascular ischemia and Raynaud's phenomenon.
- Increased blood pressure may occur.

PRECAUTIONS
- Do not exceed the recommended dosage.
- Drug abuse and dependence may occur with extended use.

DRUG INTERACTIONS
- Major substrate of CYP3A4; numerous drug-drug interactions exist. Consult a detailed reference for specific interaction.

DOSAGE AND ADMINISTRATION. See Table 43-6.

Have the patient self-administer the preparation at a lower than recommended dose when headache free. Dosing should be increased gradually until the recommended dose is achieved, or patients are troubled with side effects. The most common side effect is nausea.

OTHER DRUGS IN CLASS

Other drugs in this class are similar to the prototype except as follows.

isometheptene mucate (Midrin)

CONTRAINDICATIONS. Glaucoma, severe renal disease, hypertension, organic heart disease, hepatic disease, and concomitant use with monoamine oxidase inhibitors

WARNINGS
- *CNS effects:* The capsules contain 100 mg dichloralphenazone, which is structurally similar to chlorhydrate and increases the risk for CNS depression. Warn patients to use caution in performing tasks that require metal alertness. Warn about possible combined effects with alcohol and other CNS depressant drugs. A theoretical risk of dependence is present.

PRECAUTIONS. Use with caution in patients with hypertension and peripheral vascular disease and after recent cardiovascular attacks.

DRUG INTERACTIONS. Do not give with MAOIs because this could lead to hypertensive crisis.

dihydroergotamine (DHE-45, Migranal)

CONTRAINDICATIONS. Hypersensitivity; CAD; hemiplegic or basilar migraine; uncontrolled hypertension; peripheral vascular disease and post vascular surgery; severe hepatic or rental dysfunction; avoid use within 24 hours of triptans or ergot-like agents; avoid during or within 2 weeks of discontinuing MAO inhibitors; potent inhibitors of CYP3A4 (includes protease inhibitors, azole antifungals, and some macrolide antibiotics); pregnancy.

WARNINGS. *Fibrotic complications:* Pleural and retroperitoneal fibrosis following prolonged daily use of injectable DHE

Risk of myocardial ischemia and/or myocardial infarction and other adverse cardiac events: Do not use in patients with documented ischemic or vasospastic CAD. Do not give to patients with cardiac risk factors unless a cardiovascular evaluation shows no underlying disease. Give first dose in the office, where an ECG can be taken during administration.

Drug-associated cerebrovascular events and fatalities: Cerebral hemorrhage, subarachnoid hemorrhage, stroke, and other cerebrovascular events may occur.

Local irritation can occur.

DRUG INTERACTIONS
- Metabolized by the CYP 3A4 system, so it will interact with other drugs metabolized by the 3A4 system.

TABLE 43-4   Pharmacokinetics of Migraine Products

Drug	Absorption and Drug Availability	Onset of Action	Time to Peak Concentration	Half-life	Duration of Action	Protein Bound	Metabolism	Excretion
sumatriptan (Imitrex)								
Injectable (Imitrex)	97% available	10-60 min	12 min	2 hr	1.5-2.5 hr	15%	Liver	Renal, 60%; feces, 40%
Oral	Rapid; 16% available	1-2 hr	1.5 hr		Standard*	15%	Liver	Renal, 60%; feces, 40%
Nasal spray		15-30 min			Less	15%	Liver	Renal, 60%; feces, 40%
naratriptan (Amerge)	74% available	30 min	2-3 hr		Longer	30%	Liver	Renal, 70%
rizatriptan (Maxalt/MLT)	40% available	30-120 min	1-2 hr	2-3 hr	Longer	14%	Liver	Renal, 70%; feces, 30%
zolmitriptan (Zomig)	49% after first pass	30-60 min	1.5-3 hr	2.8-3.7 hr	Longer	25%	Liver	Urine, 60%-80%; feces, 20%-40%
Almotriptan (Axert)	80%	<1-2 hr	2.5	3 hr	Longer	35%	Liver	Urine, 40%; feces, 13%
frovatriptan	30%	2-3 hr		2.5 hr	Longer			Urine 32%; feces, 62%
eletriptan (Relpax)	50%		1.3 hr	4 hr	Longer		CYP3A4	Renal, 9%, feces, 90%
ergotamine tartrate					48 hr			
Tablets	5%	30 min	70 min	2 hr	24 hr		Liver	Feces
Suppositories	Good				24 hr		Liver	Feces
DHE 45								
Injection	50% available	15-30 min		21-32 hr	3-4 hr	90%	Liver	Biliary, 90%; renal, 10%
Migranal	Variable	15-30 min		1.5-4 hr		93%	Liver	Feces
cyproheptadine		30-60 min			8-12 hr			Renal, 65%-75%; feces, 25%-35%

*Standard: Duration of action of triptans is compared with that of sumatriptan.

TABLE 43-5   Common and Serious Adverse Effects of Migraine Medications

Drug	Common Minor Reactions	Serious Adverse Effects
Serotonin (5-HT$_1$) receptor agonists (triptans)	Dizziness, fatigue, pain, warm sensation, headache, flushing, hot or cold sensation, erythema, pruritus, chest or neck tightness, nausea, dry mouth, paresthesia, asthenia, somnolence	Chest pain, coronary artery vasospasm, MI, myocardial ischemia, ventricular fibrillation/tachycardia, agitation, TIA, seizure, elevated blood pressure
isometheptene	Transient dizziness and skin rash, drowsiness	Feeling of weakness
ergotamine tartrate	Localized edema, drowsiness, dry mouth, dizziness, nausea, vomiting	Peripheral vascular effects (numbness, tingling), tachycardia, weakness in legs
DHE	Dizziness, somnolence, paresthesia, nausea, vomiting *Nasal spray:* altered sense of taste, rhinitis	*Injection:* serious cardiac events, including vasospasm, MI, ventricular fibrillation/tachycardia, and fibrotic complications
cyproheptadine	Sedation, weight gain, GI upset, palpitations, dryness of mucous membranes, dizziness	Hypotension, increased heart rate, urinary frequency or retention, restlessness

TABLE 43-6   Dosage and Administration Recommendations of Migraine Medications

Drug	Formulation	Dosage	Administration		Maximum Dosage in 24 hr
sumatriptan	Tablets: 25, 50, 100 mg Nasal spray: 5 mg/spray Injection	25, 50, 100 mg 5, 10, 20 mg 6 mg subQ	q2h One puff each nostril q2h One injection, repeat in 1 hr		200 mg 40 mg 12 mg
naratriptan	Tablets: 1, 2.5 mg	2.5 mg	q4h	May repeat ×1	5 mg
rizatriptan	Tablets: 5, 10 mg Orally disintegrating tablets: 2.5, 5, 10 mg	5 mg 5 mg	q2h q2h		30 mg 30 mg
zolmitriptan	Tablets: 2.5, 5 mg	2.5, 5 mg	q2h		10 mg
almotriptan	Tablets: 6.25, 12.5 mg	6.25 mg	q2h		2 doses
eletriptan	Tablets: 20, 40 mg	40 mg	q2h		80 mg in 24 hr
frovatriptan	Tablets: 2.5 mg	2.5 mg	q2h		7.5 mg
isometheptene	Caplets, combination	1-2 caplet(s)	1 caplet qhr		5 caplets per 12 hr
ergotamine tartrate	Tablets, sublingual	2 mg	q30min bid		10 mg/week (6 sprays); 8 sprays/week
DHE	Nasal spray: 4 mg/ml, 0.5 mg/spray	One spray each nostril	q15min		3 mg
cyproheptadine	Tablets: 4 mg 2 mg/5 ml solution	4-8 mg	2 mg bid-qid in divided doses		24 mg

- Ingestion with grapefruit will increase serum levels and will produce overdose effects.
- DHE will decrease the therapeutic effects of nitrates.

DOSAGE AND ADMINISTRATION. See Table 43-6.

Nasal treatment: Prime the pump before administration by squeezing four times. Discard unused drug in opened ampule after 8 hours.

Prophylactic Agent

cyproheptadine (Periactin)

CONTRAINDICATIONS

- Contraindications include elderly, debilitated patients or those with angle-closure glaucoma, prostatic hyperplasia, stenosing peptic ulcer, or bladder neck obstruction.
- Do not use in children younger than 2 years of age.

WARNINGS/PRECAUTIONS

- Overdose in children may produce hallucinations, CNS depression, convulsions, or death.
- Sedation is common in adults.
- Children may experience excitement, restlessness, insomnia, and seizures.
- The drug may produce an atropine-like action, so it must be used with caution in patients treated for bronchial asthma, increased intraocular pressure, hyperthyroidism, cerebral vascular disease, or hypertension.

DRUG INTERACTIONS. This medication produces additive sedating effects when used with alcohol, other CNS depressants, hypnotics, sedatives, tranquilizers, or anxiolytic drugs. MOAIs may intensify the anticholinergic effects of antihistamine.

evolve A continually updated list of useful WebLinks may be found in the Evolve Resources at http://evolve.elsevier.com/Edmunds/NP/

44 Anticonvulsants

DRUG OVERVIEW

Class	Generic Name	Trade Name
Hydantoin	phenytoin 🔑 ✳	Dilantin
Succinimide	ethosuximide	Zarontin
GABA analogs (newer drugs)	valproic acid 🔑	Depakene
	divalproex sodium	Depakote ✳
	felbamate	Felbatol
	gabapentin ✳	Neurontin
	lamotrigine	Lamictal ✳
	pregabalin	Lyrica ✳
	tiagabine	Gabitril
	topiramate	Topamax ✳
	zonisamide	Zonegran
Barbiturates	phenobarbital ✳	Luminal
	primidone	Mysoline
Benzodiazepines	diazepam ✳	Valium
	clonazepam ✳	Klonopin
	lorazepam ✳	Ativan
Miscellaneous	carbamazepine ✳	Tegretol, Epitol
	oxcarbazepine	Trileptal ✳
	levetiracetam	Keppra ✳

✳ Top 200 drug; 🔑 key drug.

INDICATIONS

(See Table 44-1.)

- Generalized tonic, clonic, or absence seizures
- *Partial:* Simple partial, complex partial, partial with secondary generalization
- Lamotrigine, topiramate, zonisamide, and felbamate protect against partial seizures and a variety of generalized seizure types.
- Vigabatrin is effective against partial seizures (with or without secondary generalization) and infantile spasms.

- Oxcarbazepine, tiagabine, and gabapentin are mainly restricted to patients with partial epilepsy (and, in the case of oxcarbazepine, those with primarily generalized tonic-clonic seizures).
- Levetiracetam is effective in partial seizures.

TABLE 44-1   Anticonvulsants and Their Uses

Drug	Indications	Unlabeled Uses
phenytoin	Monotherapy and combination therapy for partial and generalized seizures Prevention and treatment of seizures that may occur during neurosurgery	
ethosuximide	Absence seizures	
valproic acid	Monotherapy or adjunctive therapy for absence and complex partial seizures	May be effective as monotherapy and as combination therapy for all seizure types, including generalized and myoclonic
felbamate	Only in those with severe seizures for whom other therapies have failed	Lennox-Gastaut syndrome
gabapentin	Adjunctive therapy for partial seizures with or without generalization in patients >12 yr Adjunctive therapy for partial seizures in children 3 to 12 yr	Neuropathic pain, peripheral neuropathy
lamotrigine	Adjunctive therapy for partial seizure disorder in adults and pediatric patients 2 yr or older Adjunctive therapy for patients with Lennox-Gastaut syndrome >2 yr Monotherapy in adults with partial seizures and in patients who have been on other anticonvulsants Bipolar disorder	Generalized seizure disorder Partial atonic seizures, neuropathic and chronic pain syndromes Atonic, myoclonic, and tonic seizures
pregabalin	Adjunctive therapy for adult patients with partial onset of seizures Diabetes mellitus–associated neuropathic pain and post-herpetic neuralgia	
tiagabine	Adjunctive therapy for partial seizures in patients >12 yr	
topiramate	Monotherapy for partial onset or primary generalized tonic-clonic seizures Adjunctive therapy for partial or generalized seizure disorder, and Lennox-Gastaut syndrome for patients >2 yr	Neuropathic and chronic pain syndromes Weight loss Cluster headaches
zonisamide	Adjunctive therapy for partial seizures in adults and children	Generalized seizure disorders
carbamazepine	Monotherapy and combination therapy for partial, general, and mixed seizure disorders Trigeminal neuralgia	Simple and complex partial seizures, chronic pain, restless leg syndrome, psychiatric disorders such as bipolar disorder; treatment for alcohol, benzodiazepine, or cocaine withdrawal
oxcarbazepine	Monotherapy and adjunctive therapy for partial seizure disorder in adults and children Adjunctive therapy for partial seizure disorder in children >4 yr	Atypical panic disorder Neuropathic and other chronic pain syndromes
levetiracetam	Adjunctive therapy for refractory partial seizures in adults and children 4 years or older	
phenobarbital	Generalized tonic-clonic and partial seizures	Not for myoclonic and generalized absence seizures First line for neonatal seizures
benzodiazepines (lorazepam, diazepam)	IV for status epilepticus, acute seizures for drug overdose and poison	
clonazepam	Myoclonic and atonic seizures	

Anticonvulsants, or *antiepileptic drugs* (AEDs), are the medications used to control seizures. Traditionally, these drugs were divided into five classes, including hydantoins, γ-aminobutyric acid (GABA) analogs, succinimides, barbiturates, and benzodiazepines, plus a miscellaneous class. In addition, the diuretic, acetazolamide, is used adjunctively to manage seizures. These medications may be used alone or in combination, but the different medication classes are unrelated chemically.

Over time, these drug classifications have become less popular, with many clinicians preferring to classify medications as older or newer drugs. The newer drugs are not particularly more effective, but they may have fewer side effects or drug interactions because they are involved in the induction or inhibition of hepatic P450 enzyme systems. Some of the newer drugs are also used for treating patients with problems other than seizures, such as peripheral neuropathy and pain management; many of the newer AEDs are approved for adjunctive use only.

In general, seizure disorders are managed in specialists' offices rather than in primary care settings. The primary care provider often monitors these patients once they are stable and may see them for other acute or chronic medical conditions.

THERAPEUTIC OVERVIEW

Pathophysiology and the Disease Process

A *seizure* is an alteration in behavior, function, and/or consciousness that results from an abnormal electrical discharge of neurons in the brain. Epilepsy, or the term *seizure disorder*, is used to describe chronic unprovoked recurrent seizures. Seizures are classified according to clinical presentation and EEG characteristics. The International Classification of Seizures by the Commission on Classification and Terminology of the International League Against Epilepsy is summarized in Table 44-2. The treatment chosen for seizure disorder depends on the type of seizure; thus, the correct diagnosis

of seizure disorder is imperative. Drugs appear in the table in the order in which they usually are initiated for each type of seizure.

A seizure is a symptom of an underlying brain disorder—not a disease itself. However, the origin of most seizure disorders is unknown. Underlying pathologic conditions, such as tumor, subarachnoid hemorrhage, or hematoma, must be ruled out. Not all behaviors that appear to be seizure activity are seizures. The differential diagnosis for the patient who presents with a history of "seizure" is lengthy. The practitioner must consider systemic, metabolic, and neurologic factors; trauma; brain infection; and behavioral conditions that may cause altered consciousness or behavior. These include syncope, hypoglycemia, cardiac arrhythmia, transient ischemic attack, narcolepsy, psychogenic seizures, alcohol withdrawal, and attention-deficit disorder. New-onset idiopathic epilepsy is unusual in the elderly, who are more likely to have an underlying pathologic condition or metabolic disorder. Of the neurologic disorders, seizures are most common in children. The incidence is highest in children younger than 3. In approximately one in five children who have a seizure, epilepsy will develop.

Seizure most frequently presents in a patient with a known seizure disorder who fails to take adequate suppressive

TABLE 44-2 Seizure Classification and Recommended Medication Therapy

Seizure Type	Description	Drug*
Simple partial	Focal motor or sensory symptoms; reflects area of brain affected; no change in consciousness	phenytoin carbamazepine valproic acid phenobarbital topiramate gabapentin oxcarbazepine Adjunct—lamotrigine Adjunct—pregabalin Adjunct—tiagabine Adjunct—zonisamide
Complex partial	Characterized by an aura, followed by impaired consciousness with automatisms, usually originating from temporal lobe	carbamazepine phenytoin phenobarbital valproic acid gabapentin
Secondarily generalized	Simple or complex partial seizures that progress to generalized tonic-clonic seizures	phenytoin carbamazepine phenobarbital valproic acid
Generalized tonic-clonic	Formerly "grand mal"; sudden loss of consciousness with tonic-clonic motor activity, postictal state of confusion, drowsiness, and headache	phenytoin carbamazepine phenobarbital valproic acid topiramate
Absence	Formerly "petit mal"; brief (<30 seconds) episodes of unresponsiveness characterized by staring, blinking, or facial twitching	ethosuximide valproic acid clonazepam
Myoclonic	Series of brief jerky contractions of specific muscle groups	oxcarbazepine zonisamide clonazepam
Refractory	Unable to control with other medications	felbamate levetiracetam

*Listed in order currently recommended for use, although these recommendations frequently change.

medication. Adherence issues are common with antiepileptic medications; however, concurrent illnesses, changes in medication, or addition of other medications frequently may have an impact on the metabolism of AEDs, some of which have a very narrow therapeutic window.

Assessment

Make sure the episode is actually a seizure. Question patients about what they remember before, during, and after the event. It is usually necessary to question witnesses of the seizure to gain additional information, particularly about what happens during the seizure, the length of the seizure, postictal state, and so forth. Next, try to determine the cause of the seizure. Rule out metabolic disorders, trauma, tumors or other space-occupying lesions, vascular disease, degenerative disorders, migraine with aura, tic disorders, and infectious disease. It is very clear that the origin of seizures varies by age group; the clinician should be alert to this variation when treating patients. For the initial seizure, assessment and testing may be extensive. For a patient with a known seizure disorder, the focus is on what triggered that particular seizure.

MECHANISM OF ACTION

For most of these drugs, the exact mechanism for reducing seizure activity is not clearly understood. All increase the threshold of the CNS to convulsive stimuli or inhibit the spread of seizure activity. What is known about the specific mechanisms of action for each class follows.

Hydantoins

The primary site of action appears to be the primary motor cortex, where spread of seizure activity is inhibited. Phenytoin prolongs the effective refractory period by blocking neuronal sodium channels. It stabilizes the threshold against hyperexcitability caused by excessive stimulation or environmental changes and reduces the maximal activity of brainstem centers responsible for the tonic phase of grand mal seizures. It also exhibits antiarrhythmic properties, similar to those of quinidine or procainamide. Although it has little effect on the electrical excitability of cardiac muscle, phenytoin decreases the force of contraction, depresses pacemaker action, and improves atrioventricular conduction, particularly when it has been depressed by digitalis glycosides.

GABA Analogs

The mechanism of action of valproic acid and the newer GABA analogs is not clearly understood. All of these drugs are chemically unrelated, but they increase the actions of GABA, an inhibitory neurotransmitter. They may inhibit the voltage-dependent sodium channel, thereby stabilizing the neuronal membranes. Some of the newer GABA analogs have several actions, including augmentation of GABA, blockage of voltage NA channels, antagonism of glutamate, and modulation of calcium channels.

Carbamazepine

Carbamazepine is chemically similar to the tricyclic antidepressants. It is unrelated structurally to the other anticonvulsants. Its action is similar to that of phenytoin; it limits seizure propagation by blocking postsynaptic transmission.

Barbiturates

Phenobarbital works by inhibiting depolarization of neurons by binding to the GABA receptor, which enhances the transmission of chloride ions. Barbiturates also increase the threshold for electrical stimulation of the motor cortex. Primidone is metabolized to phenobarbital and phenylethylmalonamide (PEMA), which have anticonvulsant activity. PEMA may potentiate the activity of phenobarbital.

Benzodiazepines

Benzodiazepines work similarly to barbiturates, but they also increase the number of chloride channels while facilitating transmission of chloride ions. This suppresses the spread of seizure activity but does not abolish abnormal discharge from a focus. Initiate maintenance anticonvulsant therapy after seizures have stopped.

TREATMENT PRINCIPLES
Standardized Guidelines

- French JA, et al: Efficacy and tolerability of the new antiepileptic drugs, I: Treatment of new onset epilepsy: report of the Therapeutics and Technology Assessment Subcommittee and Quality Standards Subcommittee of the American Academy of Neurology and the American Epilepsy Society, *Neurology* 62:1252-1260, 2004.

Evidence-Based Recommendations

- Little good-quality evidence has been gathered from clinical trials to support the use of newer monotherapy or adjunctive therapy AEDs over older drugs, or to support the use of one newer AED in preference to another. In general, data related to clinical effectiveness, safety, and tolerability have failed to demonstrate consistent and statistically significant differences between drugs.
- Newer AEDs, when used as monotherapy, may be cost-effective for the treatment of patients who have experienced adverse events with older AEDs, who have failed to respond to the older drugs, or in whom such drugs are contraindicated.
- *Partial epilepsy:* Beneficial—carbamazepine, phenobarbital, phenytoin, valproate
- Unknown effectiveness—other drugs
- *Generalized epilepsy:* Beneficial—carbamazepine, phenobarbital, phenytoin, valproate; unknown effectiveness—other drugs
- *Drug-resistant partial epilepsy:* Beneficial—addition of gabapentin, levetiracetam, lamotrigine, oxcarbazepine, tiagabine, topiramate, vigabatrin, or zonisamide
- Lamotrigine may be a clinical and cost-effective alternative to existing standard drug treatment—carbamazepine—for patients given a diagnosis of partial seizures.
- For patients with idiopathic generalized epilepsy or difficult to classify epilepsy, valproate remains the drug that is clinically most effective, although topiramate may be a cost-effective alternative for some patients.

Cardinal Points of Treatment

- Choose an agent appropriate to the type of seizure.
- Choose the least toxic option. Most anticonvulsants are cytochrome P450 inducers and, as such, are involved in many drug–drug interactions.

- Initiate monotherapy; start slowly and continue until steady state is reached (five times the half-life).
- Titrate the dose upward until control is achieved or adverse reactions occur.
- Choose an alternative monotherapy drug if adverse reactions to the first drug occur.

Pharmacologic Treatment

The decision to initiate anticonvulsant therapy must be made with consideration of several variables; most important are the consequences of seizure recurrence for the patient. These consequences are mainly psychosocial and may depend on age, employment, family responsibility, and access to transportation. Make the decision about drug therapy in consultation with the primary care practitioner, the neurologist, the patient, and the family.

Discontinuation of anticonvulsant medication may be considered in patients who have been seizure free for longer than 2 years. An EEG should be obtained before medication is withdrawn. The recurrence rate is usually about 40%, with most seizures occurring in the first year after medication is discontinued. The same psychosocial factors and risks of seizure recurrence for the individual patient should be considered when anticonvulsants are withdrawn as when therapy is initiated.

No evidence suggests that prophylactic anticonvulsant treatment prevents epilepsy. It is common practice to give an anticonvulsant, usually phenytoin, at the time of neurosurgery and after head trauma. Most survivors of brain surgery or head trauma do not later develop epilepsy. Phenytoin given at therapeutic doses during the week after severe head trauma does suppress seizures. This treatment is appropriate when the brain is swollen and cerebral blood flow may be compromised. A seizure could further compromise cerebral blood, leading to increased swelling and intracranial pressure. The same treatment can be applied to the perioperative period. However, no evidence indicates that anticonvulsants prevent later epilepsy; therefore, it is not necessary to give long-term anticonvulsants to these patients.

A seizure is usually self-limiting in its physical consequences unless the patient suffers physical injury during the seizure. However, research has shown that people who have seizures are at increased risk of sudden death; slowing of cognition and loss of short-term memory after a seizure; and the heavy emotional burden carried by patients who fear they suddenly may have a seizure. Patients who have seizures must live with state regulations such as those that limit their driving, require careful family planning, and control their environment for maximum safety during a seizure.

Those individuals who have status epilepticus (SE) may experience true medical emergencies that the primary practitioner must be prepared to recognize and manage. For practical purposes, SE is defined as two or more seizures that occur without complete recovery of neurologic function between seizures or as continuous seizure activity for longer than 5 minutes. Therapy should be initiated for any generalized tonic-clonic convulsive seizure activity (formerly called grand mal). Most generalized convulsive seizures last less than 2 minutes. Thus, the practitioner who witnesses a generalized convulsive seizure for longer than 2 minutes should be prepared to initiate emergency procedures. These include activating emergency medical services, such as by calling 911,

and protecting the airway. Emergency personnel should initiate intravenous access and administer intravenous benzodiazepines (lorazepam or diazepam) as protocols permit.

The goal of medical treatment is to control seizures and allow patients to return to their usual activities. Ideally, this should be done with a single medication that has no significant side effects. This is achieved in about one half of patients.

The medication to use depends on the type of seizure (see Tables 44-1 and 44-2). A neurologist generally makes this decision. The medication is started at a low dose and gradually is increased until seizures are controlled, or the patient exhibits adverse effects. If the patient continues to experience seizures despite the highest tolerated dose, a second drug is added gradually. Then the first drug is withdrawn gradually.

Phenobarbital is effective for the prevention of febrile seizures in children, although long-term prophylactic treatment for febrile seizures is not recommended by the American Academy of Pediatrics, which has concluded that the risks of long-term treatment outweigh the benefits. In general, treatment is reserved for those children at greatest risk for future neurologic problems because of seizures; these include children with febrile seizures before 18 months of age, those with neurologic dysfunction or severe developmental delays, those with complex seizures, and those who have seizures with a focal component that last longer than 15 minutes.

Although older-generation agents (AEDs) such as carbamazepine, phenytoin, and valproic acid continue to be used widely in the treatment of epilepsy, these drugs have important shortcomings, such as highly variable and nonlinear pharmacokinetics, a narrow therapeutic index, suboptimal response rates, and a propensity to cause significant adverse effects and drug interactions. Compared with older agents, some of the new AEDs offer appreciable advantages in terms of less variable kinetics and, particularly in the cases of gabapentin, levetiracetam, and vigabatrin, a lower interaction potential. Currently, new generation AEDs are used primarily as adjunctive therapy for patients who are refractory to older agents. However, because of advantages in terms of tolerability and ease of use, some of these drugs are used increasingly for first-line management in certain subgroups of patients. As the result of serious toxicity risks, felbamate and vigabatrin should be prescribed only for patients who are refractory to other drugs. In the case of vigabatrin, however, first-line use may be justified in infants with spasms.

How to Monitor

The patient who is beginning anticonvulsant therapy must be monitored frequently to confirm that the drug is in the therapeutic range, to document adverse events, and to maximize seizure control. Therapeutic levels of different drugs are given in Table 44-3.

These drugs have individual therapeutic ranges, above which most patients will experience toxic effects. If the therapeutic range is too low, most patients will not have adequate seizure control. However, individuals may do better with drug levels above or below the therapeutic range. Monitoring of serum drug levels usually must be done yearly for the patient who is being maintained on an anticonvulsant. A serum level should be checked when seizure frequency increases, if compliance is an issue, or if the patient is exhibiting toxic signs.

TABLE 44-3 Pharmacokinetics of Selected Anticonvulsant Medications

Drug	Absorption	Drug Availability After First Pass	Onset of Action	Time to Peak Concentration	Half-life	Protein Bound	Metabolism	Excretion	Therapeutic Level
phenytoin (Dilantin)	95%	70%-100% (form dependent)	3-6 hr	1.5-12 hr	7-42 hr (dose dependent)	90%	Liver	Urine	10-20 mcg/ml
valproic acid (Depakene, Depakote)	Well	90%	—	1-4 hr; ER: 4-17 hr	6-16 hr	80%-90%	Liver	Urine	50-100 mcg/ml
gabapentin (Neurontin)	50%-60%	27%-60% (inversely related to dose)	2-3 hr	1.5-4.5 hr	5-8 hr	0%-5%	None	Urine	—
lamotrigine (Lamictal)	Complete	98%	1-4 hr	1.4-4.8 hr	30 hr (monotherapy)	50%-55%	Liver	Urine, 94%; feces, 2%	—
pregabalin (Lyrica)	Well	90%	7 days (analgesic)	1.5-3 hr	6.3 hr	None	None	Urine	—
topiramate (Topamax)	Good	80%	—	2-4 hr	21 hr	15%-41% (inversely related to plasma levels)	Liver	Urine	—
carbamazepine (Tegretol)	Slow	85%	—	Unpredictable; 2-6 hr; ER: 3-12 hr	12-65 hr	70%-93%	90% liver 2D6 inducer 2C induces	Urine, 72%; feces, 28%	4-12 mcg/ml
phenobarbital (Luminal)	Well	80%-100%	0.3-1 hr	1-6 hr	52-118 hr	20%-45%	Liver	Urine	15-30 mcg/ml (children) 20-40 mcg/ml (adults)
primidone (Mysoline)	60%-80%	90%-100%	1.5-3 hr	0.5-9 hr PEMA: 8-12 hr	Parent drug: 10-12 hr; PEMA: 16 hr; phenobarbital: 52-118 hr	phenobarbital 99%	Liver	Urine	5-12 mcg/ml phenobarbital (adults)

Many medications interact with the metabolism of the anticonvulsants; therefore, serum level of the anticonvulsant should be checked when medication changes are made. Ideally, a trough level should be drawn for routine monitoring. A random level should be drawn when seizures occur. Some of the older anticonvulsant drugs have relatively long half-lives, so once steady state is achieved on a maintenance dose, little fluctuation in serum levels should occur.

Older antiseizure drugs are metabolized by the liver. However, many of the newer agents do not undergo hepatic metabolism; this allows for reduced drug–drug interactions. Hepatic enzymes should be checked before anticonvulsant therapy is initiated. It is common for hepatic enzymes to be mildly elevated in those on anticonvulsants. They should be monitored yearly and more frequently in patients with known hepatic dysfunction. Children younger than 10 years of age who are on valproic acid should be monitored closely for hepatotoxicity.

Perhaps the most clinically significant pharmacodynamic interaction is that of lamotrigine (LTG) and valproic acid (VPA); these drugs exhibit synergistic efficacy when coadministered to patients with refractory partial and generalized seizures. Because hepatic metabolism is often the cause of pharmacokinetic drug interactions, enzyme-inducing drugs such as phenytoin (PHT), phenobarbitone (PB), and carbamazepine (CBZ) readily enhance the metabolism of other AEDs (e.g., LTG, topiramate [TPM], tiagabine [TGB]). Enzyme-inducing AEDs also enhance the metabolism of many other drugs (e.g., oral contraceptives, antidepressants, warfarin) so that the therapeutic efficacy of coadministered drugs is lost unless the dosage is increased. VPA inhibits the metabolism of PB and LTG, resulting in an elevation in plasma concentrations of inhibited drugs and consequently an increased risk of toxicity. Inhibition of the metabolism of CBZ by VPA results in an elevation of the metabolite CBZ-epoxide, which increases the risk of toxicity. Other examples include inhibition of PHT and CBZ metabolism by cimetidine and CBZ metabolism by erythromycin.

The practitioner must inform the patient and assess for adverse or toxic effects. The most common reactions are rash, visual disturbances, drowsiness, and ataxia. Adverse and toxic effects specific to individual drugs are discussed later (Table 44-4).

Abnormal thyroid function tests have been reported in patients on anticonvulsants. The clinical significance of this is unknown.

Agranulocytosis is rare but has been associated with the use of carbamazepine, ethosuximide, and felbamate. Baseline and periodic blood counts must be performed, especially with felbamate; checks can be less frequent when the dose is stable. If febrile illness or anorexia occurs, blood count and liver function should be assessed. This is especially important in children.

TABLE 44-4   Common and Serious Adverse Effects of Anticonvulsants

Drug	Adverse Effects
phenytoin	Hypotension, atrial and ventricular conduction delay, ventricular fibrillation with IV administration, nystagmus, ataxia, slurred speech, confusion, drowsiness, gingival hyperplasia, increased body hair, thrombocytopenia, rash
ethosuximide	Appetite loss, ataxia, drowsiness, headache, nausea, hiccups, Stevens-Johnson syndrome, systemic lupus erythematosus, blood dyscrasias, convulsions. Children: GI upset, weight gain, headache, hyperactivity
valproic acid	GI disturbances, weight gain, irregular menses, alopecia, pruritus, rashes, including erythema multiforme, photosensitivity, hair loss anxiety, mood problems, tremor, nervousness
felbamate	Aplastic anemia, hepatic failure, GI disturbance, insomnia, headache. Children: GI upset, insomnia, lethargy, ataxia
gabapentin	Drowsiness and ataxia dose-dependent adverse effects; weight gain can occur
lamotrigine	Rash (including Stevens-Johnson syndrome), dizziness, headache, ataxia, visual disturbances, GI disturbances, drowsiness. Children: GI upset, somnolence, dizziness, headache, and diplopia
pregabalin	Dizziness, somnolence, ataxia, confusion, blurred vision, peripheral edema, abnormal thinking, dry mouth, weight gain
tiagabine	Dizziness, drowsiness, depression, confusion
topiramate	Drowsiness, inattention, anorexia, weight loss, paresthesias, renal stones
zonisamide	Drowsiness, dizziness, agitation and inattention, nausea
carbamazepine	Dizziness, drowsiness, ataxia, nausea, and vomiting; rashes, photosensitivity reactions, toxic epidermal necrolysis, and Stevens-Johnson syndrome, hypersensitivity (fever, rash, eosinophilia), pulmonary hypersensitivity (fever, dyspnea, pneumonitis)
oxcarbazepine	Dizziness, diplopia, ataxia, vomiting, nausea, drowsiness, headache, fatigue, rash, and hyponatremia
levetiracetam	Drowsiness, dizziness, fatigue, psychotic symptoms
phenobarbital/primidone	Drowsiness, confusion, dizziness, headache, nausea, vomiting, constipation. Children: hyperactivity, mood alterations, cognitive dysfunction, sleep problems
clonazepam	Children: drowsiness, ataxia, and drooling

Patient Variables

GERIATRICS. No specific guidelines have been put forth regarding the use of anticonvulsants in the elderly. All anticonvulsant therapy is individualized and must be monitored carefully when therapy is initiated. Careful attention must be paid to those patients with hepatic or renal dysfunction. Lower, less-frequent doses are needed in those with hepatic or renal dysfunction or other concomitant disease. Many of the AEDs increase the patient's risk for osteoporosis. Because many anticonvulsants are involved in the cytochrome P450 enzyme system, care must be used in giving these products to patients who are taking multiple medications.

PEDIATRICS. Patients with febrile seizures are treated with phenobarbital, benzodiazepines, or valproic acid. Phenytoin and carbamazepine are not effective for febrile seizures. Ethosuximide, valproic acid, lamotrigine, and clonazepam are considered first-line medications of choice for childhood absence epilepsy. Valproic acid, lamotrigine, topiramate, levetiracetam, and clonazepam are preferred for juvenile myoclonic epilepsy. A pediatric neurologist should be consulted before anticonvulsant therapy is initiated. Risks of recurrent seizures versus side effects of medications and compliance with long-term daily medication must be considered. The dosages of individual medications are based on the pediatric patient's weight and age.

PREGNANCY AND LACTATION

 All anticonvulsants have been associated with an increase in birth defects.

In general, the risk of birth defects in babies of mothers with epilepsy is about two to three times greater than that of the general population. The frequency of birth defects is increased in untreated epileptic mothers, but the frequency of such events in mothers treated with AEDs also seems to be higher. All epileptic women of childbearing age must be informed of the risks before pregnancy occurs. Many serious defects occur during the first trimester. The most common defects include cleft lip and palate, cardiac septal defects, and neural tube defects. A neurologist who specializes in seizure disorder should be consulted before pregnancy to determine the need for medications. The frequency of seizures may increase, decrease, or remain the same during pregnancy. Alterations in metabolism occur during pregnancy that may affect serum drug levels of anticonvulsants. Monthly follow-up and monitoring are required. Ninety-five percent of babies born to mothers on anticonvulsants are normal. Seizures and treatment with anticonvulsants are not reasons to discourage pregnancy. The woman must be made aware of the potential risks and outcomes. Care must be coordinated between the patient, the primary care provider, the obstetrician, and the neurologist to help the patient make the right decision for herself and her unborn child.

Anticonvulsants, particularly barbiturates and hydantoins, have been associated with a coagulation disorder in the neonate. Bleeding may occur in the infant during the first 24 hours after birth. Levels of vitamin K–dependent clotting factors are decreased, and prothrombin time and/or partial thromboplastin time is prolonged. It is recommended that vitamin K be given to the mother 1 month before and again during the delivery, and to the infant immediately after birth.

Some anticonvulsants are excreted in breast milk. Thus, serious adverse effects may occur in the nursing infant. Make a decision whether to discontinue the medication or discontinue breastfeeding.

The use of AEDs, therefore, has a profound influence on women in particular. In some women, seizures are triggered by the menstrual period (catamenial epilepsy). Seizures and their treatment may affect contraception, pregnancy, postpartum care, breastfeeding, and/or menopause.

RACE. No special considerations are required for the use of anticonvulsants among the races; however, most participants in studies of anticonvulsants have been white. Data on the use of anticonvulsants in other races may therefore be inadequate.

GENDER. No specific differences have been noted between male and female patients regarding the metabolism and general use of anticonvulsants. However, a few special considerations apply to women of childbearing age; in some women, an increase in seizure activity is reported around the time of the menses. If this pattern emerges, it may be helpful to increase the anticonvulsant dose at this time of the month. Numerous anticonvulsants alter the metabolism of steroid hormones, thereby influencing the effectiveness of birth control pills. This matter requires special attention in women who are taking birth control pills that contain low concentrations of hormones.

Patient Education

- Do not abruptly discontinue seizure medication because this can precipitate SE.
- Advise patients of side effects and toxic effects and monitoring of medications.
- Anticonvulsants may reduce the effectiveness of birth control pills.
- Counsel women who wish to become pregnant about the risks and outcomes. The risk of birth defects is greater in babies of mothers with untreated seizure disorder, as well as in babies of mothers who take anticonvulsant medications. Some anticonvulsant medications are excreted in breast milk.
- It is mandatory in most states for the health care provider to report to the Department of Transportation that the patient has seizures. The patient in whom seizure is newly diagnosed should be taught about state restrictions that apply to people who wish to drive cars.

 All seizure medications can cause drowsiness and can impair concentration. Advise the patient about not swimming alone and avoiding other situations that could be dangerous should the patient have an adverse medication event or seizure.

- Sleep deprivation, fever, stress, medications, and alcohol can lower the seizure threshold.
- Wear a medical alert bracelet to identify the seizure disorder.
- Advise the family about how to protect the patient from injury during a seizure: Help the patient to the floor, keeping him or her away from any objects that may be bumped; protect the airway from aspiration by using the left side-lying position if possible; do not place any objects, including fingers, into the patient's mouth.

- Advise about driving regulations within the state. Most states require a seizure-free period before driving can be resumed. Health care providers should be familiar with their state regulations or should have a contact at the Motor Vehicle Administration.
- Give information about national organizations and support groups.

SPECIFIC DRUGS

HYDANTOINS

---

phenytoin (Dilantin) 🔑

CONTRAINDICATIONS. Hypersensitivity to the drug; pregnancy

WARNINGS

💣 **Phenytoin should be discontinued if skin rash appears. Scarlatiniform or morbilliform rash, sometimes accompanied by fever, may occur. Rarely, phenytoin has produced severe dermatologic reactions such as bullous, exfoliative, or purpuric dermatitis; lupus erythematosus; Stevens-Johnson syndrome; or toxic epidermal necrolysis. A few deaths have resulted.**

- Pure absence (petit mal) seizures (because the drug may increase the frequency of these seizures)
- Sinus bradycardia, sinoatrial block, second- and third-degree AV block, and Adams-Stokes syndrome (because of its effect on ventricular automaticity)
- Acute alcoholic intake may increase phenytoin serum levels, whereas chronic alcohol use may decrease levels.
- Serum levels sustained above the optimal range may produce delirium, psychosis, encephalopathy, or cerebellar dysfunction. Hypotension occurs if phenytoin is administered rapidly via the intravenous route. The intravenous rate of administration must not exceed 50 mg/min in adults (to prevent hypotension and bradycardia).
- Occasionally, fever, lymphadenopathy, eosinophilia, arthralgia, and hepatic dysfunction, including jaundice, producing a syndrome that resembles mononucleosis, have accompanied severe cutaneous reactions.
- Adverse hematologic effects include thrombocytopenia, leukopenia, granulocytopenia, agranulocytosis, and pancytopenia. Macrocytosis and megaloblastic anemia that responds to folic acid therapy also may occur.
- Osteomalacia can occur and may be related to phenytoin interference with vitamin D metabolism.

PRECAUTIONS. Use with caution in patients with impaired liver function, elderly patients, or the gravely ill because they may show early signs of toxicity. Phenytoin can cause gingival hyperplasia, hirsutism, coarse features, and xanthemia.

Avoid improper administration, including subcutaneous or perivascular injection, to prevent soft tissue irritation. Tissue damage may range from tenderness to necrosis, which has, in rare instances, led to amputation.

PATIENT VARIABLES

- *Pregnancy:* Safe use during pregnancy has not been established. Phenytoin should be used in pregnancy only when clearly needed. In addition to fetal hydantoin syndrome, rare reports have described malignancies in children whose mothers received phenytoin during pregnancy. If it is administered during pregnancy, serum phenytoin concentrations should be monitored closely and dosage adjusted. Because of altered absorption or metabolism during pregnancy, an increased frequency of seizures may occur in pregnant women who are receiving the drug.
- Because phenytoin appears to be secreted in human milk, it is not recommended that women who are taking phenytoin breastfeed their infants.

PHARMACOKINETICS. Phenytoin is metabolized by the CYP 450 enzyme system (see Table 44-3).

Phenytoin follows nonlinear pharmacokinetics. In general, therapeutic plasma phenytoin levels are reached after 1 week of therapy with an oral dose of 300 mg daily in adults. Rapid therapeutic concentrations can be achieved in adults in 8 to 12 hours through administration of an initial oral loading dose of 1 g. Therapeutic concentrations can be attained within 1 to 2 hours after an intravenous loading dose of 1 g (at a rate not exceeding 50 mg/min).

ADVERSE EFFECTS. See Table 44-4 for common adverse effects of anticonvulsants.

DRUG INTERACTIONS. See Table 44-5 for drug interactions with anticonvulsants.

Ingestion times of antacids that contain calcium should be staggered to prevent absorption problems.

OVERDOSAGE. Most patients tolerate blood concentrations of less than 25 mcg/ml. Initial symptoms of overdosage include nystagmus, ataxia, and dysarthria.

Other signs of overdose are tremor, hyperreflexia, lethargy, slurred speech, nausea, and vomiting. Extreme lethargy, hypertension, and comatose states occur at levels greater than 50 mcg/ml. Death occurs because of respiratory and circulatory depression. No antidote is known.

DOSAGE AND ADMINISTRATION. *Treatment of adults with SE:* Loading dose of 10 to 15 mg/kg should be administered slowly intravenously at a rate not to exceed 50 mg/min, with monitoring for respiratory depression, hypotension, or ECG changes. Maintenance doses may be given orally or intravenously at 5 to 6 mg/kg/day (approximately 100 mg every 8 hours).

💣 **Shake oral suspensions well before each dose is administered, or the amount of phenytoin in each milliliter will differ at various levels of the suspension.**

Phenytoin should be given intramuscularly only as a last resort because it is erratically absorbed from intramuscular injection sites. When a patient is transferred from phenytoin to another anticonvulsant, the dosage of phenytoin should be reduced gradually over a period of 1 week, while, at the same time, therapy is instituted with a low dose of the replacement drug.

phenytoin (Dilantin) 🔑 —cont'd

HOW TO MONITOR. Because of nonlinear kinetics, poor correlation has been noted between dosage and serum level, and serum level may increase dramatically with a small increase in dose. It should be remembered that different formulations may have different bioavailability. Monitor the albumin level closely because low levels will increase the amount of available drug, leading to toxicity.

SUCCINIMIDE

ethosuximide (Zarontin)

This drug usually is considered the drug of choice in the management of absence seizures, but it is ineffective in treating most other types of seizures. It is administered orally and is titrated up or down according to patient response. The usual initial oral dose is 250 mg daily for patients 3 to 6 years of age and 500 mg for those older than 6 years. Dosage may be increased by 250 mg every 4 to 7 days until seizures are controlled and side effects are minimized. Do not exceed 1.5 g daily (given in two divided doses).

GABA ANALOGS

valproate, valproic acid, divalproex sodium (Depakene, Depakote) 🔑

CONTRAINDICATIONS. Hepatic disease or severe hepatic dysfunction; hypersensitivity to valproic acid; urea cycle disorders

WARNINGS. Potential for fatal hepatotoxicity; children younger than 2 years seem to be at increased risk, particularly those on multiple AEDs and those with severe seizure disorder, congenital metabolic disorder, mental retardation, or organic brain disease. In these groups of pediatric patients, use as the only agent with extreme caution.

The incidence of fatal hepatotoxicity decreases progressively with increasing age. Hepatotoxicity usually occurs during the first 6 months of treatment.

Liver function tests should be performed before at frequent intervals during therapy. Monitor patients closely; hepatotoxicity may be preceded by loss of seizure control, weakness, lethargy, edema, anorexia, or vomiting. Discontinue immediately if significant hepatic dysfunction is suspected.

Pancreatitis has been reported and in some cases has been life threatening. This has been seen during initial treatment and after years of therapy. Monitor for symptoms of bleeding, abdominal pain, nausea, and vomiting.

PRECAUTIONS. Valproic acid may cause thrombocytopenia and inhibition of platelet aggregation. Platelet counts and coagulation studies should be done before therapy is initiated, at regular intervals, and before any surgical procedure is performed.

Any hemorrhage, bruising, or disorder of coagulation should be investigated, and the dosage reduced or valproic therapy withdrawn.

Hyperammonemia may occur with or without lethargy or coma; it may occur in the absence of elevated liver enzymes. The drug should be discontinued if this occurs. (Also see warning related to hepatotoxicity.)

May cause drowsiness, especially if the drug is taken with other anticonvulsants. Advise the patient to be cautious when driving or swimming, and in other potentially hazardous situations that require mental alertness.

PATIENT VARIABLES

Pregnancy: *Category D:* Incidence of neural tube defects may be increased in the fetuses of mothers who receive valproic acid during the first trimester.

Lactation: Concentrations of valproic acid in breast milk are 1% to 10% of the maternal serum concentration. The effect of this on the nursing infant is unknown. Use caution when administering valproic acid to a nursing woman.

PHARMACOKINETICS. Valproate is the sodium salt of valproic acid. Divalproex sodium is a prodrug, a 1:1 compound of valproic acid and valproate in a delayed-release formulation. Valproic acid is rapidly and almost completely absorbed from the stomach. Valproate is converted to valproic acid in the stomach. Divalproex sodium dissociates into valproate in the upper small intestine. All forms of the drug are dosed as equivalent to valproic acid.

ADVERSE EFFECTS. Valproic acid usually is used in combination with other anticonvulsants; therefore, it is not possible to determine whether the adverse reactions are the result of valproic acid alone or the combination of drugs.

The common initial GI side effects usually are transient and rarely require discontinuation of the drug. Administering the drug with meals and starting with low doses and slowly increasing the dose can minimize these effects. Divalproex sodium may be better tolerated and may reduce GI effects in some patients. Table 44-4 provides common adverse effects of anticonvulsants.

Abnormal thyroid function test results have been reported; the clinical significance of these abnormal findings is unknown.

DRUG INTERACTIONS. Additive CNS depression may occur when valproic acid is administered with other CNS depressants, including other anticonvulsants and alcohol. Valproic acid and phenobarbital or primidone can produce severe CNS depression without a significant increase in the serum concentration of either drug. Patients on valproic acid and a barbiturate must be observed carefully for toxic signs, and serum levels of the barbiturate should be monitored and the dose adjusted as needed. Administration of valproic acid and clonazepam has produced absence status. It is recommended that this combination of drugs be avoided. Valproic acid has been associated with both increases and decreases in serum phenytoin level. It is important to monitor serum phenytoin levels when valproic acid is added or withdrawn. It is advisable to monitor serum concentrations of any concomitant anticonvulsants during initial valproic acid therapy.

Continued

valproate, valproic acid, divalproex sodium (Depakene, Depakote) 🔑—cont'd

Valproic acid may affect bleeding time and should be used with caution in patients who are receiving drugs that affect bleeding time such as warfarin or aspirin. Salicylates may elevate valproic acid levels; this may lead to toxicity. (See Table 44-5 for drug interactions with anticonvulsants.)

OVERDOSAGE. Overdosage may result in coma and death. Valproic acid is absorbed very rapidly; therefore, the efficacy of gastric lavage varies with time since ingestion. Naloxone may reverse CNS depression but also may reverse anticonvulsant effects; use with caution.

DOSAGE AND ADMINISTRATION. The initial dosage of 15 mg/kg/day may be increased at 1-week intervals by 5 to 10 mg/kg/day until seizures are controlled or side effects prevent further increase in dosage. The maximum recommended daily dose is 60 mg/kg/day. Administer the dosage in divided doses if the total daily dose is greater than 250 mg.

Bedtime administration may minimize CNS effects. It should be given with food to decrease GI distress. Valproic acid capsules should be swallowed whole, not chewed, to prevent local irritation to the mouth and throat. Valproate sodium oral solution should not be given with carbonated drinks; the valproic acid will be liberated, causing local irritation and an unpleasant taste. Divalproex sodium (Depakote) may be better tolerated. It may be swallowed intact, or the entire contents of the capsule(s) may be sprinkled on 1 teaspoon of semisolid food such as applesauce or pudding just before administration. Do not chew the mixture or store it for future use.

HOW TO MONITOR. Valproic acid may interact with concomitant anticonvulsants. Serum levels of the anticonvulsants should be monitored when a new drug is added and periodically.

OTHER DRUGS IN CLASS

Other drugs in this class are similar to the prototype except as follows:

gabapentin (Neurontin)

One of the more recent anticonvulsants, gabapentin is different from other anticonvulsants because it is not metabolized and is excreted by the renal system. Exert caution when administering it to elderly patients with decreased creatinine clearance, decreased muscle mass, concomitant disease, and polypharmacy.

Gabapentin does not interact with the common anticonvulsants.

Routine monitoring of clinical laboratory data is not indicated for the safe use of gabapentin. The use of serum concentration monitoring has not been established. Gabapentin does not alter the metabolism of other anticonvulsants; therefore, monitoring serum concentrations of gabapentin or other anticonvulsants is not necessary.

DOSAGE AND ADMINISTRATION. Effective dose for patients older than 12 years of age is 900 to 1800 mg/day in divided doses; start at 300 mg tid.

In children 3 to 12 years of age, give 10 to 15 mg/kg/day in three divided doses and titrate upward. Effective dose usually is reached in 3 days.

Gabapentin often is used for neuropathic pain at 300 to 1800 mg/day in three divided doses.

(See Tables 44-1, 44-4, and 44-5 for use, adverse events, and drug interactions.)

lamotrigine (Lamictal)

CONTRAINDICATIONS, WARNINGS, PRECAUTIONS. Serious rashes that require hospitalization may occur. This seems to be more frequent with rapid introduction of lamotrigine.

Instruct patients who are beginning therapy to notify the provider if a rash occurs. The rash should be promptly evaluated and a decision made whether to continue treatment. If therapy is continued, the rash must be monitored carefully. Stevens-Johnson syndrome, epidermal necrolysis, and angioedema have occurred in association with lamotrigine therapy. Fatal or life-threatening hypersensitivity reactions with clinical features of multiorgan dysfunction and disseminated intravascular coagulation have occurred.

HOW TO MONITOR. The value of monitoring serum levels of lamotrigine has not been established. Pharmacokinetic interactions between lamotrigine and concomitant anticonvulsants may occur. Monitor serum levels of other anticonvulsants, particularly when adjusting dosages.

Lamotrigine binds to melanin. This may cause toxicity in tissues such as the iris. One should be aware of the possibility of long-term ophthalmologic effects.

Photosensitization may occur; advise patients to protect against exposure to ultraviolet light or sunlight by using sunscreens and protective clothing.

Phenytoin and carbamazepine decrease plasma levels of lamotrigine. Valproic acid inhibits the excretion of lamotrigine.

See Tables 44-1, 44-4, and 44-5 for use, adverse events, and drug interactions.

BARBITURATES

phenobarbital (Luminal)

CONTRAINDICATIONS. Hypersensitivity to barbiturates, preexisting CNS depression, severe respiratory depression/disease, severe hepatic disease, uncontrolled pain, porphyria, pregnancy, and lactation

WARNINGS/PRECAUTIONS. Use with caution in patients with cardiac, renal, or hepatic impairment; hypovolemic shock; congestive heart failure; chronic or acute pain syndrome; or history of psychologic or physical drug dependence. Recommend cautious use in the elderly because of long half-life. This drug may cause paradoxical excitement in children. It cannot be withdrawn abruptly; abrupt withdrawal may cause withdrawal symptoms or SE in persons with epilepsy.

DRUG INTERACTIONS. Benzodiazepines, CNS depressants, propoxyphene, valproic acid, methylphenidate, chloramphenicol, and phenytoin enhance the effects of phenobarbital.

TABLE 44-5   Drug Interactions of Anticonvulsant Medications*

Drug	Increase Level	Decrease Level
HYDANTOINS		
phenytoin[†]	alcohol amiodarone chloramphenicol chlordiazepoxide diazepam dicumarol disulfiram Estrogens cimetidine halothane isoniazid methylphenidate Phenothiazines phenylbutazone Salicylates Succinimides Sulfonamides tolbutamide trazodone	carbamazepine Chronic alcohol abuse reserpine sucralfate
GABA ANALOGS		
valproic acid[‡]	chlorpromazine cimetidine erythromycin felbamate Salicylates Antidepressants MAOIs	carbamazepine cholestyramine lamotrigine phenobarbital phenytoin
felbamate[†‡]		carbamazepine phenobarbital phenytoin
gabapentin	cimetidine	Antacids
lamotrigine[†]	Folate inhibitors valproate acid	acetaminophen carbamazepine phenobarbital phenytoin primidone
pregabalin	Drug interactions not expected	
tiagabine	Change in concentration and clearance when administered with valproate, carbamazepine, phenytoin, or phenobarbital; clinical implications of these interactions undetermined	
topiramate[†]	acetazolamide Anticholinergic drugs digoxin, estrogens, Oral contraceptives: phenytoin	carbamazepine with topiramate; decreased concentration of topiramate valproic acid, topiramate (when given with phenytoin)
zonisamide		carbamazepine phenobarbital phenytoin
MISCELLANEOUS		
carbamazepine	cimetidine danazol diltiazem erythromycin fluoxetine	phenobarbital phenytoin primidone Succinimides theophylline

*Consult a detailed reference because drug-drug interactions with anticonvulsants are very difficult to predict and there is conflicting data on the interactions with many of these drugs (Patsalos et al, 2002; Perucca, 2006).
[†]Hepatic enzyme inducer.
[‡]Hepatic enzyme inhibitor.

Table continued on following page

TABLE 44-5   Drug Interactions of Anticonvulsant Medications* (Continued)

Drug	Increase Level	Decrease Level
carbamazepine, cont'd	isoniazid nicotinamide propoxyphene troleandomycin verapamil	valproic acid haloperidol warfarin
oxcarbazepine†		carbamazepine phenobarbital phenytoin valproic acid verapamil
levetiracetam	No clinically significant interactions with current anticonvulsant medications	

Anticoagulants, β-blockers, doxycycline, metronidazole, quinidine, verapamil, theophylline, anticonvulsants, corticosteroids, estrogens, and oral contraceptives decrease the effects of phenobarbital.

OVERDOSAGE. Confusion, hypothermia, hypotension, slurred speech, unsteady gait, jaundice, respiratory depression, or coma can result.

DOSAGE AND ADMINISTRATION. The usual oral dosage of phenobarbital is 1 to 3 mg/kg/day given in two to three divided doses.

OTHER DRUGS IN CLASS

Other drugs in this class are similar to the prototype except as follows:

primidone (Mysoline)

CONTRAINDICATIONS. Hypersensitivity to primidone, phenobarbital; pregnancy; porphyria

WARNINGS. Abrupt withdrawal of primidone or any anticonvulsant may precipitate SE. It takes several weeks to fully assess the therapeutic efficacy of primidone.

PRECAUTIONS. Manufacturers recommend performing a CBC count and chemistry panel every 6 months on patients receiving primidone.

PATIENT VARIABLES

Pregnancy. *Category D:* Primidone and the barbiturates have been associated with coagulation defects in the newborn infant.

Lactation. Primidone is excreted in breast milk in significant quantity. If increasing drowsiness occurs in the nursing infant of a mother who is taking primidone, it is recommended that the mother discontinue nursing.

ADVERSE EFFECTS. Primidone is less sedating than phenobarbital; therefore, less impairment of cognitive function is seen. Psychotic reactions are rarely seen with primidone. Nausea, vomiting, drowsiness, ataxia, and vertigo are common dose-related side effects that usually disappear with continued therapy or reduction in initial dosage.

Megaloblastic anemia is a rare idiosyncrasy that may occur with primidone therapy.

DRUG INTERACTIONS. Primidone, phenobarbital, and PEMA concentrations may increase when hydantoins are coadministered with primidone.

Concomitant use of carbamazepine and primidone may result in decreased primidone and phenobarbital levels and lower carbamazepine levels.

Concomitant use of primidone and acetazolamide may result in decreased primidone levels.

Concomitant use of primidone and the succinimides may result in decreased primidone and phenobarbital levels.

DOSAGE AND ADMINISTRATION. Primidone is given orally. When initiating therapy, slowly increase the dose to meet the individual's requirements. When primidone is replacing another anticonvulsant, decrease the anticonvulsant slowly as the primidone is being increased over at least 2 weeks.

To initiate primidone therapy in adults and children older than 8 years of age, begin with 125 to 250 mg at bedtime and increase by 125 to 250 mg per day every 3 to 7 days; the usual dose range is 750 to 1500 mg/day. The maximum dose is 2000 mg given in divided doses.

For children younger than 8 years, begin with 50 to 125 mg at bedtime and increase by 50 to 125 mg per day every 3 to 7 days; usual dose range is 10 to 25 mg/kg/day given in three to four divided doses. Do not exceed the dose of 500 mg four times a day (2 g/day).

MISCELLANEOUS ANTICONVULSANTS

carbamazepine (Tegretol, Epitol)

CONTRAINDICATIONS. Hypersensitivity to carbamazepine or any tricyclic antidepressant, concurrent use of MAOIs (discontinue MAOIs at least 14 days before initiating carbamazepine therapy), history of bone marrow depression; pregnancy

WARNINGS. Aplastic anemia and agranulocytosis, although rare, have been reported in association with carbamazepine therapy.

A benign leukopenia, which is not uncommon, is usually not progressive or associated with increased mortality from infection; it is reversible and dose related. However, any patient with a history of adverse hematologic reaction to any drug should be considered at high risk. A CBC count with white cell differential should be done before treatment is initiated. This test should be repeated every 3 months during the first year of treatment. Monitor patients carefully for white cell counts lower than 2500/mm because the drug may have to be discontinued.

Carbamazepine has mild anticholinergic activity; use with caution in patients with increased intraocular pressure.

Confusion or agitation may occur in the elderly because of the drug's relationship to tricyclic compounds.

Carbamazepine produced a dose-related increase in the incidence of hepatocellular tumor in female rats and benign interstitial cell adenoma in male rats.

PRECAUTIONS. Carbamazepine is ineffective for controlling absence seizures. Use with caution in patients with mixed seizure disorder. Carbamazepine has been associated with exacerbation of generalized seizures in these patients.

> **Baseline and periodic liver function tests should be performed. Carbamazepine should be discontinued immediately if liver dysfunction occurs or acute liver disease is suspected.**

Baseline and periodic urinalyses should be performed and blood urea nitrogen and creatinine levels determined. Carbamazepine has been associated with the syndrome of inappropriate antidiuretic hormone (SIADH), water intoxication, and hyponatremia.

Baseline and periodic eye examinations should be performed. Lens opacities have occurred rarely in patients on carbamazepine.

PHARMACOKINETICS. Carbamazepine is adequately absorbed from the GI tract. Carbamazepine suspension is absorbed more rapidly than the tablet. The liver metabolizes carbamazepine by the CYP 450 3A4 enzyme system. It can induce its own metabolism, which accounts for variability in the half-life. The initial half-life is 25 to 65 hours; after multiple dosing, this decreases to 12 to 17 hours (see Table 44-3).

ADVERSE EFFECTS. Initiating carbamazepine therapy at low doses and increasing it slowly to an effective therapeutic dose usually can minimize GI symptoms, as well as dizziness and drowsiness (see Table 44-4).

DRUG INTERACTIONS. The concomitant use of multiple AEDs (see Table 44-5) may decrease serum concentrations of carbamazepine. This is probably the result of induction of hepatic microsomal enzymes that metabolize these drugs. Loss of seizure control may not occur because the anticonvulsant activity is added. Monitor serum concentrations of AEDs given in combination, and adjust dosages accordingly. See also drug interaction discussion under the other individual anticonvulsants and in Table 44-5.

Concomitant use of carbamazepine and verapamil or diltiazem may result in increased plasma concentrations of carbamazepine, leading to toxicity. This interaction does not appear to occur with nifedipine.

Fluoxetine (Prozac) may increase plasma carbamazepine concentrations.

Increased CNS toxicity may occur with concomitant use of lithium and carbamazepine. The patient and the serum levels of both drugs are to be monitored closely.

Carbamazepine may increase the metabolism of acetaminophen, resulting in increased risk of hepatotoxicity, or it may decrease the efficacy of acetaminophen.

Concomitant use of carbamazepine and theophylline may decrease the effects of both drugs.

Concomitant use of carbamazepine and isoniazid has been reported to increase the risk of toxicity of both drugs.

The half-life of doxycycline may be decreased when it is administered with carbamazepine. If possible, use alternative antibiotic agents in patients receiving carbamazepine.

OVERDOSAGE. Signs and symptoms of carbamazepine toxicity include declining mental status, ataxia, dizziness, abnormal movements, nausea, vomiting, nystagmus, and urinary retention.

DOSAGE AND ADMINISTRATION. Individualize dosage; begin with a low daily dose and gradually increase. When adequate control is achieved, reduce the dose gradually to the minimum effective level. Administer with meals.

For management of epilepsy in adults and children older than 12 years, begin with 200 mg tablets twice daily or 100 mg suspension four times daily. Increase at weekly intervals up to 200 mg daily using a three or four times daily regimen until the desired response is obtained. Dosage should not exceed 1000 mg/day in children 12 to 15 years old or 1200 mg in those older than 15 years. Rarely, doses up to 1600 mg/day have been used in adults. Adjust maintenance dose to the minimum effective level, usually 800 to 1200 mg daily.

For children 6 to 12 years old, begin with 100 mg tablets twice daily or 50 mg suspension four times daily. Increase at weekly intervals by 100 mg/day, using a three or four times daily regimen until an optimal response is obtained. Do not exceed 1000 mg/day. You also may calculate dose on the basis of 20 to 30 mg/kg/day given in divided doses three to four times daily. Adjust maintenance dose to the minimum effective level, usually 400 to 800 mg/day.

For the symptomatic relief of pain associated with trigeminal neuralgia in adults, give 100 mg tablets twice daily or 50 mg four times daily of oral suspension on the first day. This dosage may be increased gradually up to 200 mg daily, using 100 mg increments every 12 hours with tablets or 50 mg increments four times daily for suspension until pain is relieved. The dosage needed to relieve pain may range from 200 to 1200 mg daily. The dose should not exceed 1200 mg/day. Control of pain usually can be maintained with 400 to 800 mg/day. At least every 3 months, make an attempt to reduce the dose or discontinue use of carbamazepine.

PATIENT VARIABLES

Pediatrics. Is approved for children younger than 6 years
Pregnancy and Lactation
- *Category D:* Adverse effects have been observed in human studies.
- The concentration of carbamazepine in breast milk is approximately 60% of the maternal plasma concentration. Serious adverse effects may occur in the infant. Make a decision to discontinue nursing or discontinue the drug, after considering the importance of the drug to the mother.

evolve A continually updated list of useful WebLinks may be found in the Evolve Resources at http://evolve.elsevier.com/Edmunds/NP/

Antiparkinson Agents

DRUG OVERVIEW

Class	Generic Name	Trade Name
Dopamine precursors	carbidopa/levodopa	Sinemet
	Carbidopa/levodopa (controlled-release) parcopa duodopa	Sinemet CR
Monoamine oxidase B (MAO-B) inhibitor	selegiline	Eldepryl, Zelapar
	rasagiline	Azilect
Glutamate antagonist (antiviral)	amantadine	Symmetrel
Dopamine agonists	apomorphine	Apokyn
	pramipexole	Mirapex
	ropinirole hydrochloride	Requip
Anticholinergic agents	benztropine	Cogentin
	trihexyphenidyl	Artane
Catechol-O-methyl transferase (COMT) inhibitors	tolcapone	Tasmar
	entacapone	Comtan

Top 200 drug; key drug. Another drug, rivastigmine (Exelon), has an FDA indication for Parkinson's disease dementia.

INDICATIONS

- Idiopathic Parkinson's disease (IPD)
- Management of symptoms related to parkinsonism—tremor at rest, bradykinesia, rigidity, and postural instability
- Rivastigmine approved for management of mild to moderate dementia

Unlabeled Use

- Sinemet and the dopamine agonists are used for management of the symptoms of restless leg syndrome.

Parkinson's disease (PD) is the most common neurodegenerative disorder after Alzheimer's disease. The prevalence and incidence rates of PD increase with age, and the incidence in men is significantly higher (1.5 times higher) than in women. PD is not curable; symptoms progress and worsen over time. A neuroprotective treatment that can slow or halt disease progression has not yet been established. PD treatment is complex owing to the array of motor and nonmotor features combined with early and late treatment adverse effects. Treatment for patients with PD is highly individual.

THERAPEUTIC OVERVIEW

Anatomy and Physiology

The neurotransmitters, acetylcholine and dopamine, and others in the neurons of the substantia nigra modulate movement. Damage to these neurons caused by amyloid results in excess acetylcholine and diminished dopamine in the basal ganglia. Replacement and regulation of the neurotransmitters with exogenous medications represents the hallmark of PD management; however, to improve symptoms and avoid side effects, these medications must be able to cross the blood-brain barrier without being metabolized in the periphery.

SYNTHESIS AND METABOLISM OF DOPAMINE IN THE NERVE TERMINALS. Tyrosine is converted to levodopa (L-dopa) by tyrosine hydroxylase. L-Dopa then is enzymatically decarboxylated by L-amino acid decarboxylase (L-AAD) to form dopamine. Dopamine is stored in synaptic vesicles until needed and then is released into the synapse, where it activates dopamine (D) receptors. The action of dopamine is terminated by reuptake into presynaptic vesicles or metabolism via MAO-B or COMT. This results in the formation of hydrogen peroxide, which then is metabolized to water by glutathione. If glutathione is deficient, or a surplus of hydrogen peroxide exists, hydroxyl free radicals are formed, causing lipid peroxidation and cell membrane damage.

Pathophysiology

Parkinsonism is a chronic, debilitating disease with no known cure. The goals of treatment are to relieve the symptoms of the disease and to help the patient maintain independence and mobility. By origin, PD is categorized as (1) primary or idiopathic, (2) secondary or acquired, (3) heritable, or (4) multisystem. For purposes of this text, only IPD is discussed. Practitioners are urged to consult differential diagnostic references to distinguish among the types of parkinsonism, including drug-induced cases.

PD results from a relative excess of cholinergic activity and a deficiency of dopaminergic activity in the basal ganglia. Lewy bodies (amyloid inclusion bodies) in the neurons of the pars compacta region of the substantia nigra are common in the pathophysiology of parkinsonism. Damage to these dopaminergic neurons causes loss of dopamine at their terminal projections in the caudate nucleus and putamen. Dopamine normally inhibits the action of acetylcholine in the striatum; therefore, decreased concentrations of dopamine caused by neuronal degeneration result in unopposed acetylcholine. This manifests as tremors in the patient. Clinical signs and symptoms of parkinsonism develop after approximately 80% of dopaminergic neurons are lost.

Some understanding of the origin of IPD was gained when several intravenous drug abusers developed PD after injecting a meperidine analog, methylphenyltetrahydropyridine (MPTP). The MPP ion that was formed after oxidative metabolism of MPTP by MAO-B was found to be neurotoxic to melanin-containing neurons in the substantia nigra. Inhibition of MAO-B by selegiline prevented the formation of MPP. Epidemiologic studies have shown an increased risk of developing PD with rural living and exposure to well water, pesticides, herbicides, and wood pulp mills. Discovery of a gene that could be responsible for a certain type of familial PD has brought hope for further research into the mechanism and prevention of the disease, perhaps through the use of stem cells. Stem cells represent only a very small portion of all of the neuroprotection trials and other work currently under way.

Disease Process

Dr. James Parkinson first described paralysis agitans, or shaking palsy, in 1817. Today, we know this condition as PD, Parkinson's syndrome, or parkinsonism. Age at onset of signs and symptoms varies; however, most patients first experience symptoms between the ages of 50 and 69. In up to 30% of patients, symptoms occur before age 50. Patients present with one or more of four typical clinical symptoms: tremor at rest, bradykinesia, rigidity, and postural instability. Some patients with IPD may present with only a resting tremor of 4 to 7 cycles/sec as the principal symptom. These patients usually experience a slower progression of disease and little mental status change. Patients who present with postural instability and gait difficulty, however, often have a more rapid disease progression that includes dementia and bradykinesia. Early research suggests that NSAIDs may protect against the development of PD.

Assessment

PD is a slow, insidiously progressive neurodegenerative disorder. Early signs and symptoms include paresthesias, dystonia, depression, pain, and numbness, which progress to the classic clinical features of tremor, bradykinesia, rigidity, and postural instability. Other typical problems include micrographia, hypophonia, shuffling or festinating gait, lack of facial expression (masked facies), drooling, decreased blinking, and reduced dexterity. Patients with PD may experience difficulty when initiating movement, may freeze or be unable to move when they walk in confined spaces, or may exhibit pill-rolling movements of the hands, jaw, or legs. The tremors and pill-rolling subside on initiation of voluntary movement and do not occur during sleep. Cogwheel-like rigidity, dystonic posture, and postural instability are causes of significant morbidity in patients with PD because they can lead to falls. Patients also exhibit autonomic nervous system dysfunctions such as excessive sweating, constipation, and postural hypotension. Neuropsychologic disorders such as dementia and depression may occur.

Although initially effective, dopaminergic therapies eventually are complicated in most patients by motor fluctuations, including off time (periods of return of PD symptoms when medication effect wears off) and dyskinesia (drug-induced involuntary movements such as chorea and dystonia). These motor complications can impair quality of life and cause significant disability. Risk factors for motor complications include younger age at onset of PD, increased disease severity, higher levodopa dosage, and longer disease duration. These problems often are addressed with levodopa adjustments and the addition of adjunctive medications.

Disease staging is an important step in determining drug and supportive therapy. The following scale of Hoehn and Yahr (2001) is the traditional staging tool:
- Stage I: Unilateral involvement
- Stage II: Bilateral involvement but no postural abnormalities
- Stage III: Bilateral involvement with mild postural imbalance; the patient leads an independent life
- Stage IV: Bilateral involvement with postural instability; the patient requires substantial help
- Stage V: Severe, fully developed disease; the patient is restricted to bed and chair

This tool has largely been replaced by the Unified Parkinson Disease Rating Scale (UPDRS) for following the longitudinal course of PD. This latter tool is much more cumbersome but descriptive. It consists of sections on (1) mentation, behavior, and mood, (2) ADL, and (3) motor activity. These skills are evaluated by interview. Some sections require assignment of multiple grades to each extremity. A total of 199 points is possible, with 199 representing the worst (total) disability, and 0 indicating no disability. Both of these tools may be viewed online through the Massachusetts General Hospital neurosurgical website at http://neurosurgery .mgh.harvard.edu/Functional/pdstages.htm

MECHANISM OF ACTION

Drug treatment for PD has centered on increasing the availability of dopamine in the CNS, inhibiting the effects of acetylcholine, and attempting to prevent further cell membrane damage through neuroprotective trials. The D_2-receptor subtype is the primary modulator of both clinical improvement and adverse reactions such as dystonia and hallucinations. Increased levodopa precursors and synthesis cofactors usually are not effective.

Levodopa has been the single most important drug in the antiparkinson armamentarium. Levodopa administered orally enters the blood after it is absorbed from the GI tract, and 95% of levodopa is converted to dopamine by L-AAD. The action of this enzyme can be blocked by the antagonist carbidopa, which does not cross the blood-brain barrier; therefore, levodopa in the CNS follows the synthetic path to dopamine formation and storage. Combining carbidopa with levodopa results in increased concentrations of levodopa in the CNS and decreased conversion of L-dopa to dopamine in the periphery, where it causes adverse effects.

Selegiline (also called *deprenyl*), an MAO-B inhibitor, is used early in the management of idiopathic PD in an attempt to prevent further neuronal degeneration. The mechanism of action of selegiline is not fully understood. These drugs inhibit the enzyme MAO-B, which breaks down dopamine in the brain. MAO-B inhibitors cause dopamine to accumulate in surviving nerve cells and reduce the symptoms of PD. Studies supported by the National Institute of Neurological Disorders and Stroke (NINDS) have shown that selegiline can delay the need for levodopa therapy by a year or longer. When selegiline is given with levodopa, it appears to enhance and prolong the response to levodopa and thus may reduce wearing-off fluctuations. An NINDS-sponsored study of selegiline in the late 1980s suggested that it might help to slow the loss of nerve cells in PD. However, follow-up studies cast doubt on this finding. Another MAO-B inhibitor, rasagiline, was approved by the FDA in May 2006 for use in treating patients with PD (see Table 45-3).

Selective MAO-B inhibition irreversibly blocks the metabolism of dopamine in the brain, where MAO-B is the major subtype and extends the duration of action of L-dopa. Selegiline often permits dose reductions of L-dopa and increases the duration of effect by 1 or more hours in patients who experience "wearing-off" effects of L-dopa. Selegiline may delay the use of carbidopa/levodopa in the early stages of PD via the same mechanism. Selegiline may provide neuroprotection by shunting the metabolic path of dopamine away from free radical production and oxidative stress.

Dopamine agonists: These drugs, which include bromocriptine, apomorphine, pramipexole, and ropinirole, mimic the role of dopamine in the brain. They can be given alone or in conjunction with levodopa. They may be used in the early stages of the disease, or later on to lengthen the duration of response to levodopa in patients who experience wearing off or on-off effects. They generally are less effective than levodopa in controlling rigidity and bradykinesia.

Dopamine agonists are used in the treatment of patients with IPD to increase the availability of dopamine in the CNS. These drugs work at postsynaptic dopamine receptors in the nigrostriatal system by stimulating dopamine receptors. They are being used more frequently in early parkinsonism to avoid using high doses of levodopa and in late stages of the disease to aid in the management of levodopa dose-response fluctuations.

Pramipexole is a nonergot dopamine agonist with specificity for the D_2 dopamine receptors. It binds with lower affinity D_3- and D_4-receptor subtypes. The relevance of D_3-receptor binding in PD is unknown.

Anticholinergic agents are used to control tremors caused by excessive, unopposed acetylcholine. They suppress central cholinergic activity and may inhibit reuptake and storage of dopamine in the CNS, thus prolonging the action of dopamine. They also reduce the incidence and severity of akinesia, rigidity, and tremor by about 20%, and they reduce drooling.

COMT inhibitors are central and/or peripheral blockers of dopamine metabolism. COMT stands for catechol-O-methyltransferase, another enzyme that helps to break down dopamine. Two COMT inhibitors have been approved to treat PD in the United States: entacapone and tolcapone. These drugs, which prolong the effects of levodopa by preventing the breakdown of dopamine, are used as adjuvants with levodopa to extend the therapeutic effect in patients who experience breakthrough tremors prior to their next dose. The mechanism of action of entacapone probably is related to its ability to inhibit COMT and alter the plasma pharmacokinetics of levodopa. The administration of entacapone in conjunction with levodopa and carbidopa produces more sustained plasma levels of levodopa than does the administration of levodopa and carbidopa alone. These sustained plasma levels may result in increased therapeutic effects on the symptoms of PD, as well as increased adverse effects. A decrease in the levodopa dose may be required.

Rivastigmine is available as an oral or transdermal system (*Exelon Patch*) for the treatment of patients with mild to moderate dementia associated with PD. See Chapter 41 for complete prescribing information.

TREATMENT PRINCIPLES
Standardized Guidelines

- Pahwa R et al: Guidelines: practice parameter: Treatment of Parkinson disease with motor fluctuations and dyskinesia (an evidence-based review): report of the Quality Standards Subcommittee of the American Academy of Neurology, *Neurology* 66:983-995, 2006.

Evidence-Based Recommendations

- Early Parkinson's:
  - Beneficial—immediate-release levodopa
  - Trade-off between benefits and harms—dopamine agonists, dopamine agonists plus levodopa, MAO-B inhibitors
  - Unlikely to be beneficial—modified-release levodopa
- Entacapone and rasagiline should be offered to reduce off time.
- Pergolide, pramipexole, ropinirole, and tolcapone should be considered to reduce off time.
- Apomorphine, cabergoline, and selegiline may be considered to reduce off time.
- Available evidence does not establish the superiority of one medicine over another in reducing off time.
- Amantadine may be considered to reduce dyskinesia (level C).
- Deep brain stimulation of the STN may be considered to improve motor function and reduce off time, dyskinesia, and medication usage.
- Evidence is insufficient to support or refute the efficacy of DBS of the GPi or VIM nucleus of the thalamus in reducing off time, dyskinesia, or medication usage, or in improving motor function.
- Preoperative response to levodopa predicts better outcome after DBS of the STN (level B).

Cardinal Points of Treatment

- *Initial drugs:* First line—levodopa, dopamine agonists
- *carbidopa/levodopa:* All patients will eventually need; most effective
- MAOI
  - *selegiline:* Has a modest effect; controversy continues over whether it slows the progression of Parkinson's disease
  - *rasagiline:* Recently approved; its place in treatment has not been determined
  - *Dopamine agonists:* Less likely than levodopa to cause dyskinesias or motor fluctuations
  - May be given with or before levodopa
- Pramipexole and ropinirole are effective in early and late Parkinson's.
- *amantadine:* May help patients with mild symptoms but no disability
- Apomorphine injection is used for acute treatment of episodes of immobility.
- Anticholinergics: Reduce tremor, rigidity, and drooling
  - These are older drugs with limited uses.
- *COMT inhibitors:* Reduce motor fluctuations in patients with advanced disease but increase dyskinesias; used after other adjunctive therapies have failed

Nonpharmacologic Treatment

The impact of PD treatment regimens on patients' health-related quality of life (QOL) is an important health care matter. QOL questionnaires provide insight into the management of disease from the patient's perspective and help the clinician to assess treatment efficacy. Several studies over the past few years have investigated the QOL of patients with PD; all found depression to be a significant factor in terms of QOL.

Management of PD should include programs designed to optimize the patient's general health, nutrition, and emotional and neuromuscular status. Table 45-1 provides a treatment algorithm. Refer the patient to a neurologist to confirm the diagnosis and to provide guidance with medical management.

Nonpharmacologic treatment is important. Group support, exercise, education, and nutrition can help. Patients may experience constipation and initially may gain weight if their activity level decreases. With progression of disease, patients may have trouble chewing and swallowing and may need to change their sitting position while eating, taking small bites and chewing well, drinking plenty of water between mouthfuls of food, and avoiding certain foods, such as raw vegetables and nuts, which may be more difficult to chew and swallow.

It is customary for levodopa preparations to be dispensed with instructions to take with food. In fact, they may be better and faster absorbed on an empty stomach, but it is often advised that they be taken with food if they upset your stomach. Amino acids in proteins can compete with levodopa (which is also an amino acid) for transport from the gut to the bloodstream, and from the bloodstream into the brain. Most people tolerate levodopa without nausea and are able to take their levodopa medications before meals; for some people, this may occur 1 to 2 hours before eating, whereas others find it better to take their medication 30 minutes before eating.

Some people find that avoiding high-protein foods during the day and "hoarding" them until the evening ensures better mobility during the day. Red meat, poultry, fish, milk, cheese, and eggs all are high in protein. Other individuals benefit from combining small amounts of protein with a high level of carbohydrate (e.g., fruit, bread, cereal, pasta, other grains) throughout the day. Keeping fatty foods to a minimum also may help.

Physical therapy can be very beneficial in keeping the patient mobile and keeping weight down.

Deep brain stimulation has proved effective in controlling symptoms of PD. Other surgical techniques are being used in patients who do not respond to medications, or who remain symptomatic.

Pharmacologic Treatment

The NINDS has classified medications for PD into three categories. The first category includes drugs that work directly or indirectly to increase the level of dopamine in the brain. The drugs most commonly used for PD are dopamine precursors—substances such as levodopa that cross the blood-brain barrier and then are changed into dopamine. Other drugs mimic dopamine or prevent or slow its breakdown.

The second category of PD drugs affects other neurotransmitters in the body to ease some symptoms of the disease. For example, anticholinergic drugs interfere with production or uptake of the neurotransmitter acetylcholine. These drugs help to reduce tremors and muscle stiffness, which can result from the presence of more acetylcholine than dopamine.

The third category of drugs prescribed for PD includes medications that help control the nonmotor symptoms of the disease, that is, the symptoms that do not affect movement. For example, people with PD-related depression may be prescribed antidepressants.

TABLE 45-1   Basic Treatment Algorithm for Parkinson's Disease

Stage or Problem	Therapeutic Alternatives (listed in order of use)
MILD DISEASE (STAGE I AND II)	Levodopa, immediate release Dopamine agonists
FUNCTIONALLY IMPAIRED (STAGE III): ADD	
Age younger than 65	Dopamine agonists Sustained-release carbidopa/levodopa (lowest dose possible)
Age ≥65 yr	Sustained-release carbidopa/levodopa
STAGE IV OR V	
Suboptimal peak response	Increase dose of carbidopa/levodopa or dopamine agonist. Add levodopa or dopamine agonist. Add COMT inhibitor.
Wearing off/on-off	Increase dose of carbidopa/levodopa. Increase frequency of levodopa dosing. Change to sustained-release levodopa. Add CMT (entacapone) or MAOI (rasagiline). Consider dopamine agonist (pramipexole, ropinirole) and COMT inhibitor (tolcapone); may need to decrease levodopa dose Apomorphine injection for freezing
On-off	Begin combination dopamine agonist therapy. Add levodopa to dopamine agonist. Add dopamine agonist to levodopa. Add COMT inhibitor. Modify distribution of dietary protein.
Dyskinesia/dystonia	Reduce levodopa dose. Add dopamine agonist. Change to regular-release levodopa, if dyskinesia is occurring in the late afternoon and evening.
Tremor	Anticholinergics

The timing of treatment initiation in PD generally is guided by the impact that the disease has on the individual's quality of life. Over the last decade, a paradigm shift has been noted from initiating symptomatic therapy with levodopa, the gold standard of PD treatment, to beginning treatment with a dopamine agonist (in particular for young-onset patients who are at high risk of developing motor complications) and adding levodopa as a supplement when dopamine agonist monotherapy no longer can provide satisfactory clinical control. Long-term levodopa treatment is associated with the development of motor complications that probably are initiated by abnormal pulsatile stimulation of dopamine receptors via intermittent administration of agents with short half-lives (such as levodopa). Dopamine agonists with longer half-lives can provide relatively continuous stimulation and thus possibly can diminish motor response complications. However, treatment initiation with levodopa still is preferred in patients with PD with cognitive impairment, in the elderly, and in those with atypical parkinsonism. Guidelines put forth by Bhatia et al. also recommend dopamine agonists as alternative first-line treatment options to levodopa for appropriate patients.

The Pawha et al. (2006) report, which is a systematic, evidence-based review that was prepared with the goal of improving clinicians' knowledge of presently available published clinical evidence (based mainly on randomized controlled trials), rated the different therapeutic interventions in terms of efficacy, safety, and clinical usefulness. Safety and efficacy data showed that several drug treatments can be considered as clinically useful or possibly useful for controlling motor features in early and advanced PD. Levodopa was found to be more efficacious than most other medications; orally active dopamine agonists are very similar. The authors also mention the growing consensus on the early use of dopamine agonists, especially in young patients. The choice among available treatment options depends on clinical characteristics such as patient age, disease severity, and the presence of comorbidities, as well as patients' lifestyle characteristics and preferences, costs of different medications, awareness and perception of available treatment options, and educational background of the treating physician.

An immediate-release formulation of levodopa is preferred over a controlled-release preparation for measurement of the therapeutic effect. The switch then can be made to a controlled-release preparation. Therapeutic controversy revolves around the duration of levodopa therapy. Some practitioners believe that levodopa therapy is useful for only approximately 5 years and should be withheld until disabling symptoms appear. The sustained-release formulation of carbidopa/levodopa may provide a more physiologic replacement of dopamine than is provided by other regimens. An immediate-release dose may be added to the morning dose if the patient experiences late onset or an inadequate peak response. The occurrence of blepharospasm or involuntary movement signifies that a dose reduction is needed.

Factors useful in assessing the need to start treatment include which hand is affected (dominant or nondominant), the patient's employment status, specific Parkinson's symptoms (bradykinesia is more disabling than tremor), the individual patient's sentiments, and the individual prescriber's philosophy. Other factors include the following:

- *Age.* Patients younger than 65 years of age should be started with a dopamine agonist, whereas treatment for older patients should be initiated with carbidopa/levodopa. Older patients are less likely to develop levodopa-related motor problems. Anticholinergics are contraindicated in older patients because of increased risks of cognitive impairment, blurred vision, and dry mouth.
- *Cognitive Impairment.* Treatment with carbidopa/levodopa should be initiated and polypharmacy eliminated through gradual discontinuation of drugs in the following order: sedative medications, anticholinergics, amantadine, selegiline, dopamine agonists.
- *Disease Severity.* It is acceptable to start with carbidopa/levodopa and to move to a dopamine agonist if needed.
- *Employment Status.* Dopamine agonists could be used first, especially in younger patients who are at greater risk for developing motor complications. Other experts advocate starting with carbidopa/levodopa.
- *Cost.* When financial realities outweigh the potential for future benefits, initiate treatment with the least expensive medications. Cost is a significant variable for patients. Some medications are not covered on insurance formularies; newer medications tend not to be covered by Medicare plans. Some type of prescription assistance program may help some of these patients pay for their prescriptions.
- *Combined Therapy.* When patients treated with single agents (either carbidopa/levodopa or dopamine agonists) require additional treatment, most experts agree that they should receive combination therapy rather than an increased dose of the current drug.

Levodopa Management Problems

As PD progresses, neurons lose their storage capabilities for dopamine, and patients are dependent on the rate of levodopa administration for a therapeutic response. Approximately 50% of patients treated with levodopa will experience fluctuations in their response to the drug within 5 years. These fluctuations include "wearing off," also called end-of-dose failure, as well as "on-off" effects, dyskinesias, and dystonias.

Patients may experience "wearing off" of therapeutic effect after 1.5 to 2 hours with some products. On-off effect is a sudden loss of therapeutic effect. One treatment option is to give more frequent doses of levodopa or a sustained-release formulation. If onset of action is delayed, levodopa may be given on an empty stomach before meals and crushed or chewed and taken with a full glass of water.

Other drugs: First offer entacapone or rasagiline. Consider pramipexole, ropinirole, and tolcapone. Use tolcapone with caution because of adverse reactions.

May be considered: apomorphine, cabergoline, and selegiline

Patients who experience choreiform dyskinesias during their peak levodopa effect may benefit from substituting an immediate-release for a sustained-release product, or the opposite.

Other drugs: Consider amantadine. Other alternatives include discontinuing selegiline and lowering individual doses of carbidopa/levodopa and then adding a dopamine agonist as carbidopa/levodopa doses are decreased. Patients in whom dystonias occur at the end of the dosing cycle may benefit from more frequent doses of carbidopa/levodopa or from addition of or increase in the dose of a dopamine agonist. Restriction of carbidopa/levodopa to several early to midday doses also may be of benefit.

Early morning foot dystonias may improve as the result of nocturnal administration of sustained-release carbidopa/levodopa. If this is not successful, a nocturnal dopamine agonist or an early morning carbidopa/levodopa or paracopa could be used. Patients with dystonias that occur at peak dose time may benefit from lowering the dose of carbidopa/levodopa or from addition of or increase in the dopamine agonist dose.

How to Monitor

In general, no laboratory tests are used to monitor the efficacy of antiparkinsonism drugs. Exceptions are discussed in the specific drug sections.

With the use of physical assessment measures of neurologic function, patients' responses to therapy and the presence of side effects are monitored by assessment of their functional and clinical status. Regularly assess the following: facial appearance, salivation, seborrhea, speech, tremor, rigidity/dyskinesia, finger/foot tapping, rapid alternating movement, standing up from the chair without assistance of arms/hands, posture, stability, gait, handwriting, and intellectual and psychiatric assessment.

The most common adverse effects of antiparkinsonism drugs are nausea, hypotension, and psychiatric problems; these symptoms should be monitored continually (Table 45-2).

Patient Variables

PREGNANCY AND LACTATION. Most antiparkinsonism drugs are categorized as pregnancy category C or unknown. Excretion in breast milk is unknown or does occur; therefore, avoid using any antiparkinsonism drugs during pregnancy or lactation.

PEDIATRICS. Safety in children younger than 12 years of age has not been established.

Patient Education

Support of emotional needs for both patients and caregivers is essential. Patients, families, and significant others should be educated about realistic expectations of various treatments. Encourage patients and their families to adhere to their treatment regimens and to keep a diary of their symptoms and daily medication administration times.

Patients and family members will need extensive counseling and education regarding maintaining health, nutrition, and physical activity. They also will have to devise particular strategies that they can use to deal with any psychiatric problems that may occur as the disease process worsens. The National Parkinson's Disease Association offers many resources for providers, patients, and family members.

TABLE 45-2 Adverse Effects of Antiparkinsonism Drugs

Drug	Adverse Effects*	More Frequent	Less Frequent
levodopa	After >1 yr, patient may experience on-off phenomenon or start hesitation. Neuroleptic malignant syndrome may occur upon abrupt discontinuation.	Difficult urination, dizziness, orthostatic hypotension, irregular heartbeat, depression, mood changes, nausea, vomiting, unusual body movements, anxiety, confusion, nervousness	Blepharospasm, duodenal ulcer, hemolytic anemia, hypertension, anorexia, diarrhea, dry mouth, flushing, headache, insomnia, muscle twitching, unusual tiredness, weakness
carbidopa	Allows CNS adverse effects of levodopa because of increased CNS levodopa See levodopa entry.	Anxiety, confusion, nervousness	Orthostasis, palpitations, nausea, vomiting, blurry vision, fatigue
selegiline	With doses >10 mg daily: bruxism, muscle twitches, myoclonic jerks	Dyskinesia, mood or other CNS changes, abdominal pain, dizziness, dry mouth, insomnia, nausea, vomiting	Angina, arrhythmias, asthma, bradycardia, edema, extrapyramidal effects, GI bleeding, hallucinations, headache, hypertension, orthostatic hypotension, prostatic hyperplasia, tardive dyskinesia, anxiety, apraxia, blepharospasm, diplopia, body aches, bradykinesia, chills, constipation, diarrhea, diaphoresis, drowsiness, headache, heartburn, impaired memory, urination difficulty, irritability, loss of appetite, palpitations, circumoral paresthesias, photosensitivity, tinnitus, taste changes, euphoria, tiredness, weakness
amantadine	Convulsions, leukopenia	Nausea, dizziness, insomnia	Depression, anxiety, irritability, hallucinations, confusion, dry mouth, constipation, livedo reticularis, peripheral edema, orthostatic hypotension
bromocriptine	Pulmonary infiltrates on long-term, high-dose therapy (20-100 mg daily) have occurred and slowly resolved after therapy was discontinued; rare: MI, stroke	Hypotension, nausea	Confusion, dyskinesia, hallucinations, constipation, diarrhea, drowsiness, dry mouth, nocturnal leg cramps, loss of appetite, depression, stomach pain, stuffy nose, Raynaud's phenomenon, vomiting. Some drugs may also produce pathologic gambling, sleep attacks, OCD.
pramipexole	Hallucinations, dizziness, somnolence, extrapyramidal symptoms, headache, confusion, nausea	Nausea, dizziness, somnolence, insomnia, constipation, asthenia, hallucinations, accidental injury, dyspepsia, general edema	Malaise, fever, anorexia, dysphagia, decreased weight
ropinirole	Nausea, dizziness, aggravated Parkinson's, hallucinations (dose related), somnolence, vomiting, headache	Fatigue, syncope, dizziness, dyspepsia, nausea, vomiting, somnolence	Constipation, pain, increased sweating, asthenia, leg edema, orthostatic symptoms, abdominal pain, pharyngitis, confusion, hallucinations, abnormal vision
Anticholinergic agents	Anhidrosis, hyperthermia Withdrawal symptoms: Anxiety, extrapyramidal symptoms, tachycardia, orthostatic hypotension	Anticholinergic effects: Blurred vision; constipation; decreased sweating; difficulty urinating; drowsiness; dry mouth, nose, or throat; nausea; vomiting; sensitivity to light	Euphoria, headache, memory loss, muscle cramps, nervousness, numbness in hands or feet, orthostatic hypotension, sore mouth and tongue, stomach pain, unusual excitement

*Adverse effects that led to discontinuation of treatment during clinical trials, or that occurred in more than 2% of patients.

SPECIFIC DRUGS
Dopamine Precursors

carbidopa/levodopa (Sinemet, Sinemet CR)

INDICATIONS
- *Treatment for IPD:* Used in combination because carbidopa inhibits peripheral decarboxylation of levodopa and allows higher CNS concentrations of levodopa. Allows smoother, more rapid titration; reduces nausea and vomiting; and allows concurrent pyridoxine (vitamin B₆) when needed.
- *Unlabeled use:* Management of post-herpetic neuralgia and restless leg syndrome.

CONTRAINDICATIONS
- Discontinue MAOI 2 weeks before initiation of levodopa.
- Narrow-angle glaucoma
- Undiagnosed skin lesions or history of melanoma as levodopa may activate malignant melanoma

carbidopa/levodopa (Sinemet, Sinemet CR) 🔑 —cont'd

- Risk–benefit assessment should be made if the following medical problems exist:
  - *Major significance:* Bronchial asthma, emphysema, severe pulmonary disease; severe cardiovascular disease; angle-closure glaucoma; melanoma (history or suspected); history of myocardial infarction with arrhythmias; history of peptic ulcer disease; psychosis; renal dysfunction; urinary retention
  - *Slightly less significance:* History of convulsive disorder, diabetes mellitus, endocrine disease, open-angle glaucoma, hepatic dysfunction

WARNINGS

- Use with caution in patients with severe cardiovascular, pulmonary, renal, hepatic, or endocrine disease.
- Use of this agent in patients with previous myocardial infarction with residual arrhythmias should take place only in a coronary or intensive care unit.
- Possibility exists for upper GI bleeding in patients with history of peptic ulcer disease.
- Observe patients for depression and suicidal ideation. Use cautiously in psychotic patients.
- 10 to 25 mg pyridoxine (vitamin B_6) inactivates the effects of levodopa. Patients who take carbidopa/levodopa products will not experience this inactivation until pyridoxine doses exceed 200 mg because carbidopa inhibits this action of vitamin B_6.
- Neuroleptic malignant syndrome may develop if the drug is abruptly withdrawn.
- Dyskinesias may occur at lower doses with coadministration of carbidopa/levodopa and may require dose reduction.

PRECAUTIONS

- Evaluate hepatic, hematopoietic, cardiovascular, and renal function periodically.
- Carefully monitor patients with wide-angle glaucoma for increases in intraocular pressure.
- Cautiously monitor patients on antihypertensive drugs. Lower antihypertensive dose may be required because of autonomic hypotensive effects of levodopa.

DRUG INTERACTIONS.
Antacids increase levodopa bioavailability. Anticholinergics, benzodiazepines, hydantoins, methionine, papaverine, pyridoxine, and tricyclic antidepressants decrease levodopa effectiveness. MAOIs increase the effects of levodopa and may precipitate hypertensive reactions.

Tricyclic antidepressants have caused hypertension and dyskinesia.

Dietary note: Levodopa competes directly with amino acids for absorption across the GI membrane and with amino acid transport mechanisms into the CNS. Patients should take levodopa initially with food to avoid GI adverse effects; then they should move dosing to 30 minutes before meals. Tolerance to these effects usually develops. Patients may eat 15 minutes after taking levodopa if they can tolerate the GI effects. Patients who experience suboptimal response or fluctuations with levodopa should limit protein intake at the morning and noon meals to enhance absorption and bioavailability of the drug.

DOSAGE AND ADMINISTRATION
carbidopa/levodopa Dosage

- *Initiation:* Individualize and titrate dosage. Start with one tablet of 25:100 carbidopa/levodopa three times daily or one tablet of 10:100 three times daily. Gradually increase dosage every 1 to 2 days as needed and tolerated to a maximum of 8 tablets a day.
- *Prior levodopa therapy:* Today, it is not common to have a patient taking only levodopa. In those cases, levodopa should be discontinued at least 8 hours before carbidopa/levodopa therapy is initiated.
- *Patients who require less than 1.5 g levodopa daily:* Same as no prior levodopa therapy
- *Patients who require more than 1.5 g levodopa daily:* 25 mg carbidopa/250 mg levodopa three or four times daily initially. May gradually increase dosage per day at 1- to 2-day intervals as needed and tolerated. The initial carbidopa/levodopa dose should provide 25% of the total levodopa daily dose previously required.
- An oral, rapidly disintegrating tablet is available in dosages of 10/100; 25/100; and 25/200 mg.

carbidopa/levodopa Extended-Release Dosage

- *Initial, no prior levodopa:* In mild to moderate disease, initiate therapy with 25 mg carbidopa and 100 mg levodopa twice daily at least 6 hours apart. Adjust dose every 3 days as needed. May increase to 50 mg carbidopa and 200 mg levodopa
- *Initiating, currently receiving carbidopa/levodopa:* Dosage of extended-release product should be substituted so it will provide 10% higher levodopa doses than are provided with the previous combination product. May need to increase to doses that provide 30% more levodopa per day

Total Daily levodopa Dose	carbidopa/levodopa Extended Release
300 to 400 mg	200 mg twice daily
500 to 600 mg	300 mg twice daily
700 to 800 mg	800 mg in three or more divided doses (300 mg in AM and early PM, 200 mg late PM)
900 to 1000 mg	1000 mg in three or more divided doses (400 mg AM and early PM, 200 mg late PM)

Doses always are titrated slowly according to the patient's symptoms.

PATIENT VARIABLES

Geriatrics. Older adult patients have been shown to take 2 hours to peak concentration for extended-release tablets vs. one-half hour for conventional therapy. Starting dose should be 25/100 twice daily.

MAO-B INHIBITOR

selegiline (Eldepryl)

CONTRAINDICATIONS. Meperidine or other opioids; hypersensitivity

Orally disintegrating tablet (ODT) additional contraindications: dextromethorphan, methadone, propoxyphene, tramadol, oral selegiline, other MAO inhibitors

WARNINGS. Do not exceed 10 mg per day or 2.5 mg per day of the ODT.

PRECAUTIONS. Adverse effects of levodopa may be exacerbated by the action of increased concentrations of dopamine on supersensitive dopamine receptors.

Observe patients for atypical responses because the MAO system of enzymes is not completely understood, and the quality of enzymes may vary from patient to patient.

PATIENT VARIABLES. *Stage of PD:* Selegiline may delay the need for carbidopa/levodopa by 1 year and may prolong a patient's ability to remain active.

Patients with advanced PD who take selegiline may benefit from relief from (1) "wearing off" and (2) fluctuations of L-dopa.

PATIENT EDUCATION. Patients should not exceed the recommended daily dose of 10 mg to avoid a hypertensive crisis. Describe to patients and their families the tyramine reaction that might be seen with high doses or inadvertent overdosage. Patients should report immediately any sudden, severe headache or other unusual symptoms that they have not experienced previously.

ADVERSE EFFECTS. Selegiline usually is well tolerated, although side effects may include nausea, orthostatic hypotension, or insomnia.

DRUG INTERACTIONS. Numerous interactions with MAO inhibitors have been noted and are mainly theoretical. However, it is best to avoid any combinations if possible to avoid the risk of serotonin syndrome. Meperidine is contraindicated; it should not be taken with the antidepressant fluoxetine or the sedative meperidine because of additive effects.

OVERDOSAGE. Hypotension and psychomotor agitation can occur. Doses greater than 10 mg/day are likely to inhibit both MAO-A and MAO-B, and patients may experience a hypertensive crisis similar to the tyramine or "cheese effect" crisis.

DOSAGE AND ADMINISTRATION. Parkinsonian patients receiving carbidopa/levodopa who demonstrate a deteriorating response to this treatment should take 10 mg/day in divided doses (5 mg at breakfast and lunch or 10 mg per day in the morning).

Attempt to reduce the carbidopa/levodopa dose after 2 to 3 days of selegiline therapy; 10% to 30% reductions are typical; individualize additional reductions.

GLUTAMATE ANTAGONISTS (ANTIVIRALS)

amantadine (Symmetrel)

This antiviral agent was discovered to have antiparkinsonism activity also (see Chapter 68 for antiviral uses).

WARNINGS. Prescriptions should be written for the smallest quantity needed. Suicidal ideations and successful suicides have occurred in patients with and without a prior history of psychiatric illness. Use caution in prescribing amantadine to patients who are taking other drugs with CNS effects.

Increased seizure activity is possible in patients who have a history of epilepsy.

Amantadine has been implicated in causing chronic heart failure and peripheral edema; therefore, patients with these conditions should be monitored closely on initiation of amantadine.

PRECAUTIONS

- Do not discontinue abruptly, or parkinsonian crisis may be precipitated.
- Neuroleptic malignant syndrome may occur with sudden decrease in dosage or discontinuation of therapy.
- Adjust doses of amantadine in the elderly and in patients with renal dysfunction (see chart in Dosage and Administration section).
- Closely monitor patients with liver dysfunction. Elevated concentrations of liver enzymes have occurred; these are reversible on discontinuation of the drug.

DRUG INTERACTIONS. Concurrent use with thioridazine reportedly has caused worsening tremor in elderly patients. It is unknown whether other phenothiazines may cause the same reaction.

Triamterene and hydrochlorothiazide have been reported to cause elevated amantadine concentrations.

OVERDOSAGE. Deaths have occurred with 1 g doses of amantadine. Serious cardiac, respiratory, renal, and CNS toxicity has occurred with overdosage.

DOSAGE AND ADMINISTRATION. Give 100 mg twice daily when used alone. The initial dose is decreased to 100 mg daily in patients with serious associated medical illnesses and in those receiving high doses of other antiparkinsonism agents. Onset usually occurs within 48 hours. Increase to 100 mg twice daily after 1 to several weeks. Some patients benefit from doses up to 400 mg daily; however, close monitoring is required. Patients who respond initially to amantadine therapy may experience decreased efficacy after several months.

Rapid therapeutic benefit can be attained when amantadine is added to levodopa. The dose of amantadine should be held steady at 100 to 200 mg daily while the levodopa dose is increased.

Amantadine added to optimal levodopa therapy may yield additional benefit, such as reduced fluctuation. Patients who require a decrease in levodopa dosage because of adverse effects may regain some benefit by adding amantadine to their regimen.

Dosage in renal impairment: Adjustments in dosage are required in keeping with the degree of impairment. See package insert.

pramipexole (Mirapex)

CONTRAINDICATIONS. Hypersensitivity to the drug or its ingredients

WARNINGS/PRECAUTIONS. Carefully monitor patients who are starting pramipexole therapy or are undergoing dose escalation for signs and symptoms of orthostatic hypotension.

The risk of hallucinations attributable to pramipexole is age related. This risk is 1.9 times greater than with placebo in patients with early PD who are younger than 65 years of age, and it is 6.8 times greater than with placebo in those older than 65. The risk increase vs. placebo in patients with advanced PD was 3.5 in patients younger than 65 years of age and 5.2 in patients older than 65.

Caution should be exercised when pramipexole is prescribed for patients with renal insufficiency.

Pramipexole may cause or exacerbate dyskinesias when used in conjunction with levodopa. Decreasing the levodopa dose may ameliorate this side effect.

DRUG INTERACTIONS. Carbidopa/levodopa does not influence the pharmacokinetics of pramipexole. However, pramipexole increases the levodopa C_{max} by 40% and decreases the T_{max} from 2.5 to 0.5 hour.

Cimetidine causes a 50% increase in pramipexole AUC and a 40% increase in half-life. Coadministration of drugs that are secreted by the cationic transport system (e.g., cimetidine, ranitidine, diltiazem, triamterene, verapamil, quinidine, quinine) decreases the oral clearance of pramipexole by about 20%. Drugs secreted by the anionic transport system (e.g., penicillins, indomethacin, hydrochlorothiazide, chlorpropamide) have little effect on the oral clearance of pramipexole. Pramipexole does not inhibit cytochrome P450 (CYP) enzymes, and inhibitors of CYP enzymes do not affect pramipexole elimination.

It is possible that dopamine antagonists such as neuroleptics will diminish the effectiveness of pramipexole.

PHARMACOKINETICS. Pramipexole is renally eliminated and is secreted by renal tubules via the organic cation transport system; therefore, dose adjustment is required in renal insufficiency (see Dosage and Administration following). See Table 45-3.

OVERDOSAGE. No clinical experience with intentional overdosage has been reported. One case of a patient who took 11 mg/day resulted in no adverse effects. Blood pressure remained stable while pulse rate increased to 100 to 120 beats/min.

DOSAGE AND ADMINISTRATION. Consult a neurologist. Pramipexole should be titrated gradually in all patients. Increase the dosage to achieve a maximum therapeutic effect, balanced against the principal side effects of dyskinesia, hallucinations, somnolence, and dry mouth.

Patients with normal renal function: Starting dose of 0.375 mg/day given in three divided doses. Do not increase more frequently than every 5 to 7 days. The following ascending dosage schedule of pramipexole was used in clinical trials and is suggested for use.

Week	Dosage, mg	Total Daily Dose, mg
1	0.125 tid	0.375
2	0.25 tid	0.75
3	0.5 tid	1.5
4	0.75 tid	2.25
5	1 tid	3
6	1.25 tid	3.75
7	1.5 tid	4.5

When pramipexole is used in conjunction with levodopa, a reduction in levodopa dosage should be considered. In one controlled study of patients with advanced PD, the levodopa dosage was reduced an average of 27% from baseline.

Patients with renal impairment: Adjustments in dosage are required according to the degree of impairment. See package insert.

Discontinuation: Gradual discontinuation over a period of 1 week is recommended. However, abrupt discontinuation may be uneventful.

DOPAMINE AGONISTS

ropinirole hydrochloride (Requip)

This drug is a nonergot dopamine agonist with high relative in vitro specificity and full intrinsic activity at the D_2 and D_3 dopamine receptors. It binds with higher affinity to D_3- than to D_2- or D_4-receptor subtypes. The relevance of D_3-receptor binding in PD is unknown.

CONTRAINDICATIONS. Hypersensitivity to the drug or its ingredients

WARNINGS/PRECAUTIONS. Syncope, sometimes associated with bradycardia, was observed in association with ropinirole in early PD without concomitant levodopa and in advanced PD with concomitant levodopa.

Carefully monitor patients who are starting ropinirole therapy or are undergoing dose escalation for signs and symptoms of orthostatic hypotension.

Hallucinations occurred in 5.2% of patients with PD without concomitant levodopa compared with 1.4% of placebo-treated patients. In patients with advanced PD who were receiving both ropinirole and levodopa, 10.1% of ropinirole-treated patients experienced hallucinations compared with 4.2% in the placebo group.

Ropinirole may potentiate the dopaminergic side effects of levodopa and may cause and/or exacerbate dyskinesias. Decreasing the dose of levodopa may ameliorate this side effect.

PHARMACOKINETICS. Ropinirole has a 55% absolute bioavailability, indicating a first-pass effect. Food does not affect the extent of absorption; however, the T_{max} is increased by 2.5 hours when the drug is taken with a meal. See Table 45-3.

No dosage adjustment is necessary on the basis of gender, weight, age, or moderate renal impairment (creatinine clearance, 30 to 50 ml/min). Ropinirole has not been studied in patients with severe renal impairment.

ADVERSE EFFECTS. Many potential side effects are similar to those associated with levodopa, including drowsiness, sudden sleep onset, hallucinations, confusion, dyskinesias, edema (swelling due to excess fluid in body tissues), nightmares, and vomiting. In rare cases, these can cause compulsive behavior, such as an uncontrollable desire to gamble, hypersexuality, or compulsive shopping. A related drug, bromocriptine, can cause fibrosis, or a buildup of fibrous tissue, in the heart valves or the chest cavity. Fibrosis usually goes away once the drugs are stopped.

DRUG INTERACTIONS. CYP 1A2 is the major isoenzyme responsible for metabolism in the line; therefore, the potential exists for substrates or inhibitors of this enzyme to alter the clearance of ropinirole when coadministered. Adjustment

TABLE 45-3   Pharmacokinetics of Antiparkinsonism Drugs

Drug	Absorption	Onset of Action	Time to Peak Concentration	Half-life	Duration of Action	Metabolism	Elimination	Protein Binding
carbidopa/levodopa (immediate release)	Rapid, complete	0.5 hr	0.5	1 hr	5 hr	Extensive	Renal	—
carbidopa	40%-70%		0.7 hr	1-2 hr	—	—	Renal	36%
carbidopa/levodopa (extended release)	Released over 4-6 hr; 70%-75% bioavailable	2 hr	2-3 hr	2 hr	—	—	—	—
selegiline	Good; greatly enhanced with food	1 hr	0.5 hr	1 hr	24-72 hr	Liver	Renal and feces	90%
amantadine	Rapid, complete	48 hr	1.5-8 hr	11-15 hr	—	None	Renal	—
bromocriptine	28% of oral dose	1-1.5 hr	1-2 hr	Initial: 6-8 hr Terminal: 50 hr	—	Complete	Biliary	90%-96%
pramipexole	Rapid, 90% bioavailable	2 hr	2 hr	8 hr in young; 1 hr in elderly	8 hr	Minimal	Renal	15%
ropinirole	Rapid, 55% bioavailable	<1 hr	1-2 hr	6 hr	16 hr	Extensive, inactive	Renal	40%
Anticholinergics	Well absorbed	—	—	—	—	—	—	—
benztropine	Poor	1-2 hr	—	—	24 hr	Liver	—	—
biperiden	—	2.5 hr (peak)	1-1.5 hr	18-24 hr	1-8 hr	—	—	—
diphenhydramine	Good	1-3 hr	2-4 hr	2-8 hr	4-7 hr	Liver	Renal	78%
procyclidine	Good	30-40 min	1.1-2 hr	8-16 hr	4-6 hr	Minimal	Renal	—

of ropinirole dosage may be required. Coadministration of theophylline (a CYP 1A2 substrate) did not alter the steady state pharmacokinetics of ropinirole. Coadministration of ciprofloxacin (a CYP 1A2 inhibitor) increased the AUC of ropinirole by 84% and the C_{max} by 60%.

Estrogens reduce the oral clearance of ropinirole by 36%. Dosage adjustment may not be needed for ropinirole in patients on estrogen therapy because patients must be carefully titrated with ropinirole to tolerance or adequate effect. However, if estrogen therapy is stopped or started during treatment with ropinirole, adjustment of the ropinirole dose may be necessary.

OVERDOSAGE. Side effects from inadvertent overdosage include mild orofacial dyskinesia, intermittent nausea, agitation, increased dyskinesia, grogginess, sedation, orthostatic hypotension, chest pain, confusion, vomiting, and nausea.

DOSAGE AND ADMINISTRATION. Ropinirole should be titrated gradually in all patients. The dosage should be increased to achieve a maximum therapeutic effect, balanced against the principal side effects of nausea, dizziness, somnolence, and dyskinesia.

Ropinirole may be taken with or without food. Taking ropinirole with food decreases the C_{max}; therefore, patients who take ropinirole with food may experience less nausea.

The recommended starting dose is 0.25 mg three times daily. Dosage may be titrated in weekly increments according to the patient's individual response, as described in the following ascending dose schedule of ropinirole. After week 4, if necessary, daily dosage may be increased by 1.5 mg/day on a weekly basis up to a dose of 9 mg/day and then by up to 3 mg/day weekly to a total dosage of 24 mg/day. Doses greater than 24 mg/day have not been tested in clinical trials.

Week	Dosage, mg	Total Daily Dose, mg
1	0.25 tid	0.75
2	0.5 tid	1.5
3	0.75 tid	2.25
4	1 tid	3

When ropinirole is administered with levodopa as adjunctive therapy, the dose of levodopa may have to be decreased gradually as tolerated. During clinical trials, the levodopa dose was reduced by 31% in ropinirole-treated patients.

Ropinirole should be discontinued gradually over a 7 day period. The frequency of administration should be reduced from three times daily to twice daily for 4 days. For the remaining 3 days, the frequency should be reduced to once daily before ropinirole is completely withdrawn.

ANTICHOLINERGIC AGENTS

Synthetic agents that have more selective CNS activity have replaced naturally occurring belladonna alkaloids. Peripheral anticholinergic effects may be dose-limiting factors. Antihistamines also have central anticholinergic effects, as well as a lower incidence of peripheral adverse effects than natural or synthetic alkaloids. Benztropine is most frequently used. If a patient does not respond to one anticholinergic, another may be tried. These drugs, which include trihexyphenidyl, benz-

tropine, and ethopropazine, decrease the activity of the neurotransmitter acetylcholine and help to reduce tremors and muscle rigidity. Only about half of patients who receive anticholinergics are helped by them, usually for brief periods and with only 30% improvement. Side effects may include dry mouth, constipation, urinary retention, hallucinations, memory loss, blurred vision, and confusion.

CONTRAINDICATIONS. Glaucoma, especially angle-closure; pyloric or duodenal obstruction; stenosing peptic ulcer; prostatic hyperplasia or bladder neck obstruction; achalasia; myasthenia gravis; and megacolon

WARNINGS
- *Ophthalmic:* Incipient narrow-angle glaucoma may be precipitated.
- *Elderly:* Increased sensitivity to anticholinergic drugs requires strict dosage adjustment. CNS adverse events may develop.

PRECAUTIONS
- Use with caution in patients with tachycardia, cardiac arrhythmias, hypertension, hypotension, prostatic hyperplasia (particularly in elderly), urinary retention, liver or kidney disorders, and GI or genitourinary obstructive disease.
- Mental or physical abilities may be impaired; caution is required when one is performing tasks that require alertness.
- If discontinuation of drug is required, do so gradually to avoid acute exacerbations of PD.
- Anhidrosis may occur during hot weather. Decrease dose so that thermal-regulating ability is not impaired.
- Dry mouth may cause difficulty swallowing or speaking and loss of appetite. Reduce dose, or discontinue temporarily.
- Abuse potential exists. Cannabinoids, barbiturates, opiates, and alcohol have additive effects when given with anticholinergics.

HOW TO MONITOR. Periodic intraocular pressure determinations should be made.

PATIENT VARIABLES

Geriatrics. Elderly patients may show an increased sensitivity to anticholinergic drugs, thus requiring strict dosage adjustments and monitoring. CNS adverse events may develop.

Stage of PD. Anticholinergics are helpful only in patients who present with tremor. Patients in early stages of PD who function well may not require medication. Consider adding anticholinergics as disease progresses.

DRUG INTERACTIONS
- *Amantadine, other anticholinergics, MAOIs:* Anticholinergic adverse effects may be increased; they disappear when the dose is decreased.
- *Digoxin:* Serum levels are increased when a slow-dissolution oral tablet is administered.
- *Haloperidol:* Worsening schizophrenia, decreased haloperidol concentrations, and tardive dyskinesias may develop.
- *Levodopa:* Decreased levodopa activity may result from decreased gastric motility and increased gastric deactivation of levodopa.
- *Phenothiazines:* Pharmacologic and therapeutic actions of phenothiazines reduce the effects of anticholinergics and increase anticholinergic adverse reactions.

- *Antidiarrheals:* Adsorbent produces decrease the effects of anticholinergics as the result of drug adsorption. Administer separately, 1 to 2 hours apart.

OVERDOSAGE. Serious cardiac, respiratory, or CNS symptoms, including circulatory collapse, may develop.

PATIENT EDUCATION
- Patients may take with food if GI upset occurs.
- Drowsiness, dizziness, and blurred vision may result; caution is required while driving or performing tasks that require alertness.
- Avoid alcohol and other CNS depressants.
- Dry mouth may occur. Sucking of hard candy, adequate fluid intake, and good oral hygiene may relieve symptoms. Constipation or difficulty urinating may occur; stool softeners may relieve constipation. Alert the health care provider if effects persist.
- Notify the health care provider of rapid heartbeat, confusion, eye pain, or rash.
- Use caution in hot weather; susceptibility to stroke is increased.

benztropine (Cogentin)

DOSAGE AND ADMINISTRATION. Administer 1 to 2 mg per day orally (range, 0.5 to 6 mg/day) in one to two divided doses.
- *PD:* Start with 0.5 to 1 mg at bedtime; tremor goes away with sleep, therefore medication is needed during the day, not at nighttime. Dosage of 4 to 6 mg/day may be required. Use may allow other PD symptoms to be reduced.

trihexyphenidyl HCl (Artane)

DOSAGE AND ADMINISTRATION
- Used in adjunctive therapy with levodopa and for the control of drug-induced extrapyramidal disorders.
- Give 1 to 2 mg the first day; increase by 2 mg increments at intervals of 3 to 5 days until a total of 6 to 10 mg is given daily.
- Gradually reduce or discontinue other antiparkinsonism drugs. The extended-release dosage form is used for maintenance therapy after patients' conditions have been stabilized with the use of tablets or elixir. It is tolerated best if divided into 3 doses and taken at mealtimes. High doses may be divided into four parts and administered at mealtime and at bedtime.
- If medication is given concurrently with levodopa, the usual dose of each may have to be reduced. Trihexyphenidyl 3 to 6 mg/day in divided doses usually is adequate. Do not use sustained-release forms for initial therapy because of their high doses.

COMT INHIBITOR

entacapone (Comtan)

CONTRAINDICATIONS. Hypersensitivity to the drug or its ingredients

WARNINGS. MAO and COMT are the two major enzymes that metabolize catecholamines. Do not treat patients concomitantly with entacapone and a nonselective MAOI (e.g., phenelzine, tranylcypromine) because this combination could result in inhibition of most of the pathways responsible for normal catecholamine metabolism.

Coadministration with drugs metabolized by COMT, including epinephrine, norepinephrine, dopamine, dobutamine, methyldopa, and apomorphine, may result in increased heart rate, arrhythmias, and fluctuation in blood pressure.

PRECAUTIONS. Entacapone enhances the bioavailability of levodopa; therefore; orthostatic hypotension induced by excessive dopaminergic activity is possible. Syncope also has been reported.

Ten percent of patients experienced diarrhea; 1.7% discontinued entacapone because of diarrhea. Diarrhea generally resolved on discontinuation of the drug; however, it did lead to hospitalization in two patients. Diarrhea typically presents 4 to 12 weeks after entacapone is started, but it may appear as early as 2 weeks and as late as many months after treatment initiation.

Hallucinations may present shortly after initiation of therapy, typically within the first 2 weeks. These may be responsive to levodopa dose reduction of 20% to 25% after the onset of hallucinations.

May cause or exacerbate preexisting dyskinesia. Many patients in clinical trials continued to experience frequent dyskinesias despite a reduction in their levodopa dose.

Rhabdomyolysis has been reported. This may be related to prolonged motor activity associated with dyskinesia.

ADVERSE REACTIONS. The most common side effect is diarrhea. These drugs also may cause nausea, sleep disturbance, dizziness, yellow-orange urine discoloration, abdominal pain, low blood pressure, or hallucinations.

DRUG INTERACTIONS. MAOIs given concomitantly can inhibit catecholamine metabolism. Selegiline, a selective MAO-B inhibitor, may be given concomitantly.

Drugs that interfere with bile excretion such as probenecid, cholestyramine, erythromycin, rifampicin, ampicillin, and chloramphenicol may increase the availability of entacapone.

See warnings for concomitant use with drugs metabolized by COMT.

OVERDOSAGE. COMT inhibition is dose dependent; therefore a major overdose of entacapone could inhibit COMT and prevent metabolism of catechols.

DOSAGE AND ADMINISTRATION. As an adjunct to carbidopa/levodopa therapy, administer one 200 mg entacapone tablet with each carbidopa/levodopa, up to eight times a day or 1600 mg/day.

evolve A continually updated list of useful WebLinks may be found in the Evolve Resources at http://evolve.elsevier.com/Edmunds/NP/

evolve http://evolve.elsevier.com/Edmunds/NP/

Antidepressants

DRUG OVERVIEW

Class	Generic Name	Trade Name
Selective serotonin reuptake inhibitors (SSRIs)	fluoxetine 🗝️ 🌟	Prozac, generic
	citalopram 🌟	Celexa, generic
	escitalopram	Lexapro 🌟
	fluvoxamine	Luvox, generic
	paroxetine 🌟	Paxil 🌟
	sertraline 🌟	Zoloft 🌟, generic
Serotonin/norepinephrine reuptake inhibitors (SNRIs)	venlafaxine hydrochloride SR 🗝️	Effexor XR 🌟
	duloxetine 🗝️	Cymbalta II 🌟
Norepinephrine/dopamine reuptake inhibitors (NDRIs)	bupropion 🗝️	Wellbutrin SL
Tricyclic antidepressants (TCAs)	nortriptyline 🗝️ 🌟	Pamelor, generic
	amitriptyline 🌟	Elavil, generic
	desipramine	Norpramin, generic
	doxepin 🌟	Sinequan, generic
	imipramine 🌟	Tofranil, generic
α_2-Noradrenergic antagonists	mirtazapine 🗝️ 🌟	Remeron, generic
Serotonin 2 agonists/blockers/serotonin reuptake inhibitors (SARIs/SSRIs)	trazodone 🗝️ 🌟	Desyrel, generic
	nefazodone	Serzone, generic
Monoamine oxidase inhibitors (MAOIs)	phenelzine	Nardil, generic
	tranylcypromine	Parnate, generic

🌟 Top 200 drug; 🗝️ key drug. Drugs listed in order of common use.

INDICATIONS

- Major depression (except fluvoxamine)
- Dysthymia
- *SSRIs:* Treatment of anxiety disorders

Other Indications

- *fluoxetine:* Bulimia nervosa, panic disorder, premenstrual dysphoric disorder (PMDD), OCD
- *escalitopram:* generalized anxiety disorder
- *paroxetine:* Generalized anxiety disorder, panic disorder, PTSD, OCD, social phobia, premenstrual dysphoric disorder, social anxiety disorder
- *sertraline:* Panic disorder, premenstrual dysphoric disorder, social anxiety disorder, PTSD, OCD
- *fluvoxamine:* OCD, panic disorder, bulimia nervosa, premenstrual dysphoric disorder
- *venlafaxine:* Generalized anxiety disorder
- *bupropion:* Smoking cessation

Unlabeled Uses

- *fluoxetine:* Raynaud's phenomenon, fibromyalgia, hot flashes, diabetic neuropathy
- *citalopram:* Premenstrual disorders, anorexia nervosa, bulimia nervosa, fibromyalgia, pathologic gambling
- *paroxetine:* Premenstrual disorders, pruritus, stuttering, hot flashes, diabetic neuropathy, premature ejaculation
- *sertraline:* Headache, hot flashes
- *venlafaxine:* Hot flashes, pain, autism, premenstrual dysphoric disorders
- *bupropion:* Neuropathic pain, ADHD, enhanced weight loss
- *Tricyclic antidepressants (TCAs):* Adjunct treatment of pain, panic disorder, irritable bowel syndrome
- *trazodone:* Aggressive behavior, panic disorder, insomnia, cocaine withdrawal

SSRIs represent the most commonly used first-line therapy. They produce excellent response with a good safety profile. Their use varies with the clinician's familiarity with the medication.

Venlafaxine and bupropion are also commonly used in primary care. Many of these antidepressants are reserved for use by psychiatrists.

MAOIs are used as third-line agents in cases of refractory and atypical depression. This chapter mentions MAOIs briefly but does not discuss them in detail because they generally are prescribed by a psychiatrist—not a primary care provider. Many TCAs are available, but this chapter mentions only a few. These agents produce excellent results in patients who have not responded to one of the newer antidepressants. They also are used when cost is a concern and as an adjunct treatment for depression and pain. Serzone is used only when other agents have failed; it carries a black box warning for liver toxicity. Trazodone is used largely as an adjunct or to induce sleep.

THERAPEUTIC OVERVIEW

Anatomy and Physiology

See Chapter 39 for a review of the anatomy and physiology of neurons. Table 39-1 on neurotransmitters is particularly useful. Monoamine neurons have the same structure as other neurons. The critical difference between neurons is the neurotransmitter that their receptors recognize teleologically. Three important types of monoaminergic neurons in the brain modulate mood. The first are the serotonergic neurons, also called 5-HT, which use serotonin as their neurotransmitter. The second are the noradrenergic (norepinergic) neurons, which use norepinephrine as their neurotransmitter. (This terminology is nonscholarly but the term has remained in use.) The third group consists of the dopaminergic neurons, which use dopamine as their neurotransmitter. Neurotransmitters can attach to a receptor on the same cell that they were released from (a presynaptic receptor) and affect the activity of that cell. These presynaptic receptors act as autoreceptors. They recognize when a sufficient amount of neurotransmitter is present in the synapse and inhibit further release of the neurotransmitter, operating as a brake. This works as a negative feedback system that regulates the amount of neurotransmitter in the synapse. If the presynaptic receptor is blocked, the receptor will keep the brake from functioning, allowing enhanced release of the neurotransmitter. The receptors can be blocked by an agent that occupies the receptor site but does not act on the site. This prevents the normal neurotransmitter from doing what it usually does.

Serotonergic neurons are located mainly in the area of the brainstem called the *raphe nucleus*. They regulate anxiety, movements, obsessions and compulsions, appetite and eating behavior, sleep, sexual response, and GI motility. The two major presynaptic serotonergic neuron receptors are 5-HT_{1A} and 5-HT_{1D}. Six major serotonergic postsynaptic receptors have been identified: 5-HT_{1A}, 5-HT_{1D} (the same as presynaptic), 5-HT_{2A}, 5-HT_{2C}, 5-HT_3, and 5-HT_4. Many more postsynaptic receptors are known, and new ones are being discovered. Stimulation of HT_{1A} (desirable) receptors improves mood and decreases eating disorders. HT_{2A} (undesirable) receptors are associated with anxiety, agitation, panic, decreased libido, sexual dysfunction, myoclonus, impaired sleep, and apathy. Stimulation of 5-HT_{2C} receptors causes anxiety, agitation, and panic. 5-HT_3 and 5-HT_4 receptors are located in the gut, where they control tone and motility, and their stimulation may cause nausea, vomiting, increased bowel motility, cramps, and diarrhea. Serotonergic neurons have postsynaptic autoreceptors such as 5-HT_{1A}, unlike the catecholamines norepinephrine and dopamine. Serotonergic neurons also have receptors on the cell bodies that enhance serotonin release. Norepinephrine can function as a brake for serotonin release by acting on the $NE\text{-}\alpha_2$ receptors that are found on serotonin neurons, as well as on adrenergic neurons.

Noradrenergic neurons are located primarily in the part of the brainstem called the *locus coeruleus*. The main function of the noradrenergic neurons is attention. They also have a role in control of memory, information processing, emotions, energy, psychomotor function, movement, blood pressure, heart rate, and bladder emptying.

Dopaminergic neurons are located in the substantia nigra, the medial mesencephalic tegmentum, and the hypothalamus. They control movement, primitive emotions, and visceral functions. Dopaminergic neurons have at least five types of receptors, of which D_2 receptors are the most studied. The D_2 receptor is important in Parkinson's disease and in schizophrenia. D_1 through D_4 receptors are affected by some of the atypical antipsychotic drugs. The newer antipsychotics affect mainly D_2 receptors.

Many other neurotransmitters are affected by antidepressant medications, causing numerous side effects (Table 46-1). The muscarinic system has two branches: the nicotinic and the cholinergic. Of the two, the cholinergic is by far more important. Cholinergic neurons use acetylcholine. The terms *muscarinic* and *cholinergic* often are used interchangeably. The histaminergic, α_1-adrenergic, and α_2-adrenergic systems also are involved in drug action.

Pathophysiology

Our understanding of the chemistry behind depression has grown dramatically. The neurochemical basis of depression is complex and is not the result of any one specific deficit. Depression seems to result from a gene and environment interaction. Usually, some type of severe stress produces alternation in the concentration of the neuroepinephrine transporter (the NET), or the uptake site. The function of the hypothalamic-pituitary axis and the involvement of stress-related hormones are increasingly believed to play a role in the development of depression. In reality, researchers do not know exactly what causes depression, even though the norepinephrine system has been studied intensively. Changes occur in the α- and β-adrenergic receptors—receptors that norepinephrine acts upon within the brain. Upregulation of β-receptors is thought to be due to a relative deficiency of norepinephrine at certain critical synapses in the brain. In older studies, measurements of norepinephrine metabolites, such as 3-methoxy-4-hydroxyphenylglycol (MHPG), have been reported as well. A relative lack of serotonin and decreased density of the postsynaptic 5-HT_2 receptors have been noted to produce a relative deficiency of serotonin in the brain. A relative lack of dopamine in presynaptic neurons and dopamine transporters has also been observed.

Pharmacologic research demonstrates improvement in depression when drugs are administered that increase relative amounts of these chemicals, although how this effect happens is not clear and is not as straightforward as it would seem.

Disease Process

Significant depressive symptoms are seen in nearly 40% of primary care patients, and major depression occurs in up to 10%. Major depression is a common, vastly undertreated, and potentially fatal disease. It is a heterogeneous disorder with a wide variety of presentations.

Many mood disorders must be differentiated. See Box 46-1 for the *Diagnostic and Statistical Manual of Mental Disorders, Fourth Edition (DSM-IV-TR)* diagnostic criteria for major depression. The patient with suspected major depression must have these symptoms on a daily basis for a minimum of 2 weeks. In addition, the severity of symptoms must significantly impair the patient's quality of life and ability to perform activities of daily living (ADLs). Five types of depression or basic clusters of symptoms are known. Cognitive symptoms include memory loss, slowed thoughts, decreased attention, and inability to concentrate. Vegetative symptoms include increased or decreased sleep, altered appetite or weight, psychomotor movement, and decreased sexual function. Physical symptoms consist of fatigue, muscle tension, pain—especially head and stomach, decreased sexual drive, and weakness. Behavioral symptoms include social withdrawal, loss of interest in usual activities, crying, weeping, decreased frustration tolerance, agitation and irritability, phobias, and poor attention to self-care. Emotional symptoms occur as guilt, feelings of worthlessness, suicidal ideation or behavior, disappointment with self, hopelessness, helplessness, anxiety, and delusions or hallucinations.

Another depressive disorder commonly seen in the primary care patient is atypical or "minor" depression. Symptoms of minor depression occur at the same frequency (i.e., daily, or nearly daily for at least 2 weeks) as those of major depression. However, patients with minor depression will have only two to four depressive symptoms that often include weight gain and hypersomnia. This contrasts with major

TABLE 46-1 Adverse Effects of Neurotransmitters

Neurotransmitter	Adverse Effects
Serotonin	Anxiety, agitation, anorexia, GI distress, headache, hypotension, sexual dysfunction
Norepinephrine	Tachycardia, tremors, sexual dysfunction; augments sympathomimetics
Dopamine	Extra pyramidal symptoms, ↑ prolactin levels, psychosis, insomnia, anorexia, psychomotor activation
Acetylcholine	Memory dysfunction, tachycardia, blurred vision, dry mouth, urinary retention, constipation
Histamine	Sedation, hypotension, weight gain, allergy
α_1-Adrenergic	Orthostatic hypotension, dizziness, cardiac conduction disturbance
α_2-Adrenergic	Priapism

BOX 46-1 DSM-IV Criteria for Diagnosis of Major Depressive Disorder

At least five of the following symptoms should be present nearly every day, continuously over 2 weeks. One of these symptoms must be depressed mood or anhedonia.

- Depressed mood most of the day
- *Anhedonia:* Lack of interest or pleasure in normal activities
- Appetite change or weight change
- Insomnia or hypersomnia
- Psychomotor agitation or retardation
- Fatigue, loss of energy
- Feelings of worthlessness or excessive or inappropriate guilt
- Diminished ability to think or concentrate, indecisiveness
- Recurrent thoughts of death, suicidal ideation

depression, in which weight loss and insomnia are typically seen. A total of 10% to 18% of these patients will develop major depression at 1 year.

Dysthymia is a depressive disorder in which symptoms are present for at least 2 consecutive years; these include lack of interest, low self-esteem, and low energy. It is present in approximately 3% to 5% of primary care patients.

Bereavement over the loss of a loved one is associated with symptoms of major depression. Despite the findings that 94% of these patients will meet the definition of major depression, only 17% will be treated with antidepressants. However, this apparent lack of treatment is explained by the fact that during the normal course of grief, 94% of symptoms have been found to resolve in 13 months.

Catatonic depression, comorbid anxiety disorder, and seasonal affective disorder (SAD) are other types of depressive disorder. Other diagnoses that should be considered include depression with alcohol or substance abuse or dependence, prenatal and postpartum depression, comorbid personality disorder, and the depressive phase of bipolar disorder.

The presence of bipolar disorder in the depressive stage always must be considered by the clinician. Treatment of a bipolar patient with antidepressants may induce rapid cycling to manic phase, and so careful monitoring is required, particularly if bipolar order is suspected but has not yet been confirmed.

The natural history of untreated depression is that of recurrence. Untreated depression may resolve without treatment, but recurrences are common. Risks for recurrence include increased severity and duration of the depression, psychotic symptoms, incomplete recovery between episodes, and prior episodes of depression. If a patient has had three or more episodes of depression, the chance of a relapse is greater than 90%.

Assessment

A complete history and physical examination are essential for the differential diagnosis of depression and for selection of the best medication for the patient. The discussion below is a brief review. Medical illnesses and medications also can contribute to the development of depression (see Tables 46-2 and 46-3). The diagnosis must rule out other factors such as drug or alcohol abuse, use of other medications, and medical conditions. Medical conditions that increase the risk of depression are cancer, chronic lung disease, heart disease, stroke, diabetes, end-stage renal disease, dementia, hypothyroidism, chronic fatigue syndrome, fibromyalgia, systemic lupus erythematosus, anxiety, and panic disorder. Also ask about past episodes of depression and hypomania and a family history of bipolar disorder. See Box 46-2 for a list of risk factors for depression.

Formal screening tools for depression such as the Zung Self-Assessment Depression Scale, the Beck Depression Inventory, and the General Health Questionnaire (GHQ) are available to the provider. The choice of one tool over another is a matter of preference. Two questions may elicit depression: "Over the past 2 weeks, have you felt down, depressed, or hopeless?" and "Over the past 2 weeks, have you felt little interest or pleasure in doing things?" Patients who test positive should undergo a complete diagnostic interview for a specific depressive disorder based on DSM-IV criteria.

TABLE 46-2   Illnesses Commonly Occurring With Depression

System	Examples
Autoimmune disease	Rheumatologic disorders
CNS disease	Stroke Dementia
Endocrine system disease	Diabetes Thyroid disorder
Heart disease	Chronic heart failure Myocardial infarction
Malnutrition	Vitamin deficiency Protein/calorie deficiency
Mood disorders and psychiatric conditions	Bipolar disorders Alcohol/drug dependency Eating disorders Obsessive-compulsive disorders Anxiety disorders Somatization disorders Personality disorders Psychosis
Other medical problems	Oncologic/hematologic disease Chronic fatigue syndrome Infectious disease

TABLE 46-3   Drug Classes That Produce the Side Effect of Depression

Drug Class	Specific Examples
Antihypertensives	Calcium channel blockers (diltiazem), methyldopa, nifedipine, thiazide diuretics, verapamil
Hormones	estrogen, progestins (Norplant), corticosteroids (prednisone, cortisone, ACTH), dapsone
Histamine₂-receptor blockers	famotidine (Pepcid), cimetidine, metoclopramide, nizatidine
Anticonvulsants	Barbiturates, carbamazepine, clonazepam, phenytoin, valproic acid
Antiparkinsonian	levodopa
Cardiac medications	digitalis glycosides, HMG-CoA reductase inhibitors (statins)
Antiinfectives	Fluoroquinolone antibiotics, isoniazid, metronidazole, sulfonamides
Sedative-hypnotics	Benzodiazepines
Antineoplastics	vinblastine
NSAIDs	ibuprofen, indomethacin, naproxen, sulindac

It is crucial to assess the risk of suicide in the depressed patient. The provider should pay particular attention to the presence of the following:

- Suicidal or homicidal ideation, intent, or plan
- Access to means for suicide and the lethality of those means

BOX 46-2   Risk Factors for Depression

- Female sex
- Ages 20 through 40 years, then elderly
- Family history
- *Marital status:* Unmarried men, married women
- Postpartum, within 6 months
- Negative life events, major psychosocial stressors, family distress
- Pain

- Psychotic symptoms, command hallucinations, or severe anxiety
- Alcohol or substance use
- History and seriousness of previous attempts
- Family history of or recent exposure to suicide

MECHANISM OF ACTION

Increased monoamine neurotransmitters serotonin, norepinephrine, and dopamine produce an elevated mood. All current antidepressants act on neurotransmitter systems by affecting three distinct processes: (1) neurotransmitter degradation, (2) neurotransmitter reuptake (reabsorption into the releasing cell), and (3) neurotransmitter binding.

Degradation of all three neurotransmitters is accomplished by the monoamine oxidase (MAO) enzyme. The catechol-O-methyltransferase (COMT) enzyme degrades norepinephrine and dopamine. MAO degrades neurotransmitters after reabsorption into the presynaptic neuron. MAOs occur in two forms—MAOa and MAOb—and are present in tissues throughout the body. Drugs that inhibit the enzyme and thus increase the concentrations of neurotransmitters are known as MAOIs.

The next mechanism of action of antidepressants involves inhibiting the reuptake of neurotransmitters in the synapse. Neurotransmitters are removed from the synapse by reuptake pumps on the presynaptic neuron, which takes them up and stores them for further use. Inhibiting this reuptake enhances the amount of neurotransmitter in the synapse. The third mechanism of action of antidepressants involves neurotransmitter receptor binding sensitization. This is a delayed effect.

At the same time, these antidepressants may bind themselves directly to postsynaptic receptors that produce side effects. Such receptors include histaminergic H_1, muscarinic, H_1-adrenergic, and dopaminergic D_2 receptors. The clinical effects that result when these receptors are stimulated by antidepressants may include dizziness, hypotension, tachycardia, and GI disturbances. Histaminergic H_1 antagonism has been associated with sedation and drowsiness. Muscarinic-receptor stimulation is responsible for constipation and dry mouth. Stimulation of the H_1-adrenergic receptor may be responsible for dizziness and orthostatic hypotension.

All categories of antidepressant medication have a common major mechanism of action. Slight variations within a drug category may be noted. Table 46-4 shows the antidepressants as classified according to mechanism of action. These medications are discussed in terms of the order of current usage. Older medications tend to have additional side effects. Newer antidepressants demonstrate a trend toward more specifically tailored mechanisms of action. Antidepressant therapies that are not categorized as SSRIs, TCAs, or MAOIs also have been developed; these are referred to in the literature as atypical antidepressants. The drugs include bupropion (Wellbutrin), nefazodone (Serzone), and trazodone (Desyrel).

Selective Serotonin Reuptake Inhibitors

All SSRIs work by increasing the amount of serotonin by blocking the presynaptic serotonin reuptake pump. At least 14 different postsynaptic serotonin receptors are present in humans. Each of these receptors controls a different physiologic and/or psychiatric function. The action of the SSRIs is related to which postsynaptic receptor is stimulated. It is believed that the 5-HT_{1A} receptors are primarily responsible for the antidepressant effect, and that the other receptor subtypes may be responsible for some of the side effects of SSRIs.

Serotonin/Norepinephrine Reuptake Inhibitors

Venlafaxine (Effexor) is a non–tricyclic antidepressant with dual serotonin and norepinephrine reuptake inhibition and weak reuptake inhibition of dopamine that has demonstrated efficacy in the treatment of depression and produces fewer side effects than are produced by tricyclics. Thus, it acts on all three of the monoamine neurotransmitters, as do the TCAs. Different from the TCAs and similar to the SSRIs, venlafaxine has virtually no affinity for muscarinic, histaminergic, or

TABLE 46-4   Antidepressant Classification Based on Neurotransmitter

Neurotransmitter	Tricyclics	SSRIs*	MAOIs	trazodone	bupropion	nefazodone	venlafaxine	mirtazapine
Norepinephrine uptake inhibition	+++	0	++	0	+	++	++	++
5-HT serotonin uptake inhibition	++	+++	++	++	+	+++	+++	++
Cholinergic inhibition	+++	0*	0	+	0	0	0	0
Histaminergic inhibition	++	0	0	+	0	0	0	0
α_1-Adrenergic inhibition	++	+	0	++	0	+	0	0
α_2-Adrenergic inhibition	+	+	0	++	0	0	0	++
Dopaminergic inhibition	0	0	++	0	++	0	+	0

0, No activity; +, weak activity; ++, moderate activity; +++, high activity.
*Citalopram, fluoxetine, and fluvoxamine have weak cholinergic inhibition.

α_1-adrenergic receptors. Its side effect profile is thus closer to that of the SSRIs than the TCAs. At higher doses, the risk of high blood pressure is increased. Another SNRI, duloxetine hydrochloride (Cymbalta), was approved for the treatment of major depressive disorder. Duloxetine is a potent inhibitor of serotonin and norepinephrine reuptake and a less potent inhibitor of dopamine reuptake.

Norepinephrine and Dopamine Reuptake Inhibitor (NDRI)

Bupropion is structurally similar to amphetamine and is considerably different from other antidepressants. Bupropion acts weakly as a norepinephrine and a dopamine reuptake blocker. It uniquely increases dopamine in the nucleus accumbens, which is known as the "reward area" of the brain in smokers. Therefore, bupropion is used for the treatment of smoking cessation.

Tricyclic Antidepressants

The TCAs were discovered in the 1950s and are named for their chemical structure, which contains three rings. They are subdivided further into the tertiary and secondary amines. The secondary amines (desipramine and nortriptyline) are metabolites of the tertiary amines (amitriptyline and imipramine). This results in significant differences in the pharmacokinetic and pharmacodynamic effects of each drug.

TCAs exert their therapeutic effects by blocking (inhibiting) reuptake of norepinephrine and serotonin at the presynaptic neurons. They block the reuptake of dopamine to a lesser degree. Some TCAs block serotonin$_{2A}$ receptors—an added therapeutic action. In addition, they block cholinergic, histamine, and α_1-adrenergic receptors; this effect is associated with the many side effects of TCAs. TCAs also block sodium channels in the heart and brain, which can cause cardiac arrhythmias and seizures.

Noradrenergic Antagonists

Introduced in 1997, mirtazapine is a tetracyclic compound that is unrelated to the TCAs. It is an α_2-antagonist that blocks the α_2-receptors on the adrenergic neurons. The α_2-receptors are noradrenergic receptors that act as presynaptic autoreceptors. When they detect adequate levels of norepinephrine, they stop norepinephrine release. An α_2-antagonist will block the negative feedback loop, raising norepinephrine levels. This same mechanism also will stop norepinephrine from blocking serotonin release, thus raising serotonin levels. The drug blocks three serotonin receptors (i.e., 5-HT$_{2A}$, 5-HT$_{2C}$, and 5-HT$_3$) and has antihistaminergic properties.

Serotonin 2 Agonist/Serotonin Reuptake Inhibitors

These agents block serotonin$_{2A}$ receptors and serotonin reuptake presynaptically and postsynaptically. Their most powerful action is to block serotonin$_{2A}$ receptors. This is called serotonin$_{2A}$ antagonism. They block serotonin reuptake, as do the SSRIs, but this is a less potent action. They are weak α_1-adrenergic blockers.

Nefazodone is a weak blocker of norepinephrine reuptake inhibitors. It has virtually no affinity for cholinergic, α_2-, or β-adrenergic, dopamine D$_1$, D$_2$, or histamine receptors.

Trazodone also blocks histamine$_1$ (H$_1$) receptors, and this causes sedation.

Monoamine Oxidase Inhibitors

The monoamine neurotransmitters dopamine, norepinephrine, and serotonin are broken down by the enzyme MAO. MAOIs are the medications that block this breakdown, causing increased levels of these three neurotransmitters. The first two MAOIs that blocked the MAO enzyme were irreversible, but very new ones are reversible inhibitors of MAO, known as reversible inhibitor monoamines (RIMAs).

TREATMENT PRINCIPLES

Standardized Guidelines

- The American Psychiatric Association (APA) has published guidelines on the treatment of patients with major depressive disorder. These guidelines will be included as appropriate in the discussion of these drug treatment principles. They can be accessed at www.psych.org.
- Schulberg HC et al: Treating major depression in primary care practice: an update of the Agency for Health Care Policy and Research Practice Guidelines, *Arch Gen Psychiatry* 55:1121-1127, 1998.
- Zuckerbrot RA et al: GLAD-PC Steering Group: Guidelines for Adolescent Depression in Primary Care (GLAD-PC): I. Identification, assessment, and initial management, *Pediatrics* 120:e1299-e1312, 2007.
- Cheung AH et al: GLAD-PC Steering Group: Guidelines for Adolescent Depression in Primary Care (GLAD-PC): II. Treatment and ongoing management, *Pediatrics* 120:e1313-e1326, 2007.

Evidence-Based Recommendations

The vast majority of clinical trials and meta-analyses have found that all antidepressants are considered equally effective. These conclusions are based on several factors, including effectiveness, side effects, and overall treatment costs. Thus, the choice of initial antidepressant rests with the provider. In many cases, the SSRIs are chosen as first-line agents because of their mild side effect profiles and the relative lack of danger associated with overdose.

Cardinal Points of Treatment

- Establish diagnosis.
- Assess for suicide risk.
- Institute counseling or psychotherapy.
- Offer nonpharmacologic treatment.
- Begin drug therapy as needed. See Box 46-3.

Nonpharmacologic Treatment

This chapter is focused on the primary care provider. Depression generally is treated in the primary care setting. Patients who should be referred to a psychiatrist include those who fail to achieve remission, who have symptoms of psychosis or severe symptoms, or who have depression with other comorbid psychiatric illness. Life-threatening situations such as the risk of suicide must be referred to the emergency department. Patients who are not eating or drinking should be sent urgently to psychiatry for consideration of electroconvulsive therapy (ECT). Children and adolescents often present with complex situations; all should be referred to a specialist.

BOX 46-3 Drug Choice

- *First-line drugs:* SSRIs, except fluvoxamine, SNRIs (venlafaxine), NDRIs (bupropion)
- *First line in certain conditions:* TCAs, mirtazapine
- *Second-line drugs:* SNRIs, NDRIs, TCAs
- *Third-line drugs:* SARIs, MAOIs

Patient preference is a major factor in the decision of which treatment to use. Many modalities are available for the treatment of patients with depression, including medications, psychotherapy, ECT, light therapy, and herbs. These may be used alone or in combination.

Nonpharmacologic treatment for depression is important in primary care. The primary care provider can often teach simple procedures that make important contributions to recovery, such as relaxation techniques, exercise, diet, and sleep hygiene. Exercise is especially important. Guidance on a daily routine may help get the patient moving. These requirements may be written on a prescription pad or established through a contract with the patient, if the provider believes it will be helpful in having the patient take them seriously.

Psychotherapy may be considered alone as initial therapy. Therapy is especially helpful for patients with psychosocial stressors, interpersonal difficulties, and other psychiatric illness. Psychotherapy should be recommended to all depressed patients. Often, they will refuse treatment because of the associated social stigma or lack of insurance reimbursement. Data support both psychotherapy and medications for patients with severe, chronic (longer than 2 years), or recurrent symptoms. Occasionally patients are more receptive to psychotherapy after the antidepressant has started to work. ECT is useful for patients who have severe functional impairment, such as those with catatonia; patients who refuse to eat, drink, or take medications; and those with symptoms of psychosis.

Pharmacologic Treatment

Researchers suggest that the most commonly prescribed antidepressants are similar in effectiveness to each other but differ when it comes to possible side effects. The findings, based on an Agency for Healthcare Research and Quality (AHRQ) review of nearly 300 published studies of second-generation antidepressants, show that about 6 in 10 adult patients get some relief from medications; about 6 in 10 also experience at least one side effect, ranging from nausea to sexual dysfunction. Those patients who do not respond often try another medication within the same class. About one in four of those patients recover, according to the review. Second-generation antidepressants, which include SSRIs and SNRIs, often are prescribed because first-generation antidepressants (TCAs) can cause intolerable side effects and carry high risks. Evidence is insufficient to predict which medications will work best for individual patients.

ACUTE TREATMENT PHASE. The acute phase of treatment begins when the diagnosis is established and lasts approximately 6 to 8 weeks. Remission, which is the treatment goal, is defined as a return to baseline level of symptoms and severity. The initial response rate to antidepressant drugs has been reported in the literature as ranging between 50% and 60%.

Medication should be started at a low dose that is increased gradually until the desired response is attained, or until side effects that influence compliance develop. The provider must inform the patient about what side effects are likely to occur and must help the patient cope with the side effects (see Table 46-5 for recommendations). If the patient shows a partial response in the first weeks of the trial, continue the trial of that medication for another 2 to 4 weeks. Maximum effectiveness cannot be evaluated until the patient has been on the same dosage for 2 to 6 weeks, depending on the medication. Once the patient has responded to a medication, titrate the dose until the patient has remission or experiences significant side effects. It is important to continue to adjust treatment to achieve remission instead of a partial response.

If the patient has no response after 8 to 12 weeks, gradually discontinue the drug. A second drug trial may come from the same or a different drug class. If a second drug from one category fails, choose a drug from another drug class. When the switch is made to another drug, the new drug should be started while the first drug is tapered over 2 to 4 weeks, except for fluoxetine (which does not need to be tapered because of its long half-life and active metabolite).

The first step in treatment for a person with bipolar disorder is mood stabilization. Rapid cycling may be prompted if care is not taken. If providers have little experience treating bipolar disorder, the provider should refer those patients in whom this condition is suspected.

TABLE 46-5 Recommendations to Minimize Common Adverse Effects

Adverse Effect	Antidepressant	Recommendation
Dryness of eyes and mouth	TCA	Natural tears; increase fluid intake; pilocarpine oral rinse; suck on sugar-free sour candy
Sexual dysfunction	Most	sildenafil
Sedation	trazodone, TCA, SARI, mirtazapine	Do not perform dangerous tasks; take at bedtime.
Insomnia	SSRI, venlafaxine, bupropion	Take in the morning.
Constipation	TCA	Increase fiber and fluid in the diet; get regular exercise.
Weight gain	TCA, MAOI, mirtazapine	Avoid snacking, exercise regularly; switch to SSRI, venlafaxine, bupropion.
Orthostatic hypotension	TCA, SARI, MAOI	Change position slowly; add salt to the diet; prescribe fludrocortisone.

AUGMENTATION FOR PARTIAL RESPONDERS. A second antidepressant drug is frequently added for partial responders. The provider must consider the additional risks that come with dual therapy and may opt to refer the patient to a psychiatrist. Partial responses generally can be divided into two categories; this affects the choice of augmentation. An apathetic responder may continue to have lack of pleasure, decreased libido, and lack of energy. An anxious responder may continue to have anxiety, excessive worry, insomnia, and somatic symptoms. Lithium, risperidone, and clozapine may be used for either category. Bupropion, an SSRI, methylphenidate (Ritalin), and thyroid may be used for apathetic responders. Trazodone, TCAs, mirtazapine, sedating antihistamines, and sedatives may be used for partial responders who remain anxious.

CONTINUATION PHASE. Once the patient achieves remission, the continuation phase begins; this phase lasts 16 to 20 weeks. The goal is to preserve remission and prevent relapse. *Relapse* is defined as reemergence of significant symptoms following a remission. The patient must be monitored closely during this phase.

MAINTENANCE PHASE. If the patient completes the continuation phase without remission, the maintenance phase is entered. Maintenance generally consists of continuing the medication prescribed during the treatment phase. The goal here is to prevent recurrence. Duration of treatment depends on many factors. Treatment initially provided to a patient who has simple depression that is in remission usually lasts for 1 year. Dosage reduction generally is not recommended. Those who probably will require an indefinite pharmacologic treatment maintenance phase include those who have a response without remission, those who have had more than one episode of depression, the elderly, and patients with symptoms of psychosis, depression of long duration, and severe depression. If treatment is stopped, regular follow-up with the patient continues to be necessary to monitor for relapse. In general, depression is a lifelong chronic recurrent illness that requires lifelong treatment.

In choosing which drugs should be used, consider that each neurotransmitter regulates different functions that are important to mood. To summarize briefly, *norepinephrine* tends to regulate alertness, energy, vigilance, and interaction with the environment; *dopamine* regulates motivation, pleasure, and reward; and *serotonin* usually regulates inner equilibrium, anxiety, obsessions, and compulsions.

When selecting a drug, consider the mechanism of action of the drug and the therapeutic effect of the neurotransmitters affected. Review the patient's complete history and physical examination for factors that may influence choice. See Table 46-6 for consideration of medical conditions when selecting an antidepressant. Consider the patient's age and gender, along with the history of previous response of the patient or family members because research into pharmacogenetics suggests that genes may influence response to antidepressants.

Consider the side effects associated with each drug. This is probably the most important factor that affects patient compliance with treatment. See Table 46-7 for general considerations of drug desirability for a patient. Important side effects for various drug categories are discussed below.

Dosing is also a factor in drug choice. Refer to the side effect profile of each drug for recommendations about what time of day is best to take drugs. For example, fluoxetine has the tendency to cause insomnia, so it is best taken in the morning.

Cost is important to the patient. Antidepressants tend to be expensive, and some insurance plans do not cover all medications. Generic versions generally are less expensive. However, most generic antidepressants have not been on the

TABLE 46-6   Consideration of Medical Conditions in the Treatment of Depression

Medical Condition	Drug	Implications
Asthma	MAOI	Interactions with sympathomimetics; other antidepressants are safe
Arrhythmias, conduction defects, prolonged QT interval	TCAs trazodone	May induce ventricular arrhythmias Increased risk; not recommended; contraindicated post-MI
Ischemic heart disease	All	Use with caution; do not use after acute MI
Hypertension	TCAs, trazodone TCAs venlafaxine	Drugs that block α-receptors (prazosin, etc) intensify effect; interact with diuretics to induce orthostatic hypotension Antagonize with guanethidine, clonidine, or α-methyldopa May cause usually mild, dose-dependent elevations; monitor
Dementia	Drugs with anticholinergic action	Cause ↓ memory and attention, sedation
Epilepsy	All bupropion	Monitor for drug interactions. Cause seizures in patients with eating disorders
Glaucoma	TCAs	Precipitate acute narrow-angle glaucoma in susceptible patients
Obstructive uropathy	TCAs trazodone and MAOIs	Contraindicated May retard bladder emptying
Parkinson's disease	bupropion SSRIs	Has beneficial effect on Parkinson's symptoms but may produce psychotic symptoms Increased risk of serotonin syndrome

TABLE 46-7   Considerations of Drug Desirability for a Patient

Drug	Recommended for	Potential Problems With
FIRST LINE		
SSRIs	New-onset depression; healthy, young, most patients	Early nausea, decreases sexual function
fluoxetine	Severe, anxious	Long acting
paroxetine	Atypical depression, insomnia, anxiety	Decreases sexual function, weight gain, sedation
SNRI: venlafaxine	Depression associated with psychiatric diagnoses, nonresponders to SSRIs	Anxiety, insomnia, hypertension, nonsedating
NDRI: bupropion	Overweight, psychomotor retardation, sexually active	Seizure, eating disorder, anxiety, weight loss
FIRST OR SECOND LINE		
α-NDRI: mirtazapine		
TCAs	Underweight, insomnia, agitation, anxiety	Psychomotor retardation; weight gain
amitriptyline	Healthy, young, severe, anxious, melancholic	Cardiac, thyroid, seizure; sedation
	Pain	
THIRD LINE		
nefazodone	Disturbed sleep patterns, sexually active, anxiety, agitation	Weight neutral
trazodone	Insomnia	Cardiac effects, sedation
MAOIs	Nonresponsive to other treatments; bipolar	Inability to follow strict diet

market long enough to allow for much cost reduction. TCAs tend to be less expensive than other types of antidepressants, but in patients in whom suicide may be a large consideration, TCAs are highly toxic in overdoses, whereas others, such as the SSRIs, are far less toxic.

SELECTIVE SEROTONIN REUPTAKE INHIBITORS. The SSRIs are the most commonly prescribed antidepressants for a variety of reasons. They are well tolerated and are considered safe in overdose. Symptom relief usually is seen within 3 to 6 weeks; side effects appear immediately but generally resolve in less than a week. Sexual dysfunction in both men and women is common to this class of drugs and is seen in as many as 50% of patients. If an SSRI is effective for the patient, but he or she is unwilling to cope with this, reduction of dose, addition of bupropion or buspirone, or, for men, a trial of sildenafil (Viagra) may be helpful. Another complaint that is commonly reported in approximately 10% of patients is weight gain.

Abrupt SSRI discontinuation can lead to withdrawal, characterized as "flu-like" symptoms. To avoid this, taper the drug dosage over a minimum of 2 weeks. Serotonin syndrome is potentially a lethal array of symptoms that are consistent with overactive stimulation of the CNS. It results from overstimulation of 5-HT receptors, which can be caused by coadministration of any drug that increases serotonin, including MAOIs, bupropion, lithium, dopamine agonists, tryptophan, amphetamines, and psychostimulants. The patient may display hyperactivity, tachycardia, hypertension, tremulousness, GI distress, sweating, altered mental state, fever, agitation, tremor, myoclonus, and hyperthermia. Symptoms generally appear within the first 24 hours and are treated with supportive care.

SEROTONIN AND NOREPINEPHRINE REUPTAKE INHIBITORS. Venlafaxine is a common first-line medication that often is used in patients who fail to respond to an SSRI. Nausea, dizziness, insomnia, sedation, and constipation are encountered commonly and are transient. Hypertension is associated with venlafaxine. This is dose related and usually becomes a problem when the daily dose exceeds 300 mg. All patients should have their blood pressure measured at regular intervals because this effect may be seen later in therapy. Although it is used to treat anxiety, venlafaxine also has the side effect of increased anxiety. Venlafaxine is not considered as safe in overdose as an SSRI. Duloxetine is the second drug to work via serotonin and norepinephrine reuptake inhibition. In addition to its use in major depression, duloxetine is being studied for use in pain syndromes associated with depression and in diabetic neuropathy with variable results. Common side effects are primarily GI and include nausea (most common), dry mouth, and constipation. FDA approved safety labeling revisions for duloxetine HCl delayed-release capsules (Cymbalta) to emphasize that MAOIs should not be used concomitantly or in close temporal proximity to SSRIs or SNRIs. Concomitant use of serotonergic drugs can lead to serious and sometimes fatal drug interactions. Symptoms may include hyperthermia, rigidity, myoclonus, autonomic instability with possible rapid fluctuation of vital signs, and mental status changes that include extreme agitation progressing to delirium and coma. According to the FDA, these interactions have also been reported in patients who initiated MAOI therapy following recent discontinuation of SSRIs or SNRIs. Some of these cases presented with features resembling neuroleptic malignant syndrome. There should be at least 14 days separating use of the two drugs in the same patient.

NOREPINEPHRINE AND DOPAMINE REUPTAKE BLOCKER. Bupropion is significantly different from other antidepressants. It has been shown to be a mild stimulant and has found a place among patients who present with fatigue and poor concentration. Also, bupropion also lacks the side effects associated with sexual dysfunction and is a reasonable alternative to an SSRI. Its ability to alter dopamine activity in the nucleus accumbens or the "reward area" of the brain is thought to account for its efficacy in smoking cessation. Bupropion has a very low risk of seizures. The risk of seizures is higher in patients with a history of head trauma, prior seizure, CNS tumor, or eating disorder, and in those taking concomitant medications that lower seizure threshold. Headache and mild agitation are the most common side effects.

TRICYCLIC ANTIDEPRESSANTS. TCAs typically are used as third-line agents, even though studies have shown equal efficacy in comparisons with newer agents. Patients who are tolerating TCAs and have achieved a good clinical response should remain on them. Consider a TCA when cost is paramount. TCAs are widely available in generic form and are much less expensive than SSRIs, even those available as generic agents. Their use has fallen in recent years with the advent of significantly safer and better tolerated drugs such as SSRIs. Also, substantial risk of fatal overdose can occur with doses as low as five times the therapeutic dose.

TCAs slow cardiac conduction; this may lead to heart block or arrhythmia. These agents are used with caution in patients who have preexisting cardiac dysfunction, and a baseline ECG is recommended in patients older than age 40; in addition, the QT interval should be monitored periodically. TCAs have found a niche in the treatment of patient with neuropathic pain syndromes such as trigeminal neuralgia and diabetic neuropathy (see Chapter 42 on pain management). The mechanism of action is thought to be caused by NE reuptake blockade. Amitriptyline is the TCA of first choice in pain relief, although other TCAs are also effective. The initial dose of TCA for neuropathic pain is 10 to 25 mg given at bedtime. Increase the dosage by 10 to 25 mg every 2 to 3 days. Analgesic effects usually are evident within about 1 week after an effective dosage has been reached. Patients should be informed of this delay in analgesic effects.

α_2-NORADRENERGIC ANTAGONIST/MIXED SEROTONIN BLOCKERS. Side effects of mirtazapine include sedation, fatigue, increased appetite, and weight gain. Sexual dysfunction is much less than with SSRIs. An unusual finding is that the sedation associated with mirtazapine is more common in patients who take lower (15 mg) rather than higher (30 mg) doses. Mirtazapine is very effective in alleviating depression while increasing appetite and eliminating insomnia. Anxiolytic and sleep improvements are reported to occur as early as 1 week after the drug is started, although the full antidepressant response may take several weeks, as with other antidepressants. Its use in younger patients is limited by sedation and weight gain. Another consideration in drug selection is whether potential side effects might be beneficial for a particular patient. For example, in some nursing home residents who are underweight and have a poor appetite, mirtazapine can be a good choice because the weight gain it causes is desirable.

SEROTONIN$_{2A}$ ANTAGONISTS, AND SEROTONIN REUPTAKE INHIBITORS. Trazodone and nefazodone both are included in this class, but they have different mechanisms of action. Trazodone is seldom used as a first-line agent for the management of depression because of the side effect of sedation, rare reports of cardiac arrhythmia, and priapism, which is a medical emergency. It may have a role in the treatment of patients with insomnia and may be used to augment drug therapy for patients who have a partial response but remain anxious.

Nefazodone, too, is seldom used in the treatment of depression. Twenty-five cases of liver failure and death have been reported since 1995. Close monitoring of liver transaminases (AST/ALT) has not proved to be predictive of liver toxicity. Also, nefazodone has numerous drug–drug CYP 3A4 interactions. The manufacturer withdrew the drug from the U.S. market in 2004, but generic versions are available. Nefazodone has a calming effect (with less sedation than TCAs) and may be helpful for patients with sleep disorder. Nefazodone is uniquely associated with an increase in REM sleep vs. the decrease associated with many other antidepressants. Sleep disorders and depression are so closely linked that it is theorized that the sleep disorder may be a central part of the depression. Nefazodone also may cause less sexual dysfunction than is caused by other antidepressants.

MONOAMINE OXIDASE INHIBITORS. The broad spectrum of action is inevitably associated with a broad spectrum of adverse reactions, including hypertensive crisis, which can be fatal. A hypertensive crisis can occur within several hours after ingestion of a substance that contains tyramine. Tyramine releases norepinephrine and other sympathomimetic amines, thereby raising blood pressure. Early symptoms include occipital headache, palpitations, stiff neck, nausea, vomiting, and sweating. Many medications, especially other antidepressants, and foods that contain tyramine can elicit this response. If suspected, the provider should refer the patient to the emergency department immediately. Any change of medication to or from an MAOI absolutely requires a washout period of at least 2 weeks.

> **evolve** For additional information, see the supplemental tables on the Evolve Learning Resources website.

How to Monitor

The patient should be seen weekly for the first few weeks to months until improvement is seen, then monthly until remission occurs, and periodically thereafter. Monitor for therapeutic effects and adverse reactions.

> 💣 The U.S. Food and Drug Administration requires that all antidepressants should carry the black box warning for increased risk of suicide in children/adolescents with major depressive disorder or another psychiatric disorder, especially during the first months of treatment or at times of dose change.
>
> If the patient is suicidal, the chances that the patient will commit suicide successfully are highest during the first few months of a depressive episode or shortly after an antidepressant is started.

When the medication starts to work, the patient may be energized enough to follow through on a plan. At first, limit the quantity of medication prescribed and do not use the refill option, to avoid giving the patient a method for suicide by drug overdose.

See Table 46-8 for laboratory values that must be monitored with the use of specific drugs.

> 💣 Depressed patients often require more than one medication to alleviate symptoms. There are significant drug-drug interactions among antidepressant

TABLE 46-8 Baseline and Periodic Tests Recommended

Drug	Test	Look for
All antidepressants	Weight, as indicated	Loss/gain
TCAs	ECG CBC Liver function studies Blood sugar	QT prolongation Bone marrow dysfunction ↑ AST and ALT ↑↓ Blood sugars
SSRIs	CBC, as indicated Electrolytes, as indicated	↓ Platelets ↓ Sodium SIADH
SNRIs: venlafaxine	Blood pressure Electrolytes, as indicated	Hypertension ↓ Sodium SIADH
SARIs		
trazodone	CBC, as indicated	Low WBCs
nefazodone	LFTs	Hepatotoxicity
bupropion	LFTs, as indicated	Toxic in ↓ liver function
NDRI: mirtazapine	CBC with differential, as indicated	Agranulocytosis (rare)

drugs. The following are accepted as directives to avoid drug-drug interactions:

Contraindicated Drug Combination: *Clearly contraindicated in all cases and should not be dispensed or administered to the same patient.*
SRIs/Selected MAOIs: Adverse reaction with both drugs
Antidepressants/sibutramine: Adverse reaction of the latter drug
SSRIs; nefazodone/pimozide: Adverse reaction of the latter drug
Serotoninergic Agents/sibutramine: Adverse reaction of the latter drug
Serotoninergic Agents/dexfenfluramine; fenfluramine: Adverse reaction with both drugs

Severe Interaction: *Action is required to reduce the risk of severe adverse interaction.*
SRIs/linezolid: Adverse reaction with both drugs
SSRIs; duloxetine; venlafaxine/tramadol: Decreased effect of the latter drug
SSRIs/Phentermine: Adverse reaction with both drugs
SSRIs; SNRIs/5HT-1D agonists: Adverse reaction of the former drug

Moderate Interaction: *Assess the risk to the patient and take action as needed.*
SSRIs; duloxetine/Tricyclic compounds; trazodone: Increased effect of the latter drug
SSRIs/NSAIDs; aspirin: Adverse reaction of the former drug
Selected SSRIs; SSNRIs/tamoxifen: Decreased effect of the latter drug
SSRIs; SSNRIs; venlafaxine/ampletamines: Adverse reaction with both drugs
Antidepressants/bupropion: Additive side effects from both drugs

SSRIs; Venlafaxine/lithium: Adverse reaction with both drugs
Selected SSRIs/Clozapine: Increased effect of the latter drug

Patient Variables

GERIATRICS. Elderly patients have more vegetative and cognitive symptoms and complain less of mood problems. Drug selection often is limited by medical conditions such cardiac conditions and stroke. Dehydration may lead to toxicity from antidepressants, even if low dosages are used. The elderly often have subclinical renal and hepatic dysfunction that will slow drug metabolism and excretion, raising drug levels. This is why lower dosages usually are required. Side effects are more frequent and less well tolerated, especially histaminic and anticholinergic effects. Elderly white men have the highest risk of suicide of all patients. The elderly are more sensitive to the anticholinergic side effects of TCAs, such as orthostasis, sedation, and urinary retention. This can lead to falls and worsening of urination, especially in men with benign prostatic hyperprocess.

Use of amitriptyline should be avoided in the elderly because of sensitivity to the anticholinergic side effects and cardiotoxicity.

PEDIATRIC PATIENTS AND ADOLESCENTS
- *TCAs:* Use in children older than 12 years.
- *SSRIs:* Use in patients older than 18 years; use fluoxetine in those 8 years old or older.
- *Others:* Use in patients older than 18 years.

Depression occurs in children and adolescents. Presentation can be very different than in the adult, and it varies with age. Younger children have behavioral problems such as social withdrawal, aggressive behavior, apathy, sleep disruption, and weight loss. Adolescents exhibit somatic complaints, self-esteem problems, rebelliousness, poor performance in school, or risky or aggressive behavior. Risk of suicide is relatively high, especially when accompanied by alcohol or other substance abuse. The FDA requires that a "black box" warning be added to the labeling of commonly used antidepressants that states that adolescents and young adults treated with these drugs are more likely than others to become suicidal. It should be noted that psychiatric adverse effects of SSRIs overlap with manifestations of depression itself; without knowledge of this adverse effect, clinicians may make the mistake of increasing rather than decreasing the SSRI dose of children and adolescents who are experiencing these adverse effects.

Treatment of a child or adolescent with recent onset of depression should begin with practical coping skills, family intervention, cognitive-behavioral therapy, or other forms of psychosocial treatment. Patients with depression should be treated by a pediatric specialist.

PREGNANCY AND LACTATION
- *Category C:* SSRIs (avoid paroxetine), venlafaxine, trazodone, nefazodone, mirtazapine, bupropion, amitriptyline, desipramine
- *Category D:* Imipramine, nortriptyline
- *Lactation:* All are present in breast milk; refer to the American Academy of Pediatrics (AAP) committee on

drugs (http://aappolicy.aappublications.org) for the most current information.

Risks of depression during pregnancy may involve suicide and impaired function (e.g., lack of self-care, lack of care of the fetus, inability to care for other children). Mild to moderate depression generally is treated with psychotherapy alone. The addition of an antidepressant is generally reserved for women with severe depression. The SSRIs, specifically fluoxetine and sertraline, generally are recommended because they have been studied most extensively and have shown a good safety record when used in pregnant and breastfeeding women. Fluoxetine has the advantage of long-term follow-up in infants who were exposed during pregnancy. Paroxetine carries a warning of fetal abnormalities and should not be used.

GENDER. Men often refuse to endure the sexual dysfunction that occurs with the SSRIs.

CULTURE. Culture may hamper diagnosis and hinder treatment. Many cultures do not recognize depression as an illness. The patient may have difficulty expressing his or her feelings. Depression may manifest as physical, somatic, and psychomotor symptoms. Language may be a barrier. Most patients prefer not to take medications. It is important to find out what the condition is called in the culture and to learn the causative explanation. If it is caused by evil spirits or by a frightening experience, it is unlikely that drugs will be an acceptable form of treatment. Also, many immigrants have experienced very stressful life situations, and perhaps culturally based support would be helpful (e.g., resources within immigrant communities). Some African Americans may see depression in religious terms as lack of faith or a punishment.

Patient Education

Ask about all other medications or herbs that the patient is taking.
- Side effects are seen with the first few doses but resolve in approximately 7 days.
- It may take 3 to 6 weeks before benefits are seen.
- Avoid alcohol and sedatives when taking antidepressants.
- Many antidepressants can cause sedation; patients should avoid tasks that require alertness or coordination until they know how the medication will affect them.
- Notify the primary care provider of any adverse effects.
- Notify the primary care provider if the patient intends to or becomes pregnant or is breastfeeding.
- Suggest ways to minimize adverse effects (see Table 46-5 for recommendations).

 A withdrawal syndrome may be experienced if the antidepressant is discontinued abruptly.

Notify patients of the following specific risks:
- *TCAs:* Seizures, photosensitivity
- *SSRIs:* Rash, hives or allergic phenomena, photosensitivity; swallow controlled-release form whole
- *venlafaxine:* Rash, hives, or allergic phenomena; swallow controlled-release form whole
- *trazodone:* Take with food; priapism in males

- *nefazodone:* Liver abnormalities; can cause death, rash, hives, allergic phenomena, visual disturbances, photosensitivity
- *mirtazapine:* Agranulocytosis; notify care provider if symptoms of infection are noted

SPECIFIC DRUGS
SELECTIVE SEROTONIN REUPTAKE INHIBITORS

fluoxetine HCl (Prozac)

CONTRAINDICATIONS
- Hypersensitivity
- Concomitant use with MAOIs, pimozide, or thioridazine

WARNINGS
- Suicidal thinking/behavior in children and adolescents with major depressive disorder (see Pediatrics and Adolescents previously)
- Monitor for altered platelet function.
- *Rash and accompanying events:* Approximately 7% of patients who take fluoxetine have developed rash or urticaria. Events associated with rash include fever, leukocytosis, arthralgias, edema, carpal tunnel syndrome, respiratory distress, lymphadenopathy, proteinuria, and mild transaminase elevation. Most improve quickly when the drug is discontinued. Systemic events, possibly related to vasculitis, have occurred in patients with rash. These are rare but can be serious, involving the lung, kidney, or liver. Death has occurred. Anaphylactoid events have occurred with fluoxetine. Pulmonary events have occurred rarely. Discontinue if rash appears.
- *Renal function impairment:* Use lower or less-frequent dosage.
- *Hepatic function impairment:* SSRIs are metabolized extensively by the liver. Use with caution in patients who have severe liver impairment.

PRECAUTIONS
- Anxiety, nervousness, and insomnia occur frequently.
- *Altered appetite and weight:* Weight loss may occur, especially in underweight patients; after prolonged treatment, patients tend to gain weight.
- Activation or mania/hypomania occurs infrequently.
- Seizures have occurred.
- May impair platelet aggregation, resulting in bleeding
- Hyponatremia has occurred as a result of SIADH, especially in the elderly.
- Photosensitivity may occur.
- Have patients use caution when performing hazardous tasks.

PHARMACOKINETICS. Fluoxetine has the longest half-life of any SSRI. This accounts for persistence of adverse effects after the drug has been discontinued but also allows for missed doses and minimization of discontinuation symptoms. The drug is now available in a timed-release formulation that requires only weekly administration. It is also available generically.

fluoxetine HCl (Prozac) —cont'd

DRUG INTERACTIONS. Fluoxetine is metabolized by 2D6 and is a potent inhibitor of 2D6. It is associated with many more drug interactions when compared with most other SSRIs.

OVERDOSAGE. SSRIs are considered safe in overdose.

> Overdosage is less likely than TCAs to cause death. However, patients on SSRIs are more likely to attempt suicide. Nausea and vomiting often prevent absorption.

DOSAGE AND ADMINISTRATION. Fluoxetine is the only SSRI approved by the FDA for the treatment of depression in children. Administer in the morning because of the high incidence of associated insomnia.

OTHER DRUGS IN CLASS

Other drugs in this class are similar to the prototype except as follows:

Paroxetine (Paxil) has some antihistamine actions that are more likely to cause sedation and constipation than are those of other SSRIs. Paroxetine appears to cause greater weight gain and a larger number of sexual effects and discontinuation symptoms when compared with other SSRIs; it also has many drug interactions. *Sertraline* most often is associated with nausea and vomiting. *Fluvoxamine* has the serious side effects of tardive dyskinesia, CNS depression, and psychotic symptoms. Fluvoxamine is a major inhibitor of several CYP enzymes, resulting in numerous drug–drug interactions. It is contraindicated with alosetron, pimozide, thioridazine, tizanidine, mesoridazine, or cisapride. *Lexapro* (escitalopram) is a metabolite of Celexa (citalopram).

SEROTONIN/NOREPINEPHRINE REUPTAKE INHIBITORS

venlafaxine hydrochloride (Effexor, Effexor XR)

CONTRAINDICATIONS
- Hypersensitivity
- Concomitant use with MAOIs

WARNINGS
- Sustained hypertension has occurred in patients on venlafaxine; effect is dosage dependent; blood pressure should be monitored.
- *Renal/hepatic function impairment:* Use with caution; lower dosage; monitor for effectiveness with long-term use.

PRECAUTIONS
- Anxiety, insomnia, and nervousness are commonly reported.
- *Appetite/weight changes:* Anorexia is commonly reported. Weight loss often occurs in underweight patients.
- Mania/hypomania may occur.
- Hyponatremia due to SIADH has been reported.
- Mydriasis may occur; monitor patients who have increased intraocular pressure or glaucoma.

- Seizures have been reported, especially at higher dosages.
- Abnormal bleeding, especially ecchymosis, has been associated with venlafaxine.
- *Concomitant illness:* Use with caution in patients with conditions that could affect hemodynamic response or metabolism.
- Have patient use caution when performing hazardous tasks.

DRUG INTERACTIONS. Closely monitor the effects of drugs that use cytochrome P450 2D6 and 3A4 (a weak inhibitor).

NOREPINEPHRINE/DOPAMINE REUPTAKE INHIBITORS

bupropion (Wellbutrin)

CONTRAINDICATIONS
- Hypersensitivity
- Seizure disorder
- With current or prior diagnosis of bulimia or anorexia nervosa (seizure risk)
- In combination with Zyban (contains same ingredient)
- Withdrawal from alcohol or sedatives
- Concomitant use with MAOIs

WARNINGS
- Patients with a drug abuse history may experience a mild amphetamine-like effect.
- *Hepatotoxicity:* Rare elevations in liver function tests.
- *Renal/hepatic function impairment:* Bupropion is metabolized in the liver and is excreted by the kidneys. Use with caution in patients with renal or hepatic insufficiency.

PRECAUTIONS
- *CNS:* Symptoms, including restlessness, agitation, anxiety, and insomnia, may occur.
- Neuropsychiatric signs and symptoms, including delusions, hallucinations, psychotic episodes, difficulty concentrating, confusion, and paranoia; can precipitate manic episode in bipolar disorder
- Weight loss is common.
- *Cardiac effects:* Can cause hypertension; use with caution in cardiac patients

OVERDOSAGE. Symptoms include seizures, hallucinations, loss of consciousness, and tachycardia. Deaths have been reported rarely. Treatment requires hospitalization.

TRICYCLIC ANTIDEPRESSANTS

nortriptyline (Pamelor)

Nortriptyline has lower anticholinergic and cardiovascular side effects than TCAs.

CONTRAINDICATIONS
- Hypersensitivity
- Post MI

Continued

nortriptyline (Pamelor) 🔑 —cont'd

- Pregnancy
- Concomitant use with MAOIs

WARNINGS

- *Seizure disorder:* TCAs may lower seizure threshold; use with caution in patients with a history of seizures or predisposing conditions.
- *Anticholinergic effects:* Use with caution in patients at risk for urinary retention and glaucoma.
- *Cardiovascular disorders:* Use with extreme caution in patients with cardiovascular disorders, especially arrhythmias and angina; orthostatic hypotension may occur. Obtain ECG before prescribing.
- *Hyperthyroid patients:* Monitor for cardiovascular toxicity.
- *Psychiatric:* Worsening of psychosis; possibility of suicide
- Mania/hypomania may occur, especially in patients with cyclic disorders.
- *Rash:* Drug fever may be severe; discontinue if rash appears.
- *Renal/hepatic function:* Use with caution and with reduced doses.
- *Elderly:* Low dosage; monitor for anticholinergic effects

PRECAUTIONS

- Monitor baseline and periodic leukocyte and differential counts and LFTs. Fever or sore throat may signal serious neutrophil depression; discontinue therapy.
- Monitor ECG before therapy and at appropriate intervals.
- ECT with those patients on TCAs may increase hazards of ECT therapy because of effects on the seizure threshold.
- *Elective surgery:* Discontinue TCA for as long as possible before elective surgery.
- *Blood sugar levels:* Elevated and lowered blood sugar levels have occurred.
- Weight gain has been observed.
- *Hazardous tasks:* Use caution.
- Photosensitivity may occur; have patient take protective measures.

PHARMACOKINETICS. See Table 46-9.

ADVERSE REACTIONS. Anticholinergic side effects are common with the TCAs and are associated with sedation, dry mouth, urinary retention, constipation, blurred vision, low blood pressure, and weight gain. Potentially serious effects include heart block, tachycardia, palpitations, and MI. See Table 46-10.

DRUG INTERACTIONS. See Table 46-11.

OVERDOSAGE. Overdosage is more serious in children.

Any overdose is serious and potentially fatal. Early signs include confusion, agitation, hallucinations, and coma. Cardiotoxicity depresses myocardial contractibility and causes arrhythmias.

DOSAGE AND ADMINISTRATION. See Table 46-12.

OTHER DRUGS IN CLASS

Other drugs in this class are similar to the prototype except as follows:

- *Amitriptyline* has a greater number of side effects than other TCAs; it is useful for pain treatment.
- *Desipramine* is less sedating when compared with other TCAs.
- *Nortriptyline* has fewer anticholinergic effects than does amitriptyline.

α₂-NORADRENERGIC ANTAGONISTS

mirtazapine (Remeron) 🔑

CONTRAINDICATIONS

- Hypersensitivity
- Concomitant use with MAOIs

WARNINGS

- Agranulocytosis may occur; monitor for signs of infection.
- Seizures are very rare; they have occurred only in patients who were at increased risk for seizures.
- *Cardiovascular effects:* Use with caution in patients with cardiac disease.
- Renal function impairment slows clearance of the drug; use lower dosage.
- Hepatic function impairment slows metabolism of the drug; use lower dosage.

PRECAUTIONS

- Somnolence occurs in about half of patients.
- Dizziness may occur.
- Increased appetite/weight gain is observed in many patients.
- Elevated cholesterol/triglycerides have been seen.
- Orthostatic hypotension infrequently occurs.

OVERDOSAGE. Symptoms include disorientation, drowsiness, impaired memory, and tachycardia.

SEROTONIN 2 AGONISTS/SEROTONIN REUPTAKE INHIBITORS

Trazodone and nefazodone are very different and are discussed separately.

trazodone (Desyrel) 🔑

Often used as an adjunct or for sleep. May be used as part of behavior management regimen in patients with dementia.

CONTRAINDICATIONS. Hypersensitivity

WARNINGS

- *Preexisting cardiac disease:* Trazodone may produce arrhythmias in some patients; monitor cardiac patients closely.
- *Priapism:* May require emergency treatment

PRECAUTIONS. Hypotension, including orthostatic hypotension, and syncope may occur.

OVERDOSAGE. *Symptoms:* CNS depression, seizures, and ECG changes. Death may occur when trazodone is ingested with other drugs. Hospitalize for treatment.

Text continued on page 519

TABLE 46-9 Pharmacokinetics of Antidepressant Medications

Drug	Absorption	Drug Availability (after first pass)	Onset of Therapeutic Action	Half-life	Protein Binding	Metabolism (consider for drug interactions)	Excretion	Therapeutic Serum Level (not necessarily an indicator of effectiveness)
TRICYCLIC ANTIDEPRESSANTS								
nortriptyline	Good	Significant first-pass effect	1-3 wk	28-31 hr	>90%	Liver, by 2D6 (major); metabolite of amitriptyline	Urine	50-150 mg/ml
amitriptyline	Good	Significant first-pass effect	4-6 wk	15 hr	>90%	Liver, by 2D6 (major); metabolized to nortriptyline	Urine	100-250 mg/ml
desipramine	Good	Significant first-pass effect	3 wk	14-24 hr	>90%	Liver, by 2D6 (major); inhibits 2A6 (moderate), 2B6 (moderate), 2D6 (moderate), 3A4 (moderate); metabolite of imipramine	Urine	50-300 mg/ml
SELECTIVE SEROTONIN REUPTAKE INHIBITORS								
fluoxetine	72%	—	3-4 wk	4-12 days average; 9.3 days (longer in cirrhosis)	95%	Liver, 2C9, 2D6 (major); inhibits 1A2, 2C19 (mod), 2D6 (major)	Urine	100-800 ng/ml
citalopram	Well absorbed; unaffected by food	80%	1-4 wk	33 hr	80%	Liver, 2C19 (major), 3A4 (major)	Urine, 35%; feces, 65%	
escitalopram	Well absorbed; unaffected by food	—	1-4 wk	27-32 hr	56%	Liver, 2C19, 3A4 (major); metabolite of citalopram	Urine, 35%; feces, 65%	
sertraline	Complete	—	2-4 wk	1-4 days	98%	Liver, 2C19, 2D6 (major); inhibits 2B6, 2C19, 2D6, 3A4 (mod)	Urine, 50%; feces, 50%	
paroxetine	64%	100%	2 wk	10-24 hr	95%	Liver, 2D6 (major); inhibits 2B6 (mod), 2D6 (strong)	Urine, 64%; feces, 36%	
fluvoxamine	Unaffected by food	53%	2-4 wk	15 hr	80%	Liver, 1A2, 2D6 (major); inhibits 1A2, 2C19 (major)	Urine, 95%;	
SEROTONIN/NOREPINEPHRINE REUPTAKE INHIBITORS								
venlafaxine	92%; unaffected by food	100%	2-4 wk	5 hr	20%-30%	Liver, 3A4, 2D6 (major), 2C9	Urine, 87%	
duloxetine	Well absorbed	80%	2-3 wk	12 hr	>90%	Liver, 1A2, (major); inhibit 2D6 (mod)	Urine, 70%; feces, 30%	
SARIs/SSRIS								
trazodone	60%-80%	N/A	2-4 wk	4-9 hr	89%-95%	Liver, 3A4 (major); inhibits 2D6 (mod)	Urine	0.5-2.5 mcg/ml
nefazodone	100%	20%	5-6 wk	11-24 hr	99%	Liver, 2D6, 3A4 (major); inhibits 3A4 (major)	Urine, 55%; feces, 30%	
NDRIs								
bupropion	80%	5%-20%	2-6 wk	10-21 hr	80%	Liver, 2B6 (major)	Urine, 87%; feces, 10%	50-100 mg/ml
α₂-NORADRENERGIC ANTAGONISTS								
mirtazapine	Well absorbed	50%	2-4 wk	20-40 hr; longer in women than in men	85%	Liver, 1A2, 2D6, 3A4 (major).	Urine, 75%; feces, 15%	

TABLE 46-10   Common and Serious Adverse Reactions to Antidepressants

Drug	Common Minor Effects	Serious Adverse Reactions
MAOIs	Weight gain, sedation, postural hypotension	Hypertensive crisis
TCAs	Dry mouth, constipation, blurred vision from dry eyes, sedation, urinary retention, weight gain, orthostasis, precipitation of narrow-angle glaucoma, sexual dysfunction	Cardiac arrhythmias, lower seizure threshold, psychotic symptoms, rash, bone marrow suppression
SSRIs	Headache, anorexia, nausea, diarrhea, insomnia, anorexia, weight gain, fatigue, sexual dysfunction, restlessness, anxiety, dizziness, sedation, tremor, xerostomia, diaphoresis	Serotonin syndrome, withdrawal syndrome, tachycardia, vasodilation, fever, chest pain, hypertension, palpitation, hypertension, SIADH
SNRIs: venlafaxine	Headache, insomnia, somnolence, dizziness, nervousness, nausea, xerostomia, anorexia, constipation, abnormal ejaculation/orgasm, weakness, diaphoresis	Hypertension, vasodilation, palpitation, tachycardia, chest pain
duloxetine	Sedation, dizziness, headache, insomnia, nausea, xerostomia, diarrhea, constipation, palpitations	AST/ALT increased: possibly with hyperbilirubinemia and/or increased alkaline phosphatase
SARIs		
trazodone	Dizziness, headache, sedation, nausea, xerostomia, blurred vision	Priapism, syncope, hypertension/hypotension
nefazodone	Headache, drowsiness, insomnia, agitation, dizziness, xerostomia, nausea, constipation, weakness	Hepatic failure; bradycardia, hypotension, blurred vision, abnormal vision
NDRI: bupropion	Tachycardia, headache, insomnia, dizziness, xerostomia, weight loss, nausea, pharyngitis, palpitation	Arrhythmias, chest pain, hypertension, flushing, hypotension
α_2-NE: mirtazapine	Dizziness, sedation, nervousness, dry mouth, weight gain	Agranulocytosis, cardiac effects

TABLE 46-11   Drug Interactions With Antidepressants

Antidepressant	Effects on Other Drugs
TCAs	↑ carbamazepine, anticholinergic, clonidine, dicumarol, Quinolones, grepafloxacin, sparfloxacin ↓ guanethidine, levodopa, Sympathomimetics
SSRIs	↑ Sympathomimetics, warfarin
fluoxetine	↑ hydantoin, Benzodiazepines, buspirone, carbamazepine, clozapine, cyclosporine, haloperidol, phenytoin, pimozide ↓ digoxin ↑↓ lithium
sertraline	↑ hydantoin, Benzodiazepines, clozapine, tolbutamide
paroxetine SR	↑ Phenothiazines, procyclidine, sumatriptan, theophylline ↓ digoxin
fluvoxamine	↑ Nonsedating antihistamines, cisapride, Benzodiazepines, β-blockers, buspirone, carbamazepine, clozapine, diltiazem, haloperidol, methadone, sumatriptan, tacrine, theophylline ↓↑ lithium
citalopram	↑ β-Blockers, carbamazepine ↑↓ lithium
SNRIs: venlafaxine XR	↑ desipramine, haloperidol, trazodone, sibutramine, sumatriptan
SARIs	↑ phenytoin
trazodone	↑↓ warfarin
nefazodone	2D6: ↑ Benzodiazepines, buspirone, atorvastatin, simvastatin
NDRI: bupropion SR	↑ nefazodone, 2D6
α_2-NE: mirtazapine	↑ diazepam

TABLE 46-11 Drug Interactions With Antidepressants (Continued)

Other Drugs	Effects on Antidepressant
Barbiturates, carbamazepine, charcoal, rifamycins	↓ TCAs
bupropion, cimetidine, haloperidol, histamine H₂ antagonists, SSRIs, valproic acid	↑ TCAs
venlafaxine	↑ desipramine
Barbiturates, cimetidine, L-tryptophan	↑ SSRIs
cyproheptadine, phenytoin	↓ SSRIs
cyproheptadine	↓ fluoxetine
Barbiturates	↑ paroxetine
cyproheptadine, phenytoin	↓ paroxetine
lithium	↑ fluvoxamine
Azole antifungals, erythromycin	↑ citalopram
cimetidine	↑ venlafaxine
carbamazepine	↑ trazodone
SSRIs, venlafaxine	↑ Serotonin syndrome
sibutramine, sumatriptan, carbamazepine, cisapride, cyclosporine, digoxin	↑ nefazodone
carbamazepine	↓ bupropion
amantadine, levodopa, ritonavir	↑ bupropion

TABLE 46-12 Dosage and Administration Recommendations for Antidepressants

Drug	Starting Daily Dose	Elderly	Hepatic (H) and Renal (R) Impairment	Administration	Adult Dosage Titration	Usual Daily Dose	Maximum Daily Dose
TCAs							
nortriptyline	25 mg	10-25 mg	H: Lower doses suggested	Given at bedtime or in divided doses	25 mg/day q wk	25-100 mg	150 mg
amitriptyline	50 mg	10-25 mg	R: None				
desipramine	75 mg	10-25 mg; increase by 10-25 mg weekly; usual maintenance dose: 75-100 mg/day	H: None R: None H: None R: None	Given at bedtime or in divided doses Given at bedtime or in divided doses	25 mg/day q wk 10-25 mg/day q wk	50-150 mg 100-200 mg	300 mg 300 mg
SSRIs				**WITH/WITHOUT FOOD**			
fluoxetine	20 mg	10 mg; increase by 10-20 mg q4-5wk	H: Lower dose suggested R: None suggested	Once daily in the morning	20 mg/day q4wk	20-40 mg	80 mg
Pediatric	• 8-18 years of age: 10-20 mg/day; in patients started at 10 mg/day, may increase dose to 20 mg/day after 1 wk • Lower-weight children: 10 mg/day; usual: 10 mg/day; if needed, may increase dose to 20 mg/day after several weeks • Higher-weight children and adolescents: 10 mg/day; increase dose to 20 mg/day after 2 wk; may increase dose after several more weeks, if needed; usual range: 20-60 mg/day						
sertraline	50 mg	25 mg/day; increase by 25 mg/day q2-3 days	H: Lower dose suggested R: None suggested	Once daily	25 mg/day q wk	50-100 mg	200 mg

Table continued on following page

TABLE 46-12   Dosage and Administration Recommendations for Antidepressants (Continued)

Drug	Starting Daily Dose	Elderly	Hepatic (H) and Renal (R) Impairment	Administration	Adult Dosage Titration	Usual Daily Dose	Maximum Daily Dose
paroxetine	20 mg	10 mg/day; increase by 10 mg/day q wk; maximum: 40 mg/day	H/R: Refer to elderly dosing	Once daily in the morning	10 mg/day q wk	20-50 mg	50 mg
	CR 25 mg	12.5 mg/day; increase by 12.5 mg/day q wk; maximum: 50 mg/day			12.5 mg/day q wk	12.5-62.5 mg	62.5 mg
*fluvoxamine	50 mg	Reduce dose (not specified)	H: Reduce dose (not specified) R: None suggested	Once daily in the evening	50 mg q4-7 days	150-250 mg	300 mg/day
citalopram	20 mg	10-20 mg; increase by 10 mg q wk; maximum, 40 mg/day	H: Reduce dose (not specified) R: Reduce dose in mild to moderate; avoid in severe renal impairment (ClCr <20 ml/min)	Once daily	20 mg/day q wk	20-40 mg	60 mg/day
escitalopram	10 mg	Oral: 5-10 mg/day; doses may be increased by 5-10 mg/day after at least 1 wk	H: 10 mg/day R: Reduce dose only in severe renal impairment (ClCr <20 ml/min)	Once daily	10 mg/day q wk	10-20 mg	20 mg
SNRIs							
venlafaxine	75 mg	None specific; 25-50 mg daily dose suggested; increase as tolerated by 25 mg/dose	H: Reduce total dose by 50% R: Decrease dose by 25% if ClCr 10-70 ml/min	2-3 divided doses	75 mg/day q4-7 days	225-375 mg	375 mg
	75 mg XR	37.5 mg once daily, increase by 37.5 mg every 4-7 days as tolerated	Hemodialysis: Decrease total daily dose by 50% after dialysis	Once daily with food			
duloxetine	40-60 mg	Initial dose: 20 mg 1-2 times/day; increase to 40-60 mg/day as a single daily dose or in divided doses	H: Not recommended R: Lower initial dose in mild to moderate renal impairment; not recommended in severe renal impairment (ClCr <30 ml/min or ESRD)	Once daily or in two divided doses	q2-3wk	40-60 mg	60 mg
SARIs							
trazodone	150 mg	25-50 mg q hs; increase by 25-50 mg/day q7 days; maximum dose: 150 mg/day	H: None required R: None required	Three divided doses	50 mg/day q3-7 days	150-600 mg	600 mg
nefazodone	200 mg	50 mg bid; increase by 100 mg/day in 2 wk; range, 200-400 mg/day	H: None recommended R: None required	Two divided doses	100 mg/day q2wk	300-600 mg	600 mg/day

*Not indicated in the United States for the treatment of patients with major depression.

TABLE 46-12 **Dosage and Administration Recommendations for Antidepressants** (Continued)

Drug	Starting Daily Dose	Elderly	Hepatic (H) and Renal (R) Impairment	Administration	Adult Dosage Titration	Usual Daily Dose	Maximum Daily Dose
bupropion	200 mg	37.5 mg bid; increase by 37.5 mg q3-4 days	H: Mild to moderate hepatic impairment: reduce dose or frequency	Divide into three doses	q3-4 days	300-450 mg	450 mg
	150 mg SR	100 mg once daily; increase by 100 mg q3-4 days	Severe hepatic cirrhosis: Maximum dose: Immediate release: 75 mg/day SR: 100 mg/day or 150 mg every other day	Once daily in the morning initially, then in two divided doses (PM dose should be given in the afternoon rather than at bedtime)		300-400 mg	300-400 mg
	150 mg XL	None specified	XL: 150 mg every other day R: Reduce dose (none specified)	Once daily in the morning		300-450 mg	450 mg
NDRI							
mirtazapine	15 mg	7.5 mg/day q hs; increase by 7.5-15 mg/day q1-2wk	H: None specified; dose reduction suggested R: None specified; dose reduction suggested	Once daily in the evening	q1-2wk	30 mg	45 mg/day

nefazodone (Serzone)

CONTRAINDICATIONS
- Coadministration with cisapride, pimozide, or carbamazepine
- Liver disease
- Hypersensitivity to nefazodone or other phenylpiperazine antidepressants
- Concomitant use with MAOIs
- Use in patients during the acute recovery phase of MI

WARNINGS
- *Black box warning:* Hepatotoxicity may cause liver disease, ranging from mild elevations in liver function tests to death. Hepatic disease increases levels of nefazodone and its metabolites. Use lower dosages in patients with liver impairment. Rates of hepatic failure are four times greater than anticipated.
- Do not use with MAOIs.

- Concurrent use with triazolam or alprazolam (dose reductions of 75% and 50%, respectively)

PRECAUTIONS
- Do not use in patients who have cardiac disease.
- May cause postural hypotension
- Mania/hypomania may occur; use with caution in patients with a history of mania
- Seizures occur rarely.
- *Visual disturbance:* Blurred vision, scotoma, and visual trails may occur.
- Photosensitivity can occur.

OVERDOSAGE. Symptoms of nausea, vomiting, and somnolence. Treatment is symptomatic. No deaths reported in overdosage

evolve A continually updated list of useful WebLinks may be found in the Evolve Resources at http://evolve.elsevier.com/Edmunds/ NP/

Antianxiety and Antiinsomnia Agents

DRUG OVERVIEW

Class	Subclass	Generic Name	Trade Name
Antianxiety and anti-insomnia agents	Benzodiazepines	diazepam 🗝️ ✺	Valium
		alprazolam ✺	Xanax
		chlordiazepoxide	Librium
		clonazepam ✺	Klonopin
		clorazepate	Tranxene
		estazolam	ProSom
		flurazepam	Dalmane
		lorazepam ✺	Ativan
		oxazepam	Serax
		quazepam	Doral
		temazepam ✺	Restoril
		triazolam	Halcion
Antianxiety agents		buspirone ✺	BuSpar
Antiinsomnia agents	GABA-BZ receptor agonists*	zolpidem 🗝️	Ambien ✺
		eszopiclone	Lunesta ✺
		chloral hydrate	Chloral hydrate
		zaleplon	Sonata
Melatonin receptor agonists	Melatonin	ramelteon	Rozerem

✺ Top 200 drug; 🗝️ key drug.

*GABA-BZ receptor agonists: nonbenzodiazepine benzodiazepine-receptor agonists.
See Chapter 13 for discussion of dihydramine (Benadryl), which commonly is used off-label for sleep, particularly in geriatric patients. Also see Chapter 73 for a discussion of sleep products.

INDICATIONS

- Anxiety
- Insomnia
- Benzodiazepines: See Table 47-1.
- *buspirone:* Generalized anxiety disorder; off-label: opiate addiction, panic attack
- *zolpidem:* Indication: Insomnia; off-label: Parkinson's disease
- *eszopiclone, zaleplon, ramelteon:* Insomnia only

Unlabeled Uses

The use of these drugs in the treatment of anxiety and insomnia is discussed in this chapter. Antidepressants have become a major category of drug treatment for anxiety. Their use in the treatment of anxiety is discussed in this chapter. See Chapter 46 for a detailed discussion of these medications.

In the past, barbiturates and medications similar to barbiturates were used to treat patients with anxiety and insomnia. Newer medications seem somewhat safer with minimal drug interactions and low side effect profiles that decrease the need for barbiturates. However, they should no longer be used for these purposes because of tolerance, addiction, and seizures upon withdrawal. These agents are discussed in the chapter on Anticonvulsants, Chapter 44.

Benzodiazepines still are commonly used, but their use for anxiety and insomnia should be strictly limited because of the potential for adverse effects. They remain an important class of medications and are discussed in detail in this chapter.

Three newer drug classes have improved safety profiles: Buspirone is used for anxiety, the GABA-PZ agonists (zolpidem, zaleplon, and eszopiclone) and the melatonin receptor agonist ramelteon are used for insomnia.

THERAPEUTIC OVERVIEW

Anatomy and Physiology

Fear is a normal and useful emotion when an individual is confronted with perceived danger. The sympathetic adrenergic nervous system releases epinephrine and norepinephrine, while the parasympathetic nervous system is inhibited. Serotonin and gamma-aminobutyric acid (GABA) also may be released at various levels of the neuraxis and in neurons of the brain. Stimulation of the endocrine system may result in the simultaneous release of β-endorphins that work with epinephrine and norepinephrine to produce physiologic changes such as mydriasis; pallor; increased respiratory, cardiac, and basal metabolic rates; increased blood sugar; decreased bladder, bowel, and genital functioning; and increased blood flow to the muscles. Heredity and early life experiences are thought to play a role in the development of anxiety. A 1992 analysis of 1033 female twins found that heritability was approximately 30%. This sharply contrasts with major depression, which is considered to have 70% heritability. Adverse childhood events, for example, witnessing a traumatic event,

TABLE 47-1 Indications and Unlabeled Uses of Benzodiazepines

Drug	Indication	Unlabeled Use
diazepam (Valium)	Anxiety, generalized; alcohol withdrawal, muscle spasm, tonic-clonic seizures, status epilepticus, preanesthesia	Panic disorder, IBS, insomnia, tension headache, RLS
alprazolam (Xanax)	Anxiety, generalized; panic disorder, agoraphobia	Social phobia, PMS, agoraphobia, insomnia
chlordiazepoxide (Librium)	Anxiety, acute alcohol withdrawal	IBS, tension headache
clonazepam (Klonopin)	Seizures, absence, akinetic, myoclonic, panic disorder	Periodic leg movements, parkinsonian dysarthria, manic episodes in bipolar disorder, multifocal tic disorders; adjunct in treatment of schizophrenia, neuralgias, OCD
clorazepate (Tranxene)	Anxiety, generalized; alcohol withdrawal, partial seizures	
estazolam (ProSom)	Insomnia	
flurazepam (Dalmane)	Insomnia	
lorazepam (Ativan)	Anxiety, generalized; preanesthesia	Status epilepticus, chemotherapy-induced nausea and vomiting, alcohol withdrawal, psychogenic catatonia, chronic insomnia, IBS, tension headache, muscle spasm, tremors, action
oxazepam (Serax)	Anxiety, generalized	IBS, alcohol withdrawal
quazepam (Doral)	Insomnia	
temazepam (Restoril)	Insomnia	
triazolam (Halcion)	Insomnia	

RLS, restless leg syndrome.

are associated with the onset but not the persistence of anxiety beyond childhood.

Disease Process

ANXIETY. Anxiety is characterized by excessive unease and apprehension usually in association with an event that may have an unknown outcome. It is a normal reaction and a positive motivating factor in many situations. Anxiety becomes a problem when it interferes with everyday personal, social, and/or occupational functions, or when it develops into panic attacks or compulsive behavior. This ultimately can lead to symptoms and psychologic distress that are incapacitating.

In the primary care setting, anxiety often is a symptom of an underlying disorder, such as a medical or a psychologic problem (Box 47-1). The practitioner must obtain a comprehensive history and perform a complete physical examination of the patient to assess the possible causes and effects of the anxiety. Symptoms of anxiety vary with the subtype of anxiety experienced. The physical symptoms of anxiety are listed in Box 47-2.

Elements of the history that are particularly important in evaluating anxiety include the following:

- Somatic complaints that defy remedy (e.g., stomach pains, dyspnea)
- Substance use disorders
- Complaints of a lump in the throat
- Inability to fall asleep at night—racing thoughts or worries
- These symptoms may be somewhat different in children and may vary, depending upon their age and other experiences with anxiety.
- Five major subtypes of anxiety have been identified: generalized anxiety disorder, panic disorder, phobias, obsessive-compulsive disorder, and posttraumatic stress disorder.

Generalized Anxiety Disorder. Generalized anxiety disorder (GAD) is defined as excessive anxiety and worry about life circumstances that is difficult to control. It was responsible for 12.3 million office visits to primary care providers in 1998. Twice as many women as men suffer from GAD. As many as 50% of patients with major depression will meet diagnostic criteria for GAD, and one study found this to be true in 62% of patients.

The anxiety associated with GAD is unrealistic, generalized, and persistent. It is present on more days than not for longer than 6 months. The patient often complains of somatic symptoms such as restlessness, fatigue, difficulty concentrating, irritability, muscle tension, and sleep problems. Patients generally lack the insight to connect their symptoms with their reported worries and present life stresses. A self-assessment tool called the GAD-7 has been shown to be a reliable screening tool for GAD.

Panic Disorder. A panic attack is an unexpected severe, acute exacerbation of psychic and somatic symptoms of anxiety accompanied by intense fear or discomfort that is not

---

BOX 47-1   Conditions That Can Cause Symptoms of Anxiety

MEDICAL CONDITIONS

Respiratory

COPD
Pulmonary embolism
Asthma
Hypoxia
Pulmonary edema

Cardiovascular

Angina pectoris
Arrhythmias
Chronic heart failure
Hypertension
Hypotension
Mitral valve prolapse

Neurologic

Delirium
Dementia
Benign essential tremor
Parkinson's disease
Akathisia
Postconcussion syndrome
Temporal lobe epilepsy
Vertigo

Endocrine

Hyperthyroidism
Hypercortisolism

Pheochromocytoma
Hypoglycemia

Metabolic

Hypercalcemia
Hyperkalemia
Hyponatremia

DRUGS

caffeine
amphetamine
methylphenidate
theophylline
phentermine
pseudoephedrine
Anticholinergics
Dopaminergics
cocaine

DRUG WITHDRAWAL

Alcohol
Narcotics
Benzodiazepines
Barbiturates

OTHER PSYCHOLOGIC DISORDERS

Psychosis
Manic depression
Depressive disorder

BOX 47-2   Physical Symptoms of Anxiety

RESPIRATORY

Chest pressure
Choking
Sighing
Dyspnea

CARDIOVASCULAR

Tachycardia
Palpitations
Chest pain
Faintness

AUTONOMIC

Dry mouth
Sweating
Headaches
Hot flushes

MUSCULOSKELETAL

Aches and pains
Twitching

Stiffness
Fatigue

GENITOURINARY

Frequency
Urgency
Sexual dysfunction
Menstrual problems

GASTROINTESTINAL

Swallowing difficulties
Abdominal pain
Nausea
Irritable bowel
Lump in throat

NEUROLOGIC

Dizziness
Numbness or tingling
Visual disturbance
Weakness
Tremor

---

triggered by a particular situation, and that the individual cannot "sit out." It starts abruptly and reaches a peak within 10 minutes, with at least four of the following symptoms: palpitations, tachycardia, sweating, shaking or trembling, shortness of breath, choking, chest pain or discomfort, nausea or abdominal distress, dizziness or faintness, feeling unreal or detached from oneself, fear of going crazy, fear of dying, paresthesias, and chills or hot flashes. Typical presentations include cardiovascular symptoms (40%), neurologic symptoms (40%), or GI symptoms (30%).

A panic attack becomes a panic disorder when the patient worries about having another attack and about what will happen if that should occur. Also, changes in behavior are seen with multiple attacks and result in frequent medical or emergency room visits. Because panic attacks consist of a wide array of symptoms, two thirds of patients are prompted to seek a medical rather than a mental health provider. And, in most cases, patients are unsatisfied with the lack of definitive diagnosis. This results in an enormous utilization of health care resources; one study reported that 70% (40/57) of patients saw an average of 10 physicians before receiving a diagnosis of panic disorder.

Phobic Disorders. This is the most common mental health disorder in the United States. A patient who has a phobia displays a persistent and irrational fear of a clearly definable situation, object, or activity. Exposure to the feared stimulus results in intense anxiety and avoidance that interfere with the patient's life. Three main groups of phobic disorders have been identified:

1. Agoraphobia is the fear of being in a place or situation that would elicit symptoms of a panic attack, and that would cause the patient to have difficulty leaving or that would cause him or her to be embarrassed. This often occurs in concert with a panic attack.

2. Social phobia is a fear of social situations such as public speaking.

3. Specific phobia is a fear of specific objects or situations, which may include animals, insects, heights, water, needles, and so forth.

Specific phobias can be normal in children, and many persist in a mild form in adults. Incapacity depends on the frequency with which the situation is encountered and the amount of interference with function that results.

Obsessive-Compulsive Disorder. Obsessive-compulsive disorder (OCD) is a situational preoccupation with thoughts or acts that occurs despite the patient's efforts at resistance. Obsessions are persistent thoughts, ideas, or images that intrude into conscious awareness. Compulsions are urges or impulses for repetitive intentional behaviors that are performed in a stereotyped manner in an attempt to reduce anxiety. The patient realizes that these are senseless and intrusive but is unable to stop. Insight and resistance may not be present in children who have OCD. It occurs in approximately 3% of the population in the United States. Onset in children and adults occurs around the ages of 10 and 21, respectively, and it develops earlier in males than in females. The impact on a patient's quality of life can be devastating; one study noted that 13% of patients attempted suicide.

Posttraumatic Stress Disorder. Patients with posttraumatic stress disorder (PTSD) have recurrent anxiety precipitated by exposure to or memory of some past traumatic situation. They may have recurrent dreams or suddenly may act or feel as if the event is recurring. The patient will have increased arousal and hypervigilance, leading to flashbacks and severe anxiety with an enhanced startle reaction (positive symptoms of PTSD). As a means of compensating for this intense arousal, patients may be withdrawn in an attempt to avoid reminders of the trauma. The result is a sense of numbness and emotional blunting (negative symptoms of PTSD). These patients have experienced a catastrophic event that would be clearly distressing to anyone. Onset follows the trauma after a latency period of a few weeks to months, but not longer than 6 months, and the condition lasts for at least 1 month. In a study of 368 primary care clinic patients, nearly two thirds were witnesses to or were the victims of a traumatic event; 12% of these individuals were given a diagnosis of PTSD. More than four times as many women as men develop PTSD. Traumatic events reported in women include molestation and physical assault.

Insomnia. As many as 30% of adults report problems with sleep; these are seen more commonly in women. Sleep disorders are a symptom and not a diagnostic entity; thus, a comprehensive review of the patient's history and a thorough physical examination is required to rule out all possible causes of the sleep disturbance.

Sleep disorders are categorized into the following four groups to facilitate diagnosis and management:
1. Insomnia disorders of initiating and maintaining sleep
2. *Hypersomnia:* Disorders of excessive somnolence, particularly in the daytime
3. Disorders of the sleep-wake cycle
4. *Parasomnia:* Sleepwalking, sleep tremors, enuresis

Insomnia may be associated with depression, manic disorders, alcohol or other drug abuse, heavy smoking, caffeine use, an adverse effect of many drugs, and specific medical conditions. Medications that may contribute to insomnia include the psychotropic drugs and CNS stimulants such as OTC cold medicines and theophylline. Medical conditions associated with insomnia include delirium, respiratory distress, pain, and hyperthyroidism. Certain sleep disorders such as sleep apnea are made worse by insomnia medications. The only sleep disorder discussed in this chapter is insomnia because it is the one disorder that these medications are used to treat. Insomnia generally is classified as short term, 7 to 10 days, and long term.

The practitioner must rule out all possible causes of a sleep disorder and must determine the type of disorder that is present before prescribing any type of medication. The patient should be encouraged to practice good sleep hygiene principles such as avoiding stimulating food and drink before retiring, having nighttime rituals that are relaxing, and not using the bed for reading, work, or other non–sleep-associated activities.

MECHANISM OF ACTION

Benzodiazepines

Benzodiazepines act by potentiating the action of GABA, an amino acid and an inhibitory neurotransmitter, which results in increased neuronal inhibition and CNS depression. Benzodiazepines bind to specific benzodiazepine receptor sites (e.g., BZ1, BZ2). BZ1 is involved in sleep; BZ2 is involved in memory, motor, sensory, and cognitive functions. The BZ receptor is a ligand-gated Cl^- channel, and GABA activation of the receptor results in inward flow of Cl^-, which causes increased neuronal inhibition and CNS depression. BZ1 to BZ6 refers to distinct receptor subtypes and not simply to binding sites on the same receptor molecule.

Inhibition of benzodiazepine receptors in the spinal cord causes muscle relaxation; in the brainstem, it acts as an anticonvulsant; in the cerebellum, it causes ataxia; and in the limbic and cortical area, it affects emotional behavior. Anxiolytic effects are distinct from the nonspecific consequences of CNS depression (e.g., sedation, motor impairment). Benzodiazepines act as a sedative hypnotic by acting on the limbic system and the subcortical CNS. They shorten REM sleep and stage 4 sleep but increase total sleep time. Medications have high abuse potential because they are so widely available.

Clonazepam, diazepam, and clorazepate suppress neural discharges in the patient during seizures. Seizure activity is inhibited by depressing nerve transmission in the motor cortex and suppressing the spike-and-wave discharge in absence seizures. Clonazepam has high potency and increased efficacy against absence seizures. Buspirone lacks the BZ effect.

buspirone

The exact mechanism of action of buspirone is unknown. It is not chemically related to the benzodiazepines, the barbiturates, or any other anxiolytic agents. It has a high affinity for serotonin receptors and a lesser affinity for dopamine receptors. It does not have muscle relaxation or anticonvulsant properties, and it is nonsedating.

The antianxiety effect is achieved via a partial agonist effect on CNS serotonin $5\text{-}HT_{1A}$ receptors that occurs without affecting the benzodiazepine receptors or causing CNS depression. Downregulation of postsynaptic $5\text{-}HT_2$ receptors is also possible.

GABA-BZ Agonists

The chemical structure is dissimilar from those of the benzodiazepines and other sedative hypnotics. These agents appear to act through the potentiation of GABA on benzodiazepine receptors, especially the omega-1 subunit. They are used primarily for sedation. They have exhibited some anxiolytic action but they have little effect on skeletal muscle or seizure thresholds. They appear to have minimal disruptive action on the normal sleep cycle, thus preserving deep sleep (stages 3 and 4). They have shown no potential for causing addiction. However, because they affect the benzodiazepine receptors, the potential for dependence is a matter of concern.

Ramelteon

Ramelteon is a melatonin receptor agonist with affinity for the melatonin receptors MT1 and MT2. The MT1 and MT2 receptors are acted upon by endogenous melatonin and are thought to be involved in maintenance of the normal sleep-wake cycle. This action occurs in the suprachiasmatic nucleus of the brain, which is the regulation center for circadian rhythms. Ramelteon has no affinity for the GABA-BZ receptor complex.

TREATMENT PRINCIPLES OF ANTIANXIETY AGENTS

Standardized Guidelines

- American Psychiatric Association practice guideline for the treatment of patients with acute stress disorder and posttraumatic stress disorder.
- Anxiety Disorders Association of America (ADAA; www.adaa.org, or 301-231-9350).

Evidence-Based Recommendations

- *GAD:* Cognitive-behavioral therapy; imipramine, paroxetine, sertraline, escitalopram, venlafaxine, buspirone, hydroxyzine

- *Panic disorder:* Cognitive-behavioral therapy; SSRIs, TCAs (imipramine or nortriptyline); second-line agents: venlafaxine, alprazolam, lorazepam, and clonazepam are beneficial
- *Phobic disorder:* Cognitive-behavioral therapy; agoraphobia: SSRIs (as adjunct to panic disorder treatment); social phobia: SSRIs, alprazolam and clonazepam, buspirone, atenolol, and propranolol; specific phobia: no specific drugs recommended
- *OCD:* Cognitive-behavioral therapy, SSRIs (citalopram, clomipramine, fluoxetine, fluvoxamine, paroxetine, sertraline), venlafaxine
- *PTSD:* Cognitive-behavioral therapy, SSRIs; second line: TCAs, alprazolam, olanzapine, and aripiprazole

Cardinal Points of Treatment

- Patient education/psychotherapy
- *GAD:* Acute—benzodiazepines; long term—SSRI, venlafaxine, buspirone
- *Panic disorder:* Acute—benzodiazepine; long term—SSRI
- *Phobic disorders:* Acute: β-blocker or benzodiazepine; long term: SSRI, MAOI, gabapentin
- *OCD:* SSRI (fluvoxamine), clomipramine (a TCA), buspirone
- *PTSD:* SSRI, TCA, MAOI

Patients must be reassured that they are not the victims of a terrible disease, and they can control the anxiety. Relaxation techniques and breathing exercises can be useful and may be taught by the primary care provider. Meditation also can be helpful.

Psychotherapy is an important component of the treatment provided for anxiety disorders and should be considered for every patient. Brief counseling sessions of 20 to 30 minutes have been shown to provide significant benefit. A controlled trial of 91 patients with GAD counseled by family physicians reported similar results at 3 and 6 months when compared with those treated with benzodiazepines. Patients who do not respond should be referred to a specialist for determination of appropriate psychotherapy.

Historically, the pharmacologic treatment of GAD has employed the TCAs and benzodiazepines as first-line agents. However, side effects, abuse potential, and tolerance, particularly for the TCAs, have curtailed their use over the years. Recently, the SSRIs have proved effective for GAD with minimal side effect profiles, and many providers have opted to use them as front-line agents.

Several SSRIs have been shown to be effective for GAD in clinical trials, although only a few have a formal indication. The selection of SSRI depends largely on side effect profile and cost. It is preferable to avoid those agents that have high incidences of insomnia and restlessness because these are often the subject of complaints expressed by patients with GAD. These excitatory side effects are sometimes unavoidable with the SSRIs; therefore, it is suggested that starting doses should be approximately 50% of those used in the treatment of depression.

It is frequently necessary to combine a benzodiazepine with an antidepressant in the treatment of GAD. A benzodiazepine should be used only on a short-term basis and should be tapered (by approximately 10% per week) once the antidepressant has reached its peak effect, usually after 6 to 8 weeks. Short-acting benzodiazepines are particularly difficult to discontinue because anxiety symptoms recur quickly, and this makes it difficult for patients to stop them. A longer-acting drug such as lorazepam or clonazepam is preferred. Symptoms of withdrawal normally begin to disappear within 2 weeks of a dose reduction. This can help the provider distinguish between breakthrough GAD symptoms and benzodiazepine withdrawal. These drugs have a much higher potential for abuse in patients with a history of alcohol or drug abuse and should be avoided in this population. Buspirone may be a good alternative for these patients because it lacks the potential for abuse. However, GI side effects are common, and therapeutic effects may not be seen for up to 8 weeks. The benzodiazepines may cause retrograde amnesia that will interfere with the patient's ability to learn adaptive behavior, sometimes limiting the benefit of the psychotherapy.

SSRIs are considered the drugs of choice for the treatment of panic disorder. Low initial doses and slow titration are recommended to avoid the excitatory side effects of SSRIs. The provider must counsel the patient that symptom relief may take up to 4 to 6 weeks. Venlafaxine, an SSRI, reduced the severity of symptoms but did not substantially enhance patients' quality of life in one study. TCAs are as effective as SSRIs, but bothersome side effects and increased drug interactions limit their acceptability. If a TCA is used, nortriptyline is suggested because of the relatively low incidence of side effects compared with the other TCAs. Low doses and slow titration are necessary.

Phobic disorders usually are treated according to the specific type of phobia. Specific phobias are best managed with cognitive-behavioral therapy and occasionally with short-term use of β-blockers or benzodiazepines. The SSRIs and benzodiazepines were found to be most effective in the treatment of social phobias in one meta-analysis consisting of 108 controlled trials. Clonazepam demonstrated a 78% response rate after 10 weeks of therapy in one trial vs. only 20% of patients in the placebo group. The TCAs, however, have not been shown effective for social phobias. Patients with agoraphobia are treated in the same manner as those with panic disorder.

OCD has been treated effectively for many years with clomipramine, which is a TCA with serotonin-selective properties. In addition to 5-HT, clomipramine inhibits NE reuptake via an active metabolite (i.e., desmethylclomipramine). After 10 weeks of therapy, a mean reduction of 38% and 44% in OCD score was reported in two separate studies of more than 500 patients. Placebo-treated patients reported mean reductions of only 3% and 5%. The SSRIs have been used for OCD and have proved equally effective as clomipramine in one meta-analysis of four large trials. Venlafaxine has shown efficacy comparable with that of paroxetine in a small trial of 150 patients with OCD.

Several agents are used in the management of PTSD. The 2004 treatment guidelines published by the American Psychiatric Association recommended SSRIs as first-line medications. These drugs reduce both positive and negative symptoms of PTSD, although the greatest benefit appears to result from a reduction in positive symptoms. Fluoxetine, sertraline, and paroxetine have been used for moderate to severe PTSD. One large trial of 551 patients treated with paroxetine 20 or 40 mg per day, or placebo for 12 weeks, reported statistically significant improvement in all PTSD symptoms compared with placebo. This benefit was seen in men and women with varying trauma types, time since trauma, and PTSD severity.

TCAs usually are considered second-line medications. In small studies, the TCAs have been shown to improve positive symptoms (intrusive nightmares and flashbacks) but are not as effective in reducing negative symptoms such as numbing and withdrawal. Antianxiety agents have not proved particularly useful for the management of PTSD, despite the prevalence of enhanced startle reaction and jitteriness in these patients. Patients who show little or no response to the antidepressants may be candidates for antipsychotic medications such as olanzapine and aripiprazole.

TREATMENT PRINCIPLES OF ANTIINSOMNIA AGENTS

Standardized Guidelines

- Morgenthaler T et al: Practice parameters for the psychological and behavioral treatment of insomnia: an update: an American Academy of Sleep Medicine report, *J Sleep* 2007. (Available at http://www.journalsleep.org/ViewAbstract. aspx?citationid=3076)

Evidence-Based Recommendations

- *Elderly patients:* Zaleplon and zolpidem are likely to be beneficial.

Cardinal Points of Treatment

For insomnia:
- Sleep hygiene
- Finding the cause of the insomnia is key to solving the problem.
- *Short-term insomnia:* GABA-BZ agonist, benzodiazepine
- *Long-term insomnia:* Ramelteon; GABA-BZ agonists and trazodone (sedating antidepressant) not indicated but often used

Treatment of patients with insomnia begins with sleep hygiene. It is important that the patient follow the regimen provided in Box 47-3. The patient must have reasonable expectations. Overcoming insomnia is a gradual process with no overnight success. One can move up the time of onset of sleep by only 15 minutes every 3 to 4 days.

If these measures are ineffective, a medication may be considered. It should be used in conjunction with the sleep hygiene program and should be given for a limited time to help the patient reestablish a regular sleep pattern. These

---

BOX 47-3   Sleep Hygiene

Develop a regular bedtime with lights out or dimmed.
Develop a regular waking time and avoid sleeping longer than usual.
Adjust total sleep time to fit your needs.
Avoid routine daytime naps.
Exercise regularly but not within 1 hour of bedtime.
Sleep in a cool room.
Avoid alcohol 3 to 4 hours before bedtime.
Avoid stimulants such as caffeine 8 hours before bedtime.
Avoid stressful topics, arguments before bedtime.
Try a warm bath.
Try warm milk.
Use bed only for sleeping and making love. Avoid reading, watching TV.
Learn and practice relaxation techniques.

---

medications usually move up sleep onset by 10 to 30 minutes and increase total sleep time by 20 to 40 minutes. Although the practitioner may not think this signifies much progress, the benefit perceived by the patient is substantial.

Benzodiazepines have been used for many years for the short-term treatment of insomnia. Used properly, they are safe and effective and are less expensive than the GABA-PZ agonists. Many patients become dependent on the benzodiazepine to fall asleep, and withdrawal can be difficult. Benzodiazepines must be used for a limited time and only to treat appropriate sleep disorders. Benzodiazepines are contraindicated in patients who have sleep apnea and the other hypersomnias.

The GABA-BZ agonists zolpidem, zaleplon, and eszopiclone are used frequently for the short-term treatment of insomnia. Zolpidem is used for patients who have problems with both sleep onset and maintenance. Zaleplon is more useful for onset insomnia, especially in patients who have occasional difficulty falling asleep because of time zone change or a stressful event. Eszopiclone is useful for sleep maintenance and was approved for long-term use in a study that showed effectiveness for up to 6 months. Zolpidem and zaleplon are approved only for short-term use (35 days) but are frequently used over the long term.

Ramelteon is a melatonin that is approved for chronic insomnia. The length of its use is not limited. However, it is not as effective as the GABA-BZ insomnia drugs.

Sleep hygiene remains the mainstay of treatment. Benzodiazepines and the GABA-BZ agonists are useful for short-term insomnia. Trazodone, an antidepressant with sedative effects, may be used if other therapies are not effective.

TREATMENT PRINCIPLES OF BENZODIAZEPINES

Many medications belong to the benzodiazepine class; diazepam (the prototype) was the first. Benzodiazepines share a common mechanism of action and generally have similar therapeutic effects and adverse reactions. Benzodiazepines have shown some risk for causing physiologic and psychologic dependency and are used only on a short-term basis. Specific benzodiazepines used for insomnia include temazepam, flurazepam, triazolam, estazolam, and lorazepam.

The maximum therapeutic effect may take 1 to 2 weeks to achieve, and tolerance develops in 6 to 8 weeks. Benzodiazepine use must be tapered gradually to minimize the risk of withdrawal. Patients who have a history of addiction, depression, or psychosis are not good candidates for the use of benzodiazepines. Avoid flurazepam in the elderly because of its long-acting metabolite, N-desalkylflurazepam, which greatly increases the risk of falls from oversedation.

How to Monitor

BENZODIAZEPINES

- Order periodic laboratory work to monitor liver and renal function (LFTs, BUN, CR); request CBC and urinalysis.
- Monitor for side effects such as dizziness, "hangover" effect, daytime sleepiness, ataxia, and slurred speech.
- Monitor for signs of dependence such as increased requests for medication or increased refills on prescriptions.
- Perform routine review of all medications, including OTC medications, before prescribing and at each visit.

BUSPIRONE. Monitor for dizziness.

ZOLPIDEM. Monitor for dizziness, headache.

ZALEPLON. Monitor for dizziness, light-headedness.

Patient Variables

GERIATRICS. Elderly, debilitated patients and those who have impaired liver and renal function require dosage reduction and cautious monitoring.

> ☣ The use of any CNS agent in the elderly increases the risks of oversedation and ataxia, as well as the risk of falls.

When it is necessary to use a benzodiazepine in an elderly patient, the lowest dose of a short-acting drug such as temazepam, estazolam, or triazolam is tolerated best. The nonbenzodiazepines zaleplon, zolpidem, and buspirone generally are preferred. Because of the risks associated with polypharmacy, the practitioner must examine all medications for the possibility of drug–drug interactions.

PEDIATRICS. The safety and efficacy of buspirone, zolpidem, and zaleplon in children younger than 18 years of age have not been established.
- Benzodiazepines suitable for use in children include the following:
  - *chlordiazepoxide:* Children >6 years
  - *clorazepate:* Children >9 years
  - *diazepam:* Children >6 months
  - *lorazepam:* Children >12 years (used unlabeled in children <12 years)
  - *Other benzodiazepines:* Persons over age 18 years of age

PREGNANCY AND LACTATION
- *Category B:* Buspirone; breastfeeding should be avoided
- *Category C:* Eszopiclone, zolpidem, zaleplon, ramelteon
- *Category D:* Barbiturates; fetal abnormalities occur when barbiturates are given during pregnancy. Women of childbearing age should be cautioned to use effective contraception when taking benzodiazepines or barbiturates.
- *Category D/X:* Benzodiazepines can cause fetal damage; benzodiazepines are excreted in breast milk.

Patient Education

BENZODIAZEPINES
- May cause drowsiness, dizziness, and fatigue and should be used with caution when driving or operating machinery that requires alert mental status.
- Do not use alcoholic beverages or other CNS depressants while taking these medications.
- Dependency can be a problem.
- Do not stop the medication suddenly. Withdrawal symptoms (sweating, vomiting, muscle cramps, tremors, and seizures) may occur. Dosage must be reduced gradually under the supervision of the practitioner.
- Do not take any medications, including OTC preparations, without the knowledge of your provider.
- Report the following symptoms to the provider: tremor, seizures, ataxia, dizziness, difficulty breathing, and chest tightness.

- Rise slowly from a lying or sitting position because orthostatic hypotension caused by the medication may result in dizziness.

SPECIFIC DRUGS
Benzodiazepines

---

diazepam (Valium) 🔑

CONTRAINDICATIONS
- Hypersensitivity to other benzodiazepines
- Psychoses
- Acute narrow-angle glaucoma
- Children <6 months of age (oral)
- Pregnancy
- *clonazepam:* Significant liver disease
- *alprazolam, estazolam:* Concurrent use with ketoconazole or itraconazole
- *triazolam:* Concurrent therapy with atazanavir, ketoconazole, itraconazole, nefazodone, and ritonavir

WARNINGS
- *Psychiatric disorders:* Not intended for use in patients who have a primary depressive disorder or psychosis
- *Long-term use (>4 months):* Effectiveness has not been assessed.
- *Dependence:* Prolonged use of therapeutic dosages can lead to dependence. Withdrawal syndrome has occurred in patients after as little as 4 to 6 weeks.
- Retrograde amnesia of varying severity and paradoxical reactions have occurred.
- *Renal/hepatic function impairment:* Observe for excess sedation or impaired coordination.
- Abnormal liver function tests and blood dyscrasias have been reported.

PRECAUTIONS
- *Depression:* Administer with caution; may intensify depression
- *Rebound sleep disorder:* Insomnia worse than before treatment; may occur after withdrawal
- Use with caution in patients who have respiratory disease or respiratory depression; avoid in sleep apnea.
- *Drug abuse and dependence:* High risk of dependence with prolonged use; withdrawal symptoms ranging from mild dysphoria to abdominal and muscle cramps, tremor, and convulsions. To avoid withdrawal symptoms, taper drug dosage.
- *Hazardous tasks:* Use caution while driving or performing tasks that require alertness. The ability to perform driving or other tasks may be impaired on the day after ingestion.
- Amnesia, paradoxical reactions (excitement, agitation), and other adverse behavioral effects may occur unpredictably.
- *Abnormal thinking/behavior changes:* A variety of abnormal thinking and behavior changes have been reported to occur in association with sedative-hypnotics. Use with caution.

PHARMACOKINETICS. See Table 47-2. Diazepam is the key drug because it was the first benzodiazepine and still is in common use. It has a long half-life. Lorazepam and

Continued

diazepam (Valium) 🔑 —cont'd

alprazolam, with short half-lives and a lower incidence of adverse effects, now are generally used.

ADVERSE REACTIONS. See Table 47-3.

DRUG INTERACTIONS. (Consult a more detailed reference for specific drug, if necessary.)
- Alcohol/CNS depressants, cimetidine, disulfiram, isoniazid, and probenecid enhance the effects of benzodiazepines.
- Rifampin, smoking, theophyllines, and antacids decrease the effects of benzodiazepines.
- Benzodiazepines increase the levels of digoxin and phenytoin; they enhance the actions of alcohol/CNS depressants.
- Benzodiazepines decrease the level of levodopa.
- Macrolides increase the effects of triazolam.
- Oral contraceptives decrease the effects of lorazepam and oxazepam.
- Oral contraceptives increase the effects of alprazolam, chlordiazepoxide, clorazepate, diazepam, and halazepam.
- Cimetidine, disulfiram, fluoxetine, isoniazid, ketoconazole, metoprolol, propoxyphene, propranolol, and valproic acid may increase the effects of alprazolam, chlordiazepoxide, clorazepate, diazepam, and halazepam.

OVERDOSAGE. Confusion, hypoactive reflexes, impaired coordination, slurred speech; cardiac suppression, hypotension, circulatory collapse, respiratory depression, respiratory arrest; and CNS depression somnolence, coma, and death

DOSAGE AND ADMINISTRATION. See Table 47-4.

OTHER DRUGS IN CLASS
buspirone HCl (BuSpar)

CONTRAINDICATIONS. Hypersensitivity

WARNINGS
- *Physical and psychologic dependence:* No potential for abuse has been seen; however, monitor patients for misuse.
- *Renal/hepatic function impairment:* Do not use.
- Avoid drinking with grapefruit juice.
- Avoid using with MAOI; use of SSRIs or trazodone with Buspar may cause serotonin syndrome.

PRECAUTIONS
- *Monitoring:* Effectiveness for longer than 3 to 4 weeks has not been demonstrated in controlled trials. However, patients have been treated for several months without ill effects. If used for extended periods, periodically reassess the usefulness of the drug.
- *Interference with cognitive and motor performance:* Buspirone is less sedating than benzodiazepines and does not produce significant functional impairment. However, its CNS effects may not be predictable. Use with caution.
- *Withdrawal reactions:* Will not block the withdrawal syndrome seen with benzodiazepines and other sedative-hypnotic drugs.
- *Dopamine receptor binding:* Buspirone binds to central dopamine receptors and has the theoretical potential to cause dystonia, parkinsonism, akathisia, and tardive dyskinesia. However, this has not been seen in patients.

ADVERSE EFFECTS. See Table 47-5.

DRUG INTERACTIONS
- Buspirone is metabolized primarily by CYP 3A4.
- *Calcium channel blockers:* Diltiazem and verapamil may increase serum concentrations of buspirone; consider a dihydropyridine calcium channel blocker.
- *CYP 3A4 inducers:* Decrease the effects of buspirone; examples include carbamazepine, nafcillin, nevirapine, phenobarbital, phenytoin, and rifamycins.
- *CYP 3A4 inhibitors:* Increase the effects of buspirone; examples include itraconazole, ketoconazole, fluconazole, clarithromycin, diclofenac, doxycycline, erythromycin, isoniazid, nefazodone, protease inhibitors, quinidine, and telithromycin.
- *MAO inhibitors:* Avoid using buspirone because of increased blood pressure; this includes use of traditional MAO inhibitors and the antibiotic linezolid; also, selegiline (MAO-B inhibitor; theoretical)
- *SSRIs:* Use of buspirone and SSRIs may cause serotonin syndrome.
- *Trazodone:* Concurrent use of buspirone with trazodone may cause serotonin syndrome.

OVERDOSAGE. Symptoms of overdosage include dizziness, nausea, vomiting, drowsiness, and pinpoint pupils. No antidote for buspirone overdosage is known.

GABA-BZ Recepter Agonists

zolpidem (Ambien) 🔑

CONTRAINDICATIONS. Hypersensitivity

WARNINGS
- Limit therapy to <35 days.
- Do not use for insomnia associated with a psychiatric or physical disorder.
- *Abrupt discontinuation:* Withdrawal symptoms may occur.
- *CNS depressant:* Do not engage in hazardous occupations that require complete mental alertness, motor coordination, or physical dexterity; patients should take only if they can get a full 7 to 8 hours of sleep.
- *Renal function impairment:* Use with caution; no dose adjustment.
- Hepatic function impairment increases half-life; adjust dose.
- Carcinogenesis has occurred in rats.

PRECAUTIONS
- Respiratory depression has not been observed, but use with caution.
- *Depression:* Use during depression may worsen the depression.
- *Drug abuse and dependence:* No evidence suggests that zolpidem leads to abuse and dependence, but use with caution.
- *Abnormal thinking/behavior changes:* A variety of abnormal thinking and behavioral changes have been reported to occur in association with sedative-hypnotics. Use with caution.

TABLE 47-2   Pharmacokinetics of Antianxiety Agents

Drug	Onset of Action	Time to Peak Concentration	Half-life	Duration of Action	Protein Bound	Metabolism	Excretion
Benzodiazepines		For parent compound	Parent compound/ metabolites		70%-99%	Extensively metabolized by the liver; most 3A4	
diazepam	Fast	0.5-2 hr	20-50 hr	Long	98%	Long-acting metabolite	
alprazolam	Fast	1-2 hr	6.3-26.9 hr	Intermediate	80%	Short-acting metabolite	
chlordiazepoxide	Intermediate	0.5-2 hr	5-30 hr	Long	90%-98%	Long-acting metabolite	
clonazepam	Slow	1-2 hr	18-50 hr	Long	85%	Five metabolites	Urine, unchanged, <2%
clorazepate	Fast	1 hr	40-50 hr	Long	98%	Long-acting metabolite	
estazolam	Fast	2 hr	8-28 hr	Long	93%	No long-acting metabolites	Urine, unchanged, <5%
flurazepam	Fast	0.5-1 hr; metabolite 10 hr	47-100 hr	Long	97%	Long-acting metabolite	Urine, unchanged, <1%
lorazepam	Intermediate	2-4 hr	10-20 hr	Intermediate	85%	Metabolized to inactive	
oxazepam	Slow	2-4 hr	5-20 hr	Intermediate	87%	Metabolized to inactive	
quazepam	Fast	2 hr	25-40 hr	Long	>95%	Long-acting metabolite	Trace excreted unchanged
temazepam	Intermediate	1.2-1.6 hr	9-15 hr	Intermediate	96%	No long-acting metabolites	0.2% excreted unchanged
triazolam	Fast	1-2 hr	1.5-5.5 hr	Short	78%-89%	No long-acting metabolites	2% excreted unchanged
buspirone	7-10 days	0.7-1.5 hr	2-3 hr, nonlinear	Short	95%	Oxidation	Urine, 65%; feces, 35%
zolpidem	Fast	1.6 hr	2.6 hr	6 hr	92.5%	To inactive metabolites	Renal
eszopiclone	Fast	1 hr	6 hr	Short	55%	3A4, 2E1	Inactive metabolites in urine
zaleplon	Fast	1 hr	1 hr	Short	60%	Metabolized by liver, some 3A4	Inactive metabolites in urine
ramelteon	Fast	0.75 hr	1-3 hr	Short	82%	1A2, 2C, 3A4	Inactive metabolites in urine

TABLE 47-3   Adverse Effects of Benzodiazepines by Body System

Body System	Common Minor Effects	Serious Adverse Effects
Body, general	Fever, increase or decrease in body weight, dehydration, lymphadenopathy	Behavior problems, hysteria, psychosis
Skin, appendages	Dermatitis, hair loss, hirsutism, ankle and facial edema, diaphoresis	Urticaria, pruritus, skin rash, including morbilliform, urticarial, and maculopapular
Hypersensitivity	Skin rash	
Respiratory	Nasal congestion	Respiratory depression
Cardiovascular	Palpitations, edema	Bradycardia, tachycardia, cardiovascular collapse, hypertension, hypotension
GI	Constipation, diarrhea, dry mouth, coated tongue, sore gums, nausea, anorexia, change in appetite, increased salivation, gastritis, hiccoughs	Vomiting, difficulty in swallowing
Hemic and lymphatic		Leukopenia, blood dyscrasias, including agranulocytosis, anemia, thrombocytopenia, and eosinophilia
Metabolic and nutritional	Gynecomastia, galactorrhea	

Table continued on following page

TABLE 47-3   **Adverse Effects of Benzodiazepines by Body System** (Continued)

Body System	Common Minor Effects	Serious Adverse Effects
Musculoskeletal	Muscular disturbance, joint pain	
Nervous system	CNS sedation and sleepiness, depression, lethargy, apathy, fatigue, hypoactivity, light-headedness, headache, vertigo, dizziness, nervousness, difficulty concentrating, agitation, inability to perform complex mental functions, hypotonia, unsteadiness, weakness, vivid dreams, psychomotor retardation, glassy-eyed appearance	Memory impairment; disorientation, retrograde amnesia, restlessness, confusion, crying, delirium, slurred speech, aphonia, dysarthria, stupor, seizures, coma, syncope, rigidity, tremor, dystonia, euphoria, irritability, akathisia, hemiparesis, ataxia, incoordination, extrapyramidal symptoms, paradoxical reactions, paresthesias, suicide tendencies
Special senses	Depressed hearing, auditory disturbances	Visual disturbances, diplopia, nystagmus
Hepatic		Elevated LFTs, hepatic dysfunction, hepatitis and jaundice
Genitourinary	Incontinence, changes in libido, menstrual irregularities	Urinary retention

TABLE 47-4   **Dosage and Administration Recommendations for Antianxiety and Antiinsomnia Agents**

Type of Anxiety	Drug Category	Drug	Usual Dose	Administration	Maximum Daily Dose
GAD					
Acute treatment	Benzodiazepine	alprazolam	0.25-0.5 mg	bid-tid	4 mg
		diazepam	2-10 mg	bid-qid	40 mg
		lorazepam	2-6 mg	Divide into 2-3 doses.	10 mg
		clonazepam	0.25-0.5 mg	bid-tid	3 mg
Long-term treatment	SSRIs		Usual dose, antidepressant		
	SNRI	venlafaxine	Usual dose, antidepressant		
	Miscellaneous	buspirone	7.5-20 mg	bid-tid	60 mg
PANIC DISORDER					
Acute treatment	Benzodiazepine	alprazolam and alprazolam XR and other dosage forms	0.5 mg	tid	10 mg
		lorazepam	0.5 mg	tid	Unknown
Long-term treatment	SSRIs	paroxetine; available in several dosage forms	10 mg	Daily	60 mg
		sertraline	25-50 mg	Daily	50 mg
		fluoxetine	10 mg	Daily	60 mg
	Benzodiazepines	alprazolam	0.25-0.5 mg	tid	
		clonazepam	0.125-0.25 mg	bid	
	Other (augment)	lithium, β-blocker, valproate			
PHOBIC DISORDERS					
Acute treatment	Benzodiazepines	See Anxiety.			
	β-Blocker	propranolol,	10-40 mg	prn	80 mg
Long-term treatment	SSRI	atenolol	30-100 mg	prn	100 mg
			Usual dose, antidepressant		
OBSESSIVE-COMPULSIVE DISORDER	SSRI	fluoxetine	20-80 mg	Daily (morning)	80 mg
		fluvoxamine	100-300 mg	Daily	300 mg
		paroxetine	20-60 mg	Daily (morning)	60 mg
		sertraline	50-200 mg	Daily (bedtime)	200 mg
	TCA	clomipramine	25-250 mg	Daily	250 mg
POSTTRAUMATIC STRESS DISORDER	SSRIs		Usual dose, antidepressant		

zolpidem (Ambien) 🔑

DRUG INTERACTIONS
- *Increased effect:* CNS depressants, ETOH
- *3A4 inhibitors and inducers:* 3A4 is a major metabolizing CYP.

OVERDOSAGE. Hypotension, coma

zaleplon (Sonata)

WARNINGS
- *Rapid dose decrease/discontinuation:* Signs and symptoms similar to withdrawal have been reported.
- *Renal function impairment:* No adjustment of dosage required
- *Hepatic function impairment:* Clearance is reduced in cirrhotic patients; reduce the dose. Do not use in patients with severe hepatic impairment.

TABLE 47-5   Common and Serious Adverse Effects of Other Anxiety and Antiinsomnia Agents

Drug	Common Minor Effects	Serious Adverse Effects
buspirone	CNS disturbance (headache, dizziness, insomnia, nervousness, drowsiness, light-headedness), GI effects (dry mouth, nausea, diarrhea, abdominal pain), fatigue, galactorrhea, urinary frequency	Chest pain, syncope, hypotension, hypertension, depersonalization, akathisia, hallucinations, seizures, involuntary movements, blood dyscrasias, serotonin syndrome, extrapyramidal symptoms, hostility, depression
zolpidem	Headache, drowsiness, dizziness, dry mouth, nausea, diarrhea, constipation, dyspepsia, lethargy, URI, dry mouth, myalgias, palpitations	Myalgia, dysarthria, back pain, allergy, anaphylactic shock, hypertension, arrhythmia, hypertension, ataxia, confusion, agitation, autonomic symptoms, anemia, elevated LFTs and BUN, asthenia, depression, suicidal ideation
eszopiclone	Unpleasant taste, headache, somnolence, dry mouth, dizziness, nausea/vomiting, dyspepsia, anxiety, dysmenorrhea, gynecomastia, decreased libido	Depression, worsening, suicidal ideation, aggressive behavior, hallucinations, amnesia, withdrawal if abrupt D/C, allergic reactions
zaleplon	Amnesia, anxiety, dizziness, paresthesia, somnolence, tremor, migraine, rash, constipation, dry mouth, nausea, abdominal pain, dysmenorrhea	Angina pectoris, arrhythmia, hypertension or hypotension, syncope, postural hypotension, depression, hypertonia, agitation, ataxia, confusion, anemia, leukocytosis, elevated LFTs, arthritis, depression, worsening, suicidal ideation, hallucination, withdrawal, allergy
ramelteon	Headache, somnolence, fatigue, dizziness, nausea, insomnia, diarrhea, arthralgia/myalgia, depression, taste changes, prolactin elevation, testosterone decrease, cortisol decrease	Suicidal ideation, depression, worsening hepatic tumors in animals

PRECAUTIONS. *Timing of administration:* Take immediately before bedtime or after going to bed and experiencing difficulty falling asleep. Taking zaleplon while ambulatory may result in short-term memory impairment, hallucinations, impaired coordination, dizziness, and light-headedness.

DRUG INTERACTIONS
- CYP 3A4 is a minor metabolizing enzyme of zaleplon.
- Drugs that induce CYP 3A4 may reduce zaleplon levels.
- Drugs that inhibit CYP 3A4 are not expected to affect zaleplon levels.
- Cimetidine increases the drug level of zaleplon.
- A high-fat meal may prolong drug absorption.
- Zaleplon potentiates CNS depressants.

OVERDOSAGE. Signs and symptoms of CNS depressant overdose

eszopiclone

CONTRAINDICATIONS. Hypersensitivity

DRUG INTERACTIONS
- *CYP3A4 inducers:* Decrease the effects of buspirone; examples include carbamazepine, nafcillin, nevirapine, phenobarbital, phenytoin, and rifamycins
- *CYP 3A4 inhibitors:* Increase the effects of buspirone; examples include itraconazole, ketoconazole, fluconazole, clarithromycin, diclofenac, doxycycline, erythromycin, isoniazid, nefazodone, protease inhibitors, quinidine, telithromycin, and verapamil
- *olanzapine:* Concurrent use may lead to decreased psychomotor function.

ramelteon

WARNINGS. Do not use with severe hepatic impairment.

DRUG INTERACTIONS
- Substrates of CYP 1A2 (major), CYP 3A4 (minor), and CYP 2C family (minor)
- *CYP 1A2 inhibitors:* May increase the effects of ramelteon; examples include ciprofloxacin, fluvoxamine, ketoconazole, norfloxacin, ofloxacin, and rofecoxib
- *fluconazole:* Increases the effects of ramelteon
- *ketoconazole:* Increases the effects of ramelteon; monitor for excessive somnolence
- *fluvoxamine:* Substantially increases the levels of ramelteon, leading to increased toxicity; concomitant use not recommended
- *rifampin:* May decrease levels/effects of ramelteon; monitor fluvoxamine

evolve A continually updated list of useful WebLinks may be found in the Evolve Resources at http://evolve.elsevier.com/Edmunds/ NP/

48 Antipsychotics

DRUG OVERVIEW

Class	Subclass	Generic Name	Trade Name
FIRST GENERATION			
Phenothiazine	Aliphatic	chlorpromazine 🔑	Thorazine
	Piperazine	fluphenazine	Prolixin
		perphenazine	Trilafon
		prochlorperazine	Compazine
		trifluoperazine	Stelazine
	Piperidine	mesoridazine	Serentil
		thioridazine	Mellaril
Thioxanthenes		thiothixene	Navane
Phenylbutylpiperadine	Butyrophenone	haloperidol	Haldol
SECOND GENERATION			
Dibenzepin	Dibenzodiazepines	clozapine	Clozaril
Benzisoxazole		risperidone 🔑	Risperdal ✳
	Thienobenzodiazepine	olanzapine	Zyprexa ✳
	Dibenzothiazepine	quetiapine	Seroquel ✳
		ziprasidone	Geodon ✳
Quinolinone	Dopamine system stabilizer	aripiprazole	Abilify ✳

✳ Top 200 drug; 🔑 key drug. Key drug selected because it was the first and is still in use.

INDICATIONS

- Management of psychotic disorders: Schizophrenia
- Antiemetic (see Chapter 28)
  - *thorazine:* Conduct disorders in children, bipolar affective disorder, hiccups, intractable, mania, nausea, porphyria, acute intermittent, vomiting, tetanus, adjunct
  - *prochlorperazine:* Generalized anxiety disorder, nausea, vomiting
  - *trifluoperazine:* Generalized anxiety disorder
  - *thioridazine:* Depression, behavior disorder
  - *haloperidol:* Conduct disorders in children, Tourette's syndrome, psychosis in the intensive care
  - *clozapine:* Used in schizoaffective disorder to decrease risk of chronic suicidality
  - *risperidone:* Bipolar affective disorder, mania, psychosis
  - *olanzapine:* Bipolar affective disorder, mania, agitation, psychomotor, agitation secondary to schizophrenia, agitation secondary to bipolar affective disorder
  - *quetiapine:* Bipolar affective disorder, schizophrenia

- *ziprasidone:* Bipolar affective disorder, psychomotor agitation, bipolar maintenance and bipolar depression
- *aripiprazole:* Bipolar affective disorder, mania, bipolar maintenance and bipolar depression

Unlabeled Uses

- Behavioral/psychologic symptoms of dementia (BPSD): thorazine, haloperidol
- Parenteral antipsychotics for combative patients or other serious manifestations of acute psychosis
- Control of severe nausea and vomiting, intractable: thorazine
  - *prochlorperazine:* Migraine headache
  - *risperidone:* Chronic tic syndrome, Tourette's syndrome
  - *olanzapine:* Anorexia nervosa, apathy, borderline personality disorder, nausea
  - *ziprasidone:* Autism, Tourette's syndrome

Antipsychotics, also known as major tranquilizers or neuroleptics, are used commonly in the treatment of a variety of psychotic disorders. Their use in schizophrenia and in the management of behavioral and psychologic symptoms is discussed in this chapter. Primary care providers offer general or acute care for patients who may be taking these antipsychotic drugs. This chapter provides some very general information for them. These drugs are specialty drugs, and providers who prescribe these drugs routinely will require prescribing information with much greater detail. Providers who see geriatric patients, especially in the hospital or a nursing care facility, should be prepared to use this category of drugs; they too may need more detailed information.

The first antipsychotic on the market, chlorpromazine, was introduced in the early 1950s. This is the key drug among the phenothiazine antipsychotic agents. Currently, antipsychotics are divided into two generations. The first generation includes the older, "typical" drugs that treat the positive but not the negative symptoms associated with a psychotic state. Second-generation drugs have far fewer extrapyramidal symptoms (EPS) and tardive dyskinesia (TD), and they are used to treat both positive and negative symptoms of schizophrenia. With the exception of risperidone, they are prolactin sparing.

Extrapyramidal Symptoms

Although antipsychotic drugs often are effective, almost all are associated with adverse effects. The most important adverse effects associated with antipsychotic drugs include EPS, some of which may be irreversible. EPS include parkinsonian syndrome, akathisia, dystonia, neuroleptic malignant syndrome, and TD.

TD (abnormal involuntary movements) may be progressive and irreversible, even after the drug is discontinued. It is characterized by rhythmic involuntary movement of the tongue, face, mouth, or jaw (e.g., protrusion of tongue, puffing of cheeks, puckering of mouth, chewing movements). These may be accompanied by involuntary movements of the extremities. TD has been the major limitation of first-generation antipsychotics because symptoms of TD can be disabling, preventing the patient from returning to society, even after the schizophrenia is controlled.

Neuroleptic malignant syndrome (NMS): Symptoms usually occur weeks after initiation of treatment with antipsychotics. NMS is an idiosyncratic reaction to an antipsychotic or neuroleptic drug; symptoms typically develop over a period of hours to days, and the condition is life threatening. Major symptoms include fever, catatonic stupor, muscle rigidity, autonomic instability, tachycardia, delirium, and myoglobinemia.

Parkinsonian symptoms typically occur more commonly in the elderly and with higher-potency antipsychotics, except risperidone. Symptoms include masked facies, tremor, bradykinesia, rigidity, cogwheeling, drooling, and festination.

Akathisia may be difficult to differentiate from anxiety because the two appear to be so similar. Symptoms include an intensely unpleasant need to move, restlessness, and agitation. Because of the discomfort that is felt, akathisia is often a big factor in noncompliance regarding medications.

Acute dystonia: Symptoms include muscular rigidity, usually of the tongue, neck, face, or trunk. It is most likely to occur within the first week of antipsychotic drug treatment.

Acute dystonia can be frightening, extremely uncomfortable, and life threatening if laryngeal dystonia occurs.

THERAPEUTIC OVERVIEW

It is important to understand that psychosis is not a disease. *Psychosis* is the term that is used to describe a general symptom complex in which gross impairment of reality is demonstrated. It has many causes—both organic and psychiatric. Box 48-1 lists symptoms that are commonly associated with the presentation of a clinical psychosis. Table 48-1 shows the most common medical disorders that may present with psychiatric symptoms—not all of these represent psychotic symptoms. A large number of diverse and even common medications can cause psychotic symptoms (Table 48-2). Table 48-3 lists different psychiatric disorders that may present with psychosis. Therefore, it is difficult to talk about treating the general symptoms of psychosis; it is more productive to talk about specific psychotic disorders such as schizophrenia.

Many elderly patients are particularly vulnerable to the development of psychotic symptoms. The confluence of medical disorders, psychiatric disorders, and medications may easily provoke psychotic symptoms, particularly when patients move from an unfamiliar environment to a strange setting, or when a change disturbs the tenuous balance they are maintaining while coping with medical and psychiatric problems. Geriatric patients with dementia may exhibit behavioral and psychologic symptoms, which may or may not represent psychosis. These symptoms commonly include agitation, physical aggression, delusions, and hallucinations. Other behaviors, such as refusing personal care, being unable to communicate or perform daily activities, wandering, being restless, and participating in self-destructive acts, may require the use of some of these medications, sometimes for brief intervals.

SCHIZOPHRENIA

One of the diseases that may present with psychotic symptoms is schizophrenia. Schizophrenia is a disease that is heterogeneous and complex. The pathophysiology of schizophrenia is

---

BOX 48-1   Symptoms of Clinical Psychosis

POSITIVE AXIS

Delusions
Depersonalization
Hallucinations
Illusions
Loss of reality
Paranoia
Thought disorder

NEGATIVE AXIS

Deficits of attention
Lack of grooming
Impoverished thought
Anhedonia
Lack of initiative
Alogia (absence of speech due to confusion)
Blunted affect

TABLE 48-1   Medical Conditions Associated With Psychiatric Symptoms

Causes	Example
Metabolic and endocrine	Addison's disease Calcium imbalance Carcinoid syndrome Cushing's syndrome Electrolyte abnormalities Hepatic failure Hyperparathyroidism Hyperthyroidism Hypoglycemia Hypothyroidism Hypoxia Magnesium imbalance Pheochromocytoma Porphyria Renal failure Serotonin syndrome Wilson's disease
Electrical	Complex partial seizures
Peri-ictal states (depression, hallucinations)	Postictal states (depression, dissociation, or disinhibition) Temporal lobe status epilepticus
Neoplastic	Carcinoid syndrome Carcinoma of the pancreas
Metastatic brain tumors	Primary brain tumor Remote effects of carcinoma
Arterial	Arteriovenous malformations Hypertensive lacunar state Inflammation (cranial arteritis, lupus) Migraine
Multi-infarct states	Subarachnoid bleeds Subclavian steal syndrome Thromboembolic phenomena Transient ischemic attacks
Mechanical	Concussion Normal pressure hydrocephalus Subdural or epidural hematoma Trauma
Infectious	Abscesses AIDS Hepatitis Meningoencephalitis (including tuberculosis, fungal, herpes) Multifocal leukoencephalopathy Subacute sclerosing panencephalitis Syphilis
Nutritional	Vitamin B_{12} deficiency Folate deficiency Niacin deficiency Pyridoxine (vitamin B_6) deficiency Thiamine deficiency
Degenerative and neurologic	Aging Alzheimer's disease Heavy metal toxicity Huntington's disease Jakob-Creutzfeldt disease Multiple sclerosis Parkinson's disease Pick's disease

Modified from Gabbard GO: *Gabbard's treatment of psychiatric disorders,* ed 4, New York, 2007, American Psychiatric Publishing.

TABLE 48-2   Medications That Can Cause Psychotic Symptoms

acyclovir

amantadine

Amphetamine-like drugs

Anabolic steroids

Anticholinergics and atropine

Anticonvulsants

Antidepressants, all

baclofen

Barbiturates

Benzodiazepines

β-Adrenergic blockers

Calcium channel blockers

Cephalosporins

Corticosteroids

Dopamine receptor agonists

fluoroquinolone antibiotics

Histamine H_1 receptor blockers

Histamine H_2 receptor blockers

HMG-CoA reductase inhibitors (statins)

NSAIDs

Opioids

Procaine derivatives

Salicylates

Sulfonamides

Data from The Medical Letter: Some drugs that cause psychiatric symptoms, *Med Lett* 44:1134, 2002, and Gabbard GO: *Gabbard's treatment of psychiatric disorders,* ed 4, New York, 2007, American Psychiatric Publishing.

poorly understood. Early theories involved the dopaminergic system. Recently, serotonergic pathways have been implicated. Newer theories focus on the interplay between dopaminergic and serotonergic systems, along with the involvement of muscarinic, α-adrenergic, and histaminergic systems and the presence of genetic Y chromosome disease.

Assessment

One of the diseases that may present with psychosis is schizophrenia. Schizophrenia is diagnosed by history after the patient is assessed in three areas:
1. *Characteristic symptoms:* Two of more of the following:
   a. Positive symptoms
      Delusions
      Hallucinations
      Disorganized speech (e.g., incoherence)
      Grossly disorganized or catatonic behavior

TABLE 48-3 Psychiatric Disorders That May Present With Psychosis

Type of Psychiatric Disorder	Examples
Chronic psychosis (severe)	Schizophrenia Schizoaffective disorder, bipolar type (with prominent episodes of mania) Schizoaffective disorder, depressed type (with prominent depressive episodes) Schizophreniform (<6 months' duration)
Chronic psychosis (less severe or bizarre)	Delusional disorder Shared psychotic disorder
Episodic psychosis	Depression with psychotic features Bipolar disorder (manic or depressed) Brief psychotic disorder PTSD; borderline personality disorder

Modified from Stern TA et al: *Massachusetts General Hospital handbook of general hospital psychiatry,* ed 5, St Louis, 2004, Mosby.

   b. Negative symptoms
      Impoverished thought
      Deficits of attention
      Blunted affect
      Lack of initiative
2. Social or occupational dysfunction, notably problems with work, school, interpersonal relations, or self-care
3. Duration of symptoms of 6 months or longer

Antipsychotic drugs should not be used unless the practitioner has performed a thorough physical and psychiatric assessment, the diagnosis has been ascertained, and other therapy has been ruled out. Key diagnostic questions that should be asked include the following:

1. Has a reversible organic or substance-induced cause of psychosis been ruled out?
2. Are cognitive deficits prominent? (delirium or dementia)
3. Is the psychotic illness continuous or episodic? Have psychotic symptoms (active phase) been present for at least 4 weeks? Has evidence of the illness been present for at least 6 months? Is a decline in level of functioning evident? Are negative symptoms present?
4. Are mood episodes prominent? Have episodes of major depression or mania occurred? Do psychotic features occur only during affective episodes?

Before antipsychotic drugs are initiated, take baseline vital signs. Baseline laboratory tests that should be completed include liver function tests, CBC, ECG, and UA. These tests should be repeated periodically, as dictated by the drug that is taken and the comorbidities of the patient. History of previous responses to medications, especially antipsychotics, should be noted.

MECHANISM OF ACTION

The exact mechanism of antipsychotic drug action is unknown. These drugs are thought to work by blocking postsynaptic dopamine receptors in the hypothalamus, basal ganglia, limbic system, brainstem, and medulla, and to some extent serotonin receptors. Much work has been done to elucidate which receptors each drug affects. How this receptor blocking causes specific changes in behavior and cognition is not known. See Table 48-4 for specific neurotransmitter-receptor blocking actions of individual medications. Each neurotransmitter is associated with specific side effects. However, the correlation between the two is not completely understood. A very complicated and overlapping set of mechanisms interact to produce a wide variety of effects. Another complication is that these drugs produce different effects from patient to patient. Most cause sedation in some people and agitation in others (Box 48-2).

First Generation

Typical antipsychotic drugs are more potent antagonists of D_2 dopamine receptors than of D_1 receptors. They exhibit varying degrees of selectivity among the dopamine tracts. They also have effects on cholinergic, α_1-adrenergic, and histaminic receptors.

Typical antipsychotics may be classified as of high or low potency. Low-potency (typical) antipsychotic drugs have a relatively small effect on dopamine receptors but are potent antagonists of muscarinic, α-adrenergic, and histamine H_1 receptors, resulting in side effects such as dry mouth, constipation, orthostatic hypotension, and sedation. High-potency (typical) antipsychotics have a greater effect on dopamine receptors, causing a larger number of EPS than are produced by low-potency drugs. However, they exhibit fewer muscarinic, α-adrenergic, and histaminic effects. Although exceptions are noted, in general, high-potency drugs tend to elicit fewer cardiac, sedative, seizure-promoting, and skin reactions. High-potency drugs may tend to cause diarrhea, whereas use of low-potency drugs may tend to result in constipation.

Drugs that affect dopamine D_2 receptors act as inhibitors of the synthesis and release of prolactin, thereby causing hyperprolactinemia. However, the correlation between the drugs' effects on the D_2 receptor and the frequency of their causing galactorrhea is imperfect (see Box 48-2).

Second Generation

Newer or atypical antipsychotic agents affect different receptor sites compared with first-generation antipsychotics. They bind dopamine, including D_1, D_2, D_4, and D_5 receptors, with selectivity for limbic dopamine receptors. They have an increased affinity for serotonin (5-HT_2, 5-HT_6, and 5-HT_7) receptors compared with D_2 receptors. In addition, they bind acetylcholine at α-adrenergic receptors, as well as at muscarinic, histamine H_1, and nicotinic receptors. They exhibit reduced ability or an inability to induce EPS. The FDA has required that manufacturers add a warning to the product information about these drugs regarding the incidences of hyperglycemia, obesity, and diabetes mellitus that are seen in patients who take second-generation drugs, especially olanzapine.

Aripiprazole is the first of a new class of atypical antipsychotic agents called *dopamine system stabilizers* or *dopamine partial agonists*. It combines the actions of D_2 and serotonin 5-HT_{2A} receptor antagonism.

Clozapine is specific for limbic receptors and not for striated (muscle) receptors, which explains the low incidence of EPS and TD.

TREATMENT PRINCIPLES

Standardized Guidelines

- American Psychiatric Association: Practice guidelines for the treatment of patients with schizophrenia, 2004 with updates (Available at http://www.psych.org/psych_pract/treatg/pg/Schizophrenia2ePG_05-15-06.pdf)

TABLE 48-4 Comparison of Mechanism of Action and Associated Adverse Reactions

Drug	Potency	D$_1$	D$_2$/EPS Prolactin	D$_4$	5-HT$_2$/Weight Gain	Anti-cholinergic	α$_1$/Orthostasis	α$_2$	Histamine H$_1$/Sedation
FIRST GENERATION									
chlorpromazine (Thorazine)	Low	++	++/++		+/0	++	+/+++	+	+/+++
fluphenazine (Prolixin)	High	+	+/+++		++/0	+	+/+	+++	+/+
perphenazine (Trilafon)	Low	0	++/++		+/0	+	+/+	++	0/++
prochlorperazine (Compazine)	Low		++/+++			+	+		++
trifluoperazine (Stelazine)	High		+++			+	+		+
mesoridazine (Serentil)	Low	0	++/+		+/0	+++	0/++	0	0/+++
thioridazine (Mellaril)	Low	+	++/+	+	+++/0	+++	+/+++	0	0/+++
thiothixene (Navane)	High	+++	+/+++	++	+++/0	+	+/++	++	+/+
haloperidol (Haldol)	High	++	+/+++	+	+++/0	+	+/+	+++	++/+/+
molindone (Moban)		0	+++/++	0	++++/0	+	+++/++	++	+++/++
loxapine (Loxitane)	High	0	++/++	+	+/0	+	++/+	+++	+/+
SECOND GENERATION									
clozapine (Clozaril)	High	+	+/+	+++	++/++++	+++/++	+/+++	++	+/+++
risperidone (Risperdal)	High		++/+++		++/0	0	+	++	+
olanzapine (Zyprexa)	High	+	++/+	++	+/+++	+++/++	+/++	++	+/++
quetiapine (Seroquel)	High	+++	+++/++	+++	+++/+	0/++	++/+++	+++	++/++
ziprasidone (Geodon)	High	+++	+/++	+++	+	+++	+	0	++
aripiprazole (Abilify)	High	0	Partial +++/0	D3 +++	Partial 1 and 2A +++; 2c and 7 ++	+/+	+/+	0	+/+

+ = Relative response. Additional +s indicate greater response.

BOX 48-2 Neurotransmitter and Adverse Effects

- *Antidopamine D₂*: EPS, prolactin release
- *Anticholinergic*: Blurred vision, urinary retention constipation, dry mouth
- *Antihistaminic*: Sedation
- *Antiserotonergic*: Weight gain
- *Anti–α₁-adrenergic*: Orthostatic hypotension, reflex tachycardia

- Veterans Administration, Department of Defense: *Management of persons with psychoses*, U.S. Department of Veterans Affairs, pp 1-26, Washington, DC, 2004.

Evidence-Based Recommendations

- *Psychosis*: Antipsychotic medications are effective for acute schizophrenia and schizoaffective disorder.
- Second-generation antipsychotics, which have a lower incidence of and less severe extrapyramidal symptoms, are preferred.
- Clozapine is more effective than other agents for management of aggressive behaviors and suicidality. However, it has a black box warning for leukopenia.
- *Dementia symptoms*: Olanzapine and risperidone have shown modest evidence of efficacy. However, they are associated with increased risk of cardiovascular events, including stroke, TIA, and death, in elderly patients.

Cardinal Points of Treatment

ACUTE PHASE

- Initiate pharmacologic treatment promptly as long as it does not interfere with diagnostic testing.
- Determine what the patient's response has been to other antipsychotic medications that he or she may have taken and which side effects he or she has experienced, if any.
- Begin antipsychotics at a low dose and titrate up slowly over the course of several weeks, as necessary. Do not exceed the dose at which EPS are likely to occur.
- Provide adjunctive medications, depending on comorbid conditions; these include benzodiazepines, antidepressants, mood stabilizers, and β-blockers.

STABLE PHASE

- The purpose of medication is to prevent relapse.
- Do not decrease doses of medication to limit EPS if this also causes a relapse in symptoms.

PSYCHOSIS. Typical and atypical antipsychotic drugs have been shown to be equally efficacious. However, atypical antipsychotics generally are preferred as first-line agents for long-term treatment because of the relative lack of EPS and TD—but at an increased risk of development of diabetes. Each patient will respond differently to the therapeutic and adverse effects of these drugs. There is little basis for choosing one drug over another on the basis of target symptoms. Response or lack of response to one drug does not predict response to another drug. Therapeutic effect is measured by the patient's improvement in functional abilities and reduction in psychotic symptoms.

Generally, it takes weeks to achieve the full therapeutic benefit of antipsychotic drugs. Even with initially responsive patients, relapse is possible because of drug tolerance, physical illness, comorbid conditions, or changing life circumstances. Because of the side effects, nonadherence is a big issue with almost any antipsychotic medication.

Gradually increase dosage to achieve therapeutic effect while minimizing side effects. Once therapeutic effect has been established, attempt to decrease dosage for long-term maintenance. Allow sufficient time between dosage adjustments to assess effectiveness. Guidelines do not suggest drug holidays because these were not effective in minimizing the development of TD.

The formulation used is frequently determined by the patient's willingness to take the medication. If the patient is not willing, it may be necessary to give the medication as a colorless, odorless liquid, mixed with a beverage or as an IM injection. Once the medication reaches therapeutic levels, it then may be possible to switch to an oral tablet formulation. Depot preparations are administered by injection, may be effective for up to 4 weeks, and are useful for the long-term treatment of a patient who is unwilling to take daily oral medications.

First-generation antipsychotics tend to have a greater effect on decreasing positive symptoms, with negative symptoms tending to be more chronic and refractory in nature. Second-generation agents may be more effective against the negative symptoms. Trends in psychotropic use for chronic conditions lean toward the use of second-generation drugs. First-generation drugs are available in generic form and are significantly less expensive than the newer drugs. Many drugs are currently under development.

NONPHARMACOLOGIC TREATMENT. Nonpharmacologic treatment is recommended as the initial approach. American Psychological Association (APA) guidelines suggest that the provider's actions should be directed toward preventing harm, controlling destructive behavior, reducing the severity of psychosis-associated symptoms, identifying the trigger for psychotic symptoms, affecting a rapid return to best levels, and developing family relationships to find the best after-care solution. The patient should be closely evaluated for suicide potential during this phase. Accurate diagnosis of what causes the psychotic episode is important.

PHARMACOLOGIC TREATMENT. Antipsychotic drugs are useful in treating many psychotic symptoms. For short-term treatment of an aggressive dangerous patient or a geriatric patient with delirium or dementia with agitation, haloperidol or chlorpromazine can be used IM, with results noted in 15 to 20 minutes. Use 1 mg of haloperidol for geriatric patients and 2 to 5 mg for young adults. The dose may be repeated in 20 minutes. The atypical antipsychotic, ziprasidone, may be used for the treatment of acute aggressive behavior.

Antipsychotics are useful in treating some psychiatric symptoms of dementia, including agitation, hyperactivity, hallucination, suspiciousness, hostility, and uncooperativeness. They have done much to improve the quality of life in some demented patients. However, they do not improve memory loss and may impair cognitive function. As always, use the lowest dose for the shortest possible duration. Although the use of antipsychotics in geriatric patients with dementia is a common practice, these drugs have not been granted FDA approval for this use. Studies using risperidone and olanzapine have showed increased risk of heart disease and stroke in the elderly, leading the manufacturers to declare that they are not safe and effective in the elderly population. Whether this problem can be generalized to other antipsychotics and how these study findings should affect clinical practice is not known at this time.

In other cases, antipsychotics may be used for the long-term management of behavioral/psychologic symptoms of dementia and delirium resistant to behavioral therapy. Benzodiazepines are useful for patients who have predominant anxiety. They also are useful when given on an as needed (prn) basis when a distressing event (e.g., bath, dentist visit) cannot be avoided. Second-generation antipsychotics frequently are used to decrease the occurrence of EPS symptoms. Extremely low doses should be used, often starting with the lowest dose possible. Risperidone, olanzapine, and quetiapine are used commonly in geriatric patients. No specific information is available regarding the use of other new antipsychotic agents in geriatric patients.

How to Monitor

- Monitor liver functions, CBC for blood dyscrasias, and cholesterol. The frequency of monitoring depends on the drug used and other comorbid conditions that may exist.
- *Clozapine:* Monitor weekly CBC with differential, in keeping with the manufacturer's protocol.
- Assess for extrapyramidal symptoms at each patient encounter. Use of the Abnormal Involuntary Movement Scale (AIMS) is recommended (for scale, see Goldberg et al [2007] reference in Bibliography). (See Tables 48-6 and 48-7.)
- Monitor blood glucose monthly for onset of diabetes mellitus.
- Follow weight changes, and evaluate weight loss or weight gain trends.

Patient Variables

GERIATRICS. Elderly patients have slower hepatic metabolism and increased sensitivity to dopamine antagonism. This makes them susceptible to extrapyramidal symptoms. Lower doses of antipsychotic drugs should be used. In general, use one quarter of the normal dosage. Longer waiting periods should be used before doses are increased to achieve therapeutic levels. The newer antipsychotics have been used with good results.

PEDIATRICS. In general, antipsychotics are not recommended for children younger than 12 years old. Very little information is available about this off-label practice.

Antipsychotic drugs for use in children younger than age 12 include chlorpromazine, chlorprothixene (>6 years), thioridazine, triflupromazine (low potency), prochlorperazine, trifluoperazine (>6 years), and haloperidol (high potency). Chlorpromazine should not be used in children younger than 6 months of age, except when it is potentially lifesaving. Prochlorperazine should not be used in pediatric patients who weigh less than 20 pounds and those younger

than 2 years of age. Thioridazine may be used in children older than 2 years.

Antipsychotic drugs should be used only for the treatment of acute psychosis or explosive, hyperexcitable behavior. Low doses should be used with long waiting periods before doses are increased to achieve therapeutic levels. Children, who are prone to developing EPS, tend to metabolize these drugs more quickly than adults do.

PREGNANCY AND LACTATION. Antipsychotic drugs should be avoided during pregnancy, especially during the first trimester, because significant levels of these medications are found in both fetus and amniotic fluid. The teratogenicity of antipsychotics is unclear. Infants have been born with EPS when antipsychotic drugs were administered to severely psychotic pregnant mothers. Breastfeeding should be discouraged because of the risks involved.

- *Category B:* clozapine
- *Category C:* Most other first- and second-generation antipsychotics

RACE AND GENDER. Current research has not shown that any particular race has derived greater benefit than another from the use of antipsychotic drugs. No differences in side effects or adverse effects have been documented, although elderly African American women appear to be at greater risk for TD.

It has been found that young men (<40 years) and elderly women are at increased risk for development of EPS, especially akathisia, and acute dystonia. Drug therapy should be approached cautiously and monitored carefully, especially for those patients placed on antipsychotic drugs.

Patient Education

- Hypotensive effects may be experienced during titration of dose.
- Use caution when driving or operating dangerous machinery because drowsiness may be caused by the drug.
- Inform patients of the risk of EPS, including irreversible TD.
- Use sunscreen and wear hats or protective clothing to avoid sunburn, rashes, and skin pigmentation because some antipsychotics carry labels that indicate that products may increase skin pigmentation and photosensitivity.
- If patients experience dry mouth, encourage them to drink more fluids, chew gum, or suck on hard candy.
- Immediately wash off any medication (liquid concentrate) spilled on the skin to avoid contact dermatitis.
- Smoking increases the metabolism of antipsychotic drugs and may require a dosage adjustment.
- Avoid alcohol when taking antipsychotics because it potentiates drug effects and may lead to symptoms of overdosage.
- Advise the patient to take missed doses only if remembered within 1 hour after the time the dose was due.
- Consult the provider if the patient takes any OTC medication concurrently with antipsychotic drugs.
- Take antipsychotics with food, juice, or milk, to decrease the experience of GI upset.
- Do not take antacids within 1 hour after the antipsychotic drug is taken because this may interfere with drug metabolism.

SPECIFIC DRUGS

PHENOTHIAZINES

chlorpromazine (Thorazine) 🔑

CONTRAINDICATIONS
- Hypersensitivity to any of these agents; evidence of cross-sensitivity has been found
- Coma, severe CNS depression, subcortical brain damage, concomitant use with other CNS depressants
- Bone marrow suppression, blood dyscrasias, myeloproliferative disorders
- Severe cardiovascular disease, cerebral arteriosclerosis, coronary artery disease, severe hypotension or hypertension
- Liver disease
- *thioxanthenes*: Circulatory collapse
- *haloperidol*: Parkinson's disease

WARNINGS. TD may occur with these drugs and may be irreversible. Approximately 15% to 20% of patients who are on long-term first-generation antipsychotic drugs develop TD. Symptoms may appear while the patient is on antipsychotics or may become apparent when the drug is discontinued. The only prevention is low-dose antipsychotics, administered only when necessary.

💣 **Neuroleptic malignant syndrome: Symptoms occur weeks after initiation of treatment with antipsychotics. NMS is idiosyncratic; symptoms, which typically manifest over a period of hours to days, are life threatening. (See information provided earlier in this chapter.)**

General warnings apply to the antipsychotic drugs:
- CNS effects may impair mental or physical abilities and cause drowsiness.
- *Antiemetic effects*: Drugs with an antiemetic effect can obscure signs of toxicity of other drugs or mask symptoms of disease. They can suppress the cough reflex; aspiration of vomitus is possible.
- *Pulmonary*: CNS depression may lead to decreased fluid intake, dehydration, and bronchopneumonia, which can be fatal.
- *Cardiovascular*: Use with caution in patients with cardiovascular disease or mitral insufficiency. Increased pulse rate is often noted. Orthostatic hypotension may occur. Increased activity as the result of therapy may exacerbate CAD.
- Phenothiazines are direct myocardial depressants; effects may include cardiomegaly, congestive heart failure, and refractory arrhythmias, some fatal. Quinidine-like ECG changes (increased QT interval, ST depression, and changes in AV conduction) and a variety of nonspecific ECG changes may occur; these usually are reversible, and their relationship to myocardial damage has not been confirmed.
- *Carcinogenesis*: First-generation drugs (except promazine and risperidone) elevate prolactin levels. Breast cancers may be prolactin dependent.
- Use with caution in patients who have a history of glaucoma because of the anticholinergic effects.

- These drugs may lower seizure threshold.
- Adynamic ileus occasionally occurs.
- Sudden deaths due to cardiac arrest or asphyxia or pneumonia have occurred.
- *Hyperprolactinemia*: Drugs that antagonize dopamine D_2 receptors may elevate prolactin levels.
- Jaundice is considered a hypersensitivity reaction. Monitor hepatic function according to directions issued by the drug manufacturer because of the possibility of liver damage. Use with caution in patients with liver disease.
- Use with caution in patients with renal function impairment. Monitor renal function every 3 months.
- *Thioridazine*: Pigmentary retinopathy occurs most frequently in patients receiving thioridazine.

PRECAUTIONS
- *Anticholinergic effects*: All first-generation antipsychotics have anticholinergic effects; these are strongest among low-potency drugs.
- *Cholesterol*: Some of these drugs elevate cholesterol; others decrease cholesterol. Patient response is often variable, so the clinician should monitor cholesterol levels as necessary.
- *Concomitant conditions*: Use with caution.
- *Hematologic*: Various blood dyscrasias have occurred.
- *Hyperpyrexia*: A significant rise in body temperature may indicate intolerance to antipsychotics. Discontinue.
- *Abrupt withdrawal*: These drugs are not known to cause psychic dependence and do not produce tolerance or addiction. However, the patient may experience symptoms upon abrupt withdrawal, so the medication should be slowly tapered off.
- Suicide attempt is a possibility in schizophrenia. Do not give large quantities of medication to patients at risk for suicide.
- Pigment changes and photosensitivity have occurred but are rare.
- Some drugs contain tartrazine or sulfites, which pose a risk to patients with these drug sensitivities.

PHARMACOKINETICS. These agents are lipophilic and achieve high CNS concentrations (Table 48-5).

ADVERSE EFFECTS. See Tables 48-6 and 48-7 for antipsychotic drug side effects and adverse effects related to typical and atypical antipsychotic medications.

DRUG INTERACTIONS Many; see Table 48-8

OVERDOSAGE. For all antipsychotics, overdosage may lead to increased CNS depression with resultant respiratory arrest.

DOSAGE AND ADMINISTRATION. Dosage must be individualized (Table 48-9). Liquid form usually is better absorbed than are tablets.

OTHER DRUGS IN CLASS

Other drugs in this class are similar to the prototype except as follows.

TABLE 48-5   Pharmacokinetics of Antipsychotics

Drug	Absorption	Time to Peak Concentration	Half-life	Duration of Action	Protein Bound	Metabolism	Excretion
chlorpromazine (Thorazine)	Erratic, variable	2-4 hr	24 (8-35) hr	Up to 12 hr	91%-99%	Extensive 2D6	Renal, 1%
fluphenazine (Prolixin) po	Same	2-4 hr	18 (14-24) hr		91%-99%	2D6	
perphenazine (Trilafon)	Same		12 (8-21) hr	6-12 hr		2D6	
prochlorperazine (Compazine)	Same		3-5 hr				
trifluoperazine (Stelazine)	Same		18 (14-24) hr				
mesoridazine (Serentil)	Same		30 (24-48) hr				
thioridazine (Mellaril)	Same		24 (6-40) hr	8-12 hr		2D6	
thiothixene (Navane)	Same		34 hr	34 hr			
haloperidol (Haldol)	Same		24 (12-36) hr	Up to 12 hr	92%	2D6	
molindone (Moban)	Same		12 (6-24) hr	36 hr			
loxapine (Loxitane)	Same		8 (3-12) hr	12 hr			
risperidone (Risperdal)	70%	1 hr	20-24 hr		90%	2D6	Urine, 70%; unchanged feces, 14%
ziprasidone (Geodon)	60%, increased with food	6-8 hr	7 hr		99%	Extensive liver 3A4 and 1A2	Urine, 20%; unchanged feces, 66%
clozapine (Clozaril)	27%-47%	2.5 hr	12 (4-66) hr		97%	1A2, 2D6, 3A4	Urine, 50%; unchanged feces, 30%
olanzapine (Zyprexa)	60%	6 hr	30 (20-54) hr		93%	1A2, 2D6	Urine, 57%; unchanged feces, 30%
quetiapine (Seroquel)	73%	1.5 hr	6 hr		83%	3A4	Urine, 73%; unchanged feces, 20%
aripiprazole (Abilify)	Good	3-5 hr	75-94 hr		99%	3A4 2D6	Urine, 25%; unchanged feces, 55%

TABLE 48-6   Adverse Reactions by Body System for First-Generation Antipsychotics

Body System	Common Minor Effects	Serious Adverse Reactions
Body, general	Enlarged parotid glands, polydipsia, systemic lupus erythematosus–like syndrome	Sudden death, heatstroke/hyperpyrexia
Skin	Pigment changes and photosensitivity have occurred but are rare.	
Hypersensitivity	Pruritus, dry skin, seborrhea, erythema	Urticarial (5%), maculopapular hypersensitivity reactions, angioneurotic edema, papillary hypertrophy of the tongue, photosensitivity, eczema, asthma, laryngeal edema, anaphylactoid reactions, rashes, including acneiform, hair loss, exfoliative dermatitis
Respiratory	Increased depth of respiration	Laryngospasm, bronchospasm, dyspnea, suppression of cough reflex
Cardiovascular	Hypotension, postural hypotension, hypertension, tachycardia, bradycardia, light-headedness, faintness, dizziness	Cardiac arrest, circulatory collapse, syncope, myocardial depressant, quinidine-like effect (increased QT interval, ST depression, and changes in AV conduction)
GI	Dyspepsia, increased appetite and weight, antiemetic	
Hemic and lymphatic		Agranulocytosis (rare—most occur wk 4-10), eosinophilia, leukopenia, leukocytosis, anemia, lymphomonocytosis, thrombocytopenia, granulocytopenia, aplastic anemia, hemolytic anemia, thrombocytopenic or nonthrombocytopenic purpura, pancytopenia

TABLE 48-6   Adverse Reactions by Body System for First-Generation Antipsychotics (Continued)

Body System	Common Minor Effects	Serious Adverse Reactions
Endocrine	Lactation and breast engorgement in females, galactorrhea, mastalgia, amenorrhea, menstrual irregularities, changes in libido, hyperglycemia or hypoglycemia, glucosuria, raised cholesterol levels	SIADH, hyponatremia
Central nervous system	Headache, weakness, tremor, twitching, tension, jitteriness, fatigue, slurring, insomnia, vertigo, drowsiness (80%; lasts 1 wk), CNS depression, drowsiness	NMS (0.5%-1%) with fatalities; TD, EPS: Pseudoparkinsonism (4%-40%), akathisia (7%-20%), dystonias (2%-50%), cerebral edema, staggering gait, ataxia, seizures
Autonomic	Dry mouth, nasal congestion, nausea, vomiting, paresthesia, anorexia, pallor, flushed facies, salivation, perspiration, constipation, diarrhea, frequency or incontinence, polyuria, enuresis, priapism, ejaculation inhibition, male impotence	Obstipation, fecal impaction, atonic colon, adynamic or paralytic ileus, urinary retention, bladder paralysis
Hepatic		Liver dysfunction
Behavioral effects		Exacerbation of psychotic symptoms, including hallucinations, catatonic-like states, lethargy, restlessness, hyperactivity, agitation, nocturnal confusion, toxic confusional states, bizarre dreams, depression, euphoria, excitement, paranoid reactions

TABLE 48-7   Common Drug Interactions With Antipsychotics

Antipsychotic	Drugs Affected	Drug	Antipsychotic Affected
All	↑↓ phenytoin	aluminum salts, charcoal	↓ Phenothiazines
chlorpromazine	↓ epinephrine, norepinephrine	Anticholinergics	↓ Phenothiazines
clozapine	↑ risperidone	Barbiturates, meperidine, propranolol	↑ Phenothiazines
olanzapine, quetiapine, risperidone	↓ Dopamine agonists, levodopa	Barbiturates	↓ Phenothiazines, haloperidol
Phenothiazines	↑ propranolol	carbamazepine	↓ haloperidol, olanzapine, risperidone
Phenothiazines	↓ Amphetamines, bromocriptine,	cimetidine	↑ quetiapine
Phenothiazines, haloperidol	Barbiturates	fluoxetine	↑ haloperidol
Phenothiazines, haloperidol, thioxanthene	↓ guanethidine	lithium	↑ Phenothiazines, haloperidol
pimozide	↑ Phenothiazines, TCAs, Antiarrhythmics	methyldopa	↑ haloperidol, trifluoperazine
quetiapine	↑ lorazepam	phenytoin	↓ quetiapine, thioridazine, haloperidol
thioridazine	↓ quetiapine	3A4, 2D6 inducers	↓ aripiprazole
		3A4, 2D6 inhibitors	↑ aripiprazole

fluphenazine (Prolixin, Permitil)

Start treatment with the oral formulation to determine effectiveness and dosage. The general conversion rate is 0.5 ml (12.5 mg) IM every 3 weeks for every 10 mg po.

prochlorperazine (Compazine)

Commonly used for nausea and vomiting

OTHER FIRST-GENERATION ANTIPSYCHOTICS
haloperidol (Haldol)
- Very similar to phenothiazines; high potency

SECOND–GENERATION ANTIPSYCHOTICS
clozapine (Clozaril)
INDICATIONS
- For treatment of patients who are severely ill, with refractory (to at least two other drugs) chronic schizophrenia
- The most effective antipsychotic

CONTRAINDICATIONS
- Hypersensitivity to clozapine or any other component of the drug
- Uncontrolled epilepsy

TABLE 48-8   Dosage and Administration Recommendations for Antipsychotics

Drug	Use	Initial Dosage	Dosage, Geriatric	Adjust Dosage/Usual Dosage	Maximum Daily Dose
FIRST GENERATION					
chlorpromazine (Thorazine)	Acute, long term	25 IM 10 tid-qid		May repeat in 1 hr ↑ by 20-50 mg q2wk	1000 mg
fluphenazine (Prolixin)	Oral IM/subQ	0.5-10 mg/day; divide every q6-8h intervals 12.5-25 mg q3-6wk	1-2.5 mg daily	2.5-10 mg/day ↑ 12.5 mg q3wk	40 mg
perphenazine (Trilafon)	Oral	4-8 tid		8-64 mg	64 mg
prochlorperazine (Compazine)	Psychiatric Nausea and vomiting	5-10 tid-qid Oral: 5-10 tid-qid Rectal: 25 bid		15-40 mg	150 mg 40 mg
trifluoperazine (Stelazine)	Oral	2-5 mg bid (inpatients); 1-2 mg bid (outpatients)	Lower doses bid	15-20 mg	40 mg
mesoridazine (Serentil)	Oral	25-50 mg tid		100-400 mg daily	400 mg
thioridazine (Mellaril)	Oral	50-100 mg tid	10-25 mg 1-2 times per day; maximum 400 mg/day	200-800 mg daily	800 mg
thiothixene (Navane)	Oral	2 mg tid		↑ to 15 mg daily prn	60 mg
haloperidol (Haldol)	IM acute Moderate symptoms Severe symptoms	2-10 mg 0.5-5 mg bid-tid 3-5 mg bid-tid	0.5-2 mg	q6h — —	100 mg 30 mg
molindone (Moban)	Oral	50-75 mg once daily	Not used	↑ to 100 mg daily in 3-4 days	225 mg
loxapine (Loxitane)	Oral	10 mg bid		20-100 mg in 2-4 divided doses	100 mg
SECOND GENERATION					
clozapine (Clozaril)	Oral	12.5 mg daily-bid	25 mg daily; maximum 450 mg/day	300-450 mg/day; increase by 25-50 mg daily over 2-4 wk	900 mg
risperidone (Risperdal)	Oral	1 mg bid	0.5 mg bid; increase by 0.5 mg bid q wk	4-8 mg/day; increase by 2 mg/day q wk	8 mg
olanzapine (Zyprexa)	Oral IM	5-10 mg once daily 2.5-10 mg	2.5-5 mg once daily	10-20 mg once daily; increase by 5 mg/day q wk q2-4h	20 mg 30 mg
quetiapine (Seroquel)	Oral	25 mg bid	200-500 mg/day slower titration	300-800 mg/day; increase by 25-50 mg q2-3 days	800 mg 30 mg
ziprasidone (Geodon)	Oral IM	20 mg bid with food 10-20 mg	—	40-160 mg/day; increase dose q 2 days 10-20 mg q2h or 20 mg q4h	160 mg 40 mg
aripiprazole (Abilify)	Oral	10-15 mg once daily	Same as adult	10-30 mg once daily; increase dose q2wk	30 mg

- Myeloproliferative disorders, history of clozapine-induced agranulocytosis or severe granulocytopenia, simultaneous administration with other agents that have well-known potential to cause agranulocytosis or to otherwise suppress bone marrow function
- Severe CNS depression or comatose state from any cause

WARNINGS
- Clozapine presents a significant risk for agranulocytosis, a life-threatening adverse event. Monitor leukocyte count before starting treatment, every week during treat-ment, and weekly for at least 4 weeks after discontinua-tion. Clozapine is available only through a distribution system that ensures monitoring of WBC count according to a schedule published by the manufacturer.
- Seizures have been associated with the use of clozapine.
- *Myocarditis:* Clozapine is associated with an increased risk of fatal myocarditis.
- Orthostatic hypotension with or without syncope can occur. Collapse can be profound and may be accompanied by respi-ratory and/or cardiac arrest. It also is associated with chest pain/angina, hypertension, hypotension, and tachycardia.

risperidone (Risperdal) 🔑

- Second only to clozapine as the most efficacious antipsychotic

CONTRAINDICATIONS. Hypersensitivity

WARNINGS
- Risperidone has an antiemetic effect in animals; this also may occur in humans.
- All second-generation antipsychotics may cause hyperglycemia and increased risk for diabetes mellitus.
- Risperidone and ziprasidone lengthen the QT interval, ziprasidone to a greater extent than risperidone. Other drugs that prolong the QT interval have been associated with the occurrence of torsades de pointes and sudden death.
- *Priapism:* In one patient, priapism developed.

PRECAUTIONS
- A single case of thrombotic thrombocytopenic purpura (TTP) occurred.
- Evaluate signs of risperidone misuse or abuse in patients with a history of drug abuse.
- Use with caution in patients with known cardiovascular disease and in those at risk for hypotension.
- Use lower doses in patients with renal or hepatic impairment.

- Use with caution in patients who will be exposed to extreme heat.
- May have antiemetic effect

ADVERSE EFFECTS. See Table 48-7.

DRUG INTERACTIONS. Risperidone is metabolized by the P450 system 2D6.

OTHER DRUGS IN CLASS

Other drugs in this class are similar to the prototype except as follows.

olanzapine (Zyprexa)

- Agranulocytosis and seizures have not been noted.
- Metabolized by CYP 1A2, 2D6 system
- Weight gain is common; most likely to cause diabetes mellitus
- EPS low frequency, mild

quetiapine (Seroquel)

- Causes less weight gain than clozapine or olanzapine
- Extensively metabolized in the liver; may elevate liver function tests (LFTs)
- Quetiapine oral clearance is induced by the prototype cytochrome P450 3A4 inducer, phenytoin. Use caution with potent enzyme inhibitors of cytochrome 3A4.

TABLE 48-9   Adverse Effects by Body System for Second-Generation Antipsychotics

Body System	risperidone	clozapine	olanzapine	quetiapine	aripiprazole
General	Fever	Fever	Fever	Fever	Fever
Skin	Rash Photosensitivity	Rash	Rash	Rash	Rash
Respiratory	Cough* Rhinitis		Cough* Rhinitis	Cough	
Cardiovascular	Lengthen QT interval Chest pain/angina Tachycardia	Fatal myocarditis Chest pain/angina Hypertension Hypotension* Tachycardia*	Chest pain/angina Hypotension Tachycardia	Chest pain/angina Tachycardia	
Gastrointestinal	Abdominal pain Constipation* Dyspepsia* Nausea	Constipation* Dyspepsia Nausea	Abdominal pain Constipation*	Abdominal pain Constipation* Dyspepsia	Nausea* Vomiting* Constipation*
Heme	None	Agranulocytosis	None	None	
Liver	Liver dysfunction	Liver dysfunction	Liver dysfunction	Liver dysfunction	
Endocrine	Galactorrhea	None	None	None	
CNS	Agitation* Anxiety* Dizziness Headache* Insomnia* Drowsiness Seizure	Agitation Akathisia Dizziness* Headache Seizures Somnolence* Syncope Tremor	Agitation* Akathisia Anxiety* Dizziness* Headache* Drowsiness* Insomnia* Tremor	Dizziness* Headache* Drowsiness* Insomnia* Somnolence* Akathisia* Tremor	Headache* Asthenia
Other					Blurred vision

*Highest incidence of problem.

ziprasidone (Geodon)

- Seldom causes weight gain
- More likely to cause QT interval prolongation than are other second-generation antipsychotics
- Causes EPS in 5% of patients

aripiprazole (Abilify)

- May be taken without regard to food
- Does not increase QT interval
- Has little or no effect on weight

evolve A continually updated list of useful WebLinks may be found in the Evolve Resources at http://evolve.elsevier.com/Edmunds/NP/

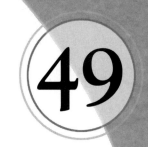

Substance Abuse

LAURA MILLER and KENNETH SAFFIER

DRUG OVERVIEW

Class	Subclass	Generic Name	Trade Name
Alcohol treatment medications	Benzodiazepines	diazepam ✴ chlordiazepoxide, lorazepam ✴	Valium, Librium, Ativan
	Opioid antagonist	naltrexone	Vivitrol, ReVia, Depade
	Gamma butyric acid analog (GABA)	acamprosate	Campral
	Aldehyde hydrogenase inhibitor	disulfiram	Antabuse
Opioid treatment medications	Opioid antagonists	naloxone	Narcan
		naltrexone	ReVia
		nalmefene	Revex
	Opioid agonist	methadone ✴	Dolophine
	Opioid partial agonists	buprenorphine	Subutex
	Opioid partial agonists (with antagonist)	buprenorphine and naloxone	Suboxone

✴ Top 200 drug.

INDICATIONS

- Alcohol use disorders
  - *benzodiazepines:* Used for withdrawal
  - *naltrexone:* ReVia; opioid antagonist; decreases intake craving
  - *acamprosate:* Decrease intake.
  - *disulfiram:* Aversive agent
- Opioid use disorders
  - *Opioid antagonists:* Overdose: naloxone, nalmefene
  - *Opioid blocking:* naltrexone
  - *Opioid agonists:* Withdrawal, maintenance: methadone
  - *Opioid partial agonists:* Withdrawal, maintenance: buprenorphine

Unlabeled Uses

- *Alcohol withdrawal and craving:* topiramate, carbamazepine
- *Alcohol dependence:* beginning studies on the use of varenicline (Chantix), which is currently approved only for smoking cessation

This chapter discusses drugs used to treat abuse of alcohol and other drugs. Evaluation of abuse of alcohol and current medical treatments are discussed. A brief listing of pharmacologic treatments for opiate dependency, as well as current research findings and interventions for cocaine and methamphetamine abuse treatment, is provided. In general, pharmacologic treatment can be especially helpful when used in conjunction with other treatment modalities for patients who are dependent on alcohol or opioids. Primary care often involves use of medications for the treatment of alcohol abuse. Treatment of opioid addiction is now within the scope of primary care by physicians who receive additional approved training in the use of buprenophine.

THERAPEUTIC OVERVIEW

Alcohol and drug addictions are chronic bio-psycho-social-spiritual diseases that profoundly affect individuals, their families, and society in general. Alcohol dependence is a serious disease that causes approximately 100,000 deaths per year in the United States. Approximately 8 million people in the United States have an alcohol dependence problem. Although not required for diagnosis, tolerance and withdrawal are frequently seen in substance use disorders. Tolerance is a central nervous system adaptation that occurs when a larger dose of alcohol or another drug of abuse is needed to obtain the desired effects. Withdrawal syndromes develop in alcohol- and drug-dependent individuals upon cessation or marked decrease. The physiologic effects of withdrawal symptoms are usually the opposite of those of the abused substance. Denial is seen invariably in individuals with substance use disorders.

Assessment

All patients should be screened at least annually and as indicated both for extent of alcohol use and any related problems. Alcoholics usually understate the amount of alcohol they consume.

Assess for use of medications that interact adversely with alcohol, including H_2-blockers, aspirin, benzodiazepines, antidepressants, narcotics, barbiturates, antihistamines, NSAIDs, metronidazole, sulfonamides, methyldopa, nitroglycerin, acetaminophen, isoniazid, antihypertensives, antidiabetic agents, warfarin, propranolol, or β-blockers. Also ask about profound drug–drug interactions that may result from alcohol-induced liver impairment and activation of CYP 2E1 metabolism.

Physical examination findings may include alcohol odor on the breath, flushed face, scleral injection, tremor, bruising, or peripheral neuropathy. Injuries from accidents such as falls may be evident. Frequently, people have severe alcohol disorders without apparent physical findings.

Laboratory tests should include CBC and LFTs. Macrocytosis is seen in more than 90% of patients (MCV 100-110 fL). This finding correlates with approximately 80 grams of alcohol consumption per day (e.g., one bottle of wine). The most sensitive laboratory tests for excessive chronic alcohol use included elevated AST and ALT, and especially GGT. When the ratio of AST to ALT becomes greater than 2, alcoholic hepatitis should be strongly suspected. A breath or blood alcohol level can also reveal the level of alcohol intake.

CLASSIFICATION LEVELS FOR ALCOHOL INTAKE

- *Low risk:* Less than 1 drink/day for women, 2 drinks/day for men; or 7 drinks/wk for women, 14 drinks/wk for men; or 3 drinks for women and 4 drinks for men on any occasion; 0 CAGE score, no dysfunction related to drinking *and* not using medications that interact adversely with alcohol.
- *Heavy and/or risky drinking:* More than 7 drinks/wk, or 3 drinks/occasion for women; for men, 14 drinks/wk or 4 drinks/occasion; score greater than 1 on CAGE, evidence of drinking-related dysfunction, or use of alcohol and medications that might adversely interact with alcohol.
- *Abuse:* More than one of the following recurring situations: drinking resulting in failure to fulfill major obligations, drinking in hazardous situations, alcohol-related legal problems, continued drinking despite persistent problems caused or worsened by alcohol.
- *Dependence:* The "3 C's" can identify dependence: (1) Compulsive use; (2) continuing use despite negative consequences, and (3) lack of control. DSM-IV criteria require three or more of the following features: tolerance, withdrawal, drinking more than intended, persistent desire to drink or unsuccessful efforts to cut down or control drinking, increased time spent in activities related to alcohol, giving up important activities because of drinking, or drinking despite knowledge of problems caused or worsened by alcohol.

Alcohol Withdrawal

Mild symptoms include anxiety, decreased mental function, tremor, depression, and insomnia. Delirium tremens is an acute organic psychosis that occurs with mental confusion, tremor, sensory hyperacuity, visual hallucinations, autonomic hyperactivity, diaphoresis, tachycardia, or seizures. Withdrawal often occurs when a patient is removed from home to the hospital or nursing home. Withdrawal symptoms generally begin about 48 to 96 hours after the last drink. Seizures occur within the first 48 hours, more likely when alcohol dependence is present. Hallucinations (i.e., visual, auditory, or tactile misperceptions) commonly occur 12 to 72 hours after the last drink. DTs usually occur about 48-96 hours after the last drink.

Screening and Assessment Tools for Alcohol Use Disorders

Alcohol Assessment Tools	Alcohol Intake Equivalents*	Interpretation and Comments
*Quantity-frequency question: Do you sometimes drink alcoholic beverages?	• Scoring: • Yes: 5 or more drinks in a day/14 wk men; 4 or more drinks in a day/7 wk women†	If positive, next screen with the CAGE, RAPS4-QF, or Audit questionnaire.
CAGE questions are as follows: C = Pt felt need to Cut down on drinking? A = People Annoyed you by criticizing your drinking? G = Felt Guilt about drinking? E = Need an Eye-opener in the morning?	Scoring: Positive if respond positive to 2 of these questions • Can adapt for pregnancy (T-ACE), asking about Tolerance; how many drinks does it take to feel high?	To distinguish those with alcoholism from those without; does not differentiate dependence from abuse
RAPS4-QF R = Do you use alcohol/drugs at Regular times? A = Use alcohol/drugs Alone, or with friends or family? P = Problems due to alcohol/drugs? S = Has alcohol/drug ever made you feel Sick? 4 = Have you had more than 4/5 drinks in one setting? More often than once a month?	Scoring: Positive if answers yes to questions; greater sensitivity and specificity over CAGE for all gender, ethnic, and service utilization groups in ERs	Eliminates many cultural terms that do not translate to other ethnic groups, such as "eye-opener"; concept of guilt, social surroundings addressed
AUDIT: 10-question bilingual written screen that can be filled out by patient	Scoring: Positive: 8 for men up to 60; 4 for women, adolescents, or men >60	Variable cutoff scores distinguish between harmful use, hazardous use, and dependence

Adapted from *Helping Patients Who Drink Too Much, A Clinician's Guide,* 2005 edition, NIAA, NIH; publication No. 05-3769.
*One standard drink = 12 ounces of beer, 5 ounces of wine, or 1.5 ounces of 80 proof spirits
†May be excessive if >65 years, with medical problems. If pregnant, advise abstinence.

MECHANISM OF ACTION AND EFFECTS OF ALCOHOL TREATMENT

For alcohol withdrawal treatment, benzodiazepines demonstrate cross-tolerance with alcohol via GABA receptors. Long-acting benzodiazepines, such as diazepam or chlordiazepoxide, generally are preferred to minimize the occurrence of breakthrough agitation and seizures. Short-acting drugs such as lorazepam and oxazepam are used in patients with severe liver disease.

Naltrexone is an opioid antagonist with highest affinity for the mu opioid receptor. Occupation of opioid receptors by naltrexone may block the effects of endogenous opioid peptides. The neurobiologic mechanisms responsible for the reduction in alcohol consumption observed in alcohol-dependent patients treated with naltrexone are not entirely understood. However, involvement of the endogenous opioid system probably has its effect on alcohol consumption. Naltrexone has little effect on cravings for alcohol. It does not cause the physical adverse effects that are produced by disulfiram.

Acamprosate is structurally related to GABA agonists and potentiates the inhibitory effects of the GABAergic system. Patients with alcohol dependence notably display an imbalance of GABA and glutamate neuronal transmission, which may be restored by acamprosate. This agent decreases glutamatergic transmission and modulates neuronal hyperexcitability during withdrawal from alcohol. It reduces voluntary intake of alcohol but does not cause a disulfiram-like reaction.

A potent alcohol dehydrogenase inhibitor, disulfiram blocks the oxidation of alcohol at the acetaldehyde stage by inhibiting the enzyme, aldehyde dehydrogenase With alcohol ingestion, disulfiram causes the patient to feel extremely unpleasant sensations ranging from flushing, dyspnea, and tachycardia, to confusion, vomiting, and syncope. Unpleasant symptoms can last from 30 minutes to 2 hours, and the intensity of the reaction depends on the amount of alcohol ingested, the dose of disulfiram taken, and the time that has lapsed between the two. The theory behind disulfiram use in the treatment of alcoholism is based on aversion. Acute reactions may be fatal.

Topiramate is a seizure medication that can help curb the craving for alcohol. This drug acts by reducing excess dopamine released through alcohol consumption. Researchers have found that patients given this drug were six times more likely than those taking a placebo to abstain from alcohol for a month.

The drugs listed above may be taken while people are still drinking, except for disulfiram. Reducing alcohol intake can significantly contribute to treatment outcomes.

TREATMENT PRINCIPLES

Standardized Guidelines

- Screening and behavioral counseling interventions in primary care to reduce alcohol misuse: Recommendation statement 2004, an update to the U.S. Preventive Services Task Force guideline.

Evidence-Based Recommendations

- VHA/DoD clinical practice guidelines for the management of substance use disorders. These can be found by going to www.guideline.gov and searching on the alcohol link.

Cardinal Points of Treatment

- The principles behind using medication for alcohol treatment involve helping patients who are dependent on alcohol reduce problematic drinking, deterring relapse back to heavy drinking, achieving and maintaining abstinence from alcohol, or a combination of these efforts.
- Pharmacologic treatment options include using the injectable forms of naltrexone (Vivitrol), which can keep blood levels elevated, to help patients control their impulse to drink. Naltrexone blocks opiate receptors that are involved in the rewarding effects of drinking alcohol and the cravings after abstinence is established. Acamprosate is possibly helpful with regenerating neurotransmitters and restoring the balance between GABA and glutamate when alcohol intake has stopped or has been significantly decreased. Disulfiram functions on the aversion model and is a significant physical deterrent to alcohol because it causes significant feelings of ill-being when alcohol is ingested or inhaled.
- Some treatment models combine alcohol treatment medications with behavioral counseling; this has been studied in the COMBINE (Combined Pharmacotherapies and Behavioral Interventions) trial.
- During the initial acute phase of alcohol withdrawal (up to 5 days), benzodiazepines help to physiologically stabilize patients.
- Medication use is successful with programs that integrate social support to motivate and educate patients on the adverse effects of alcohol, and to help them redirect their lives.

ALCOHOL ABUSE TREATMENT. Counsel all patients about safe levels of drinking. Nonpharmacologic treatment is the foundation of any therapy. Self-help groups such as Alcoholics Anonymous (www.aa.org) can be found at the National Clearinghouse for Alcohol and Drug Information website at http://ncadi.samhsa.gov. Professional counseling may help. Hospitalization is not necessary for treatment to be successful.

Pharmacologic treatment has had limited success but is helpful when patients are dependent on alcohol. Medications are used with supportive treatment to maintain sobriety when patients are unable to do so through traditional approaches. Naltrexone, an opiate antagonist, is useful as an adjunct to psychosocial therapy. It works by decreasing alcohol cravings and can be used on a long-term basis. Acamprosate can be used alone or adjunctively in therapy with naltrexone. Dangers are inherent in the use of disulfiram, and abstinence from alcohol is required.

For alcohol withdrawal, benzodiazepines play a large role in preventing seizures and other complications. For milder symptoms, clonidine, atenolol, and carbamazepine have been used successfully. The CIWA-Ar (Clinical Institute Withdrawal Assessment of Alcohol Scale, Revised), an assessment tool that was designed to evaluate the need for medical treatment for withdrawal, includes an interactive training package that is suitable for practitioners who treat patients with alcohol misuse.

OPIATE ABUSE TREATMENT. Naloxone is an opiate antagonist with a short duration of action (20 to 60 minutes); it is given subQ, IM, or by continuous IV infusion. This is generally done in the emergency department setting to counter respiratory depression due to opiate intoxication.

Naltrexone is considerably more active than naloxone and has a 24 hour duration of action. Opiate antagonist activity is related to dose. A single 50 to 100 mg oral dose of naltrexone effectively antagonizes the pharmacologic effects of 25 mg IV heroin for up to 24 hours; a single IM injection may antagonize heroin or other opiates for 2 to 4 weeks.

Nalmefene, which is structurally related to naltrexone, is indicated for the reversal of opioid effects and for opioid overdose. It has a longer duration of action than naloxone at fully reversing doses.

Methadone is dispensed both by pharmacies and by licensed narcotic treatment programs approved by the DEA and designated state authorities. Strict requirements for use are stipulated in the Federal Methadone Regulations (21 CFR 291.505). Methadone, used as an analgesic, may be dispensed in any licensed pharmacy (see Chapter 42).

Buprenorphine or a combination of buprenorphine and naloxone is sublingual treatment that is started when the patient experiences signs of withdrawal.

How to Monitor

NALTREXONE
- Monitor HR, BP, and respiratory rate.
- Monitor kidney and liver function.
- Monitor response to therapy and abstinence from alcohol.
- Risk of suicide often is increased in those with substance abuse problems.

ACAMPROSATE
- Should not be used with renal impairment with creatinine clearance <30; may be given if CrCl is 30 to 50, provided the patient is monitored regularly
- Risk of suicide is increased.

DISULFIRAM
- Monitor for liver toxicity: Check LFTs at baseline, weekly for 4 weeks, biweekly for 4 weeks, then monthly. Monitor for jaundice or for evidence of liver toxicity.
- Monitor for symptoms of optic neuritis such as eye pain or visual disturbances.
- Monitor for symptoms of peripheral neuritis such as tingling and numbness in the hands and feet.
- Monitor for headaches, drowsiness, and psychotic reactions. Assess compliance with drug therapy, abstinence from alcohol use, and progress of therapy.

Patient Variables

GERIATRICS
- *naltrexone:* Vivitrol was not evaluated specifically; use caution with renal or hepatic failure.
- *acamprosate:* Has not been evaluated; use caution when monitoring renal function
- *disulfiram:* Of limited benefit in geriatric patients because of cardiac risks

PEDIATRICS. *naltrexone, acamprosate disulfiram:* Use in pediatric population has not been evaluated.

PREGNANCY AND LACTATION. *Category C:* naltrexone, acamprosate, disulfiram; lactation safety unknown

Patient Education

NALTREXONE
- Tell patients to wear a Medic-Alert bracelet or carry ID and to notify health care providers that they are taking this medication.
- Tell patients that if they take heroin or other narcotics with this drug, they may die or sustain other serious injury, including coma.
- If patients previously used opioids, they may be more sensitive to them after using Vivitrol.
- Health care providers should monitor for signs of liver toxicity such as abdominal pain, white bowel movements, dark urine, or yellowing of the eyes.
- With Vivitrol, if patients have signs or symptoms of pneumonia or respiratory distress, they may have allergic pneumonia, which requires special medical treatment.
- With Vivitrol, if the injection site exhibits a reaction that does not resolve, patients should get medical attention. Also, once patients receive the injection, it cannot be removed.
- If they become pregnant or are lactating, patients must notify their health care provider.
- Vivitrol should be used with a treatment program that includes counseling and support.

ACAMPROSATE
- The patient may take this agent with other alcohol treatment medications but not with moderate kidney failure.
- If feeling depressed, the patient should notify the health care provider.

DISULFIRAM
- Instruct patients to avoid taking this medication if they are unwilling to make the commitment to not drink alcohol.
- Tell patients to wear a Medic-Alert bracelet and to notify their health care provider that they are taking this medication.
- A reaction can occur up to 14 days after disulfiram is taken.
- Seek medical attention and/or notify the health care provider immediately if the patient experiences chest pain, respiratory difficulty, or jaundice.
- Health care providers should monitor for signs of liver toxicity such as abdominal pain, white bowel movements, dark urine, or yellowing of the eyes.
- If feeling depressed, the patient should notify the health care provider.

SPECIFIC DRUGS

ALCOHOL TREATMENT AGENTS

naltrexone for extended-release injectable suspension (Vivitrol), naltrexone (ReVia)

CONTRAINDICATIONS
- *Active narcotic use:* Patients who receive opioid analgesics or who have current physiologic opioid dependence
- Moderate to severe renal failure
- Severe liver failure
- *Black Box Warning:* Hepatocellular injury may occur when given in excessive doses. Naltrexone is contraindicated in hepatitis or liver failure.

- The therapeutic margin of treatment is narrow; the safe dose of naltrexone and the occurrence of hepatic injury are less than five-fold separation. Vivitrol itself does not appear to act as a hepatotoxin at recommended doses.

WARNINGS

- Vivitrol may cause eosinophilic pneumonia; if the patient has pneumonia and is not responding to antibiotics, you should consider this; treatment consists of antibiotics and corticosteroids.
- Patient must be opioid free for 7 to 10 days before starting Vivitrol. Absence of opioid drug in the urine is not sufficient proof that the patient is opioid free; a naloxone challenge test can determine whether the patient is opioid free.
- Patients will respond to opioids with greater sensitivity after treatment with Vivitrol, which can sensitize them to potentially life-endangering opioid intoxication. Patients must be aware of the dangers of trying to overcome the opioid blockade by self-administering opioids; this can lead to severe, life-endangering opioid intoxication.
- If Vivitrol injections produce persistent pain or induration that continues to enlarge or does not resolve within 4 weeks, get medical attention, to prevent worsening of pain.

PRECAUTIONS

- When reversal of Vivitrol blockade is required for pain management, it is suggested that in an emergency situation, regional analgesia, conscious sedation with a benzodiazepine, nonopioid analgesics, or general anesthesia may be used. If the situation requires opioid analgesia, a rapidly acting opioid analgesic that minimizes the duration of respiratory depression is preferred. Personnel equipped and staffed for cardiopulmonary resuscitation should be kept available.
- The elimination half-life of Vivitrol is 5 to 10 days after administration.
- Monitor patients through friends and caregivers for the possibility of depression or suicidality.
- Watch for injection site reactions.
- Vivitrol does not eliminate or diminish alcohol withdrawal symptoms.

ADVERSE EFFECTS. Common adverse effects with Vivitrol include nausea, vomiting, diarrhea, injection site reactions, headache, and suicide-related events. Injection site reaction discomfort was common. In clinical studies, adverse events were described by most patients as "mild" or "moderate." On laboratory tests, an increase in eosinophil counts is returned to normal and platelets are decreased. CPK levels are increased with naltrexone without consequence.

DRUG INTERACTIONS

- thioridazine (excessive somnolence)
- Patients who are taking Vivitrol may not benefit from opioid-containing medications (e.g., antidiarrheals, cough and cold medications, opioid analgesics)

DOSAGE AND ADMINISTRATION

- Naltrexone (Vivitrol) is an IM medication; 380 mg is administered monthly to alternating buttocks. It is to be administered with the needles and diluents with which it is supplied. This agent should be refrigerated at from 36°F to 46°F and should not be exposed to freezing temperatures or temperatures greater than 77°F.
- *Naltrexone (ReVia) po 50 mg day:* Patient must be opioid free 7 to 10 days before the first dose; this may be verified by urinalysis.

acamprosate (Campral)

CONTRAINDICATIONS

- Any previously known hypersensitivity to acamprosate calcium or any of its components
- Patients with severe renal involvement (CrCl <30)

WARNINGS. Caution with depression and in elderly patients

PRECAUTIONS. Use of acamprosate does not eliminate or diminish withdrawal symptoms.

ADVERSE EFFECTS

- Diarrhea, nausea, depression, asthenia, dizziness, dry mouth, insomnia, pruritus, sweating, anxiety
- Patients should notify providers if they become pregnant or are breastfeeding; Category C drug

DRUG INTERACTIONS. Concomitant intake of alcohol and acamprosate does not affect the pharmacokinetics of either. Pharmacokinetic studies indicate that administration of disulfiram or diazepam does not affect the pharmacokinetics of acamprosate. Coadministration of acamprosate and naltrexone produced a 30% increase in acamprosate, but no adjustment of dosage is recommended.

DOSAGE AND ADMINISTRATION. Two 333 mg tablets should be given three times daily soon after alcohol withdrawal; treatment should be maintained if the patient relapses. With moderate renal impairment (CrCl, 30 to 50 ml/min), the starting dose is one 333 mg tablet given three times daily. With severe renal impairment (CrCl <30 ml/min), this treatment should not be administered.

disulfiram (Antabuse)

CONTRAINDICATIONS

- Concomitant use with alcohol
- Severe myocardial disease or coronary occlusion
- Psychosis
- Hypersensitivity to disulfiram or to other thiram derivatives used in pesticides and rubber vulcanization
- Patients who have recently received metronidazole, paraldehyde, alcohol, or alcohol-containing preparations such as cough syrups, candy-containing liqueurs, or alcohol-based flavoring extracts

BLACK BOX WARNING. Disulfiram should *never* be administered to anyone under the influence of alcohol without the patient's full knowledge and consent. A disulfiram–alcohol reaction produces an extremely unpleasant reaction that can be severe. In vulnerable patients, this may provoke respiratory depression, cardiovascular collapse, arrhythmias, myocardial infarction, acute CHF, unconsciousness, convulsions, and death.

Use with caution in patients with diabetes mellitus, hypothyroidism, seizure disorder, cerebral damage, impaired renal function, impaired liver function, a history of rubber contact dermatitis, or pregnancy.

Disulfiram plus alcohol causes the patient to feel an extremely unpleasant sensation that is manifested by flushing, dyspnea, nausea, thirst, abdominal and chest pains, palpitations, vertigo, hyperventilation, tachycardia, vomiting, hyperhidrosis, hypotension, syncope, and confusion.

PHARMACOKINETICS. In all, 70% to 90% of the dose is rapidly absorbed. The time to peak serum concentration is 1 to 2 hours. Half-life data are not available for all metabolites, but inhibition of aldehyde dehydrogenase occurs slowly for up to 12 hours and is reversible. Twenty percent of the dose remains in the body for 1 week or longer. The lungs excrete carbon disulfide, and other metabolites are excreted via the kidneys. Of each dose, 5% to 20% is excreted unchanged through the feces. Persistent effects are felt up to 2 weeks after discontinuation of the drug.

ADVERSE EFFECTS. Drowsiness is the most common side effect. Serious reactions may include respiratory depression, cardiovascular collapse, arrhythmias, acute MI, CHF, seizures, psychosis, optic neuritis, and hepatitis. Milder reactions include fatigue, headache, impotence in men, acne, metallic or garlic taste in mouth, and neuropathies. Emergency medical intervention is necessary to treat severe effects.

DRUG INTERACTIONS. Warfarin and anticoagulants increase anticoagulant effects; phenytoin levels are increased, and monitoring is needed; isoniazid can increase CNS effects—lower the disulfiram dose; avoid metronidazole because the combination may cause psychosis; capsules of amprenavir, ritonavir, lopinavir/ritonavir, diazoxide, and tipranavir include alcohol, which may cause an alcohol–disulfiram response.

DOSAGE AND ADMINISTRATION. Abstain from alcohol for at least 12 hours before beginning treatment with this product. The initial dose is 250 mg given daily (maximum dose, 500 mg) as a loading dose for 1 week.

The maintenance dose is 250 mg daily, with a range of 125 to 500 mg. Alternatively, give 500 mg daily as the initial starting dose × 1 to 2 weeks.

May be taken for months to years; tolerance does not develop, but the patient becomes more sensitive to disulfiram the longer the therapy is instituted.

topiramate (Topamax)

Topiramate has been cited as useful with alcohol treatment.

Benzodiazepines are discussed in Chapter 47. Alcohol may be potentiated by benzodiazepines, causing respiratory depression that may be life threatening.

OPIOID TREATMENT MEDICATIONS

Methadone is still the dominant medication prescribed for maintenance or withdrawal from opioids. This treatment is strictly limited to specified settings that are managed by authorized physicians. In these licensed settings, protocols are determined for dosing and management. Methadone treatment centers are listed at http://www.methadonetreatment.net.

Dosage and management for pain control are addressed in Chapter 42.

naltrexone HCl (ReVia)

BLACK BOX WARNING. Hepatotoxicity can cause hepatic injury in excessive doses: contraindicated if acute hepatitis or liver failure; caution if active liver disease: less than fivefold margin of separation between safe and hepatotoxic doses: no evidence of hepatotoxicity at recommended doses; warn patients of hepatic injury risk, discontinue treatment if acute hepatitis symptoms occur.

CONTRAINDICATIONS
- Hypersensitivity to naltrexone
- Acute hepatitis or liver failure; if used in active liver disease, must be carefully monitored for hepatotoxic effects
- Patients receiving or dependent on opioids, or in active withdrawal

WARNINGS. With mild to moderate hepatic impairment (groups A and B of Child-Pugh classification), dose adjustment is not required. Patients should be warned of the risk of hepatic injury and should seek medical attention if they have symptoms of acute hepatitis.

PRECAUTIONS
- Monitor for development of depression or suicidal thinking.
- The patient who becomes pregnant should notify the provider.

PHARMACOKINETICS. Has 96% absorption from the GI tract with peak serum levels within 1 hour; significant first-pass effect, excreted primarily by the kidneys

ADVERSE EFFECTS. Clinical studies have shown a 5% to 7% incidence of depression and 2% suicide ideation. Other adverse effects include nausea, headache, dizziness, nervousness, fatigue, insomnia, vomiting, anxiety, and somnolence.

DRUG INTERACTIONS
- Antagonizes opioid-containing products such as cough and cold remedies, antidiarrheal preparations, and opioid analgesics
- *thioridazine:* Excessive somnolence.

DOSAGE AND ADMINISTRATION
- *For treatment of opioid addiction in highly motivated patients:* 50 mg daily is recommended administered as 25 mg ×2. Wait 1 hour after first 25 mg to verify no withdrawal signs before administering second 25 mg. Alternatively, give 100 mg qod, or 150 mg every 3 days.
- Patients must be opioid free for a minimum of 7 to 10 days before beginning treatment.
- *naloxone (Narcan):* 0.4 to 2 mg subQ/IV every 2 to 3 minutes; may also give IM for opioid overdose; pure opioid antagonist. Rapidly inactivates opioids. Plasma half-life 60 to 90 minutes. Used for opiate-induced respiratory depression
- *nalmefene (Revex):* Give IV, IM, or subQ. Usual initial dose is 0.25 mcg/kg given at 2- to 5-minute intervals for opioid overdose until desired response occurs.

buprenorphine (Subutex); buprenorphine and naloxone (Suboxone)

The Drug Addiction Treatment Act of 2000 (DATA 2000) enables qualifying physicians to receive a waiver to treat up to 100 patients. Illicit and prescription opioid–dependent patients now can be treated outside of licensed narcotic treatment programs. DATA 2000 is used for both detoxification and maintenance treatment.

evolve A continually updated list of useful WebLinks may be found in the Evolve Resources at http://evolve.elsevier.com/Edmunds/NP/

50 Glucocorticoids

DRUG OVERVIEW

Class	Subclass	Generic Name	Trade Name
Glucocorticoids	Short-acting	hydrocortisone 🗝 ✸	Cortef, Hydrocortone
		cortisone	Cortisone (generic)
	Medium-acting	prednisone ✸	Deltasone, Sterapred
		prednisolone	Delta-Cortef, Prelone
		triamcinolone ✸	Aristocort, Kenacort
		methylprednisolone ✸	Medrol
	Long-acting	dexamethasone ✸	Decadron
		betamethasone	Celestone

✸ Top 200 drug; 🗝 key drug. Drugs listed in order of duration of action.

INDICATIONS

Glucocorticoids are used to treat numerous disorders, primarily through their antiinflammatory and immunosuppressive actions. In addition, they are used as replacement therapy for patients with adrenal insufficiency (Table 50-1).

Diagnostic Purposes

Long-acting glucocorticoids, particularly dexamethasone and betamethasone, are used to suppress ACTH production and allow measurement of plasma cortisol levels at specific intervals after administration. The results are useful in the diagnosis of Cushing's syndrome and in the differentiation of excess glucocorticoid secretion from a pituitary vs. an adrenal or ectopic source.

Other

Glucocorticoids are used in nephrotic syndrome to induce diuresis; in autoimmune thrombocytopenic purpura and certain hemolytic anemias; and in overwhelming infection, particularly gram-negative sepsis, to reduce inflammation. Glucocorticoids are used post transplant for immune suppression.
Unlabeled uses with application to the primary care practitioner include prevention of acute mountain sickness, treatment of the inflammatory exophthalmos of Graves' disease, and treatment of COPD.
This chapter addresses the use of glucocorticoid therapy in the treatment of inflammatory disease.

THERAPEUTIC OVERVIEW

Anatomy and Physiology

The adrenal cortex synthesizes and secretes several hormones. Among them are the glucocorticoid cortisol, the mineralocorticoid aldosterone, and a small amount of the sex steroid androgen. Aldosterone, under the influence of the renin-angiotensin system and other metabolic pathways, regulates sodium, potassium, and water retention in the body. Cortisol has a powerful antiinflammatory effect, modifies the body's immune response, and influences metabolic processes. The production of cortisol is controlled by a negative feedback loop involving the hypothalamus-anterior pituitary-adrenal cortex (HPA) axis (Figure 50-1). A low level of plasma cortisol stimulates the anterior pituitary to increase production of ACTH, which, in turn, stimulates the adrenal cortex to increase cortisol secretion. Similarly, a high level of circulating cortisol prompts downregulation of ACTH production and a resultant decrease in adrenal cortex production of cortisol.

Cortisol is naturally secreted in an uneven pattern over 24 hours, totaling 10 mg/day in normal adults. Secretion is highest during the early morning hours—2:00 to 7:00 AM—and lowest in the evening—6:00 PM to midnight.

MECHANISM OF ACTION

Glucocorticoids affect the metabolism of carbohydrates, proteins, and fats. They have direct and indirect effects on immune response, modulate inflammatory response, and play a role in the body's response to stressful stimuli (i.e., fasting states). All drugs in this class are remarkably similar and may

TABLE 50-1 Common Disorders Treated With Glucocorticoids

Disorder	Examples
Allergic conditions	Seasonal or perennial allergic rhinitis Serum sickness Drug hypersensitivity reaction
Dermatologic	Contact dermatitis Psoriasis Seborrheic dermatitis Pemphigus Erythema multiforme Stevens-Johnson syndrome Mycosis fungoides
Respiratory	Bronchial asthma Sarcoidosis Aspiration pneumonia COPD
GI	Ulcerative colitis Regional enteritis
Endocrine	Adrenocortical insufficiency Congenital adrenal hyperplasia Nonsuppurative thyroiditis
Collagen, vascular	Systemic lupus erythematosus Acute rheumatic carditis Polymyositis Polymyalgia rheumatica Temporal arteritis
Rheumatic	Rheumatoid arthritis Psoriatic arthritis Ankylosing spondylitis Acute bursitis Acute gouty arthritis Posttraumatic osteoarthritis
Neurologic	Multiple sclerosis Cerebral edema Acute stroke and spinal cord injury
Ophthalmic	Allergic conjunctivitis Uveitis Optic neuritis Herpes zoster ophthalmicus

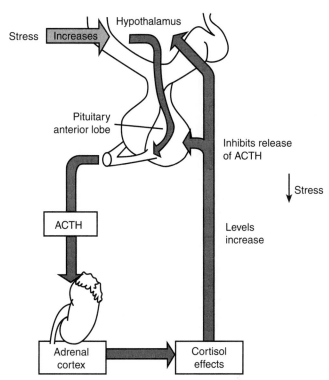

FIGURE 50-1   Adrenal-pituitary axis. (From McKenry LM et al: *Pharmacology in nursing,* ed 22, St Louis, 2006, Mosby.)

be discussed as a group; the most important differences between these drugs consist of duration of action and degree of inherent mineralocorticoid activity, which causes sodium and fluid retention (Table 50-2). Mineralocorticoid activity is needed in adrenal insufficiency but not in severe inflammation. Both cortisone and hydrocortisone have glucocorticoid and mineralocorticoid properties. Their synthetic analogs prednisone, prednisolone, and methylprednisolone have both effects as well, although glucocorticoid effects predominate. By contrast, triamcinolone, dexamethasone, and betamethasone have exclusively glucocorticoid antiinflammatory activity.

Carbohydrate and Protein Metabolism

Glucocorticoids maintain an adequate level of serum glucose by stimulating gluconeogenesis in the liver and inhibiting peripheral glucose use. They also stimulate protein breakdown, which results in increased plasma amino acid levels. In the liver, amino acids enhance enzymatic activity, which, in turn, supports increased glycogen deposition and decreased glycolysis. This action, intended to support homeostasis in the healthy body, can result in a diabetogenic state when large doses of exogenous steroids are used. Serum glucose rises in the fasting state; glucose tolerance decreases; insulin resistance develops; and glucosuria may be present. The result may be the clinical expression of latent diabetes or simply relative glucose intolerance while on steroid therapy.

Increased protein breakdown mobilizes amino acids from muscle, bone, skin, and lymph tissue. Muscle atrophy, osteoporosis, impaired wound healing, and thinning of the skin may result. In children, growth can be impaired.

Lipid Metabolism

Glucocorticoids affect the mobilization of fats from areas of deposition. Increased lipolysis occurs in areas of adipose accumulation, and serum fatty acid concentration increases. Long-term use of steroid therapy may result in increased deposition of adipose tissue in the back of the neck and in the supraclavicular area, sometimes described as a buffalo hump, and in the cheeks and the face, referred to as a moon facies. Relative loss of subcutaneous fat in the extremities may be noted.

Immune Response

Glucocorticoids mask the manifestations of both cellular and humoral immunity. Humoral immunity involves the interaction of B lymphocytes with macrophages and helper T-lymphocytes to create antibodies. Steroids do not cause a decrease in the level of circulating antibodies but may inhibit antibody creation by interfering with macrophage function and the production and activation of lymphokines. Cellular immunity is mediated primarily by T-lymphocytes. Steroids block several steps in the cascade of T-cell activation and thereby impede their ability to mount an effective

TABLE 50-2   Pharmacokinetics of Selected Glucocorticoids

Drug	Absorption	Onset of Action	Biologic Half-life	Metabolism	Excretion
hydrocortisone	GI	1 hr	8-12 hr	Hepatic	Renal
prednisone	GI	1-2 hr	12-36 hr	Hepatic 3A4	Renal
prednisolone	GI	1-2 hr	12-36 hr	Hepatic	Renal
triamcinolone	GI	1-2 hr	12-36 hr	Hepatic	Renal
methylprednisolone	GI	1-2 hr	12-36 hr	Hepatic	Renal
dexamethasone (po)	GI	1-2 hr	36-54 hr	Hepatic	Renal
betamethasone	GI	1-2 hr	36-54 hr	Hepatic	Renal

From Hardman JG, Limbird LE, editors: *Goodman & Gilman's the pharmacological basis of therapeutics,* ed 11, New York, 2007, McGraw-Hill.

cellular immune response. This action is used therapeutically to block rejection after transplant.

In addition, steroid administration has a direct effect on circulating white blood cells, causing a prompt drop in the numbers of lymphocytes, monocytes, and eosinophils in circulation and an increase in the number of circulating neutrophils. Lymphocytes are sequestered in lymph tissue, and T-cells are decreased in relatively greater numbers than B-cells. Neutrophils are released from the marrow in greater numbers and are removed from the circulation more slowly under the influence of exogenous steroids. The net result is a redistribution of white blood cell types rather than a true leukopenia.

Antiinflammatory Action

Lymphocytes, macrophages, and lymphokines all play a role in modulation of the body's inflammatory response. Thus, the impact of exogenous steroids is an interactive one between the immune response and the inflammatory response. By many of the pathways mentioned above, glucocorticoids inhibit both early manifestations of inflammation, such as local edema, capillary dilation, migration and activation of white blood cells, and phagocytosis, and the later effects, including proliferation of capillaries and collagen deposition.

It is the simultaneous inhibition of inflammation and the immune response that accounts for the effectiveness of glucocorticoids in circumstances such as acute asthma and acute allergic reactions. However, the practitioner must remain cognizant of the attendant risks of such suppression. Serious infection or illness may be masked by the absence of the characteristic signs of inflammation or immune system activation.

Stress Response

Stressful stimuli, such as surgery, fright, starvation, and abrupt physiologic challenge, prompt increased release of glucocorticoids from the adrenal cortex and release of epinephrine and norepinephrine from the adrenal medulla. Steroids potentiate the effects of the catecholamines to raise heart rate, blood pressure, and blood glucose in activating the "fight or flight" response.

Other Effects

Glucocorticoids have several indirect effects on the CNS. Changes in mood, sleep pattern, and motor activity are seen. The typical mood change involves upregulation, or euphoria, but anxiety and depression occasionally occur in some patients. Rarely, a so-called steroid psychosis occurs, which resolves with discontinuation of the medication. The precise mechanisms that underlie these effects are unknown.

Glucocorticoids increase hemoglobin concentration and increase the numbers of circulating red blood cells and platelets.

Glucocorticoids also impede the rate of growth in children. Many developing tissues, including brain, lung, liver, skin, and the epiphyses of long bones, are affected by inhibition of cell division and cell growth. Furthermore, glucocorticoid therapy may cause osteonecrosis for reasons that are poorly understood.

TREATMENT PRINCIPLES

Standardized Guidelines

See condition treated.

Evidence-Based Recommendations

See condition treated.

Cardinal Points of Treatment

- *Short-term use:* If the patient has been on the medication for a few days, it is not necessary to taper the dose before the patient stops taking it.
- *Long-term use:* Requires a very gradual reduction in dosage before the patient stops taking it.
- Critical decisions in the use of steroids revolve around length of therapy and how steroid use is stopped. The goals of treatment with glucocorticoids, other than as replacement therapy, are to control symptoms of inflammation and prevent organ damage while minimizing serious adverse effects. When possible, steroids should be added to other forms of therapy rather than given alone.

Most primary care uses of steroids call for short-term therapy (2 weeks or less). Steroid administration can suppress the hypothalamic-pituitary axis (HPA), leaving the body compromised during periods of physiologic stress because of complete or partial dependence on exogenous steroids.

Use of oral or intramuscular steroids for less than 2 weeks, even in high doses, does not require a gradual decrease in dosage to discontinue. However, it is standard that 2- to 3-week courses usually are tapered to prevent symptom recurrence.

> **Longer courses require a very gradual dosage reduction to avoid abrupt onset of the symptoms of adrenal insufficiency.**

Recovery after HPA suppression can take up to 12 months. The use of a short-acting agent and an alternate-day dosage regimen should be considered for long-term therapy. Administration of a double dose every other morning has been found to cause less suppression of the HPA axis and less growth suppression in children. However, daily therapy is indicated for acute exacerbations of disease and for a limited number of conditions such as temporal arteritis and pemphigus vulgaris.

Therapeutic administration is least likely to interfere with natural hormone production when the drug is given at the time of natural peak activity. It is generally recommended to administer the full daily dose before 9 AM. Large doses may have to be divided. Oral steroids usually are given with meals to limit GI irritation.

Prednisone is the drug of choice for most disorders seen in primary care because of its medium duration, minimal mineralocorticoid effect, and low cost. The initial dosage may have to be high to achieve rapid control of symptoms, especially in life-threatening disease. To determine the minimum dose to be given during long-term therapy, the dose should be tapered periodically to the point of worsening symptoms.

Oral preparations are the cheapest formulations; although convenience packs are available, the higher costs may not warrant their prescription. As true "miracle drugs," these products are remarkably inexpensive relative to many products on the market. Table 50-3 compares the potency of different steroid preparations.

How to Monitor

Short courses of therapy usually do not require laboratory tests. For long-term therapy, determination of baseline weight, blood pressure, serum glucose, and serum potassium levels is recommended.

Monitor for edema, weight gain, negative nitrogen balance, electrolyte imbalance, increased blood pressure, and other adverse effects, as listed in Table 50-4.

TABLE 50-4 Adverse Effects of Oral and Intramuscular Glucocorticoids

System	Adverse Effects
Dermatologic	Acne, striae, urticaria, ecchymoses, erythema, thinning of skin, impaired wound healing
Cardiovascular	Hypertension, cardiac rupture following recent MI, thrombophlebitis, thromboembolic events
GI	Peptic ulcer, pancreatitis, ulcerative colitis, perforated viscus
Endocrine	Menstrual changes, decreased carbohydrate tolerance, hyperglycemia, increased insulin need in diabetic patients, hirsutism, decreased responsiveness of HPA axis
Musculoskeletal	Loss of muscle mass, weakness, tendon rupture, osteoporosis, necrosis of femoral and humeral heads, spontaneous fractures (long bones, vertebral compression fractures)
Neurologic	Vertigo, headache, seizure, paresthesias, steroid psychosis, pseudotumor cerebri (usually after abrupt halt to therapy)
Fluid and electrolyte	Hypokalemia, hypocalcemia, sodium and fluid retention, metabolic alkalosis
Miscellaneous	Insomnia, fatigue, hypersensitivity reactions, leukocytosis, altered manifestations of infection, posterior subcapsular cataracts, glaucoma; may mask signs of infection

Additionally, monitor for signs and symptoms of disease exacerbation.

Patients whose medication is being tapered after long-term therapy should be monitored for symptoms of steroid withdrawal and adrenal insufficiency (see Adverse Effects, below).

Children on long-term therapy should be followed closely for changes in rate of growth and continued attainment of developmental milestones.

Patient Variables

GERIATRICS. Because the elderly are more prone to certain potential adverse effects of steroid therapy, caution is required with this population. Osteoporosis, susceptibility to

TABLE 50-3 Glucocorticoids: Relative Potency, Equivalent Dose, Duration

Drug	Antiinflammatory Potency	Sodium-Retaining Potency	Equivalent Dose	Duration of Action
SHORT ACTING				
hydrocortisone	1	2	20 mg	8-12 hr
MEDIUM ACTING				
prednisone	4	1	5 mg	18-36 hr
prednisolone	4	1	5 mg	18-36 hr
methylprednisolone	5	0	4 mg	18-36 hr
triamcinolone	5	0	4 mg	18-36 hr
LONG ACTING				
dexamethasone	25	0	0.75 mg	36-54 hr
betamethasone	25	0	0.6-0.75 mg	36-54 hr

From Hardman JG, Limbird LE, editors: *Goodman & Gilman's the pharmacological basis of therapeutics,* ed 11, New York, 2007, McGraw-Hill.

compression fractures, thinning of the skin, and atrophy of subcutaneous fat often are seen with aging. Steroid therapy may cause additive risks in these areas. Practitioners should use the lowest effective dose for the shortest effective time in the elderly.

PEDIATRICS. The potential for growth suppression is the greatest concern with use of glucocorticoids in children. Alternate-day dosing of intermediate-acting preparations may minimize suppression of activity of the HPA axis. A short course does not result in growth suppression.

PREGNANCY AND LACTATION. Studies have not been done in humans to fully determine the level of safety in pregnancy. Glucocorticoids cross the placenta and appear in breast milk. Long-term use during the first trimester has been associated with a 1% incidence of cleft palate. Women who have taken large doses of steroids during pregnancy should be advised to avoid breastfeeding, and their infants should be monitored closely for evidence of hypoadrenalism. Doses of 20 mg/day or less of prednisone or prednisolone or 8 mg/day or less of methylprednisolone for short periods may not cause harm to the infant. Waiting 3 to 4 hours after ingestion before breast-feeding also has been recommended.

Patient Education

- Take oral steroids with food to minimize GI upset.
- Take single daily or alternate-day doses before 9:00 AM to coincide with the timing of peak endogenous adrenal cortical activity.
- Self-monitor for signs of adverse effects, and notify practitioner if observed.
- Anticipate certain common side effects that can be troubling but not serious. These include changes in mood, insomnia, and increased appetite.
- Do not abruptly discontinue medication. Consult health care practitioner if there is a reason to stop taking the drug.
- Taper dosage down slowly as directed.
- While on long-term therapy, carry a wallet card that specifies the drug and dosage. When therapy is over, indicate date of discontinuance on the card, and carry it for an additional year to indicate the possible need for supplementation during times of severe physiologic stress.
- Learn the signs of adrenal insufficiency and report them to the practitioner if noted as dosage is tapered, or after medication is discontinued. Signs include fatigue, weakness, nausea, anorexia, weight loss, diarrhea, dyspnea, and dizziness.
- Diabetic patients must closely monitor serum glucose. Changes in dosage of insulin or an oral agent may be needed.
- Avoid immunization with a live virus such as smallpox, and avoid close contact with people who have had recent live-virus vaccinations.
- Do not use in the presence of systemic fungal infection.

SPECIFIC DRUGS

hydrocortisone (Cortef, Hydrocortone) 🔑

Hydrocortisone, a naturally occurring glucocorticoid, is the drug prototype for this class of drugs. All other drugs are compared with hydrocortisone in terms of activity. It exhibits glucocorticoid and mineralocorticoid activity, making it most useful as replacement therapy or supplementation for patients with adrenal suppression during times of physiologic stress, such as surgery.

CONTRAINDICATIONS

- Systemic fungal infection
- Known hypersensitivity
- Serious infection (except sepsis or tuberculosis)

WARNINGS

💣 Increased susceptibility to infection and potentially impaired host defense mechanisms necessitate a high index of suspicion for infection and prompt initiation of specific antiinfective therapy.

In patients with class II tuberculosis, observe closely for reactivation of active infection. Latent amebiasis also may be activated. It may be prudent to exclude amebiasis in the patient with undiagnosed diarrhea before initiating steroid therapy.

The use of live-virus vaccines is contraindicated in patients receiving long-term steroid therapy because of concerns about ineffective antibody response and the potential risk of neurologic complications.

Patients on long-term supraphysiologic doses of steroids (or whose medication has been discontinued within the past year) who anticipate a period of increased physiologic stress (e.g., surgery) may need supplementation with a glucocorticoid that also has mineralocorticoid activity. Evaluate the competency of the HPA axis through outpatient laboratory tests.

PRECAUTIONS. Use corticosteroids cautiously in the following conditions, with careful risk–benefit assessment and close monitoring during therapy: hypertension, heart failure, peptic ulcer disease, GI tract infection, diabetes, osteoporosis, osteonecrosis, seizure disorder, hepatic cirrhosis, metastatic carcinoma, Cushing's syndrome, and resistant infection.

PHARMACOKINETICS. Glucocorticoids, natural and synthetic, are well absorbed from the GI tract (see Table 50-2). Intramuscular preparations are used when oral intake is contraindicated, or when sustained action is needed. In general, the sodium esters (phosphate and succinate) are rapidly absorbed parenterally, and the acetate preparations are absorbed more slowly. Glucocorticoids are reversibly bound to both an albumin and a globulin, predominantly the latter. It is the unbound portion that is metabolically active. The liver metabolizes hydrocortisone and its synthetic analogs, and hepatic enzyme induction increases their clearance. Prednisone is a P450 3A4 substrate. Excretion occurs via the kidneys, and increased plasma levels result in increased renal clearance.

Relative potencies, dose equivalencies, and duration of action of the various agents are summarized in Table 50-3.

ADVERSE EFFECTS. Adverse effects vary in intensity and severity. Controlling factors include both dosage and length of therapy, as well as underlying physiologic factors in the patient. The decision to stop treatment rather than decrease the dosage must be individualized in each case.

hydrocortisone (Cortef, Hydrocortone) 🗝 —cont'd

Prolonged use of glucocorticoids can result in a characteristic cushingoid state. Stigmata include truncal obesity, moon facies, hirsutism, abdominal striae, acne, and the presence of a buffalo hump. Additional common adverse effects of oral and intramuscular glucocorticoids are listed in Table 50-4.

💣 Sudden discontinuation or rapid tapering of steroids in patients who have developed adrenal suppression can precipitate symptoms of adrenal insufficiency, including nausea, weakness, depression, anorexia, myalgia, hypotension, and hypoglycemia.

INTERACTIONS. Many potential drug-drug interactions are common to all corticosteroids. These are listed in Table 50-5.

DOSAGE AND ADMINISTRATION. Hydrocortisone is used for both oral and parenteral administration. The initial adult dosage range is 20 to 240 mg/day. Pediatric dosage is 0.5 to 10 mg/kg/day, usually divided into three or four doses. Dosage varies widely, depending on disease and patient variables.

OTHER DRUGS IN CLASS

Other drugs in this class are similar to the prototype except as follows.

cortisone (generic)

Used interchangeably with hydrocortisone in a wide variety of conditions

DOSAGE AND ADMINISTRATION. Start with 25 mg. Dose may be increased up to 300 mg/day po. Medication must be stored in controlled room temperatures and away from light and moisture.

prednisone (Deltasone, Sterapred)

INDICATIONS. Prednisone is the most commonly prescribed glucocorticoid. It has four times more antiinflammatory potency as hydrocortisone and exhibits minimal mineralocorticoid activity, making it the drug of choice for most disorders treated with systemic steroids in primary care.

PHARMACOKINETICS. Prednisone is an inactive substance that must be metabolized in the liver to prednisolone. This activity may be impaired in patients with liver disease.

DOSAGE AND ADMINISTRATION. Prednisone is administered orally only. Dosage varies widely, depending on the indication and patient variables. Initial dosage may range from 5 to 60 mg/day in adults. In children, dosage may range from 0.5 to 2 mg/kg/day, with a daily maximum of 80 mg/day. Dose may be given once daily or may be divided into two, three, or four daily doses.

prednisolone (Delta-Cortef, Prelone)

PHARMACOKINETICS. Prednisolone sodium phosphate oral liquid produces a 20% higher peak plasma level than is produced by tablet forms; this occurs approximately 15 minutes earlier than with oral tablets.

DOSAGE AND ADMINISTRATION. Prednisolone is administered orally, in doses of 5 to 60 mg/day. Pediatric dosage is 1 to 2 mg/kg/day, to a daily maximum of 80 mg/day. As with all glucocorticoids, dosage must be individualized.

triamcinolone (Aristocort, Kenacort, Atolone)

DOSAGE AND ADMINISTRATION. A variety of preparations are used for intraarticular, oral, topical, and inhalation therapy. The usual oral starting dose varies, based on therapeutic indication, from 4 to 60 mg/day. Slightly higher doses are used in palliative treatment for acute leukemia and lymphoma. The maximum daily dosage to avoid suppression of HPA axis is 8 mg.

methylprednisolone (Medrol)

PHARMACOKINETICS. When given concurrently with the macrolide antibiotics, methylprednisolone clearance is reduced, so a smaller dose of methylprednisolone is needed. Methylprednisolone sodium succinate has a more rapid onset of action than the acetate salt when given IM. Methylprednisolone acetate is less soluble and therefore has a longer duration of action.

DOSAGE AND ADMINISTRATION. Oral and injectable forms are long acting. Usual initial oral dose is 4 to 48 mg/day. Usual pediatric dose is 0.16 to 1.7 mg/kg/day.

dexamethasone (Decadron)

INDICATIONS. Dexamethasone is often used in acute allergic disorders. It is used to confirm the diagnosis of Cushing's syndrome and to distinguish excess glucocorticoid secretion of pituitary origin from that of adrenal or ectopic origin. It has several unlabeled uses, including the prevention and treatment of acute mountain sickness and as an antiemetic, and it may be helpful in decreasing the incidence of hearing loss in bacterial meningitis. Do not use in patients with depression.

TABLE 50-5 Corticosteroid Drug Interactions

Drug	Potential Effects of Interaction
Oral contraceptives, estrogens	Steroid half-life and concentration increased; clearance decreased
Barbiturates, hydantoins, rifampin	Steroid clearance may be increased, resulting in decreased therapeutic effect of the steroid preparation
Oral anticoagulants	Steroid may oppose or potentiate the anticoagulant effect; careful monitoring of prothrombin time is required.
digitalis	Increased potential for digitalis toxicity related to hypokalemia
Diuretics	Increased potential for electrolyte disturbance, particularly hypokalemia with potassium-depleting agents
isoniazid	Decreased concentration of isoniazid
Salicylates	Decreased concentration of salicylate; decreased therapeutic effectiveness
theophylline	Variable effect on the activity of both agents
ketoconazole	Decreased steroid clearance

PHARMACOKINETICS. Dexamethasone is well absorbed after oral administration. The acetate salt is used intramuscularly for prompt onset with a longer duration of effect.

DRUG INTERACTIONS. Ephedrine interacts with dexamethasone to decrease the half-life and increase the clearance of dexamethasone. Aminoglutethimide potentially reverses the adrenal suppression of dexamethasone.

DOSAGE AND ADMINISTRATION. Dosage varies widely and must be individualized. The usual initial adult dosage of oral dexamethasone is 0.75 to 9 mg/day. The usual pediatric dosage for airway edema is 0.5 to 2 mg/kg/day divided every 4 to 6 hours.

betamethasone (Celestone)

DOSAGE AND ADMINISTRATION. Usual oral dosage is 0.6 to 7.2 mg/day. As with all glucocorticoids, individualize the dosage.

evolve A continually updated list of useful WebLinks may be found in the Evolve Resources at http://evolve.elsevier.com/Edmunds/NP/

Thyroid Medications

$\binom{51}{}$

DRUG OVERVIEW

Class	Generic Name	Trade Name
Thyroid supplements	levothyroxine sodium (synthetic T_4) ☀	Synthroid ☀ Levoxyl ☀ Levothroid ☀
	liothyronine (synthetic T_3)	Cytomel
	liotrix (T_4:T_3 = 4:1)	Thyrolar, Euthyroid
Thyroid suppressants	propylthiouracil (PTU)	Generic
	methimazole	Tapazole
Adjunctive (diagnostic tool for thyroid cancer)	thyrotropin	Thyrogen

☀, Top 200 drug. Thyroid supplements will be discussed separately from thyroid suppressants.

Thyroid Supplements

INDICATIONS

- Hypothyroidism of any origin as replacement therapy
- Pituitary TSH suppression, treatment or prevention of euthyroid goiters, and management of thyroid cancer
  Thyroxine (T_4) is the mainstay of treatment for uncomplicated hypothyroidism. T_4 or triiodothyronine (T_3) is used for suppressive treatment for conditions such as thyroid cancer. Treatment for hypothyroidism and suppressive treatment for individuals with a history of thyroid cancer generally require lifelong replacement with thyroid hormone.

THERAPEUTIC OVERVIEW

Anatomy and Physiology

Regulation of a basal metabolism is achieved through complex coordination of the hypothalamic-pituitary-thyroid feedback control system (Figure 51-1). T_4 and T_3 are released from the thyroid gland in response to circulating serum levels of TSH secreted by the pituitary gland. In turn, TSH secretion is influenced by thyroid-releasing hormone (TRH) that is secreted by the hypothalamus. The feedback mechanism creates an inverse relationship between serum levels of T_3-T_4 and TSH-TRH. When T_3 and T_4 serum levels rise, TSH and TRH secretions are suppressed.

TRH and TSH levels can be measured directly. An elevated TSH, along with low circulating levels of free (unbound) T_3 and T_4, is diagnostic of primary hypothyroidism. Conversely, a low or undetectable TSH with high circulating levels of free T_3 and T_4 is diagnostic of thyrotoxicosis. A low TSH accompanied by low T_4 and T_3 or a high TSH with high levels of T_4 and T_3 is characteristic or a central cause (secondary or tertiary) of hypothyroidism or thyrotoxicosis, respectively.

Although rarely indicated, a stimulation test for TRH may be obtained if secondary hypothyroidism is suspected.

The thyroid gland releases T_4 (90%), T_3 (10%), and reverse T_3 (rT_3) (<1%). Elevated rT_3 may be an indication of euthyroid sick syndrome. This test usually is reserved for use when standard thyroid function tests (TFTs) yield inconclusive results.

T_3 and T_4 have a high affinity for protein. T_3 is 99.7% protein bound, whereas T_4 is 99.97% protein bound. Only the unbound portion is metabolically active. In the peripheral tissue, T_4 is converted to T_3 through the removal of iodine. Therefore, in most cases, it is necessary to administer only T_4 because the body will produce T_3 from T_4. The physiologic effects of thyroid hormones are attributed to the peripheral T_3.

Thyroid hormones exert their effect on nearly every system of the body through a variety of mechanisms. Basal metabolic rate is regulated by thyroid hormones. Thyroid hormones also influence oxygen consumption, respiratory rate, body temperature, heart rate, stroke volume, enzyme system activity, the rate of fat, protein, and carbohydrate metabolism, and growth and maturation. They are especially important in central nervous development.

Pathophysiology

In children, thyroid hormones are essential for overall normal growth and development. Without thyroid hormone, development of the central nervous system is impaired. Undetected deficiency of thyroid hormone may begin to affect children shortly after birth (as evidenced by cretinism).

Adults also may develop numerous problems related to a decreased metabolic rate. Cardiovascular, gastrointestinal, musculoskeletal, and neurologic function may be impaired by inadequate thyroid hormones.

Primary hypothyroidism, the most common form of hypothyroidism, is caused by a failure within the thyroid gland.

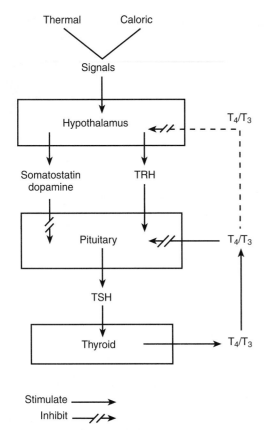

FIGURE 51-1   Regulation of thyroid-stimulating hormone secretion. Thyroxine (T_4) and triiodothyronine (T_3) from the thyroid gland exert negative feedback on the pituitary by blocking the action of TRH. Negative feedback of T_4 and T_3 at the level of the hypothalamus is less well established. Somatostatin and dopamine each tonically inhibits TSH secretion. (From Berne RM, Levy MN: *Physiology*, ed 4, St Louis, 1998, Mosby.)

Secondary hypothyroidism is caused by lack of TSH secretion from the pituitary. Tertiary hypothyroidism is caused by lack of TRH secretion from the hypothalamus.

Primary hypothyroidism has a variety of causes. One common cause is iatrogenic, that is, the result of therapy for thyrotoxicosis or other drugs such as lithium. Other causes include idiopathic thyroid atrophy and autoimmune destruction of the thyroid, such as Hashimoto's thyroiditis or postpartum thyroid disease.

Disease Process

Hypothyroidism is the metabolic state that results from deficient thyroid hormones. In adults, it is most common in women and is characterized by signs and symptoms consistent with altered energy metabolism, such as fatigue, lethargy, sensitivity to cold, dry skin, and menstrual disturbances. If untreated, it can progress to life-threatening myxedema, with characteristic appearance and physical symptoms, especially of the skin, and cardiovascular instability.

Table 51-1 lists altered laboratory findings in thyroid dysfunction. TSH is the most sensitive and useful test in the diagnosis of hypothyroidism. Free T_4 and T_3 are also useful. The amount of circulating and unbound hormones is reduced in patients with this disorder.

MECHANISM OF ACTION

A thyroid supplement serves to replace inadequate levels of endogenous T_3 and T_4. If an exogenous thyroid hormone is given to a euthyroid patient, endogenous secretion of TSH and TRH will be suppressed, as will the body's production of T_3 and T_4.

Basal metabolic rate and metabolism of carbohydrates, proteins, and fats are increased by thyroid supplements. These drugs also exert a direct effect on tissue (e.g., increased myocardial contraction).

Thyrogen is a recombinant DNA source of human TSH useful in the management and treatment of thyroid cancer patients.

TREATMENT PRINCIPLES

Standardized Guidelines

- American Association of Clinical Endocrinologists (AACE) Thyroid Task Force: Medical guidelines for clinical practice for the evaluation and treatment of thyrotoxicosis and hypothyroidism. *Endocr Pract* 8:457-469, 2002.
- American College of Obstetricians and Gynecologists (ACOG): *Thyroid disease in pregnancy*. Washington, DC, 2002, ACOG.

Evidence-Based Recommendations

- *Overt hypothyroidism:* Beneficial: levothyroxine; unknown effectiveness: levothyroxine plus liothyronine
- *Subclinical hypothyroidism:* Unknown effectiveness: levothyroxine

TABLE 51-1   Altered Laboratory Findings in Thyroid Dysfunction

Dysfunctional States	TSH	T_4/Free T_4	T_3/Free T_3	Free Thyroxine Index (FTI)	T_3 Uptake	rT_3
HYPOTHYROID STATES						
Primary	Increased	Decreased	Decreased	Decreased	Not useful	Normal
Secondary	Normal or decreased	Decreased	Decreased	Decreased	Not useful	Normal
Subclinical hypothyroidism	Increased	Normal	Normal	Normal	Not useful	Normal
HYPERTHYROID STATES						
Primary	Decreased	Increased	Increased	Increased	Increased	Normal
Secondary	Increased	Increased	Increased	Increased	Increased	Normal
EUTHYROID						
Sick syndrome	Normal or decreased	Normal or decreased	Decreased	Increased	Not useful	Increased

Cardinal Points of Treatment

- Treat hypothyroidism with levothyroxine.
- Dosage of all thyroid medication must be individualized. Dosage is based on laboratory findings and the patient's clinical response. Treatment of choice for hypothyroidism is T_4. It has a relatively slow onset of action, and its effects are cumulative over several weeks. T_3 has a more rapid onset of action and dissipation of action. T_3 may be the preferred treatment for use in rapidly correcting a hypothyroid state, in radioisotope scanning procedures, and in thyroid cancer. No evidence shows that the addition of T_3 to T_4 supplement has any benefit.
- The mean replacement dosage of levothyroxine is 1.6 mcg/kg of body weight per day, although the appropriate dosage varies among patients. The pace of treatment depends on the duration and severity of hypothyroidism and on whether other associated medical problems are present. The patient should undergo reassessment, and therapy should be titrated after an interval of 4 to 6 weeks following any change in levothyroxine brand or dose. Dosage should be titrated until a normal TSH is obtained. Adults younger than age 65 without coronary artery disease may begin with 50 to 100 mcg per day. Elderly patients and those with coronary artery disease generally should be started on a daily dose of 25 mcg. The usual maintenance dose is 75 to 150 mg po daily.
- Thyroid hormone should be administered as a single daily dose, preferably before breakfast. Levothyroxine doses are commonly measured in micrograms rather than milligrams to avoid confusion regarding the dosage. A correct dose is 75 mcg, which is the equivalent of 0.075 mg.

- The AACE emphasizes that many brands of levothyroxine are available, and these are not compared against a levothyroxine standard. Bioequivalence of levothyroxine preparations is based on total T_4 measurement and not on TSH levels; therefore, bioequivalence is not the same as therapeutic equivalence. It is recommended that patients should receive the same brand of levothyroxine throughout treatment. In general, desiccated thyroid hormone, combinations of thyroid hormones, or triiodothyronine should not be used as replacement therapy.

How to Monitor

See Tables 51-2 and 51-3.

The test for T_4 measures total thyroxine, both bound and unbound in the serum. Free thyroxine (FT_4) measures only unbound T_4. Normally, only T_4 must be measured; thyroid-binding globulin (TBG) is the protein to which thyroid hormones are bound. It can be measured directly by the TBG test. Resin T_3 uptake (T_3 RU) is an indirect measure that is no longer used. If the patient has an abnormal TBG, free T_4 may have to be evaluated.

Usually, measuring the TSH within 4 to 6 weeks is sufficient. Full therapeutic effectiveness may not be achieved for 3 to 6 weeks. TSH and symptom review usually are monitored monthly until normal and stable. Annual evaluation is recommended once maintenance therapy has been achieved. Levels also should be evaluated whenever patients experience signs and/or symptoms that could be related to underdosage/overdosage.

Children younger than 3 years of age should be maintained on the upper end of the T_4 therapeutic range with a

TABLE 51-2 Laboratory Evaluation of Thyroid Disorders

Test	Hormone Evaluated	Interpretation of Test Results
TRH (thyrotropin)	Thyrotropin-releasing hormone	Assesses the function of the hypothalamic-pituitary-thyroid axis. Most useful when other tests are inconclusive
TSH	Thyroid-stimulating hormone	Assesses the function of the hypothalamic-pituitary-thyroid axis
TBG (thyroglobulin)	Thyroxine-binding globulin	As the primary protein for hormone binding, it is most useful for evaluating discrepancies in clinical findings and other serum hormone levels
T_4 (T_4 RIA, thyroxine)	Tetraiodothyronine, thyroxine	Concentration of bound and unbound thyroid hormone (T_4) in the serum
FT_4	Free thyroxine, free T_4	Concentration of unbound thyroid hormone (T_4) in the serum. It is most helpful for diagnosis when TBG level is abnormal.
T_3 (T_3 RIA)	Triiodothyronine	Concentration of bound and unbound thyroid hormone (T_3) in the serum
FT_3	Free triiodothyronine, free T_3	Concentration of unbound, active T_3 in the serum
T_3-U (T_3 RU)	Resin T_3 uptake	Indirectly measures the concentration of thyroglobulin (TBG) by measuring the empty TBG binding sites in serum. Direct measurement of TBG may be more useful.
rT_3	Reverse T_3	A T_3 antagonist, rT_3 can be increased in euthyroid sick syndrome.
FTI (F T_4-I, T_7, T_{12})	Free T_4 index	Derived by multiplying T_4 and T_3-U, it reflects the free (unbound) T_4 in serum. This test essentially has been replaced by direct FT_3 and FT_4 measurements
LATS	Long-acting thyroid stimulator	A positive test supports the diagnosis of Graves' disease.
Antithyroid antibodies	Antithyroglobulin antibodies and/or antithyroid peroxidase antibodies	High titers in individuals with Hashimoto's thyroiditis and Graves' disease
	Anti-TSH receptor antibodies	High titers in individuals with Graves' disease

TABLE 51-3 Normal Range for Thyroid Function Laboratory Tests

Name of Test	Normal Range for Values
TRH (thyrotropin-releasing hormone)	Males: 14-24 micro units/ml Females: 16-26 micro units/ml
TSH (thyroid-stimulating hormone)	Newborn: <20 micro units/ml Adult: 0.30-5.5 micro units/ml
TBG (thyroglobulin)	16-34 micro units/ml
T$_4$ (thyroxine)	Newborn: 6.4-23.2 mcg/ml Child (1-10 yr): 6.4-15 mcg/ml Adult: 5-12 mcg/ml
FT$_4$ (free thyroxine)	0.9-1.7 ng/dl
T$_3$ (triiodothyronine)	Newborn: 32-250 ng/ml Child (1-10 yr): 94-269 ng/ml Adult: 95-190 ng/ml
FT$_3$ (free triiodothyronine)	0.2-0.52 ng/dl
T$_3$-U (resin T$_3$ uptake)	25%-35%
FTI (free thyroxine index)	1.3-4.2
Antithyroid antibodies: Anti-TBG antimicrosomal	Negative or titer <1:100
LATS (long-acting thyroid stimulator)	Negative

normal serum TSH. It is recommended that children undergo laboratory assessment of medication effectiveness every 1 to 2 months for the first year, every 2 to 3 months from 1 to 3 years old, and every 3 to 12 months thereafter.

Patients with a history of thyroid cancer who have had partial or total removal of their thyroid gland must take thyroid hormone supplements to suppress endogenous levels of TSH and to regulate their metabolism. However, a high level of TSH in a patient's bloodstream is necessary for radioiodine imaging to detect remnant thyroid tissue or metastatic disease, and for optimal sensitivity of serum thyroglobulin testing to be achieved. In the past, patients had to stop taking their hormone supplements for 2 to 6 weeks prior to testing, causing them to experience symptoms of thyroid deficiency. Thyrogen, which is a recombinant form of TSH, allows the patients to avoid hormone withdrawal and its debilitating effects while they are undergoing diagnostic testing. Specifically, thyrogen is a new diagnostic agent for adjunctive use in serum thyroglobulin testing with or without radioiodine imaging in the follow-up of patients with well-differentiated thyroid cancer.

Patient Variables

GERIATRICS. Hypothyroidism is common in the elderly. Atypical presentation includes CHF. Administration of thyroid hormone may exacerbate cardiovascular disease, particularly angina, in elderly patients. It is advisable to start low (25 mcg) and gradually increase the dosage. Absorption of the drug may increase with aging, so dosage adjustments may be required.

PEDIATRICS. Thyroid function is paramount for normal growth and development, especially of the central nervous system in children. At risk neonates should undergo FT$_4$ and

TSH screening as soon as possible after birth. Diagnosis and treatment of congenital hypothyroidism are essential in preventing cretinism. It is expected that children will require higher doses of medication to meet the metabolic demands of growth and development during the first 3 years of life. In congenital hypothyroidism, therapy may be stopped for 2 to 8 weeks after the patient reaches 3 years of age. If TSH levels remain normal, thyroid supplementation may be discontinued permanently.

PREGNANCY AND LACTATION. *Category A:* Excretion of thyroid medications in breast milk is minimal. Adjustment of thyroid hormone supplementation is common during pregnancy because of increased energy demands. Thus, close monitoring of the TSH is indicated.

Patient Education

Inform the patient and/or caregiver of the following:
- Response to this medication is not immediate. Symptoms should improve within 2 weeks.
- Thyroid deficiency generally requires lifelong therapy. Taking the medication and ensuring compliance with therapy are extremely important.
- One must not alter doses or abruptly stop the medication unless directed by the primary care provider.
- Changing the brand of medication used should be avoided because of potential variability in bioequivalence between manufacturers. (Counseling about this must be provided, so that the pharmacist will cooperate as the drug is dispensed.)
- The medication should be taken at approximately the same time each day. The preferable time of day is before breakfast or on an empty stomach to increase absorption. Taking the medication too late in the day may make it difficult to go to sleep.
- Signs and symptoms of overdosage (thyrotoxicosis) or underdosage (hypothyroidism) should be reported to the health care provider promptly. See Table 51-4 for symptoms.

SPECIFIC DRUGS

levothyroxine sodium (T$_4$) (Synthroid, Levothroid, Levo-T)

CONTRAINDICATIONS. Untreated thyrotoxicosis, uncorrected adrenal insufficiency (may precipitate adrenal crisis), recent MI, or hypersensitivity to any of the medication components

WARNINGS/PRECAUTIONS
- It is inappropriate to use any thyroid supplement for the management of obesity or fertility.
- Patients with known cardiovascular disease should be monitored carefully while taking levothyroxine. Problems also may occur in cases of occult cardiovascular disease. Therefore, this agent should be cautiously administered to patients with the potential for undiagnosed disease. Start with a low dose—25 to 50 mcg—and increase the dose slowly.
- Diabetes mellitus and diabetes insipidus may be aggravated by initiation of levothyroxine. Closely monitor and accordingly modify treatment(s) for these conditions.
- Use with caution in those patients who have had a recent MI.

TABLE 51-4   Clinical Presentation of Thyroid Dysfunction

Type of Signs/Symptoms	Thyrotoxicosis	Hypothyroidism
INITIAL		
Most frequent concerns that prompt medical care and evaluation	Amenorrhea/oligomenorrhea Frequent bowel movements Goiter Nervousness/irritability Palpitations (tachycardia) Sleep disturbance (insomnia) Unexplained weight loss Vision changes (exophthalmos) Anxious	Cold intolerance Depression and loss of concentration Dry skin (pruritus) Menorrhagia Myalgias Somnolence and fatigue
LATER		
May be evident at initial evaluation but usually develop with prolonged disease	Dependent edema Dyspnea Impaired mentation (confusion) Muscle weakness and fatigue Tremor	Constipation Goiter Memory loss/impairment Myxedema Unexplained weight gain
INCIDENTAL		
May be identified on physical examination but may not be offered as a complaint by the patient unless asked directly	Diaphoresis Heat intolerance Increased appetite	Anorexia Bradycardia Habitual abortion/sterility Impotence

Because preparations vary, make certain to write the prescription in such a way that the patient will receive the same brand of medication throughout treatment.

PHARMACOKINETICS. See Table 51-5. T_4 absorption from the gastrointestinal tract is poor (50% to 80%) but may be enhanced with fasting and reduced farther through malabsorption syndromes. A higher affinity for serum protein increases the half-life of T_4 as compared with T_3.

ADVERSE EFFECTS. See Table 51-6. Thyroid hormone absorption may be affected by a malabsorptive state and by patient age. Because levothyroxine has a narrow therapeutic range, small differences in absorption may result in subclinical or clinical hypothyroidism, or in thyrotoxicosis.

DRUG INTERACTIONS. Certain drugs, such as cholestyramine, colestipol, ferrous sulfate, sucralfate, calcium, and some antacids that contain aluminum hydroxide, interfere with levothyroxine absorption. Some anticonvulsants affect thyroid hormone bindings. Rifampin and sertraline hydrochloride may acwcelerate levothyroxine metabolism, thereby necessitating a higher replacement dose. Oral anticoagulants may have an increased effect related to vitamin K metabolism. Androgens and estrogens may reduce protein binding and decrease medication effectiveness. Insulin and oral hypoglycemic agents may be less effective upon initiation of therapy. Therefore, dosage adjustments may be required to maintain blood glucose levels. β-Blockers and digitalis preparations may become less effective as the condition of the hypothyroid patient improves.

OVERDOSAGE. Toxicity is evidenced by signs and symptoms of thyrotoxicosis and may mimic thyrotoxicosis. Decrease or temporarily discontinue levothyroxine for approximately 5 to 7 days, and then resume at a lower dose.

DOSAGE AND ADMINISTRATION. See Table 51-7.

liothyronine (T₃) (Cytomel, Triostat)

INDICATIONS. Liothyronine effectively treats hypothyroidism resulting from any cause other than transient thyroiditis. The most common uses are for thyroid suppression testing for evaluation and treatment of euthyroid goiter, myxedema nodular thyroid, and thyroid cancer.

TABLE 51-5   Pharmacokinetics of Thyroid Supplements

Drug	Absorption	Onset of Action	Time to Peak Concentration	Half-life	Duration of Action	Protein Bound	Metabolism
levothyroxine	Variable in GI (50%-80%)	3-5 days	2-4 hr	6-7 days	2-3 wk	99%	Biliary
liothyronine	Complete in GI (95% in 4 hr)	2-4 hr	1-2 hr	2-3 days	3-5 days	99%	Biliary/renal
liotrix (4 parts T₄, 1 part T₃)	Variable in GI but T₃>T₄	T₃: 12-36 hr T₄: Unknown	T₃: 24-72 hr T₄: 1-3 wk	T₃: 2-3 days T₄: 6-7 days	T₃: 3-5 days T₄: 1-3 wk	99%	Biliary/renal

TABLE 51-6   Adverse Effects of Thyroid Supplements

System	liothyronine	levothyroxine	liotrix
Dermatologic	Alopecia (children) Diaphoresis	Diaphoresis	Alopecia (children) Diaphoresis
Cardiovascular	Angina Arrhythmias Tachycardia	Angina Arrhythmias Palpitations	Angina Arrhythmias Tachycardia
GI	Abdominal cramps Diarrhea Nausea/vomiting	Abdominal cramps Diarrhea Nausea/vomiting	Abdominal cramps Diarrhea Nausea/vomiting
Endocrine	Irregular menses	Hyperglycemia Hypocholesterolemia Irregular menses	Hyperglycemia Hypocholesterolemia Irregular menses
Metabolic	Heat intolerance Weight loss	Heat intolerance Weight loss	Heat intolerance Weight loss
CNS	Insomnia Irritability Nervousness	Headache Insomnia Nervousness	Insomnia Irritability Nervousness

TABLE 51-7   Dosage and Administration of Thyroid Supplements

Thyroid Supplement	Hypothyroidism	Thyroid Suppression
liothyronine	Oral: 25 mcg/day; increase by 12.5-25 mcg/day every 1-2 weeks to a maximum of 100 mcg/day *Congenital hypothyroidism:* 5 mcg/day; increase by 5 mcg every 3-4 days until the desired response is achieved *Usual maintenance dose:* Infants: 20 mcg/day Children 1-3 yrs: 50 mcg/day Children >3 years: Adult dose	Adults: 75-100 mcg/day for 7 days

liotrix	Adults: 30 mg/day (15 mg/day if cardiovascular impairment); increase by 15 mg/day every 2-3 weeks
	Maximum of 180 mg/day
	Usual maintenance dose: 60-120 mg/day
	Congenital hypothyroidism:
	Children (dose of T4 or levothyroxine/day):
	  0-6 months: 8-10 mcg/kg or 25-50 mcg/day
	  6-12 months: 6-8 mcg/kg or 50-75 mcg/day
	  1-5 years: 5-6 mcg/kg or 75-100 mcg/day
	  6-12 years: 4-5 mcg/kg or 100-150 mcg/day
	  >12 years: 2-3 mcg/kg or >150 mcg/day	

levothyroxine	Adults: 1.7 mcg/kg/day in otherwise healthy adults <50 years old, children in whom growth and puberty are complete, and older adults who have been recently treated for hyperthyroidism or who have been hypothyroid for only a few months
	Increase every 6 weeks.
	Usual starting dose: 100 mcg
	Hypothyroidism:
	Newborns: 10-15 mcg/kg. Lower doses of 25 mcg/day should be considered in newborns at risk for cardiac failure.
	Increase dose every 4- to 6-weeks
	Infants and children:
	  0-3 months: 10-15 mcg/kg/day
	  3-6 months: 8-10 mcg/kg/day
	  6-12 months: 6-8 mcg/kg/day
	  1-5 years: 5-6 mcg/kg/day
	  6-12 years: 4-5 mcg/kg/day
	  >12 years: 2-3 mcg/kg/day	

liotrix (Thyrolar, Euthyroid)

INDICATIONS. Patients with any form of hypothyroidism may be effectively treated with liotrix. Therapy for myxedema and thyroid suppression (used in euthyroid goiter and nodular thyroid) are other common uses.

Thyroid Suppressants

INDICATIONS

- *Hyperthyroidism:* Thyrotoxicosis (in particular for primary hyperthyroidism): Long-term use may lead to disease remission. Used when surgery is contraindicated. Also used to ameliorate thyrotoxicosis before subtotal thyroidectomy or radioactive iodine therapy

Unlabeled Use

- Propylthiouracil (PTU) may prove useful in alcoholic liver disease by reducing the hepatic hypermetabolic state induced by alcohol.

THERAPEUTIC OVERVIEW

Pathophysiology

Thyrotoxicosis is the clinical state that results from an excess of thyroid hormone. The most common cause of thyrotoxicosis is primary hyperthyroidism due to, for example, Graves' disease, toxic nodular goiter, and iodide-induced hyperthyroidism (Saxe, 2004). An autoimmune process causes Graves' disease, also known as diffuse toxic goiter. Toxic nodular goiter is due to hyperfunctioning of a uninodular or multinodular goiter. Exposure to iodide is iatrogenic. Other causes of thyrotoxicosis include thyroid inflammatory diseases such as postpartum thyroiditis and subacute thyroiditis. In thyroiditis, thyrotoxicosis is usually transient.

Disease Process

The presentation of thyrotoxicosis is highly variable. See Table 51-4 for symptoms of thyrotoxicosis.

Excessive synthesis of thyroid hormone increases the individual's basal metabolism to potentially fatal levels. Cardiovascular and neurologic function may be markedly stimulated, resulting in systemic collapse.

Diagnosis is based on symptoms, physical findings, and laboratory findings. TSH will be suppressed, and T_3 and T_4 will be increased. See Table 51-1 for altered laboratory findings in thyroid dysfunction.

MECHANISM OF ACTION

Through diversion of iodine, thyroid hormone synthesis is inhibited. PTU, but not methimazole, also inhibits the conversion of T_4 to T_3 in the tissue.

Through reduced absorption of iodine, thyroid hormone synthesis is diminished. As the thyroid gland becomes depleted of hormones, tissue concentrations drop and the metabolic rate decreases. However, medications do not inhibit stored or circulating levels of T_3 or T_4. Thyroid suppressant agents do not affect oral and parenteral thyroid supplements. Normal thyroid hormone synthesis resumes rapidly with cessation of therapy. PTU also inhibits conversion of T_4 to T_3 in peripheral tissues, different from methimazole. This speeds conversion to a euthyroid state. Methimazole has the advantage of being longer acting; it therefore requires a less frequent dosage schedule, and this may enhance compliance.

TREATMENT PRINCIPLES

Standardized Guidelines

- American Association of Clinical Endocrinologists. Medical guidelines for clinical practice for the evaluation and treatment of hyperthyroidism and hypothyroidism (available at www.guideline.gov/summary/summary.aspx?doc_id =3525&nbr=002751&string=thyrotoxicosis).

Evidence-Based Recommendations

- Levothyroxine (L-thyroxine) therapy has been found to be effective in hypothyroidism.
- Antithyroid drugs (carbimazole, propylthiouracil, and thiamazole) have been found to be effective in treating patients with hyperthyroidism.
- Any antithyroid medication is likely to be effective in treating those with subclinical hyperthyroidism.

Cardinal Points of Treatment

- *First-line treatment for Graves' disease and toxic multinodular goiter:* Radioactive iodine (*Note:* Pretreatment with an antithyroid medication is indicated for elderly patients and those with cardiovascular disease.)
- *Second-line:* Surgical intervention
- *Third-line:* Antithyroid drugs
- Rest, adequate diet, and avoidance of occupational and domestic stress are other therapeutic modalities. Radioactive iodine is the usual treatment. Surgery is an option for patients who cannot tolerate or refuse radioactive iodine. Thyroid suppressants are an option for patients who cannot tolerate either option.
- Antithyroid drugs are prescribed to achieve remission of symptoms. Remission rates are variable, and symptom relapses are frequent. Remission is most likely to occur in patients with mild hyperthyroidism and small goiters. "Pretreatment" with antithyroid drugs before radioiodine therapy may be necessary for some elderly or cardiac patients. Some endocrinologists prefer antithyroid drug therapy in childhood Graves' disease. Primary hyperthyroidism during pregnancy is one clear indication for antithyroid drug treatment. These drugs will control excessive production of thyroid hormone in almost all cases of thyrotoxicosis. Up to half of patients will experience a permanent remission. However, relapses are frequent. Temporary hypothyroidism may occur with overtreatment.
- Antithyroid drugs will restore a euthyroid state in 4 to 8 weeks, although symptoms will improve sooner—usually in 1 to 2 weeks. The patient should be euthyroid before surgery. Antithyroid drugs may be required before and after radioiodine therapy.
- Titration of dosage to gain maximum therapeutic response with the lowest dosage is the objective. Generally, therapy is maintained for 12 to 18 months. Once the patient has been euthyroid for 6 to 12 months, a decision may be made to reduce dosage and ascertain whether a remission has occurred. If remission is achieved, therapy is discontinued.

Consultation and referral to a physician is warranted during treatment initiation and when the decision is made to maintain or end therapy.

- β-Adrenergic-blocking drugs such as propranolol or atenolol can be used to control the signs and symptoms of thyrotoxicosis that are related to sensitization of the sympathetic nervous system (see Chapter 18). β-Adrenergic-blocking drugs should be used cautiously in patients with asthma or heart failure.

How to Monitor

Laboratory blood work should be done before antithyroid therapy is initiated and periodically once the patient is on a maintenance dose. Serum T_4 and T_3 levels are monitored initially and after 3 to 6 weeks of therapy until a euthyroid state is achieved—usually in 3 to 5 months. Once clinical evidence of thyrotoxicosis has been resolved, an elevated TSH level indicates a need to lower the dosage.

Before treatment is initiated, a WBC count with differential is done; it is repeated with any sign of infection. Some recommend routine monitoring of the WBC for at least the first 3 months of therapy. Monitor prothrombin time during therapy, especially before surgical procedures are performed.

With the potential for hepatotoxicity, AST, ALT, alkaline phosphatase, LDH, bilirubin, and PT also may be evaluated.

During each visit, monitor for signs and symptoms of infection, as well as correction of the hypermetabolic state, seen as decreased pulse, decreased blood pressure, weight gain, elimination of nervousness, and tremor. Evaluate for hepatitis, agranulocytosis, and GI irritation (see Tables 51-2 and 51-3).

Patient Variables

GERIATRICS. Elderly individuals are less likely to experience thyrotoxicosis than hypothyroidism. Thyrotoxicosis in the elderly may have an atypical presentation consisting of symptoms such as lassitude, anorexia, and palpitations (often consistent with atrial fibrillation).

PEDIATRICS. PTU hepatotoxicity has occurred; discontinue immediately if signs and symptoms of hepatic dysfunction become apparent.

PREGNANCY AND LACTATION

- *Category D:* Thyroid suppressants cross the placenta and can induce goiter or cretinism. PTU generally is preferred if a drug is necessary. They can be effective if used judiciously. In many pregnant women, thyrotoxicosis diminishes as the pregnancy proceeds, making dosage reduction or discontinuation of the drug possible. An endocrinologist usually follows the patient.

- Thyroid suppressants should not be given while the patient is breastfeeding.

Patient Education

Inform the patient and/or caregiver to do the following:

- Avoid the ingestion of substances that contain iodine (e.g., seafood, iodized salt).
- Notify the practitioner immediately of any illness or unusual signs or symptoms. Report to the health care provider fever, sore throat, malaise, unusual bleeding or bruising, headache, skin rash, or enlargement of cervical lymph nodes.

SPECIFIC DRUGS

propylthiouracil (PTU) (Generic)

CONTRAINDICATIONS. Hypersensitivity to any of the medication components

WARNINGS/PRECAUTIONS. Agranulocytosis is potentially the most serious side effect. Individuals at greatest risk for this life-threatening condition are those over the age of 40. Bone marrow function assessed via complete blood count with differential should be closely monitored throughout therapy and up to 4 months after completion of therapy. Thrombocytopenia or aplastic anemia also may occur.

Discontinue the drug in the presence of agranulocytosis, aplastic anemia, hepatitis, fever, or exfoliative dermatitis.

Use with caution in patients older than 40 years of age. Use with caution in combination with other agranulocytosis-precipitating medications.

Carcinogenesis: Carcinoma formation has been seen in laboratory animals treated with PTU for longer than 1 year.

PHARMACOKINETICS. See Table 51-8.

ADVERSE EFFECTS. See Table 51-9. Antithyroid drug treatment is not provided without the risk of adverse reactions, including minor rashes and, in rare instances, agranulocytosis and hepatitis.

DRUG INTERACTIONS. Oral anticoagulants may decrease the efficacy of PTU. Digoxin levels may rise (especially as the patient becomes euthyroid). Thyroid uptake to ^{131}I may be reduced. Amiodarone, iodine, potassium iodide, and iodinated glycerol may decrease medication efficacy.

OVERDOSAGE. Symptoms include nausea, vomiting, epigastric distress, headache, fever, arthralgia, pruritus, edema, pancytopenia, and agranulocytosis. More rare are exfoliative

TABLE 51-8 Pharmacokinetics of Thyroid Suppressants

Drug	Absorption	Onset of Action	Time to Peak Concentration	Half-life	Duration of Action	Protein Bound	Metabolism	Excretion
methimazole	Rapid, via GI tract	12-18 hr	0.5-1 hr	6-12 hr*	1.5-3 days	None	Hepatic	Renal
propylthiouracil	Rapid, via GI tract	10-21 days*	1 hr	1-4 hr*	2 wk	80%	Hepatic	Renal

*However, thyroid hormone may begin to increase as soon as 1 hour after dose is given.

From Hardman JG, Limbird LE, editors: *Goodman & Gilman's the pharmacological basis of therapeutics,* ed 11, New York, 2007, McGraw-Hill.

TABLE 51-9 Adverse Effects of Thyroid Suppressants

System	methimazole	propylthiouracil
Dermatologic	Pruritus Rash Urticaria	Rash Skin discoloration Urticaria
GI	Hepatitis (potentially fatal) Nausea/vomiting	Diarrhea Diminished taste Hepatitis (potentially fatal) Nausea/vomiting
CNS	Headache Paresthesia Vertigo	Drowsiness Headache Vertigo
Musculoskeletal	Arthralgia	Arthralgia
Hematologic	Agranulocytosis Aplastic anemia Hypoprothrombinemia Leukopenia Thrombocytopenia	Agranulocytosis Aplastic anemia Hypoprothrombinemia Leukopenia Thrombocytopenia

dermatitis, hepatitis, neuropathy, and CNS stimulation or depression.

DOSAGE AND ADMINISTRATION
   Adult
- *Initial:* 300 to 450 mg/day in four divided doses
- *Maintenance:* 50 to 100 mg daily (Greenspan & Dong, 2007, p 630)
   Child
- *Initial:* 50 to 150 mg/day (6 to 10 years), 150 to 300 mg/day (>10 years) in divided doses every 8 hours
- *Maintenance:* Based on patient's response to therapy

methimazole (Tapazole)

DOSAGE AND ADMINISTRATION
   Adults
- *Initial:* 15 mg/day (mild disease), 30 to 40 mg/day (moderate disease), 60 mg/day (severe disease) divided into three doses
- *Maintenance:* 5 to 15 mg daily
   Children
- *Initial:* 0.4 mg/kg/day in three divided doses
- *Maintenance:* 0.2 mg/kg/day or approximately half of the initial daily dose in three divided doses. Maximum, 30 mg/day

Adjunctive (Diagnostic Tool for Thyroid Cancer)
SPECIFIC DRUGS
thyrotropin (Thyrogen)

INDICATIONS. In postsurgical evaluation of patients who require follow-up for remnant thyroid tissue, thyroid cancer recurrence, or metastasis. Used in conjunction with or without radioiodine imaging

MECHANISM OF ACTION. Significantly enhances the sensitivity of thyroglobulin testing in patients maintained on thyroid hormone therapy. Allows patients with thyroid cancer to avoid the debilitating effects of hypothyroidism when undergoing radioiodine imaging scans.

ADVERSE EFFECTS. Nausea, headache, and mild reactions of hypersensitivity, such as urticaria or rash

evolve A continually updated list of useful WebLinks may be found in the Evolve Resources at http://evolve.elsevier.com/Edmunds/NP/

Diabetes Mellitus Agents

JANE KAPUSTIN

DRUG OVERVIEW

Class	Subclass	Generic Name	Trade Name
Insulin	Rapid acting	insulin lispro	Humalog ✴
		insulin aspart	NovoLog
		insulin glulisine	Apidra
	Short acting	Regular	Humulin R Novolin R
	Intermediate acting	NPH	Humulin N ✴ Novolin N
	Long acting	insulin glargine	Lantus ✴
		insulin detemir	Levemir
	Mixtures	70/30 (70% NPH, 30% regular)	Novolin 70/30 ✴ Humulin 70/30 ✴
		70/30 (70% aspart protamine/30% aspart)	NovoLog Mix 70/30 ✴
		50/50 (50% NPH, 50% regular) 50/50 (50% lispro protamine/50% lispro)	Humalog Mix 50/50
		75/25 Humalog (75% lispro protamine, 25% lispro)	Humalog Mix 75/25
ORAL MEDICATIONS			
Second-generation sulfonylureas		glyburide ✴	Micronase, DiaBeta; Glynase (micronized)
		glipizide 🔑 ✴	Glucotrol, Glucotrol XL
		glimepiride ✴	Amaryl
Biguanides		metformin ✴ metformin ER ✴	Glucophage, Glucophage XR, Fortamet
Thiazolidinediones		rosiglitazone 🔑	Avandia ✴
		pioglitazone	Actos ✴
Non-sulfonylureas secretagogues (meglitinides)		nateglinide ✴	Starlix
		repaglinide	Prandin
α-Glucosidase inhibitors		acarbose 🔑	Precose
		miglitol	Glyset
Incretin agents	Amylin analog	pramlintide	Symlin
	Glucagon-like peptide (GLP-1)	exenatide	Byetta ✴
	DPP-4 inhibitor	sitagliptin phosphate	Januvia

✴ Top 200 drug; 🔑 key drug.

Table continued on following page

DRUG OVERVIEW (Continued)

Class	Subclass	Generic Name	Trade Name
Combination therapies		metformin/rosiglitazone	Avandamet
		metformin/glyburide	Glucovance
		metformin/glipizide	Metaglip
		metformin/pioglitazone	Actoplus Met
		rosiglitazone/glimepiride	Avandaryl
		sitagliptin/metformin	Janumet
		pioglitazone/glimepiride	Duetect

INDICATIONS

- Diabetes, types 1 and 2

Pharmacologic agents are used in conjunction with diet and exercise to control blood glucose in those with diabetes. These agents include various insulins and seven classes of oral agents. Type 1 diabetes requires the use of insulin. Type 2 diabetes is present in approximately 90% of the 21 million Americans who have diabetes. These patients are usually started on oral medication. Insulin is added when oral medications provide inadequate control. The American Diabetes Association (ADA) and the American College of Endocrinology (ACE) diagnostic and treatment criteria are used in these guidelines.

THERAPEUTIC OVERVIEW

Anatomy and Physiology

The pancreas is a gland with both endocrine and exocrine functions. The islets of Langerhans, which constitute only 1% to 2% of the gland, contain more than 1 million cells. Eighty percent of these cells are β-cells that produce and secrete insulin. α-Cells, also a component of the islets, produce glucagon, a potent hormone that promotes glycogenolysis and gluconeogenesis in the liver. The pancreas and the liver are the primary organs of glucose regulation attained via a negative feedback mechanism. When blood glucose rises, β-cells are stimulated by elevated glucose to release insulin. Insulin allows the muscle and the liver to use glucose and to store it as glycogen in the liver. Insulin also facilitates fat storage in adipose tissue, as well as uptake and conversion of amino acids to protein. As blood glucose levels fall, the cells are stimulated to release glucagon, resulting in glycogenolysis and gluconeogenesis in the liver. Glycogenolysis (conversion of glycogen into glucose) and gluconeogenesis (production of glucose from lactate and amino acids) result in increased serum glucose levels.

Insulin lowers blood glucose by enhancing glucose transport via facilitated diffusion into target tissues. Insulin binds to and stimulates receptors on each cell; this in turn fosters transport of glucose through the cell wall. Tissue insensitivity to insulin can occur when defects in receptors or defects in receptor response to insulin are present. Insulin also inhibits lipoprotein lipase, thereby preventing the release of fatty acids into the blood. Insulin promotes the transport and storage of glucose as triglycerides in fat cells.

Pathophysiology

The onset of diabetes involves a relative or absolute lack of insulin and/or insulin resistance and impaired or insufficient target cell receptors. These effects cause a lack of available glucose for cellular metabolism, resulting in glycogenolysis, lipolysis, and gluconeogenesis. Glucose uptake by the liver is impaired with a resultant increase in circulating glucagon. Protein storage is decreased. Overproduction of free fatty acids by fat cells has been noted. Elevated plasma free fatty acid levels increase hepatic glucose production by stimulating gluconeogenesis.

Type 2 diabetes is characterized by two phenomena: insulin resistance and β-cell dysfunction. The cause of type 2 diabetes is unknown, but certain factors increase the risk of development of the disease. With type 2 diabetes, secretion is impaired, hepatic glucose production is increased, and insensitivity to insulin in the tissues (insulin resistance) occurs.

Initially in type 2 diabetes, tissues become insensitive or resistant to insulin. As a compensatory mechanism, insulin release is increased so that normal glucose levels can be maintained. In fact, often, those in whom type 2 diabetes is newly diagnosed exhibit elevated insulin levels in an attempt to overcome resistance.

Insulin secretion occurs in a biphasic manner. The first phase occurs rapidly, peaks in 3 to 5 minutes, and lasts about 10 minutes. This phase is triggered by a meal or a glucose challenge. If the blood glucose concentration remains elevated, then the second phase of insulin is triggered. This involves a slow release of insulin. Persons with type 2 diabetes lose first-phase insulin release, and postprandial hyperglycemia is the first sign. As the body endures continued exposure to hyperglycemia, the β-cells become more dysfunctional; this is referred to as *glucotoxicity*. This process often begins years prior to diagnosis of type 2 diabetes. With now a relative lack of insulin, gluconeogenesis and glycogenolysis are increased in the liver because these processes are dependent not on levels of glucose but on insulin levels. This further contributes to hyperglycemia and is often responsible for elevated fasting glucose levels.

Autoimmune destruction of β-cells is implicated in the diagnosis of type 1 diabetes. Environmental and genetic predisposition also may play a role. Onset of type 1 diabetes may occur suddenly as with the onset of diabetic ketoacidosis, or slowly with less risk of ketoacidosis.

Disease Process

Testing for type 2 diabetes should be considered in all adults age 45 years and older, particularly if overweight. Testing should be repeated every 3 years. According to the ADA, risk factors for the development of diabetes that should alert the provider to screen for diabetes include the following:

- Age ≥45 years
- Overweight (BMI ≥25 kg/m²)
- Family history of diabetes (i.e., parents or siblings who have diabetes)
- Habitual physical inactivity
- Race/ethnicity (e.g., African Americans, Hispanics, Native Americans, Asian Americans, Pacific Islanders)
- Previously identified impaired fasting glucose (IFG) or impaired glucose tolerance (IGT)
- History of gestational diabetes mellitus (GDM) or delivery of a baby weighing >9 pounds
- Hypertension ≥140/90 mm Hg in adults
- HDL cholesterol ≤35 mg/dl and/or triglyceride level ≥250 mg/dl
- Polycystic ovary syndrome or acanthosis nigricans
- History of vascular disease

HISTORY OF VASCULAR DISEASE. The Expert Committee on the Diagnosis and Classification of Diabetes under the sponsorship of the ADA modified criteria for diagnosis in 1998. These criteria were adopted by the ADA and represent current guidelines for diagnosis (Box 52-1).

Complications of diabetes include microvascular disease (nephropathy, retinopathy), macrovascular disease (coronary artery disease, peripheral vascular disease, cerebrovascular disease, neuropathy), and neuropathic disease (autonomic and peripheral). Vascular and neuropathic disease contributes to the increased risk of amputation. Multiple studies, such as the Diabetes Mellitus Control and Complications Trial research

group (DCCT) and the United Kingdom Prospective Diabetes Study (UKPDS), continue to show that intensive glucose control at or below glycosylated hemoglobin (HbA1c) of 7% prevents and/or delays the onset of complications.

Assessment

Conducting a thorough history and physical examination enables the provider to obtain a baseline evaluation, identify early effects and complications of diabetes, and, together with the patient, determine individual glycemic goals. ADA clinical practice recommendations list the following:

- History should include questions about skin changes, visual problems (history of retinopathy, date of last ophthalmologic examination), thyroid function (history of hypothyroid or hyperthyroid disease), cardiac arrhythmias, hypertension, lipid abnormalities, history of CAD and/or CHF, and hematologic, pulmonary, GI (chronic diarrhea, constipation, early satiety, liver disease), GU (urinary tract infection, difficulty voiding, incontinence, erectile dysfunction), obstetric and gynecologic (history of gestational diabetes, anticipation of pregnancy, contraceptive use), neurologic (weakness, muscle wasting, paresthesias, hyperesthesia, hypoglycemic unawareness), and vascular problems (leg pain, transient ischemic attacks).
- Physical examination should include assessment of height, weight, BMI, BP, vital signs, eye, mouth, thyroid, heart, lungs, abdomen (hepatic enlargement), bruits, pulses, hands, feet, skin (acanthosis nigricans, inflammation, infection), and nervous system (reflexes, sensory examination of feet).
- Laboratory evaluation includes CBC, CMP (including creatinine, BUN, TSH, Hbg , and HbA1c), fasting lipid profile, urinalysis, test for microalbuminuria), and ECG in adults. The HbA1c reflects the state of glycemia for the past 8 to 12 weeks.

MECHANISM OF ACTION

See Tables 52-1 and 52-2.

Insulin

Insulins are proteins that bind to cell wall receptors to allow cellular utilization of glucose. Insulin lowers blood glucose levels by stimulating peripheral glucose uptake, particularly

---

BOX 52-1   Criteria for the Diagnosis of Diabetes Mellitus

Symptoms of diabetes plus casual plasma glucose concentration >200 mg/dl. (Casual is defined as any time of day without regard for time since last meal.) Classic symptoms of diabetes include polyuria, polydipsia, polyphagia, and unexplained weight loss (for type 1).
Or
Fasting plasma glucose (FPG) >126 mg/dl is elevated. Fasting is defined as no caloric intake for at least 8 hours. (Prediabetes level is 100 mg/dl.) Two fasting blood sugars >126 are needed for a diagnosis of diabetes.
Or
Two-hour plasma glucose (PG) >200 mg/dl during an oral glucose tolerance test (OGTT). The test should be performed as described by WHO, with the use of a glucose load that contains the equivalent of 75 g anhydrous glucose dissolved in water.

Taken from the American Diabetes Association (Position Statement, 2008).

TABLE 52-1   ADA Recommended Glycemic Goals

	Normal	Goal	Additional Action Suggested
PLASMA VALUES			
Average preprandial glucose, mg/dl	<100	90-130	<90 or >150
Average bedtime glucose, mg/dl	<120	110-150	<110 or >180
Peak postprandial glucose, mg/dl		<180	
WHOLE BLOOD VALUES			
Average preprandial glucose, mg/dl	<100	80-120	<80 or >140
Average bedtime glucose, mg/dl	<110	100-140	<100 or >160
HbA1c, %	<6	<7	>8

TABLE 52-2   Mechanisms of Action of Diabetic Medications

Drug	Insulin Secretion from Pancreas	Hepatic Glucose Production	Peripheral Insulin Sensitivity	Glucose Absorption from GI Tract
Insulin	Decrease	Decrease	No change	None
Sulfonylureas	Increase	Slight decrease	Slight increase	None
Thiazolidinediones	No change	Decrease	Increase	None
Meglitinides	Increase	No change	No change	None
α-Glucosidase	No change	No change	No change	Delays
metformin	No change	Decrease	Increase	None
Incretins	Increase	Decrease	No change	Delays
Amylin replacement	No change	Decrease	No change	Delays

in skeletal muscle and fat, and by inhibiting hepatic glucose production. An adequate supply of insulin is needed for transport of glucose across the cell membrane to sustain life.

Most insulin used today is produced by deoxyribonucleic acid (DNA) recombinant technology and is synthesized in a nonpathogenic strain of *Escherichia coli* bacteria or *Saccharomyces cerevisiae* fungus. Advantages of using synthetic human insulin include a decrease in the production of insulin antibodies and a diminished risk for the development of lipodystrophy at the injection site.

Insulin analogs are insulin preparations that are produced by modifying the structure of human insulin. Changing human insulin properties with amino acid substitutions improves the pharmacokinetic profile for optimal physiologic insulin replacement.

Sulfonylureas

Because most first-generation sulfonylureas are no longer used, this chapter refers to second-generation sulfonylureas simply as sulfonylureas. (Chlorpropamide is still available in the United States but is rarely used.) Sulfonylureas enhance insulin secretion primarily by binding to receptor sites on β-cells. This causes a decrease in potassium permeability and membrane depolarization. The subsequent increase in intracellular calcium ions causes exocytosis of insulin from secretory granules. Other results include suppression of hepatic glucose production through entry of insulin into the portal vein and increased muscle glucose uptake via elevated insulin levels.

Biguanides

Metformin primarily decreases hepatic glucose production. It also has minor effects on insulin sensitivity in both the liver and peripheral tissues. It has no direct effect on the pancreas and therefore does not enhance insulin secretion. Metformin also has been shown to decrease triglycerides and LDLs and to increase HDLs.

Thiazolidinediones

Rosiglitazone and pioglitazone increase sensitivity in the muscle and liver by improving control of glycemic utilization. This in turn reduces circulating insulin levels. Functioning β-cells are required for these medications to work. Specifically, these drugs are agonists for peroxisome proliferator–activated receptors-γ (PPAR-γ), which are found in adipose tissue, skeletal muscle, and liver. Activation of PPAR-γ receptors regulates the insulin-responsive genes involved in the control of glucose production, transport, and utilization and facilitates the regulation of fatty acid metabolism.

Meglitinides

Repaglinide and nateglinide lower blood sugar by stimulating the release of insulin from the pancreas in short bursts. The patient must have functioning β-cells for the medication to work. They bind receptor sites to close ATP-dependent potassium channels in the β-cell membrane. This leads to opening of calcium channels, which causes an influx of calcium that induces insulin secretion.

α-Glucosidase Inhibitors

Acarbose and miglitol act through inhibition of pancreatic α-amylase and membrane-bound intestinal α-glucoside hydrolase enzymes. These enzymes are responsible for metabolizing complex starches to oligosaccharides and for breaking down remaining saccharides to glucose and other monosaccharides. This enzyme inhibition delays glucose absorption and lowers postprandial hyperglycemia. These enzymes do not enhance insulin secretion.

Incretin Agents

AMYLIN REPLACEMENT. Pramlintide is an analog of amylin; it is an endogenous peptide that is secreted in conjunction with insulin by the pancreatic β-cells. Pramlintide produces the same physiologic effects as are caused by amylin, but it is stable enough to be used as a medication. Amylin is known to do the following:

- Suppress glucagon production, especially in the postprandial state
- Reduce postprandial hepatic glucose production
- Delay gastric emptying time
- Centrally mediate induction of satiety
- Reduce postprandial glucose levels

Pramlintide is indicated in patients with type 1 diabetes and in those with insulin-requiring type 2 diabetes. It is given by subcutaneous injection three times a day before meals. This agent must be administered as a separate subcutaneous injection but in conjunction with insulin. It is helpful for patients with wide glycemic swings. It is weight neutral or may cause weight loss. The risk of hypoglycemia is significant, and close monitoring of blood glucose followed by frequent adjustments in the dosages of other diabetes medications is required. Its ability to induce weight loss makes it an attractive option for overweight patients. Other adverse reactions include nausea, anorexia, early satiety, and vomiting.

GLUCAGON-LIKE PEPTIDE-1 (GLP-1). Incretins are hormones that are released from the gut postprandially; they often are found in low concentrations in persons with type 2 diabetes. The incretin that has received the most attention is GLP-1. Incretins stimulate insulin secretion in pancreatic β-cells and have been shown to restore both phases of insulin release. GLP-1 regulates glucose homeostasis via multiple complementary actions and along with other incretins are known to do the following:

- Stimulate glucose-dependent endogenous insulin secretion (and perhaps insulin sensitivity)
- Inhibit endogenous glucagon secretion
- Suppress appetite and induce satiety
- Reduce the speed of gastric emptying
- Possibly stimulate islet growth
- Protect β-cells from cytokine- and free fatty acid–mediated injury

EXENATIDE (BYETTA). This agent is derived from a component of the saliva of the Gila monster lizard and has been approved as adjunctive therapy for type 2 diabetes. Exenatide binds to GLP-1 receptors and stimulates insulin secretion when blood sugar is high. It is the first drug that has been shown to restore first-phase insulin secretion, which does not occur in persons with type 2 diabetes. This metabolic defect is responsible for postprandial hyperglycemia. Exenatide also acts to stimulate β-cell replication and neogenesis, increase β-cell mass, and improve glucose tolerance. It is given as an injection before the morning and evening meals. Adverse effects of exenatide include nausea, vomiting, diarrhea, and upper respiratory symptoms. It may cause a reduction in food intake that will necessitate adjustment of the patient's other diabetes drugs to prevent hypoglycemia. The risk of hypoglycemia is not increased when used with metformin, but this risk is increased when used with sulfonylureas. Exenatide is clearly associated with weight loss.

DPP-4 INHIBITORS. Endogenous GLP-1 is rapidly inactivated by the enzyme dipeptidyl peptidase-4 (DPP-4). Therefore, researchers are seeking to develop drugs that inhibit DPP-4, thus prolonging the activity of GLP-1. The first DPP-4 inhibitor, sitagliptin, was approved by the FDA in October 2006 as a once-daily oral medication. It can be used as monotherapy or can be combined with metformin or a thiazolidinedione. It reduces fasting and postprandial hyperglycemia in patients with type 2 diabetes and does not cause weight gain or hypoglycemia. Hypersensitivity to this product is the only listed contraindication for sitagliptin. The second DPP-4 drug that is awaiting FDA approval is vildagliptin.

TREATMENT PRINCIPLES

Standardized Guidelines

Generally accepted guidelines for managing diabetes have been established by the American Diabetes Association (ADA) and the American Association of Clinical Endocrinologists (ACE). Although subtle differences are evident, most guidelines are similar. See Diabetes Care, Clinical Practice Recommendations. Vol 31, Supplement 1, 2008.

Evidence-Based Recommendations

- Educational interventions are likely to be beneficial.
- Metformin is more effective than diet alone.
- Sulfonylureas reduce HbA1c further compared with placebo or diet alone.
- New sulfonylureas are better than older sulfonylureas in reducing hypoglycemia.

Cardinal Points of Treatment

- To prevent or delay onset of diabetes, patients with impaired glucose tolerance (IGT) or IFG should be advised to lose 5% to 10% of body weight and to increase physical activity to at least 150 minutes per week of moderate activity such as walking. Follow-up counseling seems to improve the likelihood of success.
- Metformin therapy should be considered in patients who are at very high risk for diabetes, based on combined IFG and IGT plus other risk factors, and who are obese and younger than 60 years of age
- Studies show that intensive glucose control improves mortality and morbidity and reduces costs.
- Because lowering A1c levels to an average of about 7% has been shown to reduce microvascular and neuropathic complications of diabetes and, possibly, macrovascular disease, the target A1c goal for nonpregnant adults is generally less than 7%
- For selected individual patients, the A1c goal is as close to normal (< 6%) as possible without significant hypoglycemia, in light of epidemiologic studies showing a small but incremental benefit to lowering A1c from 7% into the normal range.
- Because of the progressive nature of diabetes, practitioners should expect to titrate medications and augment therapy over time.
- For children, patients with a history of severe hypoglycemia, those with limited life expectancies, individuals with comorbid conditions, and those with long duration of diabetes and minimal or stable microvascular complications, less stringent A1c goals may be appropriate.
- As glucotoxicity and further β-cell dysfunction occur, the patient most likely will require higher doses of medications or the addition of new agents to maintain HbA1c at goal
- Monitoring carbohydrate intake is key to achieving glycemic control, whether by carbohydrate counting, exchanges, or experience-based estimation. For patients with diabetes, glycemic index and glycemic load use may modestly improve glycemic control vs. that observed when considering only total carbohydrate.
- People with diabetes should perform at least 150 minutes per week of moderate-intensity aerobic physical activity (50% to 70% of maximum heart rate; and unless there are

contraindications, those with type 2 diabetes should perform resistance training three times per week.

- Goals of care must be established with the patient and should reflect the individualized plan of care specifically designed for that patient. The plan of care should account for costs, side effects, preferences, and HbA1c goals.
- Evidence shows that similar guidelines for maintaining glycemic goals should be followed in treatment for the elderly. Importance is placed on maintaining optimal control to lessen the vascular and neurologic complications of the disease.

Nonpharmacologic Treatment

ESTABLISH GOALS. The first step is to establish glycemic goals for the individual patient. The patient's age, ability to provide self-care, other medical problems, social support, and financial issues all play a role in decisions regarding individual glycemic goals. (See Table 52-1 for ADA-recommended glycemic goals.) American Association of Clinical Endocrinologists Medical Guidelines for the Management of Diabetes Mellitus, *The AACE System of Intensive Diabetes Self-Management—2003 Update*, recommend a preprandial blood sugar goal <100; a 2-hour postprandial blood sugar goal <140; and an HbA1c goal of 6.5.

For patients who have type 2 diabetes, an initial physician referral or collaboration may be needed, especially if the patient's condition has been compromised. Patients with type 1 diabetes usually require a referral to an endocrinologist or a diabetes specialist.

The second step focuses on nonpharmacologic therapeutic techniques such as diet and exercise. Individuals may benefit from nutritional counseling and physical therapy.

Pharmacologic Treatment for Type 2 Diabetes

START MEDICATIONS. The third step in treatment is to administer oral medications. The choice of drug is based on the mechanism of action and patient characteristics (see Table 52-3 for treatment decision guidelines). All oral medications are indicated as first choices depending on patient characteristics. Traditionally, a sulfonylurea has been the first choice. However, metformin or a thiazolidinedione now is used frequently as a first-line choice because it reduces insulin resistance that occurs with type 2 diabetes. Sulfonylureas, metformin, and thiazolidinediones reduce overall blood sugars and are used to provide 24-hour control. Their full effects may take several weeks. The meglitinides and the α-glucosidase inhibitors generally are used as second-line treatment because of cost and side effects, respectively. Effective diabetes management requires attention to all metabolic defects associated with the disease. This often requires the use of more than one drug to target each metabolic defect. (See Table 52-2 for FDA-approved combination therapies.)

Sulfonylureas. Sulfonylureas work best early in diabetes, while the pancreas is still responsive to stimulation. They generally lose their effectiveness as diabetes progresses and β-cell function is lost. They have been found to be most beneficial in patients whose weight is normal or slightly increased. Glyburide (Micronase) is more potent than glipizide and is more likely to cause hypoglycemia. Start with long-acting glipizide (Glucotrol XL). If this is not strong enough, consider glyburide. Glimepiride may cause less

TABLE 52-3 Making Treatment Decisions in Type 2 Diabetes

BLOOD SUGARS MILDLY ELEVATED	
Trial of diet, exercise, and weight loss (if obese). If goals not reached, see below.	
NORMAL RENAL FUNCTION	
Nonobese	metformin
	Thiazolidinediones
	Second-generation sulfonylureas
	Nonsulfonylurea secretagogues (if erratic meals)
Obese	**Elevated Fasting Blood Sugar**
	Metformin
	Thiazolidinediones
	Second-generation sulfonylureas
	Incretins
	Elevated Postprandial Blood Sugar
	Nonsulfonylurea secretagogues
	α-Glucosidase inhibitors
	Second-generation sulfonylureas
IMPAIRED RENAL FUNCTION	
Nonobese	Second-generation sulfonylureas
	Nonsulfonylurea secretagogues (if erratic meals)
	Thiazolidinediones
Obese	α-Glucosidase inhibitors
	Thiazolidinediones
	Sulfonylureas
	Incretins

Adapted from Dube D, Peiris AN: Concise update in management of diabetes, *South Med J* 95:4-9, 2002.

Start at beginning dosages, and titrate every 2 to 4 weeks by monitoring preprandial and postprandial blood glucose; thiazolidinediones may take several weeks to reach maximum effectiveness; add second and third agents to achieve the goal of glycemic control.

If poor control is attained with three agents, or medical problems preclude the use of oral medications, consider insulin.

Because diabetes is progressive, additional medications and higher dosages will be needed to maintain control.

weight gain and hypoglycemia than other sulfonylureas. Maximum doses of sulfonylureas reduce HbA1c by 1.1% to 1.9% and lower blood sugar by about 20%.

Metformin. Of the oral agents, metformin is the only one that reduces hepatic glucose production. Metformin is an *anti*hyperglycemic rather than a hypoglycemic drug. Therefore, hypoglycemia is not a side effect of this drug, and it is frequently combined with a sulfonylurea in a commercially available product. Metformin also improves insulin action in muscle tissue and lowers free fatty acids but to a lesser degree than the thiazolidinediones. Additionally, it may suppress appetite, thus inducing mild weight loss. It is especially useful in patients who are obese or when given in combination with sulfonylureas or thiazolidinediones. It improves fasting, postprandial glucose, and triglycerides. It does not promote weight gain, is not implicated as a cause of hypoglycemia, and may be more likely than other treatments to decrease cholesterol. Metformin decreases HbA1c by approximately 0.9% to 1.4%

Thiazolidinediones. Thiazolidinediones reduce insulin resistance. They sensitize peripheral tissues to insulin, causing the body to better use insulin. They also affect gene transcription in adipocytes, thereby reducing free fatty acids by 20% to 40%. Decreased lipotoxicity may improve β-cell function. This makes thiazolidinediones of particular benefit in patients with the metabolic syndrome (syndrome X). The first thiazolidinedione, troglitazone, was removed from the U.S. and U.K. market because of reports of severe and sometimes fatal hepatotoxicity. The thiazolidinediones that were approved thereafter have not been found to cause liver toxicity, although spurious case reports are available in the literature. However, rosiglitazone has been implicated in adverse cardiac outcomes such as MI and now carries a black box warning to highlight a potential increased risk of myocardial ischemic events. This is thought to be a result of its increase in LDL levels (8% to 16%). This has not been shown with pioglitazone. Both drugs increase HDL by approximately 10%. Lastly, these drugs may cause a substantial increase in weight gain that is due in part to fat or fluid retention. Therefore, these drugs should not be used in NYHA Class III or IV heart failure. Thiazolidinediones reduce HbA1c by approximately 0.9% to 1.5%.

Meglitinides. Meglitinides are short-acting secretagogues that stimulate insulin secretion. They are used to decrease postprandial blood sugars. Meglitinides are taken only with meals. When taken correctly, the risk of hypoglycemia is very low. They are especially useful in patients who had fairly low fasting blood glucose levels but high postprandial glucose levels. Although they are relatively safe, they are rather weak and are used in mild diabetes and as an adjunct. Cost is another reason why these drugs are considered second-line agents. Repaglinide has a longer duration than nateglinide. Maximum doses of meglitinides reduce HbA1c by approximately 0.5% to 1.3%.

α-Glucosidase Inhibitors. α-Glucosidase inhibitors are short acting and are used to decrease postprandial blood glucose levels by binding oligosaccharides to α-glucosidase enzyme in the brush border of the small intestine. They are taken only with meals. Hypoglycemia is rare with monotherapy. By virtue of their mechanism of action, these drugs have had limited acceptance because of their GI side effects such as flatulence (41.5%), diarrhea (28.7%), and abdominal pain (11.7%). Because α-glucosidase inhibitors prevent or delay the absorption of sucrose, hypoglycemia must be treated with glucose or lactose and not with table sugar. Acarbose has fewer problems with systemic absorption than miglitol. HbA1c is reduced by 0.3% to 0.8% with this class of drugs given at maximum doses.

Amylin Replacement

AMYLIN MIMETICS. Amylin analogs reduce blood glucose levels by reducing glucagon secretion, increasing gastric emptying time, and suppressing appetite. Because it works only in the presence of glucose, amylin must be given immediately prior to meals and should be skipped if forgotten before the meal. Pramlintide and insulin have reduced HbA1c by an additional 0.4% to 0.7% vs. insulin alone at 52 weeks in patients with type 1 diabetes. Similar results were seen in patients with type 2 diabetes when pramlintide was added to insulin with or without metformin or a sulfonylurea. Side effects most commonly reported were nausea (28% to 48%), vomiting (7% to 11%), and headache (5% to 13%); these

subsided over 4 weeks. Severe hypoglycemia (1% to 17%), which was seen in patients with type 1 diabetes, resulted in an insulin dose reduction in subsequent studies. Pramlintide (Symlin) is given subcutaneously, separately from insulin, three times a day before meals that contain at least 250 calories or 30 g of carbohydrates. The insulin dose must be reduced by 50% prior to initiation if severe hypoglycemia is to be avoided. This agent is contraindicated in patients with hypoglycemia unawareness and gastroparesis. It is approved for use in patients with type 1 or insulin-requiring type 2 diabetes.

INCRETIN MIMETICS. This new class of drugs is a synthetic version of a naturally occurring hormone that increases insulin release, restores first-phase insulin secretion, suppresses glucagon secretion, and slows gastric emptying. Exenatide (Byetta) was found to reduce HbA1c at 30 weeks by 1% in patients receiving maximal doses of metformin, a thiazolidinedione, or a combination of metformin and sulfonylurea. Weight loss was approximately 1.5 kg in all groups except the metformin group, whose members lost 3 kg. Nausea (44%) was commonly reported in trials along with vomiting (13%) and diarrhea (13%). Hypoglycemia (14% to 36%) was common among patients who were given a sulfonylurea. A reduction in sulfonylurea dose is recommended. Exenatide is administered subcutaneously twice daily within an hour before meals. It is not yet approved for use with insulin, but it can be used with other oral diabetes drugs. A long-acting release formulation of exenatide is under development that is likely to be given by injection once weekly. It is approved for use only in patients with type 2 diabetes.

DIPEPTIDYL PEPTIDASE-4 (DPP-4) INHIBITORS. These agents inhibit the enzyme that breaks down endogenous GLP-1, thus prolonging its activity. Sitagliptin (Januvia), the first in this class, is given orally once daily. As monotherapy, it reduces HbA1c by 0.6% and 1.5% in patients with baseline HbA1c ≤8% and ≤9%, respectively, at 24 weeks. When given in combination with metformin, HbA1c was reduced by 0.6%. Headache (5%) and diarrhea (3%) were the only significant side effects reported. Sitagliptin is approved for type 2 diabetes when given alone or in combination with metformin as an adjunct to diet and exercise, as add-on therapy with a sulfonylurea (glimepiride) when the single agent alone does not provide adequate glycemic control, and as add-on therapy with glimepiride and metformin when dual therapy does not achieve adequate control.

ADJUST MEDICATIONS. If glycemic goals are not attained after an adequate trial of one medication, add a drug with a different mechanism of action (see Table 52-2). A third drug may be added if necessary. Combination therapy usually is required (Table 52-4). An example of this is thiazolidinedione (which decreases fasting blood sugars) combined with a meglitinide to decrease postprandial blood sugars. If fasting blood sugars are not controlled by a sulfonylurea, the addition of acarbose will improve control and diminish the insulinotropic and weight-increasing effects of sulfonylureas. Combination pills combine metformin with a sulfonylurea or a thiazolidinedione, except for Avandaryl (rosiglitazone/glimepiride), which is a thiazolidinedione/sulfonylurea combination. Another combination for

TABLE 52-4   Therapeutic Combinations: Indicated and Unlabeled

Drug	Sulfonylurea	Metformin	Thiazolidinediones	Meglitinides	α-Glucosidase Inhibitors	Incretin Agents
Insulin	Approved	FDA indication	Weight gain; pioglitazone: FDA indication; rosiglitazone: edema	Not indicated, use short-acting insulin	Not indicated, use short-acting insulin	Approved with caution (Byetta, Symlin)
Sulfonylureas		Approved	Approved	Not indicated	Not indicated	Approved with caution (Byetta, Symlin)
Thiazolidinediones	FDA indication, low risk of hypoglycemia, weight gain	FDA indication, combination product		Not indicated	Not indicated	Approved
Meglitinides	No information	FDA indication	FDA indication		Not indicated	Not indicated
α-Glucosidase inhibitors	FDA indication, beneficial	Approved, but both cause GI distress	No information	No added benefit expected		Not indicated
metformin	FDA indication, combination product		Approved	Not indicated	Not indicated	Approved
Incretin agents	Approved (with caution)	Approved	Approved	Not indicated	Not indicated	

consideration consists of exenatide combined with a sulfonylurea and metformin.

CONSIDER INSULIN. If glycemic goals are not reached, consider the addition of insulin. All oral medications may be used with insulin. Because of disease progression, treatment often requires progression to high doses of medications and the addition of other medications for control. In addition to its role in controlling HbA1c, insulin is indicated for the following reasons:

1. Patient with newly diagnosed diabetes with severe hyperglycemia (>300 mg/dL)
2. Pregnancy
3. Intercurrent illness/surgery
4. Renal or hepatic disease
5. Allergy to or intolerance of oral medications
6. Maximum doses of two oral antidiabetes drugs
7. Increased hyperglycemic symptoms, weight loss
8. Low C-peptide

When insulin is initiated for type 2 diabetes, one of the following regimens usually is ordered:

1. Basal insulin therapy in combination with oral agents
   - Start with glargine (Lantus) or detemir (Levemir) insulin 10 units or 0.2 unit/kg at bedtime. Increase dosage by 2 to 4 units every 3 to 5 days to achieve fasting blood sugar goal.
   - Start with NPH insulin 10 units at suppertime or bedtime. Increase dose by 1 to 2 units every 3 to 5 days to achieve fasting blood sugar goal.
2. Premixed insulin regimens
   - Start with 70/30 insulin at suppertime or NPH/regular insulin at suppertime. This is a good combination if bedtime and fasting blood glucose levels are elevated. Increase dose by 10% to 20% every 3 to 5 days to achieve blood sugar goals.

- Start 70/30 at breakfast and at suppertime. This is a good combination if glucoses are elevated throughout the day and if the patient is not a candidate for additional oral therapy.
3. NPH/regular insulin before breakfast and before dinner
   - Use 0.2 units per kilogram of patient's weight as total daily insulin dose.
   - Divide dose so that two thirds of total dose is given in the morning and one third of the total dose is given before dinner.
   - Divide each morning and dinner dose so that two thirds of the dose is NPH and one third is regular.
4. Basal-bolus regimens (long-acting insulin in combination with premeal rapid insulin injection)

After the patient is started on a basal dose of long-acting insulin (glargine or detemir), rapid- or short-acting insulin is added before meals. This requires that blood glucose levels be monitored frequently. One option is to add premeal rapid- or short-acting insulin to the largest meal. Then, prandial boluses of rapid-acting insulin can be added at other mealtimes. Rapid- and short-acting insulin can be added as standing doses or on a sliding scale based on blood sugar readings.

This is the most physiologic approach to insulin therapy; however, this regimen can be daunting for many diabetic patients. Consequently, twice-daily premixed insulin (given before breakfast and before dinner) is an acceptable alternative for the patient who is not willing or able to take multiple daily injections.

One inhaled insulin formulation, Exubera, was approved and several others were in clinical trials. However, very few patients were using the product and so the company elected to stop manufacturing it. Many patients with type 2 diabetes resist using insulin because of the injections. However, the amount of insulin absorbed through inhalation was variable, and this limited its usefulness.

Common Problems

When a patient whose condition is stabilized by a diabetic regimen is exposed to stress such as fever, infection, trauma, or surgery, temporary loss of glycemic control may occur. The stress response induces activation of counterregulatory hormones such as glucagon, cortisol, and catecholamines; these in turn raise glucose levels. On occasion, it may be necessary to discontinue oral medications such as metformin and to initiate insulin. Oral medications generally may be resumed when the condition has resolved.

Because corticosteroids are counterregulatory hormones, they can precipitate or worsen diabetes mellitus. Monitor glucose levels closely during steroid treatment, and adjust diabetic medications as needed.

Insulin Therapy for Type 1 Diabetes

All patients with type 1 diabetes and some with type 2 diabetes require insulin. Treatment incorporates the use of long-acting or intermediate-acting insulin to provide daily basal coverage (i.e., second-phase insulin release) and rapid-acting or regular insulin to provide bolus coverage for meals (i.e., first-phase insulin release). Multiple daily insulin injections often are used. Open-loop insulin pumps and continuous subcutaneous insulin delivery devices can be used to simplify insulin administration. When multiple daily injection programs and pumps are used, insulin administration can better mimic normal physiology.

> **Individual differences in the action of insulin have been observed; times may vary according to injection techniques used, care required for the insulin solution, and site at which the injection is given.**

A general approach to dosing theory for short- or rapid-acting insulin given prior to meals assumes that 1 unit of regular insulin covers 10 to 15 g of carbohydrate. Insulin therapy for a person who has type 1 diabetes might be started with one of the following regimens for initiation of long-acting and rapid-acting insulin:

- Insulin glargine or Lantus or Levemir insulin (long-acting)
  - Use once a day, usually at bedtime.
  - Usually, start with 50% of total daily insulin dose.
  Or
- Regular, aspart, and lispro
  - 50% of total insulin requirement is divided by 3 for each premeal bolus.
  - Premeal dosing varies with carbohydrate intake, so carbohydrate grams or servings per unit of insulin must be determined.

Currently, long-acting insulin given once a day or twice daily for basal coverage with rapid-acting insulin for premeal bolus coverage is the most promising option for good control. If the patient does not eat a meal, rapid-acting insulin should not be taken. Long-acting insulin is taken regardless of meals (Table 52-5). Use "sick day rules" to guide dosing.

Determine correct basal dosing by monitoring blood glucose levels. If all blood glucose levels are elevated throughout the day, or if the fasting blood glucose level is elevated, the basal insulin dose should be increased. Determination of correct premeal or bolus insulin is best guided by premeal and

TABLE 52-5 Insulin Characteristics and Duration of Action

Insulin	Color	Onset	Peak	Duration
RAPID-ACTING				
lispro (Humalog)	Clear	5-15 min	30-90 min	3-4 hr
aspart (NovoLog)	Clear	5-15 min	1-3 hr	3-5 hr
glulisine (Apidra)	Clear	5-15 min	30-90 min	3-4 hr
SHORT-ACTING				
Regular (R)	Clear	30-60 min	2-4 hr	6-8 hr
INTERMEDIATE-ACTING				
NPH (N)	Cloudy	2-4 hr	6-10 hr	10-16 hr
LONG-ACTING				
glargine (Lantus)	Clear	2 hr	No peak	20-24 hr
detemir (Levemir)	Clear	1 hr	No peak	6-24 hr
MIXTURES				
70/30 regular	Clear	30-60 min	2-4 hr	6-8 hr
70/30 long	Cloudy	2-4 hr	6-10 hr	10-16 hr
50/50	Cloudy	30 min	3-5 hr	10-16 hr
Humalog 75/25	Cloudy	15 min	2-3 min	18-24 hr
NovoLog 70/30	Cloudy	15 min	18-24 hr	1-4 hr

postmeal monitoring of blood sugars. For instance, if before-lunch blood glucose levels are high, an increase in prebreakfast insulin might be indicated. If 2-hour postprandial supper blood glucose level is low, then a before-supper bolus of quick-acting insulin may have to be decreased. Consistent hypoglycemia given on a presupper schedule may be an indication that the prelunch bolus should be decreased.

How to Monitor

- Follow the patient closely. The patient should be seen at least weekly for the first month. After the first month, examination should occur at monthly intervals or as indicated. In nonadherent individuals, treatment with oral agents may be unsuitable, but patients may not do well with insulin either. Teach the patient about the signs/symptoms of hypoglycemia, and caution the patient to report hypoglycemic episodes immediately. Reduce dose of oral medication or insulin if hypoglycemia occurs.
- Patients should monitor fingerstick blood sugars at home. Monitor preprandial and postprandial blood glucose levels to determine appropriate dose adjustments.
- Assess HbA1c at baseline and every 3 months to evaluate overall control. Measurements taken more frequently than every 3 months generally are not useful.
- In some areas, use of HbA1c levels to assess long-term glycemic control is being replaced by the use of average blood glucose; experts say this change will enhance clarity for diabetic patients who are looking to manage their disease.
- Monitor urine at least annually with microalbuminuria. Start patient on an ACE inhibitor or an ARB if microalbuminuria is present.
- Monitor lipids annually or more often if treatment has been initiated.

SULFONYLUREAS

- Measure baseline and at least annual renal function. Assess more frequently if patient is at risk for renal impairment.
- Monitor CBC initially and periodically.

METFORMIN. Test for lactic acidosis if patient develops laboratory abnormalities or clinical illness. Symptoms include nausea, abdominal pain, tachycardia, and hypotension. Patients with severe lactic acidosis are also tachypneic. Tests should include measurement of electrolytes, ketones, and blood glucose. Consider monitoring blood pH, lactate, pyruvate, and metformin levels as needed depending on patient levels. Serum creatinine also should be monitored. Metformin is contraindicated and must be discontinued if creatinine is >1.4 for women or >1.5 for men.

THIAZOLIDINEDIONES

- Check LFTs before administration. Do not use in patients with increased baseline liver enzyme levels (AST >3.5 times the upper limit of normal).
- Assess patients who have mildly elevated enzyme levels every 2 months during the first year of treatment and periodically thereafter.
- Monitor for symptoms that suggest hepatic dysfunction, such as unexplained nausea, vomiting, abdominal pain, fatigue, anorexia, and dark urine; check enzyme levels.
- Black box warning: May increase risk for ischemic events. Monitor for signs and symptoms of CHF, especially edema and/or dyspnea. Do not use TZDs for patients with preexisting CHF or recent MI. Patients given rosiglitazone and insulin or nitrates were at greater risk of reporting MI. Therefore, the use of rosiglitazone with insulin or nitrates is not recommended.

α-GLUCOSIDASE INHIBITORS. Monitor LFTs every 3 months during the first year of treatment and periodically thereafter.

Patient Variables

GERIATRIC

- *Sulfonylureas:* Decrease dosage in renal and hepatic impairment to avoid risk of hypoglycemia.
- *Meglitinides:* Increase risk of hypoglycemia; variable response in the elderly.
- *Biguanides:* Use with caution because of the risk of accumulation with renal insufficiency and the increased risk of lactic acidosis.

PEDIATRIC

- Sulfonylureas, thiazolidinediones (younger than age 18), meglitinides, and α-glucosidase inhibitors not recommended
- *Biguanides (children ages 10 to 16):* metformin 500 mg bid (regular-release tablets only); maximum oral dose, only 2000 mg

PREGNANCY AND LACTATION

- *Category B:* Metformin, miglitol, acarbose, sitagliptin
- *Category C:* Glipizide, glimepiride, pioglitazone, rosiglitazone, repaglinide, nateglinide, pramlintide, exenatide

- It is recommended that women who intend to become pregnant should switch to insulin. Fetal mortality and major congenital anomalies generally occur three or four times more often in the offspring of diabetic mothers.
- Metformin, glyburide, and glipizide appear to be compatible with breastfeeding. Their presence in breast milk or in other products generally is unknown, and their use is not recommended in breastfeeding mothers.
- Glyburide has been used for the treatment of patients with gestational diabetes; metformin has been used in women with PCOS who eventually became pregnant.
- Presence in breast milk is unknown; use is not recommended in breastfeeding mothers.

Patient Education

Patient education is essential for control of diabetes. Patients must understand how to take their medications correctly to avoid hypoglycemia and how to adjust medications as needed (e.g., sick days).

Avoid herbal products such as bitter melon, fenugreek, and St. John's wort, which have variable effects on blood sugar levels.

THERAPEUTIC LIFESTYLE CHANGES AND SELF-MANAGEMENT. Diet and exercise are the cornerstones of Step 2 treatment. Self-management of the disease is crucial. Patients who have diabetes need to know how to care for themselves, how to best monitor and address individual problems, and when to call a provider for assistance. Meal planning, exercise, home blood glucose monitoring (HBGM), hypoglycemia recognition and management, hyperglycemia management, sick day rules, weight management, and foot care are important. Referrals to a registered dietitian and a diabetes educator are mandatory for information and self-care. Use medication if a patient is unable to reach a glycemic goal with diet and exercise alone.

SPECIFIC DRUGS

SECOND GENERATION SULFONYLUREAS

glipizide (Glucotrol, Glucotrol XL) 🔑

CONTRAINDICATIONS
- Hypersensitivity
- Ketoacidosis

WARNINGS
- *Cardiovascular risk:* Administration of oral hypoglycemic drugs has been associated with increased cardiovascular mortality as compared with treatment with diet alone or diet plus insulin. Interpretation of this study of a first-generation sulfonylurea has been controversial.
- *Renal/hepatic function impairment:* Oral hypoglycemic agents are metabolized in the liver. These drugs and most of their metabolites are excreted by the kidneys. Hepatic impairment may result in inadequate release of glucose in response to hypoglycemia, and renal impairment may cause decreased elimination

Continued

glipizide (Glucotrol, Glucotrol XL) 🗝 —cont'd

of sulfonylureas, leading to hypoglycemia. Use these drugs with caution.

PRECAUTIONS
- Monitor closely; see "How to Monitor."
- Hypoglycemia may be severe.

PHARMACOKINETICS. See Table 52-6.

ADVERSE EFFECTS. See Table 52-7.

DRUG INTERACTIONS. See Table 52-8.

DOSAGE AND ADMINISTRATION. See Table 52-9. Patients on immediate-release glipizide may be switched to the extended-release form, which is given once a day at the same total daily dose.

BIGUANIDES

metformin (Glucophage, Glucophage XR, Glumetza, Fortamet)

CONTRAINDICATIONS
- Hypersensitivity
- Renal disease or dysfunction (creatinine >1.4 in women, >1.5 in men)
- Metabolic acidosis, including ketoacidosis, or patient who is at risk
- CHF requiring pharmacologic treatment
- Withhold therapy on the day of a procedure involving iodinated contrast media; resume no sooner than 48 hours afterward, or when renal function returns to baseline.

WARNINGS
- Lactic acidosis is a rare (≈0.03%) but life-threatening metabolic complication that can occur with metformin accumulation. It is fatal in approximately one half of cases.
- *Renal function impairment:* Metformin is excreted by the kidney. Accumulation may occur with renal function impairment; this increases the risk of lactic acidosis.
- *Hepatic function impairment:* Avoid metformin with hepatic impairment because of increased risk of lactic acid acidosis.

PRECAUTIONS
- *Hypoxic states:* Cardiovascular collapse, acute CHF, acute MI, and other conditions have been associated with lactic acidosis.
- Hold metformin for surgical procedures. Resume when oral intake is restored and renal function is normal.
- A decrease to subnormal levels of vitamin B_{12} was observed in about 7% of patients.

Hypoglycemia does not occur under normal circumstances but could occur with deficient caloric intake, strenuous exercise not compensated by caloric supplementation, or alcohol use, or during concomitant use with other glucose-lowering agents such as sulfonylureas and insulin. Metformin is available in a once-daily formulation that should prove useful for patients who have difficulty taking their medications more often than once a day.

THIAZOLIDINEDIONES

rosiglitazone (Avandia) 🗝

CONTRAINDICATIONS. Hypersensitivity

WARNINGS
- Cardiac effects and fluid retention, which may exacerbate or cause heart failure. Do not use in patients with NYHA Class III and IV cardiac status.
- Black box warning by FDA regarding increased risk for ischemic events and CHF, particularly in patients who are taking insulin or nitrates. The FDA has decided to allow the drug to stay on the market with increased warnings about the risk of cardiovascular events, while additional studies are conducted to investigate the issue.
- *Hepatotoxicity:* Available clinical data suggest that both pioglitazone and rosiglitazone offer substantially less risk of hepatotoxicity or LFT elevations. However, spurious cases have been reported. Do not use in patients with LFTs >2.5 times the upper limit of normal at baseline.
- *Ovulation:* May result in resumption of ovulation in premenopausal anovulatory patients and may introduce risk for pregnancy
- *Carcinogenesis:* Increase in incidence of adipose hyperplasia in mice
- *Fertility impairment:* Rosiglitazone reduces fertility in rats.

PRECAUTIONS
- *Hypoglycemia:* May be at risk for hypoglycemia
- *Hematologic:* May cause decreases in hemoglobin and hematocrit
- Weight gain has been seen, probably because of fluid retention and fat accumulation.

nateglinide (Starlix)

NON-SULFONYLUREAS SECRETAGOGUES (MEGLITINIDES)

CONTRAINDICATIONS
- Hypersensitivity
- Ketoacidosis

WARNINGS
- *Renal insufficiency:* Drug is safe in mild renal insufficiency but should not be used with severe renal failure.
- Patients with renal failure who were on dialysis exhibited reduced overall drug exposure (not true of repaglinide).
- Hepatic insufficiency causes increased concentration. Use lower dosages with caution.

PRECAUTIONS. Hypoglycemia is a risk. Give before a meal. If the patient skips a meal, that dose of meglitinide should not be taken.

OTHER DRUGS IN CLASS

Other drugs in this class are similar to the prototype except as follows.

TABLE 52-6   Pharmacokinetics of Oral Hypoglycemic Agents

Drug	Absorption	Drug Availability	Onset of Action	Time to Peak Concentration	Half-life	Duration of Action	Protein Bound	Metabolism	Excretion
glyburide (Micronase)	Not affected by food	Unknown	2-4 hr	2-4 hr	5-10 hr	16-24 hr	>99%	Liver	Urine, 50%; active metabolites; feces
glyburide (micronized; Glynase)	Not affected by food	Unknown	1 hr	2-4 hr	4 hr	12-24 hr	>99%	Liver	Urine, 50%; active metabolites; feces
glipizide (Glucotrol)	Delayed by food	100%	1.5-2 hr	2-3 hr	2-4 hr	12-14 hr	>98%	Liver CYP 450	Urine, 80%; no active metabolites
glipizide (Glucotrol ER)	Not affected by food	100%	1.5-2 hr	6-12 hr	2-4 hr	20-24 hr	>90%	Liver	Urine, 80%; no active metabolites
glimepiride (Amaryl)	Not affected by food	100%	1 hr	2-3 hr	5-9 hr	24 hr	>99%	Liver	Urine, 60%; active metabolites; feces
metformin (Glucophage)	Delayed by food	50%-60%	3-4 days	1-3 hr	2 hr	1.5-6 hr	Negligible	None	Urine, unchanged
rosiglitazone (Avandia)	Not affected by food	99%	Up to 12 wk (peak)	1 hr	3-4 hr	24 hr	99.8%	Liver 2C8, 2C9	Urine, 64%; feces, 23%
pioglitazone (Actos)	Not affected by food	Unknown	Up to 12 wk (peak)	3-4 hr	3-7 hr	24 hr	99%	Liver 3A4, 2C8, 1A1	Urine, 20%; feces
nateglinide (Starlix)	Not affected by food	75%	15 min	1 hr	<1 hr	4 hr	98%	Liver 3A4, 30% 2C9, 70%	Urine/feces
repaglinide (Prandin)	Completely absorbed	56%	15-60 min	1 hr	1 hr	4-6 hr	>98%	Liver 3A4, oxidation	Urine/feces
acarbose (Precose)	<2%	2%	1 hr	2 hr	3 hr	4 hr	0%	Intestines	Feces, not absorbed; urine, trace
miglitol (Glyset)	50%-70%	Dose dependent		2-3 hr	2 hr	4 hr	Negligible	None	Urine, unchanged
exenatide	Must be taken 1 hour before meals			2.1 hr	2.4 hr	Up to 10 hr		Kidney CYP 450	Urine, proteolytic degradation
pramlintide	Must be taken before meals	30%-40%		20 min	48 min	3 hr	40% unbound in plasma	Kidney CYP 450	Urine
sitagliptin	Taken with or without food	87%		1-4 hr	12 hr	24 hr	38%	Kidney CYP 450	Urine, 87%; feces, 13%

TABLE 52-7   Adverse Reactions to Diabetic Medications

Body System	Sulfonylureas	Biguanides	Thiazolidinediones	Meglitinides	α-Glucosidase Inhibitors	Incretin Agents	Insulin
Body, general	Chills, fatigue, weakness, malaise, edema, weight gain	Chills, sweating, flushing, no weight gain	Edema, weight gain, fluid retention	Weight gain	No weight gain	Hyperhidrosis	Weight gain
Skin, appendages	Rash, eczema, pruritus, erythema multiforme, sweating, exfoliative dermatitis, photosensitivity	Rash, nail disorder				Rash, injection site reaction	Rash, injection site dystrophy
Hypersensitivity	Skin reactions, urticaria						
Respiratory	Dyspnea	Dyspnea, flu syndrome		URI		URI, nasopharyngitis with Januvia	
Cardiovascular	Arrhythmia, hypertension	Chest discomfort, palpitations	↑ CHF				
GI	Anorexia, nausea, indigestion, diarrhea, GI pain, constipation, vomiting, hunger, flatulence, cholestatic jaundice	Diarrhea, nausea, vomiting, flatulence, cramping, indigestion, abdominal discomfort, abnormal stools, anorexia	Nausea, vomiting, diarrhea, elevated liver function tests	Nausea, vomiting, diarrhea	Flatulence, diarrhea, abdominal pain, rare paralytic ileus, nausea, gas	Nausea, vomiting, dyspepsia, decreased appetite, GERD	
Hemic and lymphatic	Leukopenia, thrombocytopenia, aplastic anemia, agranulocytosis, hemolytic anemia, pancytopenia, eosinophilia	B$_{12}$ deficiency	Anemia (rosiglitazone)			Antibody formation/ resistance	

Metabolic and nutritional	Hypoglycemia, syndrome of inappropriate antidiuretic hormone (SIADH)	Lactic acidosis, hypoglycemia, metallic taste, vitamin B$_{12}$ deficiency	Hypoglycemia (0.6%); rosiglitazone: ↑ LDL and HDL	Hyperglycemia, hypoglycemia; nateglinide has less hypoglycemia than repaglinide	Hypoglycemia (less than with other drugs)	Hypoglycemia (with sulfonylurea)	Hypoglycemia
Musculoskeletal	Arthralgia, myalgia, leg cramps	Myalgia	Myalgia	Arthropathy			
Nervous system	Drowsiness, asthenia, nervousness, tremor, pain, insomnia, anxiety, depression, hypesthesia, hypertonia, confusion, somnolence, abnormal gait, migraine, paresthesia, dizziness, vertigo, headache	Headache, asthenia, lightheadedness	Headache	Dizziness		Dizziness, jitteriness, headache, asthenia	
Special senses	Tinnitus, blurred vision, retinal hemorrhage	Taste disorder					
Hepatic	Hepatitis, hepatic porphyria		↑ LFTs		↑ LFTs		
Genitourinary	Decreased libido, polyuria						
Other	Disulfiram-like reaction, hyponatremia		↑ Uric acid				

TABLE 52-8   Drug Interactions of Oral Hypoglycemic Agents

Increase Drug Levels	Decrease Drug Levels
SULFONYLUREAS	
Increase sulfonylureas: Cause hypoglycemia: Androgens, anticoagulants, azole antifungals, chloramphenicol, clofibrate, gemfibrozil; History: Antagonists, magnesium salts, methyldopa, MAOIs, probenecid, salicylates, sulfinpyrazone, sulfonamides, tricyclic antidepressants (TCAs), urinary acidifiers ciprofloxacin ↑ glyburide sulfonylureas ↑ digoxin glyburide ↑↓ warfarin	Decrease sulfonylureas: Decrease effectiveness of drug: β-Blockers, calcium channel blockers, cholestyramine, corticosteroids, diazoxide, estrogens, hydantoins, isoniazid, nicotinic acid, oral contraceptives, phenothiazines, rifampin, sympathomimetics, thiazide diuretics, thyroid agents, urinary alkalinizers, charcoal
BIGUANIDES	
Alcohol, amiloride, digoxin, morphine, procainamide, quinidine, quinine, ranitidine, triamterene, trimethoprim, vancomycin, cimetidine, furosemide, iodinated contrast material, nifedipine ↑ metformin	metformin ↓ glyburide, furosemide
THIAZOLIDINEDIONES	
pioglitazone possible interaction with cyproheptadine and other CYP 3A4 drugs	troglitazone ↓ oral contraceptives
MEGLITINIDES	
3A4 inhibitors, β-blockers, NSAIDs, probenecid, MAOIs, salicylates, sulfonamides, estrogen, simvastatin ↑ repaglinide repaglinide ↑ estrogen	3A4 inducers, calcium channel blockers, corticosteroids, estrogens, isoniazid, nicotinic acid, OCPs, phenothiazines, phenytoin, sympathomimetics, diuretics, thyroid products ↓ repaglinide
α-GLUCOSIDASE INHIBITORS	
	Digestive enzymes, charcoal ↓ α-inhibitors acarbose ↓ digoxin miglitol ↓ digoxin, glyburide, metformin, propranolol, ranitidine
INCRETIN AGENTS	
sitagliptin levels increased by cyclosporine	exenatide decreases digoxin, lovastatin, acetaminophen, warfarin levels; pramlintide has potential to slow absorption of oral medications

repaglinide (Prandin)

- Increased incidence of carcinogenesis (e.g., benign adenoma of thyroid) in rats

α-GLUCOSIDASE INHIBITORS

acarbose (Precose) 🔑

CONTRAINDICATIONS
- Hypersensitivity
- Ketoacidosis
- Cirrhosis
- Bowel disease such as inflammatory bowel disease, partial or complete colonic ulceration, or predisposition to intestinal obstruction

WARNINGS
- Renal function impairment causes increased levels of the drug.
- *Carcinogenesis:* Increase in incidence of renal tumorv

PRECAUTIONS. Hypoglycemia

INCRETIN AGENTS

Symlin, Byetta, Januvia

CONTRAINDICATIONS
- Gastroparesis
- Hypoglycemia unawareness

WARNINGS
- Can cause hypoglycemia when combined with insulin or sulfonylureas
- Symlin and Byetta must be taken 1 hour before meal.

ADVERSE EFFECTS
- Hypoglycemia
- Dizziness
- Feeling jittery
- Vomiting
- Diarrhea
- Nausea most common side effect—Titrate Byetta and Symlin slowly; resolves over time

DRUG INTERACTIONS. See Table 52-8.

TABLE 52-9 Dosage and Administration Recommendations for Oral Hypoglycemic Agents

Drug	Starting Dose	Administration and Titration	Usual Daily Dose	Maximum Daily Dose
glyburide	2.5-5 mg once daily with breakfast or first main meal of the day; 1.25 mg once daily for sulfonylurea-naïve patients	Single or divided dose; ↑ 2.5 mg or less once weekly	1.25-20 mg	20 mg
glyburide, micronized	1.5-3 mg once daily with breakfast or first main meal of the day; 0.75 mg once daily for sulfonylurea-naïve patients	Single or divided dose (6 mg/day); ↑ by 1.5 mg or less once weekly	0.75-12 mg	12 mg
glipizide	5 mg before first meal once daily	30 min before meal; single or divided doses (>5 mg /day); ↑ by 2.5-5 mg q3-4 days	5 mg	40 mg
glipizide ER	5 mg before first meal once daily	↑ by 5 mg q3 months (dose adjusted according to HbA1c)	5-10 mg	20 mg
glimepiride	1-2 mg once daily with breakfast or first main meal of the day	↑ by 2 mg q1-2wk	1-4 mg	8 mg
metformin	500 mg bid *or* 850 mg once daily with meals	↑ by 500 mg q2wk; give total daily dose as three divided doses with meals	500 mg tid-850 mg bid	Child, 2000 mg; adult, 2550 mg
metformin ER	500 mg once daily with evening meal	↑ by 500 mg q week	1000-2000 mg	2000 mg
rosiglitazone	4 mg once daily without regard to meals	Single or divided dose; ↑ by 4 mg/day q8-12wk	4-8 mg	8 mg
pioglitazone	15-30 mg once daily without regard to meals	↑ to 45 mg/day q8-12wk	30 mg	45 mg
nateglinide	60-120 mg tid	1-30 min before meals	60-120 mg tid with meals	360 mg
repaglinide	0.5-2 mg tid; 0.5 mg tid for patients with HbA1c <8%; 1-2 mg tid for patients with Hb >8%	1-30 min before meals; ↑ q week	0.5-4 mg tid with meals	16 mg
acarbose	25 mg tid with first bite of meal	↑ by 50 mg tid q4-8wk	50-100 mg tid with meals	150 mg (<60 kg); 300 mg (>60 kg)
miglitol	25 mg tid with first bite of meal	↑ by 25 mg tid q4-8wk	50 mg tid with meals	300 mg
exenatide	5 mcg subQ bid within 60 minutes prior to a meal; 100 mg daily	↑ to 10 mcg subQ bid after 30 days (per patient response)	10 mcg subQ bid	20 mcg
pramlintide	Type 1: 15 mcg subQ immediately prior to meals Type 2: 60 mcg subQ immediately prior to meals	↑ by 15 mcg subQ q3days (if tolerated) ↑ to 120 mcg subQ in 3-7 days (if no significant nausea develops; if nausea develops at 120 mcg dose, then reduce to 60 mcg)	60-120 mcg subQ immediately prior to meals	180 mcg 360 mcg
sitagliptin	100 mg once daily; CrCl 30-50 ml/min: 50 mg once daily; CrCl <30 ml/min: 25 mg once daily	None	100 mg once daily	100 mg

DOSAGE AND ADMINISTRATION. See Table 52-9.

PHARMACODYNAMICS. See Table 52-6. Because these drugs act locally in the GI tract, low systemic bioavailability is therapeutically desired.

evolve A continually updated list of useful WebLinks may be found in the Evolve Resources at http://evolve.elsevier.com/Edmunds/NP/

evolve http://evolve.elsevier.com/Edmunds/NP/

53 Contraceptives

CLAIR KAPLAN

DRUG OVERVIEW

Class	Subclass	Generic Name	Trade Name
Combination estrogen and progestin	Oral monophasic	ethinyl estradiol and norethindrone	Ovcon 50
			Nortrel 0.5/35; 1/35
			Norinyl 1+35
			Ortho-Novum 1/35
			Brevicon 21
			Modicon 28
			Nortrel 0.5/35
			Ovcon-35 ✺
			Loestrin 21 1.5/30
			Loestrin FE 1.5/30
			Loestrin 1/20
			Loestrin FE 1/20
			Norethin 1/35
			Necon 0.5/35 ✺; 1.35 ✺
	ethinyl estradiol and levonorgestrel		Portia 0.15/30
			Nordette 0.15/30
			Levlen 0.15/30
			Alesse 28
			Aviane 21 ✺
			Lessina 28
			Levlite 28
			Levora 15/30 ✺
	ethinyl estradiol and norgestrel		Cryselle
			Ovral
			Ogestrel
			Lo/Ovral
			Low-Ogestrel 28 ✺
	ethinyl estradiol and ethynodiol diacetate		Demulen 1/50
			Demulen 1/35
			Zovia 1/35

✺, Top 200 drug.

Table continued on following page

DRUG OVERVIEW (Continued)

Class	Subclass	Generic Name	Trade Name
		ethinyl estradiol and desogestrel	Apri ☼
			Desogen
			Ortho-Cept 28
			Cyclessa
		ethinyl estradiol and drospirenone	Yasmin 28 ☼ Yaz
		ethinyl estradiol and norgestimate	Ortho-Cyclen Sprintec ☼
		mestranol and norethindrone	Demulen 1/35; 1/50 Norinyl 1+50 Ortho-Novum 1/50
	Oral biphasic	ethinyl estradiol and norethindrone	Jenest-28 Ortho-Novum 10/11
		ethinyl estradiol and desogestrel	Kariva 28 ☼ Mircette 28
	Oral triphasic	ethinyl estradiol and norethindrone	Tri-Norinyl Ortho-Novum 7/7/7 Estrostep Fe
		ethinyl estradiol and norgestimate	Ortho Tri-Cyclen ☼ TriNessa ☼ Ortho Tri-Cyclen Lo ☼ Tri-Sprintec ☼
		ethinyl estradiol and levonorgestrel	Enpresse Tri-Levlen Triphasil Trivora-28 ☼
	Oral extended cycle	levonorgestrel/ethinyl estradiol	Seasonale Seasonique Lybrel
	Contraceptive patch	ethinyl estradiol and norelgestromin	Ortho Evra ☼
	Intravaginal ring	ethinyl estradiol and etonogestrel ring	NuvaRing ☼
Progestin-only	Emergency contraception	levonorgestrel	Plan B
	Progestin-only oral contraceptive (POP)	norethindrone	Micronor Nor-QD
		norgestrel	Ovrette
	Progestin-only injection	medroxyprogesterone	Depo-Provera
	Progestin subdermal implants	etonogestrel	Implanon
	Intrauterine device	levonorgestrel	Mirena
Nonhormonal	Intrauterine device		ParaGard

INDICATIONS

- Prevention of pregnancy
- *Acne vulgaris:* Ortho-Tri-Cyclen, Ortho-Tri-Cyclen Lo, Ortho-Cyclin, Estrostep, Alesse, Dione-35, Yaz
- *Emergency contraception:* Plan B

Unlabeled Uses

- Anemia prevention/improvement
- Resolution of amenorrhea
- Decreased menorrhagia and dysmenorrhea
- Improved cycle control with relief of anovulatory bleeding
- Endometriosis
- Dysfunctional uterine bleeding (DUB)

- Reduction in premenstrual syndrome (PMS) symptoms
- Decreased risk of benign breast disease
- Decreased problems with ovarian cysts
- Mittelschmerz (ovulation pain) relief
- Hirsutism
- Rheumatoid arthritis control
- Perimenopausal symptom control
- Acne vulgaris
- Female hypogonadism
- Emergency contraception
- Improvement in menstrual migraines
- Reduction in endometrial and ovarian cancer risk

Agents in this class can be divided into combination agents (including both estrogen and progestin). Combined hormonal contraceptives are formulated for oral, transdermal, and intravaginal routes of administration. Progestin-only agents may be administered orally, intramuscularly, subcutaneously, in intrauterine systems, and via implants. Oral contraceptives (OCs) are commonly known as "birth control pills," or "the pill."

This chapter is intended to provide the basic information necessary to understand contraception. Because these medications are used to prevent an unwanted pregnancy and not to treat a disease, the patient is more involved in the decision making. This makes selecting the best contraceptive method somewhat of an art and a science. This is a rapidly changing field, with new information and new products. The provider will want to read farther on this topic and check for the latest information before prescribing contraceptives.

The first OC pills, which were developed in the 1950s, contained only high doses of progestin. These early pills caused significant breakthrough bleeding (BTB). During manufacture, they became "contaminated" with estrogen. The women who took the contaminated pills had less BTB, so the estrogen was left in. The first combined birth control pill, which contained much higher doses of hormones than are found in the pills used today, was released in 1960.

In the 1970s, researchers first noted a dose-response relationship between high-estrogen pills and the risk of venous thromboembolism. This was caused by the action of oral estrogen on hepatic induction of fibrinogen, which increased the tendency to form blood clots. Early pills had roughly three times more estrogen and nine times more progestin than the pills that are available today. As doses of estrogen have been decreased to below 50 mcg of ethinyl estradiol (EE), thrombus risk has markedly diminished.

The original hormonal contraceptives were monophasic (same daily dose). New progestin-only pills and phasic preparations (estrogen and/or progestin doses that change during the 21-day cycle in an attempt to mimic the typical menstrual cycle) were introduced in the 1970s. Longer-acting progestin-only methods (medroxyprogesterone, a 3-month progestin-only injection, and Norplant, a 5-year implanted rod system) were approved for the U.S. market in the 1980s. Norplant was taken off the market because of adverse publicity over litigation regarding dose standardization and removal problems. A new single-rod implant, Implanon, is now available.

In 2002, transdermal and vaginal hormone delivery systems were approved for use in preventing pregnancy. The trend for new contraceptives continues with introduction of (1) additional combination OCs with lower estrogen levels, and (2) a new progestin, drospirenone, which is derived from the diuretic spironolactone. Recently, extended-cycle contraceptives that contain levonorgestrel and an ethinyl estradiol tablet have been introduced. Women who take this product experience fewer menstrual cycles per year, or menstruation may be suppressed entirely. Other new products include formulations with more active pills and shortened placebo intervals.

THERAPEUTIC OVERVIEW
Anatomy and Physiology

THE MENSTRUAL CYCLE. The menstrual cycle, which lasts for an average 28 days, is a classic negative feedback loop involving the hypothalamus, anterior pituitary gland, and ovaries. Menstruation begins on day 1 of the cycle, with shedding of the endometrium in response to declining estrogen and progesterone levels. Cycles consist of a follicular phase and a luteal phase that are nearly equal in length. Cycle lengths vary among individuals, and variability is increased in adolescents and in women who are close to perimenopause. Most variation occurs in the follicular phase. At the end of a menstrual cycle in which a pregnancy has not occurred, the hypothalamus responds to low circulating levels of estrogen and progesterone and secretes gonadotropin-releasing hormone (GnRH). GnRH stimulates the anterior pituitary gland to secrete follicle-stimulating hormone (FSH) and luteinizing hormone (LH); these stimulate the ovaries to begin the ovulation cycle anew. The ovaries are the female gonads, which are responsible for secretion of the sex steroid hormones estrogen, progesterone, and testosterone. These gonads also store the ovarian follicles, which in turn are the home of oocytes. When a woman is born, her ovaries contain approximately 2 million follicles and, by puberty, 300,000 remain to carry her to menopause. Only about 500 follicles ovulate during the reproductive years.

FSH stimulates follicular growth and ovarian development. During each cycle, 18 to 20 follicles are stimulated; all except one dominant follicle eventually die off. The dominant follicle produces estrogen and promotes an environment favorable to healthy development of the follicle and its oocyte, in preparation for eventual ovulation. Enlargement of this dominant follicle causes estrogen levels to gradually increase. Near the middle of a cycle (around day 12 to 13 of a 28-day cycle), estrogen in the blood reaches a critical level that sends a hormonal message to the pituitary gland indicating that the follicle is mature and that ovulation is imminent. The pituitary gland responds by sending out the hormonal messenger, LH. The midcycle LH surge induces ovulation. The follicle, now a "bubble" on the side of the ovary, bursts, releasing the egg into the ampulla of the fallopian tube. At the site of ovulation, the remains of the follicle form a cyst, called the *corpus luteum*. At this time, estrogen levels drop sharply and then stabilize as the corpus luteum assumes the role of hormone production, with production of progesterone predominating over that of estrogen.

Progesterone levels are very low during the first half of the cycle but climb sharply after ovulation, with the appearance of the corpus luteum. Progesterone dominates in the second half of the cycle, or the *luteal phase*. The corpus luteum cyst, maintained by LH, is a "hormone factory" that produces large amounts of progesterone. The corpus luteum typically remains functional for approximately 12 days. If no additional hormonal message (e.g., fertilization and implantation) is sent, the corpus luteum dies and regresses on day 26 of a 28-day cycle. With the demise of the corpus luteum, blood progesterone levels drop dramatically. By the last day of the cycle, baseline progesterone and estrogen levels signal the hypothalamus to start a new menstrual cycle.

ENDOMETRIAL CHANGES. The thickness of the endometrial, or uterine, lining parallels the changing hormone levels, shedding from day 1 to about day 5 back to almost basement lining. Increasing estrogen levels in the first half of the cycle stimulate endometrial proliferation. Progesterone, which is produced in large amounts by the corpus luteum in the second half of the cycle, stabilizes the endometrium by increasing its blood supply and glycogen stores, producing a secretory endometrium that is receptive to implantation. Under the influence of progesterone, the endometrium ceases to grow in thickness but becomes significantly denser. The proliferative effects of estrogen must be present in the first half of the cycle for progesterone to produce a secretory endometrium. Without the stabilizing influence of progesterone, the endometrium would continue to thicken but, if unsupported by an adequate blood supply, would shed irregularly. This condition is seen in the woman with anovulatory cycles who, lacking the secretion of progesterone by the corpus luteum, has unpredictable, often heavy noncyclic bleeding as a result of lack of production of progesterone. Similarly, the secretion of large amounts of progesterone without adequate secretion of estrogen (unopposed progesterone) produces a thin endometrium that is not receptive to implantation.

If fertilization occurs and the egg implants, the embryo and the developing placenta produce human chorionic gonadotropin (hCG), which maintains the corpus luteum cyst for about 100 days until the placenta is advanced enough to produce its own progesterone. After the placenta matures, the corpus luteum declines.

In summary, the uterine lining proliferates in response to rising estrogen levels in the first half of the cycle. In the second half of the cycle, progesterone maintains a secretory endometrium. At the end of the menstrual cycle during which conception did not take place, progesterone and estrogen levels drop off and the unsupported uterine lining sheds (Figure 53-1).

HORMONE PHYSIOLOGY. *Hormones* are chemical messengers produced in the body that travel through the bloodstream from a gland to a distant site, where they exert their effects on specific organs or tissue.

The ovary produces three classes of sex steroid hormones: progestins, androgens, and estrogens. These steroid hormones can be synthesized in the ovaries in situ or derived from serum cholesterol that enters the ovaries. Several steps are included in the steroid biosynthesis pathway. Through a series of intermediary steps, cholesterol (a 27-carbon molecule) is broken down to progestins (21-carbon molecules), then to androgens (19-carbon molecules), and finally to estrogens (18-carbon molecules). During steroidogenesis, the number of carbon atoms can be reduced but never increased. Therefore, the metabolic breakdown of progestins can have progestational, androgenic, and estrogenic actions; the metabolic breakdown of androgens can have androgenic and estrogenic actions; but the metabolic breakdown of estrogens will have only estrogenic actions. In women, the principal circulating sex hormones—estrogen, estradiol, and the androgen, testosterone—are also directly produced by the ovary. Most estradiol and testosterone (69%) are bound to sex hormone–binding globulin (SHBG), a protein carrier. Roughly 30% is loosely bound to albumin, leaving only 1% unbound and free. It is this free 1% that determines the biologic effects of estradiol and testosterone. Estrogen administration increases SHBG levels, thereby decreasing the quantities of free, or active, sex steroids. Progestins and androgens decrease SHBG, thereby increasing the quantities of free sex steroids. All combined oral contraceptive pills (COCPs) increase SHBG, although some do so more than others, depending on the progestin component and the ratio of estrogen to progestin. Because all COCPs increase SHBG, free testosterone is always decreased by some degree in women who are taking COCPs.

Progestins. Progesterone is secreted in significant amounts (20 to 30 mg/day) in the second half of the normal menstrual cycle by the corpus luteum. During the first half of the cycle, estrogen dominates and progesterone is secreted in minute amounts (2 to 3 mg/day) by the ovaries and the adrenals. During pregnancy, the placenta secretes very large amounts of progesterone.

The plasma half-life of progesterone is only 5 to 10 minutes, after which it is degraded to other steroids that have no progestational effect. Progesterone in its natural state cannot be used in oral form because of its rapid breakdown by the liver, so chemical modifications of synthetic progestins in hormonal contraceptives were made to deliberately slow down liver metabolism, making it possible to use the oral route (Table 53-1).

Effects of progesterone in the body are limited and are seen primarily in the reproductive tract and the breast; other effects are evident as changes in metabolism. Progesterone is the dominant hormone of pregnancy; it produces a secretory endometrium, decreases uterine contractions, and stimulates alveolar epithelial growth in the breast.

Norethindrone, the progestin originally used in OCs, was derived from ethisterone, an orally active form of testosterone. The removal of a 19-carbon molecule from ethisterone

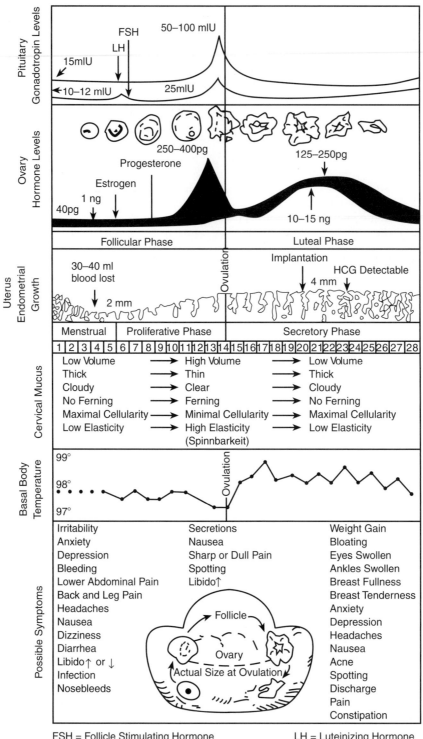

FIGURE 53-1 **Menstrual cycle events: Hormone levels, ovarian and endometrial patterns, and cyclic temperature and cervical mucous changes.** (Hatcher RA et al: *Contraceptive Technology,* ed 18 rev, New York, 2007, Ardent Media Trade, Inc.)

results in the formation of norethindrone and changes the major effect from that of an androgen to that of progesterone, but the androgenic component is never totally eliminated and the potential for anabolic and androgenic effects remains. See Table 53-2 for biologic effects of progestins and estrogen. This is a dose–effect relationship: The lower the

dose of progestins given, the lesser is the androgenic effect. At today's very low doses of progestin in COCPs, clinical effects are usually negligible. As with estrogens, serious side effects, especially adverse serum lipid changes, have been associated with high doses of progestins; therefore, the lowest effective doses available should be used. Through the

TABLE 53-1 **Synthetic Progestins and Their Characteristics**

Generation	Class	Description	Specific Drug	Comments	Progestin	Estrogen	Androgen
First	Estranes	Equivalent in actions and potency	norethindrone	Most commonly used	++	++	++
			norethindrone acetate	Converted into norethindrone	++	++	++
			ethynodiol diacetate	Converted into norethindrone	++	++	+
Second	Gonanes	Gonanes have longer half-lives than the estranes, which may translate into better cycle control	norgestrel		+++	0	+++
			levonorgestrel	Second generation	+++	0	++++
			norgestimate	In newest COCPs, converted into levonorgestrel	++	0	++
			desogestrel	In newest COCPs	+++	0	+++
Third		More selective in progestational effects	etonogestrel	In vaginal ring	+++	0	+
		Raise the SHBG more than older progestins, thereby decreasing the amount of free testosterone		Active metabolite of desogestrel	+++	0	+
			norelgestromin	In transdermal system Active metabolite of norgestimate			
Novel		Not a testosterone derivative	drospirenone	Antialdosterone activity	+++	0	0

years, changes have been made in the chemical structure of progestins in the quest to produce new progestins that have more potent progestational activity with fewer androgenic side effects.

Many different progestins are marketed in the United States for use in hormonal contraception.

Estrogens. The human body produces three estrogens: estradiol, estrone, and estriol. The major estrogen is estradiol. It is 12 times more potent than estrone and 80 times more potent than estriol. The primary source of estrogen in women with normal menstrual cycles is estradiol, which is secreted by the ovary. The ovarian follicle secretes 100 to 300 mcg of estradiol daily, depending on the phase of the menstrual cycle. Estradiol levels of greater than 200 mcg are required for ovulation to occur. The ovary also secretes small amounts of estrone, but most comes from adrenal androgens that are converted to estrone in peripheral tissues, such as adipose, skin, and muscle. Estriol is a metabolite of estrone and estradiol.

Estrogens are conjugated in the liver to form glucuronides and sulfates. About one fifth of these conjugated products are excreted in the bile; the rest are excreted by the kidneys. Synthetic estrogens, such as ethinyl estradiol (EE), are degraded very slowly in the liver and other tissues, which causes their high intrinsic potency.

Estrogens are important in the development and maintenance of the female reproductive tract. Estrogen has effects throughout the body that are most notable in the breasts, bones, liver, and urogenital structures. See Table 53-1 for estrogen effects on the body.

Two estrogenic compounds are used in COCPs in the United States: EE and mestranol. Mestranol is considered pharmacologically weaker because it must first be converted to EE. Therefore, unconjugated EE is the active estrogen in the blood in both mestranol and EE. All of the low-dose pills are low-estrogen pills. They contain ≤35 mcg of estrogen pills (EE). Mestranol is available in only a few pills in a 50-mcg dose, which is roughly equivalent to 35 mcg EE. A relatively safe dose of EE is ≤35 mcg. Pills that include 50-mcg EE are reserved for women on medications that induce liver enzymes that degrade estrogen, requiring higher initial does, and they are rarely used. It is more common practice to use other methods with women who require higher-dose pills. High-dose EE should be given under special circumstances and generally is not used in primary care. In this chapter, COCPs are assumed to contain ≤35 mcg of EE (Table 53-3).

MECHANISM OF ACTION

Hormonal contraceptive agents interfere with the hypothalamic-pituitary-ovarian negative feedback loop to inhibit ovulation. Constant, low levels of estrogen and/or progestin have suppressive effects at both the hypothalamus and the pituitary, inhibiting GnRH, FSH, and LH. Suppression of FSH and LH inhibits ovulation. Additional contraceptive effects stem from actions on the cervical mucus (thickening, to prevent passage of sperm) and the endometrium (providing a lining that is hostile to implantation). Hormonal contraceptives are not abortifacients. An implanted pregnancy will not be disrupted by their administration.

The primary contraceptive action of progestin in hormonal contraceptives is suppression of the LH surge, which inhibits ovulation. When given in supraphysiologic doses, progestins produce a decidualized endometrial bed with atrophied glands that is not receptive to implantation, as well as thick cervical mucus, which hampers sperm transport and may also impair ovum transport by slowing peristalsis and decreasing secretions in the fallopian tubes.

The contraceptive action of estrogens in hormonal contraceptives is primarily the result of suppression of FSH. Without FSH, no dominant follicle emerges and ovulation is inhibited. Estrogen contributes to endometrial stability and avoidance of irregular shedding and/or bleeding. Estrogen increases intracellular progesterone receptors, making the given dose of progestin more effective.

Emergency contraceptives (ECs) are thought to interfere with ovulation. Other possible actions include (1) disruption of the endometrium to inhibit implantation, and (2) alteration in tubal transport of sperm or ova to prevent fertilization. ECs are not effective with an existing pregnancy.

TABLE 53-2   Biologic Effects of Estrogens and Progestins

Organ and/or System Effects	Estrogenic Effects	Progestational Effects
Adrenal gland	Increases cortisol-binding globulin (transcortin) Increases free cortisol	Increases free cortisol
Bone	Promotes bone formation Stimulates osteoblasts Increases efficiency of calcium absorption Promotes calcitonin synthesis	
Breast	Stimulates ductal growth Promotes growth of estrogen receptor–positive cancers	Stimulates glandular growth Inhibits proliferation decrease in fibrocystic disease
CNS	Improves quality of sleep Antidepressant Vasomotor stability	Sedation
Gallbladder	Alteration in composition of gallbladder bile, increases cholesterol saturation Increases gallstones in women already at risk during first 2 years of estrogen use	
Hematologic effects	Increased fibrinogen; clotting factors VI, VII, IX, X, and prothrombin; ESR; transferrin Decreased antithrombin III	Increased hematocrit; fibrinolytic activity
Liver/serum lipids	Influence synthesis of hepatic DNA and RNA, hepatic cell enzymes, serum liver enzymes, and plasma proteins Increase HDL Increase triglycerides Decrease ratio of total cholesterol to HDL	Decrease HDL Increase ratio of total cholesterol to HDL Increase LDL
Metabolic effects	Fluid retention (breast discomfort, headaches) Maintenance of muscular strength Nausea Increased prolactin	Glucose intolerance (increases peripheral resistance to insulin action) Anabolic weight gain Increased appetite Depression, fatigue
REPRODUCTIVE TRACT		
Uterus	Proliferative endometrium: endometrial growth due to gland maturation and enlargement; stromal development, capillary proliferation Primes progesterone receptors	Secretory endometrium: restrained growth endometrium becomes thicker, more dense; progressive tortuosity of glands; glands become secretory
Fallopian tubes	Increase secretions, ciliary activity, and peristalsis to improve ovum transport	Slow peristalsis and decrease secretions
Cervical mucus	Increases amount, spinnbarkeit, permeability to sperm	Thick, impermeable to sperm Increases candidiasis Cervicitis
MISCELLANEOUS		
Skin	Increases secretions, lubrication Increases elasticity Chloasma (patchy increase in facial pigment)	*Oily skin, acne, sebaceous cysts, pilonidal cysts, hirsutism
Thyroid	Increases T_3, thyroxine-binding globulin, total T_4	
	Normal free T_4	
Summary: Combined effects of estrogen and progesterone	Increased angiotensin I and II, total iron binding capacity (TIBC) due to increased globulins, vitamin A (nonharmful); decreased prothrombin time, B_6 (pyridoxine), B_{12}, folic acid, ascorbic acid	

TABLE 53-3   Medications With Dosages

Generic Name	Trade Name	Estrogen, mcg	Progestin, mg
COMBINATION			
Monophasic			
ethinyl estradiol and norethindrone	Ovcon 50	50	1
	Nortrel 1/35	35	1
	Norinyl 1+35	35	1
	Ortho-Novum 1/35	35	1
	Brevicon	35	0.5
	Modicon	35	0.5
	Necon 0.5/35	35	0.5
	Nortrel 0.5/35	35	0.5
	Ovcon 35	35	0.4
	Loestrin 1.5/30	30	1.5
	Loestrin FE 1.5/30 Microgestin Fe 1.5/30		
	Loestrin 1/20	20	1
	Loestrin FE 1/20	20	1
	Microgestin Fe 1/20		
ethinyl estradiol and levonorgestrel	Portia	30	0.15
	Nordette	30	0.15
	Levlen	30	0.5
	Seasonale		
	Alesse 21	20	0.1
	Aviane 21	20	0.1
	Lessina 28	20	0.1
	Levlite 28	20	0.1
	Ovral	50	0.5
	Ogestrel	50	0.5
ethinyl estradiol and norgestrel	Cryselle	30	0.3
	Lo/Ovral	30	0.3
ethinyl estradiol and ethynodiol diacetate	Demulen 1/50	50	1
	Demulen 1/35	35	1
ethinyl estradiol and desogestrel	Apri	30	0.15
	Desogen	30	0.15
	Ortho-Cept	30	0.15
	Cyclessa	25	0.1, 0.125, 0.15
ethinyl estradiol and drospirenone	Yasmin 28	30	3
ethinyl estradiol and norgestimate	Ortho-Tri-Cyclen	35	0.18, 0.215, 0.25
mestranol and norethindrone	Demulen 1/50	50	1
	Demulen 1/35	35	1
Biphasic			
ethinyl estradiol and norethindrone	Ortho-Novum 10/11, Necon 10/11	35	0.5 × 10 day then
		35	1 × 11 day
ethinyl estradiol and desogestrel	Kariva 28	20	0.15 × 21 day then
	Mircette 28	10	0 × 5 day
Triphasic			
ethinyl estradiol and norethindrone	Tri-Norinyl	35	0.5 × 7 day then
		35	1 × 9 day then
		35	0.5 × 5 day
	Ortho-Novum 7/7/7	35	0.5 × 7 day then
		35	0.75 × 7 day then
		35	1 × 7 day
	Estrostep Fe	20	1 × 5 day then
		30	1 × 7 day then
		35	1 × 9 day

Table continued on following page

TABLE 53-3   Medications With Dosages (Continued)

Generic Name	Trade Name	Estrogen, mcg	Progestin, mg
ethinyl estradiol and norgestimate	Ortho-Tri-Cyclen	35 35 35	0.18 × 7 day then 0.215 × 7 day then 0.25 × 7 day
	Ortho-Tri-Cyclen Lo	25 25 25	0.18 × 7 day then 0.215 × 7 day then 0.25 × 7 day
ethinyl estradiol and levonorgestrel	Enpresse Tri-Levlen Triphasil Trivora-28	30 40 30	0.05 × 6 day then 0.075 × 5 day then 0.125 × 10 day
EMERGENCY CONTRACEPTION			
ethinyl estradiol and levonorgestrel	Preven	50	0.25; 2 tablets × 2 within 72 hr of intercourse, 12 hr apart
levonorgestrel	Plan B	0	0.75 × 2 within 72 hr of intercourse, 12 hr apart
PROGESTIN ONLY			
norethindrone	Ortho-Micronor Nor-QD	0 0	0.35 0.35
norgestrel	Ovrette	0	0.075
TRANSDERMAL SYSTEM			
ethinyl estradiol and norelgestromin	Ortho-Evra	20/24 hr 20 mcg/day	0.15/24 hr q wk × 3, then no patch × 1 wk
VAGINAL			
ethinyl estradiol and etonogestrel ring	NuvaRing	15/24 hr 15 mcg/day	0.12/24 hr for 3 wk, then off 1 wk, self-inserted
INTRAUTERINE			
Nonhormonal IUD	ParaGard		
levonorgestrel IUD	Mirena		52 mg q5yr
INJECTION			
Medroxyprogesterone	Depo-Provera		150 mg q12wk (IM) or 104 mg subQ q12wk

TREATMENT PRINCIPLES

Standardized Guidelines

- Brigham and Women's Hospital: *Contraception and family planning: a guide to counseling and management*, Boston, MA, 2005, Brigham and Women's Hospital.
- Contraception for women aged over 40 years, *J Fam Plann Reprod Health Care* 31:51-63, 2005.
- American Academy of Pediatrics: Emergency contraception, *Pediatrics* 116:1026-35, 2005 (available at www.managingcontraception.com/cmanagerpublish/).

Evidence-Based Recommendations

No evidence-based medicine studies regarding use of these medications for contraception have been reported. Studies have described the relative merits of these drugs for patients with dysmenorrhea, PMS, and menorrhagia.

Cardinal Points of Treatment

- Choosing a hormonal contraceptive must be individualized; the patient's wishes are integral to the selection process.
- Consider health history, experience with hormonal contraceptives, concomitant medications, and preferred mode of administration.
- Choose a method that is most likely to encourage adherence.
- Refer to the algorithm in Figure 53-2 for guidelines in choosing a product. Table 53-4 compares hormonal methods, and Table 53-5 reviews clinical considerations in contraceptive choice. Hormonal birth control methods can be used, but it is important for clinicians to be aware of the use of hormonal birth control methods for noncontraceptive benefits.

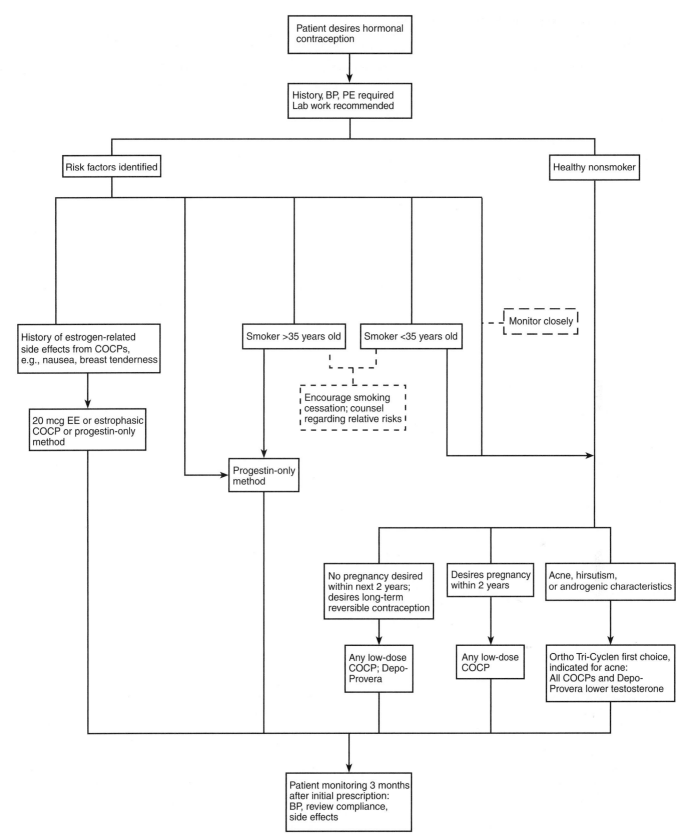

FIGURE 53-2   Algorithm for choice of a hormonal contraceptive.

TABLE 53-4 Comparison of Hormonal Methods

| | PROGESTIN-ONLY METHODS | | |
	DMPA Injection	Progestin-Only Pill (POP)	Combined OC (COCP)
ADMINISTRATION			
Frequency	Every 12 weeks	Daily	Daily
Progestin dose	High	Ultra low	Low
Blood levels	Initial peak then decline	Rapidly fluctuating	Rapidly fluctuating
First pass through liver	No	Yes	Yes
MAJOR MECHANISMS OF ACTION			
Ovary: Decreased ovulation	+++	+	+++
Cervical mucus: Decreased sperm penetrability	Yes	Yes	Yes
Endometrium: Decreased receptivity to blastocyst	Yes	Yes	Yes
FIRST-YEAR FAILURE RATE			
Perfect use	0.3%	0.5%	0.1%
Typical use	3%	1%-13%	8%
MENSTRUAL PATTERN			
Typical	Very irregular	Often irregular	Regular
Amenorrhea during use	Very common	Occasional	Rare
REVERSIBILITY			
Immediate termination possible	No	Yes	Yes
By woman herself at any time	No	Yes	Yes
Median time to conception from first omitted dose, removal	6 months	<3 months	3 months

Modified from Hatcher RA: *Contraceptive Technology,* ed 18 rev, New York, 2007, Ardent Media Trade, Inc.

- Many oral contraceptive products are available as generic formulations. Inform patients that the packaging and the "look" of their pills may change without a change in effectiveness. Although some side effects are more likely to occur with certain pills than with others, patient response is variable.
- Be sure your patients know that they can contact you to discuss any nuisance side effects, and that most of these can be eliminated by making minor changes. Stressing clinician–patient collaboration and communication can help prevent patients from simply taking themselves off a hormonal method without instituting a backup contraceptive plan.
- Stress to patients that hormonal contraception will not prevent sexually transmitted infection, and that for many patients, barrier protection is needed.

Pharmacologic Treatment

COMBINED ORAL CONTRACEPTIVE PILLS (COCPS). COCPs can be categorized as monophasic, multiphasic (biphasic, triphasic), and extended cycle pills. Monophasic pills contain identical amounts of estrogen and progestin in all 21 active pills. Multiphasic pills vary the amount of estrogen, progestin, or both over the active pill days in an attempt to mimic the normal menstrual cycle or minimize side effects. Extended cycle pills have longer treatment cycles to provide fewer menstrual periods. The basic methods used to initiate COCP are discussed in the following paragraphs.

First-Day Start. Starting COCPs within 24 hours of the onset of menses affords the best contraceptive efficacy during the first cycle. Backup or concurrent use of a second form of contraception is not necessary.

Sunday Start. Start COCPs on the Sunday of or following period onset. Backup contraception for 7 days is necessary if menses did not begin on a Sunday. The only advantages of the traditional Sunday start are avoidance of periods on the weekend and convenience, in that many manufacturers label the first pill in a pack as a "Sunday" pill.

When to Take the Pill. Take 1 pill every day at the same time. If using a 28-day pill pack, start the next pack as soon as the last pack is finished. If using a 21-day pill pack, stop pills for 7 days, then start the next pack the next day. If nausea occurs, switch to the opposite time (morning to evening) or take with food.

Missed pills, especially at the beginning or the end of the pack, may allow ovulation and unintended pregnancy to occur. Increasing the time between active pills increases the risk of ovulation. Encourage associating pill-taking with a daily

TABLE 53-5 **Clinical Considerations in Contraceptive Choice**

Condition	Considerations	Solution	Suggested Contraceptive
Age over 40	Increased cardiovascular risk	35 mcg or less of EE or POP	Low-estrogen COCPs, transdermal or vaginal ring, POPs, IUD—either hormonal or nonhormonal, implant, DMPA
Adolescent	Risk for noncompliance	Individualize to patient's needs	Low-estrogen COCPs, transdermal or vaginal ring, POPs, implant, DMPA
Cardiovascular risk	Assess risk factors, asymptomatic disease	COCP safe with superficial varicosities Mitral valve prolapse	Low-estrogen COCPs, transdermal, vaginal ring, other methods preferable: POPs, IUD—either hormonal or nonhormonal, implant, DMPA
Diabetes mellitus	Estrogen ↓ glucose tolerance Progestins ↑ glucose resistance	COCP safe with no end-stage disease	Low-dose COCP, low progestin; no POPs
Hypercoagulable; coagulation disorders	Estrogen increases coagulability	Safe if treated with anticoagulants COCPs, transdermal and vaginal ring contraindicated	POPs, DMPA, Mirena IUD, implant, barrier methods
Dysmenorrhea	Estrogens increase dysmenorrhea, flow	Low or no estrogen	POPs, continuous cycling COCPs, DMPA, transdermal, vaginal ring, implant or Mirena IUD
Hyperlipidemia	Estrogen ↑ HDL, ↓ LDL Progestin ↓ HDL, ↑ LDL	Estrogen beneficial overall, progestins are not; monitor lipids closely	Low-dose COCPs with low progestin, IUD—either hormonal or nonhormonal, barrier methods
↑ Triglycerides	Estrogen ↑ triglycerides Progestin ↓ triglycerides	Triglycerides may precipitate pancreatitis	POP, DMPA, IUD—either hormonal or nonhormonal, barrier methods
Hypertension, uncontrolled	OC ↑ blood pressure ↑ risk for MI and stroke	COCPs contraindicated	POP, IUD—either hormonal or nonhormonal, barrier methods, implant
Hypertension, controlled	With no end-organ damage, nonsmoker	Careful monitoring with repeat blood pressure readings as necessary	Low-estrogen pill, patch, or ring, POP, DMPA, IUD—either hormonal or nonhormonal, implant, barrier methods
HEADACHES			
Migraine without aura, tension	Begin during or immediately before menses because of decreased estrogen levels	Continuous OCs, contraindicated if patient smokes	Monophasic COCP used with extended or continuous cycling may be beneficial, any other methods possible Seasonale
Migraine with aura	Increased risk for stroke with COCPs (estrogen)	COCPs contraindicated	DMPA, POPs, IUD—either hormonal or nonhormonal, barrier methods, implant
POSTPARTUM			
Less than 6 weeks	Increased risk of thrombosis	Progestin-only	POP, DMPA, barrier methods
More than 6 weeks, not breastfeeding	Ovulation usually 6-8 weeks postpartum	Any hormonal method, if not contraindicated for other reasons	Low-estrogen COCP, POP, DMPA, IUD—either hormonal or nonhormonal, barrier methods, implant
More than 6 weeks, breastfeeding	Estrogen may decrease quality and quantity of milk Progestins promote milk production	Progestin-only	POP, DMPA, IUD—either hormonal or nonhormonal, barrier methods, implant; can try COCPs, but stop if breast milk is decreased
More than 14 weeks	Theoretical risk of thrombosis	Low-dose estrogen	Any method: Low-estrogen COCPs, POPs, DMPA, IUD—either hormonal or nonhormonal, barrier methods, implant

Table continued on following page

TABLE 53-5   Clinical Considerations in Contraceptive Choice (Continued)

Condition	Considerations	Solution	Suggested Contraceptive
Seizure disorder	Anticonvulsants are enzyme inducers that may increase failure rate of OCs	COCPs have drug–drug interactions with many antiseizure medications. DMPA has antiseizure benefits	DMPA preferred
Sickle cell anemia	Theoretical risk of thrombosis; progestins stabilize the red blood cell membrane Medroxyprogesterone improves the oxygen-carrying capacity of RBCs and decreases the risk of sickle cell crisis	Progestin-only	POP, DMPA preferred, implant, barrier methods, and IUDs also acceptable
SMOKING			
Younger than or equal to 35 years	Potential increased risk for thrombosis, ↑ with heavy smoking	Low-dose estrogen or progestin-only	Low-estrogen COCPs, transdermal or vaginal ring, POPs, IUD—either hormonal or nonhormonal, implant, DMPA
Older than 35 years	Greatly increased risk for vascular disease, including heart attack and stroke	Progestin-only; monitor lipid profile	POPs, DMPA, IUD—either hormonal or nonhormonal, barrier methods, implant
Systemic lupus erythematosus	Possible increased lupus flares with COCPs Vascular disease associated with lupus contraindicates estrogen	Progestin-only	POP, DMPA

routine, such as brushing teeth or mealtime, to avoid missed pills. Some women set their cell phone alarms to remind them to take their pills. See Box 53-1 for instructions on what the patient should do if she misses pills.

EXTENDED CYCLE PILLS. The FDA has approved a variety of extended cycle monophasic, continuous, 84-day active pill/7-day placebo pill regimens that contain 150 mcg levonorgestrel and 30 mcg EE. This regimen is as effective in preventing pregnancy as are conventional 21/7-day regimens. Withdrawal bleeding is comparable between the different regimens. No endometrial pathology has been found, and the side effect profile is similar in extended and conventional regimens. These drugs are predicted to be attractive to women, who will have only four menstrual periods a year. Additional manufacturers are producing new pills with shortened pill-free intervals, and many clinicians use evidence-based practice to support the practice of prescribing standard monophasic combined pills with instructions to patients that explain that they can minimize cycling by taking active pills daily without a placebo or pill-free interval. Evidence is building in support of increased contraceptive efficacy with continuous or extended cycling over traditional 21/7 regimens.

TRANSDERMAL SYSTEM. The transdermal system of hormone administration bypasses the liver, thereby eliminating the first-pass effect. It has the benefit of being convenient, requiring the weekly application of the transdermal "patch" instead of daily oral administration of contraceptive pills. The main disadvantage is that the adhesive can cause mild to moderate skin irritation. Transdermal contraceptives have up to a 99% effectiveness rate when used correctly, with a lower incidence of some side effects than is seen with OCs. The FDA has updated the labeling for the contraceptive transdermal patch to include the results of a new epidemiology study that found that users of the patch were at higher risk of developing venous thromboembolism (VTE) than women using oral contraceptive pills.

Clinical trials have suggested that transdermal systems may be less effective in women with body weight >198 pounds than in women with lower body weight.

The patch is applied once a week for 3 weeks to a different area of skin at each application; this is followed by a 1-week patch-free interval. The old patch is removed and a new one is applied. This cycle is then repeated. Patches can be applied to clean skin that is free of any lotions or other topicals on the buttock, abdomen, upper outer arm, or upper torso, where they will not be rubbed by tight clothing. If a patch becomes partly or completely detached, it should be reapplied or a new patch applied. Patients should not reapply a patch if it is no longer sticky; supplemental adhesive should not be used. Single replacement patches are available to patients from pharmacies. If a patch has been discovered to be loose or has come off, patients should use a backup method of contraception for 7 days. Patients can be switched from an OC to the patch, beginning when they would start a new pill pack

VAGINAL RING. The intravaginal ring is a delivery system whereby ethinyl estradiol and etonogestrel hormones are packaged into the ring itself, from which the medication is slowly dissipated. Its use is correlated with a pregnancy rate of 1 to 2 pregnancies per 100 woman-years.

BOX 53-1   Instructions for Patients Who Miss Pills

(APPLIES TO COMBINATION PILLS ONLY—NOT TO POPs)

Do the following if pills are missed:

- *One pill:* Take the missed pill as soon as possible. Take the next pill at the regular time. If the forgotten pill is not discovered until the next pill is due, take both pills at the same time.

Use of backup contraception for 7 days is optional.

- *Two pills in a row:* Take 2 pills as soon as possible. Take 2 pills the next day. Use a backup method for 7 days.
- *Three or more missed pills:* For first-day starters, throw out the rest of the pack and start a new one that same day. For Sunday starters, take 1 pill every day until Sunday. On Sunday, throw out the remaining pills from that pack and start a new pack that same day. The patient may or may not have a period that month. Order a sensitive pregnancy test if two periods are missed. Use backup contraception for 7 days after the missed pills.

- *Two or more missed pills at the beginning or end of a pack (total of 9 or more missed pills during pill-free interval):* Use emergency contraceptive pills, then restart new pill pack; use backup method for 7 days.
- *Backup method:* All patients should have a backup method of contraception available, such as condoms and/or spermicide, as well as Plan B ED. Sunday starters need to use a backup method for the first 7 days during their first pack of pills. First-day starters do not need a backup method during the first cycle. The backup method should be readily available in case of missed pills, vomiting or diarrhea, or discontinuation due to serious pill warning signs. New starts may be instructed to use backup for the entire first cycle while side effects, such as nausea, and missed pills are more common.

The ring is placed into the vagina by the patient. Its advantage is that it requires only monthly administration. Of the self-administered methods, this one is very convenient and private. It also avoids the first-pass phenomenon, thereby allowing for a lower dose and causing little risk of adverse reactions.

The ring is compressed and is inserted into the vagina. Its exact position in the vagina is not critical. It is removed 3 weeks later by hooking the index finger or the index and middle fingers under the ring to pull it out. The discarded ring should be placed into a foil pouch and discarded, not flushed. Patients should be switched from a combination OC to the ring by insertion within 7 days after the last active OC tablet. No backup method is needed. Switch from a progestin-only method by starting on the same day the previous method is stopped. Use an alternate method of contraception for the first 7 days.

EMERGENCY CONTRACEPTIVES. Emergency contraceptive pills (ECs) also are known as "morning after pills." These progestin-only pills, taken within 72 hours of unprotected intercourse, reduce the risk of pregnancy by at least 75%, although data suggest that efficacy may extend to 120 hours . The sooner EC is initiated, the more effective it will be. Following EC use, the next menstrual period may start a few days earlier or later than usual. Some spotting may occur before the next period. If the period does not start within 3 weeks, the patient should contact her health care provider for a pregnancy test.

Progestin-only EC is effective and has few side effects and no contraindications. It is not an abortifacient. It will not disrupt an established pregnancy. Plan B is now available over the counter to women 18 years and older. A prescription is required for women younger than 18 years. Effective emergency contraception may be obtained through the Yuzpe method, which involves the use of particular regimens of suitable monophasic pills to deliver an effective dose. Guidance for clinicians and patients on use of the Yuzpe method

based on pills that are available, along with answers to other questions, can be obtained by calling 1-888-NOT-2-LATE.

Patients should begin EC as soon as possible after unprotected intercourse. OTC labeling says to take 1 tablet and then the second 12 hours later. Many clinicians follow guidelines established by Planned Parenthood Federation of America and prescribe both doses to be taken at once. Women may use EC more often than once in a cycle, but use of EC always provides an opportunity for counseling on effective contraception.

PROGESTIN-ONLY PILLS (MINIPILLS). Benefits of progestin-only pills (POPs) include the following:

- Immediate return to fertility on discontinuation
- Avoidance of estrogen-related side effects
- Safe and effective for the lactating woman; may be started immediately postpartum
- Decreased anemia
- Decreased dysmenorrhea
- Decreased risk of endometrial and ovarian cancer
- Decreased risk of pelvic inflammatory disease (theoretical)
- Safe for patients with contraindications to estrogen

Also called minipills, POPs are used primarily in breastfeeding women and women with contraindications to estrogen. Advise the lactating woman to notify you when she stops nursing so she may be switched to COCPs. No increase in risk for thromboembolic events is seen with progestin-only pills.

POPs are more effective when they inhibit ovulation. Explain to women that the more disrupted their bleeding pattern, the more likely it is that ovulation is inhibited. If the patient cycles regularly, she probably is ovulating and should use a backup method of contraception. The patient should report to the provider any prolonged episodes of bleeding, amenorrhea, or severe abdominal pain.

Start pills on the first day of menses. Use a backup method for the first 7 days.

If changing from COCPs to POPs, omit the pill-free week and start POPs immediately after stopping active COCPs. Take pills at the same time each day. If a pill is taken more than 3 hours late, a backup method must be used for the next 48 hours.

No pill-free interval occurs. When one 28-day pack is finished, another pack is started the next day. All pills in the pack are active pills. Counseling on bleeding changes and the need to take all 28 pills helps prevent discontinuation and to enhance effectiveness.

SUBDERMAL IMPLANTS. Progestin-only contraception is also available as an implantable device in a single-rod implant that contains etonogestrel, a desogestrel metabolite that is less androgenic and exhibits more progestational activity than levonorgestrel. Insertion and removal take about 2.5 minutes.

Progestin-only subdermal implants are designed to inhibit ovulation during the entire treatment period. Although their use is approved for 3 years, they may provide contraceptive protection for up to 5 years. Follicular activity without ovulation, in the presence of nearly normal estradiol levels, has been seen with this method. Because of this, women may develop palpable, but seldom symptomatic, physiologic ovarian cysts, which usually resolve spontaneously and do not require intervention. No long-term effects on fertility have been noted in implant users. After removal of the implant, concentrations of etonogestrel are undetectable within 1 week.

Advantages of implants include their high-efficacy, long-term action; ease of use; rapid onset of action; protection against ectopic pregnancy; low relative cost; and possible protection against urogenital tract infection. Possible disadvantages include menstrual irregularities, which usually improve over time; provider-dependent difficulties with placement and removal; lack of protection against sexually transmitted infections; and side effects for some women, including headache, acne, breast tenderness, weight and mood changes, ovarian cyst formation, and galactorrhea (breast milk expression).

Contraindications for contraceptive implants include acute thrombophlebitis or thromboembolic disease, undiagnosed genital bleeding, acute liver disease, benign or malignant liver tumors, and known or suspected breast cancer. Implanon implant is an important option for women for whom combined OC hormones may not be indicated, such as cigarette smokers older than 35 years and patients with diabetes mellitus with vascular disease; hypertriglyceridemia; history of stroke, heart attack, or deep venous thrombosis; gallbladder disease; and vascular headaches or migraine headaches with neurologic symptoms.

DEPOMEDROXYPROGESTERONE INJECTION (DMPA) (DEPO-PROVERA). Depomedroxyprogesterone, sometimes referred to as "Depo" is a long-acting injectable contraceptive that may be especially useful (1) in patients who have any condition that is worsened by the menstrual cycle, such as anemia, dysmenorrhea, or menstrual migraine, (2) in those with sickle cell anemia or seizure disorder, and (3) in women with an increased risk of endometrial cancer and/or ovarian cancer. Because of its potential to suppress estrogen, some clinicians use it to manage fibroid tumors. Patients who take medroxyprogesterone experience less bleeding (many are amenorrheic), making it an excellent choice for anemic patients. Benefits include convenience and ease of compliance.

- *Few drug interactions occur:* DMPA is not affected by medications that induce liver metabolism.
- Medroxyprogesterone is available in vials and prefilled syringes for 150-mg IM injection, as well as in prefilled syringes for 104-mg subQ injection. When IM injection is given, it should be administered by Z-track technique into the gluteus maximus or the deltoid muscle. The area of the injection should not be massaged because this can lower the effectiveness of medroxyprogesterone. Although contraceptive efficacy can be ensured only when injections are given every 3 months, some DMPA may remain in the bloodstream for 6 to 9 months. The initial injection should be given during the first 5 days of menses to ensure that the patient is not pregnant.

Timing of Injections. Injections must be given every 12 weeks ± 7 days, but they can be given earlier if a woman has spotting. Although fertility may be delayed for up to a year after the method is discontinued, contraceptive efficacy cannot be guaranteed if an injection is given late. If a woman presents later than 13 weeks since her last injection, DMPA may be given if she has not had intercourse outside of the 12-week window. Otherwise, she will have to maintain abstinence for 14 days so a reliable pregnancy test can be given or must return for injection during menses, whichever is sooner.

Backup Method. If DMPA is given during the first 5 days of menses, no backup method is necessary. If it is given at any other time in the cycle, backup is necessary for the first 2 weeks.

INTRAUTERINE DEVICE. A nonhormonal mechanical copper-T IUD method is effective for 10 years. The levonorgestrel-releasing intrauterine system (LNG-IUS) combines the mechanical protection of the device with low levels of progestin that minimize menstrual bleeding. This IUD is effective for 5 years. The copper IUD also may be used for emergency contraception within 7 days of unprotected intercourse. IUDs have additional contraindications to those for OCs (see specific drug information). These must be inserted by a specially trained health care provider.

MODIFYING TREATMENT. Estrogen can be given to stabilize the endometrium if needed when significant breakthrough bleeding is reported. See Table 53-6 for a summary of common problems with contraceptive use and their solutions.

How to Monitor

- The initial visit should include assessment of weight and blood pressure, clinical breast examination, Pap smear, and pelvic examination. STD testing should be performed as part of the annual screening gynecologic examination for patients considered at risk for STD but is not necessary for monitoring. Planned Parenthood guidelines and many clinicians offer patients the opportunity to waive or defer the physical examination for a contraceptive method start.
- Some clinicians schedule follow-up visits in 3 months to check blood pressure and weight gain/loss and to review side effects and warning signs. Yearly monitoring may include

TABLE 53-6 Contraceptive Use: Problems and Solutions

Problem	Considerations	Solution	Some Suggested Contraceptives
Androgenetic symptoms	Acne, weight gain, and others	COCP with low androgen activity	Orth-Cyclen, Apri, Desogen, Ortho-Cept
Amenorrhea	Risk of pregnancy	Increase endometrial activity of COCP	Desogen, Ortho-Cept, Ortho Tri-Cyclen,
	Normal on many OCs Common with medroxyprogesterone	Change to progestin with higher endometrial activity	Ortho-Cyclen, Ovcon 35, Brevicon, or Modicon
	Treat if patient is uncomfortable	Change to COCP with higher estrogen dose for a few cycles	
		Change to COCP with lower progestin dose	
Breakthrough bleeding: OCs	Risk of pregnancy	Reassurance during first 3 months	Lo/Ovral, Nordette, Levlen, Desogen, Ortho-Cept, Ortho-Cyclen, Ortho-Tri-Cyclen
	Normal in first 3 months	Change to pill with greater endometrial activity, more potent progestin	
	More frequent with POPs Often due to missed or late pills	If on POP, add estrogen	
Breakthrough bleeding: medroxyprogesterone	Atrophy of endometrium due to hypoestrogenic state	Stabilize the endometrium with short course of exogenous estrogen	Estradiol 2 mg daily × 7 or more days, may repeat once
Estrogen sensitivity	Estrogenic effects such as nausea, edema, hypertension, heavy menses, migraines	Decrease estrogen in COCP or use progestin-only method	Loestrin 1/20, Desogen, Levlen, Loestrin 1.5/30, Lo/Ovral, Nordette, Ortho-Cept, medroxyprogesterone, POPs
Decreased libido	Decreased free testosterone levels, may occur with COCPs and with DMPA	Pill with increased androgenicity	Change COCPs to Loestrin 1.5/30, Triphasil, or Tri-Levlen; discontinue DMPA and substitute another method if side effect is pronounced

weight and blood pressure assessment, clinical breast examination, Pap smear, pelvic examination, and STD testing as indicated.

- Patients at high risk for heart disease (personal or family history) may undergo a baseline lipid profile and fasting glucose at the initial examination and yearly thereafter.
- Patients are considered at high risk for thromboembolism if they are smokers or are overweight. Counsel patients that they must not smoke while using OCPs.

Patient Variables

AGE OLDER THAN 35 YEARS. COCPs are appropriate throughout the reproductive years. Nonsmoking women may continue until menopause on any COCP that contains 35 mcg or less EE. Smoking women should not be taking COCP after the age of 35. Perimenopausal women without other contraindications are good candidates for COCPs because of their noncontraceptive benefits. COCPs help prevent some of the adverse sequelae that occur during the perimenopause, such as endometrial hyperplasia, hot flushes, and vaginal atrophy.

It is important to determine when a woman has gone through menopause and can discontinue COCPs. Beginning at age 50, FSH levels can be drawn on day 5 to 7 of the pill-free week as part of the annual examination. If FSH is greater than 20 mIU/ml, the patient can be considered menopausal and COCPs discontinued. See Chapter 54 for additional information on postmenopausal hormone therapy.

FAMILY HISTORY BREAST OR OVARIAN CANCER. Probably should describe prescriptive decision making with strong family history or knowledge of *BRCA-1* or *BRCA-2* gene

PREGNANCY AND LACTATION. Conjugated estrogen and medroxyprogesterone are designated as FDA category X; however, contradictory data indicate that no risk of birth defects is present when a woman becomes pregnant while using an estrogen-based oral contraceptive. Data regarding risks from contraceptive doses of progestins are inconclusive.

Estrogen decreases the quality and quantity of milk and is not recommended for lactating women. Progestins promote breast milk production. Progestin-only methods are recommended for lactating women who desire hormonal contraception. If COCPs are used, these should not be introduced until at least 6 weeks postpartum in a woman who is breastfeeding.

MIGRAINE. Women who have migraine with aura have a relative contraindication for COCPs. If COCPs are offered to these women, they must be closed monitored.

Patient Education

COMBINED ORAL CONTRACEPTIVE AND PROGESTIN-ONLY PILLS

- Demonstrate use of the pill package. Have the patient give a return demonstration.
  - Pills must be taken exactly as directed.
  - Use a backup method for at least 48 hours when a progestin-only OC is taken more than 2 to 3 hours late.
- For COCPs, see the drug treatment principles.
- Stress that POPs require a constant daily dose. No placebo pills or pill-free interval is provided.
- The pill does not protect against STD or human immunodeficiency virus (HIV). Stress importance of the use of male or female condoms with every act of intercourse that may pose a risk of STD.
- Instruct the patient to stop taking pills immediately and to contact her health care provider if any serious adverse reactions occur.

SPECIFIC DRUGS

COMBINATION ORAL CONTRACEPTIVE PILLS

CONTRAINDICATIONS

- Hypersensitivity
- Thrombophlebitis, thromboembolic disorders
- History of deep vein thrombophlebitis
- Cerebrovascular disease
- Myocardial infarction, coronary artery disease
- Known or suspected breast carcinoma or estrogen-dependent neoplasia
- Carcinoma of endometrium
- Hepatic adenomas/carcinomas
- Acute liver disease
- Undiagnosed abnormal genital bleeding
- Known or suspected pregnancy
- Cholestatic jaundice of pregnancy/jaundice with prior pill use
- Hypersensitivity

WARNINGS

Smoking: **Cigarette smoking increases the risk of serious cardiovascular side effects from OCs. This risk increases with age and with heavy smoking and is quite marked in women over 35 years of age. Women who use OCs should not smoke.**

Risks of OC use: **The use of OCs is associated with increased risk of thromboembolism, stroke, MI, hypertension, hepatic neoplasia, and gallbladder disease, although the risk of serious morbidity or mortality is very small in healthy women without underlying risk factors. Risk of morbidity/mortality increases significantly in the presence of other underlying risk factors such as hypertension, hyperlipidemia, obesity, smoking, and diabetes.**

Mortality associated with all methods of birth control is low and below that associated with childbirth, with the exception of women older than 35 years who smoke and women over age 40. Weigh the risk of pregnancy vs. the risk of

adverse reactions when prescribing OCs in healthy nonsmoking women older than 40 years of age, and prescribe the lowest effective dose.

- *Thromboembolism:* Be alert to the earliest symptoms of thromboembolic and thrombotic disorders.
- *Cerebrovascular disease:* OCs increase the risk of cerebrovascular events (thrombotic and hemorrhagic strokes) and vascular disease. A decline in HDL and an increase in triglycerides have been seen.
- *Ocular lesions:* Retinal thrombosis has occurred. Monitor for unexplained loss of vision, onset of proptosis or diplopia, papilledema, or retinal vascular lesions.
- *Carcinoma:* Increased incidence of breast, endometrial, ovarian, and cervical cancer has been seen.
- Hepatic benign and malignant lesions have been associated with the use of OCs, but this is rare.
- *Gallbladder disease:* This risk has decreased since the dosages of estrogen and progestin have been decreased.
- *Carbohydrate metabolism:* Glucose tolerance may decrease in relation to estrogen dose. Progestins can create insulin resistance.
- Elevated blood pressure usually begins within a few months of initiation of use.
- *Headaches:* Onset of exacerbation of migraine or development of headache with focal neurologic symptoms of a new pattern that is recurrent, persistent, or severe requires OC discontinuation.
- *Bleeding irregularities:* BTB and spotting are sometimes encountered in OC patients, especially during the first 3 months of use.
- Ectopic pregnancy may occur in cases of contraceptive failure, especially with progestin-only OCs.

PRECAUTIONS

- *Fluid retention:* OCs may cause fluid retention. Use a pill with the progestin drospirenone or use other pills with caution in patients who have conditions that might be aggravated by fluid retention, such as convulsive disorders, migraine syndrome, asthma, or cardiac, hepatic, or renal dysfunction.
- *Contact lenses:* Changes in vision or lens tolerance may develop; refer to ophthalmologist.
- Serum folate levels may be decreased by OCs. Women who become pregnant shortly after stopping therapy may have a greater chance of birth defects.
- *Acute intermittent porphyria:* OCs may precipitate attacks of acute intermittent porphyria. Use with caution.
- Vomiting or diarrhea may cause OC failure. If significant GI distress occurs, use a backup method of contraception for the remainder of the cycle.

PHARMACOKINETICS. Considerable individual variation in circulating levels of estrogen and progestin has been noted among women. EE and most oral progestins undergo a first-pass effect. A variety of other factors, such as body weight, drug interactions, and timing of medications, also affect individual variability in bioavailability.

Estrogen and progestins are rapidly absorbed from the stomach. Both undergo first-pass hepatic degradation (see Chapter 3 for more information on this process). Peak blood levels usually occur in 1 to 2 hours. Estrogen is

98% protein bound. Progestins are about 79% to 95% protein bound and are bound to SHBG (except drospirenone). The elimination half-life for the progestins is usually about 8 to 9 hours, but it varies (Table 53-7). The half-life of the metabolites is usually several days. Some metabolites are active, and others are not. Progestin metabolites are excreted in the urine. Progestin-only administration results in lower serum progestin levels and a shortened half-life than when administered with estrogens.

ADVERSE REACTIONS

- Side effects such as breakthrough bleeding, headache, nausea, and breast tenderness are most common during the first 3 months of use and should improve without intervention. Persistent problems beyond the initial 3 months of use may require a change to a different COCP. Prolonged bleeding should always be investigated.
- Serious pill warning signs that may require emergency intervention and reconsideration of whether to stop the medication are noted by the acronym ACHES:
  A: Severe Abdominal pain
  C: Severe Chest pain, cough, shortness of breath
  H: Severe Headache, dizziness, weakness, or numbness
  E: Eye problems (vision loss or blurring), speech problems
  S: Severe leg pain (calf or thigh)
- Irregular vaginal bleeding or BTB usually improves after the first 3 months of use, although it may persist or occur after a long period of use, necessitating a change to a different COCP formulation. Taking pills at the same time each day often resolves this. Pills that are very low in estrogen are more likely to be associated with BTB, as are phasic vs. monophasic pills.

- Weight gain is largely a function of diet and exercise and not of COCPs. Rarely, weight gain may be due to fluid retention (estrogen or progestin effect), increased subcutaneous fat (estrogen effect), or increased appetite (androgen effect).
- Nausea (estrogen effect) may occur with some pills and not with others. If it presents, it usually occurs during the first few pills in each cycle or the first few cycles of pill use. Taking pills with food may be helpful.
- Amenorrhea or missed periods may occur.
- Chloasma/melasma may appear and persist after COCP discontinuation.
- Depression, decreased libido, hair loss, breast tenderness, increased breast size, and mastalgia may occur.

DRUG INTERACTIONS

Drugs That Reduce Efficacy of Combined Oral Contraceptive Pills

- *Cytochrome P450 enzyme inducers:* Drugs that induce cytochrome P450 3A4 enzymes, cause the rapid breakdown of estrogen and progestin, and may decrease the effectiveness of COCPs. Patients on the following medications should consider other methods.
  - Anticonvulsants: phenobarbital, phenytoin (Dilantin), primidone (Mysoline), carbamazepine (Tegretol), ethosuximide, oxcarbazepine (Trileptal). *Note:* Patients on anticonvulsants who wish to continue on COCPs can be placed on 50-mcg pills with careful monitoring or can be switched to valproic acid, if possible. Valproic acid does not interact with COCPs.
  - *Antituberculosis:* rifampin
  - *Antifungals:* griseofulvin
  - *Other:* modafinil, protease inhibitors, St. John's wort

TABLE 53-7 Pharmacokinetics of Contraceptive Medications

Drug	Absorption	Drug Availability (After First Pass)	Time to Peak Concentration	Half-life	Metabolism	Excretion
ethinyl estradiol	Rapid	50%	6-8 hr	13-27 hr	Liver	Urine
norethindrone	Rapid, complete	65%	1-2 hr	4-13 hr	Conjugation	Urine
levonorgestrel	Rapid, complete	100% active isomer of norgestrel	1-2.5 hr	24 hr	Conjugation	Urine, feces
norgestrel	—	—	—	26-46 hr	Liver	Urine
desogestrel	Rapid, complete	84% converted into active metabolite	1.4 hr	23-50 hr	Liver	Feces, urine
norgestimate	Well	Converted to deacetylnorgestimate (active metabolite)	0.5-2 hr	37 hr	Liver	Urine, feces
norethynodrel and ethynodiol diacetate	Rapid, complete	Ethynodiol diacetate (converted to norethindrone)	1-2 hr	4-13 hr	Liver	Urine
norelgestromin	Transdermal	Converted to norgestrel	≈48 hr	29 hr	Liver	Urine, feces
etonogestrel	Intrauterine	Active metabolite of desogestrel	—	25 hr	Liver	Urine
drospirenone	Complete	76%	1-3 hr	30 hr	Liver	Urine, feces

Drugs That May Reduce Efficacy of Combined Oral Contraceptive Pills

Although the evidence is somewhat controversial, antibiotics (primarily tetracycline, amoxicillin, ampicillin, and metronidazole) may eliminate gut flora, causing a decrease in the amount of hormone absorbed from the intestine or interference with enterohepatic recirculation. Long-term antibiotic use is far less likely to be associated with this effect. Patients should be cautioned to use a barrier method during a COCP cycle when a new course of antibiotics is initiated.

Drugs That May Increase Estrogen Effects. Megadose vitamin C (2000 mg and up) has been shown to increase the amount of circulating EE by inhibiting liver enzymes that metabolize the steroids. Women who take 1000 mg or more of vitamin C per day or who are taking low-dose COCPs actually may be receiving high-dose-pill estrogen. When the patient stops taking vitamin C, she may experience spotting as estrogen levels decrease. Taking vitamin C at different times from COCP administration will not prevent this effect.

Drugs That May Have Altered Pharmacokinetics With Concomitant Combined Oral Contraceptive Pill Administration. COCPs may decrease clearance of benzodiazepines, corticosteroids, theophylline, and aminophylline. Lower doses of these medications may be indicated. The effects of tricyclic antidepressants, β-blockers, and alcohol may be increased. Analgesics such as acetaminophen may have decreased pain-relieving effect.

DOSAGE AND ADMINISTRATION. OCPs should be taken at the same time every day. The risk of pregnancy increases with each missed dose.

OTHER DRUGS IN CLASS

Other drugs in this class share the same characteristics except as follows:

ethinyl estradiol and drospirenone (Yasmin, Yaz)

Yasmin and Yaz are combined contraceptives that contain a novel progestin, drospirenone, which is not a testosterone derivative. It is chemically related to spironolactone and has antimineralocorticoid effects and antiandrogenic effects similar to progesterone. These COCPs may cause potassium retention. Caution should be used in women taking potassium-sparing diuretics, ACE inhibitors or ARBs, other aldosterone antagonists, heparin, or long-term NSAIDs. A serum potassium level should be checked during the first month of therapy in patients taking any of these drugs. With all of the other available hormonal contraceptive choices, it would be best to avoid drospirenone-containing products for women on these drugs.

CONTRAINDICATIONS (IN ADDITION TO ABOVE). Renal insufficiency, hepatic dysfunction, adrenal insufficiency, heavy smoking (15 or more cigarettes per day), and age over 35 years. Thrombohemolytic disease, breast cancer, ovarian cancer, and undiagnosed bleeding are other contraindications.

WARNINGS

Hyperkalemia. Drospirenone has antimineralocorticoid activity, including the potential for hyperkalemia in high-risk patients, comparable with those of a 25-mg dose of spironolactone.

Yasmin should not be used in patients with conditions that predispose to hyperkalemia (e.g., renal insufficiency, hepatic dysfunction, adrenal insufficiency). Women who receive daily long-term treatment for chronic conditions or diseases with medications that may increase serum potassium should have their serum potassium level checked during the first treatment cycle. Drugs that may increase serum potassium include potassium supplements, ACE inhibitors, angiotensin II receptor blockers, potassium-sparing diuretics, heparin, aldosterone antagonists, and NSAIDs.

Progestin Emergency Contraception (Plan B)

CONTRAINDICATIONS. Pregnancy (but only because of ineffectiveness, not because of teratogenicity)

Progestin-Only Oral Contraceptives

ADVERSE EFFECTS. The most common complaint with POPs is irregular bleeding, which may range from spotting to BTB to amenorrhea. This is expected and normal. Patients with amenorrhea are unlikely to be ovulating. Anticipatory counseling may help prevent discontinuation. Explain the need to take pills at the same time every day. BTB may be related to late pills.

If the patient cycles regularly, she probably is ovulating and needs to use a backup method of contraception. The patient should report prolonged episodes of bleeding, amenorrhea, or severe abdominal pain.

Other side effects include edema, abdominal bloating, anxiety, irritability, depression, and myalgia. See manufacturers' prescribing information for full information.

DRUG INTERACTIONS. Drugs that induce liver enzymes will decrease the efficacy of POPs. Patients who take the following medications should use a backup method or change to a different method: rifampin, phenobarbital, phenytoin (Dilantin), primidone (Mysoline), and carbamazepine (Tegretol). See manufacturers' prescribing information for a complete list.

Transdermal System

Risk of skin irritation, redness, or rash is increased.

Vaginal Ring

Risk of vaginal discomfort, foreign body sensation, coital problems, or device expulsion is increased.

Intrauterine Devices

ADDITIONAL CONTRAINDICATIONS. Additional contraindications include congenital or acquired uterine anomalies such as fibroids if they distort the uterine cavity; acute PID; postpartum endometriosis or infected abortion in the past 3 months; known or suspected uterine or cervical neoplasia; untreated acute cervicitis or vaginitis; women at high risk for STD, and a uterus that sounds to less than 6 cm or greater than 9 cm. Women with bleeding disorders or who are taking anticoagulants should not use the Paragard IUD, and use is contraindicated in women with copper allergy or Wilson's disease.

Depomedroxyprogesterone Injection (Depo-Provera or DMPA)

WARNINGS. Because of strong progestational effects on the endometrium, irregular bleeding and/or spotting is fairly common in the early months of use, and unpredictable bleeding and/or amenorrhea is common and expected with continued use. In contrast to COCP users, DMPA users do not have regular menstrual patterns; no cyclic withdrawal bleeding occurs. Bleeding may be heavy and prolonged initially but is usually light and sporadic. At least 50% of users become amenorrheic after the first year of use, some after the first injection. Thorough counseling regarding irregular bleeding pattern may foster method continuation.

Low estrogen levels associated with DMPA are a risk factor for osteoporosis. In 2004, the FDA added a black box warning to DMPA, stating that prolonged use of the drug may result in significant loss of bone mineral density (BMD), and that this loss is greater the longer the drug is administered. It further states that BMD loss may not be fully reversible after discontinuation of the drug. Thus, the warning suggests that women should use DMPA as a long-term method (>2 years) only if other methods are inadequate or unsuitable. Concern was initially focused on adolescence and early adulthood, critical periods of bone accretion; however, subsequent studies have shown a complete recovery of BMD within 3 years of discontinuation of DMPA, with complete recovery within 1 year in adolescents. Based on this reexamination of data, Planned Parenthood Federation of America advises affiliates that the more significant concern involves women close to menopausal age who may not have a chance to recover their BMD if they transition from DMPA to menopause. Although adequate calcium intake has not been demonstrated to prevent BMD loss, all women on DMPA should be counseled to supplement their dietary calcium and vitamin D if inadequate, and to start or continue weight-bearing exercise. This can prevent modifiable risks for future osteoporosis. With all patients, the risk of pregnancy must be weighed against known effects on BMD.

PRECAUTIONS

- *Pregnancy planned in the near future:* Median time to conception after last injection is 10 months, with a range of 4 to 31 months. A patient who desires a more rapid return to fertility should choose a different method of contraception.
- *Concern over weight gain:* Average weight gain after 1 year is 5.4 lb; after 2 years, 8.1 lb; after 4 years, 13.8 lb; and after 6 years, 16.5 lb, according to the package insert. Increased appetite is believed to be responsible for weight gain that can be seen with DMPA use.
- *Lipid effects:* Medroxyprogesterone is thought to negatively affect lipid profiles, but the extent of this effect is unclear. Progestins tend to lower HDL cholesterol and increase the ratio of total cholesterol to HDL cholesterol. Obtain baseline lipid profile and reevaluate yearly or as clinically indicated.

ADVERSE EFFECTS. Other adverse effects may include breast tenderness, allergy, headache, nervousness, dizziness, weakness, and fatigue. A prior belief that DMPA could aggravate major depression has not been substantiated.

Less common adverse effects include decreased libido or anorgasmia, vaginitis, leg cramps, alopecia, bloating, edema, rash, insomnia, acne, nausea, hot flashes, leukorrhea, and anaphylaxis.

DRUG INTERACTIONS. Antibiotics and anticonvulsants that induce liver enzymes do not affect medroxyprogesterone. Aminoglutethimide (Cytadren), a drug given for Cushing's syndrome, does lower serum concentrations of DMPA and may affect efficacy.

evolve A continually updated list of useful WebLinks may be found in the Evolve Resources at http://evolve.elsevier.com/Edmunds/NP/

54 Menopause Hormone Therapy

IVY M. ALEXANDER

DRUG OVERVIEW

Class	Subclass	Generic Name	Trade Name*
Estrogens	Conjugated estrogens	conjugated estrogens (equine)	Premarin ✸
		conjugated estrogens (synthetic)	Cenestin
		conjugated estrogens B (synthetic)	Enjuvia
	Synthesized estrogens	estrogens, esterified	Estratab, Estratest, Menest
		ethinyl estradiol	FemHrt
		estropipate (estrone)	Ogen (po), Ortho-Est
	Bioidentical	estradiol ✸	Alora, Climara ✸, Estrace, Estraderm, Estrasorb, Estring, EstroGel, Femring, Vagifem ✸, Vivelle ✸, Menostar
		estrone	Kestrone, Estrone (inj)
		estriol	Available only in compounded products in the United States (Bi-est, Tri-est)
Progestogens	Synthesized	medroxyprogesterone acetate	Provera, Cycrin, Amen
		norethindrone acetate	Norethisterone
		norgestimate	Combination: Ortho-cyclen, Ortho Tri-cyclen ✸, Prefest
	Bioidentical	micronized progesterone	Prometrium ✸
Combination agents		conjugated estrogen/ medroxyprogesterone	PremPro ✸, PremPhase
		estradiol/norethindrone acetate	Combipatch
Androgens	Synthesized Bioidentical	methyltestosterone testosterone	Combination: Estratest, Estratest HS

✸ Top 200 drug. *Examples, not comprehensive.

INDICATIONS

Hormone Therapy (HT), Estrogens, Progesterones

- Relief of moderate to severe vasomotor symptoms, postmenopausal
- Relief of vulvovaginal atrophy, postmenopausal
- Osteoporosis prevention, postmenopausal
- Dysfunctional uterine bleeding
- Secondary amenorrhea
- Primary ovarian failure and/or premature oophorectomy
- Prostate cancer (palliative treatment)

- Certain breast cancers (palliative treatment)
- Endometrial hyperplasia, prevention

Androgens

- Metastatic cancer
- Combination with estrogen for vasomotor symptom management

Unlabeled Uses

- Diminished libido in menopause

Hormones used for menopause symptom management and osteoporosis prevention are the only indications discussed in this chapter.

A variety of estrogen and progestogen formulations are available. New products frequently enter the market as hormones are reformulated, combined, and recombined. Similarly, a variety of new delivery methods are becoming available (e.g., creams and gels, and sprays).

Estrogen and progestogen are FDA approved for the treatment of moderate to severe menopause-related symptoms, including hot flashes and vulvovaginal atrophy, and for the prevention of postmenopausal osteoporosis. Many women anecdotally report improved quality of life (QOL) with HT use. These anecdotal reports are supported by findings of several research studies undertaken to evaluate QOL effects, and they are refuted by the findings of others.

Results from the Women's Health Initiative (WHI) released in 2002 changed the approach used to prescribe estrogen and progestogen. The estrogen plus progestogen (E-P) arm of the WHI randomized controlled trial was halted early because women who were taking estrogen plus progestogen (conjugated equine estrogens [CEEs] 0.625 mg and medroxyprogesterone [MPA] 2.5 mg) had an increased incidence of CHD, stroke, venous thromboembolic events (VTEs), and invasive breast cancer. The E-P arm also showed a reduced risk for colorectal cancer and a reduction in osteoporotic fracture. The estrogen-only arm of the WHI was also halted early in 2004 because of increased risk of stroke. It is interesting to note that the estrogen-only arm of the study also showed a trend toward a reduced risk of breast cancer and no change in CHD. QOL was not changed in women taking HT vs. placebo in the WHI study.

Additionally, the Women's Health Initiative Memory Study (WHIMS), a substudy of the WHI, suggested that women taking combination estrogen plus progestogen therapy had an increased relative risk of developing probable dementia compared with women in all age groups who were taking placebo. Absolute risk was greatest in the oldest group studied (women aged 75 and older). Several important limitations of the WHI have been identified: (1) The women in this study were approximately 10 years postmenopausal (average age was 63.3 years), (2) participants were not symptomatic (symptomatic women were excluded because they would have known whether they were taking active drug or placebo), (3) many participants were overweight, and (4) many had established heart disease (e.g., hypertension). However, data from the Women's HOPE (Health, Osteoporosis, Progestin, Estrogen) study suggest that lower doses of estrogen and progestogen effectively decreased vasomotor symptoms yet did not raise the risk of CHD. A more recent meta-analysis of several observational studies and a reanalysis of data from the WHI that focused on age cohorts indicate that heart disease is reduced in women who initiate HT at the time of menopause, supporting a hypothesis that the time of initiation of HT is critical. Additional research is required to further elucidate the relationship between HT and cardiovascular health. Women who took estrogen plus progestin in the WHI trial of hormone replacement therapy (HRT) have been found to remain at higher risk of breast cancer three years after the trial was stopped compared with those who took placebo. Higher risks of cardiovascular events seen in those taking the active preparation abated in the follow-up period, however, as did the beneficial effects of HRT on bone strength.

Most national organizations, such as the North American Menopause Society (NAMS), the American College of Obstetricians and Gynecologists (ACOG), the National Association of Nurse Practitioners in Women's Health (NPWH), the American Society of Reproductive Medicine (ASRM), and the U.S. Preventive Services Task Force (USPSTF), along with the FDA, support the use of HT for moderate to severe vasomotor symptoms and vaginal atrophy associated with menopause. Most of these organizations and the FDA recommend against the use of HT for prevention of chronic disease (e.g., cardiovascular disease), with the exception of osteoporosis. However, they note that other options are also available for osteoporosis prevention and should be considered in women who do not experience moderate to severe vasomotor symptoms (see Chapter 37). Additionally, current recommendations for HT use advocate using the lowest effective dose for the shortest length of time. Women who use HT should regularly review their symptoms with their clinicians to consider the need for ongoing use. The WHI results indicate that HT use for 5 years is reasonably safe. The risks vs. benefits for use, especially for longer periods, must be determined on an individual basis.

Most clinicians review use of HT with their patients annually and attempt slow weaning to determine whether therapy is still necessary, or if the woman may be able to manage her symptoms effectively at a lower dose. Therapy decisions should be individualized for each patient, with consideration of her personal and family history, symptom severity, and personal preferences. Clinicians must recognize that many women use OTC and herbal remedies to manage their menopausal symptoms. It is essential to elicit information about use of these products because they have the potential to produce adverse side effects or drug interactions. Research regarding HT use is ongoing; it is recommended that the reader consult up-to-date resources for the latest information on this topic.

THERAPEUTIC OVERVIEW OF HORMONE THERAPY

Anatomy and Physiology

See Chapter 53 for a discussion of hormone use during the reproductive years.

The menopausal transition is a natural process that all women who live long enough will experience. This transition consists of three distinct stages: perimenopause, menopause, and postmenopause. *Perimenopause* is the period that spans the 8 to 10 years prior to menopause, during which symptoms associated with changing levels of estrogen and progesterone often occur. The perimenopausal years usually occur between the ages of 42 and 55. For several years before menopause, the frequency of ovulation decreases. Hot flashes may occur and PMS may intensify. Menstrual bleeding frequently becomes irregular. Unplanned pregnancy is a risk because of the irregularity of ovulation. *Menopause* is defined as a point in time that occurs after the natural cessation of menses for 12 consecutive months. The average age of menopause in North America is 51 years. *Postmenopause*, the period following menopause, is commonly associated with symptoms such as hot flashes, sleep interruptions, and vulvovaginal changes, as well as later processes related to reduced hormone levels.

Menopause is not a disease process; rather, it is a normal transition. However, the symptoms experienced as hormone levels fluctuate and decline prior to and following menopause may require intervention.

Menses completely terminate 12 months preceding menopause, and ovarian production of estrogen ceases. The low plasma estradiol concentration that remains is the result of peripheral conversion of androgen precursors that are secreted predominantly by the adrenal glands. The precursors found in plasma become estrone rather than estradiol. The conversion of androgen precursors to estrone occurs in adipose tissue, and the adrenals provide a very small amount of progesterone.

During the perimenopausal period, as ovarian sensitivity to FSH stimulation decreases, plasma levels of FSH and LH increase. Following menopause, the lack of negative feedback from ovarian production of estradiol in the hypothalamic-pituitary-ovarian axis allows FSH and LH levels to increase to about 4 to 10 times the levels seen during the premenopausal follicular phase. Pulsatile secretion may persist, and the high levels of circulating FSH and LH stimulate the ovarian corticostromal and hilar cells to continue to produce significant levels of androstenedione and testosterone. Circulating levels of androstenedione are lower in postmenopausal women; circulating testosterone levels are similar to those found in premenopausal women.

Disease Process

IMMEDIATE-ONSET EFFECTS. Some symptoms develop while estrogen levels are changing. Vasomotor symptoms are most problematic in the first 7 years following menopause. However, they can persist for many more years. Vaginal atrophy starts early and persists throughout postmenopause, causing dryness, dyspareunia, and increased vaginal pH.

Vasomotor Tone Instability. Short-term vasomotor changes resulting from hormonal variations can cause *hot flashes* during perimenopause and postmenopause. When hot flashes are accompanied by flushing, usually at the face, neck, and upper chest, they are called *hot flushes*. Core body temperature rises, peripheral blood vessels dilate, skin conductance increases, and heart rate increases. Many women experience a prodrome before a hot flash occurs. Hot flashes or flushes also may be accompanied by dizziness, nausea, headache, palpitations, or sweating. They vary in duration and intensity, lasting from 1 to 4 minutes. The exact origin of hot flashes is poorly understood; however, they are associated with a surge in LH and declining estrogen and progesterone levels. During postmenopause, the thermoneutral zone narrows for many women, leading to sweating when the core body temperature rises above the upper limit or shivering when the core temperature dips below the lower limit. Hot flashes can be triggered by emotional stress, excitement, fear, anxiety, alcohol, caffeine, or environmental temperatures that raise the core temperature too high. Hot flashes or flushes that occur during the night are referred to as *night sweats* and interrupt sleep. Sleep interruptions frequently lead to reduced cognitive functioning and difficulty with remembering.

Vaginal Atrophy. In the postmenopausal woman, vaginal pH increases from about 5.0 to 7.0, making the tissue more susceptible to infection. Definitive changes take place at the cellular level: the cervix atrophies, the cervical os decreases in size, the superficial vaginal epithelium atrophies, the labia majora and minora shrink, and urethral tone decreases.

Muscle tone throughout the pelvic area decreases, which may lead to urinary tract infection and incontinence. The ovaries and uterus decrease in size. The vagina shortens, narrows, and loses some of its elasticity. Time for vaginal lubrication is increased, and vaginal secretions are reduced. This predisposes the woman to urinary tract infection, prolapse, dyspareunia, vaginitis, irritation, bleeding, burning, pruritus, and urinary symptoms such as frequency, urgency, and dysuria.

LONG-TERM EFFECTS. Several effects related to reduced hormone levels are not significant or identifiable until a woman is several years into postmenopause.

Cardiovascular. Women begin to develop atherosclerosis immediately following menopause; within 5 to 10 years, the incidence of cardiovascular disease in women surpasses that reported in men. Estrogen stimulates enzyme production that affects cholesterol metabolism. Without estrogen, breakdown of LDL cholesterol and production of HDL cholesterol are reduced, producing a lipid profile that contributes to the development of atherosclerosis. Estrogen also plays an important role in maintaining vascular elasticity, contributing to the increased incidence of hypertension present in postmenopausal women. Mortality rates from cardiovascular disease in women are higher than those in men; approximately 50% of all women will die from heart disease.

Breast. Breast tissue mass decreases during postmenopause. Glandular breast tissue is replaced by fat deposits and connective tissue. Breast tissue decreases both in size and in density. However, breast cancer risk increases with age.

Bone Density. Loss of bone mass is associated with postmenopause. Bone density peaks in the early to mid 30s and then begins to decline slowly over time. Loss accelerates following menopause at a rate of 1% to 5% per year for the first 4 to 8 years after menopause; it then slows again to a rate of about 1% per year. This loss of bone mass can lead to osteopenia and osteoporosis, which predispose women to fracture; it is a major cause of morbidity and mortality in the elderly. See Chapter 37, Osteoporosis Treatment, for further discussion.

Brain. Estrogen and progesterone have biochemical, neurophysiologic, and structural effects on the brain. For example, progesterone affects the regulation of GABA (an important inhibitory neurotransmitter) receptor sites. Estrogen affects cognitive function and memory, and both estrogen and progesterone aid the thermoregulatory center in maintaining normal body temperature.

Other. Menopause is associated with many additional symptoms such as dry skin, fatigue, insomnia, paresthesias, poor sleep quality, increased sleep latency, constipation, mood changes, muscle and joint pain, and decreased QOL. Now that estrogen and progesterone receptors have been identified throughout the body, systemic symptoms are beginning to be better understood.

Assessment

Monitoring FSH levels for the purpose of diagnosing menopause is no longer recommended. Identification of menopause is based on symptom patterns, menstrual changes, and age. Most clinicians do some laboratory testing to rule out other conditions that can mimic menopausal symptoms, such as thyroid abnormalities (see Chapter 51) or diabetes (see Chapter 52). If the woman is perimenopausal, FSH levels are especially unreliable because of the irregularity of hormone levels during this phase. FSH levels may be high when tested and then may fall low enough to allow for ovulation and pregnancy.

MECHANISM OF ACTION

Three classes of estrogen formulations have been identified: conjugated, synthetic, and bioidentical. Conjugated and synthetic estrogens stimulate hepatic globulins and the renin-angiotensin system to a greater extent than do bioidentical estrogens. Studies have demonstrated no clinical differences between classes. For drug action, see section "Anatomy and Physiology."

Estrogen exists in the body in three main forms: estrone (E_1), estradiol (E_2), and estriol (E_3). The active form of the most prevalent estrogen, 17β-estradiol, is not well absorbed when taken by mouth. The liver rapidly metabolizes much of the absorbed drug into inactive substances before it enters the bloodstream (first-pass phenomenon). Thus different methods of delivery have been devised. Oral estrogens are metabolized into estrone in the liver. Transdermal estrogens (creams, gels, patches, sprays) do not undergo the liver first-pass effect and can be dosed at lower levels.

In 1970, conjugated estrogens were officially defined as a mixture of sodium estrone sulfate and sodium equilin sulfate. The oldest form of estrogen is the conjugated equine estrogen (CEE), Premarin. Premarin is derived from the urine of pregnant mares and contains nine different estrogens, including sodium estrone sulfate (50% to 65%), sodium equilin sulfate (20% to 35%), and others. It received FDA approval for use in postmenopausal women in 1942 and has been included in many research studies. Multiple other estrogen formulations are also available.

Progestogens include bioidentically manufactured progesterone and a number of other synthesized compounds. Two major classes of progestogens are the 21-carbon progesterones, which are very similar to the endogenous hormone, and the 19-nortestosterone compounds, which have both progestogen effects and a variety of androgenic effects. Progestogens are lipophilic and bind to progesterone receptors throughout the body. See Chapter 53 for more information on progestogens.

Some androgens have predominantly androgenic properties, whereas others have primarily anabolic characteristics. Those androgens with highly androgenic properties are used for the treatment of patients with conditions that are hormonal in nature. Methyltestosterone is highly androgenic. Androgens with mainly anabolic effects are used to promote weight gain, increase muscle mass, or stimulate red blood cell production in certain forms of anemia.

Drug Effects in Menopause

The effects of estrogens and progestogens must be clearly separated. Estrogen, both individually and in combination with progestogens, has been studied most extensively. Progestogens most often have been studied in conjunction with estrogen for use in the management of menopause-related symptoms.

VASOMOTOR EFFECTS. Estrogen effectively treats those with hot flashes, decreasing frequency and severity. Progestogens have been used for hot flash management as well. However, because of their side effect profile, progestogens are not commonly used for this purpose.

VAGINAL ATROPHY. Use of estrogen in oral, vaginal, and transdermal forms has been shown to decrease atrophic vaginitis. Local estrogen (vaginal) provides relief more rapidly than the systemic alternatives.

CARDIOVASCULAR. Findings from the WHI study reveal a higher incidence of CHD, stroke, and pulmonary emboli risk in women taking estrogen plus progestogen. CHD was not found to be increased in women on estrogen only. Earlier studies and more recent reports evaluating effects on women close to the age of menopause describe cardiovascular benefits. Estrogen is known to increase the risk of thromboembolic disease. This risk may be dose related. Estrogen doses in HT are much lower than those in oral contraceptives (OCs).

BREAST CANCER. Data regarding estrogen and progestogen effects on breast cancer are controversial. Estrogen therapy (ET) may increase the risk of breast cancer. However, no change in mortality has been observed, and several studies have shown that women given a diagnosis of breast cancer while taking HT have a greater likelihood of survival. Evidence suggests that progestogen also may increase the risk of breast cancer. It is interesting to note that Megace (a progestogen) sometimes is used for breast cancer treatment. Some postulate that HT or ET speeds the development of breast cancer in patients who would have developed cancer at a later date. Estrogen also preserves or increases breast tissue density, making mammographic interpretation difficult in some instances.

BONE DENSITY. HT slows or halts the progression of bone loss and osteoporosis. It decreases the risk of osteoporosis-related fracture.

BRAIN. The effect of HT on brain function and on Alzheimer's disease is another area of controversy. Some studies demonstrate reduced Alzheimer's incidence, and others show an increased incidence of probable dementia. Cognitive function has been shown to improve with HT use in some studies and has not changed in others. Further research is needed in these areas.

ENDOMETRIAL CANCER. Unopposed estrogen in postmenopausal women with an intact uterus increases the risks of endometrial hyperplasia and cancer. Progestogens change the endometrium from a constant proliferative state to a secretory state, preventing endometrial hyperplasia associated with unopposed estrogen and reducing the risk of endometrial cancer.

GASTROINTESTINAL. HT predisposes users to cholecystitis. Recent data suggest that HT decreases the risk of developing colorectal cancer.

OVERALL EFFECTS OF HORMONE REPLACEMENT THERAPY. Use of HT is controversial. The benefits are that HT relieves symptoms of postmenopause, prevents osteoporosis, and provides improved QOL for women who experience moderate to severe symptoms. It also may reduce the risk of colon cancer. HT increases the risk of developing cholecystitis and may increase the risk for breast cancer. Unopposed ET in a woman who has a uterus increases the risk for developing endometrial hyperplasia and cancer. Controversy is ongoing regarding the effects of ET and HT on the cardiovascular system, coronary artery disease, stroke, thrombophlebitis, and pulmonary emboli. Clinicians must individualize their recommendations about initiating, continuing, or discontinuing HT.

TREATMENT PRINCIPLES

Standardized Guidelines

- NAMS, NPWH, ASRM, ACOG, FDA

Evidence-Based Recommendations

Meta-analyses and reviews conducted by the Cochrane Collaboration and the Agency for Healthcare Research and Quality (AHRQ) support the use of estrogen for managing menopause-related symptoms. Estrogen also has been shown to reduce the risk for colorectal cancer and osteoporosis-related fracture. Trials conducted to date support the use of estrogen for postmenopausal women who experience moderate to severe symptoms in association with menopause. Progesterone is used for the prevention of endometrial hyperplasia and cancer in postmenopausal women with an intact uterus who are using estrogen.

Cardinal Points of Treatment

- Pregnancy is possible during the perimenopausal years; these women must be counseled for appropriate selection of contraception if needed.
- Menopause-related symptom management begins with lifestyle modification.
- Use of HT must be individualized for each specific woman.
- The decision to use HT must be made in partnership with each individual woman, with consideration given to therapy risks and benefits, QOL, personal and family history, and personal preferences.
- HT should be given at the lowest effective dose and for the shortest time possible.
- The need for therapy must be regularly reevaluated.
- HT is used in conjunction with lifestyle changes to manage moderate to severe vasomotor and vulvovaginal symptoms associated with menopause in postmenopausal women. The following recommendations are supported by most national organizations and the FDA.
- Progesterone is needed for all women who have an intact uterus.

Nonpharmacologic Treatment

Lifestyle modifications are always the first step in managing perimenopausal and postmenopausal symptoms. Dietary changes include avoidance of caffeine, refined sugars, and alcohol, each of which can trigger vasomotor symptoms. In addition, midlife women should alter their diets to improve their overall health and should reduce health risks by decreasing fats, cholesterol, and salt; increasing fiber, calcium, and fluids; and attending to total caloric intake as metabolism slows with aging.

Exercise is important for moderating vasomotor symptoms, maintaining cardiovascular health, and promoting general well-being. Also, weight-bearing and resistance exercises are necessary to promote bone strength and prevent osteoporosis. Walking combined with upper body weight work generally is recommended as a safe and effective exercise. All postmenopausal women who do not have health contraindications should engage in at least 30 minutes of aerobic exercise daily. Weight-bearing and resistive exercises can be integrated and are site specific for maintaining bone strength.

Women in the United States increasingly seek complementary and alternative therapies for the management of symptoms of menopause. Data regarding efficacy are limited, and with the exception of black cohosh, few therapies have consistently demonstrated benefits. Black cohosh is an herb that has estrogen-like effects. Women who have contraindications for taking estrogen should not use Black cohosh. The exact mechanism of action of black cohosh is unclear. Recent publications suggest that no direct effect on estrogen receptors may be seen, although this is an area of controversy. Soy is a phytoestrogen, a plant substance that when ingested is metabolized into a compound that has estrogen-like properties. Complementary and alternative therapies are not regulated by the FDA in the same manner that prescription medications are. Purity, dose-to-dose or package-to-package consistency, and strength of varying forms of OTC products, herbal remedies, or soy formulations may fluctuate. Despite these potential limitations, many herbal products, soy formulations, and alternative practices (e.g., acupuncture) are used by women who experience symptoms. Research has indicated that stress management, such as deep breathing exercises similar to yoga breathing, may help to alleviate or reduce the severity of hot flashes. Herbal and OTC products can interact with prescription medications and with each other; thus information on use of these products must be elicited and documented (see Chapter 73 for additional information on alternative therapies).

Pharmacologic Treatment

Different medication regimens affect individual patients in different ways, necessitating an individualized approach to selection of therapy. Altering the medication subclass may reduce or change side effects for individual women. Similarly, altering the medication route (e.g., oral, transdermal, vaginal, injectable) may alter efficacy or tolerability of the treatment regimen. New medication delivery systems, such as the vaginal ring and transdermal routes, have been developed to increase the options available for women. Current research is under way to further elucidate the effects of route of delivery and time of HT initiation on cardiovascular disease and breast cancer risks for women.

Some women prefer medications other than HT for vasomotor symptom management. A significant body of research indicates that SSRIs such as fluoxetine, citalopram, and paroxetine and SNRIs such as venlafaxine (desvenlafaxine) can effectively reduce vasomotor symptoms in postmenopausal women. Clonidine and gabapentin have been shown to have some efficacy in vasomotor symptom relief. None of these alternative medications is as effective as ET or HT. Estrogen agonists/antagonists such as tamoxifen and raloxifene have proved ineffective in reducing hot flashes. In fact, raloxifene causes vasomotor symptoms in some women. Tamoxifen is frequently used for breast cancer treatment. Raloxifene is used for osteoporosis prevention and treatment (see Chapter 37 for additional information on osteoporosis and SERMs).

ORAL CONTRACEPTIVES DURING PERIMENOPAUSE. Oral contraceptives are not FDA approved for perimenopausal symptom management, with the exception of irregular menstrual bleeding. The woman and her clinician should make the decision together about the best treatment plan for her perimenopause-related symptoms, considering risks and benefits in view of her personal medical and family health history, symptom severity, need for contraception, and personal preferences. Informed consent is imperative.

As a woman undergoes the transition to postmenopause, her medications should be periodically reevaluated and adjusted to meet her needs. During the perimenopausal years, some women may need symptom relief, and many need protection against pregnancy. Low-dose OCs can be prescribed during the perimenopausal years to reduce symptoms while providing contraception and reducing abnormal menstrual bleeding. The dose of estrogen present in low-dose OCs is approximately four times greater than that of standard HT; thus HT is not effective for contraception in a perimenopausal woman.

Low-dose OCs during the perimenopausal years are contraindicated in smokers (Box 54-1) because of the increased risk of cardiovascular disease and VTE. OC use is associated with a reduced risk for developing ovarian and endometrial cancers. Research undertaken to evaluate the effects of OCs on breast cancer and stroke has yielded contradictory findings (see Chapter 53 for more information).

SHORT-TERM HT USE. In general, HT should be started as soon as the woman becomes postmenopausal. HT is used in the short term for the relief of menopause-related symptoms, which often are most problematic during early postmenopause. HT should be reevaluated annually and tapered as tolerated. The benefit/risk ratio for use up to 5 years is favorable.

LONG-TERM HT USE. When started during early postmenopause, HT is most effective in treating symptoms and preventing osteoporosis. The main risk associated with starting HT for women who are many years past menopause involves aggravating silent heart disease. Estrogen should be used only with caution in women with cardiovascular disease, hypertension, diabetes, or hyperlipidemia.

HT REGIMENS. Several different HT regimens can be selected (Table 54-1). Estrogen-progestogen treatment (EPT) regimens include both estrogen and progestogen and are used for women who have their uterus. Some clinicians use the intrauterine system containing progesterone to provide endometrial protection for women who are intolerant to or prefer not to take oral progesterone. The specific regimen is determined according to the woman's preference for withdrawal bleeding and tolerance of the two hormones. The estrogen-only daily regimen is used for women who do not have a uterus.

BOX 54-1   Contraindications to Use of Oral Contraceptives in Women Over 35 Years of Age

- Estrogen-dependent neoplasm
- Smoking (>15 cigarettes/day)
- Suspected pregnancy
- Untreated hypertension
- History of DVT, pulmonary embolism, stroke, ischemic heart disease
- Undiagnosed abnormal genital bleeding
- Diabetes with neuropathy, retinopathy, nephropathy, or vascular disease
- Active viral hepatitis, severe cirrhosis, benign or malignant liver tumors

---

Dosage. Oral HT is initiated at a low dose, equivalent to 0.3 mg CEE and 1.5 mg MPA. Women must be taught that full symptom relief may not be realized until 6 weeks of therapy has been completed. Vaginal treatment can be started daily or less often; usually, a half to a full applicator is used. Vaginal symptom relief usually is noticed within 1 to 2 weeks of initiation of local therapy.

Adjust Dosage as Necessary. Recheck patients after 3 months of oral therapy. Evaluate for the level of symptom control and titrate doses as needed. If the woman continues to report symptoms, increase the estrogen to the next higher dose (e.g., equivalent to 0.45 mg CEE and 1.5 mg MPA). Change the estrogen or the progestogen if specific side effects are intolerable. If a dose change is made, evaluate the woman again at 6 months. After a stable dose has been identified, annual reevaluation is appropriate. This same approach is used for transdermal and systemic vaginal products. Local vaginal product efficacy should be evaluated at approximately 2 weeks after initiation, and dose should then be titrated up or down, depending on symptom response.

ADDING ANDROGENS TO HORMONE REPLACEMENT THERAPY. Androgens are classified as Schedule III drugs because they may be misused by athletes and others who wish to enhance muscle mass and athletic performance. They are controlled under the Anabolic Steroids Control Act of 1990, and prescription and/or distribution of these drugs for nonindicated reasons can result in criminal penalties. Combination estrogen/androgen products are not Schedule III agents and can be prescribed as approved by the FDA for menopausal vasomotor symptom management.

Interest in the use of testosterone in women is growing. In the area of women's health, the only approved indication for androgen use is for treatment of severe hot flashes. The formulation is a combination of androgen with estrogen that protects against misuse and assists with compliance. Popular off-label uses of the combined products are to improve a woman's overall feeling of emotional well-being and to increase libido and energy. Testosterone has been linked with improved well-being and improved libido; combination forms may reduce the amount of estrogen needed for symptom management. Research is under way to identify androgen treatment options for women who experience low libido. Currently, in the United States, no androgen products are approved for treating women with libido problems. Use testosterone with caution in patients with cardiac, renal, or hepatic disease. It is unclear whether androgens affect cardiac risk or osteoporosis; however, they do have the potential to produce adverse effects on the patient's lipid profile. Testosterone gel 1% has been used off-label on a short-term basis for women with diminished libido. Control of menopausal symptoms should be evaluated periodically; women with an intact uterus who use combined estrogen/androgen products also need a progestogen.

How to Monitor

- Review bleeding patterns at each visit. Bleeding should not occur outside of the withdrawal period for women who use the sequential or the cyclic regimen. No bleeding or spotting should occur with the continuous regimen after 9 months. Unplanned bleeding must be evaluated.
- Schedule yearly physical examinations once the dose is stable (e.g., blood pressure, weight and height, thyroid,

TABLE 54-1   Standard Dosing Regimens for Hormone Therapy (HT)

Name	Hormone	Pattern	Comments
Continuous combined EPT	estrogen progestogen	Daily Daily	This regimen is associated with some breakthrough bleeding, which decreases over time. Many women have no bleeding after 6 to 9 months on therapy.
Continuous pulsed EPT	estrogen progestogen	Daily Take for 2 days, skip 1 day, repeat	This regimen was developed to reduce the amount of progestogen ingested and possibly progestogen side effects. It often results in more breakthrough bleeding than is seen with the continuous combined regimen.
Sequential cyclic EPT	estrogen progestogen	Daily Days 1 to 12, or days 18 to 30	This regimen causes a monthly withdrawal bleed for most women after the progestogen regimen is completed. Some women elect to use progestogen less frequently than each month to reduce the number of withdrawal bleeds. This is done off-label in a 3-month or 4-month pattern, similar to that of Seasonale or Seasonique OCs.
Intermittent cyclic EPT	estrogen progestogen	Days 1 to 21 Days 10 to 21	This regimen is rarely used because of the week without hormones. Most women who require ongoing HT cannot tolerate a full week off therapy. If the woman does tolerate a full week off therapy, weaning off HT altogether should be considered.
estrogen only	estrogen	Daily	Only women without a uterus can use this regimen.

heart and lungs, breasts, abdomen, complete pelvic and rectal examination).

- Regular, age-appropriate screening tests remain important (e.g., mammogram yearly, Papanicolaou smear every 1 to 3 years depending on history, sexually transmitted infection [STI] checks, lipid panel, thyroid function).
- *Androgen therapy:* Monitor hepatic function and cholesterol; periodically evaluate hemoglobin, hematocrit, and blood chemistry.

Patient Variables

GERIATRICS. Early studies favored starting HT within 7 years of menopause and using it for short-term symptom relief only. The newest studies favor starting HT within a few years of menopause and suggest that the lowest dose of HT should be used to control symptoms for the shortest length of time. The midlife woman may benefit from the positive effects of estrogen on the bladder and urethra, as well as from the benefits related to maintaining bone strength.

PEDIATRICS. HT is not indicated in children.

PREGNANCY AND LACTATION. *Category X:* Contraindicated

RACE/GENDER. No race effects have been reported. Except for use in the treatment of prostate cancer, estrogen and progestogen remain female gender specific.

Patient Education

- Discuss the risks vs. benefits and obtain informed consent.
- Advise women that HT may take 6 weeks to reach full efficacy. Explain that this is necessary because it takes time for the circulating estrogen and progestogen they are taking as HT to bind with the many estrogen and progesterone receptors located throughout the body. If symptoms remain, the dose can be changed. Dose titration requires time.
- Review the side effects that may occur with initiation of HT (nausea and breast swelling and/or tenderness), and explain that some side effects will wane over time.

- Take oral preparations with food or at bedtime if nausea is a problem.
- Advise women to report any signs of thromboembolic events (warm, red tender area on leg; sudden onset of chest or abdominal pain; blurred vision) or abrupt changes in headache patterns.
- Routine monitoring (e.g., mammogram, Papanicolaou smear, blood pressure, lipid levels) is essential.
- Perform monthly breast self-examination, and obtain a yearly mammogram.
- Patients on androgen replacement should be counseled on potential virilizing effects.

SPECIFIC DRUGS

ESTROGENS

conjugated equine estrogen (Premarin)

CONTRAINDICATIONS

- *Absolute contraindications:* Estrogen-dependent neoplasia (especially breast and endometrial), pregnancy (possible or confirmed), undiagnosed abnormal genital bleeding, liver dysfunction/disease, venous thromboembolism, arterial thromboembolism within 12 months, active thrombophlebitis/DVT, hypersensitivity to class/drug/component, breast cancer
- *Relative contraindications:* Cardiovascular disease, cardiovascular risk factors, hypertension, diabetes mellitus, smoker, hyperlipidemia, hypertriglyceridemia, familial hyperlipoproteinemia, obesity, age >65 years, surgery/prolonged immobilization, gallbladder disease, cholestatic jaundice with prior estrogen use or pregnancy, hypothyroidism, sensitivity to fluid retention, severe hypocalcemia, endometriosis, asthma, seizure disorder, migraine, porphyria, systemic lupus erythematosus, hepatic hemangioma

PHARMACOKINETICS. Table 54-2 provides pharmacokinetic information.

ADVERSE EFFECTS. Table 54-3 lists adverse and side effects of HT.

TABLE 54-2   Pharmacokinetics HT Delivery Systems

Drug Route	Absorption	Drug Availability (After First Pass)	Onset of Action	Time to Peak Concentration	Half-life	Duration of Action	Protein Bound	Metabolism	Excretion
ESTROGEN									
Oral	Varies (some have timed-release–style coatings)	50% ± 13%	Rapid, 0.5-3 hr	4-5 hr	1-2 hr (estradiol); 4-18 hr (estrone)	12-24 hr	50%-80%	Liver	Bile, urine
Transdermal	Slow/site-dependent: 100% abdomen, 85% thigh, arm	100% (no first-pass effect)	Rapid	Variable	1 hr	3-4 days	50%-80%	Liver	Bile, urine
Vaginal	Variable	50%-100%	3 hr	6 hr		24 hr for tablet or cream, longer for ring	50%-80%	Liver	Bile, urine
PROGESTOGEN									
Oral	Rapid	65%	Rapid	0.5-4 hr	5-14 hr	Prolonged	50%-80%	Liver	Bile, urine
ANDROGEN									
Oral	Well absorbed, undergoes first-pass effect	54%			10-100 min		98%	Liver, to active and inactive metabolites	Renal

TABLE 54-3   Selected Adverse and Side Effects of Estrogens, Progestogens, and Androgens Given With Estrogens

Body System	Estrogen	Progestogen	Androgen With Estrogen
General	Fluid retention Weight changes Libido changes	Fluid retention Weight changes Libido changes	Sodium and fluid retention Fluid retention Weight changes Libido changes Virilization Deepened voice
Skin	Chloasma or melasma Hair loss Hirsutism Acne Rash	Alopecia Rash Pruritus Acne Hirsutism	Chloasma or melasma Hair loss Hirsutism Acne Rash
Breast	Breast cancer Breast tenderness Breast enlargement	Breast tenderness Galactorrhea Breast cancer (with estrogen) Breast changes	Breast cancer Breast tenderness Breast enlargement
Pulmonary	Asthma exacerbation		Asthma exacerbation
Cardiac	Hypertension Elevated blood pressure Myocardial infarction	Hypertension Myocardial infarction (with estrogen)	Hypertension Elevated blood pressure Myocardial infarction
GI	Nausea Vomiting Abdominal cramps Bloating Cholestatic jaundice Gallbladder disease Pancreatitis	Nausea Appetite changes Weight changes Hepatic adenoma Cholestatic jaundice	Nausea Vomiting Abdominal cramps Bloating Cholestatic jaundice Gallbladder disease Pancreatitis Peliosis hepatis (rare) Hepatic cancer (rare)
Hematologic and lymphatic	Aggravation of porphyria Alteration of clotting factors Thromboembolism	Thromboembolism	Aggravation of porphyria Alteration of clotting factors Thromboembolism
Metabolic and endocrine	Reduced carbohydrate tolerance Glucose intolerance	Decreased glucose tolerance	Reduced carbohydrate tolerance Glucose intolerance Hypercalcemia Hyperlipidemia
Nervous system	Headache Migraine Dizziness Depression Mood changes Dementia Stroke	Depression Insomnia Somnolence Headache Stroke (with estrogen) Dementia (with estrogen)	Depression Headache Migraine Dizziness Mood changes Dementia Stroke
Special senses	Steepened corneal curvature Intolerance of contact lenses Vision changes Retinal thrombosis	Retinal thrombosis Optic neuritis	Steepened corneal curvature Intolerance of contact lenses Vision changes Retinal thrombosis
Genitourinary	Abnormal uterine/vaginal bleeding Endometrial cancer (without progestogen) Endometrial hyperplasia (without progestogen) Cervical secretion changes Vaginal candidiasis Uterine fibroid enlargement Ovarian cancer	PMS symptoms Withdrawal bleeding Menstrual irregularities Cancer (with estrogen)	Abnormal uterine/vaginal bleeding Endometrial cancer (without progestogen) Endometrial hyperplasia (without progestogen) Cervical secretion changes Vaginal candidiasis Uterine fibroid enlargement Ovarian cancer Clitoral enlargement

DRUG INTERACTIONS

- Some classes of drugs, such as anticonvulsant drugs (phenytoin, primidone, barbiturates, carbamazepine, rifampin), can decrease the effectiveness of estrogen (primarily through increased hepatic clearance).
- Estrogen exerts an antagonistic effect on aromatase inhibitors and ursodiol; alternatives are recommended.
- Monitoring is advised when used in conjunction with aripiprazole, dasatinid, diazoxide, hypoglycemics, insulins, lamotrigine, metformin/sulfonylurea combinations, rasagiline, ropinirole, sitagliptin, sulfonylureas, and thiazolidinediones.
- Caution is advised when used in conjunction with aminocaproic acid, aprepitant, azole antifungals, barbiturates, bexarotene, bosentan, carbamazepine, clarithromycin, systemic corticosteroids, dantrolene, delavirdine, efavirenz, erythromycins, fibric acid derivatives, fluvoxamine, griseofulvin, growth hormone, imatinib, nevirapine, omega-3 acid, oxcarbazepine, phenytoin, protease inhibitors, ramelteon, rifabutin, rifampin, tacrine, or telithromycin.

DOSAGE AND ADMINISTRATION. Table 54-4 compares different drug administration routes, and Table 54-5 provides dosage and administration information for selected products.

TABLE 54-4 Comparison of Routes for Estrogen Administration

Route	Advantages	Disadvantages
Oral	Easy to titrate dose Easy to use divided doses	Nausea Requires daily dosing First-pass liver effect
Transdermal	Simple application Enhances compliance Sustained blood levels Lower doses are effective No first-pass liver effect	Irritation at site of patch Replacement of lost patches increases cost May still require oral dosing with a progestogen
Parenteral	Once-a-month dosing Prolonged blood levels No first-pass liver effect	Pain at injection site Charge for injection May necessitate office visit May still require oral dosing with a progestogen
Vaginal	Allows local treatment Ring may enhance compliance No first-pass liver effect	Messy application if creams used May still require oral dosing with a progestogen Patient must be comfortable checking for placement

TABLE 54-5 Specific Dosage and Administration Information for Selected Estrogens, Progestogens, and Estrogen/Methyltestosterone Products*

Name	Composition	Strength	Dosage and Administration†
Alora	estradiol	0.025, 0.05 mg/day 0.075 mg/day 0.1 mg/day	Apply new patch twice/wk. Start at 0.05 mg/day. Dispensed as patient calendar pack. Apply to upper outer buttock or lower abdomen.
Climara	estradiol	0.025 mg/day 0.0375 mg/day 0.05 mg/day 0.06 mg/day 0.075 mg/day 0.1 mg/day	Apply new patch once/wk. Start at 0.025 mg/day. Dispensed as individual carton of four systems. Apply to upper outer buttock or lower abdomen.
Estraderm	estradiol	0.05 mg/day 0.1 mg/day	Apply new patch twice/wk. Start at 0.05 mg/day. Dispensed as patient calendar pack. Apply to trunk, abdomen, or buttocks.
Estrasorb	estradiol	2.5 mg/g emulsion (0.05 mg/day)	Dispensed in pouches Rub contents of two pouches onto legs (one pouch each leg) daily over a 3-minute period. Rub excess on hands into buttocks.
EstroGel	estradiol	0.06% gel (0.75 mg/1.25 g/day)	Use 1.25 g/day. Dispensed in dose pump Apply thin film wrist to shoulder. Alternate arms.
Vivelle	estradiol	0.05 mg/day 0.1 mg/day	Apply to torso.

*Oral, topical, and vaginal estrogens may require use of a progestogen for women with an intact uterus.
†Use lowest effective dose for all hormone regimens.

Table continued on following page

TABLE 54-5   Specific Dosage and Administration Information for Selected Estrogens, Progestogens, and Estrogen/Methyltestosterone Products* (Continued)

Name	Composition	Strength	Dosage and Administration†
Viville-Dot	estradiol	0.025 mg/day 0.0375 mg/day 0.05 mg/day 0.075 mg/day 0.1 mg/day	Apply new patch twice/wk. Start with 0.0375 mg/day. Apply to lower abdomen. Dispensed as patient calendar pack
TRANSDERMAL COMBINATION ESTROGEN/PROGESTOGEN SYSTEM			
Combipatch	estradiol and norethindrone	0.05/0.14mg/day 0.05/0.25mg/day	Apply new patch twice/wk. Start at 0.05 mg/0.14 mg/day. Apply to lower abdomen. Dispensed as eight systems
ORAL ESTROGENS			
Cenestin	Conjugated estrogens	0.3 mg 0.45 mg 0.625 mg 0.9 mg 1.25 mg	Given daily by mouth Start at 0.3 mg.
Enjuvia	Conjugated estrogens, B	0.3 mg 0.45 mg 0.625 mg 1.25 mg	Given daily by mouth Start at 0.3 mg.
Estrace	estradiol	0.5 mg 1 mg 2 mg	Given daily by mouth Start at 0.5 mg.
Menest tablets	Esterified estrogen	0.3 mg 0.625 mg 1.25 mg 2.5 mg	Given daily by mouth Start at 0.3 mg.
Ogen tablets	estropipate	0.625 mg 1.25 mg 2.5 mg	Given daily by mouth Start at 0.625 mg.
Ortho-Est tablets	estropipate	0.75 mg 1.5 mg	Given daily by mouth Start at 0.75 mg.
Premarin tablets	Conjugated estrogens	0.3 mg 0.45 mg 0.625 mg 0.9 mg 1.25 mg	Given daily by mouth Start at 0.3 mg.
VAGINAL ESTROGENS			
Estrace cream, 1%	estradiol	0.01% (0.1 mg/g)	Start with 2-4 g/day for 1-2 wk, then reduce to lowest effective dose.
Estring	estradiol	7.5 mcg/24 hr	Insert 1 ring to vagina q3 months.
Premarin cream	Conjugated estrogens	0.625 mg/g	Start 1-2 g/day for 1-2 wk, then reduce to lowest effective dose.
SYSTEMIC VAGINAL ESTROGEN			
Femring	estradiol	0.05 mg/day 0.1 mg/day	Insert 1 ring to vagina q3 months. Start with 0.05 mg/day ring.
ORAL PROGESTOGENS			
Aygestin tablets	norethindrone	5 mg	Off-label use
Prometrium capsule	progesterone, micronized	100 mg 200 mg	200 mg by mouth at bedtime for 12 days per cycle for women taking estrogen

TABLE 54-5 **Specific Dosage and Administration Information for Selected Estrogens, Progestogens, and Estrogen/Methyltestosterone Products*** (Continued)

Name	Composition	Strength	Dosage and Administration†
Provera, generic	medroxyproges-terone	2.5 mg 5 mg 10 mg	5-10 mg daily for 12-14 days per cycle with estrogen 2.5 mg daily if continuous
COMBINATION ORAL (ESTROGEN/PROGESTOGEN AND ESTROGEN/ANDROGEN)			
Activella	estradiol and norethindrone	0.5 mg/0.1 mg 1 mg/0.5 mg	One tablet per day Start at 0.5 mg/0.1 mg.
Estratest	Esterified estrogens and methyl-testosterone	1.25 mg/2.5 mg	One tablet/day
Estratest HS	Esterified estrogens and methyl-testosterone	0.625 mg/1.25 mg	Start with Estratest HS, increase to Estratest if needed.
Femhrt	norethindrone and ethinyl estradiol	0.5 mg/2.5 mcg 1 mg/5 mcg	One tablet/day Start at 0.5 mg/2.5 mcg.
Prefest	estradiol; estradiol and norgestimate	1 mg estradiol (3 tablets) alternating with 1 mg estradiol/0.09 norgestimate (3 tablets)	Alternating sequence of 3 tabs each; 1 tablet/day
Premphase	Conjugated estrogens; conjugated estrogens and medroxy-progesterone	0.625 mg (14 tabs) followed by 0.625 mg/5 mg (14 tabs)	One tablet/day
Prempro	Conjugated estrogens and medroxy-progesterone	0.3 mg/1.5 mg 0.45 mg/1.5 mg 0.625 mg/2.5 mg 0.625 mg/5 mg	One tablet/day Start with 0.3 mg/1.5 mg.

*Oral, topical, and vaginal estrogens may require use of a progestogen for women with an intact uterus.
†Use lowest effective dose for all hormone regimens.

PROGESTOGENS

medroxyprogesterone acetate (Provera, Cycrin, Amen)

CONTRAINDICATIONS
- Do not use in patients with hypersensitivity to the drug/class/components, undiagnosed vaginal bleeding, breast cancer, genital organ cancer, history of venous thromboembolism, arterial thromboembolism within 12 months, liver dysfunction/disease, pregnancy, missed abortion, sudden vision loss/changes, papilledema, or retinal vascular lesions.
- Use with caution in patients with cerebrovascular disease, cardiovascular disease, hypertension, diabetes mellitus, hyperlipidemia, obesity, prolonged immobilization/surgery, sensitivity to fluid retention, seizure disorder, migraine, asthma, impaired renal function, history of depression, or SLE, or in smokers or elderly patients.

DRUG INTERACTIONS. Caution is advised when MPA is used with aprepitant, bexarotene, bosentan, carbamazepine, efavirenz, griseofulvin, growth hormone, nevirapine, oxcarbazepine, phenytoin, protease inhibitors, rifabutin, rifampin, and rifapentine.

See Chapter 53 for additional information on progestogens.

ANDROGENS

methyltestosterone (Combination: Estratest, Estratest H.S.)

CONTRAINDICATIONS. See above for information on CEE; also lactation.

WARNINGS
- *Hepatic effects:* Use of long-term androgens is associated with the risk of developing hepatocellular neoplasms. Patients should be monitored for signs and symptoms of liver compromise (nausea, vomiting, jaundice, clay-colored stools, upper abdominal pain, abnormal liver function tests). Discontinue drug immediately if any of these signs or symptoms occur.
- Methyltestosterone in relatively doses can cause cholestatic hepatitis and jaundice.
- With advanced breast cancer, androgen therapy may cause hypercalcemia.
- Hypercalcemia may occur in immobilized patients.
- Edema with or without CHF

PRECAUTIONS
- Virilization (deepening voice, hirsutism, male pattern hair loss, facial acne, clitoromegaly, menstrual irregularities, and breast regression) may occur. Discontinue drug.
- *Hyperlipidemia:* Serum lipid profile may be altered.

DRUG INTERACTIONS. See above for estrogen. Also, androgens may increase sensitivity to oral anticoagulants, requiring a reduction in the dose of warfarin. Individuals with diabetes may require a decrease in insulin dose because of the metabolic effects of androgens.

evolve A continually updated list of useful WebLinks may be found in the Evolve Resources at http://evolve.elsevier.com/Edmunds/NP/

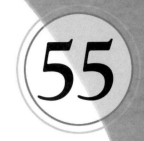

Agents Used in Treating Breast Cancer

DRUG OVERVIEW

Class	Subclass	Generic Name	Trade Name
Antiestrogens	SERM	tamoxifen ☀	Nolvadex
	Estrogen receptor downregulator	fulvestrant	Faslodex
	Estrogen receptor modulator, selective	toremifene	Fareston
Aromatase inhibitors	Aromatase inactivator	anastrozole	Arimidex ☀
		letrozole	Femara
		exemestane	Aromasin

☀ Top 200 drug.

INDICATIONS

- *tamoxifen:* Carcinoma, breast; carcinoma, breast, adjunct; ductal carcinoma in situ; carcinoma, breast, prevention
- *fulvestrant:* Carcinoma, breast
- *toremifene:* Carcinoma, breast
- *anastrozole:* Carcinoma, breast
- *letrozole:* Carcinoma, breast; carcinoma, breast, adjunct
- *exemestane:* Carcinoma, breast; carcinoma, breast, adjunct

This chapter briefly discusses the hormonal treatment of patients with breast cancer. A full discussion is beyond the scope of this book. The goal of the chapter is to familiarize the primary care provider with the medications that some patients may be taking for the treatment of breast cancer. Most of these drugs are given on a long-term daily schedule.

THERAPEUTIC OVERVIEW

The following is a very brief discussion of breast cancer.

Anatomy and Physiology

ETIOLOGY. Approximately 5% to 10% of breast cancers have a familial or genetic link. Mutations in the *BRCA* family of genes confer a lifetime risk of breast cancer that approaches 85%. *BRCA1* and *BRCA2* are the main genes involved. These genes also increase the risk of ovarian cancer. The breast cancer that occurs in women >50 years of age or in postmenopausal women is often hormone receptive.

Pathophysiology

Two main categories of breast cancer have been identified. The first is ductal carcinoma in situ (DCIS), which starts in the ductal epithelium. It is considered in situ when it has not penetrated the base membrane and is usually found in older women. Most of these cancers have infiltrated and spread by the time of discovery. This is the most common type of cancer, although the histology of these cancers is varied. The second type of cancer is lobular cancer, which consists of uniform small, round neoplastic cells that are slower to infiltrate. Among these two major categories of cancer are a variety of histologic types. For example, inflammatory cancer is rare but highly malignant. It is rapid growing and characterized by inflammation of the skin. Breast cancer is divided into four classes for optimal selection of treatment: (1) DCIS, (2) primary operable breast cancer, (3) locally advanced breast cancer, and (4) breast cancer with metastasis.

Assessment

RISK FACTORS. Much research has been related to risk factors, and new ones have been discovered. Box 55-1 lists the well-established risk factors. A breast cancer risk calculator can be found at http://www.cancer.gov/bcrisktool. It also can be obtained by calling 800-4-CANCER, or through AstraZeneca Pharmaceuticals, who manufactures tamoxifen.

Self-breast examination and mammography are effective in screening for early breast cancer. Screening mammography reduces breast cancer mortality by about 33% in women 50 to 70 years old. However, effectiveness is less well established for women younger than 50 years of age. The American Cancer Society, the American College of Radiology, and the American College of Obstetricians and Gynecologists have agreed that all women should undergo annual screening mammography beginning at age 40.

BOX 55-1   Established Risk Factors for Breast Cancer

Family history of breast cancer
Age at menarche
Age at birth of first child
Age at menopause
Benign breast disease
Radiation

MECHANISM OF ACTION

Antiestrogens

Tamoxifen is a nonsteroidal selective estrogen receptor modulator (SERM; see Chapter 37, Osteoporosis Treatment). It competes with estradiol at binding sites in the cell nucleus in breast tissue, altering gene transcription and protein synthesis. This inhibits the growth of estrogen-dependent tumor cells. Tamoxifen acts as an estrogen agonist and has a favorable effect on plasma lipid levels and bone mineral density. However, it may be linked to endometrial malignancy and thromboembolism.

Fulvestrant is an estrogen receptor antagonist that competes with estradiol by binding to estrogen receptors. This medication helps to downregulate the ER protein in human breast cancer cells.

Toremifene binds to estrogen receptors and exerts an antiestrogenic effect. It competes with estrogen for binding sites in the cancer, blocking the growth-stimulating effects of estrogen in the tumor.

Aromatase Inhibitors

Anastrozole blocks the aromatase enzyme from converting androstenedione to estrone and testosterone to estradiol. Many breast cancers also contain aromatase. Anastrozole is a potent and selective nonsteroidal aromatase inhibitor; it lowers serum estradiol concentrations.

Letrozole inhibits the aromatase enzyme by competitively binding to the heme of the cytochrome P450 subunit of the aromatase enzyme, resulting in reduction of estrogen biosynthesis in all tissues. It is a more potent inhibitor of the aromatase enzyme than is anastrozole.

Exemestane is a steroidal aromatase inactivator. It acts as a false substrate for the aromatase enzyme that binds irreversibly to the active site of the enzyme, causing its inactivation. This results in decreased circulating estrogen concentrations.

TREATMENT PRINCIPLES

Standardized Guidelines

Multiple guidelines are available. See the National Guideline Clearinghouse at www.guideline.gov, or the National Comprehensive Cancer Network Clinical Practice Guidelines at www.NCCN.org.

Evidence-Based Recommendations

LOCAL BREAST CANCER—NONMETASTATIC. (Recommendations may vary depending on whether the patient is premenopausal or postmenopausal.)

- Radiotherapy (reduced recurrence)
- Tamoxifen plus radiotherapy (reduced recurrence in women with estrogen receptor–positive tumors)
- Adjuvant aromatase inhibitors
- Adjuvant combination chemotherapy (better than no chemotherapy)
- Adjuvant tamoxifen (in women with estrogen receptor–positive tumors)
- Anthracycline regimens as adjuvant chemotherapy (better than standard CMF [cyclophosphamide, methotrexate, and fluorouracil] regimens)
- Chemotherapy plus monoclonal antibody (trastuzumab) in women with overexpressed *HER2/neu* oncogene
- Combined chemotherapy plus tamoxifen
- Less extensive mastectomy (similar survival to more extensive surgery and better cosmetic outcome)
- Ovarian ablation in premenopausal women
- Radiotherapy after breast-conserving surgery (reduced local recurrence and breast cancer mortality compared with breast-conserving surgery alone)
- Radiotherapy after mastectomy in women at high risk of local recurrence

BREAST CANCER—METASTATIC.
Beneficial:
- Hormonal treatment with antiestrogens (tamoxifen) or progestins (no significant difference in survival compared with non-taxane combination chemotherapy, so may be preferable in women with estrogen receptor–positive disease)
- Selective aromatase inhibitors in postmenopausal women (at least as effective as tamoxifen in delaying disease progression)
- Tamoxifen in estrogen receptor–positive women
Likely to be beneficial:
- Combined gonadorelin analogs plus tamoxifen in premenopausal women

Cardinal Points of Treatment

- Therapy depends on accurate, early diagnosis. SAI often is recommended now over tamoxifen.
- Therapy depends on whether or note cancer is metastatic, and whether the patient is premenopausal or postmenopausal.

Pharmacotherapeutic Treatment

All these medications have the primary effect of reducing estrogen in the body. Thus, they have many characteristics in common and are effective primarily for estrogen-sensitive cancers.

Tamoxifen was approved in 1994. The other drugs in this chapter are relatively newer. Tamoxifen is used for the prevention of breast cancer in women who are at increased risk (see Box 55-1). The benefits are weighed against the risks of drug use (see breast cancer risk calculator at http://www.cancer.gov/bcrisktool). It has a black box warning because of the risk of increased endometrial cancer, stroke, pulmonary embolism, and deep venous thrombosis. As with all drugs, the benefits should be weighed against the risks of drug use.

Tamoxifen is used for the treatment of patients with breast cancer in the following situations: when the axillary node is negative after total or partial mastectomy or radiation in tumors >1 cm, for the treatment of node-positive breast cancer in postmenopausal women after total mastectomy or after radiation, and in advanced estrogen receptor–positive metastatic disease in men or women.

The newer antiestrogen drugs have been associated with fewer adverse reactions. Currently, these are used only for the treatment of patients with breast cancer.

Aromatase inhibitors convey many of the same risks as the antiestrogens. Currently, they are used only for the treatment of breast cancer.

How to Monitor

ANTIESTROGENS
- Routine gynecologic care
- Routine eye care
- Liver enzymes, CBC; monitor lipids in patients at risk for elevated lipids
- Calcium, especially during first weeks of treatment

AROMATASE INHIBITORS
- Routine gynecologic care
- Liver enzymes, CBC, bilirubin, creatinine, bone mineral density, cholesterol (total and LDL)

Patient Variables

GERIATRICS. *tamoxifen, anastrozole:* No overall difference in tolerability

PEDIATRICS. Safety and effectiveness not studied in children. Tamoxifen and anastrozole have been used to treat precocious puberty. Long-term effects are not known.

PREGNANCY AND LACTATION. *Category D:* May cause fetal harm; it is not known whether these medications are excreted in breast milk

RACE/GENDER. Tamoxifen is used to treat both men and women with breast cancer.

Patient Education

- Report immediately abnormal vaginal bleeding or changes in vaginal discharge.

- Routine gynecologic care is essential.
- Patients should not become pregnant; this medication may cause fetal harm.
- Regular blood work, including liver function tests and total blood counts, is important.

TAMOXIFEN. Report any change in vision.

SPECIFIC DRUGS

ANTIESTROGENS

tamoxifen (Nolvadex)

CONTRAINDICATIONS
- Sensitivity to the drug
- Concomitant Coumadin therapy
- History of DVT or PE, pregnancy

WARNINGS

A black box warning has been issued for the thromboembolic effects of tamoxifen: There is an increased incidence of thromboembolic events, including deep venous thrombosis, pulmonary embolism, and stroke. These can be fatal.

- *Carcinogenesis:* Increased frequency of endometrial cancer and uterine sarcoma has been found. Increased hepatocellular carcinoma also may be seen.
- *Nonmalignant effects on uterus:* Hyperplasia, polyps, fibroid, ovarian cysts, endometriosis, menstrual irregularity or amenorrhea
- Visual disturbances, including corneal changes, cataracts, and retinopathy, have occurred.
- Hypercalcemia has occurred in patients with bone metastases.
- *Hepatic effects:* Elevated liver enzymes, hepatitis, and hepatic necrosis have occurred. Perform periodic LFTs.

PRECAUTIONS
- Leukopenia and thrombocytopenia may occur. Perform periodic CBCs.
- Hyperlipidemias have occurred infrequently. Consider monitoring.

PHARMACOKINETICS. See Table 55-1.

TABLE 55-1   Pharmacokinetics of Medications Used for Treating Patients With Breast Cancer

Drug	Absorption	Time to Steady State	Time to Peak Concentration	Half-life	Protein Bound	Metabolism	Excretion
tamoxifen	Well absorbed	4 wk	5 hr	5-7 days	99%	Extensive; substrate of 3A4, 2C9, 2D6	Feces and urine
fulvestrant	Given IM	3-6 months	7-9 days	≈6 wk	99%	Metabolized	Hepatobiliary to feces
toremifene	Well absorbed	4-6 wk	Peak plasma 3 hr	5 days	99.5%	3A4	Metabolites in feces
anastrozole	Well absorbed	7 days		50 hr	40%	85% metabolized; inhibitor of 1A2, 2C8/9, 3A4	Metabolites in urine
letrozole	Rapid and complete	2-6 wk		2 days	Weak	3A4; inhibits 2A6, 2C19	Metabolites in urine
exemestane	Rapid, 42%	7 days	1.2 hr	24 hr	90%	Metabolized	Metabolites in urine and feces

TABLE 55-2   Adverse Effects of Medications Used for Treating Patients With Breast Cancer

Body System	tamoxifen	fulvestrant	toremifene
Body, general	Disease flare, tumor pain, fatigue	Pain	
Skin, appendages	Hair thinning/loss	Injection site pain, rash	Sweating
Hypersensitivity	Erythema multiforme, hypersensitivity		
Respiratory		Dyspnea, cough	PE
Cardiovascular	Thromboembolism, peripheral edema	Thromboembolism, peripheral edema	MI, CHF, thromboembolism, edema
Gastrointestinal	Nausea/vomiting, anorexia	Nausea/vomiting, anorexia, pharyngitis, constipation, diarrhea, abdominal pain	Nausea/vomiting
Hemic and lymphatic	Thrombocytopenia, leukopenia, neutropenia, pancytopenia	Leukemia, anemia	
Metabolic and nutritional	Hypercalcemia		Hypercalcemia
Musculoskeletal	Bone pain	Bone pain, back pain	
Nervous system	Stroke, light-headedness, dizziness, headache	Headache, dizziness, insomnia	Dizziness
Special senses	Retinopathy, cataract formation, visual acuity changes		Ocular toxicity, dry eyes, abnormal visual fields
Hepatic	Elevated LFTs, hepatotoxicity, hepatic cancer		Elevated LFTs, hepatotoxicity
Genitourinary	Priapism, impotence		
Gynecologic	Endometrial hyperplasia, polyps, cancer; endometriosis, uterine sarcoma, uterine fibroids, ovarian cysts, hot flashes, vaginal discharge, menstrual irregularities, vaginal bleeding, vaginal dryness, vulvar pruritus	Hot flashes	Endometrial hyperplasia, hot flashes, vaginal discharge

ADVERSE EFFECTS. See Table 55-2. Hot flashes, nausea/vomiting, weight gain or loss, fluid retention, vaginal discharge, irregular menses, skin rash, and headaches are seen. Infrequent adverse reactions include hypercalcemia, erythema multiforme, Stevens-Johnson syndrome, bullous pemphigoid, and hypersensitivity. Changes in liver enzymes are an important adverse reaction.

DRUG INTERACTIONS. Tamoxifen is a major substrate of the cytochrome P450 3A4, 2C9, and 2D6 enzyme systems. If taken with warfarin, an increase in prothrombin time occurs and so it is contraindicated.

DOSAGE AND ADMINISTRATION. See Table 55-3.

fulvestrant

CONTRAINDICATIONS
- Hypersensitivity
- Pregnancy, bleeding diathesis

WARNINGS
- Causes fetal harm, reversible reduction in female fertility
- Has not been studied in patients with hepatic impairment

DRUG INTERACTIONS. None known; minor substrate of CYP 450 3A4

toremifene

CONTRAINDICATIONS. Hypersensitivity, pregnancy

TABLE 55-3   Dosage and Administration Recommendations for Medications Used to Treat Patients With Breast Cancer

Drug	Dosage	Administration
tamoxifen	10-20 mg	po daily-bid × 5 yr
anastrozole	1 mg	po daily
letrozole	2.5 mg	po daily
exemestane	25 mg	po daily
fulvestrant	250 mg	IM q month
toremifene	60 mg	po daily

WARNINGS
- Hypercalcemia and tumor flare may occur during the first weeks of treatment, along with diffuse musculoskeletal pain and erythema with increased size of tumor lesions that later regress, often accompanied by hypercalcemia
- Tumorigenicity has not yet been established.
- Fetal harm in pregnancy

PRECAUTIONS
- Do not use in patients with history of thromboembolic disease.

TABLE 55-4 **Adverse Effects of Aromatase Inhibitors**

Body System	anastrozole	letrozole	exemestane
Body, general	Pain, infection	Infection	Fatigue, pain, flu syndrome
Skin, appendages	Erythema multiforme, Stevens-Johnson syndrome, rash,	Sweating, rash, alopecia	Alopecia, sweating
Hypersensitivity			
Respiratory	Dyspnea, cough,	Dyspnea, cough	Dyspnea, cough
Cardiovascular	Thromboembolism, MI, angina, HTN, edema	Thromboembolism, MI, angina, chest pain, HTN, edema	Thromboembolism, MI, angina, heart failure, HTN, edema
Gastrointestinal	Nausea/vomiting, pharyngitis, abdominal pain, constipation, diarrhea	Nausea, constipation, diarrhea	Nausea, diarrhea, anorexia
Hemic and lymphatic	Anemia, leukopenia, lymphedema	Lymphopenia	Lymphopenia
Metabolic and nutritional	Weight gain, hypercholesterolemia	Weight changes, hypercholesterolemia	
Musculoskeletal	Fractures, arthralgia, arthritis, osteoporosis, bone pain	Osteoporosis, fractures, bone pain, arthralgia/myalgia, back pain, headache, insomnia, dizziness	Osteoporosis, fractures, arthralgia, elevated alk phos, osteoarthritis, carpal tunnel syndrome
Nervous system	Stroke, asthenia, headache, depression, insomnia, paresthesia	Stroke, asthenia, headache, dizziness, depression	Stroke, headache, insomnia, dizziness, depression, paresthesia
Special senses	Cataracts		
Hepatic		Elevated LFTs, elevated bilirubin	Elevated bilirubin
Genitourinary			Elevated creatinine
Gynecologic	Endometrial cancer, hot flashes, breast pain	Endometrial cancer, hot flashes	Hot flashes

- *Drug interactions, major substrate of CYP 450 3A4:* No studies have been performed.
- Thiazide diuretics may increase risk of hypercalcemia.

Aromatase Inhibitors
anastrozole
CONTRAINDICATIONS. Hypersensitivity, pregnancy

WARNINGS. Can cause fetal harm

PRECAUTIONS
- Pregnancy must be excluded.
- Use with caution in patients with elevated total and LDL cholesterol.
- Administer under the supervision of a qualified physician who is experienced in the use of anticancer agents.
- Increased incidence of hepatocellular adenoma and carcinoma and uterine stromal polyps in females and thyroid adenoma in males
- Infertility in rats

PHARMACOKINETICS. See Table 55-1.

ADVERSE EFFECTS. See Table 55-4.

DRUG INTERACTIONS
- Do not give with tamoxifen (tamoxifen reduces anastrozole levels).
- Do not give with estrogen-containing therapies.

DOSAGE AND ADMINISTRATION. See Table 55-3.

OTHER DRUGS IN CLASS
- *letrozole:* Fatigue, dizziness, somnolence; use caution when driving or using machinery
- *exemestane:* Do not administer to premenopausal women.

evolve A continually updated list of useful WebLinks may be found in the Evolve Resources at http://evolve.elsevier.com/Edmunds/NP/

56 Principles for Prescribing Antiinfectives

This chapter discusses general treatment principles applicable to most infections, with an emphasis on those of bacterial origin. Although these general guidelines cover the most common first-line primary care drugs, many exceptions are made to these recommendations. Remember to consider each patient with an infection as an individual case. Patterns of resistance change constantly and guidelines for treatment are updated at least yearly. Although these recommendations were the most current on publication, do not fail to consult the newest information from state and federal sources. The emphasis in this unit is on typical oral treatment for common primary care problems. The only exception is the use of single IM injections primarily for the treatment of sexually transmitted diseases. The first nine antiinfective chapters are focused on bacteria. Viruses and protozoa are discussed in Chapter 68; fungi are discussed in Chapter 66.

THERAPEUTIC OVERVIEW

Anatomy and Physiology

The taxonomy of bacteria is undergoing changes that reflect the new body of information about the genetic components of bacteria. See Table 56-1 for information on bacteria that are important pathogens. Bacteria are one-cell organisms with a primitive nucleus and rigid cell walls that are porous and permeable to substances of low molecular weight. Gram-negative bacteria have a more complex cell wall than gram-positive bacteria. Bacteria are called gram negative or positive according to the results of laboratory Gram stains. The difference in their cell walls is an important factor in the ability of an antibiotic to penetrate the cell walls of bacteria and kill the bacteria. Another variable that is important in decision making is whether bacteria are aerobic or anaerobic (i.e., whether or not they need oxygen). This trait will determine where in the body the organism will grow best and potentially cause infection. This information is important when one is selecting appropriate antimicrobial therapy in the absence of culture results.

Bacteria (including rickettsia and spirochetes), protozoa (chlamydia, others), fungi, viruses, and retroviruses cause infection. A rickettsia such as *Borrelia burgdorferi* (Lyme disease) is a small gram-negative obligate intracellular bacterium. Spirochetes such as *Treponema pallidum* (syphilis) are highly coiled bacteria.

Pathophysiology

Infections are among the most common reasons for primary care visits. Respiratory tract infections include acute URIs, bronchitis, pneumonia, chronic sinusitis, acute pharyngitis,

and otitis media. Other infections commonly seen in primary care are UTIs, eye infections such as conjunctivitis, ear infections such as otitis media and externa, and skin infections such as cellulitis, impetigo, and acne. See Chapter 57 for details.

More than 150 million prescriptions for oral antiinfectives are written each year in the United States. However, this number decreased, especially in children, from 1992 to 2000, because of the emergence of antimicrobial resistance and more appropriate prescribing efforts. Nevertheless, among all types of health care providers, antiinfectives rank as one of the most frequently prescribed products. Although their efficacy in decreasing mortality and morbidity is unquestioned, the overuse and abuse of these products have led to drug resistance and have raised the specter of a return to the time when clinicians were powerless to cure patients with virulent infection.

To summarize the most important general information clinicians need to know when using different types of antiinfectives, a brief review of relevant information is provided here rather than with each antibiotic chapter. Mastery of this foundational material will facilitate accurate decision making. More difficult or detailed clinical problems may require the clinician to review additional anatomic, physiologic, or microbiologic texts before making treatment decisions.

Accurate identification of the offending organism is the most critical clinical decision that must be made with any infection. This often is possible to do through simple laboratory tests, such as Gram stains, which many clinicians are able to perform in their offices. Some organisms require more extensive testing in commercial laboratories, and results may not be available fast enough to be helpful for initial treatment decisions. Knowledge of which organisms are endemic in the community during that season and which organisms seem to have developed resistance to different drugs is also important for the clinician.

Assessment

Take a thorough history, especially regarding allergies, other drugs the patient is taking, and previous antibiotic treatment. If the patient has had a previous allergic reaction, determine the type of reaction. If the infection is in the respiratory tract, inquire about smoking. Look for concomitant illness and other complicating factors. Ask about travel, work history, and exposure to high-risk environments (e.g., college and military dormitories, child care centers, patient care facilities, ill family members).

TABLE 56-1 Important Pathogens

	Morphology	Aerobe vs. Anaerobe	Organism	Most Important Pathogen	Disease Caused
BACTERIA					
Gram positive	Cocci		Staphylococcus	S. aureus	Skin and soft tissue infective endocarditis
					Osteomyelitis, bacteremia, toxic shock syndrome
			Streptococcus	S. pyogenes group A β-hemolytic (GABH)	Pharyngitis/rheumatic fever Impetigo
				S. viridans	Endocarditis
			Enterococcus	E. faecalis	Wound, UTI, endocarditis
			Pneumococcus	S. pneumoniae	Pneumonia
					Meningitis
	Rods	Anaerobe	Bacillus	B. anthracis	Anthrax
			Actinomyces	A. israelii	Cervicofacial
				A. haemolyticum	Pharyngitis
		Aerobe	Corynebacterium	C. diphtheriae	Diphtheria
		Anaerobe	Listeria	L. monocytogenes	Listeriosis
			Clostridium	C. perfringens	Gas gangrene
				C. difficile	Enteritis
				C. tetani	Tetanus
		Aerobe		C. botulinum	Botulism
Gram negative	Cocci		Neisseria	N. gonorrhoeae	Gonorrhea
		Aerobe		N. meningitidis	Meningitis
			Moraxella	M. catarrhalis	Otitis media, sinusitis, pneumonia
		Aerobe			
	Bacilli		Pseudomonas	P. aeruginosa	Bacteremia
ENTEROBACTERIA			Escherichia	E. coli	Gastroenteritis
			Shigella	S. dysenteriae	Shigellosis dysentery
			Salmonella	S. typhi	Typhoid fever
				S. enteritidis	Gastroenteritis
			Klebsiella	K. pneumoniae	UTI, various
			Proteus	P. mirabilis	UTI, various
				P. vulgaris	UTI, various
			Yersinia	Y. pestis	Plague
			Enterobacter	E. cloacae	
			Serratia	S. marcescens	
			Citrobacter	C. freundii	
			Morganella	M. morganii	
			Vibrio	V. cholerae	Cholera
			Helicobacter	H. pylori	Gastritis, PUD
	Small bacilli		Haemophilus	H. influenzae	Sinusitis, otitis, bronchitis, pneumonia
			Bordetella	B. pertussis	Whooping cough
			Pasteurella	P. tularensis	Tularemia
				P. multocida	Animal bite infections
			Campylobacter	C. jejuni	Gastroenteritis
			Gardnerella	G. vaginalis	Vaginitis
			Legionella	L. pneumophila	Legionnaire's pneumonia
		Aerobe	Nocardia	N. asteroides	Pulmonary endocarditis, systemic infection
		Anaerobe	Bacteroides	B. fragilis	
			Prevotella (formerly Bacteroides)	P. melaninogenica	URIs
Acid fast			Mycobacterium	M. tuberculosis	Tuberculosis
				M. avium	Bronchitis, etc
				M. leprae	Leprosy
Mycoplasma			Mycoplasma	M. pneumoniae	Atypical pneumonia
			Ureaplasma	M. hominis	
				M. urealyticum	
Spirochetes			Treponema	T. pallidum	Syphilis
				T. pallidum sub	Yaws
			Borrelia	B. burgdorferi	Lyme disease
Rickettsia			Rickettsia	R. rickettsii	Rocky Mountain spotted fever, typhus

Table continued on following page

TABLE 56-1   Important Pathogens (Continued)

	Morphology	Aerobe vs. Anaerobe	Organism	Most Important Pathogen	Disease Caused
PROTOZOA			Chlamydia (closely related to Gram bacteria)	C. trachomatis	Lymphogranuloma venereum, urethritis, and cervicitis
				C. psittaci	Psittacosis
				C. pneumoniae	Pneumonia
			Trichomonas	T. vaginalis	Trichomonas vaginitis
			Entamoeba	E. histolytica	Amebiasis colitis
			Cryptosporidium (spore forming)	C. parvum	Diarrhea
		Flagellate	Giardia (cyst forming)	G. lamblia	Diarrhea
			Leishmania	Many species	Skin lesions
			Plasmodium	P. falciparum	Malaria
				P. vivax	Malaria
				P. malariae	Malaria
				P. ovale	Malaria
			Toxoplasma	T. gondii	Toxoplasmosis
HELMINTHIC	Trematode				Schistosomiasis
	Cestode				
	Nematode				Anisakiasis
			Ascaris	A. lumbricoides	Ascariasis
					Enterobiasis
			Trichinella	T. spiralis	Trichinosis

Best practice is to confirm the diagnosis of bacterial infection before placing a patient on an antibiotic. Viral infections should not be treated with an antibiotic.

At least 90% of URIs are viral. When treating infection, assess whether any symptoms or signs indicate a bacterial infection. If not, consider culturing and waiting to treat until the culture results are available. If the patient has signs and symptoms that indicate probable bacterial infection, consider empirical treatment until culture results are available. Signs and symptoms that indicate bacterial infection are not always obvious and clear cut. Generally, they may include fever higher than 102° F, lymphadenopathy, swelling, and pain. Organ-specific signs and symptoms may indicate a bacterial infection of particular tissue. No formula can be given that says that if x, y, and z are present, the patient always has a bacterial infection. The clinician must have a high index of suspicion, order appropriate testing, and recognize when a patient is really ill through a blended knowledge of art and science.

Some of the red flags that suggest that serious bacterial infection may be present include the following:

- *Loss of appetite:* With fever, this can signal the presence of a significant infection. Maintenance of appetite with fever is a reliable indicator of localized or limited infection.
- *Symptoms of dehydration:* Ask about fluid intake. Consider dehydration even if illness seems minor. Look for dizziness when standing, an unsteady walk, orthostatic changes in vital signs, urine concentration of 1.025 to 1.030, and dry mucous membranes. Children and the elderly may exhibit pronounced changes in behavior or mental status.
- *Absence of fever:* Especially in patients with diabetes or those in the extremes of life, when the immune system may not cause adequate release of pyrogens, this does not exclude serious infection. High or persistent fever in children is often a sign of serious illness, and a comprehensive search for the cause is required.

Although minor infections account for most visits to primary care practices, always consider referral to a specialist for unusual symptoms or unusual responses to treatment. Infectious disease and pulmonary specialists are highly attuned to knowledge of community-acquired infections and their treatment, as well as to the more exotic presentations. Simple localized infection may progress to septic shock within hours, and the clinician must not discount the ominous symptoms of shaking chills and soaring temperatures or decreased temperature with changes in mental status that require emergency attention.

Studies show that outpatient antibiotic use, while decreasing, is still too prevalent. Currently, providers are increasingly using newer and broader-spectrum agents without rationale. Overuse of antiinfectives and resulting drug resistance not only affect the individual patient but also lead to the development of resistant strains of bacteria that then are spread throughout the community and globally. Resistant bacteria cause infections that are harder to treat, last longer, and require hospitalization with resulting increased health care costs. Future infections may also prove resistant to antiinfectives. As a result, the patient experiences more frequent infections with a narrowing range of therapeutic options. For example, otitis and sinusitis are conditions for which resistant strains have become a major problem. Administering antiinfectives for viral infection prophylaxis when not needed also places the patient at increased risk for adverse effects (including allergy, anaphylaxis, and death). Because of recent programs undertaken to educate primary care providers and patients about the dangers of overuse of antiinfectives, the inappropriate prescription of antiinfectives for viral infections has decreased for many groups in the past few years. Research documents that elderly patients still seem to have a high rate of inappropriate prescription of antiinfectives.

Despite pressures from the patient for quick relief, it is good practice to culture first and treat second. Many well-educated patients will be accepting of a "wait and see" approach. Culturing first provides results that direct definitive therapy with an antibiotic to which the organism is susceptible. If the patient is acutely ill, treat empirically until the results of the culture are available. Be sure to check the culture results to see whether the organism is susceptible to the drug prescribed. If the site cannot be cultured, treat empirically and cover the likely pathogens. If treating empirically, be sure to check with the patient in 2 to 3 days to see if he or she is improving. Determine the most likely pathogen by assessing the location of the infection and the patient setting such as community, nursing care facility, or recent hospitalization.

GRAM POSITIVE VS. GRAM NEGATIVE. Identification of an organism as gram positive or gram negative helps the clinician move to the next critical decision for choosing an antibiotic that will be effective against the specific organism.

The Gram stain is a laboratory test that is used to divide bacteria into two groups, reflecting basic differences in cell wall composition. Gram-positive bacteria retain the staining dye and appear deep violet on the microscopic slide. Gram-negative bacteria do not retain the dye and appear red on the slide. Gram-positive cell walls are low in lipids, whereas gram-negative cell walls are high in lipids. Many but not all antiinfectives exert their effects via action on cell walls, so cell wall differences determine whether certain antiinfectives will be effective.

Anaerobes are organisms that can grow in the absence of oxygen. This characteristic allows them to grow in necrotic tissue and poorly aerated portions of the respiratory tract. Mycobacteria such as the TB organism do not Gram stain; they have very tough cell walls and are difficult to kill. Yeasts are gram positive; rickettsiae are gram negative.

SENSITIVITY TESTING. Throat, blood, urine, or other specimens should be sent to hospital-based or commercial laboratories for culture and sensitivity testing. Antibiotic effectiveness against an organism is determined by exposing the organism to various antibiotics. This is the second piece of critical information needed by the clinician to make an effective treatment decision.

In vitro sensitivity tests are standardized to reflect drug concentrations in plasma. They do not reflect concentrations that can be attained at the site of infection. They also do not take into account local factors that may affect the activity of the drug, for example, the pH.

RESISTANCE TO ANTIINFECTIVES. It is very important for clinicians to pay attention to organisms that are dominant in the community and to know the local disease pattern. Patterns of resistance differ from one community to the next, and they change rapidly. Clinicians need to search for patterns in their patient population. For example, children who go to the same daycare facility are likely to have the same organisms. Keep good patient records and review them. Think about the particular patient, his or her probable exposure, and what the patient's treatment behavior has been. Take every reasonable opportunity to culture and identify organisms. Monitor all culture results and talk to other providers about what type of infections they are seeing. Group practices have an advantage over solo practitioners in this capability.

MECHANISMS OF RESISTANCE. The use of any antimicrobial agent in clinical care is associated with selective pressure for the emergence of resistant organisms. However, overuse and inappropriate use exacerbate conditions in terms of the selection of resistant bacterial strains. In the United States in 2001, Gonzales et al estimated that 55% of all antimicrobials prescribed in the primary care setting for acute respiratory infection were unwarranted. Injudicious use of antimicrobials has many root causes, including lack of knowledge of local drug resistance patterns and fear of losing patients if perceived demand for treatment is not met.

Regardless of appropriate or inappropriate drug use, bacteria exposed to antimicrobial agents can develop resistance through the following mechanisms:

1. Acquisition of genes that can produce enzymes that inactivate the antimicrobial agent. Common drug resistance–producing enzymes are collectively known as penicillinases, and the most prevalent of these is β-lactamase.
2. Acquisition of efflux pumps capable of draining the antimicrobial agent from the bacterial cell prior to any bactericidal or bacteriostatic effects. Such efflux pumps can confer multidrug resistance, such as methicillin-resistant staphylocuccus aureus (MRSA) or resistance to tetracycline due to active efflux.
3. Acquisition of several genes capable of eliminating the antimicrobial binding site during synthesis of the bacterial wall.
4. Mutations occur in the gene that encodes the target protein so it no longer binds the drug. These random events confer a selective advantage for bacteria. This mechanism does not require exposure to a particular drug. It can occur as a single-step mutation that confers a high degree of resistance, or it may be seen as a several-step mutation in which each step exhibits a slight alteration in susceptibility. Examples of resistance through mutation include *Mycobacterium tuberculosis*, *Escherichia coli*, and *Staphylococcus aureus*.
5. Bacterial mutation via transformation, conjugation, and/or transduction, with the resultant mutated form resistant to one or more classes of antimicrobials.
   a. Transduction occurs when a virus that contains deoxyribonucleic acid (DNA) infects bacteria. The virus that infects the bacteria contains plasmids of bacterial DNA that contain genes for various functions, including one that provides drug resistance. Incorporation of this plasmid makes the newly infected bacterial cell resistant and capable of passing on the trait of resistance. One plasmid carries the code for penicillinase. An example is *S. aureus*. Others contain codes for resistance to erythromycin, tetracycline, or chloramphenicol.
   b. Transformation involves transfer of DNA that is free in the environment into the bacteria. Examples include penicillin resistance in pneumococci and *Neisseria*.
   c. Conjugation is transfer of DNA from one organism to another during mating. This occurs predominantly among gram-negative bacilli such as Enterobacteriaceae and *Shigella flexneri*.

These factors together over time cause decreased penetration to the target site; alteration of the target site; and inactivation of the antibiotic by a bacterial enzyme that causes bacterial resistance. Antimicrobials are becoming less effective because of the exchange of genetic material, selection pressure, and mutations over time among pathogens. Concurrently, the total number of new antimicrobial agents under development is decreasing. Consequences that clinicians and patients face in the current antimicrobial therapy environment range from initial therapy failure to increased medical care costs associated with the management of drug-resistant infections to the ultimate crisis—patient mortality.

MECHANISM OF ACTION

Antiinfectives are classified as bacteriostatic or bactericidal in action. Bacteriostatic agents inhibit growth; bactericidal agents kill bacteria. Antiinfectives provide these effects through different mechanisms of action, including the following:

- Inhibition of cell wall synthesis, such as that seen with β-lactam antiinfectives (e.g., penicillins, cephalosporins, cephamycins, carbapenems, monobactams), vancomycin, antifungal agents, and bacitracin
- Direct action on the cell membrane to alter permeability and cause leakage of intracellular compounds, for example, the bactericidal action of polymyxin and nystatin
- Effects on function of ribosomal subunits that inhibit protein synthesis; examples include the bacteriostatic actions of tetracycline, erythromycin, clindamycin, and chloramphenicol
- Binding of ribosome subunits to alter protein synthesis and cause cell death, for example, the bactericidal action of aminoglycosides
- Changes in nucleic acid metabolism, as seen in the bactericidal actions of rifampin, quinolones, or metronidazole
- Blockage of specific essential metabolic steps by antimetabolites, for example, the bactericidal actions of sulfonamides and trimethoprim
- Inhibition of viral enzymes essential for DNA synthesis by nucleic acid analogs that produce bacteriostatic activity

TREATMENT PRINCIPLES

Standardized Guidelines

- Guidelines have been put forth for specific infections, many from the Infectious Diseases Society of America (see www.idsociety.org).
- Also consult www.guidelines.gov, the national clearinghouse for guidelines, as well as the Centers for Disease Control and Prevention and the World Health Organization.
- The CDC issues notices about changing resistance patterns and recommendations for changes in drug prescribing.

Evidence-Based Recommendations

- Will be discussed under each specific infection in the following chapters

Cardinal Points of Treatment

Select antibiotic that meets the following criteria:
- Most effective
- Narrowest spectrum
- Lowest toxicity
- Lowest potential for allergy
- Most cost-effective

PROPHYLAXIS. Cardinal to any discussion of infection is the emphasis on prevention. Knowledge of the pathogenesis of disease, including the microbiology that underlies infectious disease, reveals that many infections may be prevented by good hygiene and improved sanitation. Health care providers and people of all ages should practice the basic principles of washing hands after going to the bathroom and before eating or preparing foods, practicing good personal hygiene (taking baths or showers), avoiding polluted air and water and smoking, and eating meals that consist of fruits and vegetables with documented ability to keep the immune system strong. Together, these good health habits work to enhance resistance to disease. Clinicians send a powerful message to patients when they wash their hands before and after performing any physical examination.

On some occasions, prophylaxis is indicated. If a single effective nontoxic drug can be used to prevent an infection by a specific organism or to eradicate the organism immediately after it has been introduced, then prophylaxis may be successful. Prophylaxis often is not successful in preventing colonization or infection by microorganisms present in the environment. An example of traditional use of a prophylaxis is that used for prevention of bacterial endocarditis by group A streptococcus, but this procedure has been challenged in some studies. Treatment for a sexually transmitted disease after exposure is often effective. Attempts are being made to provide prophylaxis for HIV post exposure. Immunization when indicated (influenza, hepatitis B, HIV) and treatment after positive skin tests for tuberculosis are other examples of prophylaxis.

Prophylaxis is sometimes attempted for patients at increased risk of bacterial infection, such as those undergoing organ transplantation, cancer chemotherapy, and HIV treatment. However, prophylactic treatment may kill off normal flora of the host and allow infection to occur with drug-resistant strains, thus defeating the purpose of the prophylaxis.

evolve   See Bonus reference tables on Evolve at http://evolve. elsevier.com/Edmunds/NP/

SELECTION OF AN ANTIBIOTIC. Choose the most cost-effective antibiotic with the narrowest spectrum, lowest toxicity, and lowest potential for allergy to decrease the risk of resistance.

The idea for first-line therapy is to begin with a BB gun—not a shotgun or a cannon! Table 56-1 lists common primary care problems and the antiinfectives to which each organism is usually susceptible. Consider both drug characteristics and patient characteristics when choosing an antibiotic.

Drug Characteristics. Antibacterials tend to alter the normal flora. Normal flora help prevent overgrowth and infection by pathogenic bacteria. Change in this flora places the patient at risk for superinfection by yeast. The wider the spectrum of the antibacterial, the greater is the alteration in normal flora, and the greater is the risk of a superinfection. Choose the antibiotic with the narrowest spectrum that is effective against the organism causing the infection.

Certain antiinfectives are more likely than others to produce allergic reactions. Patients with a history of atopic allergy seem particularly susceptible to the development of allergic reactions to antiinfectives. Penicillins and sulfonamides are the most frequent causes of allergic reaction.

Certain viral infections increase the frequency of rash in response to penicillin. This often happens when amoxicillin is given to a patient with mononucleosis and is not necessarily an allergic reaction. Antiinfectives also can cause a drug fever that may be blamed mistakenly on the infection. It is important to identify the cause of the fever and to discontinue the antibiotic if drug fever is suspected.

Toxic effects resulting from the use of antiinfectives vary. Antiinfectives differ in terms of frequency and severity of adverse reactions. Gastrointestinal problems such as nausea, vomiting, diarrhea, and GI distress are almost universally caused by drugs. Sometimes, these effects discourage the patient from taking the drug. When possible, choose the least toxic of the available alternatives. See individual drug chapters for the adverse reactions associated with each particular drug.

Consider the distribution of the drug. Some antiinfectives penetrate certain sites of infection better than others such as the lungs. Antiinfectives that are extensively plasma protein bound may not penetrate to infection sites as well as others. Lipid-soluble antiinfectives will cross the blood-brain barrier. For example, tetracyclines and fluoroquinolones are effective for skin infection.

The liver metabolizes some antiinfectives. The macrolides clarithromycin, erythromycin, and troleandomycin are inhibitors of the cytochrome P450 3A4 system. Clindamycin and erythromycin are substrates of the 3A4 system. It is important to check for drug interactions before prescribing multiple products. Alterations in dosage often are required if the patient has hepatic dysfunction (see Chapter 3).

The kidney is involved in elimination of most antiinfectives. Monitor renal function and decrease dose if impaired. This is critically important when using aminoglycosides. All clinicians must know how to calculate creatinine clearance and how to reduce dosage in those patients with renal impairment (see Chapter 3).

Patient Factors That Affect Antibiotic Selection. In primary care, it usually is not important whether an antibiotic is bacteriostatic or bactericidal. If the patient is immunocompromised, a bactericidal antibiotic may be more effective than a bacteriostatic drug. This is particularly true in patients with AIDS and in those who have had organ transplants.

Local factors such as pus, hemoglobin, pH, decreased oxygen, and the presence of a foreign body (such as prosthetic valve) affect healing. The clinician must consider these variables when evaluating or starting the therapeutic regimen.

Research suggests that patient compliance decreases as the frequency of dosing increases. The clinician should not fail to ensure that the patient is able to take the medication as directed (see Chapter 7).

Severity of illness is a factor that the clinician must consider when deciding how aggressively to treat the infection and how long to treat. If patients are unable to take the medication orally or to drink enough fluids, they probably will have to be admitted to the hospital.

Concurrent illness is an important factor. Older patients tend to have more chronic illnesses. They are more susceptible to infection and are harder to treat, generally requiring longer duration of treatment. Conditions that reduce circulation, such as diabetes or congestive heart failure, may limit delivery of the antibiotic to infected sites.

The location of the infection also must be considered. The antibiotic must reach the site of the infection. If the infection is located in the brain, the antibiotic must pass the blood-brain barrier. A lipid-soluble drug may work better. Drugs that are extensively protein bound may not penetrate tissue as well.

ADMINISTER ANTIBIOTIC ACCORDING TO ACCEPTED GUIDELINES. Clinical guidelines have been developed for the treatment of many common infections. Many of these guidelines have been developed as the result of analysis of valid research and scientific studies and have been issued by federal agencies or professional groups. Evidence-based research will validate and legitimize these guidelines over time. To practice in accordance with legally defensible standards, the clinician will be expected to be knowledgeable about these guidelines and to follow them. For example, when the CDC issues a guideline that says strep throat must be treated for 10 days, clinicians must adhere to this standard of practice.

The half-life of the drug will determine the frequency of dosing. It is important to follow the appropriate dosing schedule to maintain serum and tissue concentrations of the antibiotic. The medication must be taken at regular intervals, and the clinician should write a prescription that describes precisely how the patient is to take the medication. For example, an antibiotic to be taken three times a day should be taken every 8 hours, not at each of the patient's three meals, so the clinician must be precise in writing the prescription. Stress the importance of not skipping doses.

Adequate hydration is mandatory, especially in patients with respiratory infection or any febrile infection. Forcing fluids totaling more than 2 quarts of water per day is recommended for almost all patients to thin mucous secretions and to prevent dehydration. Adequate nutrition is also important. A short course of high doses of vitamin C (2000 to 3000 mg/day) is helpful for reducing symptoms in some patients. Patients with asthma, COPD, or URI should be encouraged to stop smoking.

HOW LONG TO TREAT. Always establish a definite duration of treatment; do not begin an open-ended course. If necessary, a course of therapy can be extended if the patient evaluation reveals the need for continuation beyond the originally defined period.

Whether to discontinue a course of antiinfectives once started can be a difficult choice. If the culture shows that bacteria are resistant to the agent currently in use, it is clear that the provider must discontinue the drug and substitute one to which the bacteria are susceptible, if the patient is still ill. In general, providers should emphasize to patients that it is important to complete a course of antiinfectives, even if the symptoms are gone. This is necessary to completely eradicate the offending organism, not just the ones most susceptible to the antibiotic, while leaving resistant bacteria alive. On the other hand, the clinician should discontinue an antibiotic that was started based on empirical evidence if the culture is negative. Many providers are reluctant to do this for a variety of reasons.

Skin, eye, and vaginal infections can be treated via local application of medication. Drainage of the site, for example, in some sinus infections and in empyema, is necessary. Abscesses must be drained. Antiinfectives do not replace local treatment such as incision and drainage.

Foreign objects must be removed to achieve control of any associated infection.

The most important complication of antibiotic treatment is superinfection by an organism that is resistant to the antibiotic. This can be caused by bacteria, for example, in colitis caused by *Clostridium difficile*. Fungal infection also can be a problem. Women frequently get vaginal yeast infections when treated with an antibiotic.

Antiinfectives constitute the most commonly prescribed group of medications in primary care. The primary care provider should have a good understanding of the general principles and should be familiar with the many classes of antiinfectives that are available. Chapter 57 discusses the infections most commonly treated in primary care. In subsequent chapters, specific antiinfectives are discussed.

evolve A continually updated list of useful WebLinks may be found in the Evolve Resources at http://evolve.elsevier.com/Edmunds/NP/

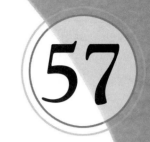

Treatment of Specific Infections and Miscellaneous Antibiotics

DRUG OVERVIEW

Class	Subclass	Generic Name	Trade Name
Antibiotics	Lincosamide	clindamycin ✺	Cleocin
	Tricyclic glycopeptide	vancomycin	Vancocin
	Synthetic nitrofurantoin	nitrofurantoin ✺	Macrobid
	Miscellaneous	fosfomycin (as tromethamine)	Monurol
Topical Preparations for Vaginal Infections			
Antifungals		clotrimazole	Gyne-Lotrimin, Mycelex (OTC and Rx)
		miconazole	Monistat (OTC and Rx)
		butoconazole	Femstat
		terconazole ✺	Terazol
		tioconazole	Vagistat
		fluconazole ✺	Diflucan
		nystatin ✺	Mycostatin
Antibiotics		clindamycin phosphate	Cleocin cream, 2%
Antiprotozoal		metronidazole	MetroGel vaginal gel, 0.75%

✺, Top 200 drug.

THERAPEUTIC OVERVIEW

The student and the beginning clinician may be overwhelmed by the numerous antibiotics that are available. Table 57-1 serves as a general summary of common offending organisms for various infections. Both the first treatment choice and the alternative treatment suggestions listed are based on a compendium of various authorities (Figure 57-1).

This chapter presents antimicrobial therapy according to disease- or site-specific recommendations. Treatments presented include recommendations for both children and adults when available. These are general guidelines for simple infections, with no complicating factors. See up-to-date specific drug information and check dosages before prescribing, especially for children and the elderly, because recommendations often vary with changing resistance patterns.

Skin and Soft Tissue Infections, Including Impetigo

Guidelines are provided by the Infectious Diseases Society of America (www.idsociety.org):

- Group A streptococci, *Staphylococcus aureus*, and group A β-hemolytic streptococci

Impetigo is a contagious infection of the skin that is common in children. The lesions are macules, vesicles, bullae, pustules, and honey-colored crusts that usually appear on the face and other exposed skin. Systemic antibiotics usually are required. However, mupirocin (Bactroban) can be used for topical treatment of mild impetigo.

CELLULITIS. Although most cellulitis seen in primary care is easily treated, the provider must rule out the following complicated patients for whom they should seek referral:

- *Cellulitis, erysipelas:* Group A strep, occasionally group B, C, or G; *Streptococcus pyogenes, S. aureus* (uncommon)
- *Necrotizing fasciitis, "flesh eating bacteria":* Usually polymicrobic with gram-positive and gram-negative and anaerobic; group A, C, G strep, *Vibrio,* enterococci, staphylococci, *Escherichia coli, Pseudomonas, Proteus, Serratia, Clostridium.* These patients require hospitalization.
- *Diabetic:* Group A strep, *S. aureus,* Enterobacteriaceae, clostridia (rare). Patients often are complicated and require hospitalization. Treatment usually is provided until 3 days after resolution of inflammation.

629

TABLE 57-1 Empirical Antimicrobial Treatment

Site of Infection	Usual Causes	First-Choice Treatment, Oral	Alternative Treatments
SKIN AND SOFT TISSUE			
Impetigo	*S. aureus* and group A strep	dicloxacillin	mupirocin topical, azithromycin, clarithromycin, erythromycin, oral cephalosporin second generation (cephalexin)
Cellulitis, extremities	Group A strep, occasionally group B, C, and G; *S. agalactiae*	TMP/SMX 250-500 mg bid po in areas where MRSA isolates account for 15% of infections	erythromycin, AM/CL azithromycin, clarithromycin, clindamycin, levofloxacin
ANIMAL BITES			
Cat	*P. multocida, S. aureus*	AM/CL 875 mg bid or 500 mg tid	cefuroxime 500 mg q12h, doxycycline 100 mg bid
Dog	*P. multocida, P. canis, S. aureus, Bacteroides* spp, *Fusobacterium*	AM/CL 875 mg bid or 500 mg tid	*Adults:* clindamycin 300 mg qid plus Cipro 500 mg bid *Children:* clindamycin 8 to 16 mg/kg/day plus TMP/SMX
Human	*S. viridans, S. epidermidis, Corynebacterium, S. aureus, Eikenella, Bacteroides*	AM/CL 875 mg bid × 5 days	clindamycin, either ciprofloxacin or TMP/SMX
Infected postoperative wound	*S. aureus,* group A strep, Enterobacteriaceae	Oral cephalosporin, first generation or AM/CL	dicloxacillin
RESPIRATORY			
Otitis media No antibiotics in past month	*S. pneumoniae, H. influenzae, M. catarrhalis,* group A strep, Enterobacteriaceae	amoxicillin	azithromycin, clarithromycin
Antibiotics in past month		amoxicillin, AM/CL, cefdinir, cefpodoxime, cefprozil, or cefuroxime	
ACUTE SINUSITIS			
No antibiotics in past month	*S. pneumoniae, H. influenzae, M. catarrhalis*	amoxicillin, AM/CL, cefdinir, cefpodoxime, cefuroxime × 10 days	clarithromycin, azithromycin, TMP/SMX, doxycycline, or fluoroquinolones
Antibiotics in past month		AM/CL or fluoroquinolones (adults) × 10 days	
Treatment failure		Mild to moderate: AM/CL + extra amoxicillin or cefpodoxime, cefuroxime, or cefdinir	*Severe:* gatifloxacin, levofloxacin, moxifloxacin
Pharyngitis	Group A, C, G strep, *C. diphtheriae, A. haemolyticum, M. pneumoniae*	penicillin V po × 10 days; oral first-generation cephalosporin in areas of high resistance	Erythromycin × 10 days, oral cephalosporin second generation × 4 to 6 days, clindamycin or azithromycin × 5 days, clarithromycin × 10 days
Acute bacterial exacerbation of COPD	*S. pneumoniae, H. influenzae, M. catarrhalis*	*Mild:* No antibiotics *Moderate:* amoxicillin, doxycycline (TMP/SMX), cephalosporin	*Severe:* AM/CL, azithromycin, clarithromycin, oral cephalosporin, fluoroquinolones with enhanced activity vs. *S. pneumoniae*
PNEUMONIA			
Age 1 to 3 months Age 1 to 24 months	*C. trachomatis,* RSV virus, *Bordetella* *S. pneumoniae, H. influenzae,* chlamydia, mycoplasma	erythromycin IV cefuroxime IV	
Age 3 months to 5 years	*S. pneumoniae,* mycoplasma, chlamydia	erythromycin, clarithromycin, azithromycin	
Age 5 to 18 years	Mycoplasma, *S. pneumoniae, C. pneumoniae*	clarithromycin 500 mg bid, azithromycin	doxycycline, erythromycin

TABLE 57-1   Empirical Antimicrobial Treatment (Continued)

Site of Infection	Usual Causes	First-Choice Treatment, Oral	Alternative Treatments
Age 18 years and older	Mycoplasma, chlamydia, *S. pneumoniae, Legionella, H. influenzae, K. pneumoniae*	azithromycin, clarithromycin, doxycycline	fluoroquinolone with enhanced activity vs. *S. pneumoniae*, oral cephalosporin second generation, AM/CL, doxycycline
PROPHYLAXIS FOR PROCEDURES			
Dental, esophageal, and URI procedures	*Streptococcus viridans*, other streptococci, enterococci, staphylococci	amoxicillin 2 g, children 50 mg/kg	1. clindamycin 600 mg, children 20 mg/kg 2. cephalexin 2 g, children 50 mg/kg 3. azithromycin or clarithromycin 500 mg, children 15 mg/kg
Gastrointestinal (excluding esophageal) and genitourinary procedures	Enteric gram-negative bacilli, anaerobes, enterococci	amoxicillin 2 g, children 50 mg/kg	IV gentamicin or vancomycin
GI INFECTIONS			
Mouth	Oral microflora infection, polymicrobial	clindamycin 300 to 450 mg q6h	AM/CL 875 mg bid or 500 mg tid
Gastroenteritis	Usually viral; amebiasis, *L. monocytogenes, V. cholerae*	Culture, treat cause	
Diarrhea, traveler's	*E. coli*, shigella, salmonella, *Campylobacter, C. difficile*, amebiasis	*Mild:* ciprofloxacin 750 mg × 1 dose *Severe:* fluoroquinolone bid × 3 days	azithromycin usual dose, or 1000 mg × 1 dose *Amebiasis, giardiasis:* tinidazole 2000 mg po × 3 days
Diarrhea, severe	*Shigella, Salmonella, C. jejuni, E. coli* 0157 H7, *E. histolytica C. difficile*	fluoroquinolone (Cipro) 500 mg q12h × 5-7 days metronidazole 500 mg tid × 10-14 days	TMP/SMX bid (resistance common) vancomycin 125 mg qid po × 10-14 days; first choice if moderately to severely ill
Diverticulitis	Enterobacteriaceae, *P. aeruginosa, Bacteroides* spp, enterococci	TMP/SMX bid or ciprofloxacin 500 mg bid metronidazole 500 mg q6h × 7 to 10 days	AM/CL 500 mg tid po × 7 to 10 days
RENAL/GU			
UTI	*E. coli, S. saprophyticus*, enterococci	TMP/SMX × 3 days, fluoroquinolone × 3 days	Nitrofurantoin, fosfomycin, oral cephalosporin, doxycycline, amoxicillin
Pyelonephritis	*E. coli, S. saprophyticus*, enterococci	fluoroquinolone × 7 days	AM/CL, oral cephalosporin, TMP/SMX DS
VAGINAL INFECTIONS			
Candidiasis	*C. albicans*	Vaginal antifungals × 3-7 days; see separate table	Immediate relief fluconazole plus azole or hydrocortisone cream; fluconazole 150 mg po × 1 dose *Severe:* fluconazole × 2 days plus 7 days azole *Chronic:* terconazole × 14 days; if resistant, switch to a more potent preparation
Bacterial vaginosis	*Gardnerella, Bacteroides*, others	metronidazole 500 mg bid × 7 days	metronidazole 2 g × 1 dose clindamycin
Trichomonas	*T. vaginalis*	tinidazole (Tindamax) 2000 mg po × 1 day	metronidazole
PROSTATITIS			
Acute	*N. gonorrhoeae* or *C. trachomatis*	Use 160 mg TMP and 800 mg SMX bid (or Septra DS bid or Bactrim DS 1 bid)	Fluoroquinolones (ciprofloxacin 250-500 mg po bid or ofloxacin 400 mg po bid)

Table continued on following page

TABLE 57-1   Empirical Antimicrobial Treatment (Continued)

Site of Infection	Usual Causes	First-Choice Treatment, Oral	Alternative Treatments
Chronic	E. coli, Klebsiella, P. mirabilis, P. aeruginosa, E. faecalis	Fluoroquinolones (ciprofloxacin 250-500 mg po bid or ofloxacin 400 mg po bid)	Use 160 mg TMP and 800 mg/SMX bid (or Septra DS bid or Bactrim DS 1 bid)
STDS			
Gonorrhea	N. gonorrhoeae	ceftriaxone 125 mg IM × 1 dose, cefixime 400 mg × 1 dose, ciprofloxacin 500 mg × 1 dose, ofloxacin 400 mg × 1 dose, levofloxacin 250 mg × 1 dose	spectinomycin 2 g IM × 1 dose, ceftizoxime 500 mg IM, cefoxitin 2 mg IM with probenecid 1 g po, cefotaxime 500 mg IM, gatifloxacin 400 mg, norfloxacin 800 po, lomefloxacin 400 mg × 1 dose
Ophthalmia neonatorum	Prophylaxis for N. gonorrhoeae	silver nitrate (1%) aqueous solution × 1 dose, erythromycin (0.5%) ophthalmic ointment × 1 dose, tetracycline ophthalmic ointment (1%) × 1 dose	
Syphilis	T. pallidum	benzathine penicillin G 2.4 million units IM × 1 dose	doxycycline 100 mg po bid × 14 days, ceftriaxone 1 g daily IM or IV × 8 to 10 days
Chlamydia	C. trachomatis	azithromycin 1 g × 1 dose, doxycycline 100 mg bid × 7 days	erythromycin base 500 mg qid × 7 days, erythromycin ethylsuccinate 800 mg qid × 7 days, difloxacin 300 mg bid × 7 days, levofloxacin 500 mg qd × 7 days
FEMALE REPRODUCTIVE			
Mastitis	S. pneumoniae, S. pyogenes, S. aureus, H. influenzae, P. aeruginosa	dicloxacillin 500 mg q6h	clindamycin 300 mg q6h
SYSTEMIC FEBRILE			
Lyme disease	B. burgdorferi	doxycycline 100 mg bid × 10 to 14 days; or amoxicillin 500 mg tid, cefuroxime 500 mg bid, × 14 to 21 days	erythromycin 250 mg qid
Rocky Mountain spotted fever	R. rickettsii	doxycycline 100 mg po bid × 7 days	chloramphenicol 50 mg/kg/day IV q6h × 7 days

AM/CL, Augmentin.
Fluoroquinolones with enhanced activity vs. S. pneumo: gatifloxacin, levofloxacin, and moxifloxacin.

- S. aureus remains a possibility and should be considered if first-line treatment is not successful. Culturing an open wound seldom produces useful information; often the report comes back with multiple organisms. Site of infection and how infection was acquired will often reveal the most likely causative organism. Community-acquired methicillin-resistant S. aureus (MRSA) infection is increasingly common; it should be diagnosed early and treated with medications such as Septra or doxycycline. Vancomycin has become the standard in areas where MRSA infections exceed 15% of the isolate. Alternatives to vancomycin also should be considered, so that widespread vancomycin resistance may be delayed, if possible. Consider levofloxacin, tetracycline, clindamycin, rifampin, gentamicin, linezolid, daptomycin, and tigecycline. Consult the latest CDC guidelines regularly for recommendations as they are issued.

ANIMAL BITES
- Cat: Pasteurella multocida, S. aureus
- Dog: P. multocida, S. aureus, Bacteroides spp, Fusobacterium

- Human: Streptococcus viridans, Staphylococcus epidermidis, Corynebacterium, S. aureus, Eikenella, Bacteroides spp, Peptostreptococcus

The location and type of the wound are important factors, as is the type of animal, in selection of appropriate treatment for the bite wound. Unprovoked animal bites should raise the suspicion of rabies. Cat bites are more likely to become infected than are human or dog bites. Human bites by children are not likely to become infected; infection is more likely with bites by adults. Dog bites are very unlikely to become infected.

Give the patient a tetanus/diphtheria booster if not vaccinated within the previous 5 years. Do not suture/glue the wound closed if it has been longer than 12 hours since the bite occurred, or if the injury is a hand wound or a cat bite. Prophylaxis is recommended for bites on the hand or in the genital region, for human or cat bites, for crush and puncture wounds, and for the treatment of patients with impaired immune systems.

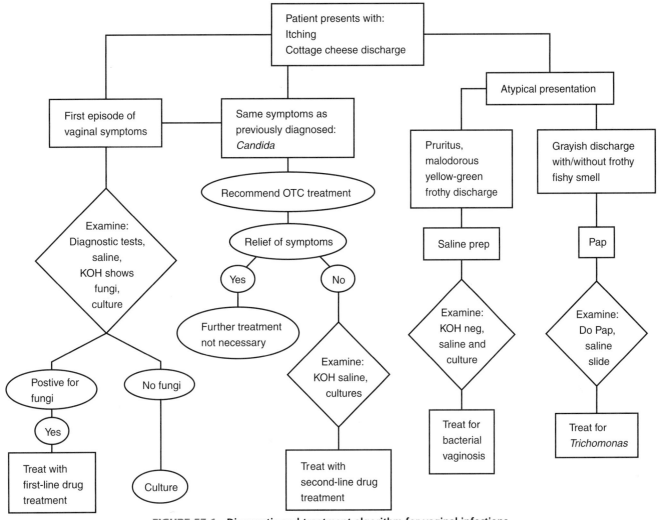

FIGURE 57-1   Diagnostic and treatment algorithm for vaginal infections.

INFECTED POSTOPERATIVE WOUND

- *S. aureus*, group A streptococci, Enterobacteriaceae
  - Superficial infected wounds usually are treated by primary care practitioner.
  - If the infection is deeper, the treatment selected will depend on the type of surgery that is required.

Respiratory Tract Infections

By far, the most common causative agent is a virus, which causes an acute self-limiting disease that should not be treated with an antibiotic. Influenza is caused by a virus and can be treated with the drugs listed in Chapter 68. Evidence suggests that antibiotics, especially broad-spectrum antibiotics, continue to be overused for adult URIs.

OTITIS MEDIA

- *S. pneumoniae, Haemophilus influenzae, Moraxella catarrhalis*, virus; group A strep; *S. aureus* and Enterobacteriaceae (uncommon)
  - Duration of treatment is generally 10 days.

Signs and symptoms that indicate a need for antibiotic treatment include otalgia, fever, otorrhea, or a bulging yellow or red tympanic membrane. Simple effusion (presence of fluid in the middle ear with no signs or symptoms of acute infection) does not have to be treated with antibiotics. Much controversy has arisen about treatment with antibiotics in the past. However, doctors and patients are becoming comfortable with the new approach of treating with an antibiotic only if clearly indicated. Patients with tympanic membrane perforation, chronic or recurrent infection, craniofacial abnormalities, or immune compromise should be referred to an ENT specialist for treatment. How recently the patient has been treated with antibiotics will affect the antibiotic choice.

SINUSITIS

- *Sinusitis, acute:* S. pneumoniae, H. influenzae, M. catarrhalis
  - *Less frequent:* Group A strep, anaerobes, *S. aureus*, Streptococcus spp, Neisseria spp, and gram-negative rods
- *Sinusitis, chronic:* Anaerobic bacteria often present (*Bacteroides* spp, *Peptostreptococcus, Fusobacterium*)
- Duration of treatment is usually 10 to 14 days.

This infection has a very similar pattern to that of otitis media, although perhaps more unusual bacteria are seen. Most sinus infections are viral. The common cold frequently involves the sinuses. Evidence of bacterial infection includes prolonged symptoms without improvement for 10 to 14 days or longer, fever higher than 102° F (39° C), unilateral pain, sinus tenderness, or tooth pain. Nasal discharge is not a reliable indicator of bacterial sinusitis. With viral URIs, the nasal discharge may change from clear to yellow during the first few days of the infection. Suspect a bacterial infection if the discharge changes to green. If the patient starts to improve and then worsens, this may indicate that a secondary bacterial infection is present.

Unfortunately, younger children may not present with the classic signs or symptoms of sinusitis. Congestion and cough that last for longer than 10 days, high fever, and purulent nasal discharge are the most likely symptoms.

Because the causative organisms are similar to those of otitis media, treatment is very similar. Decongestants and mucolytics may improve drainage. Nonpharmacologic remedies such as drinking hot fluids, applying moist heat, inhaling steam, and using saltwater nasal sprays or rinses may decrease congestion.

PHARYNGITIS. Guidelines have been provided by the Infectious Diseases Society (www.idsociety.org):
- *Pharyngitis:* Groups A and C, G strep, *Corynebacterium diphtheriae, Arcanobacterium haemolyticum,* and *Mycoplasma pneumoniae*
- Duration of therapy is at least 10 days.

Once again, virus (including mononucleosis) causes most cases of pharyngitis. The classic infection to be treated with antibiotics is group A β-hemolytic streptococci. It is extremely difficult to accurately diagnose a bacterial pharyngitis by history and physical alone. A throat culture is necessary. Symptoms such as pharyngeal pain, dysphagia, fever, tonsillar exudate, and lymphadenopathy with absence of cough increase the likelihood of a diagnosis of strep. Approximately one half of patients with these symptoms will have strep throat on culture. In areas with increased resistance to penicillin, an oral cephalosporin is more likely than penicillin to be effective.

Because of diagnostic vagueness, the provider has the option of waiting 2 days for culture results or treating empirically. Immediate empirical treatment is tempting because of symptom relief and decreased transmission but will result in substantial overtreatment. To avoid this dilemma, a rapid antigen detection test can be used. If used carefully, these tests can be very accurate. If the rapid test is positive, initiate antibiotic treatment. If it is negative, await culture results before initiating antibiotic treatment.

ACUTE BRONCHITIS
- *Infants/children* (<5): Virus is the usual cause.
- *Adolescents and adults:* Virus, M. pneumoniae, *Chlamydia pneumoniae, Bordetella pertussis*

Bronchitis is a poorly defined illness, involving a cough. A virus causes almost all cases of bronchitis. Rarely, a child older than 5 years will have bronchitis caused by M. pneumoniae or C. pneumoniae. If the child does not get better in 10 to 14 days, consider treatment with a macrolide.

ACUTE BACTERIAL EXACERBATION OF COPD
- *Streptococcus pneumoniae, H. influenzae, M. catarrhalis*
- Mycoplasma or chlamydia (rare)

Many acute exacerbations of COPD are viral. Patients may have any one of a wide variety of bacteria, depending on

previous hospitalizations, etc. These patients are likely to be frail, to have a history of smoking, and to have been previously treated with many antibiotics. A sputum culture may be difficult to obtain but will be very useful. Obtaining a sputum sample after a nebulization treatment may be necessary. Try to get the patient to stop smoking.

COMMUNITY-ACQUIRED PNEUMONIA (CAP). The Infectious Diseases Society of America has recently released guidelines for CAP (www.idsociety.org). It is helpful for the clinician to differentiate disease origins by differentiating between bacterial and atypical organisms.
- *Ages 1 to 3 months:* Chlamydia trachomatis, respiratory syncytial virus (RSV), virus, *Bordetella*
- *Ages 1 to 24 months:* RSV (bronchiolitis), viruses, *S. pneumoniae, H. influenzae,* chlamydia, mycoplasma, *S. aureus* (rare)
- *Ages 3 months to 5 years:* Viruses, *S. pneumoniae,* mycoplasma, chlamydia
- *Ages 5 to 18 years:* Mycoplasma, respiratory viruses; consider *S. pneumoniae, C. pneumoniae*
- Age 18 years and older
- *No comorbidity:* Mycoplasma, chlamydia, *S. pneumoniae, S. aureus,* group A streptococcus, *M. catarrhalis,* anaerobes, aerobic gram—bacterial, viral
- *Smokers: S. pneumoniae, H. influenzae, M. catarrhalis*
- *Postviral: S. pneumoniae,* rarely *S. aureus*
- *Alcoholic: S. pneumoniae,* anaerobes, coliforms
- *Epidemic:* Legionnaires' disease

Treatment lasts until the patient is afebrile for at least 5 days for pneumococcal pneumonia, often for 10 to 14 days. Pneumonia caused by Enterobacteriaceae, *Pseudomonas,* or *Staphylococcus* is treated for 21 to 28 days.

Because so many different bacteria can cause pneumonia, determining empirical treatment can be problematic. Mycoplasma or chlamydial infections are common, and a macrolide is recommended. However, penicillin-resistant pneumococci occur regularly and may be resistant to a macrolide or doxycycline. Frail elderly patients may require treatment with one of the fluoroquinolones.

TUBERCULOSIS. See Chapter 65.

PROPHYLACTIC REGIMENS FOR DENTAL, ORAL, RESPIRATORY TRACT, OR ESOPHAGEAL PROCEDURES. These regimens are performed for patients with risk for endocarditis or with prosthetic devices. No research findings support prophylaxis.

Many give antimicrobial prophylaxis before patients receive vascular grafts or orthopedic prostheses. Others recommend prophylaxis before dental or genitourinary procedures are performed. Prophylaxis is not recommended for dialysis catheters, ventriculoperitoneal shunts, cardiac pacemakers, and defibrillators.

GI Infections

MOUTH
- *Streptococcus mutans,* other *Streptococcus* spp, *Actinomyces* spp; oral microflora, infection often polymicrobial
- Duration of treatment is 2 to 3 weeks.

Mouth infections can be caused by a large variety of bacteria but often respond to penicillin. Because uncontaminated cultures are difficult to obtain, treatment with a broad-spectrum agent occasionally may be necessary.

GASTROENTERITIS
- *Mild:* Virus, bacterial (see below), parasitic
- Most diarrhea is viral in cause, not severe, and self-limiting.

TRAVELER'S DIARRHEA
- *Acute:* E. coli, Shigella, Salmonella, Campylobacter, Clostridium difficile, amebiasis
- *Chronic:* Cyclospora, Cryptosporidium, Giardia, Isospora
- Duration of treatment for acute diarrhea is usually 3 days.

If the patient is traveling to an area with endemic infections and may be unable to adequately observe safety precautions (e.g., bottled water), a course of antibiotics may be provided, so the patient is able to initiate treatment immediately on onset of symptoms. Treatment also may include loperamide and/or Pepto-Bismol.

SEVERE DIARRHEA
- *Diarrhea, severe:* Shigella, Salmonella, Campylobacter jejuni, E. coli 0157 H7, C. difficile, Entamoeba histolytica, and many others
- Duration of treatment is 7 to 14 days.

Symptoms of severe diarrhea include more than six liquid stools per day, temperature greater than 101° F, tenesmus, blood, and fecal leukocytes. Patients always require a stool for fecal leukocytes and culture. Treatment is based on culture results.

C. *difficile* is often a consequence of treatment with all antibiotics. The four antibiotics most likely to cause C. *difficile* infection are ampicillin, amoxicillin, cephalosporin, and clindamycin. The incidence of infection is high with these drugs because of their widespread use in children. Fluoroquinolones also are implicated in C. *difficile*–associated diarrhea, again because of widespread use. Tetracycline use is least likely to cause this problem. The presentation of C. *difficile* varies from mild illness to rapid clinical deterioration. It often is associated with copious liquid diarrhea, although it can be less acute in onset and moderate in amount of liquid stool produced. Suspect C. *difficile* in any patient who develops diarrhea after taking an antibiotic. Onset of symptoms can be delayed for weeks after treatment with an antibiotic. Because of the potential for severe symptoms, treat promptly. Vancomycin and metronidazole are discussed in detail at the end of this chapter.

DIVERTICULITIS
- *Diverticulitis:* Enterobacteriaceae, *Pseudomonas aeruginosa*, *Bacteroides* spp, enterococci
- Treatment is provided until the patient is afebrile for 3 days.

Diverticulosis is a common problem in the elderly that does not require antibiotics. Symptoms of diverticulitis include acute abdominal pain and fever, lower left abdominal tenderness and mass, and leukocytosis. Severity ranges widely from mild to severe disease. Treatment requires a broad-spectrum oral antibiotic with anaerobic activity.

PEPTIC ULCER DISEASE. *H. pylori* is implicated in many cases of peptic ulcer disease. See Chapter 24 for treatment regimens.

Renal/Genitourinary Infections

URINARY TRACT INFECTIONS
- *UTI and pyelonephritis:* E. coli, *Proteus mirabilis*, *Pseudomonas*, *Klebsiella pneumoniae*, Enterobacter, *Staphylococcus saprophyticus*, enterococci, and many others
- Duration of treatment of uncomplicated UTI is generally 3 to 10 days. In general, single-dose treatments are minimally effective in resolving UTI.
- Duration of treatment of pyelonephritis is at least 14 days.

Most resources state that a urine culture is not necessary for the management of a simple UTI. An acute uncomplicated UTI can be treated empirically. A patient who has been in the hospital or has had previous UTIs may have any one of a large number of bacteria, including *P. aeruginosa*.

For many patients, particularly the elderly, treatment is more accurately selected with urine for culture and urinalysis before treatment is initiated. Urinalysis validates culture results or shows whether the specimen was contaminated. A dipstick urinalysis will confirm the presence of a UTI, but it does not provide information about susceptibility. Culture confirms the organism and its sensitivity.

If patients have symptoms that make them uncomfortable, treat with phenazopyridine (Pyridium) or treat empirically pending culture results. If the patient's symptoms are not a problem, waiting for culture results allows the clinician to put the patient on a narrow-spectrum yet effective medication.

PROSTATITIS
- *Men with prostatitis younger than 35 years:* Consider *Neisseria gonorrhoeae* or C. *trachomatis* and look for STD. See treatment of STDs below for appropriate treatment of these organisms.

Prostatitis in older men is likely to be caused by Enterobacteriaceae. Other possible organisms include enterococci and *P. aeruginosa*.

First-line treatment for acute prostatitis consists of 160 mg TMP/SMX bid. Treatment may be required for 1 month. The problem may not resolve and prostatitis may become chronic. First-line treatment for chronic prostatitis would include any of the fluoroquinolones. Duration of treatment for chronic prostatitis is often 4 to 12 weeks.

Sexually Transmitted Diseases

Patterns of resistance to STDs are rapidly changing, and treatment recommendations change frequently. Check with the most recent CDC or state resources before treating. The local health department is a good source of information on local patterns of resistance and effective treatments.

Many patients who present with one STD will have other concomitant STDs. When gonorrhea or urethritis/cervicitis is diagnosed, treat for both *N. gonorrhoeae* and chlamydia. Concurrent treatment for syphilis also should be considered when signs indicate the possible presence of the organism.

GONORRHEA
- *Gonorrhea:* N. gonorrhoeae

Men present with urethritis with mucopurulent or purulent discharge. Women usually have no symptoms but may present with mucopurulent cervicitis. Newborn infants can get a gonococcal infection in their eyes. Because this infection can cause blindness, most states require treatment. Laboratory testing consists of Gram staining of secretions and culture.

Quinolone-resistant *N. gonorrhoeae* (QRNG) is common in Europe, the Middle East, Asia, and the Pacific. Resistance also is becoming increasingly common in the United States. The CDC now recommends a shift to the use of cephalosporins for the treatment of gonorrhea. For ophthalmia neonatorum, one of the recommended preparations should be instilled into both eyes of every neonate as soon as possible after delivery. It is not known whether this prevents chlamydial ophthalmia.

SYPHILIS

• *Syphilis: Treponema pallidum*

Syphilis is a systemic disease. Primary infection consists of an ulcer or chancre at the infection site. Secondary infection includes skin rash, mucocutaneous lesions, and lymphadenopathy. Tertiary infection syphilis consists of cardiac, ophthalmic, and auditory abnormalities and gummatous lesions. Latent syphilis lacks clinical manifestations. Darkfield examinations and direct fluorescent antibody tests of lesion exudate or tissue are the definitive methods for diagnosing early syphilis. Parenteral penicillin remains the preferred drug for the treatment of all stages of syphilis.

CHLAMYDIA

• *Chlamydial genital infection, ophthalmia neonatorum, infant pneumonia: C. trachomatis*

Men present with urethritis with mucopurulent or purulent discharge. Women present with mucopurulent cervicitis. Untreated chlamydial infection can result in pelvic inflammatory disease, ectopic pregnancy, or infertility. Because treatment for chlamydia (doxycycline) costs less than diagnostic testing, many providers treat patients given a diagnosis of gonorrhea for chlamydia also without testing.

OTHER

• *Chancroid: Haemophilus ducreyi*

Criteria for diagnosis provide a clinical picture of one or more painful genital ulcers with regional inguinal lymphadenopathy; no evidence of *T. pallidum* or herpes simplex virus (HSV) should be evident on standard laboratory testing.

• *Granuloma inguinale (donovanosis): Calymmatobacterium granulomatis*

Rare in the United States, it is common in certain tropical and developing areas. It presents as painless, progressive ulcerative lesions without regional lymphadenopathy. The ulcers bleed easily on contact.

• *Virus:* HIV, herpes simples, human papillomavirus (HPV), condyloma acuminatum

See Chapter 68 for discussion of treatment of viral disease.

Female Reproductive Infections

MASTITIS

• *Acute outpatient: S. aureus, S. pneumoniae, S. pyogenes, H. influenzae, P. aeruginosa*

Mastitis usually begins within 3 months of delivery, possibly with a sore nipple. Symptoms of cellulitis become obvious. Apply cold compresses.

VAGINITIS. *Candida, T. vaginalis,* and *Gardnerella* are the most frequent causes of vaginitis, vaginal discharge, or vulvar itching

and irritation. *N. gonorrhoeae* also can cause a vaginal discharge. *T. vaginalis* and *N. gonorrhoeae* are generally transmitted sexually; *Candida albicans* and *Gardnerella* (most common cause of bacterial vaginosis) are not. See Table 57-2.

CANDIDA INFECTIONS. *Candida* causes fungal infections of the vagina, which commonly are referred to as *yeast infections*. *Candida* is part of the normal flora of the vagina and usually is held in check by the acidic environment of the vagina. Apparent overgrowth of the organism causes symptoms. Many factors, including change in diet, poor nutrition, sleep deprivation, diabetes, use of antibiotics, pregnancy, corticosteroids, oral progestin–dominant contraceptives, and decreased host immunity (e.g., HIV infection), allow overgrowth. *Candida* may be passed between sexual partners.

Candida infection usually presents with intense pruritus and burning and copious discharge that is malodorous, white, and curd-like. Candidiasis also can cause vaginal soreness, dyspareunia, and external dysuria. Diagnosis of candidiasis is made by microscopic examination with 10% KOH showing filaments and spores. Cultures may be used when *Candida* is suspected but is not seen on microscopic examination. A patient who has recurrent or chronic candidiasis should be assessed for risk factors such as diabetes mellitus or HIV infection.

Guidelines are available from the Infection Diseases Society of America. It is safe and effective for a patient to use OTC preparations without being examined by a health care provider if she has previously been given a diagnosis of candidiasis infection and is having the same symptoms. Fluconazole tablets take about 2 to 3 days to start working. Oral treatment may be given if the patient has an aversion to vaginal products, or if she is about to start her menstrual period. In general, the patient should be examined before the oral medication is prescribed. The oral formulation may be used in conjunction with an azole or a hydrocortisone cream for more immediate relief of symptoms.

BACTERIAL VAGINOSIS. Bacterial vaginosis often occurs as an overgrowth of one or more bacteria and is not sexually transmitted. Often, the predominant organism is *Gardnerella*. Symptoms include a grayish, sometimes frothy, "fishy" smelling discharge. Vulvitis or vaginitis may be present. On saline wet mount, epithelial cells are covered with bacteria to such an extent that cell borders are obscured (clue cells). Vaginal cultures generally are not helpful.

A clinical diagnosis of bacterial vaginosis is defined by the presence of a homogeneous vaginal discharge that:
• Has a pH greater than 4.5
• Emits a "fishy" amine odor when mixed with 10% KOH solution
• Contains clue cells on microscopic examination

On laboratory examination, a Gram stain of vaginal secretions diagnostic of bacterial vaginosis will show the following:
• Markedly reduced or absent *Lactobacillus* morphology
• Predominance of *Gardnerella* morphotype
• Absence of or few white blood cells

Rule out other pathogens commonly associated with vulvovaginitis, including *C. trachomatis, N. gonorrhoeae, C. albicans,* and herpes simplex virus.

TRICHOMONAS. *Trichomonas vaginalis* is a protozoal flagellate that can infect the vagina, Skene's ducts, and the lower

TABLE 57-2 Recommended Treatment of Vaginitis

Medication	Dosage and Administration
CANDIDA	
clotrimazole cream, 1%; 100 mg, 500 mg vaginal suppository	1 applicator full intravaginally at bedtime × 7 days 100 mg vaginal tablet × 7 days; 500 mg vaginal tablet as a single dose
miconazole cream, 2%; 100 mg, 200 mg, 1200 mg vaginal suppository	1 applicator full intravaginally at bedtime × 7 days 100 mg vaginal suppository once daily × 7 days; 200 mg vaginal suppository once daily × 3 days; 1200 mg vaginal suppository once
butoconazole cream, 2%	1 applicator full intravaginally at bedtime × 3 days (Femstat-3) 1 applicator full intravaginally once (Gynazole-1)
terconazole cream, 0.4%	1 applicator full intravaginally at bedtime × 7 days
terconazole cream, 0.8%	1 applicator full intravaginally at bedtime × 3 days
tioconazole ointment, 6.5%	1 applicator full intravaginally at bedtime × one dose
BACTERIAL VAGINOSIS (GARDNERELLA)	
metronidazole	500 mg po bid × 7 days Gel (0.75%), 1 applicator full daily to bid × 5 days
clindamycin vaginal cream, 2%	1 applicator full daily before bedtime × 3 to 7 days
TRICHOMONAS	
metronidazole	250 mg po q8h × 7 days 2 g single dose *Treatment failure:* 500 mg bid × 7 days

urinary tract in women and the lower genitourinary tract in men. It is sexually transmitted. Trichomoniasis is usually asymptomatic in men, or they may have nongonorrheal urethritis. Women exhibit pruritus; a malodorous frothy, yellow-green discharge; diffuse vaginal erythema; and red macular lesions on the cervix in severe cases. Diagnosis is made by saline wet mount that shows motile organisms with flagella. *Trichomonas* may be found on a Pap smear.

Musculoskeletal Infections

It is important to aspirate the joint to obtain a culture and sensitivity for any suspected joint infection. The joint requires local aspiration often, sometimes daily. In general, these infections should be treated by a specialist.

OSTEOMYELITIS
- *Osteomyelitis:* S. aureus, gram-negative bacilli, group B streptococcus

Patients should be referred to an infectious disease specialist and an orthopedic surgeon if osteomyelitis is suspected. Blood and infected bone should be cultured. Intravenous antibiotics are required, especially for initial treatment. Occasionally, treatment for chronic osteomyelitis will be completed orally in the outpatient setting. The most common offending organism is *S. aureus*.

Infections of the Central Nervous System
MENINGITIS
- *Age younger than 1 month:* Group B streptococcus, *E. coli*, *Listeria*, miscellaneous gram negative, miscellaneous gram positive
- *Ages 1 month to 50 years:* S. pneumoniae, N meningitidis, H. influenzae (rare)

- *Age older than 50 years:* S. pneumoniae, Listeria, gram-negative bacilli, no meningococcus
- Meningitis requires hospitalization and treatment with parenteral antibiotics.

RICKETTSIAL DISEASES. Systemic febrile syndrome has many causes. Rickettsial diseases include typhus, Rocky Mountain spotted fever (RMSF), ehrlichiosis, and Q fever. Only Lyme disease and Rocky Mountain spotted fever are discussed here.

Lyme Disease. Lyme disease is caused by the spirochete *Borrelia burgdorferi* and is transmitted to humans by ticks. The tick must feed for 24 hours or longer in order to transmit the disease. Shortly after the bite occurs, the patient may experience erythema migrans and central nervous system and musculoskeletal symptoms. Confirm the diagnosis by serologic testing.

Rocky Mountain Spotted Fever. RMSF is caused by *Rickettsia rickettsii* and is transmitted by the bite of wood and dog ticks. It occurs most commonly in the middle and southern Atlantic states and in the central Mississippi valley. Symptoms include an influenza-like prodrome, followed by fever, chills, headache, myalgias, and restlessness. A red macular rash appears on the wrists and ankles and spreads centrally. It appears between the second and sixth days of the fever. Onset occurs 2 to 14 days after the tick bite.

How to Monitor
- Check culture to make sure growth is susceptible to the antibiotic chosen.
- Resolution of infection varies with severity of illness, but the patient's condition should start to improve in 2 to 3 days. Continued elevation of the patient's temperature may indicate lack of efficacy or drug fever.

- Consider monitoring the WBC count in a moderately ill patient.

Patient Variables

GERIATRICS. Geriatric patients are at considerably increased risk of infection, and their infections often are more serious than those in younger patients. Because of their low body mass, elderly patients may need a lower dose. They are particularly susceptible to the toxic effects of aminoglycosides.

PEDIATRICS. Infants are at increased risk for infection until their immune system is more mature. They are also at greater risk for toxicity until their renal and hepatic function is adequate. Tetracyclines bind to teeth, and this is a big concern during pregnancy; discolored tooth enamel may develop if tetracycline is given when the teeth are developing and can result in retardation of bone growth. Fluoroquinolones affect growth of cartilage in developing bone.

Use caution to ensure that an overweight child does not receive an overdose of antibiotics.

Children younger than 12 years of age usually need more frequent dosing with shorter dosing intervals because of increased metabolism and faster clearance.

PREGNANCY AND LACTATION. Many antibiotics are contraindicated in pregnancy. Pregnancy does affect the pharmacokinetics of antibiotics. Most antibiotics are passed into the breast milk. Again, the use of tetracyclines would be an issue during pregnancy or lactation because of the damage that they cause to the child's teeth.

GENDER. Certain antibiotics interact with oral contraceptive pills. Use an alternative method of contraception. Rifampin is the most frequent cause. Tetracycline and penicillins also have been implicated. Use extra caution in patients on low-dose contraceptives. This interaction is due to alteration of the normal first-pass mechanism seen with OCP therapy.

Women are at risk for vaginal yeast infection when treated with an antibiotic. If this is a frequent problem, the patient may use an OTC vaginal antifungal cream concomitantly.

Patient Education

- Take all of the medication even if the condition improves.
- Call the provider if no improvement is seen within 2 to 3 days.
- Warn the patient of the most common side effects of the specific antibiotic. Caution patients about adverse effects such as vaginal yeast infection and C. *difficile* infection–induced diarrheal illness.
- Stop the medication if an allergic reaction occurs, and notify the provider.
- Most antibiotics should be taken on an empty stomach with a full glass of water, 1 hour before or 2 hours after eating.
- Lemon yogurt, other citrus flavors, or chocolate masks the bitter flavor of many medications. Gum can be used to mask the aftertaste.
- Certain antibiotics may interfere with the effectiveness of oral contraceptives. Use an alternative method of contraception during the month in which antibiotics are taken.
- Be specific about when the patient should take the medication. Evenly spaced dose intake should be emphasized to maintain therapeutic blood levels.

- Antibiotics should never be shared with others or kept and taken for another occasion of illness.
- Daily ingestion of yogurt with active cultures or acidophilus may help prevent some of the diarrheal effects of certain antibiotics and may decrease overgrowth of yeast infections.
- Report to the provider if the patient is not getting better within a few days of administration of the antibiotic.
- Report any rash, fever, or chills, or any other sensitivity to the drug.

SPECIFIC DRUGS

clindamycin phosphate (Cleocin)

INDICATIONS. Reserve this drug for cases of serious infection, when less toxic antimicrobial agents are inappropriate. Used for serious infections caused by susceptible strains of streptococci, pneumococci, and staphylococci. This drug also has great utility in anaerobic infections.

In primary care, clindamycin is combined with tretinoin gel formulations and is used in the topical treatment of noninflammatory and inflammatory lesions of acne vulgaris. The addition of clindamycin to tretinoin enhances the comedolytic efficacy of tretinoin in moderate to severe acne of the face, maintaining at the same time its antiinflammatory efficacy, thus accelerating resolution of all types of acne lesions without affecting the safety of response to both components.

CONTRAINDICATIONS. Hypersensitivity; previous pseudomembranous colitis; regional enteritis, ulcerative colitis

WARNINGS
- Can cause severe and possibly fatal colitis. Symptoms include severe persistent diarrhea, severe abdominal cramps, and passage of blood and mucus. May be aggravated by antiperistaltic agents
- Reserve for serious infections for which less toxic antimicrobial agents are inappropriate.
- *Hypersensitivity reactions:* Use with caution in patients with a history of asthma or significant allergies.
- *Hepatic function impairment:* Use with caution in patients with severe hepatic disease. Dose adjustment is recommended.

PRECAUTIONS
- Monitor liver/kidney function, blood counts with prolonged therapy.
- Use caution in patients with GI disease, particularly colitis.
- Superinfection is a risk.

PATIENT VARIABLES

Geriatrics. Older patients may not tolerate the diarrhea; monitor carefully.

Pediatrics. Use with caution.

Pregnancy and Lactation. *Category B:* Safety has not been established; appears in breast milk. The American Academy of Pediatrics considers clindamycin to be compatible with breastfeeding.

MECHANISM OF ACTION. Clindamycin binds exclusively to the 50S subunit of bacterial ribosomes and suppresses protein synthesis.

ADVERSE EFFECTS
- *Cardiovascular:* Hypotension
- *GI:* Diarrhea (2% to 20%), pseudomembranous colitis (0.01% to 10%), nausea, vomiting, abdominal pain, esophagitis, glossitis, stomatitis
- *Hematologic:* Neutropenia, leukopenia, agranulocytosis, thrombocytopenic purpura, aplastic anemia
- *Hepatic:* Increased transaminases
- *Renal:* Dysfunction characterized by azotemia, oliguria, and proteinuria
- *Dermatologic:* >10%: Dryness, burning, itching, scaliness, erythema, or peeling of skin (lotion, solution); oiliness (gel, lotion)

DOSAGE AND ADMINISTRATION
- May be taken without regard for meals
- Take each dose with a full glass of water.

vancomycin (Vancocin)

INDICATIONS. Vancomycin IV is used most often in serious or life-threatening staphylococcal or streptococcal infections. The colonization of vancomycin-resistant enterococci has substantially increased. Many hospitals are now restricting use of the drug unless prescribed under strict guidelines and approved by a pharmacist.

The primary care use of vancomycin is for pseudomembranous colitis caused by C. *difficile.* It is given in oral form when treatment with metronidazole is contraindicated or ineffective. Metronidazole is preferred because of the high cost of vancomycin and the increase in incidence of vancomycin-resistant enterococcal infections when it is used. However, vancomycin remains the drug of choice for severe cases of C. *difficile.*

WARNINGS
- Ototoxicity has occurred; may be permanent.
- Hypotension, reversible neutropenia, nephrotoxicity, and renal failure are among the warnings. Must be monitored closely.
- The "red man" syndrome may be stimulated by too rapid IV infusion. It is not an allergic reaction. It is characterized by a sudden and profound fall in blood pressure with or without a maculopapular rash over the face, neck, upper chest, and extremities.

MECHANISM OF ACTION. It works by preventing synthesis of the bacterial cell wall by blocking peptidoglycan strand formation.

ADVERSE EFFECTS. Anaphylaxis, drug fever, nausea

DOSAGE AND ADMINISTRATION
- Give 500 mg to 2 g/day po in three or four divided doses for 7 to 10 days.
- Alternatively, give 125 mg po three or four times daily for 7 to 10 days.

nitrofurantoin (Macrobid, Macrodontic, generic)

INDICATIONS. Used in treating UTIs caused by susceptible strains of *E. coli,* enterococci, and *S. aureus* and by some strains of *Klebsiella* and *Enterobacter* spp. Least expensive antibiotic

CONTRAINDICATIONS
- Renal function impairment (CrCl <60 ml/min)
- Pregnancy (term; 38 to 42 weeks)

WARNINGS/PRECAUTIONS
- Pulmonary reactions may be seen with acute, sudden onset of dyspnea, chest pain, cough, fever, and chills. Chronic pulmonary reactions may be associated with prolonged therapy.
- Hemolytic anemia may be induced.
- Hepatic reactions, including hepatitis and cholestatic jaundice, occur rarely with fatalities.

PATIENT VARIABLES
Pediatrics. Contraindicated in infants younger than 1 month of age
Pregnancy and Lactation. *Category B:* Product is excreted in milk.

ADVERSE EFFECTS
- Peripheral neuropathy may occur and may be severe or irreversible.
- Superinfection may occur.
- The most common problems are anorexia, nausea, and emesis.

DRUG INTERACTIONS
- Anticholinergics increase nitrofurantoin bioavailability.
- Magnesium salts decrease absorption of nitrofurantoin.
- Uricosurics such as probenecid increase serum levels of nitrofurantoin.

PATIENT EDUCATION
- May cause GI upset; take with food or milk
- May cause brown discoloration of the urine
- Notify health care provider if patient experiences fever, chills, cough, chest pain, difficulty breathing, skin rash, or numbness or tingling of the fingers or toes, or if intolerable GI upset occurs.

DOSAGE AND ADMINISTRATION
- *Adult:* 50 to 100 mg qid for 7 to 10 days
- *Children:* 5 to 7 mg/kg/day divided every 6 hours

fosfomycin (Monurol)

INDICATIONS. Used in treatment of UTIs in women

PATIENT VARIABLES
Pediatrics. Contraindicated in children
Pregnancy. Category B
Lactation. Concurrent use not recommended

ADVERSE EFFECTS. Main adverse effects are diarrhea, nausea, dyspepsia, vaginitis, headache, dizziness, and asthenia.

DRUG INTERACTIONS. Serum level may be lowered by drugs that enhance GI motility.

DOSAGE AND ADMINISTRATION. Mix 3 g packet with 4 oz cold water and drink immediately. Give one dose per episode of UTI.

evolve A continually updated list of useful WebLinks may be found in the Evolve Resources at http://evolve.elsevier.com/Edmunds/NP/

58 Penicillins

DRUG OVERVIEW

Class	Subclass	Generic Name	Trade Name
Natural penicillins		penicillin G	Bicillin (IM)
		penicillin V ✳	Veetids, Pen-Vee K generic 🔑
Aminopenicillins	Second generation (activity against gram-negative bacilli)	ampicillin	Principen, generic
		amoxicillin ✳	Amoxil ✳, Trimox, generic
		amoxicillin and potassium clavulanate (AM/CL) ✳	Augmentin ✳
		ampicillin/sulbactam	Unasyn
Penicillinase-resistant penicillins	Antistaphylococcal penicillins (active against penicillinase-producing staphylococci)	dicloxacillin nafcillin oxacillin	Dynapen, Dicloxacil Unipen, Nafcil (IV) Prostaphlin, (IM<IV)
Carboxypenicillins	Third generation (anti-pseudomonal penicillin)	ticarcillin ticarcillin/potassium clavulanate	Ticar (IV) Timentin (IV)
Ureidopenicillins	Fourth generation (anti-pseudomonal penicillin)	piperacillin piperacillin sodium and tazobactam sodium	Pipracil (IM<IV) Zosyn (IV)

✳,Top 200 drug; 🔑, key drug.

INDICATIONS

See Table 58-1 for specific indications.
- Otitis media
- Streptococcal pharyngitis
- Sinusitis
- Pneumococcal pneumonia
- Urinary tract infection in pregnancy
- Animal bite
- Impetigo
- Syphilis
- Gonorrhea

Sir Alexander Fleming, a British scientist, discovered penicillin in 1928, and the medicine has been available since the 1940s. Since that time, penicillins have remained an extremely important class of antibiotics for treating most gram-positive bacteria; some penicillins can treat gram-negative bacteria. Penicillins are considered the safest antibiotics. Important penicillins for the primary care provider include penicillin VK, amoxicillin, amoxicillin/clavulanate, and dicloxacillin. These generally are indicated in the treatment of mild to moderately severe infections caused by penicillin-sensitive microorganisms.

They are used extensively for empirical therapy and for treatment determined by culture. Different penicillins exhibit different antimicrobial activity. This chapter focuses on the outpatient use of oral penicillins. Nafcillin is available as IV treatment only and is not discussed further. The carboxypenicillins and the ureidopenicillins are active against a large number of infectious diseases. These generally are given IV in a hospital setting and are not discussed further. Other β-lactam drugs, the carbapenems (ertapenem, imipenem, and meropenem), are similar in chemical structure to the penicillins. These drugs are used in hospitals and are given IM or IV for severe infections; these also will not be discussed further.

THERAPEUTIC OVERVIEW

Allergy

Before prescribing any penicillin, check for drug allergy. The incidence of penicillin allergy is unknown but is probably between 5% and 10%. Life-threatening anaphylaxis is estimated at 0.01% to 0.05%. A patient's report of penicillin allergy correlates poorly with a positive skin test. A patient with a negative skin test has a very low probability of an allergic reaction to penicillin. Among patients with a positive skin test for penicillin, less than 5% will have an immediate

TABLE 58-1 **Penicillin Indications With Dosage and Administration Recommendations**

Drug	Bacteria	Site/Disease	Dosage (oral)
penicillin G benzathine (IM only)	Group A streptococcus	Tonsil, URI, skin, soft tissue	*Adult:* 1.2 million units as a single dose *Child (<60 lb):* 300,000-600,000 units as a single dose
	T. pallidum	Syphilis (venereal and congenital; not indicated as a single dose for neurosyphilis but can be given weekly × 3 weeks following IV treatment)	*Adult, child >12 years:* 2.4 million units as a single dose *Child <2 years old:* 50,000 units/kg as a single dose
penicillin V	*Streptococcus*	URI, scarlet fever, erysipelas	*Adult and child >12 years:* 125-250 mg q6-8h × 10 days
	Streptococcus	Pharyngitis in children	*Child <12 years old:* 25-50 mg/kg/day divided q6h × 10 days
	Pneumococcus	URI, otitis media	250-500 mg q6-8h until afebrile × 2 days minimum
	Staphylococcus	Skin and soft tissue	250-500 mg q6-8h
	Group A streptococcus	Prevention of recurrence following rheumatic fever	250 mg bid continuous
dicloxacillin	Penicillinase-resistant *Staphylococcus*	Mild to moderate infection	*Adult:* 125 mg q6h *Child:* 12.5 mg/kg/day in divided doses q6h
		Severe infection	*Adult:* 125-500 mg q6h *Child:* 25 mg/kg/day divided doses q6h
oxacillin	Penicillinase-resistant *Staphylococcus*	Mild infection	*Adult:* 500 mg q4-6h *Child <40 kg:* 50 mg/kg/day in divided doses q6h
		Severe infection (following parenteral therapy)	*Adult:* 1 g q4-6h *Child <40 kg:* 100 mg/kg/day in divided doses q4-6h
ampicillin	*H. influenzae, Staphylococcus, S. pneumoniae,* spp. *Shigella, E. coli, Salmonella, P. mirabilis,* enterococci *N. gonorrhoeae*	URI, soft tissue GI, GU infections	*≤20 kg:* 50 mg/kg/day in divided doses q6-8h *>20 kg:* 250 mg q6h *Adult, child >20 kg:* 500 mg q6h *Child ≤20 kg:* 100 mg/kg/day q6h 3.5 g as a single dose plus 1 g probenecid
amoxicillin	ENT: *Streptococcus* α- and β-hemolytic, *S. pneumoniae, Staphylococcus* spp, *H. influenzae*	Mild/moderate Severe	*Adult, child >40 kg:* 500 mg q12h or 250 mg q8h *Child >3 mo and <40 kg:* 25 mg/kg/day in divided doses q12h or 20 mg/kg/day in divided doses q8h 875 mg q12h or 500 mg q8h 45 mg/kg/day in divided doses q12h or 40 mg/kg/day in divided doses q8h
	Skin: *Streptococcus* spp, α- and β-hemolytic, *Staphylococcus* spp, *E. coli*	Mild/moderate Severe	500 mg q12h or 250 mg q8h 25 mg/kg/day in divided doses q12h or 20 mg/kg/day in divided doses q8h *Adult, child >40 kg:* 875 mg q12h or 500 mg q8h *Child >3 mo and <40 kg:* 45 mg/kg/day in divided doses q12h or 40 mg/kg/day in divided doses q8h
	GU tract: *E. coli, P. mirabilis, Enterococcus faecalis*	Mild/moderate	*Adult:* 500 mg q12h or 250 mg q8h *Child:* 25 mg/kg/day in divided doses q12h or 20 mg/kg/day in divided doses q8h *Severe, Adult, child >40 kg:* 875 mg q12h or 500 mg q8h *Severe, Child:* 45 mg/kg/day in divided doses q12h or 40 mg/kg/day in divided doses q8h
	Streptococcus spp, α- and β-hemolytic, *S. pneumococcus, Staphylococcus* spp, *H. influenzae*	Lower respiratory tract (mild/moderate/severe)	*Adult:* 875 mg q12h or 500 mg q8h *Child >3 mo and <40 kg:* 45 mg/kg/day in divided doses q12h or 40 mg/kg/day in divided doses q8h
	N. gonorrhoeae	Gonorrhea	*Adult:* 3 g as single oral dose *Prepubertal children >2 yr:* 50 mg/kg with probenecid 25 mg/kg as single dose

TABLE 58-1   Penicillin Indications With Dosage and Administration Recommendations (Continued)

Drug	Bacteria	Site/Disease	Dosage (oral)
amoxicillin and potassium clavulanate	H. influenzae, M. catarrhalis	Otitis media, sinusitis	*Adult, child >40 kg:* 500 mg q12h or 250 mg q8h *Child <3 mo:* 30 mg/kg/day divided q12h (duration otitis media 10 days) *Child >3 mo:* 200 mg/5 ml suspension: 25 mg/kg/day divided q8h; 125 mg/5 ml suspension: 20 mg/kg/day divided q8h
	H. influenzae, M. catarrhalis	Severe infection, lower respiratory tract	*Adult:* 875 mg q12h or 500 mg q8h *Child >3 mo:* 200 mg/5 ml suspension: 45 mg/kg/day divided q8h; 125 mg/5 ml suspension: 40 mg/kg/day divided q8h
Augmentin XR	H. influenzae, M. catarrhalis, H. parainfluenzae, K. pneumoniae or methicillin-susceptible S. aureus, S. pneumoniae	Pneumonia, sinusitis	4000/250 mg/day given as two tablets q12h × 10 days; sinusitis, × 7 to 10 days for pneumonia

reaction to a cephalosporin. Current recommendations are that if a penicillin skin test is positive, the patient should avoid β-lactam antimicrobials or should be considered for penicillin or cephalosporin desensitization. Cross reactivity to carbapenems is also possible; therefore, a carbapenem may not be a reasonable choice for penicillin-allergic patients.

Resistance

Microbial resistance to the penicillins, now common, has become a major limitation to their use. Resistance of bacteria to penicillins and other β-lactam antibiotics occurs through three mechanisms. The most important mechanism involves bacteria-producing β-lactamase, which breaks down the β-lactam ring and renders the penicillin inactive. *Staphylococcus aureus* is one of the most important of these organisms. Methicillin-resistant *Staphylococcus aureus* (MRSA) is now resistant to most antibiotics and is very difficult to treat. Methicillin is no longer marketed in the United States because of resistance and toxicity. Inhibitors of the β-lactamases such as clavulanic acid, sulbactam, and tazobactam often are used in combination with certain penicillins, to prevent their inactivation.

The second mechanism of resistance is diminished permeability of the drug through the bacterial outer cell membrane. The antibiotic is unable to penetrate the cell wall, especially of gram-negative bacteria. The last mechanism involves decreased binding of the drug at its target sites on the inner bacterial membrane.

MECHANISM OF ACTION

Penicillin is a derivative of 6-aminopenicillanic acid that is composed of a distinct four-membered β-lactam ring fused to a five-membered thiazolidine ring; this constitutes the chemical structure. Penicillin subclasses have additional chemical constituents that bestow differences in antimicrobial activity, susceptibility to acid, enzyme hydrolysis, and biodisposition. Many biosynthetic types of penicillin have been created through the introduction of diverse acids, amines, or amides into developing penicillin molds, to render products superior to the natural penicillins.

Penicillins, which are bactericidal against susceptible organisms, disrupt synthesis of the bacterial cell wall and compete for and bind to specific enzyme proteins that catalyze transpeptidation and cross-linking. The enzymes to which they bind are called penicillin-binding proteins (PBPs). They consist of transpeptidases, transglycosylases, and D-alanine carboxykinases and are implicated in the final phases of building and reshaping of the bacterial cell wall while it is growing and dividing. This action interferes with the biosynthesis of mucopeptides and prevents linkage of structural components of the cell wall. After the penicillin molecules bind and inhibit the transpeptidase enzymes, susceptible bacteria are no longer able to lay protein cross-links across the peptidoglycan backbone of the cell wall. In addition to being structurally weak, this formation is thought to catalyze the activation of autolytic enzymes in the cell wall that cause progressive bacterial lysis.

TREATMENT PRINCIPLES

- Oral penicillins generally are indicated for the treatment of mild to moderately severe infection caused by penicillin-sensitive microorganisms. These broad-spectrum antibiotics are used as empirical treatment for many infections, according to the site of infection, in some cases while the results of a culture are awaited.
- All penicillins, with the exception of amoxicillin, are absorbed better when taken on an empty stomach.
- Many penicillins, including penicillin G (IM), penicillin V, cloxacillin, dicloxacillin, amoxicillin, and amoxicillin and potassium clavulanate (AM/CL), are indicated as first-choice empirical treatment for many infections, including skin infections, animal bites, otitis media, sinusitis, pharyngitis, acute exacerbation of COPD, syphilis, mastitis, and Lyme disease (see Table 58-1). Penicillin V remains the drug of choice for group A β-hemolytic streptococcus. Penicillin G remains the drug of choice for syphilis.
- A minimum of 10 days of treatment is recommended for any infection caused by group A β-hemolytic streptococci, to prevent the occurrence of acute rheumatic fever or acute glomerulonephritis. In severe staphylococcal infection, continue therapy with penicillinase-resistant penicillins for at least 14 days.
- The natural penicillins are generally active against non–penicillinase-producing staphylococci and streptococci and most gram-positive organisms. They also are active against some gram-negative cocci such as *Neisseria* and against most anaerobic bacteria. Natural penicillins, if the bacteria are not resistant, are more effective against gram-positive bacteria

than are semisynthetic penicillins. Penicillin V (oral) can be used instead of penicillin V (IM, IV), except against gram-negative species such as penicillinase-producing *Neisseria gonorrhoeae* and *Haemophilus*.

- The aminopenicillins are active against all of the bacteria that penicillin G is active against, along with non–penicillinase-producing staphylococci, some streptococci, and some gram-negative cocci and enterococci. The addition of a β-lactamase inhibitor product to the treatment regimen expands the spectrum to include greater numbers of gram-positive and gram-negative bacteria and anaerobes. The combination of amoxicillin and clavulanate is commonly used intravenously and increases the spectrum of amoxicillin effectiveness to cover *S. aureus*, *Moraxella catarrhalis*, *Haemophilus influenzae*, *Salmonella*, and *Shigella*.
- Penicillinase-resistant penicillins are used for the treatment of infections caused by penicillinase-producing staphylococci and some streptococci that have demonstrated susceptibility to the drug. They may be used to initiate therapy in suspected cases of resistant staphylococcal infection prior to the availability of susceptibility test results. Do not use in infections caused by organisms susceptible to penicillin G.
- The carboxypenicillins are less active than the ureidopenicillins against streptococci and *Haemophilus* spp.
- The ureidopenicillins have increased the activity of penicillin against gram-negative and anaerobic bacteria, including *Pseudomonas*. Together, the third- and fourth-generation agents are known as the antipseudomonal penicillins.
- Extended-spectrum penicillins are effective in treating *Pseudomonas aeruginosa*; this is commonly seen in patients with cystic fibrosis.

How to Monitor

- Monitoring is particularly important in newborns and infants, and when high dosages are used.
- Perform bacteriologic studies to identify causative organisms and to determine their susceptibility, so that appropriate therapy is administered.
- Monitor for resolution of the infection and for resistance, especially to community-acquired MRSA.
- *Clostridium difficile* infection of the bowel may develop.
- Penicillin G potassium can cause hyperkalemia.
- *Penicillin G with procaine:* Monitor for sensitivity to procaine.
- *Penicillinase-resistant penicillins:* Obtain blood cultures, WBC, and differential cell counts prior to initiation and at least weekly during therapy with penicillinase-resistant penicillins. Measure liver transaminase AST and ALT levels during therapy to monitor for liver function abnormalities. Perform periodic urinalysis, BUN, and creatinine determinations during therapy, and consider dosage alterations if these values become elevated. If renal impairment is known or suspected, reduce the total dosage and monitor blood levels to avoid possible neurotoxic reactions.
- When administering penicillin parenterally, the practitioner should monitor the patient for at least 30 minutes post-administration to rule out any allergic or anaphylactic reaction to the drug.

- Avoid subcutaneous and fat layer injections; pain and induration may occur.
- Inadvertent intravascular administration of IM injections has resulted in severe neurovascular damage. Damage has occurred after injections into the buttock, thigh, and deltoid areas. These reactions occur most frequently in infants and small children.
- Some products contain tartrazine and sulfites.

Patient Variables

GERIATRICS. Oral penicillins generally are well tolerated. Ask specifically about a penicillin allergy because the patient may have difficulty remembering old allergies. The high sodium content of certain parenteral penicillins such as carbenicillin disodium and ticarcillin disodium may pose a danger for patients with cardiac and renal conditions.

PEDIATRICS. For infants younger than 3 months old, investigate the history of penicillin allergy in the mother. Pediatric renal tubular function appears to mature more slowly than the glomerular filtration rate and reaches adult levels at approximately 7½ to 8 months of age. Penicillins are secreted by the renal tubules; therefore, clearance is reduced at birth but appears to increase swiftly during the first year of the child's life.

The safety and efficacy of carbenicillin, piperacillin, and the β-lactamase inhibitor/penicillin combinations have not been established in infants and children younger than 12 years old.

PREGNANCY AND LACTATION. *Category B:* No adequate studies. Use during pregnancy only if clearly needed. Penicillin crosses the placenta and is excreted in breast milk; it may cause diarrhea, candidiasis, or allergic response in the nursing infant. Use of ampicillin by nursing mothers may lead to sensitization of infants.

GENDER. Women who are taking ampicillin, bacampicillin, and penicillin V should be educated to use an alternative method of contraception if they are using estrogen-containing contraceptives because OCP effectiveness is believed to be compromised during antibiotic usage.

Patient Education

Patients should take medication on an empty stomach 1 hour before or 2 hours after meals, with a full glass of water. Penicillin V may be given with meals, although drug levels may be higher when given on an empty stomach. Ampicillin should be given on an empty stomach to enhance absorption. Amoxicillin may be given without regard for meals. AM/CL is best given with a meal to minimize GI upset.

Patients should notify the health care provider if skin rash, itching, hives, severe diarrhea, shortness of breath, urticaria, black tongue, sore throat, nausea, vomiting, fever, swollen joints, or any unusual bleeding or bruising occurs.

Those patients with penicillin allergies or hypersensitivity should be urged to wear some type of emergency identification, to inform others of their allergy.

Patients or family members should report any symptoms that suggest a developing allergic reaction. Intradermal skin tests may detect previous drug sensitivity.

Store tablets at 15° to 30° C (59° to 86° F). Reconstituted solutions remain stable for 14 days when refrigerated.

SPECIFIC DRUGS

Penicillin VK 🔑

All penicillins share the following characteristics, except as noted.

CONTRAINDICATIONS
- History of hypersensitivity to penicillins, cephalosporins, or imipenem
- Severe infection with an oral penicillin during the acute stage
- AM/CL: History of AM/CL-associated cholestatic jaundice or hepatic dysfunction

WARNINGS. Hypersensitivity reactions often are serious and occasionally fatal. The incidence of anaphylactic shock is between 0.015% and 0.04%. Accelerated reactions (urticaria and laryngeal edema) and delayed reactions (serum sickness) also may occur. These are more likely in patients with a history of atopic conditions. Hypersensitivity myocarditis may occur at any time. Initial symptoms include rash, fever, and eosinophilia.

An urticarial rash (nonallergic) occasionally occurs with ampicillin. This is common in patients with mononucleosis.

A risk of cross-sensitivity of penicillins with cephalosporins has been noted. Estimated incidence is between 3% and 5%. Skin testing and desensitization are available. Desensitization is used most often in the treatment of syphilis.

Treatment of allergy includes antihistamines and, if necessary, corticosteroids and epinephrine. Anaphylaxis requires emergency measures.

The dosage of penicillin G should be reduced in patients with severe renal impairment; additional modifications are needed when hepatic disease accompanies the renal impairment.

PRECAUTIONS
- Patients who receive continuous prophylaxis for various reasons may harbor increased numbers of penicillin-resistant organisms.
- Probenecid increases serum concentrations of penicillin.
- Patients with cystic fibrosis have a higher incidence of side effects.
- With streptococcal infection, therapy must be sufficient to eliminate the organism within 7 to 10 days, to prevent sequelae (endocarditis, rheumatic fever).
- Resistance may occur.
- Pseudomembranous colitis has been reported.
- Superinfection may result.
- Some products contain tartrazine or sulfites that also may provoke hypersensitivity reactions.
- Other products contain aspartame, which is contraindicated in patients with PKU.

PHARMACOKINETICS. See Table 58-2. Absorption is variable. Penicillins are widely distributed into body fluids and into the pleural and pericardial cavities; they are passed into joints, into bile, to the placenta, and to breast milk. Adequate penicillin levels are attainable in the cerebrospinal fluid when the meninges are inflamed.

Oral penicillins reach peak concentrations about 1 to 2 hours after ingestion. They are well distributed to most tissues, including lung, liver, muscle, bone, placenta, abscess, middle ear, pleura, peritoneum, and synovium. They are not lipid soluble and do not cross the blood-brain barrier well.

Most penicillin products undergo rapid renal elimination; approximately 85% to 90% are excreted by tubular secretion. The half-life of penicillin in serum varies from approximately 0.4 to 1.3 hours and can last as long as 20 hours in the anuric patient. Nafcillin, oxacillin, cloxacillin, and dicloxacillin levels usually do not increase in anuric patients because compensation is increased for diminished urinary elimination by hepatic metabolism or biliary excretion. The amount of penicillin excreted by the liver is minimal except for nafcillin and oxacillin.

ADVERSE EFFECTS

Hypersensitivity occurs in about 5% to 10% of patients receiving penicillins, depending on the type of preparation and the route of administration. The risk of anaphylaxis is approximately 0.05%. The frequency of reaction is least when the penicillin is given orally (po), is somewhat higher with IV administration, and is distinctly higher when it is combined with procaine and is administered IM.

Table 58-3 lists important adverse reactions by body system. Elevated levels of BUN and creatinine occur very rarely, and photosensitivity does not occur with penicillins.

DRUG INTERACTIONS. The penicillins interact with many other drugs. Table 58-4 lists major drug interactions.

OVERDOSAGE. Symptoms include neuromuscular hyperexcitability, convulsions, agitation, and confusion.

DOSAGE AND ADMINISTRATION
- Dosage and administration recommendations vary according to the age of the patient. Table 58-1 provides general recommendations. Dosage and administration must be adjusted according to individual conditions.
- Because penicillin absorption is affected by food, these agents should be taken on an empty stomach. However, penicillin V, amoxicillin, bacampicillin, and AM/CL can be given without regard for meals.

OTHER DRUGS IN CLASS

Other drugs in this class are similar to the key drug except as follows:

NATURAL PENICILLINS
- *Penicillin G (Crysticillin AS)* is the only parenteral penicillin in common use in the outpatient setting.
- *Penicillin V (Veetids, Pen-Vee K)*, despite increasing resistance, remains an important medication. *Unlabeled uses:* prophylactic treatment of children with sickle cell anemia; anaerobic infection

TABLE 58-2 Pharmacokinetics of Penicillin

Drug	Absorption	Onset of Action	Time to Peak Concentration	Half-life	Protein Bound	Metabolism	Excretion
penicillin G (IM benzathine salt)	20% decreased with food	po, 0.5-1 hr IM, 15-30 min	po, 30-60 min IM, 30 min	0.5 hr	55%	20%	Renal
penicillin V	60%	0.5-1 hr	0.5-1 hr	1 hr	80%	55%	Renal
amoxicillin	75% not decreased with food	2 hr	1-2 hr	1.7 hr	20%	10%	Renal, 86%
ampicillin	40% decreased with food	1.5-2 hr	1.5-2 hr	1 hr	20%	10%	Renal, 60%
dicloxacillin	50% to 85% decreased with food	0.5-1 hr	0.5-1.5 hr	0.8 hr	98%	Liver, 10%	Renal
nafcillin	erratic, decreased with food	1-2 hr	1-2 hr	0.5 hr	90%	Liver	Renal/bile
oxacillin	30%	0.5-1 hr	0.5-1 hr	0.4 hr	94%	Liver, 45%	Renal/bile

TABLE 58-3 Adverse Effects of Penicillin

Body System	Common Minor Effects	Serious Adverse Reactions
Skin, appendages	Maculopapular and erythematous rashes, local pain at site of injection, ecchymosis, phlebitis	
Hypersensitivity	Urticaria, pruritus, fever	Serum sickness–like reactions with chills, fever, edema, arthralgia, prostration Serious and sometimes fatal anaphylaxis, and laryngeal edema, with fever, rash, joint swelling, myocarditis
GI	Anorexia, nausea, vomiting, diarrhea, epigastric distress, glossitis, hoarseness, black hairy tongue, abnormal taste, dry mouth	Entercolitis, pseudomembraneous colitis
Hematologic		Anemia, hemolytic anemia, thrombocytopenia, thrombocytopenic purpura, eosinophilia, leukopenia, granulocytopenia, reduction of hemoglobin or hematocrit, prolongation of bleeding and prothrombin time, decrease in WBC and lymphocyte counts, increase in lymphocytes, monocytes, basophils, and platelets
CNS	Dizziness, fatigue, insomnia, reversible hyperactivity and prolonged muscle relaxation, neuropathies, headache, anxiety, confusion, agitation, depression, lethargy	Transient myopathy, neurotoxicity, neuromuscular hyperirritability, hallucinations, convulsions and seizures
CV	Tachycardia, vasovagal reaction	Cardiac arrest, pulmonary emboli, syncope
Renal	Elevation of creatinine or BUN, vaginitis	Interstitial nephritis, neuropathy

TABLE 58-4 Drug Interactions With Penicillin

Penicillin	Drug Acted On
Penicillins ampicillin may reduce bioavailability	↓ Oral contraceptives atenolol
Drug	**Action on Penicillin**
β-Blockers	May potentiate anaphylactic reaction to penicillin
tetracycline	↓ penicillins
aspirin, sulfonamides, indomethacin, thiazides, furosemide	↑ penicillin G
probenecid	↑ penicillins renally excreted
allopurinol	↑ Rate of ampicillin-induced rash

evolve See Bonus tables on http://evolve.elsevier.com/Edmunds/NP/

AMINOPENICILLINS

- *Ampicillin (Principen)* and amoxicillin (*Amoxil, Trimox*) are commonly used. Amoxicillin has better absorption than ampicillin. Ampicillin produces a higher rate of adverse GI effects than the other penicillins
- *Amoxicillin (Amoxil, Trimox)* is the most commonly used penicillin; it has largely replaced ampicillin and is available in several formulations. The suspension, 250 mg/5 ml (1 bottle, 150 ml), is inexpensive and appropriate for children. It also is available in chewable tablets at 125 and 250 mg. The tablets are provided in many strengths.

• *Amoxicillin and potassium clavulanate (AM/CL) (Augmentin):* The 12-hour dosing regimen causes less diarrhea than is caused by amoxicillin alone. The 200 and 400 mg suspension and chewable tablets contain aspartame. AM/CL comes as 250, 500, and 875 mg amoxicillin and 125 mg clavulanic acid. This means that two 250 mg tablets are not equivalent to one 500 mg tablet (has more potassium clavulanate). AM/CL also is available in tablets, chewable tablets, and powder for oral suspension in different strengths. Augmentin XR comes as 1000 mg amoxicillin and 62.5 mg potassium clavulanate.

PENICILLINASE-RESISTANT PENICILLINS

• *dicloxacillin (Dynapen), oxacillin (Prostaphlin):* Dicloxacillin is the only drug in this category that is in common use.

evolve A continually updated list of useful WebLinks may be found in the Evolve Resources at http://evolve.elsevier.com/Edmunds/NP/

Cephalosporins

DRUG OVERVIEW

Class	Subclass	Generic Name	Trade Name
Cephalosporins	First generation	cephalexin 🗝 ☀	Keflex
		cefadroxil ☀	Duricef
	Second generation	cefprozil ☀	Cefzil
		cefaclor	Ceclor
		cefpodoxamine	Vantin
		cefuroxime	Ceftin
		loracarbef	Lorabid
	Third generation	cefixime	Suprax
		ceftibuten	Cedax
		ceftriaxone	Rocephin (IM, IV)
		cefdinir	Omnicef ☀
		cefditoren	Spectracef

☀, Top 200 drug; 🗝, key drug.

INDICATIONS

First-Generation Drugs

- Skin and soft tissue
- Urinary tract infection (UTI)

Second- and Third-Generation Drugs

- Otitis media
- Gonorrhea
- Acute bronchitis or pneumonia in patients with COPD
- Pneumonia, community-acquired
- Pharyngitis
- Sinusitis
- Lyme disease

Cephalosporins comprise a large category of antimicrobials with a wide spectrum of activity that are superior to penicillin (Table 59-1). The generations are loosely based on antimicrobial spectrum of activity. This chapter discusses the most common oral cephalosporins with one exception, ceftriaxone, which can be given IM in the primary care setting. Many first-, second-, third-, and fourth-generation cephalosporins are used IM or IV for serious infections and are not discussed. The primary care provider should be familiar with one oral cephalosporin from each generation. The most widely used cephalosporins for the primary care provider

consist of cephalexin (Keflex), cefprozil (Cefzil), cefuroxime (Ceftin), and ceftriaxone (Rocephin).

The cephalosporins represent the most commonly used antibiotic class because of their broad spectrum, ease of administration, safety and efficacy, and favorable pharmacokinetic profile with minimal side effects. All cephalosporins are active against most gram-positive cocci, such as *Staphylococcus aureus*, and many strains of gram-negative bacilli, such as *Escherichia coli*. Cephalosporins are classified by "generation," with each successive generation boasting broader activity against gram-negative organisms, although at the expense of action against gram-positive organisms. The mold cephalosporin acremonium (now *Acremonium chrysogenum*) was discovered in sewage in Sardinia, Italy, in 1945. In 1964, the first cephalosporin, cephalothin, was marketed.

THERAPEUTIC OVERVIEW

Allergy

It is widely believed that many individuals with a true penicillin allergy may also be allergic to cephalosporins. However, less than 5% of patients with a positive skin test for penicillin will react to a cephalosporin. Evidence-based guidelines of the American Academy of Pediatrics endorse the use of cephalosporin antibiotics for pediatric patients with reported allergy to penicillin for sinusitis and otitis media.

TABLE 59-1   Cephalosporin Indications With Dosage and Administration

Drug	Bacteria	Site/Disease	Dosage
FIRST GENERATION			
cephalexin (Keflex)	GABHS, *S. pneumoniae*, staph, *H. influenzae*, *E. coli*, *Klebsiella*, *Proteus*	URI, UTI, skin	*Adult:* 250-500 mg q6h *Child:* 25-50 mg/kg/day in divided doses *Otitis media:* 75-100 mg/kg/day in 3 or 4 divided doses
cefadroxil (Duricef)	GABHS, *S. pneumoniae*, staph, *H. influenzae*	Pharyngitis, tonsillitis	*Adult:* 1 g/day in single or two divided doses × 10 days *Child:* 30 mg/kg/day in single or two divided doses × 10 days
	E. coli, *Klebsiella*, *Proteus*	UTI, skin	*Adult:* 1-2 g/day in single or two divided doses (2 g/day complicated UTI) *Child:* 30 mg/kg/day in single or two divided doses
SECOND GENERATION			
cefuroxime (Ceftin)	GABHS, staph	Pharyngitis, tonsillitis	*Adult:* 250 mg bid × 10 days *Child (3 mo-12 yr):* 20 mg/kg/day (maximum, 500 mg/day) divided bid × 10 days
	GABHS, *S. pneumoniae*, *H. influenzae*, *M. catarrhalis*	Otitis media, impetigo	*Child:* 30 mg/kg/day (maximum, 1 g/day) divided bid × 10 days
	S. pneumoniae, *H. influenzae*, *M. catarrhalis*; strep, staph	Acute exacerbation of COPD, skin, soft tissue	*Adult:* 250-500 mg bid × 10 days
	E. coli, *Klebsiella*, *Proteus*, *Morganella*, *Citrobacter*	UTI	*Adult:* 125-250 mg bid × 7 to 10 days
	N. gonorrhoeae	Gonorrhea	*Adult:* 1 g single dose
	B. burgdorferi	Early Lyme disease	*Adult:* 500 mg bid × 20 days
cefprozil (Cefzil)	GABHS	Pharyngitis, tonsillitis	*Adult (>13 yr):* 500 mg once daily × 10 days *Child (2-12 yr):* 7.5-15 mg/kg (maximum, 1 g/day) q12h × 10 days
	S. pneumoniae, *H. influenzae*, *M. catarrhalis*	Otitis media	*Child (>6 mo-12 yr):* 15 mg/kg q12h × 10 days
	Same	Sinusitis	*Adult:* 250-500 mg q12h × 10 days *Child:* 7.5-15 mg/kg q12h × 10 days
	Same	Exacerbation of COPD	*Adult:* 500 mg q12h × 10 days
	Strep, staph	Skin, soft tissue	*Adult:* 250-500 mg q12h × 10 days *Child (2-12 yr):* 20 mg/kg (maximum, 1 g) q24h × 10 days
cefaclor (Ceclor)	Strep, staph	Mild to moderate infection Acute exacerbation of COPD Pharyngitis, tonsillitis	*Adult:* 250-500 mg q8h *Adult:* 500 mg q12h × 7 days *Adult:* 375 mg (ER) q12h × 10 days *Child:* 20 mg-40 kg/day (maximum, 1 g/day) in divided doses q8h
cefpodoxime (Vantin)	*S. pneumoniae*, *H. influenzae*, *M. catarrhalis*, *S. pyogenes*	Pneumonia, bronchitis Pharyngitis, tonsillitis Skin Otitis media Pharyngitis/tonsillitis	*Adult:* 200 mg q12h × 14 days *Adult:* 100 mg q12h × 5 to 10 days *Adult:* 400 mg q12h × 7 to 14 days *Child (2 mo-12 yr):* 10 mg/kg/day (maximum, 400 mg/day) divided q12h × 5 days *Child (2 mo-12 yr):* 10 mg/kg/day (maximum, 200 mg/day) in two divided doses × 5-10 days
loracarbef (Lorabid)	*S. pyogenes*, *S. pneumoniae*, *H. influenzae*, *M. catarrhalis*	Pharyngitis/tonsillitis Sinusitis Lower respiratory tract	*Adult:* 200 mg q12h × 10 days *Adult:* 400 mg q12h × 10 days *Adult:* 400 mg q12h × 7-14 days
	Strep, staph	Skin	*Adult:* 200 mg q12h × 7 days
	Same	UTI	*Adult:* 200-400 mg q12h × 7 days
THIRD GENERATION			
cefixime (Suprax)	*H. influenzae*, *M. catarrhalis*, *S. pyogenes*	Otitis media, pharyngitis, tonsillitis, acute exacerbations of COPD	*Adult:* 400 mg/day as single dose or 200 mg bid × 10 days *Child (<50 kg or <12 yr):* 8 mg/kg/day suspension as single daily dose or a 4 mg/kg q12h × 10 days
ceftriaxone (Rocephin)	*S. pneumoniae*, *S. aureus*, *H. influenzae*, *H. parainfluenzae*, *K. pneumoniae*, *S. marcescens*, *E. coli*, *E. aerogenes*, *P. mirabilis*, *S. pyogenes*	Lower respiratory, skin and skin structure, UTI	*Adult:* 1-2 g once daily × 4-14 days IM *Child:* 50-75 mg/kg/day in divided doses q12h IM × 10-14 days
	N. gonorrhoeae	Gonorrhea	Single IM dose of 250 mg

Table continued on following page

TABLE 59-1 **Cephalosporin Indications With Dosage and Administration** (Continued)

Drug	Bacteria	Site/Disease	Dosage
cefdinir (Omnicef)	Same	Pharyngitis, tonsillitis, sinusitis	*Adult:* 300 mg q12h or 600 mg once daily × 10 days *Child (6 mo-12 yr):* 7 mg/kg q12h or 14 mg/kg once daily × 10 days (maximum, 600 mg/day)
		Acute exacerbation of COPD	*Adult:* 300 mg q12h or 600 mg once daily × 10 days
		Pneumonia, skin, soft tissue	*Adult:* 300 mg q12h × 10 days *Child (6 mo-12 yr):* 7 mg/kg q12h × 10 days (maximum, 600 mg/day)
		Otitis media	*Child (6 mo-12 yr):* 7 mg/kg q12h or 14 mg/kg once daily × 10 days (maximum, 600 mg/day)
cefditoren (Spectracef)	*S. pyogenes, S. aureus*	Pharyngitis, tonsillitis, skin, soft tissue	*Adult:* 200 mg bid × 10 days
	H. influenzae, H. parainfluenzae, S. pneumoniae, M. catarrhalis	Acute exacerbation of COPD, pneumonia	*Adult:* 400 mg bid × 10 days; pneumonia: 14 days

GABHS, Group A β-hemolytic *Streptococcus pyogenes.*

Resistance

The disadvantage of cephalosporins is that the broad-spectrum capacity of these drugs encourages rapid overgrowth of resistant bacteria, limiting their usefulness. Three general mechanisms of resistance have been identified for cephalosporins—the same ones as for penicillin. Again, the most common mechanism of resistance to cephalosporins is destruction by hydrolysis of the β-lactam ring by β-lactamase. Also important is the ability of the drug to penetrate the walls of the bacteria. If the drug can penetrate quickly, less of the drug is broken down by β-lactamase.

MECHANISM OF ACTION

The basic structure of the cephem nucleus includes a β-lactam ring fused to a six-member sulfur-containing dihydrothiazine ring. This is different from penicillins, which have a five-member thiazolidine ring.

Cephalosporins are β-lactam antibiotics that have the ability to resist bacterial enzymes, specifically, β-lactamase. They have a similar mechanism of action to that of penicillin and interfere with cell wall synthesis through inhibition of the synthesis of the bacterial peptidoglycan in the cell wall. The antibiotic binds to the enzymes that build/maintain the cell wall. This makes the cell wall osmotically unstable. Cephalosporins are bactericidal and usually are effective against rapidly growing organisms. Cephalosporins differ in terms of which enzymes they affect.

TREATMENT PRINCIPLES

Cephalosporins have a very wide spectrum of activity. They generally are useful for empirical treatment of many of the most common infections seen in primary care.

First-generation agents are the most active against gram-positive cocci, including β-lactamase–producing *S. aureus,* group A β-hemolytic streptococci (GABHS), and *Pneumococcus.* However, penicillin remains the drug of choice for treating GABHS pharyngitis. Cephalosporins have moderate activity against gram-negative bacilli, including *E. coli, Klebsiella,* and *Proteus mirabilis.* They are inactive against *Bacteroides fragilis, Citrobacter, Enterobacter, Pseudomonas, Serratia,* and all other *Proteus* spp. First-generation cephalosporins are not effective against *Neisseria, Haemophilus influenzae,* and *Moraxella catarrhalis.* Two first-generation cephalosporins available as oral products are commonly used. Cephalexin (Keflex) must be given every 6 hours, whereas cefadroxil (Duricef) may be dosed twice daily.

Second-generation cephalosporins continue to exhibit efficacy against gram-positive organisms, with the added advantage of increased gram-negative activity and β-lactamase stability. These drugs generally are active against some strains of *Acinetobacter, Citrobacter, Enterobacter, Klebsiella, Neisseria, Proteus, Providencia,* and *Serratia* spp. In addition, second-generation products have good activity against *E. coli.* They are effective against most strains of *M. catarrhalis* and *H. influenzae,* including those strains that produce β-lactamase. Many second-generation cephalosporins have been developed. The manufacturers suggest that second-generation cephalosporins may be appropriate for twice-daily dosing; however, an examination of their half-life suggests that this may not be appropriate (Table 59-2).

Third-generation cephalosporins have the broadest spectrum of activity of all the cephalosporins and are extremely effective against gram-negative organisms. The gram-positive activity, as a whole, is sharply reduced. Their activity against anaerobes varies with the agent. Third-generation drugs are more active against *E. coli, Klebsiella pneumoniae, P. mirabilis, Enterobacter, Serratia, Citrobacter, Morganella, Salmonella,* and *Shigella.* Some are active against *Pseudomonas aeruginosa.* This generation of antibiotics is able to achieve excellent penetration into blood and body fluids, including the cerebrospinal fluid. Because of their lack of toxicity, even at high doses, these antibiotics are an excellent alternative to aminoglycosides, which require therapeutic drug monitoring.

The third-generation cephalosporins cefixime (Suprax) and cefuroxime (Ceftin) are available in oral form. Although ceftriaxone (Rocephin) is available only in IM and IV forms, it is used in primary care as a once-daily IM injection. Ceftriaxone IM is used in outpatient settings as a one-time dose for the treatment of sexually transmitted diseases and sometimes as adjunct therapy in Lyme disease. When this agent is used for gonorrhea, the patient generally is also positive for *Chlamydia,* so a macrolide is prescribed concurrently.

Clinicians must be aware of the limitations of cephalosporin effectiveness. Cephalosporins do not exhibit activity against a

TABLE 59-2   Pharmacokinetics of Common Cephalosporins

Drug	Absorption	Time to Peak Concentration	Half-life	Protein Bound	Excretion
cephalexin (Keflex)	Well absorbed, 90%	1 hr	1 hr	14%	Urine
cefadroxil (Duricef)	Rapid	12 hr	1.5 hr	20%	Urine
cefuroxime (Ceftin)	Give IM, IV, or po; dosage forms not bioequivalent; absorption better after food	2-3 hr	1.3 hr	33%-50%	Urine; give with probenecid to slow clearance
cefprozil (Cefzil)	Well absorbed	1-2 hr	1.25 hr	36%	Urine
cefaclor (Ceclor)	With or without food	30-60 min	To 1 hr	25%	Urine
cefpodoxime (Vantin)	Slowed with food; use film-coated tablet	2-3 hr	2-3 hr	21%-29%	Urine
loracarbef (Lorabid)	Well absorbed	0.8-1.2 hr	1 hr	25%	Urine
cefixime (Suprax)	40% to 50% absorbed; reduced with food; oral suspension absorbed better than tablet	2-6 hr	3-4 hr	65%	Urine
ceftriaxone (Rocephin)	Given IM or IV	2-3 hr	6-8 hr	85%-95%	Urine
cefdinir (Omnicef)	With or without food	2-4 hr	1.7 hr	60%-70%	Urine
cefditoren (Spectracef)	Absorbed faster with high-fat meal	2-4 hr	1.5-3 hr	85%	Urine

number of common organisms, including penicillin-resistant *Pneumococcus*, methicillin-resistant *Staphylococcus aureus* (MRSA) and *Staphylococcus epidermidis*, *Enterococcus*, *Listeria*, *Mycoplasma*, clostridia, *Campylobacter*, *Chlamydia pneumoniae*, and *Chlamydia trachomatis*.

How to Monitor

These drugs have a wide safety margin and do not require routine monitoring of drug levels.

Treatment with antibacterial agents, such as ciprofloxacin (Cipro) and cefadroxil (Duricef), can alter the colon's normal flora, leading to overgrowth of *C. difficile* and subsequent release of toxins A and B that contribute to the development of CDAD, which may range in severity from mild diarrhea to fatal colitis. Because hypertoxin-producing strains of *C. difficile* can be refractory to antimicrobial therapy, they are associated with increased morbidity and mortality. The FDA advises that CDAD be considered in all patients who present with diarrhea after antibiotic use. Cases of CDAD have been reported more than 2 months after completion of an antimicrobial course of therapy. Current antibiotic therapy for the primary infection may need to be discontinued in patients with known or suspected CDAD.

Patient Variables

GERIATRICS. Products generally are safe and effective. Renally adjusted dosing based on creatinine clearance may be necessary.

PEDIATRICS. These products generally are safe and effective. In neonates, accumulation of cephalosporins has occurred. Each cephalosporin has a different age for established safety, ranging usually from 1 to 9 months. Cefaclor extended-release tables

and cefonicid, cefmetazole, cefoperazone, cephalexin, and cefotetan are not indicated for children.

PREGNANCY AND LACTATION. *Category B:* Cephalosporins appear safe for pregnant patients, but relatively few controlled studies have been conducted. Use only when potential benefits outweigh potential hazards to the fetus. These products cross the placenta and are excreted in breast milk.

Patient Education

- Take these products with food or milk to prevent GI upset.
- Notify the provider of any nausea, vomiting, or diarrhea that might develop.
- Notify the provider of any response that would suggest an allergic reaction.

SPECIFIC DRUGS

cephalexin (Keflex) 🔑

All cephalosporins share the following characteristics, except as noted.

CONTRAINDICATIONS. Hypersensitivity to any cephalosporin

WARNINGS
- Some patients may experience cross-sensitivity with penicillin.
- Serum sickness–like reactions (erythema multiforme, skin rash with polyarthritis, arthralgia, fever) have been reported.
- Products have triggered seizures in some patients.

Continued

TABLE 59-3 Adverse Effects of Cephalosporins

Body System	Common Minor Effects	Serious Adverse Effects
Body, general	Malaise, asthenia, dysgeusia	Fever, chills, pain/tightness in chest
Dermatologic	Diaphoresis, flushing	Urticaria, cutaneous moniliasis
Hypersensitivity		Fever, maculopapular rash, anaphylaxis, angioedema, Stevens-Johnson syndrome, erythema multiforme, toxic epidermal necrolysis
Respiratory		Asthma, dyspnea, interstitial pneumonitis, bronchospasm, pneumonia, rhinitis (loracarbef)
Cardiovascular	Palpitations, tachycardia	Hypotension, chest pain, vasodilation, syncope
GI	Nausea, vomiting, diarrhea, constipation, dyspepsia, anorexia, thirst, glossitis, abdominal pain, flatulence, stomach cramps	Melena, bleeding peptic ulcer, ileus, gallbladder sludge, colitis, including pseudomembranous colitis
Hemic and lymphatic		Eosinophilia, neutropenia, thrombocytopenia, agranulocytosis, hemolytic anemia, decreased platelet function, aplastic anemia
Metabolic and nutritional	Glucosuria	
Musculoskeletal	Muscle cramps, stiffness, neck spasms	Myalgia, arthralgia, rhabdomyolysis
Nervous system	Headache, dizziness, vertigo, lethargy, fatigue	Paresthesia, confusion, anxiety, hyperactivity, nervousness, insomnia, hypertonia, somnolence
Hepatic		↑ LFTs, hepatomegaly, hepatitis, jaundice, cholestasis
Genitourinary	Dysuria	Transitory elevations in BUN, creatinine, reversible interstitial nephritis, hematuria, toxic nephropathy, acute renal failure (rare), ceftriaxone—casts in urine

cephalexin (Keflex) 🔑 —cont'd

- Coagulation abnormalities have been reported with moxalactam, cefamandole, cefoperazone, ceftriaxone, and cefotetan.
- Pseudomembranous colitis may occur because of *Clostridium difficile*.
- Immune hemolytic anemia has been observed; however, it is rarely serious.
- *Renal function impairment:* Products may be nephrotoxic; use with caution in patients with renal impairment.
- *Hepatic function impairment:* Cefoperazone is excreted in bile. Half-life is increased in hepatic disease.
- Hypersensitivity reactions range from mild to life threatening.

PRECAUTIONS
- Inject intramuscular preparations deep IM.
- Superinfection may occur.

PHARMACOKINETICS. Most cephalosporins are excreted by the kidneys and thus require moderate dosage adjustments in patients with renal insufficiency. There is no need, however, for routine monitoring of renal function. See Table 59-2 for a comparison of product pharmacokinetics.

ADVERSE EFFECTS. See Table 59-3. Most symptoms are GI, including nausea, vomiting, and diarrhea. These are usually mild and only rarely require discontinuation of the drug. Cefixime (Suprax) is the exception to the rule; diarrhea severe enough to require discontinuation of the drug may occur in as many as 10% of patients taking this

cephalexin (Keflex) 🔑 —cont'd

drug. Cefaclor may cause serum sickness. No photosensitivity reactions have been reported.

DRUG INTERACTIONS. See Table 59-4.

OVERDOSAGE. The symptom most commonly associated with overdosage is development of seizures. Treatment is supportive.

Generalized tonic-clonic seizures, mild hemiparesis, and extreme confusion have occurred after large doses in renal failure with cefazolin.

DOSAGE AND ADMINISTRATION. Virtually all cephalosporins can be administered with food with no effect on total amount of drug absorption, although delays in absorption and peak concentration may result.

TABLE 59-4 Drug Interactions With Cephalosporins

Cephalosporin	Action on Other Drugs
Cephalosporins cefazolin, cefoperazone, cefotetan	May ↑ aminoglycoside nephrotoxicity May ↑ action on ethanol, anticoagulants
Drug	**Action on Cephalosporin**
probenecid, loop diuretics Antacids H₂-antagonists Iron supplements	↑ cephalosporins ↓ cefaclor, cefdinir, cefpodoxime cefpodoxime, cefuroxime ↓ cefdinir

OTHER DRUGS IN CLASS

FIRST GENERATION

- *Cefadroxil (Duricef)* offers the advantage of twice-daily dosing; however, cephalexin (Keflex) is more commonly used.
- *Cephradine (Velosef)* offers no advantages over cephalexin.

SECOND GENERATION

- *Cefuroxime (Ceftin)* is available in IM, IV, and oral formulations.

- *Cefprozil (Cefzil)* in many cases is the least expensive of the oral second-generation cephalosporins.

THIRD GENERATION

Of the oral third-generation medications, cefditoren (Spectracef) is the least expensive.

> **evolve** A continually updated list of useful WebLinks may be found in the Evolve Resources at http://evolve.elsevier.com/Edmunds/NP/

Tetracyclines

DRUG OVERVIEW

Class	Subclass	Generic Name	Trade Name
Natural	Short acting	tetracycline 🗝️ ☀️	Panmycin, Sumycin
Semisynthetic	Intermediate acting	demeclocycline	Declomycin
	Long acting	doxycycline ☀️	Vibramycin, Doryx, DoxyCaps, VibraTabs
		minocycline ☀️	Minocin Arestin, Dynacin, Vectrin

☀️, Top 200 drug; 🗝️, key drug.

INDICATIONS

See Table 60-1 for specifics.
- Acute exacerbation of COPD
- Sinusitis
- Pneumonia
- Chlamydia
- Rickettsial infections
- UTIs
- Demeclocycline has an unlabeled use to treat syndrome of inappropriate antidiuretic hormone (SIADH).
- Minocycline microspheres, tetracycline, fiber, and low-dose doxycycline are used in adjunctive treatment of periodontitis.

The two tetracyclines seen in primary care are tetracycline and doxycycline. Doxycycline is by far the most commonly used tetracycline. Tetracyclines are active against a wide range of aerobic and gram-positive and gram-negative bacteria (*Haemophilus ducreyi, Yersinia pestis*). Most gram-positive bacteria are now resistant to tetracyclines. These are not the drugs of choice for *Streptococcus* or *Staphylococcus*. Their greatest usefulness is against rickettsia, mycoplasma, protozoa, and chlamydia. Tetracyclines are not active against fungi or viruses. Tetracyclines are being used increasingly for malaria as mefloquine-resistant strains are increasing. They have few major side effects, except on the teeth of children and pregnant women, and possibly diarrhea, which can be a symptom of superinfection or a side effect. In the 1950s, tetracyclines were discovered to be produced by *Streptomyces aureofaciens*.

THERAPEUTIC OVERVIEW

Allergy

Allergies are not common. Anaphylaxis, urticaria, periorbital edema, fixed drug eruptions, and morbilliform rashes may occur. A systemic lupus erythematosus–like syndrome has been seen, along with positive antinuclear antibody.

Resistance

Resistance to tetracyclines is plasmid mediated and occurs via decreased influx into the cell, decreased access to the ribosome, and enzymatic inactivation. *Campylobacter* and *Shigella* have become largely resistant. A total of 15% to 60% of pneumococci have become resistant. No known protozoa, chlamydia, or rickettsia have become resistant.

All of the tetracyclines exhibit similar antimicrobial activity, and cross-resistance is common. Resistance has reduced their usefulness in recent years. Another major restriction is the contraindication for use in children younger than 8 years old and in pregnant women. If used in children or in pregnant women, the drug may permanently stain teeth. The severity of staining is determined by timing, duration, and the form of tetracycline administered. The traditional method used to repair the staining required aggressive tooth preparation. Recently, conservative preparations for porcelain veneer have been used with success.

MECHANISM OF ACTION

The basic tetracycline structure is a hydronaphthacene nucleus that contains four fused six-carbon rings. Tetracyclines differ in terms of substitutions on the fifth, sixth, or seventh position of the basic tetracycline structure. These substitutions affect lipid solubility, serum half-life, and the effect that food has on bioavailability of the drug.

The tetracyclines are bacteriostatic antibiotics. Their mechanism of action is to inhibit protein synthesis in the susceptible organism by binding to the 30S ribosome subunit, thereby impeding the binding of aminoacyl tRNA to the receptor site on the messenger RNA ribosome complex. Tetracyclines also may reversibly bind to 50S ribosomal subunits and may alter cytoplasmic membranes of susceptible organisms, resulting in leakage of cytosolic nucleotides. This action requires active microbial growth that distinguishes tetracyclines as bacteriostatic rather than bactericidal agents.

TABLE 60-1   Tetracycline Indications With Dosage and Administration Recommendations

Drug	Bacteria/Organism	Site/Disease	Dosage
tetracycline	*S. pneumoniae, M. catarrhalis, H. influenzae, Brucella, Legionella, Mycoplasma*	Mild to moderate Acute exacerbation COPD Severe acne, long term	*Adult:* 500 mg q6h × 10-14 days *Child (>8 yr):* 25 to 50 mg/kg in four equal doses (preferably q6h) *Child (>8 yr):* Initially, 1 g/day in divided doses. Maintenance, 125-500 mg/day
doxycycline	Same as tetracycline, anthrax *(Bacillus anthracis)* *B. burgdorferi*	Mild to moderate Acute exacerbation COPD Gonorrhea Lyme disease	*Adult:* First day 100 mg q12h *Child (>8 yr):* <45 kg: 4.4 mg/kg divided into two doses on first day, then 2.2 mg/kg one or two divided doses bid 100 mg q12h × 7 days or 300 mg as single dose and 300 mg 1 hr afterward 100 mg bid × 14-21 days
minocycline	*Chlamydia trachomatis, Ureaplasma urealyticum* *N. meningitidis*	Urethritis Asymptomatic carriers	100 mg bid for at least 7 days 100 mg q12h × 5 days

TREATMENT PRINCIPLES

Little difference in microbial activity is noted between the different tetracyclines. Tetracyclines are wide-spectrum antibiotics that are useful for empirical therapy. They are one of the drugs of first choice for acute bacterial exacerbation of COPD, chlamydia, and rickettsial infection, and they provide a second-line consideration for many other infections, especially in a patient with allergy to other antibiotics.

The choice between tetracyclines is made by determination of drug characteristics. Doxycycline and minocycline are the two most commonly used tetracyclines. Most tetracyclines must not be taken with milk or antacids; however, minocycline and doxycycline do not have this complicating facto so it is easier to get the patient to take them correctly. Also, doxycycline has a longer half-life than tetracycline. Doxycycline produces less gastrointestinal disturbance than the other tetracyclines, although it can cause diarrhea. Overall, doxycycline is the most useful tetracycline in primary care; however, it is imperative that pregnant women not take doxycycline.

Nonantibiotic actions of tetracyclines result in antiinflammatory processes, immunosuppression, inhibition of lipase and collagenase, enhancement of gingival fibroblast cell attachment, and wound healing.

How to Monitor

- Obtain baseline tests for renal and hepatic function and a CBC every 3 months for patients on long-term therapy. May cause increased AST, ALT, serum alkaline phosphatase, bilirubin, and amylase concentrations. Additionally, all tetracyclines except doxycycline may increase serum BUN.
- Loss of appetite, jaundice, or abdominal pain may indicate possible hepatotoxicity.
- *minocycline:* A change in mental status could indicate possible intracranial hypertension.

Patient Variables

GERIATRICS. Tetracyclines are well absorbed in the elderly, even in patients with achlorhydria or low gastric pH. With the exception of doxycycline and minocycline, serum levels of tetracyclines are increased by impaired renal function, and dosages should be reduced. Because the primary routes of excretion with doxycycline and minocycline are biliary, and the serum half-life of these agents is unaffected by renal insufficiency, either doxycycline or minocycline would be a good choice of a tetracycline in the elderly, particularly if deteriorating renal function is a matter of concern.

PEDIATRICS

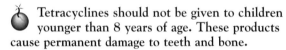

Tetracyclines should not be given to children younger than 8 years of age. These products cause permanent damage to teeth and bone.

PREGNANCY AND LACTATION

- *Category D:* Tetracyclines cross the placenta; because of the chelating effect, they bind with calcium, resulting in discoloration of deciduous teeth, enamel hypoplasia, and inhibition of fetal skeletal growth. The period for greatest risk of discoloration of the anterior deciduous teeth ranges from the middle of the second trimester up to 6 months of age in the newborn. Tetracyclines should never be given to pregnant patients.
- Relatively high concentrations of tetracyclines are excreted in breast milk. Therefore, these agents are contraindicated during lactation.

GENDER. Tetracyclines may decrease the pharmacologic effects of oral contraceptives; breakthrough bleeding or pregnancy may occur. Use an alternative form of contraception as backup protection during antibiotic therapy.

Patient Education

All tetracyclines should be taken with the patient sitting upright with a full glass of water (240 ml) to avoid esophagitis or esophageal ulceration. The patient should not lie down for approximately one-half hour after taking each dose because most reported cases of esophageal ulceration involve patients' lying down immediately after taking a tetracycline dose.

All tetracyclines, with the exceptions of doxycycline and minocycline, should be taken on an empty stomach (i.e., 1 hour before or 2 hours after meals) to maximize absorption.

With the exceptions of doxycycline and minocycline, the use of iron preparations, antacid products, or other products that contain aluminum, magnesium, calcium, zinc, and milk products substantially decreases absorption via oral administration.

Because of the potential for tetracycline-induced photosensitivity, the patient should avoid unnecessary exposure to the sun. If sun exposure is unavoidable, sunscreens with a minimum sun-protection factor (SPF) of 30 should be used.

Patients should report any signs and symptoms of hepatotoxicity (e.g., persistent nausea, vomiting, anorexia with or without yellow coloring of the skin or eyes, dark urine, pale stools) and should stop taking the medication.

evolve See Bonus tables at http://evolve.elsevier.com/Edmunds/NP/

SPECIFIC DRUGS

tetracycline 🔑

All tetracyclines share the same characteristics, except as noted.

CONTRAINDICATIONS
- Hypersensitivity
- Pregnancy, lactation, use in children, except doxycycline can be used to treat children and lactating women with anthrax.

WARNINGS

 Photosensitivity may manifest as an exaggerated sunburn reaction.

- Demeclocycline long-term therapy has resulted in diabetes insipidus syndrome (polyuria, polydipsia, and weakness).
- Minocycline has caused light-headedness, dizziness, and vertigo. Patients should use caution during hazardous tasks.
- Except for doxycycline and minocycline, tetracyclines will accumulate in patients with renal function impairment. Except for doxycycline, tetracyclines may cause an increase in BUN levels.
- High doses of tetracyclines can cause liver failure.

PRECAUTIONS
- Benign intracranial hypertension with severe headache and blurred vision has occurred.

Unused tetracyclines should be discarded to prevent Fanconi-like renal toxicity on proximal renal tubules, resulting from ingestion of outdated and degraded tetracycline.

- Superinfection may occur.
- Some products contain sulfites that may provoke a reaction in sensitive individuals.

PHARMACOKINETICS. See Table 60-2. Tetracyclines are incompletely absorbed when patients are fasting; absorption is decreased with food, except with use of doxycycline and minocycline. Doxycycline is the best absorbed tetracycline.

Doxycycline and minocycline are highly lipid soluble and readily penetrate into the cerebrospinal fluid, brain, eye, and prostate. The other tetracyclines are intermediate in their lipid solubility.

Tetracyclines are concentrated by the liver in the bile and are excreted unchanged in the urine and feces. Reduction in dosing and/or interval is required in renal impairment, except with doxycycline and minocycline.

Because tetracycline is excreted unchanged in the urine via glomerular filtration and through a secondary biliary excretion route, reduction in dosing and/or interval is required in renal impairment. See Table 60-2 for a comparison of tetracycline pharmacokinetics.

ADVERSE EFFECTS. Hypersensitivity is rare. Doxycycline is believed to be associated with less nephrotoxicity than the other tetracyclines, even though associated renal failure has been reported. Tetracyclines can cause esophagitis. See Table 60-3.

DRUG INTERACTIONS. See Table 60-4.

OVERDOSAGE. If overdosage has just occurred with oral administration, antacids or milk products may be administered in an attempt to prevent or at least minimize absorption.

DOSAGE AND ADMINISTRATION

With the exception of doxycycline and minocycline, tetracyclines interact with divalent and trivalent cations to form insoluble and nonabsorbable chelate. Therefore, it is critical that tetracyclines not be taken together with products that contain calcium, magnesium, zinc, or iron (e.g., antacids, milk products, calcium- or iron-containing supplements, iron preparations).

Bismuth subsalicylate, kaolin, and pectin reduce absorption of oral tetracyclines and should be avoided. Food inhibits the absorption of tetracyclines, again with the exceptions of doxycycline and minocycline. Therefore, except for doxycycline and minocycline, the tetracyclines should be taken on an empty stomach, 1 hour before or 2 hours after meals or any other medication that contains divalent or trivalent cations.

OTHER DRUGS IN CLASS

- *Tetracycline* is the only drug in this class that must not be taken with food and requires dosing adjustment in renal impairment.
- *Doxycycline* (*Vibramycin, Doxy Caps*) is associated with fewer reports of renal failure than the other tetracyclines. It also offers the advantage of twice-daily dosing. Doxycycline is recommended for the treatment of patients with

TABLE 60-2   Pharmacokinetics of Tetracycline

Drug	Percent	Oral Absorption	Lipid Solubility	Half-life	Half-life in Anuria	Usual Adult Oral Daily Dosage	Protein Binding	Metabolism	Routes of Excretion
tetracycline HCl	60-80	Slowed	Intermediate	8 hr	57-108 hr	250-500 mg q6h	20%-67%	Minimal	Renal, 60%
demeclocycline HCl	66	Slowed	Intermediate	10-17 hr	40-60 hr	150 mg q6h; increase up to 300 mg q12h		None	Renal/biliary
doxycycline	90-100	Reduced by 20%, not clinically significant	High	12-22 hr	12-22 hr	100 mg q12h-100 mg q24h	80%-93%	50%	Biliary, 75%; renal, 25%
minocycline HCl	90-100	Not significant	High	11-23 hr	11-23 hr	100 mg q12h	76%	Principally hepatic	Biliary/renal, hepatic, 10%

TABLE 60-3   Adverse Effects of Tetracyclines

Body System	Common Minor Effects	Serious Adverse Reactions
Body, general	Deposition in teeth	Superinfection
Skin, appendages	Maculopapular and erythematous rashes, photosensitivity, onycholysis and discoloration of nails	Exfoliative dermatitis (minocycline): blue-gray pigmentation, Stevens-Johnson syndrome
Hypersensitivity	Photosensitivity	Urticaria, angioneurotic edema, anaphylaxis, anaphylactoid purpura, pericarditis, exacerbated systemic lupus erythematosus (SLE), polyarthralgia, serum sickness–like reactions (fever, rash, arthralgia), pulmonary infiltrates with eosinophilia
Gastrointestinal	Anorexia, nausea, vomiting, diarrhea, epigastric distress, bulky loose stools, stomatitis, sore throat, glossitis, hoarseness, black hairy tongue	Esophageal ulcers, dysphagia, enterocolitis, inflammatory lesions in anogenital region
Hemic and lymphatic		Hemolytic anemia, thrombocytopenia, thrombocytopenic purpura, neutropenia, eosinophilia
Central nervous system	Headache; minocycline—light-headedness, dizziness, vertigo	Transient myopathy
Hepatic		Fatty liver, hepatotoxicity, hepatitis (rare), ↑ LFTs, hepatic cholestasis (rare, with high levels)
Renal		↑ BUN, creatinine

TABLE 60-4   Drug Interactions With Tetracycline

Tetracycline	Action on Other Drugs
tetracycline	Anticoagulants: ↑ hypoprothrombinemia effects ↑ Serum levels of digoxin ↓ Insulin requirements ↓↑ Lithium levels ↓ Pharmacologic effects of oral contraceptives ↓ Effects of penicillins

Drug Acting	Action on Tetracycline
Antacids Barbiturates, carbamazepine, and hydantoins cimetidine Iron salts sodium bicarbonate	↓ Absorption (except doxycycline and minocycline) ↓ Levels of doxycycline ↓ GI absorption ↓ GI absorption ↓ GI absorption

community-acquired methicillin-resistant *Staphylococcus aureus* (MRSA).

- *Minocycline (Minocin)* is almost completely absorbed when taken orally. With its long half-life, minocycline can be taken twice a day. It has good tissue penetration because of high lipid solubility.

evolve A continually updated list of useful WebLinks may be found in the Evolve Resources at http://evolve.elsevier.com/Edmunds/NP/

61 Macrolides

DRUG OVERVIEW

Class	Subclass	Generic Name	Trade Name
Macrolides	Erythromycins 🔑	erythromycin base	E-Mycin, Ery-Tab, Eryc
		erythromycin estolate	Ilosone, Erythrozone
		erythromycin stearate	Erythrocin
		erythromycin ethylsuccinate	EryPed, E.E.S.
	Newer macrolides	azithromycin ✸	Zithromax 🔑 ✸, Z-Pack Oral Suspension
		clarithromycin ✸	Biaxin, Biaxin XL ✸
Ketolide		telithromycin	Ketek ✸

✸, Top 200 drug; 🔑, key drug.

INDICATIONS

See Table 61-1 for specifics.
- Otitis media
- Acute bronchitis or pneumonia in patient with COPD
- Community-acquired pneumonia
- Pharyngitis
- Sinusitis

Erythromycin, azithromycin, and clarithromycin are commonly used in primary care. They have primary indications and are used as an alternative to penicillin in sensitive patients. Erythromycin was derived from *Saccharopolyspora erythraea* (originally *Streptomyces erythreus*), found in the Philippines in 1952. Erythromycin is active against most pneumococci and group A β-hemolytic strep. It is also useful for atypical infections such as *Legionella pneumophila*, *Mycoplasma pneumoniae*, *Corynebacterium diphtheriae*, *Chlamydia trachomatis*, *Listeria monocytogenes*, *Ureaplasma urealyticum*, and some rickettsia. Susceptible gram-negative bacteria include *B. pertussis*, *Neisseria gonorrhoeae*, and meningitis. The ketolide telithromycin was approved in 2004. Severe hepatotoxicity has been reported (with one fatality and one liver transplant), indicating that ketolide must be used with caution. For additional FDA information, see http://www.fda.gov/cder/drug/advisory/telithromycin.htm

A major limitation to erythromycin use is the frequent occurrence of GI side effects and drug interactions. However, the newer macrolides (azithromycin and clarithromycin) rarely cause problematic GI side effects. Macrolides affect the cytochrome P450 3A4 system, thereby inhibiting the metabolism of certain drugs. A careful patient history of concurrent medications will prevent potentially adverse drug interactions.

Allergy

Reactions include skin rash, fever, and eosinophilia. Cholestatic hepatitis, which occurs rarely, most often with the estolate compound, may be an allergic reaction to the estolate.

Resistance

As macrolide use has increased, macrolide resistance also has increased. Three major mechanisms of resistance to the macrolides have been identified. The most common one is decreased permeability of the cell wall to macrolides. Some bacteria are able to pump the antibiotic out. The second mechanism, target site alterations, results from a genetic ability to decrease binding of the antibiotic to targets on the ribosome. Decreased binding confers a high degree of resistance. The third major mechanism is drug inactivation by enzymes. Use of macrolides increases the nasopharyngeal presence of macrolide and penicillin-resistant pneumococci. Macrolide-resistant *streptococcus* is a problem in the treatment of community-acquired pneumonia and middle ear infections. About half of patients with macrolide-resistant infections had not taken antibiotics in the past 6 months. Group A strep resistance is increasing to up to 15% to 35% in some geographic areas. *Strep pyogenes*, *Staph aureus*, *Strep viridans*, *Clostridium perfringens*, and *Haemophilus influenzae* are developing increased resistance to macrolides.

MECHANISM OF ACTION

Macrolides consist of a large lactone ring to which sugars are attached. Structural modifications in clarithromycin and azithromycin make them more acid stable, improve tissue penetration, and broaden the spectrum.

Macrolides may be bacteriostatic or bactericidal. The mechanism of action involves inhibition of protein synthesis that results from binding specifically to the 50S ribosomal

TABLE 61-1   Macrolide Indications With Dosage and Administration Recommendations

Drug	Bacteria	Site/Disease	Dosage
erythromycin	GABHS, *S. pneumoniae*	URI mild to moderate, lower respiratory infection	*Adult:* 250-500 mg qid × 10 days *Child:* 20-50 mg/kg/day in divided doses × 10 days
	M. pneumoniae	Respiratory tract	*Adult:* 500 mg qid × 5-10 days
	S. pyogenes, S. aureus	Skin and skin structure	*Adult:* 250-500 mg qid × 10 days *Child:* 20-50 mg/kg/day in divided doses × 10 days
	B. pertussis	Whooping cough	*Adult:* 500 mg qid × 14 days *Child:* 40-50 mg/kg/day in divided doses × 14 days
	C. diphtheriae	Diphtheria; eradicate carriers	500 mg q6h × 10 days
	GABHS	Prevention	250 mg bid
clarithromycin	GABHS	Pharyngitis, tonsillitis	250 mg q12h × 10 days
	H. influenzae, M. catarrhalis, S. pneumoniae	Acute sinusitis	500 mg q12h × 14 days
	H. influenzae	Acute exacerbation of COPD	500 mg q12h × 7-14 days
	H. parainfluenzae	Acute exacerbation of COPD	500 mg q12h × 7 days
	H. influenzae	CAP (pneumonia)	250 mg q12h × 7 days
	S. pneumoniae, M. pneumoniae, C. pneumoniae	CAP (pneumonia)	250 mg q12h × 7-14 days
	Streptococcus, Staphylococcus	Skin	250 mg q12h × 7-14 days
azithromycin	*S. aureus, S. pyogenes, S. pneumoniae, H. influenzae, M. catarrhalis, Legionella*	Acute exacerbation of COPD, CAP, pharyngitis, tonsillitis, skin	*Adult:* 500 mg × 1 day, then 250 mg × 4 days
		Otitis media	*Child (>6 mo):* 30 mg/kg (maximum, 1500 mg) × one dose, or 10 mg/kg (maximum, 500 mg) once daily × 3 days, or 10 mg/kg × 1 day, then 5 mg/kg (maximum, 250 mg) × 4 days
		CAP	*Child:* 10 mg/kg × 1 day, then 5 mg/kg × 4 days
telithromycin	*S. aureus, Strep pneumoniae, H. influenzae, M. catarrhalis, Chlamydophila (Chlamydia) pneumoniae, Mycoplasma pneumoniae*	CAP	800 mg (two 400 mg tablets) once daily × 10 days
		Sinus	800 mg (two 400 mg tablets) once daily × 5 days
		Bronchitis, chronic or acute exacerbation	800 mg (two 400 mg tablets) once daily × 5 days

CAP, Community-acquired pneumonia; GABHS, group A β-hemolytic *Streptococcus pyogenes.*

subunit. This causes the RNA to dissociate from the ribosome and prevents protein synthesis. Macrolides inhibit a specific step in protein synthesis whereby the new tRNA moves from the ribosome to the new site. Telithromycin blocks protein synthesis by binding to a specific location of the RNA on the 50S ribosome.

Other effects of the macrolides occur as gastrointestinal stimulation; they also appear to modulate inflammation by inhibiting production of the cytokine interleukin-8. In addition, macrolides may be used as prokinetic agents in hospitalized patients.

TREATMENT PRINCIPLES

Most practitioners consider the macrolides to be a safe first-line choice for patients with uncomplicated infection. Erythromycin products are relatively inexpensive; however, the newer macrolides are more expensive. When a macrolide is prescribed, caution should be taken with dosing in the presence of severe renal or hepatic impairment.

Erythromycin is a first-choice drug for the treatment of children with pneumonia (ages 3 months to 5 years) or ophthalmia neonatorum. Erythromycin is an alternative treatment for impetigo, cellulitis, otitis media, pharyngitis, chlamydia, and Lyme disease. Erythromycin also provides alternative treatment for the prevention of bacterial endocarditis in patients allergic to penicillin. Azithromycin is another first-choice drug for the treatment of pneumonia in children (ages 6 months to 5 years and older). Azithromycin also is a first-choice drug for the treatment of chlamydia in adults and is used alternative treatment for patients with impetigo, cellulitis, sinusitis, pharyngitis, acute exacerbations of COPD, and traveler's diarrhea. Clarithromycin is used in adults for pharyngitis, sinusitis, otitis media, acute exacerbation of COPD, pneumonia, and skin infection.

The major differences between erythromycin and the newer macrolides include GI tolerability, a broader spectrum of activity, and dosing frequency. Erythromycins must be taken three or four times a day. Azithromycin offers the advantage of once-daily dosing. Clarithromycin requires twice-daily dosing. The longer drug action of azithromycin can make a critical difference in patient adherence.

The strength of each erythromycin product is expressed as erythromycin base equivalents. As a result of differences in absorption and biotransformation, varying quantities of each erythromycin salt form are required to produce the same free erythromycin serum levels. Erythromycin base is acid labile and usually is formulated in enteric- or film-coated forms for oral administration. Acid-stable salts and esters (estolate, ethylsuccinate, and stearate) are well absorbed.

The macrolides are active primarily against gram-positive organisms, including *Streptococcus pyogenes* (GABHS) and *S. pneumoniae*. The newer macrolides have added effectiveness against gram-negative bacteria and anaerobes. Macrolides are of value for their unique ability to treat atypical pathogens such as *M. pneumoniae*, which are seen in community-acquired pneumonias.

Azithromycin and clarithromycin have significantly increased potency against gram-negative bacteria and anaerobes and generally are reserved for more complicated infections such as community-acquired pneumonia, exacerbation of COPD, and sinusitis.

How to Monitor

When used long term, monitoring of hepatic function is prudent, especially for erythromycin estolate.

Patient Variables

GERIATRICS. Lower doses of macrolides generally are not necessary in the elderly, provided they do not have severe renal or hepatic impairment.

Check renal and hepatic function before beginning treatment with the drug.

PEDIATRICS. Age, weight, and severity of illness are important factors in determining dosage for children when erythromycin, azithromycin, and clarithromycin are prescribed.

PREGNANCY AND LACTATION
- *erythromycin: category B.* Erythromycin estolate has been associated with elevated liver function tests in 10% of pregnant women and should be used cautiously in pregnancy.
- *azithromycin: category B.*
- *clarithromycin, telithromycin: category C.* These drugs should not be used in pregnancy except in clinical circumstances when no alternative is available.
- Erythromycin is considered compatible with breastfeeding. However, the drug is transferred via breast milk, and the nursing woman should be aware that the nursing child will be exposed to the drug as well. Azithromycin and clarithromycin may be excreted in breast milk, and caution should be exercised when these drugs are administered to a nursing woman.

Patient Education

- Do not chew, cut, or crush the tablets.
- Most erythromycin products should be taken with food.
- Clarithromycin may be taken with or without food.
- Azithromycin tablets can be taken without regard to food. The oral suspension should be given on an empty stomach.
- Clarithromycin suspension should not be refrigerated. It should be shaken well before each use.
- Patients who use oral contraceptives for birth control should be advised that macrolides can reduce their efficacy, and that they should consider using a backup method of contraception.
- *telithromycin:* Visual disturbances may occur, particularly a delay in accommodation; pseudomembranous colitis has been seen; this agent has the potential to prolong the QTc interval of the ECG, which may place patients at increased risk for ventricular arrhythmia; myasthenia gravis may be exacerbated.

SPECIFIC DRUGS

erythromycins

All macrolides share the following characteristics except as noted.

CONTRAINDICATIONS
- Hypersensitivity to any macrolide
- *erythromycin estolate:* preexisting liver disease

WARNINGS
- Superinfection has occurred.
- Pseudomembranous colitis (*Clostridium difficile*) has occurred.
- *Cardiac effects:* Ventricular arrhythmia, including ventricular tachycardia and torsades de pointes in individuals with prolonged QT intervals, has been reported with macrolide antibiotics; however, this has not occurred with azithromycin.
- Rare serious allergic reactions, including angioedema, anaphylaxis, and Stevens-Johnson syndrome, as well as toxic epidermal necrolysis, have occurred rarely.
- *Hepatotoxicity:* Erythromycin, especially erythromycin estolate, has been associated with infrequent cholestatic hepatitis. Findings include abnormal hepatic function, peripheral eosinophilia, and leukocytosis.
- Erythromycin may aggravate the weakness of patients with myasthenia gravis.
- *Renal/hepatic function impairment:* Erythromycin is excreted by the liver. Exercise caution in administering to patients with impaired hepatic function. Hepatic dysfunction without jaundice has been reported. Because azithromycin is eliminated principally via the liver, exercise caution when administering to patients with impaired hepatic function. Clarithromycin is excreted principally via the liver and kidney and may be administered without dosage adjustment to patients with hepatic impairment and normal renal function. However, in severe renal impairment, the dosage should be halved or dosing intervals doubled.
- *azithromycin:* Do not use for pneumonia in patients judged as inappropriate for oral therapy for pneumonia.
- *clarithromycin:* Do not use with ranitidine bismuth citrate in patients with a history of acute porphyria.

PRECAUTIONS. Superinfection may result.

PHARMACOKINETICS. See Table 61-2. Erythromycin often is inconsistently absorbed; many preparations are enteric coated to protect their destruction by gastric acid and to facilitate absorption.

Food delays the onset of effects of clarithromycin. Azithromycin is absorbed faster when taken with food. Erythromycin stearate and certain formulations of erythromycin bases must be taken 3 hours before or after a meal. Because the erythromycins can cause GI upset, compliance may be an issue. Macrolides are readily distributed into body tissues and fluids. Tissue levels are higher than

TABLE 61-2   Pharmacokinetics of Macrolides

Drug	Absorption	Drug Availability (After First Pass)	Onset of Action	Time to Peak Concentration	Half-life	Protein Bound	Metabolism	Excretion
erythromycin	30%-50%	Varies, depending on formulation, food presence, and gastric emptying	Varies, depending on formulation	Varies between 1 and 4 hr	1.4 hr	70%-96%	Hepatic; demethylation 1A2 inhibitor 3A4 substrate and inhibitor	Urine, 5%-15%; significant quantity in bile
azithromycin	37%, decreased with food	40%	2 hr	2-3 hr	68 hr	12%-50%	Small amount demethylated	Primarily feces, unchanged
clarithromycin	50%	50%	1-3 hr	Tabs: 2 hr Susp: 3 hr	250 mg: 3-4 hr; 500 mg: 5-7 hr	65%-70%	3A4 small amount; oxidized to active metabolite	Urine, 20%-30%
telithromycin	57%, not affected by food			1 hr	10 hr	60%-70%	50% 3A4, 50% CYP 450 independent	Unchanged in feces, 7%; unchanged in urine, 13%

erythromycins 🔑 —cont'd

serum levels; thus, they are effectively delivered to the site of infection. Macrolides are one of the many drugs that depend on P450 3A4 as a major route of metabolism; toxicity may occur when this route is blocked.

ADVERSE EFFECTS. See Table 61-3. Allergic reactions are rare. Erythromycin has significantly more adverse GI effects than the newer macrolides.

💣 **Erythromycin also has a wider range of adverse effects. It is more likely to cause serious allergic reactions and cardiac arrhythmias. Cardiac effects occur mainly in patients who have a prolonged QT interval.**

Of the erythromycin salts, erythromycin estolate is most commonly associated with hepatotoxicity. Clarithromycin and azithromycin have not been associated with jaundice; however, they also are principally excreted via the liver and kidney, and caution should be taken regarding dosing of these drugs in the presence of severe renal or hepatic impairment.

DRUG INTERACTIONS. See Table 61-4. The macrolides are metabolized by the CYP450 3A4 system and interact with drugs also metabolized by that system.

OVERDOSAGE. Symptoms include nausea, vomiting, epigastric distress, and severe diarrhea. Hearing loss may occur with erythromycin, especially in patients with renal insufficiency.

DOSAGE AND ADMINISTRATION. See Table 61-1. Erythromycin base is available in enteric-coated tablets 250 mg for every 6-hour use, and 333 mg for every 8-hour use. It also is available in delayed-release 250 mg capsules. Erythromycin estolate comes in tablets (500 mg), capsules (250 mg), and suspension, 125 or 250 mg/5 ml. Erythromycin stearate comes in 250 and 500 mg tablets. Erythromycin ethylsuccinate comes in chewable 200 mg tablets and 400 mg tablets and in suspension (200 and 400 mg/5 ml).

OTHER DRUGS IN CLASS

Other drugs in this class are similar to the key drug except as follows:
- *Erythromycin* is much less expensive than the newer macrolides.
- *Erythromycin estolate* has a lower rate of GI side effects than ethylsuccinate.

Newer Macrolides

All have a much lower incidence of GI side effects than erythromycin.

azithromycin (Zithromax, Z-Pack): It is important to give a loading dose, without which minimum plasma concentrations may take 5 to 7 days to reach steady state. A new formulation of azithromycin (Zmax) may be taken in a single dose of 2 g.

Azithromycin and clarithromycin have better absorption, longer half-lives, and a greater spectrum of activity than erythromycin.

Telithromycin is not used a great deal in primary care because of the risk of hepatotoxicity, and because other available drugs confer less risk.

CONTRAINDICATIONS. Macrolide hypersensitivity, history of hepatitis and/or jaundice associated with telithromycin or other macrolide antibiotic use

WARNINGS
- Hepatic dysfunction and severe hepatitis resulting in death have been reported (see http://www.fda.gov/cder/drug/advisory/telithromycin.htm).
- Pseudomembranous colitis has been reported.
- Telithromycin has the potential to prolong the QT interval, which may lead to increased risk for ventricular arrhythmias, including torsades de pointes; exacerbations of myasthenia gravis have been reported.

PRECAUTIONS
- May cause visual disturbances such as lower accommodation, blurred vision, difficulty focusing, and diplopia

TABLE 61-3   Adverse Effects of Macrolides

Body System	Common Minor Effects	Serious Adverse Reactions
Body, general		Superinfections
Skin, appendages	*erythromycin:* rash; *azithromycin:* photosensitivity	
Hypersensitivity		*erythromycin:* urticaria; Stevens-Johnson syndrome, anaphylaxis; *azithromycin:* angioedema
Cardiovascular		↑ QT interval, ventricular arrhythmias, torsades de pointes (not with azithromycin)
GI	Abdominal distress, diarrhea, dyspepsia, nausea, vomiting	
Hemic		Neutropenia, thrombocytopenia
CNS	*erythromycin:* insomnia, headache, dizziness, asthenia	*erythromycin:* seizures
Hepatic		↑ ALT, AST, hepatotoxicity; *erythromycin:* cholestatic hepatitis
Genitourinary		↑ BUN, creatinine

TABLE 61-4   Drug Interactions of Macrolides

Macrolide	Action on Other Drugs
Macrolides	↑ Oral anticoagulants, benzodiazepines, buspirone, carbamazepine, cyclosporine, digoxin, disopyramide, ergot alkaloids, statins, tacrolimus, theophylline
erythromycin	↑ bromocriptine, felodipine, grepafloxacin, sparfloxacin, methylprednisolone ↓ lincosamide
Newer macrolides	↑ omeprazole
clarithromycin	Increase digoxin, 3A4 drugs
azithromycin	Increase cisapride, phenothiazine, pimozide
Drug	**Action on Macrolide**
pimozide	↑ Macrolides
rifampin, theophylline	↓ Macrolides
clarithromycin, fluconazole	↑ Newer macrolides

- Syncope, usually associated with vagal syndrome, has been reported.
- Use caution when operating hazardous machinery.

ADVERSE EFFECTS. See Table 61-3.

DRUG INTERACTIONS
- Erythromycin and clarithromycin interact with other CYP3A medications. Azithromycin does not.
- *clarithromycin:* Contraindicated because it increases levels of belladonna, ergotamine, phenobarbital, cisapride, eletriptan, phenothiazines, pimozide, and ranolazine. Avoid concurrent use with most antiarrhythmics, TCAs, some hypertensives, statins, theophylline, warfarin, and many other agents because of the tendency to increase drug levels.
- *3A4 inhibitors, ketoconazole, and itraconazole:* increase telithromycin
- *3A4 substrates:* cisapride increases risk of increased QT interval; simvastatin and midazolam levels increased
- *2D6 substrates:* metoprolol level increased
- *Others:* digoxin and theophylline levels increased; sotalol levels decreased; no effect on warfarin, contraceptives, ranitidine, or antacids

DOSAGE AND ADMINISTRATION. See Table 61-1.

evolve A continually updated list of useful WebLinks may be found in the Evolve Resources at http://evolve.elsevier.com/Edmunds/NP/

Fluoroquinolones

62

DRUG OVERVIEW

Class	Generic Name	Trade Name
Fluoroquinolones	ciprofloxacin 🗝 ✹	Cipro
	norfloxacin	Noroxin, Ofloxacin, Ciloxan
Fluoroquinolones with enhanced activity against *Streptococcus pneumoniae*	levofloxacin	Levaquin ✹
	moxifloxacin	Avelox ✹
	gemifloxacin	Factive

✹, Top 200 drug; 🗝, key drug.

INDICATIONS

See Table 62-1 for specifics.
- Lower respiratory infections
- Skin and skin structure infections
- Bone/joint infections
- Infectious diarrhea
- Sexually transmitted diseases
- Complicated urinary tract infections
- Prostatitis
- Otitis media, otitis externa
- Conjunctivitis, corneal ulcers

Quinolones were discovered in 1962 as a byproduct of chloroquine synthesis. The earliest drugs were called quinolones. Later, a fluorine radical was added to the structure, and these newer drugs were called fluoroquinolones, to distinguish them from the earlier drugs. Currently, all quinolones on the market are fluoroquinolones. Many texts now use the terms *quinolone* and *fluoroquinolone* interchangeably.

The fluoroquinolones are a group of potent antibiotics with a wide spectrum of action against gram-positive and gram-negative organisms. The primary care provider should be familiar with ciprofloxacin, moxifloxacin, and levofloxacin. Fluoroquinolones have a good safety profile and excellent absorption after oral administration. Headache and dizziness occur in up to 11% of patients and are the most commonly reported adverse events. The newer fluoroquinolones offer expanded coverage of gram-positive pathogens, and one agent, moxifloxacin, is active against anaerobes. However, three fluoroquinolones introduced after 2001 have been taken off the market because of adverse events.

Quinolones are active against aerobic gram-negative bacilli, especially Enterobacteriaceae, *Haemophilus*, and gram-negative cocci such as *Neisseria* and *Moraxella catarrhalis*. They are active against *Staphylococcus* and *Mycoplasma*. Ciprofloxacin and levofloxacin are the only quinolones active against *Pseudomonas aeruginosa*.

THERAPEUTIC OVERVIEW

Allergy

Allergic reactions occur in 0.5% to 3% of patients. Rashes are the most common allergic reaction. The newest fluoroquinolone, gemifloxacin, causes rashes in 14% of young women. More serious reactions such as anaphylaxis, drug fever, vasculitis, interstitial nephritis, and serum sickness have been uncommon. If patients demonstrate any of these reactions, it is recommended that they not take any of the fluoroquinolones.

Resistance

Resistance occurs by mutation. No quinolone-modifying abilities have been seen in bacteria. Spontaneous mutations that result in resistance alter the target enzymes or alter drug transport across the cell wall. Plasmid-mediated quinolone resistance has been seen. These mutations produce efflux pumps to remove the antibiotic from the cell. *Pseudomonas* and *staphylococci* are the two most troublesome. Recently, resistance to *N. gonorrhoeae*, *C. jejuni*, and *E. coli* has been noted. Underdosing caused by failure to finish the prescribed course of medication should be avoided to prevent resistance.

MECHANISM OF ACTION

Quinolones have a dual ring structure. Substitutions on the dual rings determine the type of quinolone. Ofloxacin is a racemic mixture (right- and left-handed molecules) that contains the active ingredient, levofloxacin. The mechanism of action of the fluoroquinolones is inhibition of deoxyribonucleic acid (DNA) gyrase, an enzyme that is essential in the transcription, replication, and repair of bacterial DNA. The blocking of DNA gyrase that occurs at concentrations of 0.1 to 10 g/ml promotes superhelical formation of bacterial DNA, resulting in destruction of the DNA.

TABLE 62-1   Fluoroquinolone Indications With Dosages and Recommendations

Drug	Bacteria	Site/Disease	Dosage and Administration
ciprofloxacin	E. coli, Klebsiella, Proteus, Enterobacter	Uncomplicated UTI Cystitis (mild/moderate) Cystitis (severe)	250 mg bid × 3 days 250 mg bid × 7-14 days 500 mg bid × 7-14 days
	M. catarrhalis, H. influenzae, M. pneumoniae, Listeria, Legionella, Staphylococcus	Lower respiratory tract, skin, and skin structure Sinusitis	500-750 mg bid × 7-14 days 500 mg q12h × 10 days
	Shigella, Serratia, Salmonella	Infectious diarrhea; intraabdominal	500 mg bid × 5-7 days (Salmonella) 500 mg bid × 3 days (Shigella) 500 mg bid × 7-14 days (intraabdominal)
norfloxacin	Same as ciprofloxacin	Uncomplicated UTI	400 mg q12h × 3 days
levofloxacin	Same plus GABHS, many gram negative	Acute exacerbation of COPD CAP Sinusitis Skin, soft tissue Uncomplicated UTI	500 mg once daily × 7 days 500 mg once daily × 7-14 days 500 mg once daily × 10-14 days 500 mg once daily × 7-10 days 250 mg once daily × 3 days
moxifloxacin	Same as ciprofloxacin plus anaerobic activity (Bacteroides spp)	Uncomplicated UTI Sinusitis Acute exacerbation of COPD CAP Skin and soft tissue (uncomplicated)	400 mg once daily × 3 days 400 mg once daily × 10 days 400 mg once daily × 5 days 400 mg once daily × 7-14 days 400 mg once daily × 7 days
gemifloxacin	Same plus GABHS, many gram negative	CAP Acute exacerbation of COPD	320 mg po once daily × 7 days 320 mg po once daily × 5 days

CAP, Community-acquired pneumonia; GABHS, group A β-hemolytic Streptococcus pyogenes.

TREATMENT PRINCIPLES

Fluoroquinolones should not be considered first-line antibiotics for mild infection; however, they are often the agent of first choice for UTIs and pyelonephritis because of the frequency of resistant bacteria with these conditions. In general, they should be reserved for moderate infections and bacterial infections that are resistant to other antibiotics. Because fluoroquinolones have good tissue penetration, they provide effective treatment for skin, bone, and genital infections. CNS penetration, however, is poor and is not considered clinically effective. Always give fluoroquinolones orally when possible because oral absorption is excellent.

Fluoroquinolones are considered first-choice drugs for empirical treatment of complicated sinusitis, severe diarrhea, UTIs, pyelonephritis, and prostatitis. The CDC advises that fluoroquinolones should not be used any longer for gonorrhea. They are acceptable as an alternative treatment for dog bite, acute sinusitis, severe sinusitis, and chlamydia. Fluoroquinolones with enhanced activity via S. pneumoniae provide alternative therapy for acute exacerbation of COPD and pneumonia in adults.

Fluoroquinolones are active against many gram-positive organisms; gram-negative organisms, including Moraxella catarrhalis, Haemophilus influenzae, Escherichia coli, chlamydia, and Mycoplasma pneumoniae; and anaerobes. They are not active against Clostridium difficile.

How to Monitor

- Monitor renal, hepatic, and hematopoietic function during prolonged therapy.
- Patients on warfarin anticoagulation should be monitored closely for prothrombin times and INR at baseline—daily for the first week of therapy, and weekly thereafter. The patient should be instructed to report immediately any sign of bleeding.
- Patients on any theophylline product (e.g., theophylline, oxtriphylline, aminophylline) should have serum theophylline levels monitored because theophylline clearance may be decreased with concomitant fluoroquinolone use.
- Evaluate renal and hepatic function at baseline and every 6 weeks if therapy is to be continued.
- Monitor hematology parameters periodically for evidence of leukopenia, hemolytic anemia, and thrombocytopenia.
- Monitor for CNS side effects such as headache, weakness, shaking, dizziness, drowsiness, and confusion.

Patient Variables

GERIATRICS. Elderly patients are more likely than others to have reduced renal function, which increases the half-life of the fluoroquinolone. Dosages should be adjusted in patients with impaired renal function. Also, older adults are more prone to develop tendon rupture and adverse CNS reactions.

PEDIATRICS. These agents are not recommended for use in the pediatric age group (<18 years of age) because permanent articular damage has been documented in young experimental animals (i.e., dogs, rats, and rabbits), and transient arthropathies have been reported in children. However, data acquired over the past 10 years have shown a lack of effect in humans. This has led to the use of ciprofloxacin for the treatment of children with cystic fibrosis, for whom the benefit outweighs the risk. Ciprofloxacin has been approved by the FDA for the treatment of patients with UTI, including pyelonephritis. Ofloxacin and Ciloxan are drugs that are commonly used in children.

PREGNANCY AND LACTATION

- *Category C:* No adequate studies have been conducted. Use during pregnancy only if the potential benefit justifies the potential risk to the fetus.
- Fluoroquinolones reach breast milk concentrations equal to serum levels within 2 hours of administration. Because of the association of fluoroquinolones with articular damage, these agents are not recommended for use in nursing mothers.

DOSAGE IN RENAL IMPAIRMENT. Even though the fluoroquinolones are metabolized in the liver, elimination depends on renal function. Fluoroquinolones are excreted primarily through the renal system; adjustment of the dose is essential in patients with impaired renal function.

Patient Education

- The patient should be instructed to drink plenty of fluids while taking these products.
- Norfloxacin should be taken on an empty stomach. Ciprofloxacin and levofloxacin tablets can be taken without regard to meals. Levofloxacin solution should be taken on an empty stomach.

  Fluoroquinolones should not be taken with milk, antacids, iron preparations, or any product that contains aluminum, magnesium, calcium, iron, or zinc. Sucralfate, an aluminum salt of a sulfated glyceride, also should be avoided. Absorption of the fluoroquinolone can be reduced by as much as 98% by chelation; therefore, the drug should be taken at least 2 hours before or 6 hours after divalent or trivalent cation–containing products.

- Use caution when driving, operating machinery, or performing any task that requires attentiveness because fluoroquinolones can cause dizziness, drowsiness, or confusion.
- Avoid undue exposure to the sun, or use a sunscreen to prevent the occurrence of a photosensitivity reaction.

SPECIFIC DRUGS

ciprofloxacin (Cipro)

Cipro is the most commonly used fluoroquinolone in primary care. All fluoroquinolones share the following characteristics, except as noted.

CONTRAINDICATIONS

- Any indication of hypersensitivity to any of the fluoroquinolones
- Tendinitis or tendon rupture associated with quinolone use
- Patients receiving QT-prolonging drugs or drugs reported to cause torsades de pointes

WARNINGS

Phototoxicity: Moderate to severe phototoxic reactions have occurred in patients exposed to direct or indirect sunlight or to artificial ultraviolet light during or following treatment with all quinolones. These reactions have occurred with light through glass and with the use of sunblocks.

- Drugs with enhanced activity have been shown to prolong the QT interval in some patients.
- *Convulsions:* Increased intracranial pressure, convulsions, and toxic psychosis have occurred. CNS stimulation also may occur, and this may lead to tremor, restlessness, light-headedness, confusion, dizziness, depression, hallucinations, and, rarely, suicidal thoughts or acts. Use with caution in patients with known or suspected CNS disorders or other factors that predispose to seizures or lower the seizure threshold.
- *Tendon rupture/tendinitis:* Ruptures of the shoulder, hand, and Achilles tendons that required surgical repair or resulted in prolonged disability have been reported. Discontinue therapy if the patient experiences pain, inflammation, or rupture of a tendon.
- *Syphilis:* Ciprofloxacin, norfloxacin, and gatifloxacin are not effective for syphilis. High doses to treat gonorrhea may mask or delay symptoms of incubating syphilis. Test for syphilis before treating for gonorrhea.
- Pseudomembranous colitis has been reported.
- *Hypersensitivity reactions:* Serious and occasionally fatal reactions have occurred in patients—in some, after the first dose. Some reactions were accompanied by cardiovascular collapse, loss of consciousness, tingling, pharyngeal or facial edema, dyspnea, urticaria, and itching.
- *Renal function impairment:* Alteration in dosage regimen is necessary.

PRECAUTIONS

- *Crystalluria:* Needle-shaped crystals were found in the urine of patients on norfloxacin and ciprofloxacin. Ensure proper hydration to reduce the chance of renal irritation.
- *Hemolytic reactions:* Rarely, hemolytic reactions have occurred in patients with G6PD activity.
- *Myasthenia gravis:* Fluoroquinolones may exacerbate the signs, leading to life-threatening weakness of the respiratory muscles.
- Blood glucose abnormalities have been reported, most frequently in diabetic patients.
- Superinfection can occur.

PHARMACOKINETICS. Fluoroquinolones are well absorbed after oral administration and are widely distributed to most body tissues and fluids. High tissue concentrations are achieved in the kidneys, gallbladder, liver, lungs, cervix, endometrium, prostate, and phagocytes. High concentrations are achieved in the urine, sputum, and bile. Ciprofloxacin and ofloxacin also are distributed to skin, fat, muscle, bone, and cartilage and have been found to penetrate into the cerebrospinal fluid. See Table 62-2 for a comparison of pharmacokinetics in the fluoroquinolones.

ADVERSE EFFECTS. Fluoroquinolones generally are well tolerated. The most common adverse effects are GI (e.g., nausea, vomiting, diarrhea, abdominal pain), CNS (e.g., headache, dizziness, confusion, restlessness, sleep disorders, seizures), and dermatologic (e.g., rash, pruritus). Hypersensitivity is rare (Table 62-3). Levofloxacin offers a lower risk of phototoxic, cardiac, or hepatic adverse events than are seen with the other quinolones.

Continued

TABLE 62-2   Pharmacokinetics of Fluoroquinolones

Medication	Absorption	Time to Peak Concentration	Half-life	Protein Bound	Metabolism, %	Excretion
ciprofloxacin	60%-70%	0.5 hr	3-5 hr	20%-40%	20	Renal, 50%; bile, 20%-35%
norfloxacin	35%		3-4 hr	10%-15%	20	Renal, 30%; bile, 30%
levofloxacin	99%	1.5 hr	7 hr	30%		Renal, 75%
moxifloxacin	86%	2 hr	1-5 hr	40%		Renal, 22%
gemifloxacin	71%	1-2 hr	7 hr	60%-70%	Minimal liver; CYP none	Feces, 60%; renal, 40%

TABLE 62-3   Adverse Effects of Fluoroquinolones

Body System	Common Minor Effects	Serious Adverse Reactions
Body, general	Fever, edema	Superinfections
Skin, appendages	Rash, pruritus, phototoxicity	
Hypersensitivity		Anaphylaxis, urticaria, toxic epidermal necrolysis, Stevens-Johnson syndrome, exfoliative dermatitis
Cardiovascular	Palpitations	Enhanced activity against *S. pneumo*—prolong the QT interval
GI	Nausea, abdominal pain, diarrhea, vomiting, dry/painful mouth, dyspepsia, constipation, flatulence	Pseudomembranous colitis
Hemic and lymphatic		Leukopenia, eosinophilia, G6PD—hemolytic reactions
Metabolic and nutritional		Hypoglycemia
Musculoskeletal		Rupture of shoulder, hand, and Achilles tendons
CNS	Headache, dizziness, fatigue/lethargy/malaise, somnolence/drowsiness, insomnia, paresthesias, light-headedness	Seizure, increased intracranial pressure, toxic psychosis, CNS stimulation, tremor, restlessness, confusion, depression, hallucination
Special senses		Visual disturbances
Hepatic		↑ LFTs
Genitourinary		↑ BUN, creatinine, renal failure, crystalluria (rare)

ciprofloxacin (Cipro) 🗝 —cont'd

DRUG INTERACTIONS. See Table 62-4. Antacids, vitamins, enteral formulas, sucralfate, and other medications that contain divalent or trivalent cations (e.g., magnesium, calcium, aluminum, zinc) significantly reduce the absorption of fluoroquinolones. Fluoroquinolones should be given 2 hours before or 6 hours after administration of these products. Ciprofloxacin is available in an extended-release form to be given once a day. Levofloxacin may be given once a day at a 750-mg dose. Levofloxacin 750 mg po daily × 5 days has been shown to be as effective in sinusitis as 500 mg po × 10 days.

OVERDOSAGE. Overdosage of the fluoroquinolones may result in confusion, hallucinations, seizures, and renal failure.

OTHER DRUGS IN CLASS

Other drugs in this class similar to the key drug except in the following ways:

- Fluoroquinolones with enhanced activity against *S. pneumoniae:* All are useful for moderate to severe respiratory infection. Oral dosing can prevent hospitalization for IV antibiotics.
- All have risks of cardiac adverse effects such as QT prolongation and torsades de pointes—levofloxacin less than the others.
- *Levofloxacin* has less risk of hepatic adverse events than do the other quinolones.
- *Levofloxacin* and moxifloxacin have less potential to cause seizures and less phototoxicity.
- *Gatifloxacin* can cause hyperglycemia and hypoglycemia, usually in diabetic patients; the risk of *C. diff* is increased. This agent is no longer commonly used.

TABLE 62-4 Drug Interactions With Fluoroquinolones

Fluoroquinolone	Action on Other Drugs
Fluoroquinolones moxifloxacin ciprofloxacin, norfloxacin ciprofloxacin, norfloxacin	↑ theophylline ↓ Antiarrhythmic agents ↑ caffeine ↑ cyclosporine

Drug	Action on Fluoroquinolone
cimetidine	↑ fluoroquinolones
sucralfate, iron salts	↓ fluoroquinolone
probenecid	↑ norfloxacin
nitrofurantoin	↓ norfloxacin

- *Gemifloxacin* causes a higher incidence of rash than do the other fluoroquinolones, especially in young women; it is more expensive than the other fluoroquinolones.

evolve A continually updated list of useful WebLinks may be found in the Evolve Resources at http://evolve.elsevier.com/Edmunds/NP/

NOTE

Warnings have been issued for some fluoroquinolone antibiotics for the increased risk of tendon ruptures of shoulder, hand, Achilles, and other tendons in people older than 65 years, especially those receiving concomitant treatment with corticosteroids. These may occur during therapy or up to several months after discontinuation of drugs. There also may be rare risk for serious and potentially fatal adverse events that may occur after repeated doses. Patients should be advised to discontinue therapy if they experience related symptoms and to rest and avoid exercise until tendonitis and tendon rupture have been ruled out. The products identified with increased risk are second-generation quinolones ciprofloxacin (*Cipro* [tablets/oral suspension], intravenous injection [*Cipro IV*], and extended-release tablets [*Cipro XR*]; and ofloxacin [*Floxin* tablets] and the third-generation quinolone levofloxacin [*Levaquin* tablets, oral solution, injection, and injection in 5% dextrose]).

There is the risk for serious and occasionally fatal hypersensitivity reactions that may often occur after the first dose of a quinolone. These have included cardiovascular collapse, hypotension or shock, seizure, loss of consciousness, tingling, angioedema, airway obstruction, dyspnea, urticaria, and other serious skin reactions. There is a rare risk for serious and sometimes fatal events after multiple doses. Clinical manifestations may include one or more of the following: fever, rash, or severe dermatologic reactions (e.g., toxic epidermal necrolysis and Stevens-Johnson syndrome); vasculitis, arthralgia, myalgias, and serum sickness; allergic pneumonitis; interstitial nephritis and acute renal insufficiency or failure; hepatitis, jaundice, acute hepatic necrosis or failure; and anemia (including hemolytic and aplastic), thrombocytopenia (including thrombocytopenic purpura), leukopenia, agranulocytosis, pancytopenia, and other hematologic abnormalities. Treatment should be discontinued at the first sign of a skin rash, jaundice, or any other sign of hypersensitivity, and supportive measures should be instituted.

Treatment with antibacterial agents, particularly ciprofloxacin, ofloxacin and levofloxacin, can alter the colon's normal flora, leading to overgrowth of *C. difficile* and subsequent release of toxins A and B that contribute to the development of CDAD. Nearly all antibiotics have been implicated in CDAD, which may range in severity from mild diarrhea to fatal colitis. Because hypertoxin-producing strains of *C. difficile* can be refractory to antimicrobial therapy, they are associated with increased morbidity and mortality and may require colectomy. The FDA advises that CDAD be considered in all patients who present with diarrhea after antibiotic use. Careful examination of medical history is required because of the potential for late-onset disease; cases of CDAD have been reported more than 2 months after completion of an antimicrobial course of therapy. The FDA notes that current antibiotic therapy for the primary infection may need to be discontinued in patients with known or suspected CDAD. Appropriate fluid and electrolyte management, protein supplementation, antibiotic therapy for *C. difficile*, and surgical evaluation also may be required.

63 Aminoglycosides

DRUG OVERVIEW

Class	Subclass	Generic Name	Trade Name
Aminoglycosides	Gentamicin	gentamicin 🔑	Garamycin, G-Mycin
	Kanamycin	amikacin	Amikin
		kanamycin	Kantrex
		tobramycin	TobraDex, Nebcin
	Neomycin	neomycin	Cortisporin, Neosporin, Mycifradin
		paromomycin	Humatin
	Streptomycins	streptomycin	Generic

🔑, Key drug.

INDICATIONS

Oral

- Suppression of oral bacterial flora

Topical

- Irrigation of infected wounds

Parenteral

- Complicated UTIs
- Complicated respiratory infections
- Skin/bone/soft tissue infections
- CNS infection
- GI infection (peritonitis)

Susceptible Organisms

- *Acinetobacter*
- *Enterobacter*
- *Escherichia coli*
- *Klebsiella*
- *Proteus*
- *Pseudomonas*
- *Serratia*
- *Staphylococcus aureus*
  - *P. aeruginosa*

Streptomycin and amikacin also active against *Mycobacterium.*

Aminoglycosides generally are reserved for the treatment of patients with serious gram-negative infections that are resistant to other antibiotics. They normally are not used in primary care, but they are important antibiotics, and all providers should be familiar with their use. They are more potent than other antibiotics and are used systemically for serious infections. Aminoglycosides have a narrow therapeutic window, so careful dosing based on the pharmacokinetics of the drug is required. These agents are associated with significant nephrotoxicity (10% to 20%), ototoxicity (3% to 14%), and neuromuscular blockade (extremely rare). Aminoglycosides interact with β-lactam antibiotics, destroying the β-lactam ring, an amino group that renders both antibiotics inactive. They are excreted renally, so patients with impaired renal function are at increased risk for toxicity. Their use in treatment of infection is either IV or IM. Oral aminoglycosides are not absorbed; their only use is for suppression of intestinal bacteria in GI preoperative surgical preparation. Table 63-1 provides a summary of indications for each product. Aminoglycosides are used extensively in topical

preparations. Topical aminoglycosides are discussed in Chapters 11 and 12 for localized treatment of the eye, skin, ear, and so forth. Nine aminoglycosides are available in the United States. Aminoglycosides were derived from a soil actinomycetes bacterium that had been systematically screened for antimicrobials. Gentamicin is a mixture of three closely related constituents.

THERAPEUTIC OVERVIEW

Allergy

Allergic reactions are rare but may include anaphylaxis, toxic epidermal necrolysis, erythema multiforme, and Stevens-Johnson syndrome.

Resistance

Resistance is rare but can occur through enzymatic inactivation. As is described in Chapter 56, mutations can result in resistance, such as resistance of *Mycobacterium tuberculosis* to streptomycin. A mutation has allowed many *E. coli* to

TABLE 63-1 Indications for Aminoglycoside Agents

Indications	amikacin	gentamicin	kanamycin	neomycin	streptomycin	tobramycin
Systemic infections*	+	+				
Gram-negative bacteremia/sepsis	+	+				
Peritonitis	+	+				+
Meningitis	+	+				+
Pneumonia	+	+				+
Urosepsis	+	+			+	+
Tuberculosis	+				+	
Endocarditis	+	+			+	
MRSA/penicillinase-resistant strains						
Infectious diarrhea			+	+		
GI sterilization			+	+		
Pyoderma		+		+		
Superficial *Staphylococcus, Streptococcus, Pseudomonas* infections		+		+		

*Aminoglycosides are not first-line drugs and are used only in patients with life-threatening infection.

become resistant. Resistance also may result from decreased drug uptake or efflux pump activity.

MECHANISM OF ACTION

Aminoglycosides have a six-membered ring with amino group substituents. The term *aminoglycoside* refers to the glycosidic bonds between the ring and amino-containing sugars. Aminoglycosides are bactericidal antibiotics that strongly and irreversibly bind to the 30S subunit of bacterial ribosomes, blocking the recognition step in protein synthesis and causing misreading of the genetic code. The ribosomes separate from messenger RNA; cell death ensues.

TREATMENT PRINCIPLES

Oral Use

Aminoglycosides are used for suppression of GI bacterial flora and in the treatment of patients with hepatic coma.

Topical Use

Aminoglycosides have a wide variety of topical uses.

Clinically significant serum levels have occurred following topical use of aminoglycosides for surgical procedures (e.g., gut sterilization).

> **Irreversible deafness or renal failure may result from extremely high concentrations of aminoglycosides in the blood. Death may occur as the result of neuromuscular blockade following irrigation of small and large surgical fields with an aminoglycoside preparation.**

Consider potential toxicity when ordering aminoglycoside irrigation of a wound.

Parenteral Use

These medications are reserved for short-term treatment (<10 to 14 days) of patients with serious infection caused by susceptible strains of gram-negative bacteria, to minimize the risk of toxicity. Bacteriologic studies should be performed to identify causative organisms and their susceptibility to specific aminoglycosides. They may be considered as initial therapy in patients with suspected gram-negative infection; therapy may be instituted before the results of susceptibility testing are obtained. Clinical trials have demonstrated that some of these products are ineffective in infections caused by gentamicin- and/or tobramycin-resistant strains of gram-negative organisms. The decision to continue therapy with a particular drug should be based on the results of susceptibility tests, the severity of infection, the response of the patient, and the important additional considerations of state of hydration, renal status, and other medications that may be taken concomitantly.

How to Monitor

- Serum peak (drawn approximately 30 to 45 minutes after IV dosing; 60 minutes after IM dosing) and trough (drawn immediately before dosing) levels should be monitored after the second or third dose and every 3 to 4 days thereafter for the duration of therapy.
- During treatment, collect urine specimens for examination during therapy.
- Monitor serum calcium, magnesium, and sodium.
- Test eighth cranial nerve function by serial audiometric testing. Hearing loss in the high frequency range usually occurs.
- Monitor kidney function through creatinine and BUN values.

TABLE 63-2   Pharmacokinetics of Aminoglycoside Antibiotics

Drug	Absorption	Onset of Action	Time to Peak Concentration	Half-life	Duration of Action	Protein Bound	Metabolism	Excretion	Therapeutic Serum Level
gentamicin	Tissues good; CNS poor	1-2 hr	IV 30 min; IM 30-90 min	2-3 hr	8 hr	0%-30%	100% excreted unchanged	Renal	Peak, 5-10 mcg/ml; trough, 0.5-2 mcg/ml
amikacin	Tissues good; CNS poor	1-2 hr	IV 30 min; IM 1-2 hr	2-3 hr	8 hr	1%-10%	100% excreted unchanged	Renal	Peak, 15-30 mcg/ml; trough, 5-10 mcg/ml
kanamycin	Tissues good; CNS poor	Rapid	30 min-2 hr	2-4 hr		1%-10%	>90%	Renal	Peak, 15-30 mcg/ml; trough, 5-10 mcg/ml
neomycin	Tissues good; CNS and GI poor		2-3 hr	3 hr		0%-30%	Fecal	97% unchanged; renal, 3%	Not applicable
streptomycin	Tissues good; CNS poor	1-2 hr	IM: 1 hr	2-5 hr	24 hr	34%	100% excreted unchanged	Renal	Peak, 20-30 mcg/ml; trough, <5 mcg/ml
tobramycin	Tissues good; CNS poor	1-2 hr	IV: 30 min; IM: 30-60 min	2-3 hr	8 hr	<30%	100% excreted unchanged	Renal	Peak, 4-10 mcg/ml; trough, 0.5-2 mcg/ml

Patient Variables

GERIATRICS. Diminished glomerular filtration rate related to aging may prolong the drug's half-life and increase the risk of toxicity.

PEDIATRICS. Premature infants and neonates have immature renal systems, resulting in a prolonged half-life of aminoglycosides.

PREGNANCY AND LACTATION
- *Category C:* gentamicin, tobramycin, and amikacin
- *Category D:* neomycin, streptomycin, and kanamycin

Patient Education

- It is necessary to monitor blood values during therapy to ensure effectiveness and prevent toxicity.
- If any visual, hearing, or urinary problems develop, the health care provider should be contacted immediately; discontinue aminoglycosides if tinnitus or subjective hearing loss occurs.
- When IM injections are given, the injection site may be uncomfortable for a short time. Warm, moist heat to the area and mild analgesics may reduce localized pain.

SPECIFIC DRUGS

Because these medications generally are not used in primary care, only the more important information is presented. Dosage and administration are not discussed.

gentamicin (Garamycin)

CONTRAINDICATIONS
- Hypersensitivity

WARNINGS
- Aminoglycosides are associated with significant nephrotoxicity and ototoxicity.
- Carefully monitor BUN, creatinine, and creatinine clearance values. Recovery of renal function occurs if the drug is stopped at the first sign of renal impairment.
- Electrolyte imbalance may be seen as decreased serum levels of sodium, potassium, calcium, and magnesium.
- Superinfection (especially by fungi) may occur.
- It is essential to maintain adequate hydration, especially with children and the elderly.
- Hypomagnesemia occurs in more than one third of patients whose oral diet is restricted or who are eating poorly.
- Neuromuscular blockade can occur and may result in respiratory paralysis.

PHARMACOKINETICS. Table 63-2 compares the pharmacokinetics of aminoglycoside products.

ADVERSE EFFECTS. See Table 63-3. Serious adverse reactions are common, and their incidence varies for each aminoglycoside. Impaired renal function occurs in 10% to 20% of patients, ototoxicity in 3% to 14%, and

gentamicin (Garamycin) 🔑 —cont'd

vestibular toxicity in 4% to 6%. Muscle paralysis can occur with high parenteral doses.

DRUG INTERACTIONS. Drug serum levels are the best indication of toxicity. See Table 63-4.

TABLE 63-3   Adverse Effects of Aminoglycosides

Body System	Common Minor Effects	Serious Adverse Reactions
Body, general		Drug fever, ↓ calcium, sodium, potassium, magnesium
Skin, appendages		See Hypersensitivity
Hypersensitivity		Rash, urticaria, itching, anaphylaxis/anaphylactoid reaction
Respiratory		Apnea
Cardiovascular		Hypotension
GI	Nausea vomiting, diarrhea	
Hemic and lymphatic		Anemia, eosinophilia, leukopenia, thrombocytopenia, granulocytopenia
Musculoskeletal		Acute muscular paralysis
CNS	Headache	Encephalopathy, confusion, lethargy, disorientation, neuromuscular blockade, paresthesia, seizures, numbness, peripheral neuropathy
Special senses	Dizziness, tinnitus, vertigo, roaring in ears	Hearing loss/deafness, loss of balance, visual disturbances/blurred vision
Hepatic		↑ LFTs
Genitourinary		↓ Renal function

TABLE 63-4   Drug Interactions With Aminoglycosides

Aminoglycosides	Action on Other Drugs
Aminoglycosides	↑ Neuromuscular blockers, polypeptide antibiotics
Drugs	**Action on Aminoglycoside**
cephalosporins, vancomycin, loop diuretics, penicillins	↑ Aminoglycosides

OTHER DRUGS IN CLASS

Other drugs in this class are similar to the prototype except as follows:

• *neomycin (ingredient in Cortisporin, Neosporin):* Oral administration of neomycin decreases intestinal bacterial levels and may be useful in treating patients with bacterial diarrhea or preoperative bowel sterilization. It is used topically, otically, and ophthalmologically for superficial infection of the skin, ears, and eyes. Irrigation of the urinary bladder with neomycin is effective in preventing bacteriuria in patients with indwelling urinary catheters. Patients with UTIs should have a urine culture and sensitivity done for determination of appropriate antibiotic therapy. Superinfection (especially fungi) may occur. An irrigant is intended only for genitourinary use because irrigation of other wounds or sites increases the risk of systemic absorption. The risk of systemic absorption of the irrigating solution is increased when therapy exceeds 10 days, or when the patient has open wounds or mucosal excoriation. Poor absorption from the GI tract decreases the risk of systemic toxicity and negates the need for serum peak and trough levels. Neomycin and polymyxin antibiotic (Neosporin) combinations have a cumulative toxic effect when absorbed systemically.

evolve A continually updated list of useful WebLinks may be found in the Evolve Resources at http://evolve.elsevier.com/Edmunds/NP/

64 Sulfonamides

DRUG OVERVIEW

Class	Subclass	Generic Name	Trade Name
Sulfonamides	Short to medium acting	sulfisoxazole	Generic, Gantrisin
		sulfamethoxazole	Gantanol, generic
		sulfadiazine	Generic
		trimethoprim and sulfamethoxazole ([TMP/SMX]) 🔑 ✹	Bactrim DS, Septra DS
	Active in gut	sulfasalazine	Azulfidine, see Chapter 29
	Topical	sulfacetamide	See Chapter 12
		silver sulfadiazine	Silvadene

✹, Top 200 drug; 🔑, key drug.

INDICATIONS

See Table 64-1 for specifics.
- UTIs
- Acute exacerbation of COPD
- Pneumonia
- Traveler's diarrhea
- Diverticulitis
- Sinusitis

The sulfonamides have a wide antibacterial spectrum that includes both gram-positive and gram-negative organisms; they are most commonly used for UTIs. Sulfonamide therapy continues to have a place in the treatment or prophylaxis of specific clinical conditions such as *Pneumocystis* pneumonia, toxoplasmosis, isosporosis, typhoid fever, pertussis, nocardiosis, and listeriosis. Strains of community-acquired methicillin-resistant *Staphylococcus aureus* (CA-MRSA) have emerged as an important group of pathogens. Sulfonamides and tetracycline antibiotics remain valuable low-cost agents for use with most CA-MRSA soft tissue and skin infections.

Frequent allergic reactions and drug resistance limit the more extensive use of sulfonamides. Sulfamethoxazole is combined with trimethoprim (TMP/SMX) for its synergistic effect and is the most commonly used of the sulfonamides. Silver sulfadiazine is frequently used in wound infections and burns. Sulfonamides are divided into four classes. Two are systemic antibiotics (short acting and long acting); for topical infections and bowel problems. Short-acting agents are rapidly absorbed and rapidly eliminated. Long-acting agents are rapidly absorbed but are excreted slowly. No long-acting sulfonamides are currently available in the United States because of associated toxicity, especially seen as Stevens-Johnson syndrome.

Poorly absorbed sulfonamides are use to treat infections of the bowel and to prepare individuals for surgery. Topicals include sulfonamides that are not absorbed systemically; these are used topically, particularly in the eye and ear. The first antibiotic was a sulfonamide that was developed by the German dye industry; it was first used in 1932 against streptococcal infection.

THERAPEUTIC OVERVIEW

Allergy

Sulfonamide or "sulfa" allergy is fairly common, occurring in about 6% of the general population. Allergic reactions to sulfonamides are divided into type 1 (immediate hypersensitivity) and types 2 to 4 (IgG and IgM antibody, and T-cell mediated). Allergies occur to sulfonamide metabolites at the N1 and N4 amino nitrogen on the heterocyclic ring. Only the antibiotic sulfonamide drugs have this structure. Nonantibiotic sulfonamide drugs do not contain this structure. Although much concern has been expressed about cross-allergy with other drugs that contain a sulfonamide functional group, research has shown that this does not occur. A theoretical possibility remains that a T-cell–mediated allergy could possibly be related to the sulfonamide compound. This has not yet been demonstrated. The fact that people who have an allergy to a drug often have many allergies confuses the picture. For example, some patients have an allergy to penicillin and an allergy to cephalosporins that are not related. The data suggest that patients who are allergic to sulfonamide antibiotics do not need to avoid nonantibiotic sulfonamides.

Type 1 immediate sensitivity reactions include anaphylaxis, urticaria, angioedema, and hypotension that occur within 30 minutes of drug administration. Type 2 hypersensitivity (cytotoxic) reactions cause hemolytic anemias, neutropenias, thrombocytopenias, and vasculitides, which generally become

TABLE 64-1   Sulfonamide Indications With Dosage and Administration Recommendations

Drug	Bacteria	Site/Disease	Dosage
sulfisoxazole	*H. influenzae, S. pneumoniae, Pneumocystis jiroveci, Pneumocystis pneumoniae,* toxoplasmosis, isosporosis, typhoid fever, pertussis, nocardiosis, and listeriosis	UTI, otitis media, bronchitis, pneumonia, traveler's diarrhea, diverticulitis, sinusitis, dog bite	*Adult:* Loading dose 2-4 g, maintenance 4-8 g/day in four to six divided doses *Child (>2 mo):* Initial dose 75 mg/kg, then 120-150 mg/kg/day (maximum, 6 g/day) in four to six divided doses
sulfamethoxazole	Same	Same	*Adult:* 2 g initially, maintenance dose 1 g bid *Child (> 2 mo):* Initially 50-60 mg/kg, maintenance dosage 25-30 mg/kg bid
sulfadiazine	Same	Same	*Adult:* Loading dose 2-4 g, then 2-4 g/day in three to six divided doses *Child (> 2 mo):* Loading 75 mg/kg, maintenance 150 mg/kg/day in four to six divided doses; see detailed reference for further dosing information for infants and newborns
TMP/SMX	Same plus *Shigella flexneri*	UTI and otitis media, shigellosis (× 5 days)	*Adult:* 160 TMP/800 SMX q12h × 10-14 days; see detailed reference for further dosing information on other infections *Child (>2 mo):* Dose based on TMP component. Doses vary according to severity and location of infection. *Usual range:* 6-12 mg/kg/day TMP in two divided doses × 10 days

apparent within 7 to 14 days of administration. Type 3 hypersensitivity reactions affect entire organs. Skin, joints, and kidneys often are affected. Classic serum sickness syndrome (i.e., fever, vasculitis, lymphadenopathy, rashes, and urticaria) is also included in this category. These symptoms occur days to weeks after initiation of administration. Type 4 (cell-mediated or delayed hypersensitivity) is mediated by cytokines released by T cells. Maculopapular rashes, Stevens-Johnson syndrome, and toxic epidermal necrolysis are examples. These conditions usually take 48 to 72 hours to develop.

Resistance

Resistance is a common problem that limits the usefulness of sulfonamides. Streptococci, staphylococci, Enterobacteriaceae, *Neisseria,* and *Pseudomonas* are resistant. The single mechanism of resistance is random mutation, which results in overproduction of para-aminobenzoic acid (PABA) or structural changes in an enzyme. Transfer of resistance occurs through plasmids. Plasmid-mediated resistance has become more common, especially with trimethoprim. Resistance also is decreased by bacterial permeability.

MECHANISM OF ACTION

Sulfonamides are derived from sulfanilamide, which has a structure similar to that of PABA. PABA is necessary for bacteria to produce folic acid. Sulfonamides exert bacteriostatic activity. These are competitive antagonists that inhibit the enzyme responsible for the utilization of PABA in the synthesis of folic acid. This mechanism prevents reproduction of bacteria that synthesize folic acid. Those bacteria that do not require folic acid and those that can use folic acid absorbed from the GI tract are unaffected by the sulfonamides. Human cells are not affected by this mechanism because they do not synthesize folic acid. Trimethoprim bonds to dihydrofolate reductase, the required enzyme of dihydrofolic acid, to produce tetrahydrofolic acid, another enzymatic pathway that involves folate production.

TREATMENT PRINCIPLES

The increasing frequency of resistant organisms has limited the usefulness of the sulfonamides. Resistance develops quickly to sulfonamide alone, and cross-resistance is common. The addition of trimethoprim improves sulfonamide activity somewhat. Sulfonamide allergy is fairly common and can be serious with severe skin reactions. This also limits its usefulness. One advantage is low cost.

TMP/SMX is a first-line treatment for acute bacterial exacerbation of COPD and diverticulitis. It is an alternative treatment for dog and human bites, acute sinusitis, diarrhea, UTIs, and pyelonephritis.

Sulfonamides are active against some gram-positive and some gram-negative bacteria, but not against anaerobes. These agents may be effective against *Streptococcus pneumoniae, Moraxella catarrhalis, Escherichia coli, Klebsiella* spp, *Enterobacter,* and *Legionella* organisms.

How to Monitor

- Wide variation in blood levels may be seen with identical doses. Blood levels should be measured in patients receiving sulfonamides for serious infection.
- Patients should be observed very carefully for the development of severe adverse effects.
- Symptomatic evaluation should provide an indication of effectiveness.

Patient Variables

GERIATRICS

The use of TMP/SMX in the elderly results in an increased risk of severe reactions, especially when used in conjunction with other drugs or in those with impaired renal or liver function.

The most frequently reported severe adverse reactions in the elderly include skin reactions, bone marrow depression, and decreased platelets, with or without purpura. The elderly patient who is also taking certain diuretics, especially thiazides, may have an increased incidence of thrombocytopenia with purpura.

PEDIATRICS. Limited data are available on the safety of repeated courses of TMP/SMX in children younger than 2 months of age. Sulfonamides are not recommended in children younger than 2 months.

PREGNANCY AND LACTATION. *Category C/D:* Do not use at term (*category D*). Because TMP/SMX may interfere with folic acid metabolism, use during pregnancy only if the potential benefits outweigh the potential hazards to the fetus. Although it is not first-line therapy for asymptomatic bacteriuria or cystitis, TMP/SMX can be used during the second trimester.

Lactation: Excreted in breast milk

Patient Education

- Patients should be instructed to drink one 8-ounce glass of water with each dose and several times a day to prevent crystalluria.
- Take on an empty stomach with a full glass of water.
- Patients should avoid prolonged exposure to sunlight because photosensitivity may occur.
- Patients should notify the provider if hematuria, rash, tinnitus, dyspnea, fever, chills, or sore throat develops.
- *For patients taking the oral suspension:* Product should be shaken well and refrigerated after opening.

SPECIFIC DRUGS

trimethoprim and sulfamethoxazole (TMP/SMX) (Bactrim DS, Septra DS) 🔑

CONTRAINDICATIONS
- Hypersensitivity to SMX or TMP
- Megaloblastic anemia due to folate deficiency
- Pregnancy at term and lactation; infants younger than 2 months of age

WARNINGS
- Do not use to treat patients with streptococcal pharyngitis because of the greater incidence of resistance than with penicillin.
- *Hematologic effects:* Agranulocytosis, aplastic anemia, and other blood dyscrasias. Both TMP and SMX can interfere with hematopoiesis. In patients with G6PD deficiency, hemolysis may occur.
- *Hypersensitivity:* Although rare, fatalities associated with the sulfonamides have occurred as the result of hypersensitivity of the respiratory tract.
- Stevens-Johnson syndrome, toxic epidermal necrolysis
- Fulminant hepatic necrosis may occur.

☀ **Rash, sore throat, fever, arthralgia, cough, shortness of breath, pallor, purpura, and jaundice may be early signs of serious reactions. The drug should be discontinued at the first sign of any adverse reaction.**

TMP/SMX should be used with caution in patients with impaired renal or liver function and in those with chronic folate deficiency, asthma, or severe allergy.

Treatment with antibacterial agents, such as TMP/SMX can alter the colon's normal flora, leading to overgrowth of *C. difficile* and subsequent release of toxins A and B that contribute to the development of CDAD. Nearly all antibiotics have been implicated in CDAD, which may range in severity from mild diarrhea to fatal colitis. Because hypertoxin-producing strains of *C. difficile* can be refractory to antimicrobial therapy, they are associated with increased morbidity and mortality and may require colectomy. The FDA advises that CDAD be considered in all patients who present with diarrhea after antibiotic use. Careful examination of medical history is required because of the potential for late-onset disease; cases of CDAD have been reported more than 2 months after completion of an antimicrobial course of therapy. The FDA notes that current antibiotic therapy for the primary infection may need to be discontinued in patients with known or suspected CDAD. Appropriate fluid and electrolyte management, protein supplementation, antibiotic therapy for *C. difficile*, and surgical evaluation also may be required.

PRECAUTIONS. Use with caution in patients with possible folate deficiency (elderly, chronic alcoholics, anticonvulsant therapy, malabsorption, malnutrition), severe allergy, or bronchial asthma.

Superinfection may occur.

PHARMACOKINETICS. Sulfonamides are readily absorbed from the GI tract. They are distributed throughout the body tissues, entering the CSF, pleura, synovial fluids, and eye. Different patients bind sulfonamides to plasma proteins to varying degrees, resulting in wide interpatient variation in serum levels. These agents are not metabolized by the cytochrome P450 enzyme system in the liver but are metabolized in the liver via conjugation and acetylation. Patients who are slow acetylators have an increased risk of toxicity. Renal excretion occurs mainly by glomerular filtration. Table 64-2 provides information on pharmacokinetics.

ADVERSE EFFECTS. Hypersensitivity reactions are common. Although blood dyscrasias are relatively rare, they can be fatal.

The incidence of adverse effects due to sulfonamides is higher in patients with acquired immunodeficiency syndrome. Table 64-3 lists common adverse effects.

DRUG INTERACTIONS. In elderly patients receiving diuretics, especially the thiazides, the incidence of thrombocytopenia with purpura is increased. See Table 64-4.

OVERDOSAGE. Symptoms of overdose of TMP/SMX have not been reported. Signs and symptoms of overdose with the sulfonamides include anorexia, colic, nausea, vomiting, dizziness, headache, drowsiness, and unconsciousness.

Continued

TABLE 64-2   **Pharmacokinetics of Sulfonamides**

Drug	Absorption	Time to Peak Concentration	Half-life	Protein Bound	Metabolism	Excretion
sulfisoxazole	96%	1.5-3 hr	5-6 hr	90%	Liver	Kidney, 50%
sulfamethoxazole	100%	2 hr	11 hr	70%	Liver	Kidney, 14%
sulfadiazine	100%	3-6 hr	10 hr	40%	Liver	Kidney
trimethoprim and sulfamethoxazole	90%-100%	1-4 hr	SMX: 9 hr; TMP: 6-17 hr	SMX: 68%; TMP: 45%	Liver, 15%-40%	Kidney

TABLE 64-3   **Adverse Effects of Sulfonamides**

Body System	Common Minor Effects	Serious Adverse Reactions
Body, general		Chills, fever, lupus erythematosus phenomenon
Skin, appendages	Photosensitivity	Morbilliform, scarlatinal, erysipeloid, pemphigoid, purpuric, petechial
Hypersensitivity		Stevens-Johnson–type erythema multiforme, generalized skin eruptions, epidermal necrolysis, urticaria, periarteritis nodosum, serum sickness, pruritus, exfoliative dermatitis, anaphylactoid reactions, periorbital edema, conjunctival or scleral injection
Respiratory		Allergic decreased pulmonary function
Cardiovascular		Allergic myocarditis
GI	Nausea, vomiting, abdominal pain, diarrhea, anorexia	Pancreatitis, stomatitis, pseudomembranous enterocolitis, glossitis
Hemic and lymphatic		Agranulocytosis, aplastic anemia, thrombocytopenia, leukopenia, hemolytic anemia, purpura, hypoprothrombinemia, neutropenia, eosinophilia, methemoglobinemia
Musculoskeletal		Allergic arthralgia
CNS	Headache, insomnia, apathy, drowsiness	Peripheral neuropathy, mental depression, convulsions, ataxia, hallucinations, tinnitus, vertigo, polyneuritis, neuritis, optic neuritis, transient myopia
Hepatic		Hepatitis, hepatocellular necrosis
Genitourinary		Crystalluria, elevated creatinine, toxic nephrosis with oliguria and anuria

trimethoprim and sulfamethoxazole (TMP/SMX) (Bactrim DS, Septra DS) 🔑 —cont'd

DOSAGE AND ADMINISTRATION
- Total daily dose should not exceed 320 mg TMP and 1600 mg SMX.
- Decrease dosage in patients who have impaired renal function.
- See Table 64-1.

TABLE 64-4   **Drug Interactions With Sulfonamides**

Sulfonamide Product	Action on Other Drugs
Sulfonamides	↑ Oral anticoagulants, hydantoins, methotrexate, sulfonylureas, tolbutamide, uricosuric agents ↓ cyclosporine
TMP/SMX	↑ Diuretics, zidovudine

Drugs	Action on Sulfonamide Product
Thiazide diuretics, indomethacin, methenamine, probenecid, salicylates	↑ Sulfonamides

evolve A continually updated list of useful WebLinks may be found in the Evolve Resources at http://evolve.elsevier.com/Edmunds/NP/

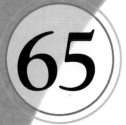

65 Antitubercular Agents

DRUG OVERVIEW

Class	Generic Name	Trade Name
Antitubercular	isoniazid (INH)	Generic (Laniazid)
	rifampin (RIF)	Rifampin, Rifadin, Rimactane
	rifabutin	Mycobutin
	rifapentine	Priftin
	pyrazinamide (PZA)	Generic
	ethambutol HCl (EMB)	Myambutol
	streptomycin (SM)	Generic
	cycloserine	Seromycin
	ethionamide	Trecator
	p-aminosalicylic acid (PAS)	Paser
Aminoglycoside	amikacin/kanamycin	Generic
	capreomycin	Capastat
Fluoroquinolones	levofloxacin	Levaquin ✸
	moxifloxacin	Avelox ✸
	gatifloxacin	Tequin

✸, Top 200 drug.

INDICATIONS

- Prevention and treatment of tuberculosis (TB)

This chapter discusses antibiotics commonly used in the prevention and treatment of tuberculosis. Their mechanisms of action differ and are discussed in the specific drug sections. No key drug is indicated for this chapter because all antibiotics differ from one other in many ways. The focus here is on the drugs used to treat patients with latent tuberculosis infection because this is an important component of primary care.

TB is a highly contagious, reportable disease whose treatment should be initiated by an infectious disease specialist. The primary care provider should be attentive to the possibility that patients may have TB, especially if they come from a high-risk population such as those with HIV/AIDS. These patients should be referred for initial workup and treatment. The primary care provider frequently follows the patient throughout the course of therapy.

THERAPEUTIC OVERVIEW
Pathophysiology

TB is caused by *Mycobacterium tuberculosis*, a thick-walled bacterium. The primary route of infection is inhalation of infectious particles. The bacilli are also spread to the lymphatic system and may lodge in bone or other organ systems such as the bone, bladder, or central nervous system. A cell-mediated immune response results in tubercle formation.

Disease Process

TB is an infection that has been known for centuries. Its incidence in the United States decreased between 1953 (84,000 cases) and 1985 (22,000 cases). This fall in statistics resulted from reactivation of old infections and the fact that TB became a disease of elderly persons. In 1992, however, more than 26,000 new cases were reported; this represented an 18% increase from 1985. Since 1992, the incidence of TB has slowly decreased, and in 2005, it slipped to its lowest since 1953 (14,000 cases). The current increase in incidence is linked to the increased prevalence of HIV infection and the increase in foreign-born immigrants in the United States. A nonimmunocompromised adult exposed to the disease (reacts positively to a tuberculin skin test) has a 10% risk of developing clinical illness or active TB. Patients infected with HIV, however, are significantly more likely to develop active disease and account for 30% to 50% of new cases. In 2006, the TB rate among foreign-born persons in the United States was 9.5 times that of those born in the United States.

Clusters of patients with TB are considered recently transmitted cases that occur within geographic localities, in demographic groups, or among individuals who share certain behaviors and lifestyles. Neighborhoods associated with clustered cases and recent transmissions tend to be characterized by low socioeconomic status, inadequate housing, and high rates of drug abuse, poverty, and crime. Unclustered cases are those most likely associated with reactivation of old infection; these usually are found in middle-class neighborhoods.

The most common site of TB infection is the pulmonary system. TB can also infect the bone, causing bone pain, and the urinary tract, causing UTI symptoms. It then can become disseminated, causing systemic symptoms. Pulmonary TB is seen predominantly in urban areas, whereas rural areas have an increased incidence of urinary and bone TB.

Reactivation disease occurs in a patient who was infected in the past. When the patient becomes old or immunocompromised, the disease may reactivate. This can occur in a patient with COPD who is taking prednisone (see Box 65-1 for risk factors for TB).

Assessment

Clinical symptoms of primary pulmonary TB include fever (70%), cough, pain in the chest when breathing or coughing, and cough productive of sputum or blood. General symptoms of TB, either pulmonary or disseminated, include weight loss, fatigue, malaise, fever, and night sweats. A child is likely to be asymptomatic or to present with a systemic infection rather than with pulmonary symptoms. In patients who have a history of TB, the clinician should always suspect reactivation; this accounts for approximately 90% of TB cases among non-HIV patients with TB.

TESTING FOR EXPOSURE TO TB. A patient with a positive test is considered to have a latent tuberculosis infection. The Mantoux tuberculin skin test is the preferred test for TB because it is the most accurate. The tine test should no longer be used. With the Mantoux tuberculin skin test, 0.1 ml of purified protein derivative (PPD) tuberculin containing 5 tuberculin units (TU) is injected intradermally to produce a discrete, pale elevation of skin 6 to 10 mm in diameter.

Criteria used for interpretation of the PPD are listed in Box 65-2. The test should be read 48 to 72 hours after the injection is given. Positive reactions may still be measurable up to 1 week after testing. If the patient returns after more than 3 days and the results appear negative, the test must be repeated. The test site is measured crosswise to the axis of the forearm. Only the induration (hardness) is measured. Erythema is not measured. The result is recorded in millimeters, not as positive or negative.

Candidates for testing include all high-risk patients (as indicated in Box 65-1) plus employees or residents in congregate settings, such as hospitals, prisons and jails, homeless shelters, and nursing homes, or people from areas of the world with a high prevalence of TB. Close contacts of someone with infectious TB who has a negative PPD should be retested 10 weeks after the contact. Previously, it was taught that the clinician should never give a PPD to a patient who had received a bacille Calmette-Guérin (BCG) vaccination. However, previous vaccination with BCG usually should not influence the need for tuberculin skin testing. Most patients who have received BCG have been told that they must never have a PPD because of the risk for a serious adverse reaction, thus they will refuse the PPD. Previous vaccination with BCG does not change the need for treatment or testing.

Patients who are immunocompromised should be evaluated for anergy prior to receiving the PPD. When a clinician elects to use anergy testing as part of a multifactorial assessment of

---

BOX 65-1 Patients at Risk for Tuberculosis

- Persons with HIV infection
- Close contacts of a person with infectious TB
- Persons with certain medical conditions that decrease resistance to infection, such as diabetes mellitus, lymphoma, certain GI surgeries, 10% below ideal body weight, chronic renal failure, certain cancers, silicosis, and immunosuppressive therapy
- Persons who inject drugs
- Foreign-born persons from areas where TB is common
- Medically underserved, low-income populations
- Residents and employees of long-term care facilities such as nursing homes and correctional facilities
- Locally identified high-prevalence groups such as migrant workers and the homeless
- Health care workers at risk for exposure to TB in the workplace

---

BOX 65-2 Criteria for a Positive Tuberculin Skin Test

- More than or equal to 5 mm induration
  - X-ray or clinical evidence of TB
  - Close contact of person with active disease
  - Evidence of old, healed TB lesions
  - Persons with HIV infection
  - Recipients of organ transplant
  - Persons with immunosuppression
- Greater than 10 mm induration
  - Children younger than 4 years old; children or adolescents exposed to adults at high risk
  - Foreign-born persons from high-prevalence countries
  - HIV-seronegative IV drug users
  - Persons with medical conditions known to increase risk
  - Employees and residents of long-term and health care facilities
  - Persons who inject drugs
  - Personnel of a mycobacteriology laboratory
- Greater than 15 mm induration
- All others

a person's risk for TB, FDA-approved methods include the Mantoux-method tests (mumps and *Candida*), which are used together and have cut-off diameters of 5 mm of induration (see http://www.cdc.gov/mmwr/preview/mmwrhtml/00049386. htm). Other protocols suggest that the mumps skin test antigen (MSTA) and tetanus toxoid (fluid) may be used. Give 0.1 ml of the antigen intradermally. Read at 48 to 72 hours. Any induration greater than 2 mm is considered positive (reactive), so PPD testing can proceed. Causes of a false-negative skin test include HIV, lymphoma, and recent live vaccinations.

The two-step method should be used in patients who may have diminished skin test reactivity, such as geriatric patients. The procedure is to give a PPD, which is followed by a second PPD in 1 to 3 weeks if the first is negative. Yearly administration of the PPD obviates the need for further two-step testing. If the first test is negative but the second is positive, the patient is considered to have a positive PPD. This reaction is commonly called "boosted." Evaluate elderly patients and high-risk employees with the two-step procedure. It is important to know whether a patient has truly converted from negative to positive, or if he or she was boosted by a two-step PPD to avoid the false impression of a conversion.

DIAGNOSIS OF TUBERCULOSIS. The chest radiograph is no longer a good screening tool for TB disease among low-risk persons, such as the Caucasian population born in the United States. However, in high-risk environments, such as a homeless shelter with a recent history of infectious TB among its residents, the radiograph may be a useful tool for screening contacts and symptomatic persons. A chest x-ray (CXR) examination should be obtained on all patients who have a positive PPD. Posteroanterior and lateral views should be obtained. An apical lordotic view should be obtained if the history is suggestive of TB and initial films are normal. A person with a normal x-ray is unlikely to have pulmonary TB, making the chest x-ray a very sensitive test. The diagnosis of tuberculosis in a child, especially a young child, presents many challenges.

X-ray examination is performed to detect lung abnormalities that indicate active disease. However, the films do not confirm that TB causes any detected abnormalities. A biopsy showing caseation granulomas would confirm the diagnosis. Previously, an annual chest x-ray was required for all persons with a positive PPD. Although state policies may vary, most people are considered cleared of TB indefinitely if their chest x-ray is clear, and another chest x-ray is required only if they again develop signs or symptoms of TB.

Culturing of the TB organism takes 6 weeks. Thus, for diagnosing TB and determining the severity of a patient's illness, TB control programs worldwide rely on the acid-fast bacilli (AFB) smear. In this test, a sample of sputum is inspected under a light microscope for the presence of tuberculosis bacteria. It is a fast, inexpensive, and simple method of diagnosing TB. Gastric aspiration also can be used to obtain specimens of swallowed sputum. Although this procedure is uncomfortable, it is more cost-effective and less invasive then bronchoscopy. It is the best way to obtain specimens from infants and from some young children who cannot produce sputum even with aerosol inhalation. When gastric aspiration is used to obtain specimens from children, the procedure should be done in the morning, before the patient gets out of bed or eats.

Positive results mean that a patient should immediately be placed in isolation in a hospital, because every cough could launch enough bacteria to infect many other people. Negative results must be interpreted in view of other findings or test results. Both theoretical and experimental results have cast doubt on the ability of the AFB smear to detect infected patients. Although as few as five TB bacteria in the lungs can start a new infection, a sample must contain 5000 to 10,000 bacteria per milliliter to reach the test's threshold of detection. Epidemiologic investigations confirm an elevated rate of TB among those exposed to patients who tested negative. Thus, awareness is growing worldwide that persons with negative smears but positive cultures of sputum cause a significant number of infections.

Direct examination of sputum samples reveals the presence of acid-fast bacilli. Patients with a positive smear are considered contagious. Culturing sputum, which takes 6 weeks, yields the classic definitive diagnosis. A sputum test, the *Mycobacterium tuberculosis* Direct Test, can give results in 4 to 5 hours. However, this test misses TB in about 5% of cases, so a culture is still required.

In conclusion, the presumptive diagnosis of active TB is made when the patient has any of the following:
- Recent conversion to positive PPD associated with characteristic signs/symptoms
- Positive sputum smear
- Characteristic chest x-ray
- Biopsy showing caseating granulomas
- Some clinicians add HIV/AIDS to this list because of the high rate of concurrent infection of these patients with TB.

The confirmed diagnosis of active TB is made by a positive culture from any body fluid or biopsy specimen.

MECHANISM OF ACTION

All drugs used in the treatment of TB are antibiotics. Each drug is quite different. See section on a specific drug for its specific mechanism of action.

TREATMENT PRINCIPLES

Standardized Guidelines

- Centers for Disease Control and Prevention, Division for Tuberculosis Elimination: Targeted tuberculin testing and interpreting skin test results and treatment of tuberculosis, *CDC Fact Sheets* (available at www.cdc.gov/nchstp/tb).
- American Thoracic Society, Centers for Disease Control and Prevention, and the Infectious Diseases Society of America: *MMWR* 52(RR11):1-77, 2003 or reprinted in Treatment of tuberculosis, *Am J Respir Crit Care Med* 167:603, 2003.

Evidence-Based Recommendations

To prevent TB in high-risk people without HIV infection, isoniazid is given for 6 to 12 months (6 months was as effective as 12 months). Isoniazid increases the risk of hepatotoxicity compared with placebo.

For patients with newly diagnosed pulmonary tuberculosis, a 6-month course of chemotherapy with at least two drugs is recommended. Several regimens are available. Each regimen has an initial phase, which includes three or four drugs given for 6 to 8 weeks, followed by a continuation phase, with two drugs given for 18 weeks.

Cardinal Points of Treatment

TREATMENT OF LATENT INFECTION

- Isoniazid is the treatment of choice.
- In patients who are HIV infected, treatment generally begins as soon as TB is suspected and is modified according to the status of HIV disease.
- In patients who are not HIV infected, treatment usually is reserved until a definitive diagnosis has been made.

TREATMENT OF ACTIVE INFECTION

- Report all cases to local and state health authorities.
- Test and treat close contacts.
- Monitor closely to ensure that the patient is compliant and is responding to prescribed drugs.
- DOT (direct observed therapy) has the highest success rate.
- Administer multiple drugs to which organisms are susceptible.
- Add at least two new antitubercular agents when treatment failure is suspected.

Drug resistance to the medications commonly used to treat TB is a major problem. Over the past 40 years, many inner-city patients have frequently taken inadequate amounts of medication or have discontinued therapy prematurely, leading to bacilli that are resistant to many antitubercular drugs in these geographic areas. These resistant organisms then infect other people. The tubercle bacilli may be resistant to several of the standard antitubercular drugs, such as isoniazid, rifampin, and ethambutol. Some strains are resistant to all known antitubercular drugs. The incidence of resistance is high, and the patterns of resistance are different in different geographic locations. Thus, patterns of resistance determine local treatment, which continually changes in response to the development of new resistance.

TREATMENT OF LATENT TUBERCULOSIS. It is important to clarify who should receive preventive treatment. See Box 65-3 for risk factors for progression of latent tuberculosis. Anyone who has a risk factor should be considered for treatment.

Individuals at risk should be evaluated to rule out active TB. The health care provider should assess for a history of hepatitis, heavy alcohol ingestion, liver disease, or age older than 35—factors that will affect treatment choices. If the history is positive, LFTs should be performed to determine whether the patient has any contraindications to therapy. Risk vs. benefit must be weighed for each patient.

Treatment Options
- First-line drugs:
  - isoniazid, rifampin, rifabutin, rifapentine, pyrazinamide, ethambutol
- Second-line drugs:
  - cycloserine, ethionamide, streptomycin, amikacin/kanamycin, capreomycin, p-aminosalicylic acid (PAS), levofloxacin, moxifloxacin, gatifloxacin
- Dispense 1 month's supply of medication at a time. Monitor patient monthly.

If the patient has been exposed to TB that is known to be resistant, consult the local health department for treatment recommendations.

TREATMENT OF ACTIVE DISEASE. Report all presumptive or confirmed TB cases within 24 hours to your health department. Maintain respiratory isolation.

> **BOX 65-3** **Risk Factors for Progression from Latent to Active Tuberculosis Infection**
>
> Recent skin test converters
> Close contacts of individuals with infectious, clinically active TB
> HIV infection
> Radiographic evidence of previous TB
> Low body weight (10% below ideal)
> Chronic lung disease
> Diabetes mellitus
> Chronic renal failure
> Jejunoileal bypass
> Impaired immune system from disease
> Immunosuppressive agents—prednisone, TNF-α antagonists

A patient is assumed to be contagious in any of the following circumstances:
- Cough is present.
- The patient is undergoing cough-inducing procedures.
- Sputum smear is positive and until three negative sputum smears are obtained.
- The patient has been on therapy for at least a week.
- The patient is showing poor response to therapy.

To prevent the spread of TB in patients who are seen in a clinic setting, health care providers should (1) maintain a high suspicion for TB, (2) isolate suspected cases immediately, (3) see patients with TB when no patients who are at increased risk for TB are present in the clinic setting, (4) maintain proper ventilation in the facility, and (5) maintain a TB isolation room if patients with TB are seen frequently in the clinic.

Inpatient treatment guidelines were established by the CDC. Many states have introduced these treatment guidelines into law in order to protect the public safety.

Multidrug regimens are required for the treatment of TB. Initial therapy for TB usually consists of four drugs: isoniazid, rifampin, pyrazinamide, and ethambutol or streptomycin. It is essential to never add single drugs to a failing regimen. Generally, an infectious disease specialist initiates treatment and follows the patient.

Compliance is the key to successful treatment of tuberculosis. Direct observed therapy (DOT) is now the standard of care in many areas, including Maryland and New York City. In DOT, every dose of antitubercular medication taken by the patient is observed and supervised by a health care worker. Patients who are not compliant with medication therapy may be sent to prison to ensure that DOT is carried out. Emerging results from numerous state health departments suggest that DOT programs for TB reduce the prevalence of multidrug-resistant disease, cut the cost per case of individuals treated, and improve the rate of treatment completion.

 Health care providers and institutions that fail to recommend and register patients with TB for DOT when resources are available are probably unnecessarily putting their community at increased risk for TB.

How to Monitor

ISONIAZID PROPHYLAXIS. See patients on a monthly basis and ask about signs/symptoms of liver damage or other toxic effects, such as anorexia, nausea or vomiting, fatigue, weakness, new and persistent paresthesias of the hands and feet, persistent dark urine, icterus, rash, or elevated temperature. Obtain routine LFTs monthly for patients at high risk of developing INH hepatitis. These include patients older than 35 years, daily drinkers, those with concomitant medications toxic to the liver, and those with a history of liver disease. Discontinue INH immediately if a patient develops signs or symptoms of toxicity.

PATIENTS WITH ACTIVE TB. Obtain chest x-ray at baseline and at 6 months. Collect sputum smear and culture at baseline and monthly until negative. Measure levels of hepatic enzymes, as well as bilirubin, serum creatinine, CBC, platelets, and serum uric acid, at baseline and monthly in those patients who are taking INH, RIF, and EMB therapy for active TB.

Routine measurements of platelet count and hepatic and renal function are not necessary during treatment unless the patient has a baseline abnormality or is at increased risk of hepatotoxicity (e.g., hepatitis B or C virus infection, alcohol abuse). At each monthly visit, patients who are taking EMB should be questioned regarding possible visual disturbances such as blurred vision or scotomata; monthly testing of visual acuity and color discrimination is recommended for patients who are taking doses that on a milligram-per-kilogram basis are greater than those recommended, and for patients receiving the drug for longer than 2 months.

Patients who are taking specific drugs should be monitored for specific problems. For patients who are taking INH, obtain periodic ophthalmologic examinations; for those taking pyrazinamide, collect blood glucose levels (may be particularly difficult to control glucose levels of patients with diabetes mellitus [DM]); with ethambutol, monitor color vision for red-green at baseline and at 2 and 3 months; with streptomycin (second-line drug), obtain an audiogram before beginning the drug and at 2 and 3 months, and monitor drug serum concentrations of streptomycin; with cycloserine, monitor blood levels weekly in patients with reduced renal function.

Patient Variables

GERIATRICS. Patients are at increased risk for toxic effects, especially on the liver and the CNS.

PEDIATRICS. Treatment of infants, children, and adolescents with TB is similar to that provided for adults, with one exception. Ethambutol is not recommended unless routine eye examination can be performed.

INH, rifampin, and pyrazinamide are commonly used with children. Ethambutol is not recommended for use in children younger than 13 years unless benefit outweighs risk. Streptomycin is not recommended for use in children. Safety and dosage of cycloserine and ethionamide have not been established for pediatric use.

PREGNANCY AND LACTATION
- *Category C:* Treatment for TB with a three-drug regimen is recommended. Isoniazid, rifampin, and ethambutol are preferred. The risks of TB pose a greater risk to the fetus than do the side effects of drug therapy. Despite crossing the placenta, these drugs do not appear to exert a teratogenic effect.
- *Category D:* Aminoglycosides
  - *ethionamide:* Teratogenic effects demonstrated in animals
- INH, rifampin, pyrazinamide, ethambutol, and cycloserine all appear in breast milk. Breastfeeding should not be discouraged in women receiving isoniazid, rifampin, and ethambutol.

Patient Education

Patients should be given extensive education about the nature of the disease and the need to follow instructions exactly. The most important points are summarized as follows:

Compliance
- Take medication exactly as directed.
- Keep all appointments for follow-up.
- Adequate testing will be required to determine whether TB is being halted.
- Maintain respiratory isolation while contagious.
- Avoid intimate contact with others.
- Cough into tissue, and dispose of tissue in closed plastic bags.
- Do not share utensils or drinking glasses.
- Use good hand washing technique.
- Adhere to proper hydration, diet, rest, and exercise.

SPECIFIC DRUGS

isoniazid (INH) (generic, Laniazid)

CONTRAINDICATIONS
- Known contact with an isoniazid-resistant TB case
- Previous INH-associated hepatotoxicity
- Acute liver disease, severe chronic liver disease

WARNINGS
- Watch for hypersensitivity reactions.
- Monitor patients with renal or hepatic function impairment.
- *Carcinogenesis:* INH induces tumors in mice.
- Patients with seizure disorder who are being treated with isoniazid and malnourished patients or those predisposed to peripheral neuropathy should receive pyridoxine (10 to 50 mg/day). Peripheral neuropathy, characterized by paresthesias in the hands and feet, is a frequent dose-related adverse effect. Up to 44% of patients can develop this complication on a dosing regimen of 16 to 24 mg/kg/day. This reaction occurs more frequently in malnourished patients, diabetic patients, and alcoholics. Concomitant administration of pyridoxine is recommended in these patients to reduce the risk of neurotoxicity. Neurotoxic effects that are much less frequently reported include toxic encephalopathy and optic neuritis; these may occur in patients who are alcoholic and diabetic, those with seizure disorders, pregnant patients, and infants who are breastfed while the mother is taking INH.
- Ophthalmic examinations are recommended annually or with any visual symptoms.

PHARMACOKINETICS. Table 65-1 compares pharmacokinetics for all antitubercular products. INH is metabolized primarily by acetylation and dehydrazination. The rate of

TABLE 65-1 Pharmacokinetics of Major First-Line Antitubercular Medications

Drug	Absorption	Time to Peak Concentration	Half-life	Protein Bound	Metabolism	Excretion	Therapeutic Serum Level
isoniazid	Food may interfere with rate of absorption	1-2 hr	Variable (0.5-5 hr)	15%	Hepatic: acetylation; rate of metabolism genetically determined (slow/fast acetylators)	Urine (>75%)	1-7 mcg/ml
rifampin	Readily absorbed	2-4 hr	3-4 hr	80%	Hepatic	Bile, 70%; urine, 30%	3-41 mcg/ml
pyrazinamide	Well absorbed	2 hr	9-10 hr	Most tissues	Hepatic	Renal	9-12 mcg/ml
ethambutol	75%-80%	2-4 hr	2-4 hr	Most tissues	Hepatic oxidation	Renal, 50%; feces, 20%	Requires special assay
streptomycin	PO poor; IM rapid	1 hr (IM)	3-5 hr	34%	Renal glomerular filtration	Urine, 90%	*Peak:* 20-30 mcg/ml; *Trough:* <5 mcg/ml
cycloserine	70%-90%	3-4 hr	10 hr		Hepatic	Urine, 60%	25-30 mcg/ml
ethionamide	80%, rapid	1 hr	2-3 hr	30%	Hepatic	*Renal:* Active drug and metabolites	

acetylation is genetically determined, with approximately 50% of blacks and whites being "slow acetylators" and the rest rapid acetylators; most Eskimos and Asians are "rapid acetylators."

MECHANISM OF ACTION. INH is bacteriostatic for resting organisms and bactericidal for dividing organisms. It interferes with lipid and nucleic acid biosynthesis in growing organisms.

ADVERSE EFFECTS. Table 65-2 summarizes major side effects of all anti-TB products according to body system affected.

The most frequent adverse effects to INH involve the nervous system and the liver.

DRUG INTERACTIONS
- Isoniazid is a major CYP450 3A4 inhibitor and 2C19 inhibitor.
- Concomitant use of alcohol is associated with a higher incidence of hepatitis.
- Benzodiazepine activity may be increased.
- *disulfiram:* Acute behavioral and coordination changes
- *phenytoin:* Increased levels
- *carbamazepine:* Toxicity or INH hepatotoxicity may result.
- *ketoconazole:* Serum concentration decreased
- *Anticoagulants, oral:* Activity may be enhanced.
- *cycloserine:* Increased CNS side effects, especially dizziness
- *meperidine:* Hypotension or CNS depression
- *rifampin:* High rate of hepatotoxicity
- *Aluminum-containing antacids:* Reduce oral absorption, administer separately
- INH has some MAOI activity and may cause interactions with tyramine-containing foods. Diamine oxidase also may be inhibited, causing reactions to foods that contain histamine.

OVERDOSAGE. Symptoms of nausea, vomiting, dizziness, slurring of speech, blurring of vision, and visual hallucination are early signs. Later symptoms, including respiratory distress and CNS depression, can be fatal.

PATIENT EDUCATION
- Take on an empty stomach 1 hour before or 2 hours after a meal.
- Minimize alcohol consumption.
- Avoid foods that contain tyramine (see MAO inhibitors) and histamine (tuna, sauerkraut, and yeast extract).
- Notify health care provider if fatigue, weakness, nausea/vomiting, loss of appetite, yellowing of skin or eyes, darkening of urine, or numbness and tingling in hands or feet occur.

DOSAGE AND ADMINISTRATION. Table 65-3 indicates dosage, administration, and available formulations for all antitubercular products.

rifampin (RIF) (Rifadin, Rimactane)

CONTRAINDICATIONS
- *Hypersensitivity:* The use of rifampin to treat active TB was discussed in *MMMR*, March 2000, and is specifically contraindicated for patients who take any of the protease inhibitors or NNRTIs; rifabutin was contraindicated for patients taking the protease inhibitor ritonavir or the NNRTI delavirdine. New data indicate that rifampin can be used for the treatment of active TB in three situations: (1) in a patient whose antiretroviral regimen includes the NNRTI efavirenz and two NRTIs; (2) in a patient whose antiretroviral regimen includes the protease inhibitor ritonavir, and one or more NRTIs; and (3) in a patient whose antiretroviral regimen includes the combination of two protease inhibitors (ritonavir and either saquinavir hard gel capsule [HGC] or saquinavir soft gel capsule [SGC]). In addition, updated guidelines recommend that the dose of rifabutin should be substantially reduced (150 mg two or three times per week) when it is administered to patients who are taking ritonavir with or without saquinavir HGC or saquinavir

Continued text on page 684

TABLE 65-2   Adverse Effects of Major First-Line Antitubercular Agents

Body System	isoniazid	rifampin	pyrazinamide	ethambutol	streptomycin	cycloserine	ethionamide
Body, general		Stains urine orange-red		Fever, malaise, dizziness, headache			
Skin, appendages				Dermatitis, pruritus		Rash	Rash, alopecia
Hypersensitivity	Fever, rash, vasculitis				Rash, fever		
Cardiovascular						CHF	Postural hypotension
GI	Nausea, vomiting	Distress	Disturbances	Nausea, vomiting, anorexia, abdominal pain			Anorexia, nausea/vomiting, diarrhea, metallic taste, jaundice
Hematologic and lymphatic	Agranulocytosis, thrombocytopenia	Thrombocytopenia	Thrombocytopenia	Thrombocytopenia			Thrombocytopenia
Metabolic and nutritional			↓ DM control			Anemia: B_{12}, folic megaloblastic	
Musculoskeletal		Gout, myalgias, arthralgias	Gout, joint pain				
Nervous system	Peripheral neuropathy, numbness, tingling of extremities		Mental confusion			Drowsiness, somnolence, dizziness, headache, lethargy, depression, tremor, paresthesia, anxiety, vertigo, memory loss, seizures, possible suicidal tendencies	Depression, drowsiness, asthenia, peripheral neuritis, neuropathy, headache, tremors, psychosis
Special senses				Optic neuritis, loss of acuity, loss of red-green discrimination	Ototoxicity		
Hepatic	Jaundice, abnormal LFTs	Hepatic toxicity	Hepatic toxicity			Elevated LFTs	
Genitourinary		Hyperbilirubinemia			Nephrotoxicity		

TABLE 65-3   Dosage and Administration Recommendations for Antitubercular Drugs

Drug	Dosage	Administration
isoniazid	*Route:* PO, IM *Active TB (Adult):* 5 mg/kg once daily (10 mg/kg/day in one or two divided doses for disseminated disease); *Twice weekly*:* 15 mg/kg (maximum, 900 mg) *Three times weekly*:* 15 mg/kg (maximum, 900 mg) *Latent TB:* *Once daily:* 300 mg for 6 months (HIV negative); 9 months (HIV positive) *Twice weekly*:* 900 mg *Pediatric dose:* Active TB: *Once daily:* 10-15 mg/kg (maximum, 300 mg) *Twice weekly*:* 20-30 mg/kg (maximum, 900 mg) *Latent TB:* 10-20 mg/kg/day in one or two divided doses (maximum, 300 mg/day) *Twice weekly*:* 20-40 mg/kg (maximum, 900 mg) for 9 months Give as a single daily dose; may be divided Give pyridoxine (15-50 mg a day) while patient is on INH.	Take on an empty stomach, 1 hr before or 2 hr after a meal. Minimize alcohol consumption. Avoid foods that contain tyramine (see MAO inhibitors) and histamine (tuna, sauerkraut, and yeast extract).
rifampin	Oral and IV *Active TB:* *Once daily:* 10 mg/kg/day (maximum, 600 mg/day) *Twice weekly*:* 10 mg/kg (maximum, 600 mg) *Three times weekly*:* 10 mg/kg (maximum, 600 mg) *Latent TB:* as an alternative to isoniazid *Once daily:* 10 mg/kg (maximum, 600 mg) for 4 months *Active/Latent:* Pediatric (<12 yr): 10-20 mg/kg (maximum, 600 mg). May be given once daily or twice weekly	Take on an empty stomach, 1 hr before or 2 hr after meals. Avoid missing doses. May cause red-orange discoloration of body fluids.
rifabutin	*Adults:* 5 mg/kg (300 mg) Not approved for children 150 mg once daily OR 300 mg weekly in combination with amprenavir, idinavir, or nelfinavir 150 mg every other day OR 150 mg ORALLY three times weekly in combination with ritonavir 450 mg ORALLY once daily OR 600 mg three times weekly in combination with efavirenz 150 mg every other day OR 150 mg three times weekly in combination with saquinavir/ritonavir 300 mg once daily OR 300 mg three times weekly in combination with nevirapine	
rifapentine	*Adults:* 10 mg/kg continuation phase (600 mg) Intensive phase: 600 mg twice weekly × 2 months in combination with other antitubercular drugs (i.e., daily isoniazid pyrazinamide, and ethambutol) Continuation phase: 600 mg once weekly × 4 months in combination with isoniazid or appropriate agent *Child:* Appropriate dosing not established	
pyrazinamide	Oral (dose based on lean body weight) *Once-daily dose:* 15-30 mg/kg/day (maximum, 2 g/day) *Twice weekly*:* 50 mg/kg (maximum, 4 g) *Three times weekly*:* 25-30 mg/kg (maximum, 3 g) *Pediatric:* 15-30 mg/kg/day (maximum, 2 g/day); divide dose	Stress importance of not missing any doses. Store medication at 59°-86° F.
ethambutol	Initial treatment: (dose based on lean body weight) *Once daily dose:* 15-25 mg/kg/day (maximum, 1.6 g/day) *Twice weekly*:* 50 mg/kg (maximum, 4 g) *Three times weekly*:* 25-30 mg/kg (maximum, 2.4 g) *Pediatric dose (≥13 yr):* 15-20 mg/kg daily (1.0 g) See once-daily and twice-weekly dosing regimens above. *Re-treatment:* 25 mg/kg/day once daily; after 60 days of therapy, decrease dose to 15 mg/kg/day.	May cause GI upset; take with food. Aluminum-containing antacids may interfere with absorption; separate administration by several hours.
streptomycin	IM route only *Usual dose:* 15 mg/kg/day (maximum, 1 g/day) *Twice weekly*:* 25-30 mg/kg (maximum, 1.5 g) *Three times weekly*:* 25-30 mg/kg (maximum, 1.5 g) Adjust dosage according to renal function. *Pediatric dose:* *Once daily:* 20-40 mg/kg/day (maximum, 1 g/day)	Watch for symptoms of ototoxicity and nephrotoxicity.

Table continued on following page

TABLE 65-3   Dosage and Administration Recommendations for Antituberculosis Drugs (Continued)

Drug	Dosage	Administration
cycloserine	*Initial:* 250 mg twice daily for first 2 wk; 500 mg to 1 g daily in divided doses for 18-24 months (maximum, 1 g/day) *Pediatric dose:* 10-20 mg/kg/day (maximum, 1 g/day) in two divided doses for 18-24 months	Avoid alcohol consumption. Monitor blood levels.
ethionamide	*Oral:* 250 mg once daily × 2 days, then 250 mg bid × 2 days *Usual dose:* 750-1000 mg/day in three or four divided doses Concomitant administration of pyridoxine is recommended *Pediatric dose:* 15-20 mg/kg/day; take in two divided doses	May cause stomach upset, metallic taste, or loss of appetite. Take with food to minimize GI upset. Notify practitioner if GI effects persist. Keep in tightly closed containers.
amikacin/kanamycin	Adult and child: 15 mg/kg/day either daily or 2-3 times weekly *Child:* 15-30 mg/kg/day (1 g) IV or IM in one dose	Give IV or IM; monitor infusion or injection site.
capreomycin	Adult: 1 g daily Child: 15-30 mg/kg/day (1 g) daily	
p-aminosalicylic acid (PAS)	*Adult:* 8-12 g/day in two or three divided doses *Child:* 150 mg/kg/day in three divided doses (max 12 g daily)	
levofloxacin	*Adult:* 500-1000 mg daily *Child:* No information	
moxifloxacin	*Adults:* 400 mg daily *Child:* No information	
gatifloxacin	*Adults:* 400 mg daily *Child:* No information	

*Directly observed therapy.
For complete prescribing details, see *MMWR,* June 20, 2003 (available at http://www.cdc.gov/mmwr/preview/mmwrhtml/rr5211a1.htm) (Table 3).

SGC), and that the dose of rifabutin should be increased (either 450 mg or 600 mg daily or 600 mg two or three times per week) when rifabutin is used concurrently with efavirenz.

WARNINGS
- Hepatotoxicity with fatality has developed. Monitor liver function carefully. In patients with hepatic impairment, dosage should not exceed 8 mg/kg/day po or IV.
- Hyperbilirubinemia may occur.
- Porphyria may be exacerbated.
- Meningococcal resistance may emerge rapidly.
- Hypersensitivity reactions may occur during intermittent therapy, or if therapy is resumed after interruption.
- The drug may be associated with carcinogenesis.
- Monitor CBC and LFTs monthly, or as symptoms suggest that hepatotoxicity may be developing.
- Urine, feces, saliva, sputum, sweat, and tears may be colored red-orange. Soft contact lenses may be permanently stained.
- Thrombocytopenia has occurred, primarily with high-dose intermittent therapy or after resumption of interrupted treatment. It occurs rarely during well-supervised daily therapy. The condition is usually reversible, but fatalities have occurred.

MECHANISM OF ACTION. Rifampin inhibits DNA-dependent RNA-polymerase activity, thereby suppressing RNA synthesis. It can be bacteriostatic or bactericidal and is most active against bacteria undergoing cell division.

ADVERSE EFFECTS. GI symptoms and rash are common adverse effects. High doses may cause flulike syndrome, hematopoietic reactions, and other serious side effects.

DRUG INTERACTIONS
- *P450:* Rifampin is a strong inducer of 1A2, 2A6, 2B6, 2C8, 2C9, 2C19, and 3A4.
- Rifampin may decrease the therapeutic effects of the following drugs: acetaminophen, oral anticoagulants, barbiturates, benzodiazepines, β-blockers, oral contraceptives, corticosteroids, cyclosporine, disopyramide, estrogens, phenytoin, methadone, quinidine, sulfonylureas, theophyllines, and verapamil. (Consult a detailed drug prescribing reference to review the numerous drug interactions that can occur with rifampin.)
- Digoxin serum concentrations may be decreased by rifampin.
- Rifampin inhibits assays for folate and vitamin B_{12}.

OVERDOSAGE
- *Symptoms:* Nausea, vomiting, and lethargy. Liver toxicity may occur; patient must be hospitalized.

PATIENT EDUCATION
- Take on an empty stomach 1 hour before or 2 hours after meals.
- Avoid missing doses.
- May cause red-orange discoloration of body fluids
- Notify practitioner if flulike symptoms, yellow discoloration of skin or eyes, skin rash, or itching occurs.

DOSAGE AND ADMINISTRATION. See Table 65-3.

pyrazinamide (PZA)

CONTRAINDICATIONS. Hypersensitivity, liver damage, or acute gout

WARNINGS/PRECAUTIONS

- Inhibits renal excretion of urates and may cause hyperuricemia and gout
- Use with caution in patients with renal function impairment. Reduction in dosage is not usually necessary.
- Closely monitor patients with hepatic function impairment. Order liver function tests monthly or when any symptoms suggest the possibility of hepatotoxicity.
- In patients with diabetes, blood sugar control may be more difficult to attain.

MECHANISM OF ACTION. The mechanism of action is unknown. It may be bacteriostatic or bactericidal against M. *tuberculosis*, depending on the concentration.

ADVERSE EFFECTS. Mild arthralgia and myalgia are frequent. The most common serious adverse reactions are gout and hepatic toxicity.

DRUG INTERACTIONS. No P450 interactions are known.

OVERDOSAGE. Experience is limited. Liver toxicity may develop.

PATIENT EDUCATION. Patient reports fever, loss of appetite, malaise, nausea and vomiting, darkened urine, yellowish discoloration of skin or eyes, and pain or swelling of joints.

DOSAGE AND ADMINISTRATION. See Table 65-3.

ethambutol HCl (EMB) (Myambutol)

CONTRAINDICATIONS. Hypersensitivity or known optic neuritis; use in children, unconscious patients, or any other patients who may be unable to discern and revport visual changes.

WARNINGS/PRECAUTIONS. Renal impairment requires dose adjustment.

- *Patients with renal impairment:*
  - *CrCl >50 ml/min:* No dosage adjustment is needed.
  - *CrCl 10 to 50 ml/min:* Extend dosing interval to every 24 to 36 hours.
  - *CrCl <10 ml/min:* Extend dosing interval to every 48 hours.
- *Intermittent hemodialysis:*
  - 15 mg/kg po three times per week after hemodialysis

> **Visual testing should be conducted before ethambutol therapy is initiated and periodically while on therapy. Vision testing should be done on each eye individually and on both eyes together. It should include visual acuity, ophthalmoscopy, peripheral fields, and color discrimination.**

Hyperuricemia, with or without precipitation of gout, can occur with ethambutol therapy.

MECHANISM OF ACTION. Ethambutol impairs cellular metabolism, causing cessation of cell multiplication and cell death. It is bactericidal and is active[[[[[[only against *Mycobacterium*.

ADVERSE EFFECTS. See Table 65-2.

DRUG INTERACTIONS. At least 4 hours should elapse between doses of aluminum hydroxide–containing antacids and ethambutol. Aluminum salts may delay and reduce the absorption of ethambutol.

PATIENT EDUCATION

- May cause GI upset; take with food
- Aluminum-containing antacids may interfere with absorption; separate administration by 4 hours.
- Notify practitioner if changes in vision, blurring, red-green color blindness, or skin rash occurs.

DOSAGE AND ADMINISTRATION. See Table 65-3.

streptomycin (SM)

See Chapter 63, Aminoglycosides, for complete information.

MECHANISM OF ACTION. Streptomycin is a bactericidal antibiotic. It acts by interfering with normal protein synthesis.

ADVERSE EFFECTS. Ototoxicity and nephrotoxicity are serious adverse effects.

DOSAGE AND ADMINISTRATION. See Table 65-3. The drug is given by IM injection.

cycloserine (Seromycin)

WARNINGS/PRECAUTIONS

- CNS toxicity, dysarthria, or allergic dermatitis warrants discontinuation or reduction in dosage.
- Toxicity is related to high blood levels; the therapeutic index is narrow.
- In renal function impairment, cycloserine will accumulate and toxicity will develop.
- Anticonvulsant drugs or sedatives may be effective in controlling symptoms. Pyridoxine also may help.
- This agent has been associated with B_{12} and folic acid deficiency, megaloblastic anemia, and sideroblastic anemia.
- Monitor CBC, serum creatinine/BUN, and serum cycloserine concentrations monthly or as necessary to follow or confirm adverse effects.

MECHANISM OF ACTION. Cycloserine inhibits cell wall synthesis and can be either bacteriostatic or bactericidal.

ADVERSE EFFECTS. CNS symptoms such as convulsions, psychosis, somnolence, depression, confusion, hyperreflexia, headache, tremor, vertigo, and paresis are the most problematic.

DRUG INTERACTIONS

- isoniazid (increase in dizziness)
- Alcohol (increases risk and possibility of epileptic episodes)

- ethionamide
- pyridoxine, vitamin B$_6$

OVERDOSAGE
- *Symptom:* CNS depression

PATIENT INFORMATION
- Notify practitioner if signs of dizziness, mental confusion, skin rash, or tremor occur.
- Avoid alcohol consumption.
- May cause drowsiness; use caution when operating dangerous machinery

DOSAGE AND ADMINISTRATION. See Table 65-3.

ethionamide (Trecator-SC)

INDICATIONS. Treatment of tuberculosis when first-line therapy (INH, rifampin) has failed

CONTRAINDICATIONS. Hepatic impairment (severe) or hypersensitivity

WARNINGS/PRECAUTIONS
- Hepatitis occurs more frequently; monitor LFTs.
- Management of diabetes may be more difficult.
- Patients with a history of psychiatric illness such as depression should be closely monitored during ethionamide treatment. Psychotic disturbances, including mental depression, have been reported in patients taking ethionamide.

- Patients with a history of thyroid disease such as hypothyroidism should be closely monitored during ethionamide treatment. Ethionamide may cause or exacerbate hypothyroidism. Periodically monitor thyroid function tests of all patients during ethionamide treatment.

MECHANISM OF ACTION. Ethionamide probably inhibits peptide synthesis and is bacteriostatic or bactericidal, depending on concentration attained and susceptibility of the organism. It is highly specific against *Mycobacterium*.

DRUG INTERACTIONS. Temporarily raises serum concentrations of INH. May potentiate the adverse effects of other antitubercular drugs if administered concomitantly, especially with cycloserine. Avoid excessive ethanol ingestion because it may produce psychotic reaction.

PATIENT EDUCATION
- May cause stomach upset, metallic taste, or loss of appetite
- Take with food to minimize GI upset.
- Notify practitioner if these effects persist.

DOSAGE AND ADMINISTRATION. See Table 65-3.

evolve A continually updated list of useful WebLinks may be found in the Evolve Resources at http://evolve.elsevier.com/Edmunds/NP/

Antifungals

DRUG OVERVIEW

Class	Subclass	Generic Name	Trade Name
Azoles	Imidazoles	clotrimazole*	Lotrimin, Mycelex, Lotrisone
		econazole*	Spectazole
		ketoconazole* ✹	Nizoral
		miconazole*	Monistat
		oxiconazole*	Oxistat
	Triazoles	fluconazole ✹	Diflucan
		itraconazole	Sporanox
		voriconazole	Vfend
		posaconazole	Noxafil
	Allylamine	terbinafine*	Lamisil ✹
		naftifine	Naftin
	Benzylamine derivative	butenafine*	Mentax
	Polyenes	nystatin* ✹	Nystatin
		amphotericin B	Mycostatin
	Echinocandins	caspofungin	Cancidas
		micafungin	Mycamine
		anidulafungin	Eraxis
	Hydroxypyridine	ciclopirox*	Loprox
	Other	griseofulvin microsize and ultramicrosize	Gris-PEG, Grifulvin V

*Covered in Chapter 11, Dermatologic Agents.
✹, Top 200 drug.

INDICATIONS

- Onychomycosis
- Tinea
- Candida
- Histoplasmosis
- Blastomycosis
- Pneumocystosis
- Cryptococcosis
- Aspergillosis

A growing number of antifungals are now available for topical or oral use. This chapter discusses the oral antifungals most commonly used in the primary care treatment of two types of fungal infection: (1) endemic fungal infection, such as blastomycosis, histoplasmosis, and sporotrichosis, and (2) superficial fungal infection not responsive to topical therapy. Chapter 11 discusses the treatment of superficial fungal infections with topical antifungal agents. Several of the newer antifungals are administered parenterally and are used in specialty practice; these are not discussed here. Ketoconazole and itraconazole have black box warnings—itraconazole for CHF and 3A4 drug interactions, ketoconazole for hepatotoxicity and 3A4 drug interactions.

All antifungals are associated with a significant risk of serious adverse reactions and should be used with caution. The azoles are synthetic compounds with broad antifungal activity that are effective against most yeast and filamentous fungi. Many new antifungals are available for the treatment of invasive aspergillosis and other serious fungal infections refractory to other therapy, particularly in patients with HIV; these are used primarily by dermatologists or other specialists and are not discussed in this chapter. Amphotericin B is an older drug that is not discussed in this text because it is used primarily by specialists for progressive and potentially fatal fungal infections.

THERAPEUTIC OVERVIEW

Anatomy and Physiology

Fungi can be divided into two broad categories based on morphology: yeasts and molds. Yeasts are unicellular fungi that are typically round or oval and reproduce by budding. When buds do not separate, they form long chains of yeast cells known as *pseudohyphae*. Molds are multicellular colonies that are composed of tubular structures called *hyphae* that grow by branching and longitudinal extension. Some fungi are dimorphic and can grow as either yeast or molds, depending on environmental conditions.

Fungal and mammalian cells are eukaryocytes. In contrast to bacteria, which are prokaryocytes, eukaryocytes have a distinct nucleus, specialized organelles, and a protective cell membrane. A key difference between fungal and mammalian cells is the sterol used in the synthesis of their respective cell membranes—ergosterol in fungi, and cholesterol in mammals.

Pathophysiology

Mycosis is the presence of parasitic fungi in or on the body. Most fungi that are pathogenic in humans grow as yeast, are nonmotile, and with rare exceptions are not transmissible. Fungal infections can be superficial (confined to the keratinous layers), subcutaneous, or deeply invasive.

Disease Process

Fungal infections have increased dramatically over the past 20 years. This increase is associated with the widespread use of broad-spectrum antibiotics, a rise in the number of invasive procedures, immunosuppression associated with organ transplants and chemotherapy, the treatment of autoimmune disorders, and HIV. The HIV epidemic has radically altered the spectrum and frequency of fungal infections. Fungal infections in transplant patients and those with HIV tend to be severe and usually require treatment for a prolonged period of time.

TOPICAL FUNGI. Fungal infections of the nails remain prevalent, and the demand for treatment has increased as safer drugs have been developed. A factor that limits this treatment is the refusal of many health insurance companies to reimburse for these medications, which are expensive and must be used for an extended period. Infections of the nails are generally impervious to superficial treatment. Ciclopirox (Penlac) is a new topical medication that is effective for skin and nail infections; however, it is expensive (see Chapter 11).

Some tinea infections require systemic treatment. Tinea capitis (most commonly caused by *Trichophyton tonsurans*) usually requires systemic treatment. Tinea corporis (usually caused by *T. rubrum*) usually responds to topical therapy but may require systemic treatment. Tinea versicolor is caused by *Malassezia furfur* (also known as *Pityrosporum orbiculare*) and frequently requires systemic treatment.

Candida albicans is part of the normal flora of the mouth, vagina, and feces of most people. Overgrowth of candida organisms causes mucosal candidiasis, which may affect the mouth, esophagus, and vulvovagina. It is also frequently found on the skin, especially in skin folds. Vulvovaginal candida is discussed in Chapter 57. Topical candida is discussed in Chapter 11. Risk factors for invasive candidiasis (fungemia and endocarditis) include neutropenia, recent surgery, broad-spectrum antibiotic therapy, indwelling catheters (IV or bladder), and immunodeficiency. HIV infection should be suspected if the patient has invasive candidiasis.

ENDEMIC MYCOSES. The primary care provider should be aware of endemic fungal infections in rural and regional populations and should maintain a high index of suspicion. Some types of diagnostic cytology, such as skin scraping smears, are inexpensive and are easily done in the outpatient setting. Most of these fungi do not result in systemic infection in immunocompetent persons. Individuals who are immunocompromised, especially those with HIV, are at higher risk for infection. Other groups at risk include infants, young children, and the elderly. Although many fungal species have been identified, only the most common are discussed here.

Endemic mycoses are fungi that cause disease in healthy hosts. Infection is caused by inhalation of the organism from the environment during the mold phase. The clinical presentation is generally a nonspecific or atypical pulmonary infection. Many fungi are associated with geographic regions, and these patterns assist clinicians in making a clinical diagnosis. However, because many individuals travel, this information has become less reliable. The severity of disease depends on the amount inhaled and the immune response of the patient.

Histoplasmosis is caused by *Histoplasma capsulatum*, which is prevalent in eastern and central United States. It can be found in bird droppings and bat exposure along river valleys, especially the Ohio and Mississippi River valleys. Locations with a large bat population and many flocks of birds are more likely to be affected. It is common to find human infection in these areas. Most cases are asymptomatic or mild and go unrecognized. More severe infections present as atypical pneumonia. Progressive disseminated infections can be severe and may be fatal. Severe symptoms include marked prostration, fever, dyspnea, and loss of weight.

Coccidioidomycosis is caused by *Coccidioides immitis*, a mold that grows in soil in arid regions of southwestern United States, Mexico, and Central and South America. Few immunocompetent people get these infections, but among those who do, chronic pulmonary disease or death may occur. Clinical findings include respiratory tract symptoms with fever, chills, and arthralgia.

Blastomycosis is caused by *Blastomyces dermatitidis*. It is endemic to the south-central states that border the Mississippi and Ohio River basins, southeastern and midwestern United States, and Canada. Infection occurs primarily in healthy individuals during occupational or recreational contact with soil from streams and rivers. Although many may be asymptomatic, disseminated infection can cause lesions on the lungs, skin, and bones, and in the urogenital system. Patients may have primarily cutaneous symptoms, including papules, nodules, or plaques.

Pneumocystosis is caused by *Pneumocystis jiroveci*. This fungus is found in the lungs of many domesticated and wild mammals and is distributed worldwide in humans. It seldom causes illness in immunocompetent people. It causes an acute pneumonia in premature or debilitated infants in hospitals and underdeveloped countries, as well as in older children and adults who have weakened cellular immune systems, most commonly HIV. It is a frequent cause of death in patients with AIDS.

Cryptococcosis is caused by *Cryptococcus neoformans*, a yeast that is found worldwide in soil and in dried pigeon dung. It is acquired by inhalation. Immunocompetent people rarely develop clinically apparent pneumonia. Progressive lung disease and dissemination occur in patients with immunodeficiency, including HIV.

Aspergillosis is caused by *Aspergillus fumigatus*. The fungus can be found in soil and decaying vegetation and may invade items of food and water. This fungus often colonizes in burn eschar and detritus in the external ear canal. Clinical symptoms include bronchospasm and pulmonary infiltrates. It can become invasive, again most commonly in patients who are immunocompromised, such as those with HIV.

MECHANISM OF ACTION

The azoles are primarily fungistatic rather than fungicidal. They are classified as imidazoles or triazoles, depending on whether the azole has two or three nitrogens in the five-membered azole ring.

The primary antifungal effect of the azoles is inhibition of ergosterol synthesis. This is accomplished by disrupting C-14 α-demethylase, an enzyme dependent on cytochrome P450. Without ergosterol, fungal cell membranes become more permeable and leak cell contents. Cell growth and replication are thereby inhibited.

Terbinafine blocks the biosynthesis of ergosterol, an essential component of fungal cell membranes.

Griseofulvin is derived from a species of *Penicillium*. It is deposited in the keratin of diseased tissue, making it resistant to fungal infection. The diseased tissue is gradually exfoliated and is replaced by noninfected tissue. See Table 66-1 for a comparison of the mechanisms of action of commonly used antifungals.

TREATMENT PRINCIPLES

Standardized Guidelines

The Infectious Diseases Society of America has put forth guidelines for the treatment of patients with coccidioidomycosis or candidiasis (www.idsociety.org).

Evidence-Based Recommendations

- Onychomycosis
  - *Effective:* Oral terbinafine more than oral itraconazole
  - *Likely to be beneficial:* fluconazole (modest results), topical ciclopirox (mild cases involving the very distal nail plate)

Cardinal Points of Treatment

- Topical fungi are often resistant to oral treatment; in order of effectiveness, treatment may consist of terbinafine, itraconazole, or fluconazole
- *Endemic fungal infections:* In order of effectiveness, itraconazole and fluconazole
- Culture or microscopy should be performed whenever possible to confirm a diagnosis of fungal infection. A wide variety of tests are available, including the following:
  - Potassium hydroxide preparation (KOH), interpreted by both a dermatologist (KOH-CLINIC) and a laboratory technician (KOH-LAB)
  - KOH with dimethyl sulfoxide (KOH-DMSO); when combined with chlorazol black E (KOH-CBE), interpreted by a dermatologist
  - Culture with dermatophyte test medium or with mycobiotic and inhibitory mold agar (Cx)
  - Histopathologic analysis with the use of periodic acid–Schiff stain (PAS)
- If infection is unresponsive to empirical therapy, cultures must be obtained to confirm the diagnosis and rule out resistant organisms. Table 66-2 summarizes the drugs of choice for treatment of patients with fungal infection, depending on the identified organism. Use the least toxic drug possible for the particular infection. It is clear that these drugs have the potential for serious adverse reactions, and drug interactions are a problem.

TABLE 66-1   Classification and Mechanism of Action of Selected Antifungal Antibiotics

Class	Representative Drugs	Mechanism of Action and Antifungal Effects
Azoles	clotrimazole	Inhibition of fungal lanosterol 14-α demethylase, resulting in depletion of ergosterol and accumulation of toxic sterols in the fungal cell membrane; fungistatic
Triazoles	voriconazole	*Candida:* Time-dependent fungistatic *Aspergillus:* Time-dependent slow fungicidal
Polyenes	nystatin	Interaction with ergosterol, formation of aqueous channels, increased membrane permeability, and subsequent leakage of intracellular components; fungistatic and fungicidal properties
	amphotericin B	Fungicidal
Hydroxypyridine	ciclopirox	Inhibition of essential enzymes by creation of a large polyvalent cation through chelation, thus interfering with mitochondrial electron transport processes and energy production; fungicidal and fungistatic properties
Other antifungals	griseofulvin	Inhibition of fungal cell mitosis and nucleic acid synthesis and interference with the function of spindles and cytoplasmic microtubules by binding to α- and β-tubulin; fungistatic

Modified from Zhang AY et al: Advances in topical and systemic antifungals, *Dermatol Clin* 25:165-183, 2007.

TABLE 66-2 Oral Antifungals: Indications With Dosage and Administration Recommendations

Drug	Site/Disease	Dosage and Administration
ketoconazole	Candidiasis, histoplasmosis, severe tinea, onychomycosis	Adult: 200-400 mg po once daily Child (>2 yr): 3.3-6.6 mg/kg/day as single daily dose × 1-2 wk Candida × 2 wk; systemic 6 mo
fluconazole	Candidiasis	Adult vaginal: 150 mg as single oral dose Adult oral: 200 mg × 1 day, then 100 mg daily × 2 wk Adult esophageal: 200 mg × 1 day, then 100 mg daily × 3 wk
itraconazole	Onychomycosis Blastomycosis/histoplasmosis Aspergillosis	200 mg once daily for 12 wk 200-400 mg/day × 3 mo or longer 200-400 mg/day × 3-4 mo
terbinafine	Onychomycosis	Fingernail: 250 mg/day × 6 wk Toenail: 250 mg/day × 12 wk
griseofulvin	Tinea corporis, tinea cruris, tinea capitis Tinea pedis, tinea unguium	Adult: 500-1000 mg as a single or divided daily dose (microsize) (330-375 mg ultramicrosize) × 2-4 wk (tinea corporis); 4-8 wk (other uses) Adult: 750-1000 mg (microsize) or 660-750 (ultramicrosize) per day in divided doses for 4-8 wk (tinea pedis) and 4-6 mo (tinea unguium)

- The optimal duration of treatment with antifungal therapy is not clear. Depending on the infection, it may be continued for weeks, months, or, as is frequently the case in patients with AIDS, indefinitely.
- Fluconazole has been approved for single-dose treatment of vulvovaginal candidiasis, although the CDC continues to recommend that topical therapy with an imidazole-derivative antifungal is preferable because of the appearance of fluconazole-resistant candidiasis in patients with and without HIV.
- Terbinafine is not effective against *Epidermophyton floccosum*, *C. albicans*, or *Scopulariopsis brevicollis*.
- Griseofulvin is used for tinea infections of the skin, hair, and nails that are not responsive to topical therapy caused by *Trichophyton*, *Microsporum*, and *Epidermophyton* fungi. It is ineffective against other organisms, such as candidiasis, blastomycosis, coccidioidomycosis, and histoplasmosis. Griseofulvin used for tinea requires lengthy treatment, and recurrences are common. Topical treatment of tinea capitis is usually ineffective because the fungus invades the hair shaft. A once-daily dose of griseofulvin given for 4 to 6 weeks is usually effective.

How to Monitor

ALL ANTIFUNGALS
- Perform initial cultures. Assess response to therapy with repeat cultures as necessary.
- Assess for signs or symptoms of hepatitis such as fatigue, anorexia, nausea, vomiting, jaundice, dark urine, or pale stools.
- Perform LFTs before initiating therapy and periodically thereafter. In healthy individuals, testing should be done every 4 to 6 weeks. Patients at risk must be monitored carefully and may require biweekly testing.

AZOLES. Assess for inhibition of synthesis in patients treated with high-dose ketoconazole (androgen synthesis inhibitor) for prostate cancer. Patients receiving itraconazole 600 mg/day may experience adrenal suppression. High doses and/or prolonged therapy with itraconazole have been associated with hypokalemia and secondary ventricular fibrillation. In healthy individuals, single-dose therapy with fluconazole does not require LFTs prior to initiation.

TERBINAFINE. *Immunodeficiency:* Consider monitoring CBC in patients receiving treatment for longer than 6 weeks.

GRISEOFULVIN. Check baseline and periodic renal, liver, and hematopoietic function.

Patient Variables

GERIATRICS
- Elderly patients tend to be susceptible to hepatotoxicity and are likely to be on other medications that may interact with these drugs. Lower dosages of these products are required in patients with reduced renal function.
- Itraconazole oral solution is formulated with hydroxypropyl-β-cyclodextrin, which is eliminated by the kidneys. It should be not be used in patients with a creatinine clearance lower than 30 ml/min.

PEDIATRICS
- *ketoconazole, griseofulvin:* The safety of use in children younger than 2 years has not been established.
- *fluconazole:* Has been used in immunocompromised children 6 months and older.
- *itraconazole:* Has been used in children 6 months to 12 years of age with serious systemic infection. Safety and efficacy have not been established.
- *terbinafine:* Safety and efficacy have not been established.
- *griseofulvin:* >2 years; may produce estrogen-like effects in children, including enlarged breasts and hyperpigmentation of areolae, nipples, and external genitalia

PREGNANCY AND LACTATION
- *Category B:* terbinafine, not recommended; present in breast milk
- *Category C*
  - *ketoconazole, fluconazole (known teratogen), itraconazole (no studies to date), griseofulvin:* Teratogenic effects have been seen in animals.

- Women taking ketoconazole, fluconazole, itraconazole, or griseofulvin should use contraception during and for 2 months after therapy because of possible teratogenic effects.
- Women using oral contraception should be advised to use supplemental contraception, such as a barrier method, during and for 2 months after antifungal therapy.
- Excreted in breast milk; do not prescribe to nursing women

Patient Education

ALL ANTIFUNGALS

- Take as prescribed. Inadequate treatment periods may result in a poor response or early recurrence of symptoms.
- Immediately report any signs or symptoms of hepatitis such as fatigue, anorexia, nausea, vomiting, jaundice, dark urine, or pale stools.
- Griseofulvin and ketoconazole many cause photosensitivity.
- During treatment, avoid alcohol consumption and medications that contain acetaminophen.

AZOLES

- Do not take ketoconazole or itraconazole within 2 hours of taking antacids.
- Take fluconazole without regard for food or gastric acidity restrictions.
- Women of childbearing age should use contraception or abstain from sexual intercourse while on azole therapy.

GRISEOFULVIN

- Bioavailability improves when given with food.
- Headaches, if they occur, usually disappear with continued therapy or when griseofulvin is taken with food.
- Notify provider if skin rash or sore throat appears.
- May potentiate effects of alcohol

SPECIFIC DRUGS

AZOLES

Individual azoles have unique differences and are discussed separately.

Imidazoles

ketoconazole (Nizoral)

CONTRAINDICATIONS

- Hypersensitivity
- Fungal meningitis due to poor penetration into the CSF
- Concomitant use with oral triazolam, ergot derivatives, and cisapride

WARNINGS

- *Hepatic toxicity:* Asymptomatic elevations of plasma aminotransferase occur in less than 10% of patients on azole therapy.

> 💣 **Ketoconazole and rarely the triazoles can cause clinically significant and even fatal hepatitis. Therapy must be stopped immediately if signs or symptoms of hepatitis develop, or if laboratory evidence suggests persistent or progressive hepatic dysfunction.**

- In one series, the median time for development of symptomatic hepatitis associated with ketoconazole therapy was 28 days, but it sometimes occurred in as few as 3 days. Toxicity is usually hepatocellular, but a cholestatic or mixed pattern of injury may occur and is associated with an elevated alkaline phosphatase. Hepatic injury is usually reversible with recovery in several weeks to months after discontinuation of the drug.
- *Hypersensitivity reactions:* Anaphylaxis occurs rarely after the first dose. Other hypersensitivity reactions, including urticaria, have been reported.

PRECAUTIONS

- *Steroidogenesis:* Ketoconazole can directly inhibit adrenal cortisol and testosterone synthesis. Testosterone levels (and therefore levels of estradiol) are lowered by ketoconazole doses greater than 400 mg/day and are eliminated altogether with 1600 mg/day. A variety of hormonal disturbances, including low sperm counts, decreased libido, impotence, gynecomastia, and menstrual irregularities, may occur. High doses may inhibit adrenal cortisol production and, in rare cases, may cause adrenal insufficiency. These effects have been exploited therapeutically in the treatment of patients with prostate cancer or Cushing syndrome (hypercortisolism).
- These products require gastric acidity for dissolution and absorption. They should not be taken with antacids, anticholinergics, or H_2-blockers.

PHARMACOKINETICS. See Table 66-3.

ADVERSE EFFECTS. See Table 66-4. Ketoconazole is associated with the least favorable toxicity profile among the azoles.

DRUG INTERACTIONS. See Table 66-5.

DOSAGE AND ADMINISTRATION. See Table 66-6.

Ketoconazole: Bioavailability depends on an acidic pH for absorption. Administration with food may decrease absorption.

Triazoles

fluconazole (Diflucan)

CONTRAINDICATIONS

- Hypersensitivity; use with caution in patients with hypersensitivity to other azoles
- Pregnancy

WARNINGS

- *Hepatotoxicity:* See ketoconazole; incidence and severity are less with fluconazole.
- *Allergic/dermatologic reaction:* Anaphylaxis and exfoliative skin disorders have occurred rarely in patients with serious underlying conditions such as AIDS or malignancy while on fluconazole. In some cases, these problems have resulted in death.
- *Carcinogenesis:* Hepatocellular adenomas have been observed in rats.
- Fertility impairment has occurred in rats. This hormone change has not been observed in women treated with fluconazole.

TABLE 66-3 Pharmacokinetics of Selected Common Antifungals

Drug	Absorption	Drug Availability (After First Pass)	Time to Peak Concentration	Half-life	Protein Bound	Metabolism	Excretion
ketoconazole	Variable	—	1-2 hr	2 hr, then 8 hr	99%	Liver, 3A4 potent 1A2, 2C	Bile
fluconazole	100%	90%	1-2 hr	30 hr	10%	Liver, 2C and 3A4 inhibitor	Renal, 80%
itraconazole	*Solution:* give on empty stomach *Capsules:* give with food	55%-70%	2-5 hr	21 hr	99.8%	Liver 3A4	Renal; inactive metabolites
terbinafine	70%	40%	2 hr	36 hr	99%	Liver 2D6	Renal; inactive metabolites
griseofulvin	Variable	—	4 hr	—	—	No P450	—

PRECAUTIONS
- Reduce dose for patients with renal dysfunction.
- *Single-dose use:* Carries a higher incidence of adverse reactions (26%) when compared with intravaginal agents (16%)

PHARMACOKINETICS
- Food or gastric pH does not affect fluconazole.
- Fluconazole is excreted renally with therapeutic concentrations achieved in the urine.
- Fluconazole is unique among the azoles in that it crosses the blood-brain barrier and has good penetration into the CSF.

ADVERSE EFFECTS. See Table 66-4. Systemic side effects (26%) are more common than local symptoms associated with intravaginal imidazole or triazole (17%). Gastrointestinal side effects, which are the most common type (2% to 7%), may include transient nausea, vomiting, diarrhea, and abdominal pain. Headache (2% to 13%) and anaphylaxis (rare) have been reported with a single dose of fluconazole.

DOSAGE AND ADMINISTRATION. See Table 66-6. Administration of a loading dose on day 1 (give twice the usual daily dose) results in steady state concentration in 1 or 2 days instead of 5 to 10 days.

itraconazole (Sporanox)
CONTRAINDICATIONS
- *CHD:* Patients with evidence of ventricular dysfunction such as CHF or a history of CHF
- Coadministration of pimozide, dofetilide, quinidine, cisapride, triazolam, or oral midazolam, HMG-CoA reductase inhibitors metabolized by the CYP 3A4 system (lovastatin, simvastatin)
- Pregnant women or women contemplating pregnancy
- Hypersensitivity to azoles

WARNINGS
Cardiac dysrhythmia: Life-threatening cardiac dysrhythmia or sudden death has occurred in patients using pimozide or quinidine concomitantly with itraconazole or other CYP3A4 inhibitors.

- *CHF:* Itraconazole has a negative inotropic effect. Risk factors for CHF, including ischemic and valvular disease, COPD, and renal failure, should be taken into consideration.
- *Hepatotoxicity:* Hepatitis, including liver failure and death, has been reported. Monitor hepatic enzymes.
- *Hepatic function impairment:* Itraconazole is predominantly metabolized in the liver. The half-life is prolonged in patients with liver failure.
- *Bioequivalency:* Do not use itraconazole capsules and oral solution interchangeably. Drug exposure is greater with the oral solution.
- Patients with HIV may have decreased absorption of drug as a result of hypochlorhydria.
- *Renal function impairment:* Use with caution; monitor serum potassium.
- Itraconazole injection should not be used in patients with severe renal impairment or renal failure with a creatinine clearance <30 ml/min. Although itraconazole concentrations are not affected by changes in renal function, clearance of the vehicle hydroxypropyl-β-cyclodextrin) used in the injection is significantly decreased.
- Absorption is decreased with decreased gastric acidity. Do not take at the same time as drugs that decrease acidity.
- *Carcinogenesis:* Rats had a slightly increased incidence of soft tissue sarcoma. It has not been found in humans.

PHARMACOKINETICS. See Table 66-4. Absorption is reduced when administered with drugs that decrease gastric acidity. Therapeutic concentrations may persist in fingernails and toenails for up to 6 months after discontinuation of the drug.

ALLYLAMINE
terbinafine (Lamisil)
CONTRAINDICATIONS. Hypersensitivity

WARNINGS
- *Hepatic failure:* Rare cases of liver failure, some leading to death, have occurred. The severity of hepatic events may be worse in patients with liver disease.
- *Ophthalmic:* Changes in the ocular lens and retina have been reported. The clinical significance of these changes is unknown.

TABLE 66-4   Adverse Effects of Antifungals

Body System	ketoconazole	fluconazole	itraconazole	terbinafine	griseofulvin
Body, general	Fever, chills	—	Edema, fatigue, fever, hypokalemia	—	Fatigue
Skin, appendages	Photophobia, pruritus	Exfoliative dermatitis, Stevens-Johnson syndrome, alopecia	Rash, alopecia	Rash, pruritus, exfoliative, dermatitis, Stevens-Johnson syndrome	Photosensitivity
Hypersensitivity	Urticaria, anaphylaxis	Angioedema, anaphylaxis	—	Urticaria	Rash, urticaria, angioneurotic edema, erythema multiforme
Respiratory	—	—	Bronchitis/bronchospasm, cough, dyspnea	—	—
Cardiovascular	—	—	Arrhythmias, CHF, pulmonary edema	—	—
GI	Nausea, vomiting (5%), abdominal pain, diarrhea	Nausea, abdominal pain, diarrhea, dyspepsia, vomiting	Nausea, diarrhea, vomiting, abdominal pain, dyspepsia	Diarrhea, dyspepsia, abdominal pain	Oral thrush, nausea, vomiting, epigastric distress, diarrhea
Hemic and lymphatic	Thrombocytopenia, leukopenia, hemolytic anemia	Leukopenia	—	Neutropenia	Leukopenia
Metabolic	Lower serum testosterone	—	—	—	—
CNS	Headache, dizziness, somnolence	Headache, dizziness, seizures	Headache, dizziness, neuropathy	Headache	Headache, dizziness, insomnia, mental confusion, impairment of performance
Special senses	—	Taste perversion	Taste perversion	Ophthalmic changes, taste disturbance	—
Hepatic	Hepatic toxicity	Hepatic toxicity (less than other antifungals)	Hepatic toxicity	Hepatic toxicity	Hepatic toxicity
Genitourinary	Impotence	—	—	—	Proteinuria, nephrosis
Other	Suicidal tendencies, severe depression, gynecomastia, bulging fontanels	—	—	—	—

TABLE 66-5   Drug Interactions With Antifungal Agents

Antifungal	Action on Other Drugs
ketoconazole	↑ benzodiazepines, buspirone, carbamazepine, corticosteroids, cyclosporine, donepezil, nisoldipine, protease inhibitors, quinidine, sulfonylureas, tacrolimus, TCAs, warfarin, zolpidem ↓↑ Oral contraceptives ↓ theophylline
fluconazole	↑ alfentanil, zolpidem, benzodiazepines, buspirone, corticosteroids, cyclosporine, losartan, nisoldipine, phenytoin, sulfonylureas, tacrolimus, theophylline, TCAs, warfarin, zidovudine ↓↑ Oral contraceptives
itraconazole	↑ alfentanil, benzodiazepines, buspirone, calcium channel blockers, carbamazepine, cisapride, corticosteroids, cyclosporine, digoxin, haloperidol, HMG-CoA reductase inhibitors, hydantoins, oral hypoglycemic agents, pimozide, protease inhibitors, quinidine, rifampin, tacrolimus, tolterodine, warfarin, zolpidem
terbinafine	↑ caffeine, dextromethorphan ↓ cyclosporine
griseofulvin	↑ Anticoagulants, oral contraceptives, cyclosporine, salicylates
Drugs	**Act on Antifungals**
Antacids, didanosine, sucralfate, proton pump inhibitors, H$_2$-antagonists, isoniazid, rifampin	↑ ketoconazole ↓ ketoconazole
hydrochlorothiazide	↑ fluconazole
cimetidine, rifampin	↓ fluconazole
Hydantoins, antacids, proton pump inhibitors, H$_2$-antagonists	↓ itraconazole
cimetidine	↑ terbinafine
rifampin	↓ terbinafine
Barbiturates	↓ griseofulvin

TABLE 66-6   Oral Treatment of Selected Fungal Infections

Disease	First-Line Treatment	Alternative
Onychomycosis, fingernail	terbinafine 250 mg once daily × 6 wk	itraconazole 200 mg po daily × 3 mo fluconazole 150-300 mg po qwk × 3-6 mo
Onychomycosis, toenail	terbinafine 250 mg po once daily × 12 wk	itraconazole 200 mg po daily × 3 mo OR 200 mg bid × 1 wk/mo × 3-4 mo fluconazole 150-300 mg po every wk × 6-12 mo

Tinea capitis	terbinafine 250 mg po daily × 4 wk
	Child (10-20 kg): 62.5 mg once daily × 4 wk
	Child (20-40 kg): 125 mg once daily × 4 wk
	Child (>40 kg): 250 mg once daily × 4 wk
		itraconazole 3-5 mg/kg/day for 4-6 wk
		fluconazole 6 mg/kg/day for 3-6 wk
		griseofulvin:
		    Adult: 250 mg (ultramicrosize) po bid × 6-12 wk
		    Child: 20-25 mg/kg × 6-12 wk

Tinea corporis, cruris, or pedis	Oral therapy reserved for chronic or extensive disease
	Tinea pedis
	    fluconazole 6 mg/kg daily (child)
	    terbinafine 10-20 kg: 62.5 mg once daily × 4 wk; 20-40 kg: 125 mg once daily × 4 wk; >40 kg: 250 mg once daily × 4 wk; 250 mg once daily (adult)
	    itraconazole 5 mg/kg daily × 2 wk
	    griseofulvin 10-15 mg/kg daily × 4-6 wk (child); 250-500 mg (microsize) bid (adult) × 4-8 wk
	Tinea cruris
	    Oral therapy not necessary
	Tinea corporis
	    See above; treatment duration generally 2 wk	

TABLE 66-6 Oral Treatment of Selected Fungal Infections (Continued)

Disease	First-Line Treatment	Alternative
Tinea versicolor	ketoconazole 400 mg po single dose OR 200 mg daily × 5 days OR fluconazole 400 mg po single dose OR itraconazole 400 mg po single dose	
Histoplasmosis	itraconazole 200 mg once daily; may increase dose by 100 mg increments to a maximum 400 mg/day (divide doses); duration of therapy varies (1 day to >6 mo)	
Coccidioidomycosis, primary pulmonary	Severe—amphotericin B	ketoconazole/fluconazole 400 mg/day or itraconazole 200 mg bid; duration of therapy ranges from 3-6 mo for primary uncomplicated infection and up to 1 yr for pulmonary (chronic and diffuse) infection
Blastomycosis	itraconazole 200 mg once daily; may increase dose by 100 mg increments to a maximum 400 mg/day (divide doses); duration of therapy varies (1 day to >6 mo)	fluconazole (less effective) 800 mg/day × 6 mo
Cryptococcosis	itraconazole: *Pneumonia:* HIV positive (unlabeled use): Induction: 400 mg/day for 10-12 wk; maintenance: 200 mg bid lifelong *Meningitis:* Mild to moderate (unlabeled use): 200-400 mg/day for 6-12 mo (lifelong for HIV positive)	
Aspergillosis	itraconazole 200-400 mg/day	
Candida, esophageal	fluconazole 200 mg on day 1, then 100-200 mg/day for 2-3 wk; *Child:* 6 mg/kg × 1, then 3-12 mg/kg × 2 wk	itraconazole 100-200 mg once daily × 3 wk; continue dosing for 2 wk after resolution of symptoms; *Child:* 5 mg/kg daily × 2 wk (unlabeled)
Candida, oral thrush	fluconazole 200 mg once daily *Child:* 6 mg/kg × 1, then 3-12 mg/kg × 2 wk minimum	itraconazole oral solution: Vigorously swish 10 ml in the mouth for several seconds at a time once daily (20 ml total daily dose), or 10 ml bid × 1-2 wk in patients refractory to oral fluconazole; *Child:* Not recommended
Candida, vaginitis	fluconazole 150 mg po single dose; may repeat dose in 3 days if severe symptoms present	

- *Neutropenia:* Isolated cases of severe neutropenia have been reported but were reversible with discontinuation.
- *Dermatologic:* Isolated reports of Stevens-Johnson syndrome, toxic epidermal necrolysis
- *Renal function impairment:* Do not use with significant renal impairment because use of this drug in this population has not been studied.
- *Hepatic function impairment:* Not recommended for patients with chronic or active liver disease; assess liver function before prescribing

griseofulvin (Gris-PEG, Grifulvin V)

CONTRAINDICATIONS
- Hypersensitivity (5% to 7%)
- Hepatocellular failure, porphyria

WARNINGS
- Hypersensitivity has been reported in 5% to 7% of patients. It may include skin rashes, urticaria, and angioneurotic edema and necessitates withdrawal of therapy.
- *Prophylaxis:* The safety and efficacy of griseofulvin prophylaxis for fungal infection have not been established.
- *Carcinogenesis:* Liver tumors in mice, but not in other species
- *Fertility impairment:* Men should wait 6 months after completing therapy before attempting to father a child;

women should avoid risk of pregnancy while receiving therapy.

PRECAUTIONS
- *Prolonged therapy:* Renal, hepatic, and hematopoietic functions must be monitored periodically.

> **Penicillin cross-sensitivity: Because griseofulvin is derived from a species of penicillin, cross-sensitivity is possible; however, patients with known sensitivity to penicillin have been treated without adverse effects.**

- *Lupus erythematosus:* Exacerbation of lupus erythematosus and lupus-like syndromes has occurred in patients receiving griseofulvin.
- *Photosensitivity:* Patients on griseofulvin should take protective measures against the sun (i.e., sun block or protective clothing).

DOSAGE AND ADMINISTRATION. Absorbed better when taken with meals high in fat content. The ultramicrosize griseofulvin is better absorbed than conventional microsize griseofulvin.

> **evolve** A continually updated list of useful WebLinks may be found in the Evolve Resources at http://evolve.elsevier.com/Edmunds/NP/

The Immune System and Antiretroviral Medications

DRUG OVERVIEW

Class	Subclass	Generic Name	Trade Name
Antiretrovirals	Nucleoside reverse transcriptase inhibitors (NRTIs)	zidovudine (ZDV, AZT) 🔑	Retrovir
		lamivudine (3TC)	Epivir
		abacavir (ABC)	Ziagen
		didanosine (ddI)	Videx, Videx EC
		stavudine (d4T)	Zerit
		tenofovir disoproxil fumarate (TDF)	Viread
		zalcitabine (ddC)	Hivid
		zidovudine/lamivudine	Combivir
		zidovudine/lamivudine/abacavir	Trizivir
		emtricitabine (FTC)	Emtriva
	Nonnucleoside reverse transcriptase inhibitors (NNRTIs)	delavirdine (DLV) 🔑	Rescriptor
		efavirenz (EFV)	Sustiva
		nevirapine (NVP)	Viramune
	Protease inhibitors (PIs)	ritonavir (RTV) 🔑	Norvir
		amprenavir (APV)	Agenerase
		indinavir (IDV)	Crixivan
		nelfinavir (NFV)	Viracept
		saquinavir (SQV)	Invirase, Fortovase
		lopinavir/ritonavir (LPV/RTV)	Kaletra
		atazanavir	Reyataz
		fosamprenavir (f-APV)	Lexiva
	Second-generation PI	darunavir	Prezista
	Fusion inhibitor	enfuvirtide 🔑	Fuzeon, T-20
	HIV integrase inhibitor	raltegravir	Isentress

🔑, Key drug.

INDICATIONS

Nucleoside Analog Reverse Transcriptase Inhibitors (NRTIS)

- NRTIs in general are used in combination with nonnucleoside reverse transcriptase inhibitors (NNRTIs) or protease inhibitors for the treatment of patients with HIV infection.
- *zidovudine:* Reduces neonatal transmission of HIV and provides postexposure prophylaxis
- *lamivudine:* Treatment of patients with chronic hepatitis B
- *tenofovir:* In combination therapy with abacavir in newly treated HIV-infected patients and in those who have failed other antiretroviral regimens; for hepatitis B, some new studies suggest that these agents are not quite as effective.

Nonnucleoside Reverse Transcriptase Inhibitors (NNRTIS)

- Usually used in combination therapies for the treatment of patients with HIV infection

Protease Inhibitors (PIs)

- Usually used in combination therapies for the treatment of patients with HIV infection

Entry (Fusion) Inhibitors

- Enfuvirtide can be used as part of a medication regimen in patients with limited treatment options. Enfuvirtide should be used only in patients who have previously used other anti-HIV drugs and have ongoing evidence of viral replication.

The pandemic of HIV emerged approximately 25 years ago, and AIDS now has claimed more than 25 million lives worldwide. The recommended use of antiretroviral agents in clinical practice will continue to evolve as new information from clinical trials and research becomes available. Infectious disease specialists generally provide treatment for patients with symptomatic HIV infection because of the difficulty involved in keeping current with the latest treatment protocols. Primary care providers generally are concerned with prevention of transmission of the virus. Yet having knowledge of current drug therapies and their side effects is necessary because HIV-infected patients rely on their primary care provider to help them evaluate their complaints and to provide treatment to some of them even to a limited extent.

THERAPEUTIC OVERVIEW OF HIV AND RETROVIRUSES

Anatomy and Physiology

HIV is a retrovirus from the family of viruses referred to as lentiviruses. Retroviruses are viruses that replicate through the use of the reverse transcriptase enzyme, which allows the virus to incorporate its genome into that of certain host cells. This key enzyme transcripts the RNA into double-stranded DNA, and this results in insertion of the viruses' genomes into CD4 receptor–containing cells. The primary CD4 receptor–containing cells are tissue-based macrophages and helper T-cells. Three primary categories of human retroviruses have been identified: T-cell leukemia retroviruses, endogenous viruses, and human immunodeficiency viruses (HIV-1 and HIV-2). This chapter discusses in detail only HIV-1

Pathophysiology

The HIV virus attaches to the CD4 protein with the help of co-receptors (CXCR4 or CCR5) found on T-helper lymphocytes and other cells such as macrophages and dendritic cells. The HIV then fuses its membrane with that of the host cell and inserts its genetic material into the cytoplasm. The viral genetic material then is transcribed into double-stranded DNA called proviral DNA (Figure 67-1). The HIV enzyme, reverse transcriptase, is responsible for creating double-stranded DNA from viral RNA. Once produced, this DNA often becomes integrated into the chromosomal DNA of the host cell. The HIV DNA is expressed by the host cell's genetic machinery. Expression of HIV DNA creates new HIV RNA genetic material and messenger RNA. The messenger RNA codes for the development of HIV polyproteins that must be cleaved, or separated, into individual proteins by the HIV enzyme protease if infectious virions are to be produced. Once this occurs, new virions are assembled and bud from the host cell's membrane; they are able to infect new cells.

Disease Process

The defining stages of HIV infection through progression to AIDS have changed over the years as drug treatments have become extremely effective in preventing the opportunistic infections that once led to severe debilitation and death. The natural history of the disease follows this course: primary infection then early, middle, and advanced or late-stage HIV infection or AIDS (Figure 67-2).

The disease seems to be divided into a primary phase, which includes initial acute infection that almost always presents with a mild to moderate viral syndrome that often mimics such infections as infectious mononucleosis. This stage includes the development of antibody production and the stabilization of viral load levels. Early and middle stages of HIV infection can be fairly asymptomatic and represent the time when the virus entrenches itself in the architecture of the host's immune system. The virus during this time destroys normal lymphoid architecture and creates reservoirs that are difficult to eradicate despite the best drug treatment. CD4 and CD8 cells too undergo immunologic changes that render them useless in effectively killing and/or controlling HIV infection, leading to rapid HIV replication and mutation. It is during this stage that CD4 counts decrease dangerously to 200 to 300 cells/mm^3.

Advanced or late stages of HIV infection show continued falling of CD4 counts, with drops to 50 cells/mm^3. The patient experiences neurologic changes that are heralded by dementia, peripheral neuropathy, and myelopathy. Further immune system collapse occurs with the onset of recurrent opportunistic infections such as *Pneumocystis jiroveci, Cryptosporidium* diarrhea, *Mycobacterium avium* complex, and multiple viral primary or reactivated infections such as herpes simplex or varicella zoster. Chronic illness leads to constitutional disease with muscle wasting, weight loss, fevers, and

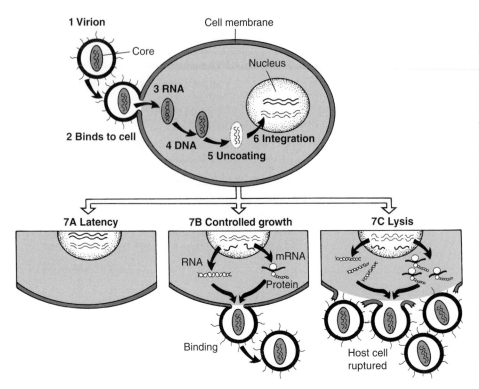

FIGURE 67-1 **Infection and cellular outcomes of HIV.** HIV infection begins (1) when a virion, or virus particle, (2) binds to the outside of a susceptible cell and fuses with it, (3) injecting the core proteins and two strands of viral RNA. Uncoating occurs, during which the core proteins are removed and viral RNA is released into the cytoplasm of the infected cell. (4) The double-stranded DNA (provirus) migrates to the nucleus, (5) uncoats itself, and (6) is integrated into the cell's own DNA. The provirus then can do a couple of things; it can (7A) remain latent or (7B) activate cellular mechanisms to copy its genes into RNA, some of which is translated into viral proteins or ribosomes. The proteins and additional RNA then are assembled into new virions that bud from the cell. The process can take place slowly while sparing the host cell (7B), or so rapidly that the cell is lysed or ruptured (7C). (From McCance KL, Huether SE: *Pathophysiology*, ed 2, St Louis, 1994, Mosby.)

severe fatigue. Malignancy with Kaposi's sarcoma is also seen. The compilation of AIDS and the sequelae of opportunistic infections results finally in death.

Assessment

The following baseline information should be obtained before a patient is started on antiretrovirals:

- Documentation of all medications and dosages
- Past history and current medical problems, including hepatitis, pancreatitis, and alcohol use
- Helper T-lymphocyte count (CD4) and plasma HIV RNA measurement. These studies help to assess a patient's immunologic status and severity of infection. They also provide a means of measuring the efficacy of therapy.
- CBC, including WBC with differential; also, evaluation of folate, vitamin B_{12}, ferritin, iron, and percentage of iron saturation
- LFTs and hepatitis B, C, and A serologies
- Rapid plasma reagin or VDRL test for syphilis
- *Amylase:* Triglyceride and lipase levels may be warranted in cases in which antiretrovirals that may cause pancreatitis are used (Table 67-1). An isoamylase fractionates the amylase into pancreatic and salivary amylase. This should be examined in patients with elevated amylase levels to differentiate salivary from pancreatic because some patients with an elevated amylase level are found to have elevated salivary amylase with normal pancreatic amylase. An elevated salivary amylase is not an indication of pancreatitis and therefore is not an indicator for stopping medication.
- *Triglyceride levels:* Hypertriglyceridemia often is seen in HIV infection. Elevated triglyceride levels have been reported in some patients before the development of pancreatic symptoms.
- *Pregnancy testing:* This will determine specific antiretroviral treatment choices.

- *Peripheral neuropathy:* A vitamin B_{12} level should be checked because vitamin B_{12} deficiency is common in HIV-infected patients. Use a 128-cycle/second tuning fork to obtain a timed vibratory sensation at the metatarsal joints of both great toes. A normal timed vibratory sensation is the ability to feel the vibration for longer than 10 seconds. Documenting a patient's timed vibratory sensation before starting an antiretroviral agent allows the practitioner to evaluate whether any changes in vibratory sensation may be due to antiretroviral agents that cause peripheral neuropathy.

MECHANISM OF ACTION

In the two decades since zidovudine (formerly known as AZT) was introduced, 21 additional agents in five drug classes have been approved; potent combination therapy has become a worldwide standard of care; morbidity and mortality in the developed world have been substantially reduced, and major antiretroviral regimens have been initiated throughout the developing world. Balanced against the progress that has been made is the identification of a surprising number of major toxic effects and recognition of drug class cross-resistance and the restrictions this places on alternate treatment regimens in the setting of treatment failure. Strict adherence is essential to prescribed therapy because nonadherence allows virus(es) to replicate to resistant strains.

Antiretroviral agents act to stop the production of new retroviruses by interfering with the ability of the retrovirus to replicate (see Figure 67-1). NRTIs disrupt replication of the virus at the point at which the virion is replicating its RNA to make DNA via the reverse transcriptase, the enzyme that copies viral RNA into DNA. NNRTIs resemble false nucleotides by binding within a mechanism to inhibit the reverse transcriptase enzyme activity. PIs prevent the protease enzyme from cleaving essential proteins into the HIV virion (see Figure 67-2). Fusion inhibitors prevent HIV

HIV life cycle

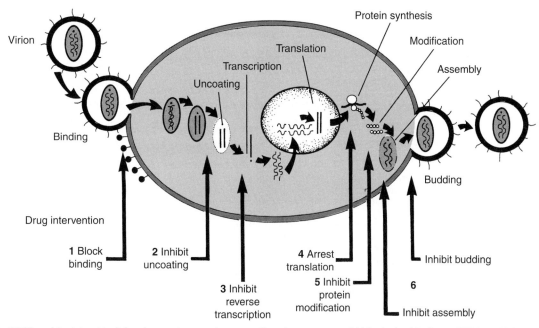

FIGURE 67-2 **HIV is subject to attack by drugs at several stages.** Certain agents could block the binding of HIV to CD4 receptors on the surfaces of helper T-cells (1). Other agents might keep viral RNA and reverse transcriptase from leaving their protein coat (2). Drugs such as AZT and other dideoxynucleosides prevent the reverse transcription of viral RNA into viral DNA (3). Later, antisense oligonucleotides could block the translation of mRNA into viral proteins (4). Certain compounds could interfere with viral assembly by modifying such processes (5), and finally, antiviral agents such as interferon could keep the virus from assembling itself and budding out of the cell (6). (Modified from Yarchoan R et al: AIDS therapies. In: *The Science of AIDS: Readings from* Scientific American, New York, 1989, WH Freeman.)

from entering target cells. Integrase inhibitors are also called *strand transfer inhibitors*. This refers to the process of DNA strand transfer from the viral genome to the host genome.

Highly Active Antiretroviral Treatment

The great progress that has been demonstrated in the treatment of HIV has been made through the use of different drug combinations or drug cocktails or highly active antiretroviral treatment (HAART). HAART therapy is used to describe the combination of multiple antiretrovirals to achieve the maximum effect in viral load suppression to a goal of undetectable viral load levels. When HAART treatment is given, the following management strategy is recommended when therapy must be changed:

1. Base changes on drug regimen on the following:
   - CD4 decline measured on two occasions
   - Virologic failure demonstrated by increases in HIV RNA viral load
   - Toxicity
   - Patient tolerance
   - Inability to comply with the regimen
2. Perform genotypic or phenotypic resistance testing while the patient is still on the old regimen, and use the results to help choose a new regimen.
3. Always change at least two of the antiretrovirals in the regimen.
4. Avoid choosing agents with resistance patterns that overlap those the patient has failed.
5. Avoid choosing agents with side effects similar to those to which the patient is intolerant.
6. Try to make the next regimen simpler if at all possible.

Genotypic or phenotypic testing is available as an in vitro tool to examine resistance of HIV to antiretroviral agents. Genotypic assays detect drug resistance mutations that are present in reverse transcriptase and protease genes. Phenotypic assays measure the ability of the virus to replicate within concentrations of the antiretrovirals. These assays facilitate selection of antiretroviral agents when drug regimens are changed. It is best to consult with an expert who can assist with interpretation of these results. The U.S. Department of Health and Human Services (DHHS) antiretroviral guidelines are a comprehensive reference for changing medications.

Individual drugs included in HAART therapy are discussed in the following paragraphs.

Reverse Transcriptase Inhibitors

Reverse transcriptase inhibitors prevent the HIV enzyme reverse transcriptase from creating HIV proviral DNA from viral RNA. This in turn prevents production of new viruses. Two primary categories of reverse transcriptase inhibitors have been identified: (1) nucleoside reverse transcriptase inhibitors (NRTIs) and (2) nonnucleoside reverse transcriptase inhibitors (NNRTIs).

NNRTIs must be phosphorylated within target cells to their active triphosphate form. It is important to note that the nucleotide analog reverse transcriptase inhibitor, tenofovir, is included in the same category as a nucleoside subclass. However, the structural difference between nucleotides and nucleosides is that the nucleotides already have a phosphate group, so only two steps of phosphorylation are required instead of three. Once these medications are in the active

TABLE 67-1 Baseline and Screening Laboratory Studies for HIV/AIDS

Laboratory Test	Frequency, Indication
CD4 count	At diagnosis, every 3-6 months, monitor response to antiretroviral
HIV viral load	At diagnosis, before treatment, 2-8 wk after start of new treatment
Complete blood count with differential	Every 3-6 mo, more frequently for low values and bone marrow toxicities (AZT)
Vitamin B_{12}	As needed for evaluation of B_{12} deficiency, neuropathy vs. HAART therapy–induced neuropathy
Serum chemistries	Every 3-6 mo, glucose monitoring every 3-4 mo. More frequently for abnormal values and those that cause hyperglycemia (all PIs, NRTIs, and NNRTIs). Lipodystrophy syndrome may be associated with increased lactate and alanine aminotransferase and lower levels of albumin, cholesterol, triglycerides, glucose, and insulin.
LFTs	Every 3-6 mo, more frequently for abnormal values and elevated LFTs (D4T, delavirdine, nevirapine, PIs). Increased bilirubin (indinavir). LFTs should be closely monitored with nevirapine at baseline, 2 wk × 1 mo, then monthly × 12 wk, and then every 1-3 months thereafter
Amylase/lipase	Every 3-6 months, monitor closely for pancreatitis
Lipid profile	Every 3-4 mo, monitor for patients taking PIs or NNRTIs. If increased at baseline, monitor within 1-2 mo of HAART initiation
Serum lactate	No current recommendations because of significant technical blood drawing difficulties. If patient symptomatic of lactic acidosis seen with NNRTIs, experts suggest evaluation will reveal hypercalcemia, increased anion gap, and elevated aminotransferase, CPK, LDH, amylase, and lipase.
Urinalysis	As indicated for indinavir, monitor for nephrolithiasis; UA may show crystalluria, increased urine pH, proteinuria, hematuria, and pyuria.

triphosphate form, they work through at least two mechanisms: chain termination and competitive inhibition.

Chain termination occurs when reverse transcriptase adds the reverse transcriptase inhibitor into the growing chain of HIV proviral DNA. Antiretroviral nucleoside analogs all have a modification in their sugar ring that prevents additional nucleotides (the building blocks of DNA) from being added. This stops the production of HIV proviral DNA, thereby preventing the formation of new HIV viruses.

Competitive inhibition of the endogenous nucleoside-5′-triphosphates is a process by which the phosphorylated reverse transcriptase inhibitor competes with and replaces the endogenous nucleoside-5′-triphosphates. The endogenous nucleoside-5′-triphosphates are necessary for the production of HIV proviral DNA. By competing with and replacing the nucleoside-5′-triphosphates, neither HIV proviral DNA nor new HIV viruses are produced.

NNRTIs do not require phosphorylation or intracellular processing to be activated. They are noncompetitive, binding to reverse transcriptase and inhibiting the function of this enzyme by binding at sites distinct from nucleoside binding sites.

Protease Inhibitors

One of the final stages of the HIV life cycle is the production of HIV polyproteins, for which coding is provided by the viral messenger RNA. These polyproteins must be cleaved or separated into individual proteins by the HIV enzyme known as protease if infectious virions are to be produced. Protease inhibitors block the HIV enzyme protease and thereby prevent certain HIV polyproteins from being cleaved or separated into the individual proteins necessary for the production of new infectious virions. This causes production of noninfectious HIV virions.

Fusion Inhibitors

Enfuvirtide is the first in a new class of medications called *fusion inhibitors* that work by preventing the AIDS virus from invading the white blood cells that are the primary targets of HIV. Entry fusion inhibitors work by attaching themselves to proteins on the surfaces of T-cells or proteins on the surfaces of HIV cells. For HIV to bind to T-cells, the proteins on the outer coat of the HIV must bind to the surface receptors on T-cells. Fusion inhibitors prevent this from happening. Some fusion inhibitors target the gp120 or gp41 or the CD4 protein or the CCR5 or CXCR4 receptors. If entry inhibitors are successful, HIV is unable to bind to the surfaces of T-cells and to gain entry into the cells. Enfuvirtide, the only FDA-approved fusion inhibitor, binds to the glycoprotein 41 molecule, which is involved in viral entry and prevents the folding mechanism or fusion required for entry into the cell.

HIV Integrase Inhibitors

The first of a new pharmacologic class of antiretroviral agents was approved at the end of 2007. Accelerated approval was given for raltegravir tablets (400 mg) used in combination with other antiretroviral agents for the treatment of HIV-1 infection.

New products are constantly under development and extensive research is in progress. A good deal of experimentation on effective drug combinations has been conducted. It will be essential for any clinician who treats HIV+ patients to consult the latest sources for prescribing and treatment information.

TREATMENT PRINCIPLES

Standardized Guidelines

- Guidelines from the International AIDS Society USA were updated for antiretroviral therapy in adults and were published in the August 13, 2006 issue of JAMA. (Hammer SM et al, International AIDS Society–USA Panel: Treatment for adult HIV infection: 2006 recommendations of the International AIDS Society–USA panel, JAMA 296:827-843, 2006.)
- The revised recommendations highlight four clinical issues: (1) when to start antiretroviral therapy, (2) which drugs to use in initial treatment, (3) when and how to change a treatment regimen, and (4) use of antiretroviral therapy in special circumstances.
- Monitor the National Guideline Clearinghouse for new recommendations at http://www.guidelines.gov/

Evidence-Based Recommendations

What are the effects of different antiretroviral drug treatment regimens in HIV infection?
- Beneficial
  - Boosted protease inhibitor–based regimens are at least as effect as standard protease–based triple regimens at reducing viral load.
  - Dual NRTI regimens are more effective than NRTI monotherapy but less effective than protease inhibitors or NNRTI-based triple regimens.
  - NNRTI-based triple regimens increase viral suppression compared with dual-NRTI regimens or protease inhibitor–based triple regimens.
  - Protease inhibitor–based triple regimens are more effective than dual-NRTI regimens and less effective at achieving viral response than NNRTI-based triple regimens.
  - Triple-NRTI regimens provide similar viral suppression to dual-NRTI regimens.
- Unknown effectiveness
  - Early vs. delayed treatment
  Monitor new EB findings, which are updated monthly at www.clinicalevidence.com

Cardinal Points of Treatment

- The latest guidelines continue to recommend initiation of therapy in all symptomatic persons and in asymptomatic persons after the CD4 cell count falls to below 350/mcl and before it declines to 200/mcl.
- Although the choice of specific antiretroviral agents should be based on the individual patient profile, guidelines recommend an NNRTI or a PI boosted with low-dose ritonavir, each combined with two NRTI inhibitors. Since the guidelines were last revised, available data have confirmed that four drugs generally are no better than three drugs when treatment with currently available NRTIs are used and PIs should be used in treatment-naive patients not infected with drug-resistant virus.
- Drug toxicity or intolerance or treatment failure mandates a change in therapy. The virologic target for patients with treatment failure is now a plasma HIV-1 RNA level lower than 50 copies/ml.
- Viral suppression to undetectable levels is the goal of treatment; current tests measure only to 50 copies on the ultrasensitive assay (or 75 on the common assay).

HAART generally should achieve this goal in 16 to 24 weeks. If viral load increases after initial suppression, patient adherence to HAART must be questioned. If viral resistance is suspected, genotypic testing is favored over phenotypic testing because of cost and ease of testing. The presence of resistance should be answered by inclusion of at least two medications active against the resistant HIV strain.

- If a patient is intolerant of a certain medication in HAART, it is reasonable to try to change only the offending agent, particularly in previously treatment-naive patients. Treatment interruptions or intermittent therapy is not recommended because of an increased risk for resistance.
- Special populations of patients infected with HIV include the following:
  - *Pregnancy:* Initiation of antiretroviral therapy should be avoided in the first trimester when possible, although women with HIV who are receiving stable regimens usually should continue treatment throughout pregnancy. Zidovudine, lamivudine, and emtricitabine are preferred NRTIs in pregnancy.
  - *tenofovir and emtricitabine:* Recommended in cases in which patients require treatment for both HIV and hepatitis B
  - *Infection with tuberculosis in patients with HIV:* Should be treated with a rifamycin-based regimen, and HAART should be selected with the prospect of drug interactions with antituberculosis agents in mind.
  - Adherence to antiretroviral therapy over the short term and the long term is crucial for treatment success and must be continually reinforced.

PROPHYLAXIS/PREVENTION. As given by the primary care provider, counseling regarding risks for HIV and AIDS should include providing patients with accurate information regarding prevention and prophylaxis. The patient should be made aware of the disease, its route of transmission, and, most important, how to prevent infection. Regimens change frequently, and the latest information should be followed.

Prevention of HIV infection, according to the CDC, is best accomplished by abstaining from sexual intercourse or by maintaining a long-term, mutually monogamous relationship with a partner who has been tested and who is confirmed uninfected (CDC HIV/AIDS Prevention Fact Sheet). Otherwise, the *correct* and *consistent* use of a male latex condom and the use of latex dental dams during oral sex with a female are other ways to reduce the risk of transmission. Eliciting information on sexual habits and counseling male and female patients on how to use a condom are effective ways to promote safe sexual behavior.

Antiretrovirals are used as prophylaxis to prevent HIV seroconversion in health care workers who recently have been exposed to HIV (≤72 hours). A multicenter study sponsored by the CDC revealed that the use of postexposure prophylaxis (PEP) with zidovudine was associated with a 79% decrease in the risk of HIV seroconversion. PEP should be initiated within 1 to 2 hours after exposure. Currently, PEP guidelines recommend the use of zidovudine, in addition to lamivudine and a protease inhibitor. These recommendations vary according to the type of exposure and the patient population; CDC bulletins should be consulted for information on the very specific regimens that should be followed.

Use in the case of exposure of a non–health care worker is controversial because risk exposure is difficult to assess. No current data suggest that PEP in this setting is safe or effective. The decision should be made carefully and should be based on circumstances of the exposure, and the patient should be well informed of the regimen's risks and benefits.

TREATMENT. Once infection has been identified, the patient should be referred to an infectious disease specialist or a center that provides care to HIV-infected individuals. Consideration regarding insurance is an unfortunate but realistic concern because care and treatments are costly. The patient should be reassured that the infectious disease experts are partners to primary care providers, and that the patient's relationship with the primary care provider will continue. Patients should be counseled on what tests they can expect and what types of treatments may be recommended. Patients also should be counseled about the risks of transmission of their infection, and they should be instructed that all past and present partners should be notified of the infection. The infection should be reported in keeping with state guidelines.

The decision to start antiretroviral agents in a patient who is not being treated in a "prophylactic" manner is controversial. However, almost all experts agree that starting therapy is necessary in those patients with symptomatic disease, those with decreasing CD4 T-cell counts and a high viral load, and those who experience acute primary HIV infection. Treatment for patients who do not fall into this category remains controversial and is based on open discussion between the patient and his or her health care providers.

Guidelines have been developed for the clinical management of HIV-infected adults and adolescents that provide details of treatment strategies and adverse effects, information on initiation of therapy, and other treatment principles. The current treatment method is based on the use of multiple antiretrovirals with the goal of suppressing HIV replication for months or perhaps even years. This concept is the driving force in today's treatment of a patient with HIV infection who is in need of antiretroviral treatment (Table 67-2).

How to Monitor

Baseline laboratory studies and screening testing should be performed as described in the initial evaluation section. If patients are symptomatic or have comorbidities, then more scrupulous testing may be indicated. After antiretroviral therapy has been initiated, monitor responses through laboratory tests as outlined in Table 67-1. (It is important to note that this table is a general reference.)

Patient Variables

SPECIAL POPULATIONS. Patients with renal and hepatic insufficiency can pose a therapeutic challenge to the practitioner who is caring for HIV-infected patients. Renally impaired patients may require dose modifications because of decreased drug clearance of most antiretrovirals. See specific reputable product information for details.

Patients with severely impaired liver function may be at greater risk of toxicity and should be monitored closely.

TABLE 67-2   International AIDS Society—U.S. Guidelines for Initiation of Antiretroviral Therapy in Adults

Category	CD4/mcl	Recommendations
Symptomatic	Any	Treatment mandatory
Asymptomatic	<200	Treatment mandatory
Asymptomatic	200-350	Treatment recommended

From Hammer SM et al: Treatment for adult HIV infection: 2006 recommendations of the International AIDS Society–USA Panel, *JAMA*, 296:827-843, 2006.

GERIATRICS. Except for geriatric patients, the life expectancy of HIV-infected persons who are receiving HAART now has been extended, most likely because of the immune reconstitution that results from potent antiretroviral therapy. Limited available data on combined antiretroviral therapy in the elderly seem to show a similar virologic success rate but slower immune recovery compared with younger patients. When selecting an antiretroviral, the practitioner should be cautious in dosing for an elderly patient because of the greater risk for decreased hepatic, renal, or cardiac function, and because of the likelihood of concomitant disease or other medication therapy. As an increasing number of HIV-infected individuals become older than 50 years of age, additional studies should begin to explore their tolerance to antiretroviral agents, as well as details on pharmacokinetics, drug–drug interactions, and toxicities. Each of the drugs used in treating HIV infection may demonstrate adverse effects with sustained therapy. Already, reports have described increased coronary artery disease in individuals who have been taking protease inhibitors.

PEDIATRICS. As of March 2004, 20 antiretroviral agents were approved for use in HIV-infected adults and adolescents in the United States; 12 of these have an approved pediatric treatment indication. Of available agents, the following have been approved for pediatric use: NRTIs (zidovudine, didanosine, stavudine, lamivudine, and abacavir), NNRTIs (nevirapine and efavirenz), and PIs (ritonavir, nelfinavir, amprenavir, and lopinavir/ritonavir). No current treatment guidelines are available for NRTIs (zalcitabine and tenofovir), NNRTIs (delavirdine), or PIs (saquinavir hard and soft gel capsules, and indinavir). Fusion inhibitor (enfuvirtide) safety profile has not been established for patients younger than 6 years of age, and doses are based on weight for patients between 6 and 16 years of age.

PREGNANCY AND LACTATION. Clinicians who care for HIV-infected women should provide family planning services and counseling to optimize medications and health prior to a pregnancy. Before any HIV-positive pregnant woman is treated with an antiretroviral, the practitioner is highly encouraged to enroll the patient in the Antiretroviral Pregnancy Registry by calling 800-258-4263, or by checking the website at www.agregistry.com. This registry for professional and patients was established to monitor maternal-fetal outcomes among pregnant women who receive antiretrovirals. Fatal lactic acidosis occurred in pregnant women treated with a combination of stavudine and didanosine.

All HIV-positive women should be warned of the high risk of HIV transmission via breast milk. The CDC advises all HIV-infected women not to breastfeed.

- *Category B:* nelfinavir, ritonavir, tenofovir, didanosine, enfuvirtide, saquinavir, emtricitabine, atazanavir, darunavir
- *Category C:* abacavir, amprenavir, fosamprenavir, delavirdine, efavirenz, indinavir, lamivudine, lopinavir, nevirapine, stavudine, zalcitabine, zidovudine, rattegravir
- *Category D:* hydroxyurea

Patient Education

Adherence is an essential aspect of antiretroviral therapy (ART) in that even a few missed doses may result in the emergence of resistance patterns. Given the limited number of available agents and associated resistance patterns, patients must be made to understand the certainty of this phenomenon with missed doses.

Patients should be instructed to take their medications as prescribed. Some strategies such as providing a written schedule, pill boxes, alarm clocks, pagers, and other mechanical devices aid adherence. Underdosing, partial adherence, or nonadherence may result in the development of a resistant strain(s) of HIV that will not be susceptible to treatment. Taking less than the prescribed dose can be more harmful than not taking the drug at all.

Patients should be informed that antiretrovirals do not cure HIV infection, and that the use of these medications does not preclude the ongoing need to prevent transmission through safe sex practices and universal precautions.

Patients also should be instructed about drinking bottled water, ensuring good nutrition, and seeking therapy promptly for signs of infection or systemic disease.

SPECIFIC DRUGS

ANTIRETROVIRALS

Reverse Transcriptase Inhibitors

Zidovudine and lamivudine, which are used in prophylaxis, are discussed in detail here.

zidovudine (ZDV, AZT) (Retrovir)

- Reduces neonatal transmission of HIV and used as postexposure prophylaxis

CONTRAINDICATIONS. Life-threatening allergic reactions

WARNINGS

- *Hypersensitivity:* Rare events, including anaphylaxis, have occurred. If rash develops, careful evaluation is warranted.
- *zidovudine:* Should be used with particular caution in patients who have an absolute granulocyte count lower than 1000 cells/mm³ or a hemoglobin level less than 9.5 g/dl because of worries about bone marrow suppression.
- Myalgias and inflammatory frank myositis may occur with long-term zidovudine therapy.
- Rare occurrence of lactic acidosis/severe hepatomegaly with steatosis. Close monitoring is required, especially in obese women with risk factors for liver disease.
- Use caution in combination with interferon-α with or without ribavirin. Monitor closely for hepatic

decompensation, anemia, or neutropenia; dose reduction or discontinuation of interferon and/or ribavirin may be necessary.
- Zidovudine is eliminated by renal excretion after the liver metabolizes it. In patients with renal impairment, dose reduction is recommended (see "Dosage and Administration"). Patients with very severely impaired liver function may be at greater risk of toxicity.

PRECAUTIONS. Be particularly cautious about other medications that cause myelosuppression such as ganciclovir and interferon-α. Be aware of other underlying causes of bone marrow suppression in AIDS. Patients who take zidovudine generally have an elevated mean corpuscular volume (MCV).

ADVERSE EFFECTS. See Table 67-3.

DRUG INTERACTIONS. Ribavirin and interferon-α may increase the risk of hepatic decompensation or other signs of mitochondrial toxicity such as pancreatitis or lactic acidosis. Also may decrease the antiviral activity of zidovudine. Pyrazinamide efficacy is significantly reduced and alternative therapy may be warranted. Probenecid may increase zidovudine levels. Use of dapsone has resulted in neutropenia. Trimethoprim increases serum levels of zidovudine; however, dosage adjustment is not indicated. Phenytoin levels may be altered with concomitant use of zidovudine. Zidovudine and acyclovir given in combination may cause drowsiness and lethargy in some patients. Methadone increases the AUC of zidovudine by approximately 43%, thereby increasing the possibility of zidovudine-related toxicities.

DOSAGE AND ADMINISTRATION. Zidovudine may be taken with or without food. Zidovudine (AZT) monotherapy is *not* recommended. Because these dosing recommendations are constantly being revised by infectious disease specialists, consult the latest product information. For a summary of general dosing information, see the supplemental tables on the Evolve Resources website. **evolve**

If a patient's hemoglobin is less than 7.5 g/dl or decreases by more than 25% from baseline, and/or the granulocyte count is less than 750/mm³ or decreases by more than 50% from baseline, interruption of zidovudine may be necessary until bone marrow recovery is indicated. If less severe anemia or granulocytopenia occurs, reducing the dose may be adequate. Many practitioners have chosen to place their patients on cytokines such as epoetin alfa (Epogen) and G-CSF to treat anemia and/or granulocytopenia.

Nausea associated with the use of zidovudine may improve if taken on a full stomach or with the syrup formulation. Patients with poor tolerance can start at a low dose that is gradually escalated (by 100 mg every few days) until full dosage is achieved (600 mg daily).

Results of the ACTG 076 clinical trial showed that treating women with zidovudine during pregnancy significantly decreased perinatal transmission from 25% to approximately 8%. Based on these important data, the USPHS guidelines currently recommend specific zidovudine dosing for this population. Practitioners should call the Antiretroviral Pregnancy Registry at 800-258-4263.

TABLE 67-3 **Adverse Effects of Antiretroviral Agents**

Drug	Important Adverse Reactions
NRTIs	Lactic acidosis/hepatic steatosis/failure, hypersensitivity
zidovudine (ZDV, AZT)	Myelosuppression (macrocytic anemia or granulocytopenia, myalgias, and malaise), headache, nausea, myopathy/myositis, hepatic steatosis, lactic acidosis/hepatic steatosis, elevated creatine phosphokinase, excessive eyelash growth, and nail hyperpigmentation
lamivudine (3TC)	Neutropenia, amylasemia, headache, nausea, malaise, fatigue, peripheral neuropathy, insomnia, pancreatitis in children
abacavir	Systemic hypersensitivity reaction, nausea, vomiting, transaminitis, anemia, neutropenia
didanosine (ddI)	Pancreatitis, peripheral neuropathy, retinal depigmentation, diarrhea, headache, dry mouth, insomnia, nervousness, amylasemia, transaminitis, hyperuricemia, lactic acidosis/hepatic steatosis, hepatic dysfunction, retinal changes, and optic neuritis
stavudine (d4T)	Lactic acidosis/hepatic steatosis/failure, peripheral neuropathy, diarrhea, nausea, vomiting, transaminitis, hypersensitivity, pancreatitis, headache, fat redistribution
tenofovir (TDF)	Lactic acidosis/hepatic steatosis/failure, GI symptoms (nausea, diarrhea, flatulence, vomiting, abdominal pain, anorexia), headache
zalcitabine (ddC)	Lactic acidosis/hepatic steatosis/failure, pancreatitis, peripheral neuropathy, rash, esophageal ulceration, pancreatitis (rare) amylasemia, transaminitis, lactic acidosis/hepatic steatosis, GI symptoms (nausea, diarrhea, flatulence, stomatitis, and aphthous esophageal ulcers), maculopapular rash, cardiomyopathy, fevers
emtricitabine (FTC)	Lactic acidosis, hepatic steatosis
NNRTIs	Hepatotoxicity
delavirdine (DLV)	Transaminitis, rash, pruritus, headache, bilirubinemia, myalgia, arthralgia, headache, nausea, diarrhea, fatigue, neutropenia, anemia
efavirenz (EFV)	Transaminitis, rash, CNS and psychiatric disturbances
nevirapine (NVP)	Transaminitis, hepatotoxicity, rash (Stevens-Johnson), hypersensitivity, fever, nausea, headache
PIs	Hepatotoxicity, insulin resistance/hyperglycemia, hyperlipidemia and bleeding episodes in hemophiliac patients
ritonavir	Nausea, diarrhea, taste perversion, circumoral paresthesias, transaminitis, elevated triglycerides, thrombocytopenia, granulocytopenia
amprenavir	Rash, nausea, perioral paresthesias, diarrhea, transaminitis, elevated triglycerides
indinavir	Nephrolithiasis, nausea, abdominal pain, fat redistribution. Crix belly,* indirect bilirubinemia, hematuria, sterile pyuria, crystalluria
nelfinavir	Diarrhea, nausea, neutropenia, increased creatine phosphokinase, vomiting
saquinavir	Diarrhea, nausea, abdominal pain, ataxia, neutropenia, hemolytic anemia, transaminitis
lopinavir/ritonavir	Pancreatitis, nausea, diarrhea, elevated triglycerides
fosamprenavir (f-APV)	Skin rash, diarrhea, nausea, headache, transaminase elevation, hyperglycemia, fat maldistribution, lipid abnormalities, bleeding episodes in hemophiliacs
atazanavir	Indirect hyperbilirubinemia, prolonged PR interval, fat maldistribution, hyperglycemia, increased bleeding episodes in hemophiliacs
ENTRY INHIBITOR	
enfuvirtide	Hypersensitivity, local site reaction, diarrhea, nausea, fatigue
HIV integrase inhibitor	Diarrhea, nausea, and headache

*Crix belly is characterized by elevated levels of triglycerides, cholesterol, and plasma glucose with a weight gain of 40 pounds or greater. Fat accumulates in the lower abdomen and flanks, and tissue in the arms and legs often is lost. Named after Crixivan; however, it may be associated with other protease inhibitors.

OTHER DRUGS IN CLASS

Other drugs in this class are similar to the prototype except as follows.

lamivudine (3TC) (Epivir)

Lamivudine can be combined with emtricitabine, zidovudine, or abacavir to maximize potency and tolerability in an NRTI combination.

It also is used in the treatment of patients with chronic hepatitis.

CONTRAINDICATIONS. Hypersensitivity

WARNINGS. Lactic acidosis and severe hepatomegaly with steatosis have been reported with the use of nucleoside analogs alone or in combination, including lamivudine and other antiretrovirals. Rare cases of pancreatitis have been reported. Dose adjustment is required with renal impairment.

Important Differences Among Lamivudine-Containing Products. Epivir tablets and oral solution contain a higher dose of the same active ingredient (lamivudine) than is found in Epivir-HBV, which is used for patients with chronic hepatitis B. The formulation and dosage of Epivir-HBV are not appropriate for patients dually infected with HIV and HBV. If a decision is made to administer lamivudine to these patients, Epivir or Combivir (lamivudine/zidovudine) tablets should be used.

PRECAUTIONS. Reduction in dosage is recommended for patients with renal impairment.

ADVERSE EFFECTS. See Table 67-3. Lamivudine has limited toxicities compared with the other antiretrovirals.

DRUG INTERACTIONS. Few drug interactions have been reported with lamivudine. Trimethoprim/sulfamethoxazole significantly increases the AUC of lamivudine by 43%, and it decreases renal clearance by 35%.

DOSAGE AND ADMINISTRATION
- Epivir is available in 150 mg and 300 mg tablets and oral solution 10 mg/ml and is administered with or without food.
- *Adults (>16 years):* Dosage is based on weight in kilograms (kg): ≥50 kg: 150 mg twice daily or 300 mg once daily; <50 kg: 4 mg/kg twice daily (maximum, 150 mg per dose)
- *Pediatric dosage (3 months to 16 years):* 4 mg/kg (maximum, 150 mg per dose) every 12 hours up to 300 mg once daily
- *Combination therapy:* AZT 300 mg/3TC 150 mg, one tablet twice daily
- *Renal impairment (Clcr <50 ml/min):* These patients should have dose modifications because of decreased drug clearance. Consult package insert.

abacavir (Ziagen)

ADVERSE EFFECTS. Hypersensitivity syndrome (5%). Symptoms include fever, rash, fatigue, respiratory distress, abdominal pain, headache, and nausea. This is a key feature that can occur within hours following exposure to the drug.

DOSAGE AND ADMINISTRATION
- *Oral:* 300 mg twice daily or 600 mg once daily given in combination with other antiretroviral therapy. Dosing adjustment is necessary in patients with liver impairment.
- Patients should carry a wallet medication card to notify emergency personnel of the use of abacavir in case of a hypersensitivity reaction.
- Patients should be warned that interruption in abacavir therapy for reasons other than hypersensitivity could result in a hypersensitivity reaction once the drug is restarted.
- All patients should be registered (1-800-270-0425).

didanosine (ddI) (Videx)

DOSAGE AND ADMINISTRATION
- To be taken on an empty stomach (>½ hour before or >2 hours after meals)
- Space apart from all protease inhibitors (except for Videx EC, which can be taken with indinavir).

- To be taken with water or apple juice
- Can be taken with light meal if taken with tenofovir; still must be spaced apart from protease inhibitors

tenofovir disoproxil fumarate (Viread)

DRUG INTERACTIONS
- Acyclovir, cidofovir, ganciclovir, valacyclovir, and valganciclovir may increase the serum concentrations of tenofovir.
- Tenofovir will increase levels of ddI; dose adjustment is required.
- Tenofovir may decrease the levels of atazanavir, resulting in a loss of response. Specific dosing recommendations are available for atazanavir.

Nonnucleoside Reverse Transcriptase Inhibitors (NNRTIs)

delavirdine mesylate (DLV) (Rescriptor) 🔑

CONTRAINDICATIONS
- Hypersensitivity
- Concurrent use of alprazolam, cisapride, ergot alkaloids, midazolam, pimozide, rifampin, or triazolam

PRECAUTIONS. Diffuse, maculopapular, pruritic skin rash. When a severe rash occurs, or a rash is noted with other symptoms such as fever, blistering, oral lesions, conjunctivitis, swelling, myalgias, or arthralgias, delavirdine must be discontinued immediately.

DRUG INTERACTIONS. Certain NRTI components should not be combined, for example, zidovudine and stavudine are antagonistic to each other, stavudine and didanosine have overlapping toxic effects, and tenofovir and didanosine should not be used in treatment-naive patients with wild-type virus because of dampened CD4 cell responses and toxic effects. Abacavir and tenofovir should not be used as the dual-NRTI components of an initial regimen because of genetic fragility.

💣 Administration of delavirdine with certain medications may result in potentially serious and/or life-threatening events. See the latest manufacturer information.

Delavirdine is a strong inhibitor of the cytochrome P450 enzymes 2C9, 2C19, 2D6, and 3A4. It is also a substrate for 3A4; therefore, it is not recommended for concurrent use with astemizole, alprazolam, terfenadine, midazolam, cisapride, rifabutin, rifampin, triazolam, ergot derivatives, amphetamines, calcium channel blockers (nifedipine), and anticonvulsants (phenytoin, carbamazepine, phenobarbital).

Delavirdine increases levels of dapsone, clarithromycin, quinidine, warfarin, indinavir, and saquinavir. A reduction in indinavir to 600 mg three times a day should be considered when it is combined with delavirdine. H_2-receptor antagonists may reduce the absorption of delavirdine. Consult a detailed drug reference for further information on these important drug interactions.

OTHER DRUGS IN CLASS

Other drugs in this class are similar to the prototype except as follows.

efavirenz (Sustiva)

Efavirenz is recommended because of its efficacy and tolerability, but it is teratogenic (category D); *must* not be used as a single agent to treat patients with HIV

PRECAUTIONS. Efavirenz plus 2 NRTIs has become the standard-of-care comparator in clinical trials. Because of teratogenic risk during the first trimester, the use of efavirenz requires adequate contraception in women of childbearing potential. Efavirenz is now available in a fixed-dose formulation with tenofovir and emtricitabine, allowing patients to take only 1 pill a day.

DRUG INTERACTIONS. Because of strong cytochrome P450 3A4 inhibition and substrate, this medication may affect levels of numerous drugs, including indinavir, amprenavir, lopinavir, or saquinavir. Dose adjustment may be necessary; use with caution with these antiretroviral medications. Consult a detailed drug reference for further information on these important drug interactions.

nevirapine (Viramune)

Nevirapine has virologic activity similar to that of efavirenz, with the advantage of safety for the fetus at all stages of pregnancy. However, a risk of potentially fatal hepatotoxicity is noted in women with CD4 cell counts higher than 250/mcl and in men with counts higher than 400/mcl. Nevirapine is also recommended as an alternative NNRTI in patients in whom the central nervous system toxicity of efavirenz is not tolerated or does not decrease within 2 to 3 weeks of treatment initiation. This drug should be avoided as initial therapy in women with CD4 cell counts higher than 250/mcl and in men with CD4 cell counts higher than 400/mcl.

ADVERSE EFFECTS

- Hepatotoxicity occurs in >10% of patients with or without clinical hepatitis. Increasing reports of serious, even life-threatening, hepatic necrosis. Two thirds occur in the first 12 weeks of therapy. Liver function testing includes baseline, 2 weeks prior to dose escalation, 2 weeks post dose escalation, and monthly during first 12 weeks or beyond.
- Severe life-threatening skin rash—Stevens-Johnson syndrome—has been reported, more commonly in females. When a severe rash occurs, or a rash presents with other symptoms such as fever, blistering, oral lesions, conjunctivitis, swelling, myalgias, or arthralgias, nevirapine must be discontinued immediately.

PROTEASE INHIBITORS

A protease inhibitor may be used in prophylaxis of HIV.

ritonavir (Norvir) 🔑

Among the ritonavir-boosted PIs, recommended components include lopinavir, atazanavir, fosamprenavir, or saquinavir. More data are available for lopinavir and ritonavir, but hyperlipidemia and other metabolic adverse effects also support the use of atazanavir and ritonavir.

Recommended NRTI components in the initial regimen are tenofovir and emtricitabine, zidovudine and lamivudine, or abacavir and lamivudine. Although tenofovir is well tolerated, it should be used cautiously or avoided altogether in patients with preexisting renal insufficiency.

Ritonavir-boosted lopinavir offers the convenience of once-daily dosing among treatment-naive patients. Ritonavir-boosted atazanavir may not increase lipid levels as extensively as other ritonavir-boosted PIs, but it is associated with hyperbilirubinemia.

CONTRAINDICATIONS

- Hypersensitivity
- Concurrent alfuzosin, amiodarone, cisapride, dihydroergotamine, ergonovine, ergotamine, flecainide, methylergonovine, midazolam, pimozide, propafenone, quinidine, triazolam, and voriconazole (when ritonavir 800 mg/day)

WARNINGS

- Because ritonavir is metabolized primarily by the liver, it should be used with extreme caution in patients with moderate or severe hepatic impairment.

PRECAUTIONS

- Tobacco decreases the AUC of ritonavir.

DRUG INTERACTIONS

- Concurrent use with amiodarone, astemizole, bepridil, cisapride, dihydroergotamine, ergonovine, ergotamine, flecainide, lovastatin, methylergonovine, midazolam, pimozide, propafenone, quinidine, simvastatin, St John's wort, terfenadine, or triazolam is contraindicated. Ritonavir may also cause large increases in the levels of hypnotic and sedative drugs. These drugs include alprazolam, clorazepate, diazepam, estazolam, flurazepam, triazolam, and zolpidem. Because these drugs compete for the CYP3A, life-threatening reactions may occur.
  Ritonavir contains alcohol in its formulation; therefore, coadministration of disulfiram (Antabuse) or metronidazole can cause Antabuse-type reactions.
  Many drug interactions have been noted with ritonavir, and it is highly recommended that the clinician should review pharmaceutical information prior to initiation of any new medication. Ritonavir decreases levels of ethinyl estradiol, theophylline, sulfamethoxazole, and zidovudine. Ritonavir decreases levels of rifabutin to one quarter of standard dose and increases levels of clarithromycin and desipramine. Those patients taking ritonavir and clarithromycin with renal impairment should have further dose reduction; reference to a pharmaceutical source is warranted.
  Consult a detailed drug reference for additional information on these important drug interactions.

DOSAGE AND ADMINISTRATION

- Administer 600 mg twice daily when used as a single PI or 100 to 400 mg twice a day when used with another PI by mouth. The medication should be taken with meals if possible. Oral solution may be mixed in chocolate milk or nutritional supplements such as Ensure or Advera within 1 hour of dosing, for improved taste.
- Adult dosage is 600 mg twice daily
- *Dose escalation regimen to improve GI tolerance:* 300 mg every 12 hours for 1 day, 400 mg twice a day for

ritonavir (Norvir) 🔑 —cont'd

2 days, 500 mg twice a day for 1 day, and then 600 mg twice a day

- Pediatric dosage is 400 mg/m^2 twice daily by mouth and should not exceed 600 mg twice daily. Dose escalation is as follows: Start at 250 mg/m^2 twice daily on day 1, then increase at 2- or 3-day intervals by 50 mg/m^2 twice daily until 400 mg/m^2 twice-daily dosing is achieved.
- *Renal impairment:* Dose reduction is not necessary.

In pediatric patients, ritonavir should be used as combination therapy with other antiretrovirals. For patients who are also taking other antiretroviral medications, refer to product information for specifics on antiretroviral dosage adjustments. Ritonavir may be better tolerated when used in combination with another antiretroviral; ritonavir should be initiated alone before the second agent is subsequently added.

OTHER DRUGS IN CLASS

Multiple drugs are now included in this class. Refer to recent dosing information because food affects absorption of some drugs in this class.

FUSION INHIBITOR

enfuvirtide (Fuzeon, T-20) 🔑

CONTRAINDICATIONS
- Hypersensitivity

WARNINGS
- Medication must be taken by subcutaneous injection twice daily, rotating among the abdomen, thigh, and upper arm. Local injection site reaction is the most common adverse effect; symptoms may include pain, induration, erythema, nodules, cysts, pruritus, and ecchymosis.
- An increased rate of bacterial pneumonia was observed in trials. It is unclear whether a relationship exists, but patients on this medication should be carefully monitored for signs and symptoms of pneumonia.
- Hypersensitivity reactions have occurred and may occur on rechallenge. Patients who develop symptoms that are suggestive of a systemic hypersensitivity reaction should discontinue enfuvirtide.

HIV INTEGRASE INHIBITOR

raltegravir (Isentress)

Raltegravir is indicated for use in combination with other antiretroviral agents to treat patients with HIV-1 infection. Raltegravir is the first agent in this new pharmacologic class of antiretroviral agents.

Raltegravir targets integrase, an HIV enzyme that integrates the viral genetic material into human chromosomes—a critical step in the pathogenesis of HIV. Raltegravir and other integrase inhibitors are often referred to as *strand transfer inhibitors.* This term refers to the process of DNA strand transfer from the viral genome to the host genome. The drug is metabolized away via glucuronidation.

INDICATIONS. Raltegravir is approved only for use in individuals whose infection has proved resistant to other HAART drugs. As with any HAART medication, raltegravir cannot be used as monotherapy.

ADVERSE EFFECTS. Adverse events most commonly reported with raltegravir were diarrhea, nausea, and headache. Blood tests showed abnormally elevated levels of a muscle enzyme in some patients receiving raltegravir.

DOSAGE AND ADMINISTRATION. Raltegravir is taken 400 mg orally twice daily. Doses of 200, 400, and 600 mg have been studied. The medication can be taken without regard for food.

At the 2007 conference on retroviruses and Opportunistic Infections, researchers presented phase 3 data showing that 77% of patients taking the 400 mg dose of raltegravir plus other antiretroviral drugs reached HIV viral loads below 400 copies—nearly twice that of a control group.

Combination Drug Therapies

DHHS Panel guidelines recommend an initial regimen for treatment-naive patients that consists of a combination of two NRTIs with an NNRTI, or two NRTIs with a single PI or a PI boosted with low-dose ritonavir (Table 67-4).

Other options are considered acceptable and may be used in certain circumstances. These options are considered alternatives in cases of antiviral activity, intolerability, or drug interaction potential.

After starting a therapeutic regimen, the patient should follow up with the clinician within 1 to 2 weeks to discuss

TABLE 67-4   DHHS Panel HAART Recommendations

Drug	COLUMN A		COLUMN B
	NNRTI	PI	2 NRTI
PREFERRED REGIMEN SELECTION			
Select NNRTI or one PI combination from Column A + one 2 NRTI combination from Column B	efavirenz	atazanavir + ritonavir, fosamprenavir + ritonavir bid, lopinavir-ritonavir bid	renofovir-emtricitabine* (co-formulated), zidovudine-lamivudine (co-formulated)
ALTERNATE REGIMEN SELECTION			
Select NNRTI or one PI combination from Column A + one 2 NRTI combination from Column B	nevirapine	atazanavir (unboosted), fosamprenavir (unboosted), fosamprenavir + ritonavir bid, lopinavir-ritonavir qd	abacavir-lamivudine* (co-formulated), didanosine + (emtricitabine or lamivudine)

*Emtricitabine may be used in place of lamivudine and vice versa.
U.S. Department of Health and Human Services (DHHS): *Guidelines for the Use of Antiretroviral Agents in HIV-Infected Adults and Adolescents,* Rockville, MD, 2006, DHHS.

symptoms related to HIV, any adverse effects of the drugs, and the patient's degree of adherence to the therapeutic plan.

Determining appropriate HAART therapy and whether change is needed is both an art and a science and should be within the domain of HIV and infectious disease specialists. HAART drug regimen medications might have to be changed based on the following:

- Virologic failure shown by increases in HIV RNA viral load
- Medication toxicity
- Patient tolerance
- Drug adherence or inability to comply with the regimen
- Pregnancy
- Drug resistance

The combination of medications also may be altered in the presence of coexisting disease such as hepatitis C or tuberculosis.

evolve A continually updated list of useful WebLinks may be found in the Evolve Resources at http://evolve.elsevier.com/Edmunds/NP/

Antivirals and Antiprotozoal Agents

DRUG OVERVIEW

Class	Subclass	Generic Name	Trade Name
Antivirals	Antiherpes	acyclovir ✻	Zovirax ✻
		famciclovir	Famvir
		valacyclovir	Valtrex ✻
		penciclovir	Denavir
Antivirals	Antiinfluenza	amantadine	Symmetrel
		rimantadine	Flumadine
	Neuraminidase inhibitors	oseltamivir	Tamiflu ✻
		zanamivir	Relenza
Antiprotozoal		metronidazole ✻	Flagyl
		tinidazole	Tindamax
		chloroquine	Plaquenil

✻, Top 200 drug.

INDICATIONS

- acyclovir, famciclovir, valacyclovir, and penciclovir
  - *Herpes simplex (types 1 and 2):* Treatment of acute infection and chronic suppression
  - Varicella-zoster viruses (chickenpox and shingles)
  - Epstein-Barr virus (mononucleosis)
- *amantadine, rimantadine:* Influenza A
- *zanamivir, oseltamivir:* Influenza A and B
- *metronidazole, tinidazole:* Many protozoa, *Clostridium difficile*, amebiasis, trichomoniasis, giardiasis, bacterial vaginosis
- *chloroquine:* Malaria

This chapter discusses the use of antiviral drugs and common antiprotozoal medications in primary care. This chapter does not discuss the use of antiviral drugs in the treatment of patients with HIV. The antiherpetic drugs acyclovir, famciclovir, and valacyclovir are closely related. They are used in the treatment of initial and recurrent (more than six outbreaks per year) mucosal and cutaneous herpes simplex types 1 and 2, and for the treatment of acute herpes simplex virus (HSV) infection. Acyclovir has the greatest antiviral activity in vitro against herpes simplex virus type 1, followed in decreasing order of potency by HSV type 2 (HSV-2), varicella-zoster virus, Epstein-Barr virus, and cytomegalovirus.

Penciclovir is structurally similar but is used only topically (see Chapter 11).

Amantadine, rimantadine, zanamivir, and oseltamivir are used for the prevention and treatment of influenza virus infection. Amantadine is also used in Parkinson's disease (see Chapter 45). Amantadine and rimantadine are similar, as are oseltamivir and zanamivir. Oseltamivir currently is being stockpiled in preparation for an avian influenza pandemic and is not generally available.

Metronidazole has several uses in addition to the treatment of protozoa, including treatment of bacterial and amebic infections. Chloroquine is used for malaria; however, many strains of malaria are now resistant to chloroquine. Many antiparasitic and antiprotozoal medications are important in international travel but are only rarely encountered in primary care. These are not discussed here.

THERAPEUTIC OVERVIEW OF VIRUSES AND PROTOZOA

Anatomy and Physiology

VIRUS. A virus is a single- or double-stranded DNA or RNA molecule enclosed within a protein coat. Some may also have a lipoprotein envelope. They may contain proteins that cause antigenic reactions or enzymes that initiate viral replication. The virus lacks metabolic functions and must rely on the host cell for the metabolism or synthesis of chemicals. According to the definition of life, viruses are not alive. They do not eat or produce waste. They do not reproduce independently.

DNA viruses include herpesviruses (chickenpox, shingles, herpes), adenoviruses (conjunctivitis, pharyngitis), hepadna viruses (hepatitis B), and papillomaviruses (warts). RNA viruses include rubella (German measles), rhabdoviruses (rabies), picornaviruses (poliomyelitis, meningitis, colds), arboviruses (yellow fever), orthomyxoviruses (influenza), and paramyxoviruses (measles and mumps). The retroviruses are a subgroup of RNA viruses that are discussed in the chapter on the immune system and antiretroviral medications (see Chapter 67). Several other viruses are discussed in the chapter on immunization and immunity (see Chapter 69). Some of the less common viruses are not described in this text.

PROTOZOA. The word *parasite* is used to refer to protozoa, helminths, and arthropods. Parasites are metabolically dependent on a host. This chapter discusses only a few of the many protozoa that are most commonly seen in the United States. Malaria is included in this discussion because it is such an important disease worldwide.

Protozoa, which are small and unicellular, are the simplest organisms in the animal kingdom. They are divided into categories based on their type of locomotion. Important protozoal diseases include amebiasis, caused by *Entamoeba histolytica;* giardiasis, caused by *Giardia lamblia;* and trichomoniasis, caused by *Trichomonas vaginalis.*

Protozoa also cause malaria. These organisms include *Plasmodium falciparum, P. vivax, P. malariae,* and *P. ovale.*

Viral Disease Process

HERPES SIMPLEX. Herpes simplex virus type 1 (HSV-1) causes infections of the mouth and face (herpes labialis), and of the skin, esophagus, and brain. Vesicles form moist ulcers after several days and epithelialize over 2 to 3 weeks. In some geographic locations, HSV-1 infection is a common cause of first episodes of genital herpes. These may occur in stable, monogamous relationships and are less likely to recur than genital infections caused by HSV-2.

HSV-2 causes infection of the genitals, rectum, skin, hands, and meninges. Asymptomatic shedding of the virus is commonly the mechanism of transmission. Thus the disease can be transmitted sexually. Recent serologic surveys, which employs type-specific antibody assays, show a rising prevalence of previous HSV-2 infection in postadolescent populations in developed countries; many of these infections were asymptomatic.

Herpes simplex can be a primary infection (which can be asymptomatic) or can result from activation of a latent infection. It is unknown what triggers activation. Type 2 is latent in the presacral ganglia. Both type 1 and type 2 can cause keratitis, encephalitis, recurrent meningitis, disseminated infection, and Bell's palsy.

The varicella-zoster virus (VZV) is the human herpesvirus 3. This virus causes chickenpox in children, which is highly contagious and is spread by inhalation of infective droplets or contact with lesions. In older adults or immunocompromised patients, the virus can cause shingles. Shingles is caused by reactivation of the virus that is latent in the nerve ganglion. It causes a vesicular rash that appears on an erythematous base in a dermatome pattern, accompanied by pain and systemic symptoms.

INFLUENZA. Influenzavirus causes epidemics of acute illness that is transmitted by the respiratory route. Influenza is diagnosed by association with an epidemic that is confirmed by viral cultures. The standard trivalent influenzavirus vaccine provides partial immunity to certain strains of influenza A and B that vary from year to year.

Protozoal Disease Process

GIARDIASIS (*GIARDIA*). This is the most common cause of waterborne diarrheal disease in the United States. It is transmitted by fecal-oral spread of cysts via contaminated food or water. It is resistant to chlorination levels found in water supplies and can survive freezing for several days. Symptoms include diarrhea, fatigue, malaise, abdominal cramps, and weight loss. A diagnostic test is available to detect antigens in the stool.

MALARIA. Malaria is the most significant protozoal disease in the world, causing 1.5 to 2.7 million deaths annually. Symptoms of malaria include periodic attacks of chills, fever and sweating, headache, myalgia, splenomegaly, anemia, and leukopenia. Increasing drug resistance has caused treatment of malaria to be problematic. An additional complication is the fact that plasmodia go through distinct stages that affect their susceptibility to different agents. For example, chloroquine is active against asexual blood stages but not against sexual blood stages or asexual liver stages. Prophylaxis of malaria in travelers depends on risk factors, including the area to be visited and the type of malaria that is active in that area. Chloroquine and primaquine are used in non–chloroquine-resistant areas.

MECHANISM OF ACTION
Antivirals

If it is to be effective, an antiviral drug must enter infected cells and act at the site of infection. Effective agents have a narrow spectrum of activity, inhibiting replication but not killing the virus. They target a specific viral protein, usually an enzyme that is involved in viral nucleic acid synthesis. Resistance may develop quickly, but the time frame is influenced by many factors. The difference between in vitro sensitivity testing and in vivo effectiveness is not clear. The human patient must have a good immune system to recover from infection.

Acyclovir is a synthetic purine nucleoside analog. Valacyclovir is a prodrug of acyclovir, and famciclovir is a prodrug of penciclovir. (See Chapter 3 for a discussion of prodrugs.) Both have similar mechanisms of action as acyclovir. They work by inhibiting viral DNA synthesis. These drugs are activated by the enzyme thymidine kinase, which is found only in cells that are infected by the virus. Consequently, they are relatively nontoxic to cells that are not infected by the virus. In chemical terms, activation of the antiviral first occurs in the infected cells and is followed by phosphorylation by the enzyme thymidine kinase. Finally, acyclovir triphosphate (the active derivative obtained from monophosphate by host cell enzymes) inhibits viral DNA polymerase, thereby blocking viral replication.

Amantadine and rimantadine are structurally similar tricyclic amines. They both inhibit an early step in viral replication, and they have an effect on the viral assembly. The locus of action is the influenza A virus M2 protein, which is an integral membrane protein.

Zanamivir and oseltamivir are thought to inhibit the virus neuraminidase; this alters virus particle aggregation and release.

Antiprotozoals

METRONIDAZOLE. Metronidazole is considered a cytotoxic agent, but its exact mechanism of action is not well understood. Metronidazole damages DNA synthesis, resulting in cell death. Most probably, metronidazole initially enters cells by passive diffusion and then is activated by an enzymatic system that is present only in certain cells, such as anaerobic cells and protozoa. A reaction occurs, and a nitrogen group is reduced. The metabolites are toxic substances that bind to DNA and RNA and interrupt synthesis.

CHLOROQUINE. The exact mechanism of action is unknown. Chloroquine raises the internal pH of parasites. It also may influence hemoglobin digestion or interfere with parasite/nucleoprotein synthesis.

TREATMENT PRINCIPLES

Standardized Guidelines

See World Health Organization at www.worldhealth/int for specific diseases treatment guidelines.

Evidence-Based Recommendations

- Oral antivirals are effective in herpes.
- Neuraminidase is effective in influenza.

Cardinal Points of Treatment

- Herpes simplex and zoster
  - Start treatment as soon as possible.
  - Acyclovir, famciclovir, and valacyclovir all are effective for short-term treatment, long-term suppression, and treatment of recurrences.
  - Treatment of acute infection does not eliminate chronic infection.
- Antiinfluenza
  - Resistance to amantadine and rimantadine has made them largely ineffective.
  - Oseltamivir and zanamivir are effective against most strains of influenza A and B but generally are not available.
  - Zanamivir must be given by inhalation.
- Antiprotozoals
  - Metronidazole is effective for many infections—bacterial, trichomoniasis, amebiasis, giardiasis, and *Clostridium difficile*.
  - Tinidazole is similar to metronidazole but is not used for *C. diff* infections.

Pharmacologic Treatment

HERPES SIMPLEX TREATMENT. Acyclovir, famciclovir, and valacyclovir all are useful in the treatment of herpes viruses. They are used as treatment for acute infection and for chronic suppression and recurrences. Systemic therapy for initial episodes does not prevent the establishment of latency or the development of future recurrences, even when given in high or prolonged dosage. Oral acyclovir is the most useful and effective form of the drug for the treatment of herpes simplex virus and varicella infection. In patients with frequent recurrences, oral acyclovir has prevented or reduced the frequency or severity of recurrences in more than 95% of patients. Topical acyclovir is significantly less effective but will shorten healing time and the duration of viral shedding and pain in patients with an initial outbreak of herpes. No clinical benefit was found when the topical form was given in recurrent episodes of genital herpes. Topical acyclovir is effective against herpes labialis; it reduces the duration of the condition by about half a day.

When prescribing these drugs, the practitioner should understand two important principles. First, the peak of viral activity and reproduction occurs prior to the appearance of any symptoms. Therefore, therapy is prescribed late in the disease process. Second, viral agents work by inhibiting reproduction without eradicating latent viruses. Elimination of the virus is not complete, but these agents can assist in reducing and suppressing symptoms. The effectiveness of the drug depends on how early treatment is initiated.

Almost all persons with initially symptomatic HSV-2 infection have symptomatic recurrences. More than 35% of such patients have frequent recurrences. Recurrence rates are especially high in persons with an extended first episode of infection, regardless of whether or not they receive antiviral chemotherapy with acyclovir. Men with genital HSV-2 infection have about 20% more recurrences than do women—a factor that may contribute to the higher rate of HSV-2 transmission from men to women than from women to men and to the continuing epidemic of genital herpes in the United States.

These antiviral drugs are indicated for the treatment of genital herpes in the following circumstances: initial episode of genital herpes, frequently recurring episodes (more than six per year), immunocompromised patients (treatment or long-term suppression), and severe genital herpes. Antivirals should not be used in mildly affected patients because resistance to the medication can occur. Although resistance is rare, it is more likely to occur with prolonged or repeated therapy in severely immunocompromised patients. Use of acyclovir, valacyclovir, and famciclovir in the nonpregnant and the pregnant woman can significantly alter the disease and influence transmission rates, along with decreasing morbidity and mortality associated with HSV infection. The three oral antiherpes medications are equally effective; acyclovir is less expensive than the others.

HERPES ZOSTER TREATMENT. Antiviral drugs have been shown to enhance the healing of lesions and to decrease or stop the pain frequently associated with zoster lesions (paresthesia, dysesthesia, hyperesthesia), particularly in the generally more severe cases of shingles that occur in patients 50 years of age or older. Treatment has been more successful when started within the first 48 hours following the onset of rash.

ANTIINFLUENZA DRUGS. Many strains of influenza A have developed resistance to amantadine and rimantadine. These drugs are not recommended for prophylaxis of seasonal influenza.

Considerable concern has arisen about the possibility of an avian influenza pandemic. Preparation for a pandemic has produced many problems. Oseltamivir is the most effective drug, but production problems have been reported. It is made from the seed of star anise, which has limited availability, and is thus an expensive medication. The federal government is stockpiling the medication, and it is not available to the general public.

Because zanamivir is inhaled, concern has been expressed about its effectiveness against systemic influenza. However, one study showed 70% to 90% effectiveness for prophylaxis before or after exposure to influenza A or B. Neuraminidase inhibitors can decrease the severity and duration of symptoms in patients with influenza if treatment is started within 48 hours after the onset of illness; the earlier treatment is started, the better is the outcome. Resistance to oseltamivir has started to occur in Vietnam.

There have been reported neuropsychiatric symptoms following administration of these drugs. Symptoms of delirium and abnormal behavior have prompted new warnings regarding use.

ANTIPROTOZOAL DRUGS

Metronidazole. Metronidazole has both antibiotic and antiprotozoal actions. It is useful for a wide variety of infections. Metronidazole has excellent activity against most gram-negative and gram-positive anaerobes and is indicated for use in many serious infections. Because metronidazole reaches high concentrations in most body tissues, it is very successful in the treatment of intraabdominal, intrapelvic, and cerebral infections, as well as endocarditis, bone and joint infections, and head and neck infections caused by susceptible anaerobes. Metronidazole also reaches high concentrations in abscesses (e.g., cerebral, hepatic, abdominal abscesses) and often is indicated in their treatment. Metronidazole does not cover gram-positive cocci or aerobic organisms; hence it usually is used in combination with another drug for the treatment of complicated infections.

In primary care settings, metronidazole is the drug of choice for the treatment of *T. vaginalis*. Because trichomonas is a sexually transmitted disease, both partners have to be treated for a cure to be achieved (i.e., to prevent reinfection of the other partner). The practitioner has the option of prescribing a 1- or 7-day course of treatment. A single oral dose (2 g) usually is as effective as the 7-day course. Although some evidence has shown that the 7-day treatment may have a slightly higher cure rate, the 1-day treatment may be justified if patient compliance is in question. Metronidazole also is indicated for the treatment of bacterial or nonspecific vaginitis.

Metronidazole is the current treatment of choice for symptomatic intestinal infection caused by *G. lamblia* and *E. histolytica*. Both parasites are found worldwide, and they usually are contracted by ingesting contaminated water or food. Sporadic outbreaks of *Giardia* occur throughout the United States and occasionally are seen in the primary care setting.

Metronidazole is the recommended first-line treatment of patients with *C. difficile*. Studies have shown that metronidazole is effective in most cases of *C. difficile*. However, vancomycin remains the drug of choice for severe cases.

Much attention has been focused on the use of metronidazole in the treatment of patients with *Helicobacter pylori,* an organism involved in the development of gastritis and peptic ulcer disease. Metronidazole, when given in conjunction with bismuth (and sometimes omeprazole or a histamine blocker), appears to be effective in treating *H. pylori*. The addition of tetracycline may increase the length of remission (see Chapter 25).

Chloroquine. Chloroquine is used for chemoprophylaxis of malaria. It is effective against *P. falciparum* and *P. malariae* infections that are not resistant. Chloroquine is given weekly starting 1 week before travel, during travel, and continuing for 4 weeks after leaving. Chloroquine also is used for the treatment of malaria.

How to Monitor

ANTIVIRALS. Monitor closely for toxicity and adverse effects, especially in patients with renal impairment.

ANTIPROTOZOALS

- *metronidazole:* Perform total CBC with differential leukocyte counts before and after therapy.
- *chloroquine:* Perform baseline and periodic ophthalmologic examinations every 3 months or with any eye symptoms.
- Monitor for muscular weakness, question and examine the patient, and test knee and ankle reflexes.
- Monitor CBC every 3 months.

Patient Variables

GERIATRICS

- Medications generally are very effective and well tolerated.
- *Antiherpes agents:* Reduce dosage in the elderly and in those with decreased renal function. The elderly are more likely to have renal or CNS adverse events.
- *amantadine, rimantadine:* Reduce dosage in patients older than 65 years.
- *zanamivir, oseltamivir:* No dosage adjustment is necessary.
- *metronidazole:* Decreased dosage adjustment may be necessary.

PEDIATRICS

- *famciclovir, valacyclovir:* Safety and efficacy in children younger than 18 years have not been established.
- *acyclovir:* Safety and efficacy in children younger than 2 years have not been established.
- *amantadine, rimantadine:* Safety and efficacy in children younger than 1 year have not been established.
- *zanamivir:* Safety and efficacy have not been established in patients younger than 7 years (treatment) and 5 years of age (prophylaxis).
- *metronidazole:* Safety and efficacy have not been established, except in the treatment of amebiasis.
- *chloroquine:* Children are especially sensitive to these drugs. Fatalities following accidental ingestion of relatively small doses and sudden deaths from parenteral chloroquine have been recorded. Do not exceed a single dose of 5 mg chloroquine *base* per kilogram in infants or children.
- *oseltamivir phosphate, zanamivir.* Children and adolescents with influenza may have neuropsychiatric symptoms, many of which may be significant.

PREGNANCY AND LACTATION

- *Category B:* acyclovir, famciclovir, valacyclovir, and metronidazole: Do not use metronidazole during first trimester.
- *Category C:* amantadine, rimantadine, zanamivir, chloroquine

- *acyclovir, amantadine, rimantadine, metronidazole, chloroquine:* Appear in breast milk; use is not recommended.
- *famciclovir, valacyclovir, zanamivir:* Safety and use in lactation are unknown.

Patient Education

ANTIVIRALS

Antiherpes Agents. Avoid sexual intercourse when visible herpes lesions are present.

Amantadine, Rimantadine

- Blurred vision or impaired mental acuity may occur. Use caution in performing tasks that require acute vision or physical coordination.
- Avoid excessive alcohol use because it will exacerbate CNS effects.

Zanamivir

- Instruct patients on use of the delivery system.
- Use of zanamivir for the treatment of influenza has not been shown to reduce the risk of transmission of influenza to others.
- Stop use of the drug if the patient experiences bronchospasm.

ANTIPROTOZOALS

Metronidazole

- May cause GI upset; take with food
- May cause darkening of the urine or metallic taste
- Avoid alcohol use; results in severe nausea and vomiting

Avoid alcoholic beverages and any products that contain alcohol because together, they may cause severe nausea, vomiting, flushing, and/or heart palpitations—a disulfiram-like reaction.

Chloroquine

- May cause GI upset; take with food
- Report visual disturbances or difficulty in hearing or ringing in ears, diarrhea, vomiting, muscle weakness, or rash.
- Keep out of reach of children; overdosage is especially dangerous in children.
- Medication may cause diarrhea, loss of appetite, nausea, stomach pain, or vomiting. Notify provider if effects are pronounced or bothersome.

SPECIFIC DRUGS

ANTIVIRALS

Antiherpetic Agents

acyclovir (Zovirax), famciclovir (Famvir), valacyclovir (Valtrex)

CONTRAINDICATIONS. Hypersensitivity or intolerance to the drug or any of its components

WARNINGS

- *acyclovir, famciclovir:* Testicular toxicity has occurred in rats.
- *famciclovir:* Carcinogenesis—increase in incidence of mammary adenocarcinoma was seen in rats.
- Famciclovir caused chromosomal aberrations in mice.
- Valacyclovir does not appear to be mutagenic.
- *valacyclovir:* Thrombotic thrombocytopenic purpura/hemolytic-uremic syndrome has occurred in patients with advanced HIV.

PRECAUTIONS

With some conditions, it may be prudent to obtain a viral culture to prove the identification of the virus when one is treating herpes simplex. Other conditions (e.g., poison ivy) may cause similar lesions.

- *Renal function impairment:* Reduce dosage according to the guidelines given in the package insert. Drugs are excreted mainly through the kidneys. Use caution in patients with decreased renal function (creatinine clearance less than 60 ml/min). Use with caution in patients who are poorly hydrated or are on other nephrotoxic medications, because these predispose the patient to acute renal failure.
- Ensure that the patient drinks fluids and does not become dehydrated.
- Use cautiously in patients who have underlying neurologic disorders, or who have had prior neurologic reactions to drugs. A small percentage (1%) of patients receiving parental acyclovir have had major neurologic symptoms such as lethargy, obtundation, tremors, confusion, hallucinations, agitation, seizures, or coma.
- Use can result in emergence of resistant viruses. HSV and varicella-zoster virus strains resistant to one drug generally have been cross-resistant to other drugs in this class.

PHARMACOKINETICS. See Table 68-1. The drug is widely distributed in body tissues and fluids, including brain, kidney, lung, liver, muscles, spleen, uterus, vaginal mucosa and secretions, cerebrospinal fluid, and herpetic vesicular fluid.

ADVERSE EFFECTS. See Table 68-2. Side effects commonly experienced with oral acyclovir include GI symptoms such as nausea, vomiting, and diarrhea. In general, more side effects have been noted with long-term or chronic use of the drug.

DRUG INTERACTIONS. See Table 68-3.

DOSAGE AND ADMINISTRATION. Table 68-4 provides recommendations for common primary care usage. Parenteral dosages for acute or severe infections are not included. Medication may be taken without regard to meals. Begin as soon as a diagnosis is made. These drugs are most effective if given within 24 to 48 hours of onset of signs and symptoms. Give reduced dose with any indication of renal impairment.

Antiinfluenza Agents

amantadine (Symmetrel), rimantadine (Flumadine)

Amantadine and rimantadine are similar and are discussed together.

CONTRAINDICATIONS. Hypersensitivity to either drug

WARNINGS

- Deaths have been reported from overdose with amantadine. Suicide attempts have been reported, some of which have been fatal in patients without a history of psychiatric illness.

TABLE 68-1   Pharmacokinetics of Antivirals and Antiprotozoals

Drug	Absorption	Time to Peak Concentration	Half-life	Protein Bound	Metabolism	Excretion
acyclovir	15%-30%	1.5-2 hr	2.5 hr	9%-33%	Liver	Urine, 60%-90%
famciclovir	77%	1 hr	2.3 hr	~20%	Liver	Urine, 73%
valacyclovir	54%	2-3 hr	2.5-3.3 hr	15%	Liver	Urine, 45%
amantadine	Well	3.3 hr	17 hr	60%	Not appreciable	Urine, >80%
rimantadine	Well	6 hr	25 hr		Liver	Renal, 25%
zanamivir	Inhaled, 4%-17% systemically absorbed	1-2 hr	2.5-5 hr	<10%	None	Urine
oseltamivir	Well		1-3 hr	3%	Liver	Urine
metronidazole	Well	1-2 hr	8 hr	<20%	Liver	Urine
tinidazole	PO, rapid, complete	1-2 hr	12-14 hr	12%	Liver, 3A4	Liver, renal 25% unchanged

💣 **Amantadine can exacerbate emotional problems in patients with a history of psychiatric disorder or substance abuse.**

- *Seizures and other CNS effects:* Observe patient with a seizure history carefully for increased seizure activity. Reduced dosage may be required. Caution patients who note CNS effects or blurring of vision against performing tasks that require alertness and motor coordination.
- Use with caution in patients with history of recurrent eczematoid rash, or psychosis or severe psychoneurosis not controlled by chemotherapeutic agents.
- Chronic heart failure may occur. Use caution in patients with cardiac history.
- Use amantadine with caution in patients with liver disease.
- Renal function impairment may require a reduced dose because amantadine accumulates in plasma.
- Safety and pharmacokinetics of rimantadine in renal and hepatic insufficiency have been evaluated only after single-dose administration. In renal failure, the half-life was increased. In hepatic failure, apparent clearance was decreased.

PRECAUTIONS
- Do not discontinue abruptly in patients with Parkinson's disease because it may precipitate a parkinsonian crisis.
- Sporadic cases of possible neuroleptic malignant syndrome have been reported with dose reduction or withdrawal. Observe carefully when dosage is reduced or discontinued.
- Notify primary care provider if patient develops mood or mental changes, swelling of the extremities, difficult urination, or shortness of breath.

OVERDOSAGE. Symptoms include cardiac, respiratory, renal, and CNS toxicity. Death has occurred from overdose with amantadine; the lowest reported acute lethal dose was 1 g. Acute toxicity may be attributable to the anticholinergic effects of amantadine.

zanamivir (Relenza), oseltamivir (Tamiflu)

CONTRAINDICATIONS. Hypersensitivity

WARNINGS. Oseltamivir phosphate and zanamivir now have strong warnings regarding the risk for neuropsychiatric adverse events. Symptoms of delirium and abnormal behavior leading to sometimes fatal self-injury have been reported with use of oseltamivir for the treatment of influenza.

PRECAUTIONS
- *zanamivir:* Allergic reactions, including oropharyngeal edema and serious skin rashes, have been reported.
- Bacterial infections may begin with influenza-like symptoms, may coexist, or may be a complication of influenza. These agents do not prevent such complications
- *Underlying respiratory disease:* Safety and efficacy have not been demonstrated in patients with underlying COPD. Some patients with underlying respiratory disease have experienced bronchospasm or decline in lung function with zanamivir. Zanamivir generally is not recommended for the treatment of patients with underlying airway disease such as asthma or COPD.
- Zanamivir has not been shown to prevent influenza and should not replace annual influenza immunizations.
- Safety and efficacy have not been demonstrated in patients with high-risk underlying medical conditions.

DOSAGE AND ADMINISTRATION
- *Prophylaxis:* Therapy should begin within 2 days of exposure. The duration of protection lasts for as long as dosing is continued.
- *Treatment:* Begin within 2 days of onset of symptoms.
- May be taken without regard to food, although tolerability may be enhanced with food

ANTIPROTOZOALS

metronidazole (Flagyl)

CONTRAINDICATIONS
- History of hypersensitivity to metronidazole or other nitroimidazole derivatives
- Pregnancy
- Disulfiram use

TABLE 68-2 Adverse Effects of Antivirals and Antiprotozoals

Body System	acyclovir	famciclovir	valacyclovir	amantadine	rimantadine	zanamivir	oseltamivir	metronidazole	chloroquine
Body, general	Malaise	Fatigue, pain, fever		Fatigue	Fatigue	Malaise, fatigue, fever	Fatigue	Bacterial infection, influenza-like symptoms, moniliasis	
Skin, appendages	Rash	Pruritus		Photosensitivity, rash	Rash	Urticaria			Hair loss, pruritus, rash, pigment changes
Hypersensitivity				Anaphylaxis					
Respiratory		Pharyngitis, sinusitis		Respiratory failure	Dyspnea	Nasal symptoms, bronchitis, sinusitis	Cough	Rhinitis, sinusitis, pharyngitis	
Cardiovascular				Orthostatic hypotension, CHF, hypertension, arrhythmias	Hypertension, CHF, heart block				Hypotension, ECG changes, cardiomyopathy
GI	Nausea, vomiting, diarrhea, constipation	Nausea, vomiting, diarrhea, abdominal pain, dyspepsia, constipation, anorexia	Nausea, vomiting, abdominal pain	Nausea, anorexia, dry mouth, constipation, diarrhea, vomiting	Nausea, vomiting, anorexia, dry mouth, abdominal pain	Diarrhea, nausea, vomiting, abdominal pain	Nausea, vomiting, diarrhea, abdominal pain	Nausea, abdominal pain, diarrhea, dry mouth	Anorexia, nausea, vomiting, diarrhea, abdominal cramps
Genitourinary								Vaginitis, genital pruritus, dysmenorrhea	
Hemic and lymphatic			Leukopenia, thrombocytopenia	Leukocytosis					Agranulocytosis, blood dyscrasias
Musculoskeletal		Back pain, arthralgia	arthralgia			Myalgia, arthralgia			Neuromyopathy
CNS	Headache	Headache, dizziness, insomnia, somnolence, paresthesia	Headache, dizziness	Dizziness, insomnia, depression, anxiety, restlessness, irritability, hallucinations, ataxia, headache, psychosis	Insomnia, dizziness, headache, asthenia, nervousness, ataxia, somnolence, agitation, hallucination, confusion, seizure	Headache, dizziness, peripheral neuropathy	Headache, dizziness, insomnia, vertigo	Headache, dizziness	
Special senses				Visual disturbance	Tinnitus, eye pain			Metallic taste, disulfiram-like reaction	Irreversible retinal damage, blurred vision, scotoma

TABLE 68-3   Drug Interactions With Antivirals and Antiprotozoals

Antiviral/Antiprotozoal	Action on Other Drugs
famciclovir	↑ digoxin
amantadine	↑ CNS stimulants
metronidazole	↑ hydantoins, lithium
chloroquine	↓ kaolin or magnesium trisilicate

Other Drugs	Action on Antivirals/ Antiprotozoals
probenecid, zidovudine	↑ acyclovir
cimetidine, probenecid, theophylline	↑ famciclovir
cimetidine, probenecid	↑ valacyclovir
Anticholinergic agents, quinidine, quinine, triamterene, thiazide diuretics, trimethoprim/sulfamethoxazole	↑ amantadine
cimetidine	↑ rimantadine
acetaminophen, aspirin	↓ rimantadine
cimetidine	↑ chloroquine

 This medication should not be given to patients who will ingest any type of alcohol. This includes alcoholic drinks, alcohol-based cough syrups, flavorings, and other products. Although the extent of risk is unknown, in sensitive individuals the product will cause a severe and immediate disulfiram (Antabuse)-like reaction if the patient has drunk alcohol while taking the medication.

WARNINGS
- *Neurologic effects:* Seizures and peripheral neuropathy have been reported in patients treated with metronidazole. Administer metronidazole with caution to patients with CNS disease.
- Patients with severe hepatic disease may experience an accumulation of metronidazole and its metabolites; therefore, the dose prescribed for these patients may have to be adjusted. A 50% dose reduction has been recommended in cases of severe liver failure.

Black Box Warning: Carcinogenesis has been found in rodents with long-term oral administration.

PRECAUTIONS
- Patients with Crohn's disease are known to have an increased incidence of GI and extraintestinal cancers. It is not known whether metronidazole increases the risk.
- Known or previously unrecognized candidiasis may present more prominent symptoms during therapy and requires treatment with a candidacidal agent.
- *Caution:* Evidence or history of blood dyscrasia. Mild leukopenia has been seen during administration; however, no persistent hematologic abnormalities attributable to the drug have been observed. Perform complete blood count with differential leukocyte counts before and after therapy with metronidazole.
- *Caution:* CNS disorder
- *Caution:* Impaired liver function

PHARMACOKINETICS. Metronidazole is well absorbed orally, with peak serum levels occurring 1 to 2 hours after adminis-

tration. Food does not alter the oral bioavailability of the drug but can delay peak serum levels by 1 to 2 hours. Plasma concentrations are proportional to the administered dose for both oral and intravenous use. For instance, oral administration of 250 mg and 500 mg tablets produces peak serum levels of 6 and 12 mcg/ml. The half-life of metronidazole is approximately 8 hours.

Metronidazole has a large volume of distribution. Less than 20% of the drug is bound to plasma proteins. It is well absorbed and concentrated in all body tissues and fluids, including bone, pelvic tissue, cerebrospinal fluid, meninges, bile, saliva, seminal fluid, breast milk, placenta, abscesses (including brain and hepatic), empyema fluid, and middle ear fluid.

Metabolism of metronidazole occurs in the liver. The metabolites of the drug have very strong bactericidal activity against most strains of anaerobic bacteria and *Trichomonas*. Plasma clearance of metronidazole is decreased in patients with decreased liver function; consequently, such patients may require altered doses. A 50% dose reduction has been recommended in patients with severe liver failure.

The major route of elimination of metronidazole and its metabolites is through the urine. Although some of the drug's metabolites may accumulate in patients with renal failure, it is unlikely to cause toxicity. Therefore, a dose reduction usually is not required in patients with decreased renal function. However, the literature does suggest a reduced dose in patients with severe renal failure.

DRUG INTERACTIONS. The most severe reaction may occur with concurrent ingestion of alcohol, which produces a disulfiram-like reaction. In sensitive individuals, this is a violent reaction that causes immediate nausea, vomiting, diarrhea, and cardiovascular effects. Table 68-3 lists other common drug interactions.

OVERDOSAGE. Single oral doses of up to 15 g have been reported with symptoms such as nausea, vomiting, and ataxia. Neurologic symptoms (including seizures and peripheral neuropathy) have been reported after 5 to 7 days of doses of 6 to 10.4 g every other day.

DOSAGE AND ADMINISTRATION. See Table 68-4. The pharmacokinetics of metronidazole may be altered in elderly patients or patients with hepatic failure. Therefore, monitoring of serum levels in certain cases may be necessary for adjusting the dosage properly. The metronidazole tablet (Flagyl ER) should be taken while fasting. Reduce dosage in patients with hepatic disease. Dosage reduction is not needed in renal insufficiency.

chloroquine (Plaquenil)

CONTRAINDICATIONS
- Hypersensitivity
- Retinal or visual field changes
- Long-term therapy in children (hydroxychloroquine)

WARNINGS
- Resistance to this product develops easily. Certain strains of *P. falciparum* are resistant. Treat with other therapy if resistance develops.
- May cause irreversible retinal damage; monitor vision frequently during treatment
- Use with caution in patients with G6PD deficiency.

TABLE 68-4 Dosage and Administration Recommendations for Antivirals and Protozoals

Drug	Disease	Stage	Dosage and Administration	Max Dose
acyclovir	Herpes simplex, genital	Initial	200 mg po q4h (5 times per day) × 10 days; 400 mg po tid for 5-10 days (unlabeled)	
		Chronic suppressive	400 mg bid or 200 mg tid-qid (up to 12 months)	
		Recurrent episode	200 mg po q4h (5 times per day) × 5 days; 400 mg po tid for 5 days (unlabeled)	
	Herpes simplex, labialis	Treatment	*Topical:* Apply 5 times per day × 4 days	
	Herpes zoster	Acute	800 mg q4h (5 times per day) × 7-10 days	
		Chickenpox	20 mg/kg qid × 5 days. Initiate within 24 hr of symptom onset.	800 mg
famciclovir	Herpes simplex, genital	Initial	250 mg tid × 7-10 days	
		Chronic suppressive	250 mg bid (up to 1 yr)	
		Recurrent episode	1 g bid × 1 day. Initiate treatment within 6 hours of symptom onset.	
		Recurrent episode, HIV+	500 mg bid × 7 days	
	Herpes simplex, labialis	Treatment	1.5 g as a single dose. Initiate at sign or symptom onset.	
	Herpes zoster	Acute	500 mg every 8 hours × 7 days. Initiate treatment within 72 hr of rash onset.	
	Renal impairment	All indications	Dosing adjustment is necessary; see detailed drug reference for specific dosing for each indication and the corresponding degree of renal impairment.	
valacyclovir	Herpes simplex, genital	Initial	1 g bid × 10 days	
		Suppressive	1 g once daily; 500 mg once daily in patients with <9 recurrences/yr	
		Suppressive, HIV+	(CD4 ≥100 cells/mm^3): 500 mg bid	
		Recurrent episode	500 mg bid × 3 days	
	Herpes zoster	Acute	1 g tid × 7 days	
amantadine	Influenza A	Prophylaxis and treatment	13-64 yr: 100 mg bid × 3-5 days. Initiate within 24-48 hr of symptom onset.	
			≥10 yr and >40 kg: See adult dosing	150 mg/day
			≥10 yr and <40 kg: 5 mg/kg once daily	
			1-9 yr: 5 mg/kg/day in two divided doses	
			65 yr: 100 mg once daily	100 mg/day
		Clcr 30-50 ml/min	200 mg on day 1, then 100 mg/day	
		Clcr 15-29 ml/min	200 mg on day 1, then 100 mg on alternate days	
		Clcr <15 ml/min	200 mg every 7 days	
		Hemodialysis	200 mg every 7 days	
rimantadine	Influenza A	Prophylaxis, treatment	Adult: 100 mg bid	
			Child (1-10 yr): 5 mg/kg/day once daily	150 mg/day
		Clcr <10 ml/min		100 mg/day
oseltamivir	Influenza A and B	Prophylaxis	Adult and child (>12 yr): 75 mg once daily × 10 days. Initiate within 2 days of exposure.	
			Child (1-12 yr):	
			15 kg: 30 mg once daily	
			15-23 kg: 45 mg once daily	
			23-40 kg: 60 mg once daily	
			>40 kg: 75 mg once daily	
		Clcr 10-30 ml/min	75 mg every other day or 30 mg once daily	
		Treatment	Adult and child (>12 yr): 75 mg bid × 5 days; initiated within 2 days of exposure	
			Child (1-12 yr):	
			15 kg: 30 mg bid	
			15-23 kg: 45 mg bid	
			23-40 kg: 60 mg bid	
			>40 kg: 75 mg bid	
		Clcr 10-30 ml/min	75 mg once daily for 5 days	
zanamivir	Influenza A and B	Prophylaxis	2 inhalations (10 mg) once daily × 10 days beginning 24-36 hr after onset of symptoms	
			Child (≥5 yr): See adult dosing.	
		Treatment	Adults and child (≥7 yr): 2 inhalations (10 mg) bid × 5 days	
metronidazole	Bacterial vaginosis	Treatment	500 mg twice daily or 750 mg ER once daily × 7 days	
			250-500 mg tid-qid × 7-14 days	
	C. difficile		Child: 30 mg/kg/day divided every 6 hr × 7-10 days	
tinidazole	Giardiasis, amebiasis, trichomoniasis	Treatment	2 g po × 1 with food as a single dose (giardiasis; trichomoniasis [both partners]); continue for 3-5 days (amebiasis [3 days]; amebiasis, liver abscess [3-5 days])	
			Child (>3 yr): 50 mg/kg (up to 2 g). See above for treatment duration.	

- Muscular weakness may occur; discontinue if symptoms develop.
- May exacerbate psoriasis or porphyria
- Use with caution in hepatic disease or alcoholism or with other hepatotoxic drugs.

PRECAUTIONS. Monitor CBC; see "How to Monitor."

ADVERSE EFFECTS. See Table 68-2. Cardiovascular events, ophthalmic retinal damage, and agranulocytosis are some of the more important severe adverse effects.

OVERDOSAGE. Headache, drowsiness, visual disturbances, cardiovascular collapse, convulsions, and death can occur. Treatment is symptomatic.

DOSAGE AND ADMINISTRATION. See CDC recommendations for use of chloroquine.

evolve A continually updated list of useful WebLinks may be found in the Evolve Resources at http://evolve.elsevier.com/Edmunds/NP/

evolve http://evolve.elsevier.com/Edmunds/NP/

Immunizations and Biologicals

LAURIE SCUDDER

IMMUNIZATION AND BIOLOGICAL AGENTS COMMONLY USED IN PRIMARY CARE

Disease	Active Immunity	Passive Immunity	Testing
Hepatitis A	Hepatitis A vaccine, inactivated	Immune globulin, Ig	Antibody levels
Hepatitis B	Hepatitis B vaccine	Hepatitis B immune globulin	Antibody levels
Diphtheria	DTaP	Diphtheria antitoxin	
Tetanus/pertussis	DPT-HIB vaccine, DTaP, Td, tetanus toxoid	Tetanus immune globulin	
Haemophilus pneumonia	*Haemophilus influenzae* B vaccine		
Human papillomavirus	Human papillomavirus vaccine		
Polio	Poliovirus vaccine, inactivated		
Rubeola (measles)	MMR, measles (rubeola) vaccine	Immune globulin, IM	Rubella titer
Mumps	Mumps vaccine, rubella and mumps vaccine, MMR		
Rubella (measles)	MMR (rubella vaccine)		
Varicella-zoster	Varicella virus vaccine	Varicella-zoster immune globulin	
Influenza	Influenzavirus vaccine		
Pneumococcal pneumonia	Pneumococcal polysaccharide vaccine, polyvalent and pneumococcal conjugate vaccine		
Meningitis	Meningococcal polysaccharide vaccine		
Rabies	Rabies vaccine (HDCV)	Rabies immune globulin, human	
Rotavirus			
Tuberculosis	BCG vaccine		Tuberculin tests
Yellow fever	Yellow fever vaccine		
Typhoid	Typhoid vaccine		

INDICATIONS

The individual immunizations mentioned in the above table are not discussed in equal detail; emphasis is placed on immunizations recommended in the pediatric and adult schedules of the CDC Advisory Committee on Immunization Practices (ACIP). Maintaining the patient's vaccination status is a major component of primary care. Nurse practitioners should keep up-to-date with the latest recommendations and keep their patients' immunizations up-to-date. (For recommended immunizations schedules, go to www.cdc.gov.)

THERAPEUTIC OVERVIEW

The goal of immunization is the eradication of disease. Numerous infectious diseases, many of which are potentially fatal, have been sharply curtailed worldwide through vigilant adherence to immunization strategies and public health control measures. In the United States, diphtheria, measles, polio, and tetanus are almost unknown. Children who are not vaccinated for religious, cultural, or other reasons are at risk for disease and increase societal risk by contributing to the pool of unvaccinated individuals who are capable of transmitting infection to susceptible and high-risk individuals. The 2004 National Immunization Survey documented that the percentage of children aged 19 to 35 months who received all doses of recommended vaccines, which includes four doses of diphtheria, tetanus, and pertussis (DTaP), three or more doses of polio vaccine, one or more doses of measles-containing vaccine, three or more doses of Hib vaccine, three doses of hepatitis B vaccine, and one dose of varicella, increased to 80.9%, compared with 72.7% in 1998, the first year of the survey (http://www.ahrq.gov/qual/nhqr06/nhqr06report.pdf).

Despite this success, however, it is estimated that 5% to 15% (National Committee for Quality Assurance, http://web.ncqa.org/) of all 2-year-olds in the United States have not received vaccines that should be completed by that time. State and national statistics suggest the need to improve public education on the importance of immunization.

Anatomy and Physiology: The Immune System

The first line of defense against disease consists of the skin, mucous membranes, body hair, and body secretions. The second line of defense is the inflammatory response, which is critical for the body's survival when faced with stressors from the environment and is increasingly recognized as an important factor in a variety of acute and chronic diseases. The immune system is the third line of defense against the invasion of antigens.

The main function of the immune system is to protect the body from damage caused by the introduction of a foreign substance. A number of stimuli can trigger the inflammatory response. These include infectious agents, ischemia, antigen–antibody interactions, and thermal or other injury. In many conditions, the cause of the inflammation is not known. The inflammatory response includes three phases: (1) acute, transient, local vasodilation and increased capillary permeability; (2) delayed, subacute infiltration of leukocytes and phagocytic cells; and (3) chronic proliferative tissue degeneration and fibrosis.

Organs of the immune system consist of primary and secondary organs. Primary organs are responsible for the development and storage of lymphocytes. The bone marrow and the thymus gland are the primary organs of the immune system. Secondary organs include lymph nodes, spleen, and Peyer's patches. These secondary organs of the immune system entrap foreign substances, produce antibodies, and stimulate T-cell production, all with the main objective of destroying the antigen. All WBCs originate from a stem cell in the bone marrow. Stem cells first differentiate into myeloid and lymphoid cells. Myeloid cells differentiate into polymorphonuclear (PMN) leukocytes and into monocytes/macrophages. Lymphoid cells differentiate into B- and T-lymphocytes (Figure 69-1).

Two types of nonspecific WBCs and two types of specific WBCs have been identified.

NONSPECIFIC WBCs. The first type of WBC includes polymorphonuclear leukocytes, also called granulocytes (neutrophils, eosinophils, basophils, and mast cells). These are the most active cells and contain the largest number of immune cells in the body. They arrive first at a site of injury, infection, or inflammation and function in several ways. They phagocytize foreign substances and release chemotaxic substances that encircle the area of invasion, killing and preventing contamination by foreign substance into other areas; they also stimulate the release of antimicrobial substances that aid in the destruction of foreign material.

- *Neutrophils* contain large granules. These granules degranulate when they come in contact with antigens and release enzymes that destroy foreign substances and can injure surrounding tissue. Debris from this destructive action produces an exudate/pus. Enzymes that are secreted from these granules are known as chemotaxic factors; they include leukotrienes, vasoactive kinins, and toxic metabolites.
- *Eosinophils* are very similar to neutrophils. They contain granules and engage in the process of phagocytosis. They seem to congregate in the respiratory and gastrointestinal tracts. They are especially prominent during allergic reactions and parasitic infections, and they carry certain enzymes that neutralize chemicals responsible for allergic responses. They release potent chemotaxic factors that cause inflammation, bronchospasm, and tissue damage.
- *Basophils* also contain granules that produce histamine and heparin, which play a role in the immune response. The basophil is not a strong structure, and it is easily damaged, which causes the granules to release histamine and heparin. Vasospasm, increased vascular permeability, and increased inflammation are the major effects seen when this occurs. This reaction increases the severity of allergic responses.
- *Mast cells*, the guardians of the immune system, are found in cutaneous and mucosal tissue. They can immediately recognize invasive non-self (foreign) antigens without the aid of macrophages or lymphocytes. They are the effectors of immediate hypersensitivity reactions and contain most of the body's IgE. When this IgE and an antigen meet, there is immediate degranulation and release of histamine, prostaglandin, and leukotrienes, as well as arachidonic acid metabolism, which potentiates the hypersensitivity response.

The second type of nonspecific WBC is the monocyte/macrophage. When monocytes are released into the bloodstream, they migrate to various tissue sites, where they differentiate (mature) and become macrophages. Macrophages serve three functions in the immune response. The first is to secrete biologically active compounds/molecules such as prostaglandins, interleukins, interferons, tumor necrosis factors, growth factors, proteins, and enzymes, which serve to provide host defense from specific antigens. The second is to remove excess dead or damaged antigens. The third is to engulf and present antigens to lymphoid cells for elimination. Macrophages are found in connective tissue (histocyte), the liver (Kupffer's cells), alveolar tissue in the lung, and microglial cells in the nervous system. They are also found in the spleen, lymph nodes, and other organs.

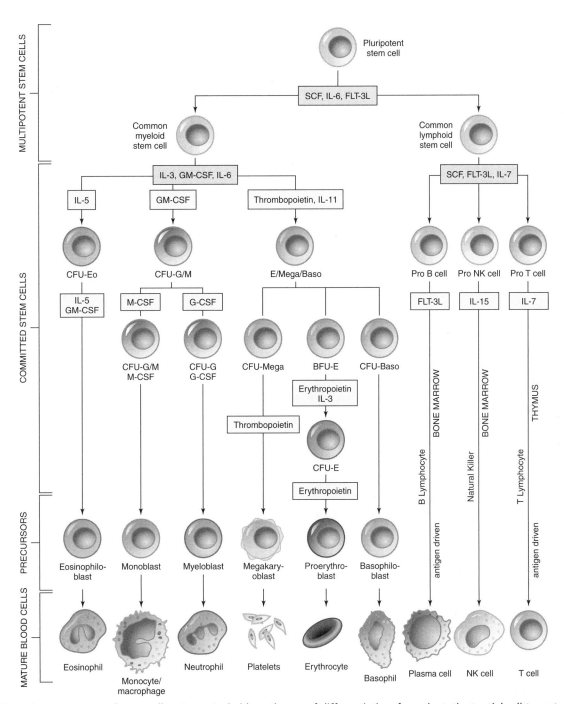

FIGURE 69-1   Bone marrow and stem cell systems. Probable pathways of differentiation, from the totipotential cell to mature blood cells. (PMN, Granulocytes.) (From McCance KL, Heuther SE: *Pathophysiology,* ed 4, St Louis, 2002, Mosby.)

SPECIFIC WBCs. The specific WBCs consist of the two lymphocytes (B- and T-cells). These cells react with antigens to produce reactions that create a specific response that will destroy the antigen. These do not participate in nonspecific inflammatory responses.

- The B-lymphocytes are those cells that produce antibodies. They undergo specific differentiation when exposed to an antigen and become plasma cells that are the major secretors of antibodies (Figure 69-2). The major function of these antibodies is to destroy a specific antigen and remove it from the body. In response to a specific antigen, a single antibody is produced (each antigen has a specific antibody). The

antibodies are grouped into five different classes known as immunoglobulins. These classes contain formed chains of immunoglobulins expressed on the cell surface and labeled IgG, IgA, IgM, IgE, and IgD. Table 69-1 describes the features of these antibodies. B-lymphocytes provide humoral immunity through the secretion of these immunoglobulins.

- *T-cell lymphocytes* make up 65% to 80% of all lymphocytes in the blood. Three different types of T-cells are known: helper, suppressor, and cytotoxic. *Helper cells* aid in initiation of the immune response by helping B-cells synthesize antibodies for action. *Suppressor cells* help keep B-cell antibody production in check. They hold

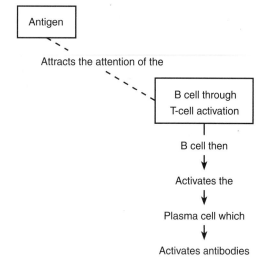

FIGURE 69-2 Immune response—humoral.

back the immune response or restrict antibody production because, if left unchecked, these B-cells can do more harm than good. *Cytotoxic cells,* or *killer cells,* circulate to kill cells not recognized as self cells (such as tumor cells). Activation of these cells occurs through interaction of antigens with macrophages. Through secretion of the special products produced by macrophages, T-cell proliferation occurs. These activated T-cells release substances known as lymphokines that influence the growth of other cells necessary for body defense, thus amplifying the immune reaction (Figure 69-3).

The lymphokine interferons are active against viruses.

OTHER IMMUNE SYSTEM COMPONENTS. Three plasma protein systems are located in the plasma of blood, not inside a cell. These include the complement, clotting, and kinin systems. Each initiates a cascade of reactions, ending with potent biochemical mediators of the inflammatory response. The complement system is a nonspecific mediator of inflammation that is potent against bacterial infection. IgG or IgM usually initiates the cascade by forming an immune complex. The kinin system begins with bradykinin, which causes dilation of vessels, acts with prostaglandins to induce pain and increase vascular permeability, and is important in the prolonged phase of inflammation. Platelets stop bleeding and release serotonin, which has vascular effects

similar to histamine. The clotting system is discussed in Chapter 23. Cytokines are glycoproteins, which are chemical messengers that modulate the immune response

THE NONSPECIFIC INFLAMMATORY RESPONSE. Two basic antiinflammatory actions occur: phagocytosis (ingestion of unwanted material) and secretion of cytokines that mediate the inflammatory response. A bewildering array of these substances with overlapping sources and functions have been identified.

Macrophages, mast cells, T-helper cells, natural killer cells, and others secrete many cytokines, including colony-stimulating factor interleukins, tissue necrosis factor, and interferon.

The inflammatory response begins when circulating proteins and blood cells come into contact with a stimulus. Neutrophils arrive at the site first and phagocytose (ingest) the particles that are causing the inflammation. The mast cells are already present in the loose connective tissues close to blood vessels. Monocytes and macrophages arrive and begin phagocytosis. Mast cells, monocytes, and macrophages release many substances called collectively mediators or facilitators of inflammation. The mast cell is the most important activator of the inflammatory response.

Mast cells immediately release substances from their granules, which cause immediate inflammation. These substances include histamine, neutrophil chemotactic factor, and eosinophil chemotactic factor. The mast cell also synthesizes then releases leukotrienes and prostaglandins, which causes long-term inflammation (see Figure 34-2). These facilitators start a chain of reactions, thereby producing exudate that defends against infection and facilitates tissue repair and healing.

Whereas many mediators of inflammation are known, this discussion focuses on the prostaglandins, which are affected by aspirin and NSAIDs.

Prostaglandins cause increased vascular permeability and neutrophil chemotaxis (movement), and they induce pain. Increased vascular permeability allows diffusion of large molecule inflammatory substances across cell walls into the site of inflammation. Prostaglandins are made within the mast cell from arachidonic acid through the action of the enzyme cyclooxygenase (COX) and are classified into groups according to their structure. Prostaglandins E_1 and E_2 are active in the inflammatory response. Aspirin and NSAIDs act to block the enzyme COX from producing prostaglandins, thereby inhibiting inflammation (see Chapter 34 and Figure 34-2).

TABLE 69-1 Characteristics and Functions of Immunoglobulins

Immunoglobulins	Amount in Serum	Location of Concentration	Stimulated By	Functions
IgG	Most abundant in the blood, 75%	Intravascular Extravascular	Allergic response Second immunoglobulin	Provides immunity against bloodborne infection (i.e., bacteria, viruses, some fungi)
IgA	15%	Intravascular Secretions	Presence of antigens Antiviral antibody	Most common antibody in secretions, where it protects mucous membranes Bactericidal with lysosome
IgM	10%	Intravascular	Presence of antigens	First immunoglobulin produced during an immune response Activates complement
IgD	1%	On the surface of B-cells	Presence of antigens	Antigen-specific receptor on B-cells

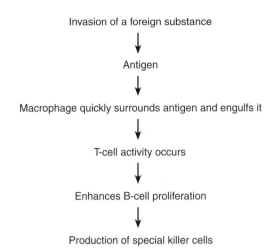

Invasion of a foreign substance

↓

Antigen

↓

Macrophage quickly surrounds antigen and engulfs it

↓

T-cell activity occurs

↓

Enhances B-cell proliferation

↓

Production of special killer cells

FIGURE 69-3   Immune response—cell mediated.

THE SPECIFIC IMMUNE RESPONSE. The immune response is activated through generation of humoral or cellular immunity. *B-lymphocytes* are the cells involved in antibody-mediated or humoral immunity. *T-lymphocytes* are the effectors for cell-mediated immunity. This response can be summarized as follows:

- A foreign substance (the antigen) invades.
- A macrophage engulfs it and presents it on its cell surface.
- The expressed antigen stimulates T-cell activity.
- T-helper cells are activated to enhance B-cell differentiation into plasma cells and the production of antibodies/immunoglobulin (IgG, IgM, IgA, IgE, IgD).
- Proliferation of B- and T-cells produces clones with a memory that enables them to recognize a returning invader. This memory produces a more potent and rapid immune response should the invader return.

MECHANISM OF ACTION

Immunizations act to confer immunity to a particular disease. There are two types of immunity: active and passive.

THERAPEUTIC OVERVIEW

ACTIVE IMMUNITY. Active immunization involves the administration of all or a part of a microorganism to evoke a response. Antigens are taken from living or dead organisms, and small amounts are given intradermally or subcutaneously. This process stimulates the body's immune response, and antibodies are stimulated to protect the immunized person from greater exposure to this particular disease-producing antigen. This immunity is retained for a prolonged period, thereby protecting the person from the disease whenever he or she may be exposed to that antigen. This immunity can be "boosted" at specific intervals.

Active immunization is accomplished with three different types of agents:

1. *Inactivated vaccines (killed agents):* Most bacterial vaccines, and some viral, involve the use of inactivated agents. These agents are not capable of replicating within the host and thus present little risk to the recipient. Maintenance of life-long immunity requires the administration of multiple doses. Mucosal protection after the use of killed vaccines is less than with the use of live vaccines. Thus, local infection or colonization with the agent can occur, along with potential for transmission, although systemic disease is prevented.

2. *Live vaccines (attenuated):* Most viral vaccines involve the use of live virus that has been chemically changed to decrease its virulence. Active infection, with replication of the virus, occurs in the host following administration of the product, although few adverse effects occur. This route generally produces a superior response, including mucosal immunity, and does not require the use of multiple doses.

3. *Active immunization:* This may be accomplished with use of a modified product of an organism, such as a toxoid, which consists of modified bacterial toxins and retains the ability to stimulate antibody formation but is nontoxic. This route of immunization is used against diphtheria and tetanus. Maintenance of protective titers of antitoxin requires periodic administration of booster doses of toxoid.

PASSIVE IMMUNITY. Passive immunity occurs when antibodies that one acquired from a human or an animal (with acquired immunity to a specific organism) are given to people who do not have immunity to the organism. Newborn infants achieve this naturally from their mothers through the placenta and through breastfeeding. It can also be achieved through injections of gamma globulins (for hepatitis protection) or antisera or antitoxins. This process temporarily provides the same protection as that given to a person who has achieved active acquired immunity. These antibodies naturally break down and are eliminated from the body. See Table 69-1 for a summary of the characteristics and function of immunoglobulins.

Antisera (antibodies of animal origin used to counteract the effects of a toxin) and human plasma are used after exposure. Very specific indications and guidelines govern the use of these products. They are not discussed in detail in this chapter. Contact your local health department or the CDC for guidelines concerning the use of antisera.

Incompetent immune systems do not develop active immunity in response to vaccines and toxoid. These patients need protection from infection. This protection can be accomplished through passive immunity, identification of the deficient immune mediators, and replacement of those mediators, or by giving these patients antiinfective drugs. Agents that are classified as immune mediators are agents such as interferon, interleukins, and immunoglobulin.

All immunizations contain several different components, such as the following:

- *Immunizing agent:* This active component of the product may be a killed or attenuated vaccine or a toxoid.
- *Suspending fluid:* This may be either sterile water or saline or a complex tissue-culture fluid. It may contain proteins derived from the medium in which the vaccine was produced, such as egg antigen in inactivated influenza vaccine. Individuals who experience anaphylactic reactions to egg may be allergic to influenza vaccine; studies of MMR vaccine have demonstrated that egg-allergic children may be safely vaccinated.
- *Preservatives:* Trace amounts of preservatives, stabilizers, or antibiotics often are added to prevent bacterial overgrowth in multiuse vials of vaccines. Individuals may have allergic reactions to products such as neomycin that may be present in minute amounts. Thimerosal, a mercury-containing organic compound widely used as a preservative, was removed from or was reduced to trace amounts in all vaccines in 2001 because of concerns about potential neurodevelopmental

pathology in infants who may receive multiple vaccines that contain thimerosal and may be unable to adequately clear this product because of hepatic immaturity (see http://www.fda.gov/cber/vaccine/thimerosal.htm). In 2004, the Institute of Medicine released a report that rejected a causal link between vaccines and developmental disorders, including autism, in children. The FDA is continuing its efforts to reduce the exposure of infants, children, and pregnant women to mercury from various sources.

- *Adjuvants:* This is often an aluminum-based compound that is added to enhance the immunogenicity of an agent and prolong its stimulatory effects. This is necessary for some inactivated vaccines and for toxoids.

Comparable vaccines made by different manufacturers may be used interchangeably, if used according to recommended guidelines. Available data suggest that adequate response occurs even when products from different manufacturers are used during the same series. Figure 69-4 shows the recommended childhood immunizations generally used in primary care.

> **evolve**   See Bonus tables at http://evolve.elsevier.com/Edmunds/NP/

TREATMENT PRINCIPLES

Standardized Guidelines

- Recommended childhood, adolescent, and adult immunization schedules: United States, 2008
- Centers for Disease Control Advisory Committee on Immunization Practices
  - Schedule for Children 0-6 Years
  - Schedule for Persons 7-18 Years
  - Catch-up Schedule for Persons 4 Months to 18 Years
  - Adult Immunization Schedule

All are available at http://www.cdc.gov/vaccines/recs/schedules/default.htm

Evidence-Based Recommendations

- ACIP: General recommendations on immunization, *MMWR* 55(RR15):1-48, Dec 1, 2006 (Available at http://www.cdc.gov/mmwr/preview/mmwrhtml/rr5515a1.htm?s_cid=rr5515a1_e)

Cardinal Points of Treatment

- General principles for vaccine administration:
  - The Recommended Childhood and Adolescent Immunization Schedule and the Recommended Adult Immunization Schedule are revised annually. Health care providers should ensure that they are following the most up-to-date schedules, which are available on the CDC website.
  - Vaccination providers should adhere as closely as possible to recommended vaccination schedules. ACIP recommends that vaccine doses for all products with the exception of rabies vaccine should be administered 4 or fewer days before the minimum interval or age to be counted as valid. Longer-than-recommended intervals between doses do not reduce final antibody concentrations, although protection might not be attained until all doses have been administered. With the exception of oral typhoid vaccine, an interruption in the vaccination schedule does not require restarting the entire series of a vaccine or toxoid or addition of extra doses.

- Health care providers should simultaneously administer all vaccines for which a person is eligible because simultaneous administration increases the probability that an individual will be vaccinated fully at the appropriate age. Administration of each preparation at a different anatomic site is desirable. Simultaneous administration of the most widely used live and inactivated vaccines has produced seroconversion rates and rates for adverse reactions similar to those observed when the vaccines are administered separately. An inactivated vaccine can be administered simultaneously or at any time before or after a different inactivated vaccine or live vaccine. Live vaccines also may be administered simultaneously. However, live vaccines such as measles, mumps, and rubella should not be administered after receipt of an antibody-containing product such as immunoglobulin until the passive antibody response to the product has degraded. This process is dependent on dose and specific product. Exceptions to this rule are yellow fever vaccine, oral typhoid vaccine, and live-attenuated influenza vaccine, which may be administered after immunoglobulin.
- Use of combination vaccines can reduce the number of injections required at a visit. Licensed combination vaccines can be used whenever any components of the combination are indicated, and its other components are not contraindicated.
- Vaccines made by different manufacturers are generally interchangeable. Although it is preferable to complete a series with a single product, vaccination should not be deferred because the brand used for previous doses is not available or is unknown
- Persons without documentation of vaccine receipt should be considered non-immunized if a reasonable effort to locate records is unsuccessful. These individuals should be started on the age-appropriate vaccination schedule. Serologic testing for immunity is an alternative to vaccination for certain antigens (e.g., measles, rubella, hepatitis A, tetanus).

Guidelines concerning the use of immunizations are one of the most carefully studied areas of pharmacology. Joint guidelines for adults are promulgated by the ACIP and the American Academy of Pediatrics (AAP). Guidelines are revised yearly as new products are introduced and recommendations for use of older products change; these guidelines determine the standard of care that all primary care providers are expected to provide. With the increase in the immunocompromised population and the increasing numbers of immigrants living in the United States who require catch-up vaccination, the greatest challenge for primary care providers is to master the exceptions to the recommended schedule. Figure 69-4 provides the recommendations for pediatric immunizations from the ACIP and the AAP. The latest updates are available on the CDC website. In addition, a catch-up schedule for children up to the age of 18 years is available.

Critical decisions to be made in immunizations include which products to give and when to give them. Before using any biological, the health care provider should take all precautions known for the detection or prevention of allergic or any other adverse reaction. This should include a review of the patient's history regarding possible sensitivity, the ready availability of epinephrine 1:1000 and other appropriate

Recommended Immunization Schedule for Persons Aged 0–6 Years—UNITED STATES • 2008

For those who fall behind or start late, see the catch-up schedule

Vaccine ▼ Age ▶	Birth	1 month	2 months	4 months	6 months	12 months	15 months	18 months	19–23 months	2–3 years	4–6 years
Hepatitis B[1]	HepB	HepB		see footnote 1		HepB					
Rotavirus[2]			Rota	Rota	Rota						
Diphtheria, Tetanus, Pertussis[3]			DTaP	DTaP	DTaP	see footnote 3	DTaP				DTaP
Haemophilus influenzae type b[4]			Hib	Hib	Hib[4]	Hib					
Pneumococcal[5]			PCV	PCV	PCV	PCV				PPV	
Inactivated Poliovirus			IPV	IPV		IPV					IPV
Influenza[6]						Influenza (Yearly)					
Measles, Mumps, Rubella[7]						MMR					MMR
Varicella[8]						Varicella					Varicella
Hepatitis A[9]						HepA (2 doses)				HepA Series	
Meningococcal[10]										MCV4	

Range of recommended ages

Certain high-risk groups

This schedule indicates the recommended ages for routine administration of currently licensed childhood vaccines, as of December 1, 2007, for children aged 0 through 6 years. Additional information is available at www.cdc.gov/vaccines/recs/schedules. Any dose not administered at the recommended age should be administered at any subsequent visit, when indicated and feasible. Additional vaccines may be licensed and recommended during the year. Licensed combination vaccines may be used whenever any components of the combination are indicated and other components of the vaccine are not contraindicated and if approved by the Food and Drug Administration for that dose of the series. Providers should consult the respective Advisory Committee on Immunization Practices statement for detailed recommendations, including for **high-risk conditions:** **http://www.cdc.gov/vaccines/pubs/ACIP-list.htm.** Clinically significant adverse events that follow immunization should be reported to the Vaccine Adverse Event Reporting System (VAERS). Guidance about how to obtain and complete a VAERS form is available at **www.vaers.hhs.gov** or by telephone, **800-822-7967.**

1. Hepatitis B vaccine (HepB). *(Minimum age: birth)*
At birth:
- Administer monovalent HepB to all newborns prior to hospital discharge.
- If mother is hepatitis B surface antigen (HBsAg) positive, administer HepB and 0.5 mL of hepatitis B immune globulin (HBIG) within 12 hours of birth.
- If mother's HBsAg status is unknown, administer HepB within 12 hours of birth. Determine the HBsAg status as soon as possible and if HBsAg positive, administer HBIG (no later than age 1 week).
- If mother is HBsAg negative, the birth dose can be delayed, in rare cases, with a provider's order and a copy of the mother's negative HBsAg laboratory report in the infant's medical record.

After the birth dose:
- The HepB series should be completed with either monovalent HepB or a combination vaccine containing HepB. The second dose should be administered at age 1–2 months. The final dose should be administered no earlier than age 24 weeks. Infants born to HBsAg-positive mothers should be tested for HBsAg and antibody to HBsAg after completion of at least 3 doses of a licensed HepB series, at age 9–18 months (generally at the next well-child visit).

4-month dose:
- It is permissible to administer 4 doses of HepB when combination vaccines are administered after the birth dose. If monovalent HepB is used for doses after the birth dose, a dose at age 4 months is not needed.

2. Rotavirus vaccine (Rota). *(Minimum age: 6 weeks)*
- Administer the first dose at age 6–12 weeks.
- Do not start the series later than age 12 weeks.
- Administer the final dose in the series by age 32 weeks. Do not administer any dose later than age 32 weeks.
- Data on safety and efficacy outside of these age ranges are insufficient.

3. Diphtheria and tetanus toxoids and acellular pertussis vaccine (DTaP). *(Minimum age: 6 weeks)*
- The fourth dose of DTaP may be administered as early as age 12 months, provided 6 months have elapsed since the third dose.
- Administer the final dose in the series at age 4–6 years.

4. *Haemophilus influenzae* type b conjugate vaccine (Hib). *(Minimum age: 6 weeks)*
- If PRP-OMP (PedvaxHIB® or ComVax® [Merck]) is administered at ages 2 and 4 months, a dose at age 6 months is not required.
- TriHIBit® (DTaP/Hib) combination products should not be used for primary immunization but can be used as boosters following any Hib vaccine in children age 12 months or older.

5. Pneumococcal vaccine. *(Minimum age: 6 weeks for pneumococcal conjugate vaccine [PCV]; 2 years for pneumococcal polysaccharide vaccine [PPV])*
- Administer one dose of PCV to all healthy children aged 24–59 months having any incomplete schedule.
- Administer PPV to children aged 2 years and older with underlying medical conditions.

6. Influenza vaccine. *(Minimum age: 6 months for trivalent inactivated influenza vaccine [TIV]; 2 years for live, attenuated influenza vaccine [LAIV])*
- Administer annually to children aged 6–59 months and to all eligible close contacts of children aged 0–59 months.
- Administer annually to children 5 years of age and older with certain risk factors, to other persons (including household members) in close contact with persons in groups at higher risk, and to any child whose parents request vaccination.
- For healthy persons (those who do not have underlying medical conditions that predispose them to influenza complications) ages 2–49 years, either LAIV or TIV may be used.
- Children receiving TIV should receive 0.25 mL if age 6–35 months or 0.5 mL if age 3 years or older.
- Administer 2 doses (separated by 4 weeks or longer) to children younger than 9 years who are receiving influenza vaccine for the first time or who were vaccinated for the first time last season but only received one dose.

7. Measles, mumps, and rubella vaccine (MMR). *(Minimum age: 12 months)*
- Administer the second dose of MMR at age 4–6 years. MMR may be administered before age 4–6 years, provided 4 weeks or more have elapsed since the first dose.

8. Varicella vaccine. *(Minimum age: 12 months)*
- Administer second dose at age 4–6 years; may be administered 3 months or more after first dose.
- Do not repeat second dose if administered 28 days or more after first dose.

9. Hepatitis A vaccine (HepA). *(Minimum age: 12 months)*
- Administer to all children aged 1 year (i.e., aged 12–23 months). Administer the 2 doses in the series at least 6 months apart.
- Children not fully vaccinated by age 2 years can be vaccinated at subsequent visits.
- HepA is recommended for certain other groups of children, including in areas where vaccination programs target older children.

10. Meningococcal vaccine. *(Minimum age: 2 years for meningococcal conjugate vaccine (MCV4) and for meningococcal polysaccharide vaccine (MPSV4))*
- Administer MCV4 to children aged 2–10 years with terminal complement deficiencies or anatomic or functional asplenia and certain other high-risk groups. MPSV4 is also acceptable.
- Administer MCV4 to persons who received MPSV4 3 or more years previously and remain at increased risk for meningococcal disease.

The Recommended Immunization Schedules for Persons Aged 0–18 Years are approved by the Advisory Committee on Immunization Practices (www.cdc.gov/vaccines/recs/acip), the American Academy of Pediatrics (http://www.aap.org), and the American Academy of Family Physicians (http://www.aafp.org).
DEPARTMENT OF HEALTH AND HUMAN SERVICES • CENTERS FOR DISEASE CONTROL AND PREVENTION • SAFER • HEATHIER • PEOPLE™

CS103164

FIGURE 69-4 **Recommended childhood immunization schedule for children 0 to 6 years.** Schedules for persons 7 to 18 years, catch-up for persons 4 months to 18 years, and adult immunizations are available at http://www.cdc.gov/vaccines/recs/schedules/default.htm. (From Centers for Disease Control and Prevention, National Immunization Program: Recommended childhood and adolescent immunization schedule: United States, 2008. http://www.cdc.gov/vaccines/recs/schedules/child-schedule.htm Accessed April 30, 2008.)

agents used for control of immediate allergic reactions, and a knowledge of the recent literature pertaining to the biological to be used, including the nature of side effects and adverse effects that may follow its use.

Individuals with impaired immune responsiveness, whether because of the use of immunosuppressive therapy, a genetic defect, HIV/AIDS, or other causes, may have a reduced antibody response to active immunization procedures. Deferral of the administration of live vaccines may be considered in individuals receiving immunosuppressive therapy. Other groups should receive vaccines according to the usual recommended schedule.

SCHEDULE FOR IMMUNIZATION OF CHILDREN. Both the CDC's ACIP and the AAP Committee on Infectious Disease have issued immunization guidelines for children that are revised annually and published each January. Recommendations from these two bodies may vary slightly, and these variances are noted in a joint Recommended Vaccine Schedule, which was last issued in January 2008.

IMMUNIZATION OF ADULT AND ELDERLY PERSONS. Although significant emphasis has been placed on the subject of childhood immunizations, recommendations for adult immunization have been lacking. However, with the recognition of increased pertussis, pneumococcus, and other vaccine-preventable diseases in adults, the CDC issued the first schedule for adult immunizations in October 2002; this was most recently updated in October 2006.

AT RISK AND POSTEXPOSURE PATIENTS. Certain populations are considered to be at risk and require modification of the routine vaccination schedule. Details for these exceptions may be found on the CDC website.

Some of the important exceptions are summarized as follows:
1. In compliance with recommendations for all individuals, it is particularly important that all health care workers be immunized against hepatitis B. In addition, health care workers in emergency department settings and on emergency response teams, such as emergency medical technicians and paramedics, may elect to be vaccinated against smallpox. Specific recommendations for the use of smallpox vaccine are discussed later in this chapter.
2. Travelers to many underdeveloped nations may require specific immunizations depending on where they are traveling. The CDC publishes information on vaccine recommendations for travel. These can be found by calling (800)-CDC-SHOT, or by looking online.
3. A guide to contraindications for vaccination has been produced by the National Immunization Program and is available on the CDC website.
4. Immunosuppressed individuals, including those with HIV, individuals receiving chemotherapy, and those on corticosteroids, will require modifications of the recommended immunization schedule. Where possible, efforts should be made to appropriately vaccinate individuals prior to beginning regimens such as chemotherapy.

PRINCIPLES OF ADMINISTRATION OF VACCINES. Numerous myths exist about contraindications to administration of vaccines. For all currently available products, the following principles apply:
- Minor upper respiratory infection or gastroenteritis, with or without fever, is not an appropriate indication for withholding a scheduled vaccine dose.
- Concurrent administration of an antibiotic is not a contraindication to immunization.
- In most cases, preterm infants should be immunized at the usual recommended chronologic age and with the recommended dose.
- Pregnancy is a contraindication to administration of live vaccine. However, pregnancy in a household member is not a reason to withhold vaccine from a child or adult
- Women who are breastfeeding may be immunized with all products with the exception of smallpox vaccine. No evidence suggests that trace amounts of a vaccine present in breast milk are harmful to infants.
- A lapse in the recommended immunization schedule does not require that the entire series be restarted. Needed doses should be given at the first opportunity as though the usual interval had occurred.
- Half-doses of vaccine are *never* indicated in individuals who had a significant reaction to a previous dose. In addition, reduced or divided doses are not recommended for preterm or low birth weight infants.
- Family history of an adverse event with an immunizing agent, family history of seizures, and family history of sudden infant death are not appropriate indications for withholding recommended immunizations.
- Soreness, redness, or swelling in the area of the immunization or fever lower than 40.5° C (105° F) following a previous vaccine is not an indication to withhold subsequent doses.

All immunizing agents have specific contraindications that will be discussed separately.

NOTIFICATION OF RISKS AND BENEFITS OF THE VACCINE. The National Childhood Vaccine Injury Act of 1986 mandates the notification of patients and parents of the risks and benefits of individual vaccines. This legislation requires the distribution of standardized information to these individuals. A simplified version of information pamphlets was approved by federal legislation in 1993 and is available from vaccine manufacturers, the CDC, and most state health departments.

The legislation requires health care providers who administer vaccines to keep permanent records of all immunizations given, along with specific information about the manufacturer of the product and the lot number of all doses. In addition, the provider is required to report occurrences of events suspected to be the result of vaccine by using a mechanism titled the Vaccine Adverse Event Reporting System (VAERS). Reports may be made online at http://vaers.hhs.gov. The specifics of reportable events for each agent are discussed separately. In addition, this act established a Vaccine Injury Compensation Table that determined the injuries, disabilities, and conditions for which compensation may be made.

How to Monitor

Vaccines that are administered as recommended induce protective immunity in more than 95% of recipients. It is not recommended or necessary to obtain serum titers to document immunity.

Patient Variables

GERIATRICS. The immune systems of the elderly are less active.

PEDIATRICS. Immunizations are an integral part of the primary health care of children.

PREGNANCY AND LACTATION
- Live vaccines usually are contraindicated in pregnancy (see individual drugs).
- It is usually safe to give vaccines while the mother is breastfeeding.

Patient Education

With most vaccines, the arm in which the vaccine is given may become sore; this can be treated with a warm compress. Some patients develop generalized flu-like symptoms. For any feeling of malaise or flu, the patient often is instructed to take acetaminophen. Most symptoms are mild and self-limited. Reactions that should be reported to the health care provider are discussed separately.

Notify patients, parents, or guardian of the risks and benefits of each individual vaccine, and give them the standardized information pamphlets.

SPECIFIC VACCINES

IMMUNIZATIONS

Hepatitis B Vaccine

Currently available vaccine is produced through recombinant DNA technology. Plasma-derived vaccine is not available in the United States. Although the amount of HBsAg protein varies among vaccine products, completion of the series induces protective antibody in 90% to 95% of adults and children with no evidence of different rates of seroconversion, and these products may be used interchangeably. Pediatric formulations contain no or only trace amounts of thimerosal. Long-term studies indicate that protection appears to be long lasting even in the face of low or undetectable anti-HBs concentrations.

CONTRAINDICATIONS, WARNINGS, AND PRECAUTIONS. Because of the long incubation period for hepatitis B, it is possible for unrecognized infection to be present at the time the vaccine is given. The vaccine may not prevent hepatitis B in such patients.

Epinephrine should be available for immediate use should a rare anaphylactoid reaction occur. Any serious active infection is cause for delaying use of the vaccine, except when, in the opinion of the health care provider, withholding the vaccine entails a greater risk.

Caution should be exercised in administering the vaccine to those who have a severely compromised cardiopulmonary status or to others in whom a febrile or systemic reaction could pose a significant risk.

ADVERSE EFFECTS. Pain at the injection site (<25%) and low-grade fever are the most frequently reported side effects, with an incidence of 1% to 3%. Allergic reactions are infrequent; anaphylaxis is uncommon.

DOSAGE AND ADMINISTRATION. Two vaccines are available and in different strengths. However, the dose volume is the same for each product. The dose is 0.5 ml for persons younger than 20 years of age and 1 ml for those older than 20 years, when given intramuscularly.

Children. Hepatitis B vaccination is recommended for all infants, regardless of their mothers' hepatitis status. The recommended three-dose schedule should be begun prior to hospital discharge; the second dose is given 1 to 2 months later, and the final dose at age 6 months. It is acceptable to administer four doses when combination vaccines are used after the birth dose. In infants born to HBsAg-positive mothers or those of unknown status, the newborn dose should be administered by 12 hours of age, along with hepatitis B immunoglobulin (HBIG).

Preterm infants should be immunized after they reach a weight of 2 kg or by 2 months of age. Older children and adolescents not vaccinated as infants may be vaccinated with doses given at 0, 1 to 2, and 4 to 6 months. A two-dose schedule of Recombivax HB (Merck & Co Inc, Whitehouse Station, NJ) may be given to persons 11 to 15 years of age, with doses given at 0 and 4 to 6 months.

Adults. Routine immunization of all adults is not currently recommended, except in settings in which a high proportion of adults have risks for HBV infection; these include drug abuse treatment facilities, correctional facilities, and clinics that provide care for men who have sex with men (MSM), intravenous drugs users, and clients at high risk for sexually transmitted infection. In these settings, universal hepatitis B vaccination for all unvaccinated adults is recommended. Outside of these high-risk settings, adults with specific risk factors who were not previously immunized should receive immunization. These groups include the following:
- Health care and public safety workers, including trainees, custodians, and others with potential occupational exposure to blood and blood-contaminated body fluids
- Residents and staff of institutions for the developmentally disabled, long-term correctional facilities
- Hemodialysis patients
- Patients with bleeding disorders who receive blood products
- Household contacts and sexual partners of HBV carriers
- Immigrants, adoptees, and family members from countries where HBV is endemic
- International travelers who will be visiting countries with moderate or high rates of HBV infection (a list of these countries can be found at www.cdc.gov/)
- Individuals with more than one sexual partner in the previous 6 months, persons with a recent sexually transmitted infection, clients in sexually transmitted infection (STI) clinics, and men who have sex with men
- Injecting drug users

Pregnancy and Lactation. Routine screening for HBV is recommended for all women early in pregnancy; it should be repeated late in pregnancy for negative women who are at high risk for infection. No adverse effects on the developing fetus have been noted when vaccine is administered during pregnancy. Pregnancy and lactation are not contraindications to HBV vaccination.

HOW SUPPLIED. Two commercially available monovalent recombinant preparations in the United States contain between 10 and 40 mcg/ml of HBsAg protein. The immune response of the two is interchangeable; therefore, an individual who begins a series with one brand may safely complete treatment with the second.

A Combination. In addition, a *Haemophilus* B conjugate–hepatitis B combination is available (Comvax, Merck & Co Inc) and a DTaP-IPV–hepatitis B combination is available (Pediarix, GlaxoSmithKline, Research Triangle Park, NC). Neither may be used for the birth dose of hepatitis B, but they may be used for subsequent doses if all components are indicated.

Only monovalent vaccine should be used if the first dose is given in the newborn period; four doses of hepatitis B may be given if the schedule is completed with combination vaccine at 2, 4, and 12 months.

Diphtheria-Tetanus-Pertussis Vaccine (DTP, DP, DT, DTaP, TdaP)

Although the incidence of all of these infections has decreased dramatically since the introduction of vaccine, pertussis continues to be a serious concern, with an annual incidence in the United States of approximately 25,000 cases. Diphtheria and tetanus preparations both are toxoids that are made by treating toxins with formaldehyde. The pertussis component is available as an acellular preparation that contains detoxified pertussis toxin and pertussis proteins. The five commercially available pertussis preparations available in the United States vary in formulation of pertussis antigen; immunogenicity is similar.

CONTRAINDICATIONS, WARNINGS, AND PRECAUTIONS. When the pertussis component is contraindicated, primary series should be completed with DT. In addition, unstable, changing neurologic disorders (e.g., uncontrolled epilepsy, infantile spasms, progressive encephalopathy) are reasons to delay immunization until the condition has been clarified. Stable neurologic disorders (e.g., well-controlled epilepsy, cerebral palsy, developmental delay) are not contraindications. Absolute contraindications to administration of pertussis-containing preparations are the following effects noted after previous doses of DTP or DTaP:

- *Allergic hypersensitivity reactions:* Anaphylaxis, if it occurs at all, is extremely rare. Urticaria may follow pertussis vaccine. If the appearance is delayed, it is unlikely to represent an IgE-mediated process and is not a contraindication to subsequent doses.
- Encephalopathy within 7 days of its administration

The following conditions were previously considered to be contraindications but have not been demonstrated to cause permanent sequelae and now are listed as precautions to further administration of DTaP:

- Temperature of 40.5° C (104.8° F) within 48 hours
- Collapse or shock-like state within 48 hours
- Persistent, inconsolable crying that lasts longer than 3 hours after vaccine administration
- Unusual, high-pitched crying within 48 hours
- Seizures with or without fever within 3 days

Vaccination with pertussis should be delayed in children with progressive neurologic disorders associated with developmental delay and/or neurologic findings, conditions known to be associated with progressive neurologic deterioration such as tuberous sclerosis, or a history of recent onset of seizures of unknown origin. A decision to vaccinate these children should be made on a case-by-case basis and will have to be reevaluated with changes in their condition.

ADVERSE EFFECTS. Localized redness, induration, and tenderness at the injection site are common, especially as the doses in a series increase. Significant swelling involving the entire thigh or upper arm also can occur, especially after the fourth or fifth dose; this reaction does not increase risk for the same reaction with subsequent doses and should not preclude administration of subsequent required doses. Temperature greater than 38° C (100.4° F), drowsiness, fretfulness, and anorexia are common; they occur significantly more often after DTaP than after DT and are self-limited; their likelihood decreases as the number of doses increases. The pertussis component of the vaccine is responsible for most of these reactions. None of these reactions results in sequelae, and they are not contraindications to subsequent doses.

Moderate to severe systemic reactions are infrequent. The *2006 Red Book* (American Academy of Pediatrics Committee on Infectious Disease, 2006) indicates that these may include the following:

- Fever (temperature >40.5° C or >105° F) occurring in less than 0.3% of recipients
- Persistent, inconsolable crying that lasts longer than 3 hours was reported to occur in 1:100 doses of older whole-cell preparations of DTP; incidence following acellular pertussis preparations is significantly less.
- Seizures were reported to occur in 1:1750 doses of older whole-cell preparations. The incidence with DTaP is substantially less; seizures that do occur are usually of the febrile type.
- Hypotonic-hyporesponsive episodes were known to occur with older preparations. The incidence with DTaP is unknown but is significantly less.
- Acute encephalopathy and permanent neurologic deficit had been reported in a few cases following whole-cell DTP. However, numerous studies have not supported a causal relationship between DTP vaccine and neurologic injury. A survey of Canadian health centers found no cases after administration of more than 6.5 million doses of DTaP.

Side effects often can be managed with acetaminophen or ibuprofen. In addition, warm tub baths and ice packs may relieve local side effects.

DOSAGE AND ADMINISTRATION. Give 0.5 ml intramuscularly according to the primary immunization schedule.

Children. Children should receive a first dose of DTaP at between 6 and 8 weeks of life, with subsequent doses at 4 and 6 months. At least 6 weeks should pass between doses. A fourth dose should be given after the age of 15 months; at least 6 months should pass between the third and fourth doses. A fifth dose is indicated after the age of 48 months.

Subsequent booster doses of Tdap, a preparation that contains a lower dose of diphtheria toxoid and pertussis toxin, should be given every 10 years.

Adults. Pertussis accounts for up to 7% of coughs in adults. Although the disease is milder in adults, adults are recognized to be the source of infection for children. In 2006, the ACIP added routine pertussis vaccination to the adult schedule. Specifically, adults aged 19 to 64 years should receive a single dose of Tdap to replace tetanus and diphtheria toxoids vaccine (Td) for booster immunization against tetanus, diphtheria, and pertussis. Emphasis should be placed on vaccinating adults who have close contact with infants and health care personnel. An interval as short as 2 years from the last Td is suggested; shorter intervals can be used (see http://www.cdc.gov/mmwr/preview/mmwrhtml/rr5517a1.htm?s_cid=rr5517a1_e).

Pregnancy and Lactation. When possible, women should receive Tdap before becoming pregnant. Women who have not previously received Tdap should receive a dose of Tdap during the immediate postpartum period. Tdap may be given to lactating women.

HOW SUPPLIED

- *DTaP:* Diphtheria, tetanus toxoids combined with acellular pertussis vaccine
- *DT:* For infants and children older than 7 years in whom pertussis is contraindicated
- *Td:* Tetanus and diphtheria toxoids for persons older than 7 years. The diphtheria component is reduced in concentration because adverse effects are age and dose related.
- *Tdap (Adacel, Sanofi Pasteur, Swiftwater, PA):* Tetanus toxoid, reduced diphtheria toxoid, and acellular pertussis vaccine approved for use in persons 11 to 64 years of age
- *DTaP-Hib (TriHIBit, Sanofi Pasteur):* DTaP combined with *Haemophilus influenzae* type b vaccine
- *DTaP-IPV–Hepatitis B (Pediarix, GlaxoSmithKline):* Approved by the FDA in 2003, the vaccine combines DTaP, injectable polio vaccine, and hepatitis B vaccine and may be given at 2, 4, and 6 months of life.

Haemophilus B Conjugate Vaccine (Hib)

This product is a polysaccharide that is conjugated with a carrier protein coat to increase immunogenicity. This protein is more antigenic because of its ability to invoke a T-cell response. T-cells allow a "memory" response, and successively increased antibody production occurs after each exposure. The carrier protein alone invokes this T-cell response. Carrier proteins include diphtheria toxoid, a nontoxic mutant diphtheria toxin, an outer membrane protein complex of *Neisseria meningitidis*, or tetanus toxoid that is used for the immunization of children against *Haemophilus* type b.

CONTRAINDICATIONS, WARNINGS, AND PRECAUTIONS. Children with impaired immune systems, such as those infected with HIV, may not mount sufficient immunity with the recommended vaccine schedule and may require an additional dose.

ADVERSE EFFECTS. Very few side effects occur with any of the conjugate preparations. Localized swelling, tenderness, and redness occur in less than 25% of recipients. Systemic effects such as fever are very uncommon. No serious side effects are known.

DOSAGE AND ADMINISTRATION. The product is a suspension that must be shaken vigorously to obtain a uniform suspension before each dose is withdrawn from a multidose vial. Dose is 0.5 ml given intramuscularly.

Children. Immunize all children beginning at 2 months with subsequent doses (boosters) at 4, 6, and 12 to 15 months. Children aged 12 to 14 months require at least two doses; infants older than 2 months but younger than 12 months should receive two doses, with a booster given at 12 to 15 months. Children who were not immunized as infants who are now older than 15 months need only one dose. PRP-OMP, which contains an outer membrane protein complex, is recommended as the first dose in Native American children because of the increased risk of early disease in that population.

Children who have had invasive Hib disease when younger than 24 months of age may, despite this illness, have low antibody concentrations and are at risk for a subsequent episode. Any vaccine given before this disease occurs should be ignored, and conjugate vaccine should be readministered beginning within 1 month according to the recommended schedule for nonimmunized children of the same age. Children who are older than 24 months at the time of disease do not require immunization, irrespective of previous status.

Adults. Vaccine is not indicated in those older than 60 months of age.

HOW SUPPLIED. Five commercial preparations are available in the United States, and recommendations for each vary. All contain an Hib capsular polysaccharide that is covalently linked to a carrier protein. HbOC Hib (oligosaccharides conjugated to diphtheria CRM197 toxin protein, HibTITER, Wyeth Pharmaceuticals Inc, Philadelphia, PA) and PRP-T Hib (polyribosylribitol phosphate polysaccharide conjugated to tetanus toxoid, ActHIB, Sanofi Pasteur) require three doses in the primary series, with a booster given at 12 to 15 months. PRP-OMP, a purified capsular polysaccharide (PRP) conjugated to the outer membrane protein (OMP) of *Neisseria meningitidis* serotype B (PedvaxHIB, Merck & Co Inc), requires only three doses at 2, 4, and 12 to 15 months. Vaccines may be used interchangeably. In such cases, the number of doses recommended to complete the series is determined by the HbOC or PRP-T product, not by the PRP-OMP vaccine. PRP-OMPHib is also available in combination with hepatitis B vaccine (Comvax, Merck); this product may be given at 2, 4, and 15 months but may not be used in infants younger than 6 weeks of age. PRP-T is available in combination with DTaP (TriHIBit, Sanofi Pasteur) and may be used only for the fourth dose of the Hib and DTaP series.

Polio Vaccine (IPV, OPV)

The poliovirus is an *Enterovirus* that is classified as type 1, 2, or 3. Thus vaccines are trivalent, that is, they provide protection against all three subtypes. Inactivated, or killed, polio vaccine (IPV) is administered parenterally and is now the only type of vaccine available in the United States.

CONTRAINDICATIONS, WARNINGS, AND PRECAUTIONS. IPV contains trace amounts of streptomycin, neomycin, and polymyxin B; thus allergic reactions to one of these three antibiotics may rarely occur.

ADVERSE EFFECTS. No serious adverse events are known to occur as the result of administration of IPV.

DOSAGE AND ADMINISTRATION. The dose is 0.5 ml given intramuscularly.

Children. Children should be vaccinated with four doses, beginning at 2 months of life; subsequent doses are administered at 4 months, 6 to 18 months, and 4 to 6 years. When accelerated protection is indicated, the first dose may be administered as early as 6 weeks, with a second dose given a minimum of 4 weeks later. Giving the third dose at 6 months may lead to increased compliance.

Adults. Most adults in the United States are immune as a result of childhood vaccination or exposure to wild virus. Vaccine should be considered for adults who travel to endemic areas, for laboratory workers handling wild virus, or for health care workers in close contact with patients who may be shedding virus. Unimmunized adults should receive two doses at intervals of 4 to 8 weeks, with a booster dose given 6 to 12 months later. Incompletely immunized adults who previously received OPV may complete the series with IPV.

Pregnancy and Lactation. Administration during pregnancy should be avoided, although no risks are known to be associated with administration of IPV during pregnancy. If immediate protection is indicated, pregnant women may receive IPV. IPV may be given to lactating women.

HOW SUPPLIED. Preparations are available in two formulations.
- *Inactivated polio virus (IPV):* This killed virus preparation is administered parenterally, either subcutaneously or intramuscularly. This preparation provides excellent systemic immunity; current IPV preparations are of enhanced potency and produce seroconversion rates equal to or better than those of OPV or DTaP–hepatitis B–IPV (Pediarix, GlaxoSmithKline). This combination vaccine may be used for the primary series (2, 4, 6 to 18 months).
- *Oral polio virus (OPV):* This live virus is administered orally. Although it is not available in the United States, because of lower cost and ease of administration, OPV is the vaccine of choice in areas with known circulation of wild virus. Additionally, it provides a mucosal barrier that is protective against spread of the virus as a result of inadequate sanitation.

Measles-Mumps-Rubella Vaccine

MMR vaccine is a live-attenuated vaccine that is prepared in chick embryo cell culture. After administration of a single dose of live-virus vaccine, 95% of individuals develop adequate serum antibody.

CONTRAINDICATIONS, WARNINGS, AND PRECAUTIONS. MMR vaccination is contraindicated in the following situations:
- Pregnancy
- Immediate anaphylaxis to a previous dose is a contradiction to receipt of subsequent doses.
- Significantly immunocompromised individuals or those receiving immunotherapy should not be given live-virus vaccines. HIV infected persons, with the exception of severely ill, immunocompromised individuals, should be vaccinated. Individuals on high-dose corticosteroid therapy should not be vaccinated until 1 month after discontinuation.
- Individuals who have received immunoglobulin antibody–containing blood products within the preceding 3 months should not be vaccinated until at least 3 months after receipt. If these products are given less than 14 days after MMR, the vaccine should be repeated in 3 months.
- The tuberculin skin test may be performed at the time of immunization; otherwise, it should be postponed until 4 to 6 weeks later because immunization can temporarily suppress the tuberculin reaction.

ADVERSE EFFECTS. Many side effects to these preparations have been reported; most problems are not serious. They include the following:
- From 5% to 15% of vaccinated patients experience body temperature of at least 103° F, which begins 7 to 12 days

after vaccination and commonly lasts 1 to 2 days; fever has been reported to last up to 5 days. Most individuals are otherwise asymptomatic.
- Five percent of recipients may experience transient rashes on days 7 to 12.
- Frank arthritis rarely occurs in children, although 10% to 15% of adult women may experience significant joint pain, particularly in peripheral small joints. No permanent joint destruction has been reported.
- Transient thrombocytopenia has been reported, although the incidence is unknown.
- Side effects are markedly less common with second doses, presumably because most individuals are already immune.
- No side effects have been reported in immune persons who were inadvertently vaccinated.
- Seizure risk is slightly elevated following measles vaccination, although a known seizure disorder is not a contraindication to vaccine administration.
- Measles vaccine is not causally linked to the risk of developing autism spectrum disorders.

Rarely, side effects that are more serious may occur. Allergic reactions occur rarely and are usually attributable to trace amounts of neomycin; children with known anaphylaxis to topical or systemic neomycin should receive vaccine in settings where such a reaction can be treated. A history of contact dermatitis to neomycin is not a contraindication. The measles component of the vaccine is produced in chick embryo cell culture but does not contain a significant amount of egg protein. Children with egg allergy are at low risk for anaphylactic reactions to measles-containing vaccine, and skin testing for egg allergy is not indicated. The incidence of subacute sclerosing panencephalitis (SSPE) after vaccine is significantly lower than the risk of acquiring this condition from measles infection.

DOSAGE AND ADMINISTRATION

Children. The first dose is recommended at 12 to 15 months of age with a booster dose given at elementary school entry. Children who have had physician-diagnosed measles or who have laboratory evidence of immunity do not require vaccinations.

Adults. In response to a significant increase in cases of mumps in 2006, the ACIP revised recommendations for mumps vaccine in adults. It is now recommended that health care workers with no history of mumps vaccination and no other evidence of immunity should receive two doses (at a minimum interval of 1 month between doses). Health care workers who previously have received only one dose should be given a second dose. Because birth before 1957 is considered to be only presumptive evidence of immunity, health care institutions should routinely recommend a single dose of mumps vaccine for unvaccinated workers born before 1957 who do not have a history of physician-diagnosed mumps or laboratory evidence of mumps immunity; a second dose should be strongly considered if an outbreak occurs.

Pregnancy and Lactation. Live-virus vaccines should not be administered during pregnancy. In addition, women of childbearing age who receive a rubella-containing preparation should be counseled to defer pregnancy for 3 months. If vaccination should occur during the first trimester, the pregnant woman should be counseled on possible risks to the fetus. It is currently suggested that inadvertent rubella vaccination during pregnancy is not sufficient reason to recommend termination of the pregnancy. MMR preparations may be given to children with pregnant mothers. MMR may be given to women who are breastfeeding.

HOW SUPPLIED. Monovalent preparations of measles, mumps, and rubella are available. In epidemic areas, it may be indicated to immunize infants younger than 12 months with one of these preparations. For routine use, however, a trivalent preparation (MMR) or a quadrivalent preparation containing varicella (MMRV) should be used.

MMRV (ProQuad, Merck) is identical and of equal titer to the measles, mumps, and rubella (MMR) vaccine. MMRV may be given for any dose between the ages of 12 months and 12 years; it is not indicated for younger or older patients.

Varicella Vaccine

Varicella vaccine was licensed for general use in March 1995. Preparations contain cell-free live-attenuated varicella-zoster virus; trace amounts of neomycin are also found. In well children older than 12 months of age, a single dose results in a seroconversion rate of greater than 95%. An age-related decrease in the ability of the immune system to mount and maintain a primary response is seen after the age of 12 years. In adolescents older than 12 years and in adults, seroconversion rates after one dose range from 79% to 82%; two doses produce a seroconversion rate of 94%. The rate of disease after immunization appears to be about 1% to 3% per year. Even more important, a very high rate of protection from severe varicella disease is apparent. In those individuals who do contract the virus after vaccination, disease is reported to be much milder. In 2006, a zoster vaccine containing a live-attenuated form of varicella-zoster virus (Zostavax, Merck) was approved by the FDA for use in adults older than 60 years. The zoster vaccine contains the same live-attenuated strain as is found in the varicella vaccine but at a 14-fold higher concentration. It has been demonstrated to prevent zoster in 50% of recipients and the more serious complication of postherpetic neuralgia in approximately two thirds of recipients.

CONTRAINDICATIONS, WARNINGS, AND PRECAUTIONS. Varicella vaccine may be given simultaneously with MMR; however, if it is not given simultaneously, the interval between administrations should last at least 1 month. Varicella vaccine does not appear to have any effect on the administration of any other vaccine.

Varicella vaccine should not be given routinely to immunocompromised individuals. This includes those with malignancies or congenital immunodeficiency, or those who are receiving immunosuppressive therapy or long-term systemic steroids. Children with acute lymphocytic leukemia who have been in remission for at least 1 year may be immunized if they have documented adequate lymphocyte and platelet counts.

HIV-infected children ≥ 1 year with CD4+ T-lymphocyte counts $\geq 15\%$ should receive two doses of single-antigen varicella vaccine at a minimum interval of 3 months. MMRV should not be used in these children because safety data with this newer product are not yet available.

Varicella virus should not be given to those individuals who are receiving high-dose systemic corticosteroids (>2 mg/kg/day of prednisone); after discontinuation of steroids, vaccination should be delayed for 1 month. In children who are on lower doses (1 to 2 mg/kg/day of prednisone), the risk of vaccination with a live-attenuated virus must be weighed against the risk of infection with wild virus. Some experts recommend vaccination of these children if steroid use is discontinued for a period of 1 or more weeks both before and after administration. Decisions to vaccinate these children must be made after consultation with appropriate physicians. Inhaled steroid use is not a contraindication to use of the vaccine.

As with other live virus vaccines, administration should be withheld if an individual has received immune globulin during the preceding 5 months.

The association between wild virus varicella, salicylate use, and the development of Reye's syndrome is well known. No such association has been found with the use of varicella vaccine; however, the manufacturer recommends that salicylates should not be given for 6 weeks after administration of the vaccine.

Vaccine should not be given to individuals who have had an anaphylactic reaction to neomycin. As with other vaccines, moderate to severe illness is reason to withhold vaccination.

ADVERSE EFFECTS. Adverse effects are minimal. Less than 25% of children and adults report mild pain and erythema at the injection site. Approximately 7% to 8% of vaccinees develop a mild maculopapular or morbilliform rash within 1 month of receiving vaccine. Rarely, varicella virus has been recovered from these skin lesions. No disease has been reported in susceptible individuals who have had contact with vaccinees with a rash.

DOSAGE AND ADMINISTRATION

Children. Beginning in 2007, a two-dose schedule for children is recommended. Children should be routinely vaccinated at 12 months and at 4 to 6 years. The second dose can be administered at an earlier age, provided the interval between the first and second doses is at least 3 months. A second dose catch-up varicella vaccination is recommended for children and adolescents through college age who previously had received only one dose.

Adults. Previously, adults born before 1966 were considered most likely to be immune. Beginning with the 2007 schedule, that date was changed to 1980. It is now recommended that adults born after 1980 who lack a reliable history of varicella vaccine should be vaccinated at the earliest opportunity; two doses spaced 4 to 8 weeks apart are necessary. For health care workers and pregnant women, birth before 1980 should not be considered adequate proof of immunity, and further testing and/or vaccination should be considered. No adverse sequelae have been noted in immune individuals who receive vaccine.

Additionally, ACIP has recommended that a single dose of zoster vaccine be given to adults 60 years of age or older, whether or not they report a prior episode of herpes zoster. The full text of the CDC ACIP guidelines may be viewed at: www.cdc.gov/mmwr/preview/mmwrhtml/rr5705al.htm?s_cid_rr5705al_e.

Pregnancy and Lactation. As with all live viruses, pregnancy is a contraindication to administration of the vaccine. Pregnancy should be avoided for 1 month following vaccination. A pregnant household member is not a contraindication to the administration of vaccine to susceptible individuals. Breastfeeding is not a contraindication to receipt of *varicella vaccines*.

HOW SUPPLIED. Varicella vaccine is available in three formulations.

- *Varicella-zoster vaccine (Varivax, Merck)*: A monovalent live-attenuated preparation of the wild Oka strain of varicella; recommended dose is 0.5 ml given subcutaneously
- *MMRV (ProQuad, Merck)*: The titer of Oka varicella-zoster virus is higher in MMRV vaccine than in single-antigen varicella vaccine (a minimum of 3.13 $\log_{10}$ plaque-forming units [pfu] vs. 1350 pfu [approximately 1.13 $\log_{10}$], respectively).
- *Zostavax (Merck)*: For use in adults older than 60 years for the prevention of shingles; approved by the FDA in 2006

Influenza Vaccine (Various Strains)

Although *Healthy People 2010* set a goal of 90% vaccination rates in older and other high-risk individuals, success in meeting this goal has been mixed, with minority populations and adults older than 65 not residing in nursing homes less likely to be immunized. Although influenza vaccination rates for whites were 66% in 1997, rates for African Americans and Hispanics were only 45% and 53%, respectively (*Healthy People, 2010*). Despite rising vaccination rates, continuing epidemics of influenza occur during the winter months and are responsible for an average of approximately 20,000 deaths per year in the United States. Rates of infection are highest among children, but rates of serious illness and death are highest among persons older than 65 years and persons of any age who have medical conditions that place them at increased risk for complications from influenza.

Two vaccine types are available: inactivated influenza vaccines (TIV) and live-attenuated influenza vaccine (LAIV). Both vaccines are produced in embryonic egg and both are multivalent, containing three different viral subtypes; the composition changes annually in anticipation of expected prevalent influenza strains. The efficacy of vaccines is difficult to document because of yearly variations in circulating strains and the similarity of symptoms between true influenza disease and other viral respiratory illnesses. Thus influenza vaccine is not effective against all possible strains of influenza virus, and protection is afforded only against those strains of virus from which the vaccine is prepared or against closely related strains. The impact of immunization is most noticeable in adult populations, probably because of the lower frequency of colds and other viral disease. Protection against disease is probably in the range of 70% to 80%, with duration of efficacy of less than 1 year.

CONTRAINDICATIONS, WARNINGS, AND PRECAUTIONS. Influenza vaccine should be withheld in the following conditions:

- Individuals receiving chemotherapy should not receive vaccine until at least 4 weeks after discontinuation of therapy.
- The effect of steroid therapy on influenza vaccine immunogenicity is unknown. Steroid therapy should not necessarily delay the administration of vaccine, particularly in those individuals in whom influenza can be expected to be particularly severe.
- The AAP recommends that influenzavirus vaccine should not be administered within 3 days of immunization with a pertussis-containing vaccine because both vaccines may cause febrile reactions in young children.
- The effects of steroid therapy on influenza vaccine immunogenicity are unknown. Steroid therapy should not necessarily delay the administration of vaccine, particularly in those individuals in whom influenza can be expected to be particularly severe.

ADVERSE EFFECTS. TIV contains only noninfectious viruses and therefore cannot cause influenza. Occasional cases of respiratory disease following vaccination represent coincidental illnesses unrelated to influenza vaccination. LAIV may be transmitted rarely to unimmunized contacts of the recipient.

Febrile reactions in children younger than 13 years old are uncommon with TIV; adults and children older than 13 years infrequently experience fever. Malaise and local soreness and erythema occur in approximately 10% of cases. Rates of fever, rhinitis, and nasal congestion in recipients of LAIV appear to be the same as with placebo. However, a threefold risk of asthma attacks has been noted in children who were given LAIV.

The risk of developing Guillain-Barré syndrome, or other temporary neurologic disorders, is slightly increased after vaccination with TIV.

Individuals with severe anaphylactic reactions to eggs or chickens or gentamicin sulfate may, on rare occasions, experience similar reactions after TIV. In view of the need for yearly administration and the availability of chemoprophylaxis against influenza A, it is recommended that these individuals should not receive vaccine. Individuals who would benefit from the vaccine should be given a skin test or other allergy-evaluating test, with the influenzavirus vaccine used as the antigen.

Immunocompromised individuals may have a reduced antibody response to active immunization procedures.

Influenza vaccine often contains one or more antigens used in previous years. However, immunity declines during the year after immunization. Therefore, revaccination on a yearly basis is necessary to provide optimal protection for the current season.

DOSAGE AND ADMINISTRATION. Providers should begin vaccination efforts in October and should continue to offer vaccine until circulating influenza is no longer present in the community. Children younger than 9 years who are receiving vaccine for the first time require a booster dose 1 month after receiving the initial dose.

Children. Efficacy has not been evaluated in children younger than 6 months of age. Yearly immunization is recommended for all children between the ages of 6 and 59 months, their caregivers, and household contacts.

Children older than 59 months of age from the following high-risk categories also should be vaccinated:

- Children with chronic pulmonary, renal, metabolic, neurologic, or cardiovascular disorders, including asthma and diabetes mellitus
- Hemodynamically significant cardiac disease
- Hemoglobinopathies, including sickle cell disease
- Any disease that requires the use of immunosuppressive therapy
- HIV infection
- Those receiving long-term aspirin therapy
- Children with spinal cord injury or conditions that can increase the risk for aspiration

Vaccination also should be considered for children in living situations where rapid transmission of disease is likely. These include residents of group homes or college dormitories and those who are members of athletic teams that live and travel together. In addition, children who live in close contact with an at-risk child should be considered for immunization, to decrease the potential for spread to others.

Two doses spaced at least 1 month apart are recommended for those individuals receiving vaccine for the first time. If strains have not changed significantly, immunization may be achieved in subsequent years with the administration of only one dose.

Adults. Adults in the following categories should be considered for routine administration:

- Persons older than 50 years
- Residents of nursing homes and other long-term care facilities
- Adults with chronic pulmonary, cardiovascular, metabolic, or renal disorders
- Adults with hemoglobinopathies or immunosuppression (including immunosuppression caused by medications or by HIV)
- Health care workers, employees of long-term care facilities, child care workers, and household members of individuals in high-risk categories

Two doses spaced 1 month apart are recommended for those individuals receiving the vaccine for the first time. If strains have not changed significantly, immunization in subsequent years may be achieved with the administration of only one dose.

Pregnancy and Lactation. Women who will be in their second or third trimester during influenza season should be vaccinated. Women who are breastfeeding may be vaccinated safely.

HOW SUPPLIED

- Inactivated whole-virus vaccines prepared from purified virus particles
- Subvirion vaccines, which are prepared by another step of disrupting the lipid-containing outer membrane of the virus
- Purified surface antigen vaccines

These last two preparations are called *split-virus vaccines*; they are the only TIV products licensed for use in children younger than 13 years. They are equally safe and immunogenic.

A limited amount of thimerosal-free vaccine began to be available during the 2002 influenza season; these products currently are licensed for use only in children older than 4 years of age.

A nasal spray flu vaccine (FluMist, Aviron, MedImmune, Gaithersburg, MD), a cold-adapted, live-attenuated, trivalent influenzavirus vaccine, is now available for use in well individuals between the ages of 5 and 49 years; testing is under way to assess safety in younger children.

Pneumococcal Vaccine

Two types of pneumococcal vaccine are available. The first, PPV23, is a polyvalent product that is a mixture of highly purified capsular polysaccharides from the 23 most prevalent or invasive pneumococcal types. It is recommended for use in adults and children older than 2 years of age. A pneumococcal conjugate vaccine, PCV7, which conjugates the capsular polysaccharides from the seven most invasive types of pneumococci with diphtheria protein, is approved for use in children between the ages of 2 months and 10 years.

CONTRAINDICATIONS, WARNINGS, AND PRECAUTIONS. In patients who require penicillin (or other antibiotic) prophylaxis against pneumococcal infection, such prophylaxis should not be discontinued after vaccination with this vaccine.

The polysaccharide vaccine is a pregnancy category C product and should be given to a pregnant woman only if clearly needed.

ADVERSE EFFECTS. Although both of these agents are polysaccharide and conjugate vaccines, local reactions are the most common side effect, and they include local injection site soreness, erythema, and swelling, usually lasting no longer than 2 days; local induration occurs less frequently. Rash, urticaria, arthritis, arthralgia, adenitis, and serum sickness occasionally have been reported. Malaise, myalgia, headache, and asthenia have also been seen. Fever is more common following administration of conjugate vaccine and occurs in about one fourth of all children; older children are less likely to experience fever.

DOSAGE AND ADMINISTRATION. Infants should be vaccinated using the pneumococcal conjugate product at 2, 4, 6, and 12 to 15 months. Children receiving their first pneumococcal vaccination between 2 and 6 months of age should receive three doses, 6 to 8 weeks apart, with a booster at 15 to 18 months. Children who do not receive their first dose at between 7 and 11 months of age should be given two doses, 6 to 8 weeks apart, with a booster at the recommended age. Children who receive their first dose at between 12 and 23 months of age should be administered two doses, 6 to 8 weeks apart, and will not require a booster dose. High-risk children at between 24 and 59 months of age should receive two doses of PCV7 spaced 2 months apart. Additionally, they should receive two doses of PPV23 within the first 2 months after the second PCV7, and the second 3 to 5 years later. High-risk categories include the following:

- Children with anatomic asplenia or who have splenic dysfunction from sickle cell disease or other causes
- Children with chronic illnesses with an increased risk of pneumococcal disease, such as those with functional impairment of cardiorespiratory, hepatic, and renal systems
- Children with immunosuppression, including HIV infection

Children in high-risk groups who are older than 59 months of age should be vaccinated with a single dose of PPV23. However, PCV7 also may be used in children up to the age of 9 years; in some cases, children may benefit from receiving a dose of PCV7 followed by PPV23 8 weeks later.

In addition, adults in the following categories should be considered for vaccination with PPV23:

- Persons 50 years of age or older
- Patients with other chronic illnesses may be at greater risk of developing pneumococcal infection or having more severe illness as a result of alcohol abuse or coexisting disease.
- Patients undergoing splenectomy should be vaccinated, if possible, 8 weeks prior to surgery.
- Patients beginning immunosuppressive therapy should be vaccinated, if possible, at least 2 weeks before initiation of therapy.
- Patients with Hodgkin's disease if immunization can be given at least 10 days before treatment

Vaccine also should be considered for adults residing in closed-group communities such as residential schools and nursing homes, groups epidemiologically at risk in the community, and patients at high risk of influenza complications.

Both products should be administered as a single 0.5 ml dose. PCV7 should be given intramuscularly; PPV23 may be administered subcutaneously or intramuscularly.

HOW SUPPLIED. The polysaccharide product comes in multi-dose vials of 14-or 23-valent vaccines.

PPV7 (Prevnar, Wyeth) is available as a single-dose vial or a prefilled syringe.

Respiratory Syncytial Virus Prophylaxis

A monoclonal antibody product, palivizumab (Synagis, MedImmune), for use in high-risk children younger than 24 months of age, was approved by the FDA in 1998. Although not a vaccine but rather an antibody that is given to high-risk infants younger than 24 months of age, it is included in this discussion because it is now part of the routine recommendations for these infants.

Respiratory syncytial virus (RSV) is recognized to be the most significant causative agent in acute respiratory tract illness in infants and young children, causing significant morbidity in high-risk infants, including preterm babies. The AAP recommends that high-risk infants and children should receive prophylaxis for RSV at the start of the anticipated RSV season, which typically extends from winter to early spring in temperate climates. Infants born at less than 32 weeks' gestation and preterm infants born at 32 to 35 weeks with at least two additional risk factors (e.g., day care attendance, exposure to environmental pollutants, school-aged siblings, congenital abnormalities of the airways, neuromuscular disease) should receive prophylaxis during their first RSV season. Children younger than 2 years of age with chronic lung disease that has required medical therapy within 6 months of RSV season onset and those with hemodynamically significant heart disease may require therapy in their second RSV season.

CONTRAINDICATIONS, WARNINGS, AND PRECAUTIONS. Because of the significant costs associated with palivizumab, use should be considered carefully in infants born at between 32 and 35 weeks who do not have other risk factors for severe infection. Risk factors include child care attendance, school-aged siblings, congenital neurologic or musculoskeletal disease, and exposure to significant air pollutants or congenital abnormalities of the airway.

ADVERSE EFFECTS. Administration of palivizumab does not require alteration in the routine vaccination schedule and does not interfere with immunologic response to these agents. The incidence of adverse effects after the administration of palivizumab is similar to that of placebo.

DOSAGE AND ADMINISTRATION. RSV prophylaxis should be begun at the start of RSV season—between October and December in most parts of the United States—and should be terminated at the end of the season, typically from March to May.

Dose is 15 mg/kg of body weight, administered intramuscularly once a month for a total of five doses.

HOW SUPPLIED. Palivizumab is supplied in 50 mg and 100 mg single-dose vials, and opened vials must be used within 6 hours.

Meningococcal Vaccine

Neisseria meningitides is the second most common cause of bacterial meningitis in the United States; it has a case-fatality rate of approximately 10% to 20% despite therapy with anti-microbial agents, to which all strains remain highly sensitive. For uncertain reasons, a significant increase in outbreaks of infection has occurred over the past 10 years; more than one third of these outbreaks have occurred in the college dormitory setting. Two vaccines are available in the United States; both are tetravalent and protect against serogroups A, C, and Y, and W-135 antigens from *N. meningitidis*. Historically, most disease outbreaks have been the result of serogroup C; however, recent outbreaks resulting from serogroups Y and B have been reported. Approximately half of infections in infants younger than 1 year of age are the result of infection with serogroup B, for which no vaccine is available. Antibodies against the serogroup A and C polysaccharides declined markedly over the first 3 years after a single dose of vaccine, with the decline being most pronounced in the youngest children. In 1997, the American College Health Association recommended that college health centers proactively inform entering college students who would be residing in dormitories and their parents about the risk of disease and offer vaccine. In 2000, both the AAP and the ACIP issued their own recommendations that these students be offered vaccine. In 2005, with licensure of a conjugate vaccine, recommendations were issued for routine use in school-age children.

CONTRAINDICATIONS, WARNINGS, AND PRECAUTIONS. Since licensure of meningococcal conjugate vaccine (MCV4), there have been 17 reports of Guillain-Barré syndrome (GBS), including 15 in teenagers, with onset within 6 weeks of receipt of vaccine, indicating a slightly increased risk. As a result, the CDC has recommended that the product not be used routinely in individuals with a history of GBS, although GBS history is not an absolute contraindication and vaccination may be considered in high-risk individuals

MCV4 is pregnancy category C, although vaccination should be considered for pregnant women at high risk of infection.

ADVERSE EFFECTS. Adverse effects are mild and infrequent, consisting of localized erythema, pain, headache, and fatigue lasting 1 to 2 days. Young children may have transient mild fever.

DOSAGE AND ADMINISTRATION. A single dose of MCV4 is recommended at 11 to 12 years of age or prior to high school entry. Additionally, individuals older than 11 years of age who are at high risk of meningococcal disease and were not previously immunized should be immunized. These include college freshmen living in dormitories, military recruits, individuals traveling to or living in endemic areas, such as parts of Africa, and those with asplenia or terminal complement component deficiency. Additionally, family members or others potentially exposed to meningitis during an outbreak and microbiologists routinely exposed to meningococcal bacteria should receive vaccine. Included are those who were previously vaccinated with meningococcal polysaccharide vaccine (MPSV4), provided 3 to 5 years have lapsed since receipt of the polysaccharide product.

MCV4 is the preferred agent for individuals aged 11 to 55 years; MPSV4 may be used in children between the ages of 2 and 10 years and in adults older than 55 years. MCV4 is not licensed for use in persons older than 55 years. The immunizing dose is a single injection of 0.5 mg given subcutaneously. The vaccine may be given at the same time as other immunizations.

Routine use of MPSV4 has not been recommended. No products are licensed for use in children younger than 2 years of age. Because antibody levels decrease very rapidly after administration of MPSV4, usually within 3 to 5 years after vaccination, revaccination may be warranted for individuals at increased risk of meningococcal disease; these decisions should be made on an individual basis.

HOW SUPPLIED
- MCV4 (Menactra, Sanofi Aventis)
- MPSV4 (Menomune, Sanofi Pasteur)

Hepatitis A Vaccine

Hepatitis A is highly contagious, and the predominant mode of transmission is person-to-person via the fecal-oral route. Infection has been shown to be spread by contaminated water or food, by infected food handlers, after breakdown in usual sanitary conditions after floods or natural disasters, by ingestion of raw or undercooked shellfish from contaminated waters, and during travel to areas of the world with poor hygienic conditions. Increased incidence is also seen among institutionalized children and adults, especially in day care centers where children have not been toilet trained. Hepatitis also can be spread through parenteral transmission and by blood transfusions or by needle sharing with infected people. The incubation period for hepatitis A averages 28 days, and its course is extremely variable. Although many children may have asymptomatic infection, most older children and adults are symptomatic, with a self-limiting course characterized by fever, malaise, nausea, and jaundice. Recovery is usually complete and is followed by protection against hepatitis A virus (HAV) infection.

CONTRAINDICATIONS, WARNINGS, AND PRECAUTIONS. Because hepatitis A has a relatively long incubation period (15 to 50 days), this vaccine may not prevent hepatitis A infection in individuals who have an unrecognized hepatitis A infection at the time of vaccination.

The vaccine may be given at the same time as other immunizations.

Safety data in pregnancy are limited, but there appears to be little risk associated with administration of this inactivated product.

ADVERSE EFFECTS. Generally, the vaccine is associated with only mild and short-term effects: 1% to 10% of patients may have local reactions at the injection site with induration, redness, and swelling. Patients also may experience headache, fatigue, mild fever, malaise, anorexia, or nausea. Serious side effects have not been reported.

DOSAGE AND ADMINISTRATION. Prior to 2006, vaccination was recommended only for high-risk groups, including intravenous drug users, men who have sex with men (MSM), individuals living in or traveling to areas with higher rates of endemic disease, and those with liver disease. In 2006, the ACIP recommended routine administration of hepatitis A vaccine to children older than 12 months of age. A first dose is given at 1 year, and a second is given 6 to 12 months later. Dose is 0.5 ml given intramuscularly in children 1 to 18 years; a dose of 1 ml is recommended for those 19 years of age and older.

Previous recommendations for administration in high-risk individuals remain unchanged. States with a higher rate of disease that had previously been routinely vaccinating children should continue with these programs In states without preexisting programs for vaccination against hepatitis A, catch-up vaccination of older, previously unvaccinated children is encouraged. Individuals traveling to developing countries with high rates of infection, including Mexico, should be considered for vaccination. In addition, MSM, individuals using intravenous drugs, and those who work in high-risk settings such as research settings where hepatitis A is present or with infected animals should be considered for vaccination. Finally, individuals at high risk for fulminant liver disease, such as those with chronic liver disorders or recipients of clotting factors, should be considered for immunization.

Although it is preferable to complete the series with the same product, products may be used interchangeably.

HOW SUPPLIED. Hepatitis A vaccine, inactivated (Havrix, GlaxoSmithKline; Vaqta, Merck), is a whole-cell, purified sterile suspension of inactivated viral proteins.

Combination hepatitis A, inactivated, and hepatitis B, recombinant (Twinrix, GlaxoSmithKline), contains hepatitis A antigen (half of the Havrix adult dose) and 20 mcg of recombinant hepatitis B surface antigen protein (the same as the Engerix-B [GlaxoSmithKline] adult dose). It is licensed for use in individuals older than 18 years of age who have not previously been immunized against either virus. It is administered in the same way as single-antigen hepatitis B vaccine, that is, with three doses given on a 0-, 1-, and 6-month schedule.

Rotavirus Vaccine

Rotavirus is the most common cause of severe diarrheal disease worldwide. In U.S. children who typically are able to access quality medical care, the virus accounts for 70,000 hospitalizations and 100 deaths per year, and it is the causative agent in 5% to 10% of all gastroenteritis infections in children younger than 5 years of age. Although children in developed countries are likely to recover with oral rehydration therapy, worldwide this accounts for more than half a million deaths annually in children under the age of 5 years. Almost all children have become infected by the age of 3 years, and although initial infection protects against subsequent severe gastroenteritis, asymptomatic infection with spread to nonimmune children occurs. Symptoms are variable but may last as long as a week and consist of vomiting, watery diarrhea, fever, and abdominal pain. The mode of transmission is fecal-oral with a winter seasonal pattern. A rapid antigen test of stool samples is available. Multiple serotypes of rotavirus are in circulation, and regional and year-to-year variations have been noted. However, four strains make up 96% of the globally identified strains. A tetravalent vaccine was licensed by the FDA in 1998 but was withdrawn in 1999 after reports of an association with intussusception.

In February 2006, a bovine pentavalent rotavirus vaccine (PRV) containing four reassortant rotaviruses was licensed for use and incorporated into the routine childhood immunization schedule in 2007.

CONTRAINDICATIONS, WARNINGS, AND PRECAUTIONS. The current vaccine has not been associated with an increased risk for intussusception, although the manufacturer has committed to postvaccine studies, which are ongoing. PRV is a live-virus vaccine that should not be given to infants with known or suspected weakened immune system disorders, including HIV. Infants born to mothers with HIV should not receive a first dose unless it has been established that the infant is not infected with HIV. Infants with a suspected severe allergic reaction to a first dose should not receive subsequent doses. Rotavirus vaccine may be coadministered with other childhood vaccines. Vaccine should be deferred until 6 weeks after receipt of an antibody-containing product such as immunoglobulin. However, if this delay would cause the first dose to be administered after 13 weeks of age, a shorter deferral interval should be used.

ADVERSE EFFECTS. Rates of adverse effects are similar to those reported with placebo. Diarrhea and vomiting are slightly more common in the week following receipt of vaccine. Preterm infants may receive PRV according to the routine schedule.

DOSAGE AND ADMINISTRATION. Infants should receive three doses of pentavalent rotavirus vaccine administered orally at 2, 4, and 6 months of age. The first dose should be administered at 6 to 12 weeks of age; immunization should not be initiated for infants older than 12 weeks of age. Subsequent doses should be administered at 4- to 10-week intervals, and all three doses of vaccine should be administered by 32 weeks of age. The product is not approved for use in children older than 32 weeks of age.

HOW SUPPLIED. PRV (RotaTeq, Merck) is provided in a squeezable plastic tube with a twist-off top that contains a single 2 ml dose. The vaccine is stored in the refrigerator and should be administered as soon as possible after removal from refrigeration.

Human Papillomavirus Vaccine

Approximately 20 million people in the United States are infected with human papillomavirus (HPV), and as many as 5 million new cases of HPV infection occur every year. HPV infection can result in visible genital warts, subclinical infection, and, most seriously, cervical cancer. An estimated 5000 deaths/year occur in the United States as the result of cervical cancer. HPV types are categorized according to their relative risk of specific clinical events, and more than 100 types have been identified. Although most infections with HPV are benign and self-resolving with high-risk HPV types, most commonly, types 16 and 18 can cause low- and high-grade cervical cell abnormalities that are precursors to invasive cervical cancer, accounting for more than 65% of cervical cancer cases in the United States. A quadrivalent vaccine with protection against four HPV subtypes (6, 11, 16, and 18) was licensed by the FDA in June 2006. Clinical trials conducted in women 16 to 26 years old have demonstrated 100% efficacy in preventing cervical precancers and nearly 100% efficacy in preventing vulvar and vaginal precancers and genital warts caused by the targeted HPV types. The combined immunization schedule now recommends routine use of the vaccine in girls and women ages 9-26 years

CONTRAINDICATIONS, WARNINGS, AND PRECAUTIONS. Vaccination should be deferred in individuals who have experienced an allergic reaction to a previous dose. An acute minor illness is not an indication for deferral, although vaccination should be withheld for more serious illness. HPV vaccine may be administered with other routine childhood vaccines. It may be administered to immunocompromised individuals and women who are lactating; it is not recommended during pregnancy.

ADVERSE EFFECTS. The only reported adverse event is mild injection site pain, which is common.

DOSAGE AND ADMINISTRATION. A 0.5 ml intramuscular dose of HPV vaccine is recommended to be given on a three-dose schedule, with initial dose followed by doses 2 and 6 months later. Routine vaccination is recommended for females aged 11 to 12 years; the vaccination series can be started in females as young as 9 years of age, and a catch-up vaccination is recommended for females aged 13 to 26 years who have not been vaccinated previously or who have not completed the full vaccine series. Ideally, vaccination should begin prior to initiation of sexual activity, although the vaccine should still be given even to women with a history of genital warts, a positive HPV test, and an abnormal Pap smear. Routine screening, including the recommendations for Pap smear, is unchanged in women who have been vaccinated.

HOW SUPPLIED. Quadrivalent HPV vaccine (Gardasil, Merck) is available in single-dose and multidose vials. It should be stored refrigerated.

Rabies Vaccine and Rabies Immune Globulin (RVA, RIG)

Rabies vaccine is given prophylactically to individuals at high risk of exposure to rabid animals, including veterinarians, animal handlers, and certain laboratory workers. It should be given as a series and should be started immediately after any bite from a suspicious animal. Rabies immunoglobulin gives passive protection when started immediately after exposure to rabies virus. It takes approximately 1 week for antibodies to develop.

Rabies vaccine is available as a human diploid-cell vaccine (HDCV) and as a purified chick embryo cell (PCEC).

CONTRAINDICATIONS, WARNINGS, AND PRECAUTIONS. No contraindications to administration of rabies IG or vaccine are known. Pregnancy is not a contraindication. The product does not pose a risk for nursing infants or children.

ADVERSE EFFECTS. Although adverse reactions are less common with currently available products, 15% to 25% of adults may experience local reactions, such as pain and swelling, as well as systemic reactions, including headache, muscle pain, nausea, and dizziness. Reactions are much less frequent in children. Severe reactions, including several cases of a Guillain-Barré–like syndrome, do not appear to be causally linked to vaccine.

DOSAGE AND ADMINISTRATION. Postexposure prophylaxis should begin as soon as possible, preferably within 24 hours, and requires administration of both RIG and vaccine. Vaccine dosing varies for children and adults.

For both adults and children, RIG at a dose of 20 IU/kg should be given as soon as possible, with as much of the dose as possible used to infiltrate the wound; RIG may be diluted with saline to increase volume and allow penetration of the entire wound. The remaining volume should be given intramuscularly at a distant site. Vaccine should be given at the same time; the dose is 1 ml, given intramuscularly, of the three available vaccines on days 0, 3, 7, 14, and 28. The same product should be used for all doses. Adults should receive an intramuscular injection in the deltoid; the anterolateral thigh may be used in young children. In individuals who have been previously vaccinated, RIG is not given. Two doses of vaccine should be given; the first should be given on the day of exposure, and the second dose should be given 3 days later.

Both adults and children should be given a three-dose regimen consisting of a 1 ml dose of any available product on days 0, 7, and 21 or 28. Booster doses at 2-year intervals may be necessary, as determined by serum antibody levels.

A preexposure rabies vaccination is now available. The regimen consists of three doses. The second dose is given 7 days after the first vaccination; the third dose is given 21 or 28 days after the first vaccination. Booster doses are indicated with frequent or continuous risk of exposure to rabies virus, and when blood testing indicates absent or low levels of immunity against rabies.

HOW SUPPLIED
- Vaccine:
  - Human diploid cell vaccine (HDCV) (Imovax, Sanofi Pasteur)
  - Purified chicken embryo cell (PCEC) (RavAvert, Chiron Corporation, Emeryville, Calif)

  Both preparations are available in single-dose vials.
- Rabies immune globulin:
  - Imogam Rabies HT (Sanofi Pasteur)
  - BayRab (Bayer, Elkhart, Ind)

Yellow Fever Vaccine

This vaccine is a live-attenuated virus preparation that provides immunity in 7 to 10 days with continued efficacy for about 10 years. It is indicated for travelers to areas where yellow fever is endemic. Updated information on endemic areas can be found at Travelers' Health on the CDC website (http://www.cdc.gov/), and the A live-attenuated vaccine is available at state-approved immunization centers.

CONTRAINDICATIONS, WARNINGS, AND PRECAUTIONS. Children younger than 9 months of age should not be vaccinated, although in special, high-risk cases, vaccination may be considered for children aged 4 to 9 months. Vaccination should never be given to children younger than 4 months of age. The safety of yellow fever vaccination during pregnancy has not been established, and vaccination should be considered only when travel to endemic regions, with an associated high risk of exposure, is unavoidable. The seroconversion rate after vaccination in pregnant women is uncertain, and serologic testing to determine immunity should be considered. Although no cases of transmission through breast milk have been reported, vaccination of nursing women should be avoided unless there is a high risk of exposure. Vaccinated patients should continue to take precautions to avoid mosquito bites. Recommendations for use in children younger than 9 months of age, pregnant women, or immunocompromised individuals may be obtained from the Division of Vector-Borne Disease on the CDC website.

ADVERSE EFFECTS. Fever or malaise usually appears 7 to 14 days after administration. Myalgia and headache also may develop. Anaphylaxis or encephalitis may occur rarely; most yellow fever vaccine–associated cases of neurotropic disease, formerly known as postvaccinal encephalitis, have occurred in children younger than 6 months of age.

DOSAGE AND ADMINISTRATION. *Adults and children:* Administer a single immunizing dose of 0.5 ml subcutaneously. A single dose is recognized to provide immunity for 10 years and may provide lifelong protection.

Limited available data suggest that vaccine may be safely administered at the same time as other commercially available vaccines.

HOW SUPPLIED. 17D-204 strain (YF-VAX®, Sanofi Aventis) is packaged in one-dose and five-dose vials. The vaccine should be refrigerated until it is reconstituted by the addition of diluent supplied by the manufacturer.

Typhoid Vaccine

Typhoid or enteric fever is caused by *Salmonella* serotype typhi. Although it is uncommon in the United States, this infection, which is transmitted via food or water infected by feces from an infected individual, is endemic in many parts of the world. Of the 400 cases of typhoid fever that occur in the United States each year, 70% are reported to be acquired outside of the United States. Currently available vaccines are estimated to be about 70% effective in preventing typhoid fever, depending in part on the degree of exposure. Vaccine is available as a live-attenuated oral product (Ty21a) and a polysaccharide preparation that is delivered by intramuscular injection (ViCPS). Researchers at the National Institute of Child Health and Human Development have recently developed an oral product that reportedly has 91% efficacy and may be given to children as young as 2 years.

Typhoid vaccine is indicated (1) for those traveling to areas where typhoid fever is endemic, notably India and neighboring countries, the Middle East, and Central Africa, (2) when contact with infected individuals is expected, and (3) in laboratory workers who handle organisms.

CONTRAINDICATIONS, WARNINGS, AND PRECAUTIONS. Do not give the oral formulation to immunocompromised individuals because it contains live virus. Administration of the antimalarial proguanil should be delayed until 10 days after the final dose of oral vaccine is received. Similarly, administration of oral vaccine should be delayed until 24 hours after use of any antimicrobial drugs. Because the oral vaccine requires replication in the gut, it should not be administered during an acute gastroenteritis.

ADVERSE EFFECTS. Oral vaccine is associated with minimal systemic adverse reactions, including nausea, abdominal pain, fever, and rash. Polysaccharide products may cause fever, headache, and local induration or erythema at the injection site.

DOSAGE AND ADMINISTRATION

- *Oral:* Vaccine may be given to individuals older than 6 years of age. Take one enteric-coated capsule on alternate days (days 1, 3, 5, and 7) for four doses. Swallow capsule whole 1 hour before a meal with cool or lukewarm water. Complete at least 1 week before travel or contact. Current recommendations are to repeat the entire four-dose course every 5 years for booster protection as indicated.
- *Polysaccharide:* Vaccine may be given to individuals older than 2 years of age. Give a single 0.5 ml dose intramuscularly, with a booster dose every 2 years if the risk of exposure remains high.

HOW SUPPLIED

- *Oral:* Single, foil blister containing four doses in a single package
- *Parenteral:* Available as a single-dose injectable vaccine in vials of 5, 10, 20, and 50 ml, depending on the suspension

Smallpox Vaccine

Routine administration of smallpox vaccine was discontinued in the United States in 1972, when the virus was declared to be eradicated in the wild. Current concerns about its use as a weapon of mass destruction have led to reinstitution of immunization in selected at-risk populations. The smallpox vaccine currently available in the United States (Dryvax, Wyeth) is a live-virus preparation of infectious vaccinia virus. Smallpox vaccine does not contain smallpox (variola) virus.

CONTRAINDICATIONS, WARNINGS, AND PRECAUTIONS. Because of the incidence of potentially severe reactions, routine immunization is not recommended. Vaccine is contraindicated in the following situations:

- Individuals and household contacts who have ever been diagnosed with eczema or atopic dermatitis or acute or chronic skin condition such as atopic dermatitis, wounds, burns, impetigo, or varicella-zoster should not be vaccinated, even if their skin condition is well controlled. These individuals are at high risk of developing eczema vaccinatum, a potentially severe and sometimes fatal complication.
- Individuals with diseases or conditions that cause immunodeficiency or immunosuppression, including HIV/AIDS, organ transplant, and malignancy, or recipients of radiation, chemotherapy, or high-dose corticosteroids, should not be vaccinated because of the higher risk of developing progressive vaccinia, a condition that results in dangerous replication of the vaccine virus. Household contacts of individuals undergoing such treatment should not receive smallpox vaccine until they or their household contacts have been off immunosuppressive treatment for 3 months.
- Live-virus vaccines should not be given during pregnancy. Pregnant women who receive the smallpox vaccine are at risk of fetal vaccinia, a very rare condition that results in stillbirth or death of the infant shortly after delivery. Women who are pregnant or intend to become pregnant in the next month and their household contacts should not be vaccinated.
- Previous allergic reaction to smallpox vaccine or any of the vaccine's components

- Moderate or severe acute illness should prompt a delay until the illness is resolved.
- Smallpox vaccine is contraindicated for children younger than 12 months of age and should not be administered in nonemergency settings in persons younger than 18 years of age.
- Breastfeeding mothers should not receive the smallpox vaccine because it is not known whether vaccine virus or antibodies are excreted in human milk.
- Following rare reports of cardiac events after vaccination, it is currently recommended that individuals with known cardiac disease such as previous myocardial infarction, angina, chronic heart failure, or cardiomyopathy should not be vaccinated. It is unknown whether these events are causally linked to vaccination; this association is being studied.

During a smallpox emergency, such as a weapons of mass destruction attack, all contraindications to vaccination would be reconsidered in light of the risk of smallpox exposure.

ADVERSE EFFECTS. Smallpox vaccination, although generally safe, has been associated with a significant incidence of adverse reactions. Most are benign, but they may be alarming in appearance and occasionally serious and life threatening. Severe adverse reactions are more common in persons receiving primary vaccination than in those being revaccinated.

Local reactions, such as local edema, satellite lesions, pain, and swelling of regional lymph nodes, may occur 3 to 10 days after vaccination and may persist for up to 4 weeks. The resultant viral cellulitis may be confused with bacterial cellulitis. In up to a third of recipients, these reactions may be severe enough to prompt the individual to seek treatment.

Systemic reactions include fever in up to 70% of primary vaccinees, malaise, myalgia, and erythematous or urticarial rashes. As with local reactions, up to a third of these recipients are ill enough to miss work.

The lesion produced at the vaccination site contains high vaccinia virus titers and is frequently pruritic. The itching that results may lead to transfer of the virus to the face, eyes, genital area, and rectum as secondary lesions, which usually heal without treatment. Successful vaccination produces a lesion at the vaccination site. Beginning about 4 days after vaccination, the florid site contains high titers of vaccinia virus. This surface is easily transferred to the hands and to fomites, especially because itching is a common part of the local reaction. The most severe manifestation is vaccinia keratitis, which may result in lesions of the cornea and, if untreated, corneal scarring with resultant visual impairment. Vaccinated health care workers should avoid contact with patients, particularly those with immunodeficiency, until the scab has separated from the skin at the vaccination site.

Generalized vaccinia results in vesicles or pustules on normal skin distant from the vaccination site; this generally resolves without specialized treatment and without residual effects. Progressive vaccinia, also known as vaccinia necrosum, is a severe, potentially fatal illness that is characterized by progressive necrosis in the area of vaccination, often with distant lesions. Prompt hospitalization and aggressive use of massive doses of VIG are required.

As of May 2003, 30 cardiac events, including myopericarditis and ischemia, had been reported to the VAERS among 36,217 persons who had been vaccinated as part of the civilian smallpox preevent program. An investigation is in progress, and surveillance for adverse cardiac events continues.

Eczema vaccinatum results in localized and systemic spread of vaccinia virus, which produces extensive lesions. This may occur even in those individuals who do not have active dermatitis at the time of vaccination. Treatment includes hospitalization and vaccinia immunoglobulin.

The FDA has recommended that vaccinees be deferred from donating blood for 21 days, or until the scab has separated.

DOSAGE AND ADMINISTRATION. ACIP recommends vaccination of laboratory workers who directly handle cultures or animals contaminated or infected with virus. The Armed Forces vaccinates selected personnel. Additionally, vaccination can be considered for health care workers who have contact with virus through patients or fomites. Vaccination is achieved with a single-use bifurcated needle through a technique called *multiple puncture vaccination*. Three insertions are necessary for primary vaccination, and 15 insertions are necessary for revaccination. A trace of blood should appear at the site of vaccination within 15 to 20 seconds. During primary vaccination, if no trace of blood is visible after three insertions, an additional three insertions should be made using the same bifurcated needle without reinserting the needle into the vaccine vial.

HOW SUPPLIED. Licensed Dryvax vaccine for civilians (Wyeth) is available only through the CDC.

evolve A continually updated list of useful WebLinks may be found in the Evolve Resources at http://evolve.elsevier.com/Edmunds/NP/

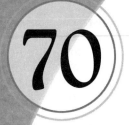

Weight Management

DRUG OVERVIEW

Class	Subclass	Generic Name	Trade Name
Anorexiants	Mixed neurotransmitter reuptake inhibitor	sibutramine	Meridia
	Sympathomimetic	phentermine ☀	Fastin, ProFast, Adipex-P, Lonamin
Lipase inhibitors		orlistat	Xenical; Alli (OTC)

☀, Top 200 drug.

INDICATIONS

Obesity

▪ Sibutramine and orlistat currently are the dominant medications used in helping patients lose weight. Phentermine can be used in the short term only.

THERAPEUTIC OVERVIEW

Pathophysiology

Obesity involves both genetic and environmental factors. A segment of the population is genetically predisposed to obesity. Another segment of the population succumbs to adverse environmental conditions, such as fast food, sedentary jobs, and few opportunities to exercise. These individuals phenotypically express obesity.

Taking in more calories than are expended causes obesity. Overweight individuals tend to eat too many grams of fat and to consume too many calories. Although decreasing fat intake is important in reducing cardiovascular risk factors and lowering cholesterol, it is calories that really count with weight gain.

An individual's energy expenditure must be closely examined. This is divided into three categories. First, resting energy expenditure is what the body consumes when just resting; this is about 60% of energy used in a day and depends on the amount of lean body mass and the individual's age. Resting energy goes down with age and up with lean body mass. A person who has more muscle will have higher resting energy expenditure. It is very difficult to change this level to any significant degree. However, it does determine most of the energy that a person burns.

The second category of energy expenditure is the exercise or activity energy expenditure. This is about 30% of the energy burned and is highly variable. For example, a person who is relatively sedentary but who wiggles and fidgets burns about 600 more calories a day than the sedentary bradykinetic individual. Given this basic principle, patients who wish to lose weight should be more physically active.

The third category of energy expenditure comes from the thermic effect of food and is responsible for about 10% of energy expenditure. In obese individuals, small decreases occur in their thermic-effect-of-food rates, but these do not explain the obese state.

Adipose tissue in the body is used primarily to store energy in the form of triglyceride. During periods when food is not eaten, the body draws from the adipose tissue reservoir to find what is needed to help the individual survive. When the individual eats too much, the adipose tissue reservoir is over-filled. The store of triglycerides remains available to be broken down into fatty acids for use as energy. Considerable interest has been expressed in pursuits undertaken to enhance understanding of whether obese individuals are more efficient at storing triglycerides than lean people. It has been observed that an obese person who takes in 100 g of fat might be more likely to deposit that as adipose tissue, whereas a lean person might oxidize it and burn it off as heat.

When obesity is discussed at the cellular level, two factors must be considered: (1) how many fat cells the individual has, and (2) to what extent these fat cells are filled with fat. To answer these questions, it is important for one to understand that fat storage consists of two components: (1) the fat cells, and (2) the stromal vascular or supporting connecting tissue. Fat cells start out as preadipocytes. These are fibroblast-like cells that do not respond to insulin, and they do not store fat. They are small, spindle-like cells that are found within the fat cell; they divide and can turn into fat cells with excessive stimulation of nutrients. These fat cells also can enlarge and make huge fat cells. There is a limit to how stretched these fat storage cells can become. After fat cells reach a certain level, they recruit additional preadipocytes to make more fat cells.

When the number of fat cells an individual has is determined, it can be seen that there are two critical times in life when many preadipocytes are made, and thus the person will develop a larger pool of fat cells for the body to use. The first time is at age 2, and the second is at puberty. An individual who becomes obese at 2 or at puberty has a bigger supply of precursor cells and thus may be more resistant to long-term weight loss. It is not correct to say that at puberty people have all the fat cells they will ever have, and that they will die with that number. People can accumulate fat cells throughout life if they give in to the environmental stimulus, which is overeating. Some metabolic diseases also contribute to the increased development of fat cells.

The reason why it is very difficult to lose weight, once an individual has formed extra fat cells, is that fat cells do not divide once they are differentiated, but they also do not die. In a process called *programmed cell death*, or *apoptosis*, cells get rid of excess cells. However, adipocytes, as a rule, do not go through apoptosis and die; they are around for life. Obesity must be prevented because once the individual has accumulated fat, it is very difficult to lose. Even if fat cells contain no fat, they remain prepared and are waiting to take up more triglycerides.

Obesity and adipose tissue mass are tightly regulated. Patients complain, "I just get so hungry, I start eating again, and then I gain weight back." If individuals have a certain mass of adipose tissue, the body does whatever it can to defend that mass. As soon as patients start to reduce adipose tissue through diet and exercise, the body thinks it is starving, so it makes these individuals hungry. Many physiologic mechanisms kick in. Neuropeptides in the brain and enzymes in the lining of the stomach help to accomplish this. They stimulate the body to say it is hungry and to eat. All of these factor interactions in brain, environment, and adipose tissue work to try to restore fat mass to its previous level.

HAZARDS OF OBESITY. Obesity, or the state of being overweight, is associated with increased morbidity and mortality. Obesity is an independent risk factor for coronary heart disease and diabetes. Hypertension and diabetes mellitus are more difficult to control in the obese patient. The patient is at increased risk for CAD, CHF, stroke, gallbladder disease, osteoarthritis, and sleep apnea or other respiratory problems. Levels of triglycerides, total serum cholesterol, and LDL are elevated and levels of HDL are decreased. Obesity is associated with increased risk of certain cancers such as endometrial, breast, colon, and prostate. Obesity is associated with gynecologic problems such as complications of pregnancy, menstrual irregularities, hirsutism, and stress incontinence. In addition, patients who are obese are at increased risk for depression and have higher surgical risks.

Disease Process

Obesity is an excess of body fat relative to lean body mass. *Overweight* is defined as BMI of 25 to 29.9 kg/m². *Obesity* is defined as BMI of 30 kg/m² or greater, according to the Clinical Guidelines on the Identification, Evaluation, and Treatment of Overweight and Obesity in Adults, published by the National Heart, Lung, and Blood Institute (NHLBI) in June 1998. These guidelines provide basic information underlying the diagnosis and management of obesity and should be consulted by all clinicians.

> **evolve** See list of resources on the Evolve website to obtain copies through the Internet.

Obesity is increasing in prevalence, both in this country and throughout the world, in all segments of the population. The prevalence of obesity increases with age. In the United States, obesity is more prevalent in some minority groups and in patients with lower income and less education.

The economic costs associated with people who are overweight or obese are tremendous. The total cost attributable to obesity was over $99 billion in 1995. One half of these costs were direct medical costs resulting from diseases attributed to obesity. Indirect costs represent lost productivity due to obesity and are similar to those associated with smoking. Because obesity is associated with the development of other chronic diseases such as diabetes, coronary heart disease, and arthritis, additional indirect costs associated with obesity increase dramatically. Thus costs are both individual and societal.

Assessment

The most useful estimate of body fat is the BMI. The BMI is a powerful indicator of health risk that should be included in the comprehensive evaluation of any patient.

When patients are considered for a weight reduction program, one should assess their BMI, weight, waist circumference, overall risk status, and motivation to lose weight.

The BMI is a number that is derived by dividing the weight in kilograms by the height in meters squared. The easiest way for most individuals to do the calculation is to multiply 704.5 by the patient's weight in pounds. Divide that number by the patient's height in inches multiplied by itself. Conversion charts are easily available.

$$BMI = 704.5 \times \text{Weight in pounds}/(\text{Height in inches})^2$$

Normal BMI is considered to be 19 to 24.9 kg/m². By way of reference, the average fashion model has a BMI of about 16.5. Tiger Woods has a BMI of 21.

Persons with a BMI of 20 to 25 have the lowest mortality. For the most part, increasing BMI is associated with increasing mortality. If BMI is less than 25, the health risk is minimal. Patients with BMI above 27 are in the moderate range; with BMI above 40, it is more likely that they will develop diabetes or some other obesity-related condition. Obese geriatric patients have less upper and lower body function. The incidence of obesity does not change, but functional status changes in the geriatric population.

In individuals who are overweight, where the fat is located is also an important consideration. Waist circumference is an independent predictor of risk factors and morbidity and is correlated with abdominal fat content. Men at high risk have a waist greater than 102 cm (40 in). Women at high risk have a waist greater than 88 cm (35 in). The Nurses' Health Study has documented that women whose waist measurement is 38 inches or more have 3 times the risk of heart disease as do women whose waists measure 28 inches or less. Women who are apple-shaped and who have a high waist-to-hip ratio are at greater risk for heart disease than are pear-shaped women, whose weight is concentrated in their hips and thighs. A large waist correlates with the metabolic syndrome.

The metabolic syndrome, formerly known as syndrome X, has been identified as an important risk factor in obese patients for diabetes and cardiovascular disease. In this process, fat cells release substances such as free fatty acids, complement D and cytokines (which promote inflammation), prothrombic agents, and angiotensinogen. Free fatty acids increase insulin resistance, raising insulin levels and leading to increased sodium reabsorption. Elevated sodium levels are associated with higher blood pressure. Insulin resistance may result in elevated blood sugar levels and diabetes mellitus, and free fatty acids and increased lipids raise the risk of CAD. Diagnostically, metabolic syndrome must consist of three or more of the following:

Abdominal fat (waist circumference)	>35 inches (men, 40)
Insulin resistance (fasting sugar)	110 mg/dl
Triglycerides	150 mg/dl
HDL cholesterol	<50 (men, 40)
High blood pressure	135/85 mm Hg

Evaluation of overall patient risk requires consideration of all conditions that might be caused by obesity or overweight. These include cardiovascular risk factors, CAD, atherosclerosis, diabetes mellitus (DM), sleep apnea, osteoarthritis, gallstones, physical inactivity, and high levels of serum triglycerides. Their presence increases the importance of weight reduction for that patient.

The clinician also must evaluate the patient's reasons and motivation for weight loss, previous weight loss attempts, understanding of the problem, physical activity, diet, and financial constraints. Patient motivation is essential to weight loss success.

MECHANISM OF ACTION

Anorexiants are indirect-acting sympathomimetic amines. They are thought to provide a direct stimulant effect on the satiety center in the hypothalamus. Different anorexiants act through different pathways.

Sibutramine, a class IV controlled substance, is a member of a new class of antiobesity drugs that work by increasing levels of serotonin and norepinephrine in the brain. It is known as a serotonin and norepinephrine reuptake inhibitor (SNRI). In addition to its actions on serotonin and norepinephrine, it exerts a minor effect on dopamine levels. Serotonin works in the hypothalamus, the center that regulates food intake. Sibutramine increases serotonins, reduces appetite, and increases satiety. Patients are less hungry, and they get full faster. Lower levels of serotonin are also associated with depression, which may explain why people eat to improve their mood. A desirable side effect of sibutramine is reduced depression.

Phentermine is a class IV controlled substance that acts by modulating central norepinephrine and dopamine receptors through the promotion of catecholamine release.

Orlistat works through a completely different mechanism. Orlistat blocks approximately 30% of fat absorption within the GI tract. It acts locally and is minimally absorbed. The GI tract enzyme, lipase, together with a colipase, breaks down fat molecules before they can be absorbed. Orlistat interferes with lipase and works in the jejunum to inhibit pancreatic lipase.

TREATMENT PRINCIPLES
Standardized Guidelines

- U.S. Preventive Services Task Force Guidelines for Screening for Obesity in Adults, revised 2003.
- National Heart, Lung, and Blood Institute at NIH Clinical Guidelines on the Identification, Evaluation, and Treatment of Overweight and Obesity in Adults, 2003.

- Institute of Medicine Committee on Prevention of Obesity in Children and Youth, Food and Nutrition Board, Board on Health Promotion and Disease Prevention, 2005. In Koplan JP et al, eds: *Preventing Childhood Obesity: Health in the Balance*, Washington, DC, The National Academies Press.

Evidence-Based Recommendations

- *Trade-off between benefits and harms:* diethylpropion, mazindol, orlistat, phentermine, rimonabant, sibutramine
- Orlistat, sibutramine, and rimonabant modestly reduce weight, with differing effects on cardiovascular risk profiles and specific adverse effects

Cardinal Points of Treatment

- Diet essential
- Phentermine for short-term use only
- Orlistat and sibutramine for long-term use

Treatment goals in working with the overweight or obese individual are to (1) prevent further weight gain, (2) reduce body weight, and (3) maintain a lower body weight over the long term. An initial goal is to reduce body weight by about 10% from baseline. A reasonable time frame for this loss is 6 months. A treatment algorithm from the NHLBI addresses the management of patients who are obese or overweight. A stepped-care model has also been devised by Shape Up America, a group organized by C. Everett Koop, and a new group called the American Obesity Association.

Nonpharmacologic Treatment

No single treatment modality is independently effective in the management of obesity. Intervention is unlikely to be effective if it is not tempered with strategies designed to enable the patient to make permanent lifestyle changes. It is a common misconception that drug therapy alone will control this problem.

To place weight loss strategies in the proper perspective, it is important to view all weight loss options. Blackburn and colleagues (2007), in a compelling discussion, argue that lifestyle modifications help modify the external environment to help the patient lose weight. These strategies are designed to decrease the patient's exposure to food, decrease cues for eating, increase dietary restraint, and increase physical activity. They suggest that pharmacologic modifications help control the patient's internal environment to decrease hunger, decrease food preoccupation, increase satiation, and decrease nutrient absorption. These two strategies have potential additive effects.

Randomized controlled trials have compared different diet and activity interventions for inducing and maintaining weight loss, as well as different methods of providing lifestyle modifications, including on-site vs. Internet-based delivery. A summary of the literature on comprehensive lifestyle modification programs reported that they induce a loss of approximately 10% of initial weight over 16 to 26 weeks of group or individual treatment, delivered on-site. Comparable comprehensive Internet programs induced a weight loss of approximately 5% of initial weight. Patients' consumption of portion-controlled diets (including liquid meal replacements) was associated with significantly greater short-term weight loss than was the eating of isocaloric diets of conventional foods. Factors found to be associated with long-term weight control included continued contact between patient and practitioner (whether on-site or by e-mail), high levels of physical activity, and long-term use of pharmacotherapy combined with lifestyle modifications (Wadden et al, 2007). Goals that include enough weight loss to reduce cardiovascular risk for the patient are particularly useful.

For children who are overweight, the practitioner should calculate and monitor the BMI to track weight changes and should work with the parent and the child at each visit to establish reasonable dietary and exercise plans. It is essential that attention be focused on achieving weight loss for children as early as possible to decrease costs and problems associated with prolonged obesity.

Helping patients to lose weight begins with assessment of the patient's motivation to lose weight. Even with patients who are very motivated, the clinician must spend time to understand their concerns and to tailor a program to fit their situation. Individuals who have always been overweight by 100 lb or more may never be able to get to their ideal body weight. Most will not lose weight at the rate they would desire. Helping them to develop realistic expectations is foundational to success.

How do you determine what is an appropriate weight for an individual? The answer to this question has changed over the years. The normal weight chart developed from actuarial data of the Metropolitan Life Insurance Company was the standard that was used for years. These charts have been modified over time to reflect heavier weights caused by better nutrition and changing views of what a "normal" person weighs. National guidelines stipulate that BMI is a better indication of obesity than is weight; therefore, many clinicians now use the weight needed for a normal BMI as the goal.

It is important to set specific weight loss goals. An overall target goal and a time period within which to accomplish this goal are helpful. More meaningful for both monitoring and motivational purposes are monthly goals of a 2- to 4-lb weight loss. A successful strategy included in many weight loss programs is a system of built-in rewards that patients give themselves when they reach the goal, for example, new haircuts or cosmetic makeovers. Some patients may do better when they meet their goals through an organized program such as Weight Watchers; others do better alone.

Any successful weight loss regimen is based on reduction of caloric intake and an increase in physical exercise. Without both of these, weight loss is generally transient. Medications may be helpful in both foundational areas in suppressing appetite and helping to keep energy levels high, so the patient feels like exercising.

DIET. Lowering of caloric intake every day will result in a reasonable, slow, steady weight loss. Several valid methods may be used to arrive at the proper dietary prescription for an individual.

Total daily allotment of calories is based on the requirements of the patient and depends on his or her nutritional status when the diet is instituted and on an estimate of daily activity. During their peak growth period, active adolescent boys need 3100 to 3600 cal/day, and adolescent girls need 2400 to 2700 cal/day. Children generally require 1000 cal/day plus an additional 100 calories for every year of age. Accordingly, a 10-year-old child should receive approximately 2000 calories daily.

A general rule of thumb is that it takes approximately 10 calories to support each pound of weight. For example, a 150 lb woman is probably eating 1500 calories. To lose weight, the patient must decrease intake to below the level needed to maintain weight. The patient must decrease daily intake by 500 calories for each pound he or she wishes to lose weekly. Weight loss of about 1 to 2 lb/week commonly will occur for up to 6 months. After 6 months, the rate of weight loss will often plateau. This occurs because the patient has lower energy expenditure at the lower weight. Once a patient has plateaued, evaluate whether he or she needs to lose more weight. If so, reevaluation of diet and exercise is required. The patient must further decrease calories and/or increase physical activity to achieve this.

Three major types of diets are used: balanced, low fat, and low carbohydrate. Much controversy has arisen about diets for obesity. Although patients may lose more weight initially on a low-carbohydrate diet, the weight lost after 1 year is about equal for low-carbohydrate and low-fat diets, but the low-carbohydrate or Mediterranean diets have more favorable effects on lipids and/or glycemic control. Thus, whatever the diet, patients should be encouraged to make reasonable eating changes that they can live with for years, to avoid extremes, and to have balanced nutrition in what they eat.

Rapid weight loss is not advisable. Studies have shown that regaining weight almost always follows rapid weight reduction. Also, the risks for gallstones and electrolyte abnormalities are increased when weight loss is excessive.

Once the patient has reached a particular weight loss goal, the goal is changed to weight maintenance at the lower weight. It is important to continue to monitor these patients to help them stay at the lower weight.

In 2008, a new system for scoring the nutritional value of some foods will become available in a limited number of grocery stores. This should provide a standardized way to make healthier food choices. The Overall Nutritional Quality Index (ONQI) was developed by a group of nutrition and health experts and takes into account a number of factors in assigning a score of 1 to 100 for each food, including negatives like the amount of saturated fat, sugar and cholesterol in a food, and positives like fiber, nutrients, omega-3 fatty acids and the quality of the proteins. The grocers are not obligated to use the scoring system, but it will be made available to them. The scoring system will let consumers compare different types of the same food, so they will be able to tell which are more or less healthy.

EXERCISE. An increase in physical activity is the second essential component of weight reduction. Exercise leads to increased expenditure of energy, inhibits food intake, and reduces overall CAD risk. Efforts to lose weight by exercise alone without calorie reduction usually produce a 2% to 3% weight decrease. Exercise may be useful in decreasing abdominal fat as well as weight. A regular exercise program such as walking is something almost every patient can tolerate, and patients can integrate more activity into their lives by walking up stairs, parking at the far end of the lot, and so forth.

BEHAVIOR. To achieve long-term weight loss, the patient must change basic eating and activity patterns. Specific strategies include keeping a food diary, managing stress, controlling stimuli (e.g., avoiding situations that precipitate overeating), solving problems (self-correcting problems), and providing contingency management, cognitive restructuring (setting realistic goals), and social support.

These three components of weight reduction (i.e., treatment diet, exercise, and behavior therapy) work best when used together under the supervision of a health care provider.

SURGERY. Surgery is the treatment of choice for extremely obese individuals with comorbid problems. Surgery is used after pharmacologic therapy has proved ineffective. Several surgical procedures are currently being used. These include bariatric surgery, vertical banded gastroplasty, gastric banding, and gastric bypass. Patients who require surgical intervention should find a surgical specialist who has had experience with the extremely obese. Currently used techniques include vertical banded gastroplasty, wherein the stomach is stapled into a small pouch, and gastric bypass roux-en-Y, in which a small pouch is made before the proximal jejunum is transected.

For patients who undergo gastric surgery, the clinician may have to deal with surgically created malabsorption or physical restriction. Regurgitation is a significant problem with restrictive surgery in many patients. These people may have a high level of intolerance to food; they will need to make major changes in diet. Malabsorption syndromes may lead to micronutrient or macronutrient deficiency, anemia, protein malnutrition, dumping syndrome, and so forth. Gastric leaking may also be a problem at the site of anastomosis; this leads to peritonitis. Patients need medical and psychologic monitoring.

Pharmacologic Treatment

Overall, the use of medications in treating obesity has not proved to be an effective long-term solution for most individuals. However, initial weight loss may encourage the patient to make other changes regarding exercise or eating behavior that will lead to more lasting weight loss.

Critical decisions that must be made relate to whether it is appropriate to use pharmacologic therapy and, if so, whether the patient has any conditions that contraindicate use of these products. Clinical trials have shown that use of these drugs, in combination with a sensible diet, results in approximately a 6- to 12-pound mean weight loss. Weight loss drugs should be used only for patients who are at increased medical risk because of their weight and should not be used for "cosmetic" weight loss. The NHLBI guidelines state that these drugs may be useful for a patient with BMI of 30 or greater with no concomitant obesity-related risk factors or diseases, or for a patient with BMI of 27 or greater with concomitant obesity-related risk factors or diseases.

Medications work by helping the patient stay on a diet and exercise plan. A drug will not cause weight loss if the patient continues to eat at the same level. Most of the weight loss will occur during the first 6 months of treatment with the drug. If the patient does not respond within the first month of therapy, the likelihood of response is very low.

Sibutramine generally is used for no longer than 6 months. It should be stopped after 1 month if it is not effective. Safety and efficacy beyond 2 years have not been determined at this time. It can help with modest weight loss and can help keep weight off. Sibutramine can cause increases in blood pressure and pulse. People with a history of high blood pressure, CAD, CHF, arrhythmias, or stroke should not take this medication, and blood pressure should be monitored regularly.

Phentermine is used as a short-term adjunct in weight reduction. It should not be used for longer than a few weeks. It may be tried if sibutramine is not effective. However, significant serious risks are associated with its use.

Orlistat (Xenical) acts to increase fecal fat excretion. The extent of drug activity may be determined by measuring the amount of fat in the stool. The maximum amount of fat excretion is around 25% to 30%. (If 100 g of fat is consumed in a day, 30 g will end up in the stool.) Once the medication is stopped, fecal fat excretion goes back down to normal.

Orlistat has been shown to be about as effective as, or perhaps a little less effective than, the sympathomimetics. In a short-term study, an approximate reduction in initial weight of 10% was reported. In long-term studies, most of the weight loss occurred during the first months and was maintained for up to 2 years.

Orlistat is associated with irritating GI side effects, such as soft liquid stools and oil in the stool. Some people have had oily stool spotting, necessitating the use of minipads. These symptoms appear to be dose dependent. Long-term use might be associated with the development of vitamin deficits. Levels of vitamin D and beta carotene were decreased by 20% to 24% but remained within the normal range. Fat-soluble vitamin supplementation may be required (to be taken at a different time than orlistat).

Also, the patient may ask about many herbal and OTC products that are advertised to help with weight loss. The lay literature is filled with information about fat substitutes such as Olestra (currently limited to snack foods). Patients might ask about medications derived from the exoskeletons of shrimp and lobsters (Chitosan). These products absorb fat and have been used for the cleanup of oil spills; these fat absorbers are available in some health food stores. No data can be found in the professional literature regarding these products. OTC products used for weight loss have often contained ephedrine, which was available in herbal form. Ephedrine can be very dangerous, causing stroke, headache, tachycardia, hypertension, and catecholamine-like symptoms, such as restlessness, dry mouth, insomnia, fatigue, and other central nervous system effects. Ephedrine use should be discouraged. Adverse effects from ephedrine have caused the FDA to remove this product from most preparations. (Consult the FDA website for the best information about herbal supplements and their safety, at www.fda.gov.)

A variety of other medications have been used off-label to help with weight loss. The antidepressant bupropion plus an antiepileptic agent zonisamide has been found to be more effective than placebo. Bupropion was started at a dose of 100 mg/day, which was increased to 200 mg/day after 2 weeks. Zonisamide was started at 100 mg/day, with gradual titration to 400 mg/day by week 4.

EVALUATING PATIENTS WHO HAVE TAKEN DEXFENFLURAMINE OR FENFLURAMINE. Dexfenfluramine (Redux) and fenfluramine (Pondimin) were effective anorexiants that acted centrally to suppress appetite. These were the first drugs to be successfully associated with weight loss, and the public demand for them was enormous. Clinicians and patients began to use fenfluramine in combination with phentermine—the "phen-fen" regimen. The combination was very effective in depressing appetite; however, these medications were not intended to be used together.

Fenfluramine (Ionamin, Fastin) and dexfenfluramine (Redux) were voluntarily removed from the market in 1997 because of growing complaints of pulmonary hypertension and valvular heart disease in patients who had used these products. Approximately 5% to 25% of patients who used the combination developed valvular heart disease.

Patients with pulmonary hypertension or valvular disease exhibit the following signs and symptoms: dyspnea, shortness of breath, decreased exercise tolerance, angina, syncope, and lower extremity edema. If the patient has symptoms, he or she should be referred to a cardiologist. It is a wise precaution to have all patients who are taking these drugs, even those who are asymptomatic, undergo echocardiography.

How to Monitor

- Monitor the patient's progress at least monthly. The patient may benefit from weekly weight assessments during the first 3 months and then monthly.
- *sibutramine:* Monitor blood pressure periodically.

Patient Variables

GERIATRICS

- *sibutramine, phentermine:* Use with caution in the elderly because of the possibility of reduced hepatic or cardiac function.
- *orlistat:* Monitor nutritional status for vitamin E, D, or B deficiency.

PEDIATRICS. *Do not use sibutramine* (younger than age 16), *phentermine, or orlistat;* safety and **efficacy have not been established.**

PREGNANCY AND LACTATION

- *Category B:* orlistat not recommended
- *Category C:* sibutramine, phentermine not recommended

Patient Education

SIBUTRAMINE

- Patient must keep regular monthly follow-up visits.
- Notify the primary care provider if a rash or hives develops.
- Avoid taking any OTC cold preparations that may contain decongestants.
- Blood pressure must be monitored closely.

PHENTERMINE

- The drug may cause insomnia; avoid taking this medication late in the day.
- Avoid alcohol or other CNS active drugs and anorectic agents.
- Notify primary care provider if the patient experiences palpitations, nervousness, or dizziness.
- The drug may cause dry mouth and constipation.
- It also may produce dizziness or blurred vision, which may interfere with driving or performing other tasks that require alertness.
- Take on an empty stomach.

ORLISTAT

- Take with a meal.
- Take multiple vitamins at a different time from when orlistat is taken.
- May cause leakage of stool

SPECIFIC DRUGS

ANOREXIANTS

sibutramine (Meridia)

CONTRAINDICATIONS

- MAOIs (during or within 14 days)
- Hypersensitivity
- Anorexia/bulimia nervosa
- Other centrally acting appetite suppressant drugs

WARNINGS

- Sibutramine substantially increases blood pressure in some patients. Regular monitoring of blood pressure is required when this product is prescribed.
- Use caution when prescribing sibutramine with other agents that may raise blood pressure or heart rate, including decongestants and cough, cold, and allergy medications that contain agents such as ephedrine or pseudoephedrine.
- Serotonin syndrome is a rare but serious constellation of symptoms. It is especially likely to occur if the patient is taking sibutramine along with an SSRI or triptans for migraine, certain opioids, or tryptophan. Symptoms include excitement, hypomania, restlessness, loss of consciousness, confusion, myoclonus, tremor, ataxia, and dysarthria. Emergency medical attention is required.
- Treatment with sibutramine has been associated with increased heart rate or blood pressure. Do not use in patients with a history of CAD, CHF, arrhythmia, or stroke.
- *Glaucoma:* Because sibutramine can cause mydriasis, use with caution in patients with narrow-angle glaucoma.
- Exclude organic causes of obesity before prescribing sibutramine.
- *Renal/hepatic function impairment:* Do not use in patients with severe renal impairment or severe hepatic dysfunction.

PRECAUTIONS

- *Abuse/physical and psychologic dependence:* Evaluate patient for history of drug abuse, and follow closely for signs of misuse or abuse (development of tolerance, incremental increase in doses, drug-seeking behavior).
- *Primary pulmonary hypertension (PPH):* Certain centrally acting weight loss agents that cause release of serotonin have been associated with PPH, a rare but lethal disease. No cases of PPH have been reported with sibutramine. However, it is not known whether or not sibutramine may cause this disease.
- *Seizures* were reported in less than 0.1% of patients. Use with caution in patients with a history of seizures.
- *Gallstones:* Weight loss can precipitate or exacerbate gallstone formation.
- *Interference with cognitive and motor performance:* Although sibutramine does not affect psychomotor or cognitive performance, any CNS active drug has the potential to impair judgment, thinking, or motor skills.

PHARMACOKINETICS. See Table 70-1.

ADVERSE EFFECTS. See Table 70-2.

DRUG INTERACTIONS. See Table 70-3. The product is extensively metabolized by the cytochrome P450 3A4 system.

TABLE 70-1   Pharmacokinetics of Weight Loss Agents

Drug	Absorption	Drug Availability (after first pass)	Time to Peak Concentration	Half-life	Protein Bound	Metabolism	Excretion
sibutramine	Rapid, 77%	Metabolized to active form	3-4 hr	14-16 hr	95%	Liver 3A4	Renal, 85%
phentermine	Slow	—	8 hr	20 hr	—	—	Renal
orlistat	Minimal	—	8 hr	—	99%	In GI wall	Feces

DOSAGE AND ADMINISTRATION
- Take once a day without regard to meals.
- Initial dose is 10 mg po once daily; may be increased to 15 mg po once daily after 4 weeks

phentermine (Adipex-P, Fastin, ProFast, Lonamin)

CONTRAINDICATIONS. Advanced arteriosclerosis, symptomatic cardiovascular disease, moderate to severe hypertension, hyperthyroidism, known hypersensitivity to the sympathomimetic amines; or glaucoma, highly nervous or agitated states, or history of drug abuse during or within 14 days following MAOIs and coadministration with other CNS stimulants.

WARNINGS
- Indicated for short-term use only. Tolerance to the anorexic effect usually develops within a few weeks. When this occurs, the recommended dose should not be exceeded in an attempt to increase the effect; rather, the drug should be discontinued.

- Valvular heart disease has been reported in chemically related anorexiants. Monitor closely for development of symptoms.

 PPH is a rare, frequently fatal disease of the lungs that has been reported in chemically related anorexiants. Monitor closely for development of symptoms.

PRECAUTIONS
- Psychologic disturbances have occurred in patients who received an anorectic agent together with a restrictive diet.
- *Cardiovascular disease:* Exercise caution in patients with even mild hypertension.
- The least amount feasible should be prescribed or dispensed at one time to minimize the possibility of overdosage.
- Insulin requirements in DM may be altered.
- These drugs are chemically and pharmacologically related to the amphetamines and have abuse potential. Intense psychologic dependence and severe social dysfunction may

TABLE 70-2   Adverse Effects of Weight Loss Agents

Body System	sibutramine	phentermine	orlistat
Skin, appendages	Rash, sweating	Hair loss, excessive sweating, ecchymosis, flushing	
Hypersensitivity		Urticaria, rash, erythema	
Respiratory	Rhinitis, pharyngitis	Dyspnea	
Cardiovascular	Tachycardia, vasodilation, migraine, hypertension, palpitations	Palpitations, tachycardia, arrhythmias, including ventricular, precordial pain, PPH, valvular disease, ↑ BP	
GI	Anorexia, constipation, increased appetite, nausea, dyspepsia, dry mouth	Dry mouth, nausea, vomiting, abdominal discomfort, diarrhea, GI disturbances, constipation, stomach pain	Oily spotting, flatus with discharge, fecal urgency, fatty/oily stool, oily evacuation, increased defecation, fecal incontinence, abdominal pain, gingival disorder, nausea, rectal discomfort
Hemic and lymphatic		Bone marrow depression, agranulocytosis, leukopenia	
Musculoskeletal	Arthralgia, myalgia	Muscle pain	
Nervous system	Headache, insomnia, dizziness, nervousness, anxiety, depression, paresthesia, somnolence, CNS stimulation, emotion lability	Malaise, overstimulation, CVA, nervousness, restlessness, dizziness, insomnia, anxiety, euphoria, drowsiness, depression, agitation, dysphoria, dyskinesia, tremor, headache, psychosis, agitation, jitteriness, depression following withdrawal	
Special senses	Taste perversion	Unpleasant taste, mydriasis, blurred vision	
Genitourinary	Dysmenorrhea	Dysuria, polyuria, urinary frequency, impotence, menstrual upset, gynecomastia, changes in libido	Menstrual irregularity

TABLE 70-3   Drug Interactions With Weight Loss Agents

Medications	Acts on Other Drugs
Sibutramine (major substrate of CYP 3A4; see detailed drug reference for specific interaction)	↑ Other agents that ↑ BP, MAOIs, SSRIs, ergot, lithium, opioids, triptans, tryptophan
phentermine	↑ TCAs, SSRIs
orlistat	↓ Fat-soluble vitamins ↓ cyclosporine
Other Drugs	**Act on Weight Loss Agents**
alcohol	↑ sibutramine
cimetidine, erythromycin, ketoconazole	↓↑ sibutramine
MAOIs	↑ phentermine

occur. If either of these occurs, gradually reduce the dosage to avoid withdrawal symptoms (extreme fatigue, sleep EEG changes, mental depression). Chronic intoxication is manifested by severe dermatoses, marked insomnia, irritability, hyperactivity, and personality changes and psychosis.

• The drug may impair the ability of the patient to engage in potentially hazardous activities such as operating machinery or driving a motor vehicle.

ADVERSE EFFECTS. The adverse effects can be serious (see Table 70-2).

DOSAGE AND ADMINISTRATION. Give 8 mg tid one-half hour before meals, or 15 to 37.5 mg as a single dose before breakfast or 10 to 14 hours before retiring.

LIPASE INHIBITORS

orlistat (Xenical, Alli [OTC])

CONTRAINDICATIONS
• Chronic malabsorption syndrome
• Cholestasis
• Hypersensitivity to the product

WARNINGS. Organic causes of obesity should be excluded before orlistat is prescribed.

PRECAUTIONS
• *Diet:* Advise patients to adhere to dietary guidelines.
• When taken with meals, orlistat blocks the absorption of about one quarter of any fat consumed. That fat—about 150 to 200 calories' worth—is passed out of the body in stools, which can be loose as a result.
• Adverse GI reactions may increase when orlistat is taken with a diet that is high in fat. About half of patients experience gastrointestinal side effects.
• Patients should take a multiple vitamin to ensure adequate nutrition because orlistat reduces the absorption of some fat-soluble vitamins and beta carotene. Do not take at the same time as orlistat.
• Some patients may develop increased levels of urinary oxalate with treatment.
• Diabetic patients with weight loss may improve metabolic control, which might require a reduction in oral hypoglycemic medication.
• As with any weight loss agent, the potential exists for misuse of orlistat, especially with anorexia nervosa or bulimia.

OVERDOSAGE. Single doses of 800 mg and multiple doses of up to 400 mg tid for 15 days have caused no significant adverse reactions.

DOSAGE AND ADMINISTRATION
• 120 mg tid with or 1 hour before or after a fat-containing meal
• The new OT drug contains half the dose of the prescription capsules.

evolve A continually updated list of useful WebLinks may be found in the Evolve Resources at http://evolve.elsevier.com/Edmunds/NP/

Smoking Cessation

DRUG OVERVIEW

Class	Generic Name	Trade Name	Formulation
Nicotine replacement therapy	nicotine polacrilex	Nicorette	Gum
	nicotine	Nicoderm CQ	Transdermal
		Habitrol	Transdermal
		Nicotrol	Transdermal
		ProStep	Transdermal
		Nicotrol NS	Nasal spray
		Nicotrol inhaler	Oral inhaler
		Commit	Lozenge
Antidepressant	bupropion ✺	Zyban, Wellbutrin ✺	Tablet
Nicotine receptor agonist	varenicline	Chantix	Tablet

✺, Top 200 drug.

Many pharmacologic approaches have been used to help people stop smoking. In current use are the nicotine replacement therapy (NRT) products and bupropion (Zyban, GlaxoSmithKline; Wellbutrin, GlaxoSmithKline). This chapter discusses methods for assisting the patient to stop smoking. The only drugs that are discussed in detail in this chapter are the NRT products because bupropion is discussed in Chapter 46. Many NRTs are now available OTC, but the patient still benefits from professional guidance on how to use these products.

THERAPEUTIC OVERVIEW

Results of a 2006 national survey show that about 1 in 5 U.S. adults smoke cigarettes, a number unchanged since 2004, making it the leading preventable cause of disease and death in the nation. This contrasts with the decline in smoking seen between 1997 and 2004. Smoking is strongly correlated with age. An estimated 27.9% of those aged 18 to 24 smoke, followed by 27.3% of those aged 25 to 44, 23.3% of those aged 45 to 64, and only 10.5% of people who are 65 or older. (The relatively low number of older smokers may be due to the fact that many smokers die prematurely as a result of their smoking.) There is an inverse relationship with increased years of education.

Smoking has been associated with more than 420,000 deaths annually, causing risk for cancer of the lung, larynx, esophagus, and others. Cigarette smoking is associated with coronary artery disease/myocardial infarction, COPD, peripheral artery disease, and cerebrovascular disease. Cancer and respiratory diseases have also been associated with passive (environmental) smoking.

Nicotine and other tobacco-related components (tar and aromatic hydrocarbons) are probable causative factors for the psychologic and pathologic sequelae of smoking. Individuals, especially children, who are subjected to passive smoke have a higher risk of developing asthma. Current research suggests that children already in danger of developing heart disease because of high cholesterol blood levels face a triple jeopardy if they live in smoke-filled homes, because the passive smoke lowers by about 10% the level of the child's HDL, or the good cholesterol that protects against heart attacks.

Primary care is an ideal setting in which to institute smoking cessation measures. Most smokers see a primary care provider each year. The provider should screen all patients for smoking behaviors and should recommend that all patients stop smoking. In fact, some third-party payers or insurance companies now require preferred providers to ask about tobacco use and to document recommendations to quit. Some companies are starting to raise health insurance premiums if the purchaser is a smoker, and most life insurance companies already have higher rates for smokers.

Research suggests that many health care providers fail to take advantage of opportunities to recommend that the patient stop smoking. Primary care clinicians especially should be knowledgeable about the components of successful smoking cessation programs.

Although most smoking cessation therapy is aimed at cigarette smokers, cigars and chewing tobacco also contain nicotine and place the patient at risk. These smoking cessation products are helpful in patients who get nicotine from these other products.

MECHANISM OF ACTION

Nicotine is rapidly absorbed across the pulmonary capillary membrane and is delivered to the brain in high concentration within seconds of inhalation. The typical smoker (10 to 15 cigarettes/day) delivers 200 to 300 boluses of the addictive drug nicotine to the brain each day.

Nicotine increases heart rate, elevates blood pressure, causes peripheral vasoconstriction, enhances platelet aggregation and fibrinogen levels, decreases nitric oxide, and blunts its vasodilatory effects. It also increases carbon monoxide levels, and this reduces oxygen delivery to the myocardium. Nicotine activates the sympathetic nervous system and can induce coronary vasospasm. A risk of blood clots has been documented for young women on hormonal contraception and who smoke. Research has demonstrated that smokers may lose their cognitive abilities, such as remembering, thinking, or perceiving, more rapidly than elderly nonsmokers.

Cigarette smoking has been found to be particularly hazardous for those who already have some pathologic condition. The risk of vasospasm following subarachnoid hemorrhage is increased in smokers. Cigarette smoking exaggerates risk factors for cardiovascular disease by significantly increasing a protein known as thromboglobulin, which increases the activity and clotting functions of platelets in hypertensive smoking patients. Smoking also increases epinephrine, stimulating the heart and blood pressure in hypertensive patients who smoke.

Even patients who suffer from the results of smoking continue to engage in the behavior. Among smokers who undergo angioplasty or coronary artery bypass surgery, almost three in five continue to smoke after their procedure.

Nicotine, the chief alkaloid in tobacco products, binds stereoselectively to acetylcholine receptors at the autonomic ganglia, in the adrenal medulla, at neuromuscular junctions, and in the brain. Two types of CNS effects are believed to form the basis of nicotine's positively reinforcing properties: (1) a simulating effect (exerted mainly in the cortex via the locus coeruleus), which increases alertness and cognitive performance, and (2) a reward effect via the "pleasure system" in the brain in the limbic system. At low doses, the stimulant effects predominate, whereas at high doses, the reward effects predominate.

Regular nicotine consumption through smoking is associated with neuroadaptation of nicotinic receptors, which results in increasing numbers of receptors and the development of tolerance and drug dependence. Symptoms from abrupt withdrawal include irritability, restlessness, anxiety, difficulty concentrating, lethargy, depression, increased appetite, weight gain, and minor somatic complaints (headache, myalgia, constipation, fatigue). These symptoms may be reduced through the use of nicotine-containing smoking deterrents, which produce lower nicotine plasma concentrations (approximately 3 to 17 ng/ml) than those achieved through smoking (approximately 20 to 50 ng/ml).

When the drugs that are helpful in nicotine addiction are examined, the mechanism of action for bupropion cannot be identified. Bupropion is an inhibitor of the neuronal uptake of norepinephrine, serotonin, and dopamine. Another product, varenicline, partially stimulates nicotine receptors but to a lesser degree than nicotine does. It blocks the ability of nicotine to stimulate the dopamine system, which mediates the pleasurable effects of nicotine. It provides sufficient nicotine effects to decrease the urge to smoke and to ease withdrawal symptoms. If a patient restarts smoking while on varenicline, he or she will not experience the pleasurable effects of nicotine.

TREATMENT PRINCIPLES
Standardized Guidelines
- U.S. Preventive Services Task Force Counseling to Prevent Tobacco Use and Tobacco-Caused Disease, 2003.

Evidence-Based Recommendations
- *Beneficial:* Nicotine replacement therapy, varenicline, antidepressants (bupropion or nortriptyline), not SSRIs

Cardinal Points of Treatment
- Brief advice on smoking cessation can be successful.
- Pharmacotherapy is recommended unless contraindicated.
- *First line:* Nicotine replacement therapy, bupropion, varenicline
- *Second line:* clonidine, nortriptyline

Table 71-1 lists actions and strategies for the primary care clinician from the Agency for Healthcare Research and Quality (AHRQ) guidelines. Research from the National Ambulatory Medical Care Surveys of 1991 through 1995 has documented that physicians reported counseling patients about smoking or prescribing nicotine replacement far less often than is called for by current practice guidelines, thus missing many opportunities to help their patients quit smoking.

PREVENTION AND EARLY INTERVENTION. With each visit to a health care provider, it is critical to ask patients if they smoke. If patients do not smoke, praise them for their wisdom and encourage them not to start. This is very important in children and adolescents and former smokers. Emphasize the immediate effects of tobacco, such as bad breath, stains on the fingers and teeth, reduced exercise performance, and dry skin and hair. Early research on addiction suggests that patients are not fully addicted for 3 years after starting to smoke, so this is the time to encourage them to stop.

Pharmacotherapy reduces the physical effects of nicotine withdrawal but does not address the psychologic aspects of smoking cessation. The highest rate of smoking cessation is seen in those individuals who are able to just stop smoking "cold turkey" and avoid replacement therapy. However, many are not able to do this. Pharmacotherapy should be used in conjunction with a behavioral modification program. Brief advice (5 minutes) has been shown to be helpful. The five A's model is recommended as a foundation for counseling (see Table 71-1). Also, a GETQUIT Support Plan is available to assist all patients who are taking varenicline.

COMPONENTS OF SMOKING CESSATION. For all patients who do smoke, the provider should assess their willingness to attempt to quit (Figure 71-1). If they are unwilling or unready to quit, the provider should focus on motivational issues. The negative consequences of smoking also should be emphasized. Patients are not influenced often by remote events such as COPD or lung cancer but may be motivated by immediate effects such as fewer and milder respiratory infections or asthma. They may particularly respond to suggestions that they are hurting their family, particularly small or unborn children. Discuss the positive consequences of smoking

TABLE 71-1   Actions and Strategies for the Primary Care Clinician to Use in Smoking Cessation

Action	Strategies for Implementation
STEP 1. ASK: SYSTEMATICALLY IDENTIFY ALL TOBACCO USERS AT EVERY VISIT	
Implement an office-wide system that ensures that for *every* patient at *every* clinic visit, tobacco-use status is queried and documented.*	This action should be implemented using preprinted progress note paper or, for computerized records, an item that assesses tobacco-use status. Alternatives are to place tobacco-use status stickers on all patients' charts or to indicate smoking status via computerized reminder systems.
STEP 2. ADVISE: STRONGLY URGE ALL SMOKERS TO QUIT	
In a *clear, strong,* and *personalized* manner, urge every smoker to quit.	Advice should be *Clear:* "I think it is important for you to quit smoking now, and I will help you." "Cutting down while you are ill is not enough." *Strong:* "As your clinician, I need you to know that quitting smoking is the most important thing you can do to protect your current and future health." *Personalized:* Tie smoking to current health or illness and/or the social and economic costs of tobacco use, motivational level/readiness to quit, and the impact of smoking on children and others in household. Encourage clinic staff to reinforce the cessation message and support the patient's attempt to quit.
STEP 3. ASSESS: IDENTIFY SMOKERS WILLING TO ATTEMPT TO QUIT	
Ask every smoker if he or she is willing to make an attempt to quit at this time.	If the patient is willing to attempt to quit at this time, provide assistance (see Step 4). If the patient prefers more intensive treatment, or if the clinician believes that more intensive treatment is appropriate, refer the patient to interventions administered by a smoking cessation specialist, and follow up with the patient regarding quitting (see Step 5). If the patient clearly expresses an unwillingness to attempt to quit at this time, provide a motivational intervention.
STEP 4. ASSIST: AID THE PATIENT IN QUITTING	
Help the patient to devise a plan for quitting.	*Set a quit date:* Ideally, the quit date should be within 2 weeks, with patient preference taken into account. *Help the patient prepare for quitting:* The patient must *inform* family, friends, and coworkers about quitting and must request understanding and support. *Prepare* the environment by removing cigarettes from it. Prior to quitting, the patient should avoid smoking in places where he or she spends a lot of time (e.g., home, car). *Review* previous attempts at quitting. What helped? What led to the relapse? *Anticipate* challenges to the planned quit attempt, particularly during the critical first few weeks.
Encourage drug therapy except in special circumstances. Give key advice on successful quitting.	Encourage drug therapy for smoking cessation. *Abstinence:* Total abstinence is essential. "Not even a single puff after the quit date." *Alcohol:* Drinking alcohol is highly associated with relapse. Those who stop smoking should consider limiting or abstaining from alcohol use during the quit process. The presence of other smokers in the household, particularly a spouse, is associated with lower success rates. Patients should consider quitting with their significant others and/or developing specific plans to maintain abstinence in a household where others still smoke.
Provide supplementary materials.	*Source:* Federal agencies, including the National Cancer Institute and the Agency for Healthcare Research and Quality nonprofit agencies (American Cancer Society, American Lung Association, American Heart Association); or local or state health departments *Selection concerns:* The material must be culturally, racially, educationally, and age appropriate for the patient. *Location:* Readily available in every clinic office
STEP 5. ARRANGE: SCHEDULE FOLLOW-UP CONTACT	
Schedule follow-up contact, either in person or via telephone.	*Timing:* Follow-up contact should occur soon after the quit date, preferably during the first week. A second follow-up contact is recommended within the first month. Schedule additional follow-up contacts as indicated. *Actions during follow-up:* Congratulate success. If smoking occurred, review the circumstances and elicit a recommitment to total abstinence. Remind the patient that a lapse can be used as a learning experience and is not a sign of failure. Identify the problems already encountered, and anticipate challenges in the immediate future. Assess nicotine replacement therapy use and problems. Consider referral to a more intense or specialized program.

From The Smoking Cessation Clinical Practice Guideline Panel and Staff: The agency for Health Care Policy and Research smoking cessation clinical practice guideline, *JAMA* 275:1270, 1996.
*Repeated assessment is not necessary in the case of the adult who has never smoked or has not smoked for many years, and for whom this information is clearly documented in the medical record.

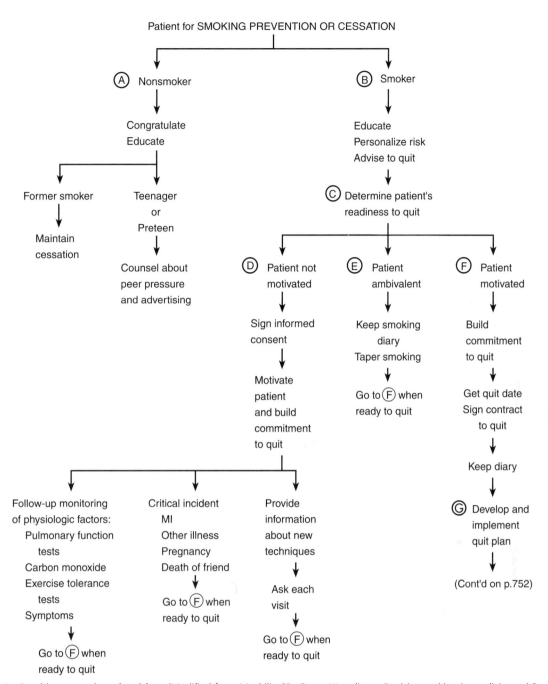

FIGURE 71-1 **Smoking cessation algorithm.** (Modified from Mushllin SB, Green HL, editors: *Decision-making in medicine,* ed 3, St Louis, 2008, Mosby.)

cessation, such as saving money, tasting food better, and feeling better physically.

Once the patient is ready to try to quit, the provider should help the patient plan to quit and monitor his or her progress. The patient should be offered specific help on how to quit successfully. Brief interventions are often successful.

Most patients have tried unsuccessfully to quit. They should be encouraged to try again through reminders that most people who succeed in stopping smoking make several attempts before their final successful attempt. Each attempt should not be seen as a failure but as a trial for the next attempt. They should try to find out what went wrong the last time they tried and determine how they can plan to avoid the problem situation.

Nonpharmacologic therapies are the mainstay of therapy. How to encourage the patient to explore these strategies is the first critical treatment decision. Patients should have a realistic idea about the difficulty of smoking cessation. They probably will experience withdrawal symptoms such as craving, irritability, restlessness, and increased appetite. With a clear understanding of the difficulties, the patient should set a realistic quit date.

Find out why the patient uses nicotine. Is it for stimulation, handling, pleasure, stress reduction, or weight reduction, or does it result from feelings of social pressure, craving, or habit? The patient then should develop specific strategies to cope with reasons for smoking. Patients for whom smoking is a habit should plan to alter their patterns of behavior to avoid

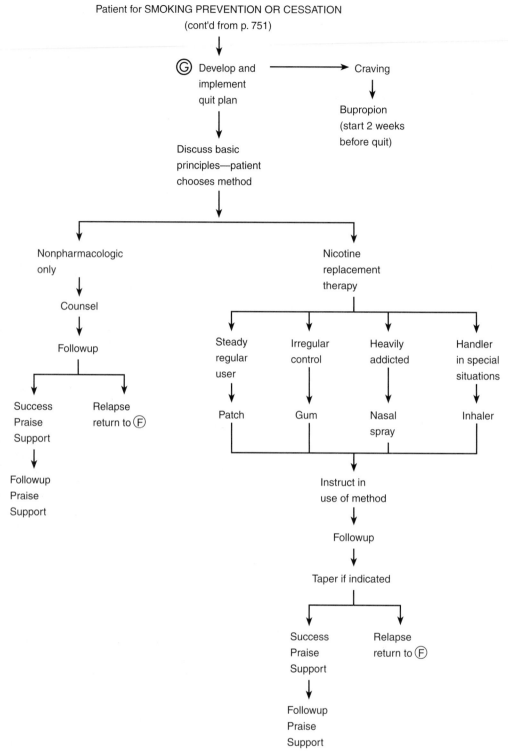

FIGURE 71-1, cont'd Smoking cessation algorithm.

common cues to light a cigarette. Those who like to handle cigarettes need to find something to keep their hands busy to replace handling cigarettes. Patients who use cigarettes for stimulation should replace cigarettes with another stimulating exercise, such as walking, and should avoid fatigue. Other methods of stress reduction such as deep breathing or other relaxation exercises should be encouraged.

All patients should make plans for how to handle difficult situations. Exercise such as walking can promote a feeling of

well-being. Patients should set up a reward system for staying nicotine free, such as using the money saved to buy something they have been wanting.

Many patients are concerned about weight gain if they stop smoking. They should be warned that they may gain weight, but that watching their diet and increasing their exercise can minimize this. They should prepare themselves by having healthful, low-calorie meals and snacks available.

Specific nonpharmacologic approaches include aversive conditioning, hypnosis, acupuncture, behavior modification, and multicomponent programs. Intensive treatment programs are often necessary for patients who have great difficulty stopping and have failed several times.

evolve See the resources listed at the end of the chapter and on the Evolve Website for places that patients can go for support programs and smoking cessation assistance.

Pharmacologic Treatment

NICOTINE REPLACEMENT THERAPY. When patients commit to stopping smoking, they often feel a loss of control of their lives. It may be helpful to describe different forms of smoking cessation therapy and to have them help select the mechanism. Nicotine replacement therapy (NRT) is often especially good for patients who are heavily dependent on nicotine and who smoke more than two packs a day. However, NRT may be offered to most patients as an option.

Make sure the patient receives an adequate dose; one of the main reasons for failure of nicotine treatment is underdosing. Another cause of failure is incorrect use of the product.

First, help the patient choose the dosage form that will work best for him or her. The patch is usually best for patients who smoke at regular intervals. Gum may work better for patients who smoke at irregular intervals. The patch offers a more convenient, once-a-day application. Gum offers more direct control of the amount of nicotine the patient receives. The gum can be used when the patient has a craving. The nasal spray is useful for responding quickly to a craving. The nasal spray is especially beneficial for highly dependent smokers. The inhaler mimics the act of smoking and will be useful for patients who enjoy handling cigarettes. Conversely, this technique may interfere with the need to change behavior, and patients eventually will have to learn to break the habit of handling something if they are to be successful. The inhaler is also useful when gum will not work because of concomitant consumption of acidic foods or beverages, alcohol, or coffee. Social occasions involving alcohol are often especially difficult, and the inhaler might be most acceptable in this situation. Gum might be more acceptable at work. Patients who have a stomach ulcer or diabetes should not use gum or lozenges but may use patches. However, patients who have an allergy to adhesive tape or preexisting skin problems should not choose NicoDerm CQ or Nicotrol. All replacement products are meant for those who smoke more than 10 cigarettes a day. Nicorette 2 mg is used for those who smoke fewer than 25 cigarettes daily; Nicorette 4 mg is best for those who smoke 25 or more cigarettes daily. Commit Lozenges use a different index for the initial choice. Those who smoke their first cigarette more than 30 minutes after waking should begin with the 2 mg lozenge, and those who smoke their first cigarette within 30 minutes of waking should begin by using the 4 mg lozenge.

Although many NRT products are now available OTC, certain patient populations should seek the advice of a health professional before starting therapy, particularly with the patch. These include people younger than 18 years, those with heart disease or an irregular heartbeat or who have had a recent heart attack, people with high blood pressure that is not controlled with medication, those taking prescription medicine for depression or asthma, and people with skin problems or who are allergic to adhesive tape. Pregnant or nursing women first should try to stop smoking without the nicotine patch and should seek the advice of a health professional before using a nicotine patch. Previously, no health insurance plan covered these medications. However, recently, Medicare has been paying for smoking cessation counseling for patients who have health problems caused by their smoking.

Many people are concerned about the safety of using NRT. The risk of using NRT must be weighed against the risk of continued smoking, as well as the risk of using the patch while smoking. Cigarette smoking is known to promote myocardial ischemia. This can be seen on an ECG in patients with CAD who smoke a cigarette. Patients with CAD may be especially vulnerable to the ischemic effects of nicotine. Studies have shown that patients with CAD who use NRT to stop smoking do not have an increased incidence of adverse cardiac effects. NRT has been shown to have no platelet activation effects and no clinically meaningful effects on heart rate and blood pressure. It is especially important that patients with CAD stop smoking for their health, and NRT has proved safe and effective in this population.

> Whatever method is chosen, the patient should use only one particular product. Patches cannot be combined with gum or lozenges. While using any product, the patient must not use nicotine in any form (e.g., cigars, cigarettes, dip, snuff, pipes). Additional use of any of these products may cause serious nicotine toxicity.

Nicotine replacement products are meant to help patients stop smoking. They are not meant to help get a patient through a long flight or an all-day meeting in a nonsmoking building. Additionally, when the length of time labeled for use is over, the patient should stop using these products (e.g., 10 to 12 weeks per manufacturer labeling). Any patient who experiences symptoms of nicotine overdose (nausea, vomiting, dizziness, weakness, rapid heartbeat, diarrhea) should stop using the product immediately and should see a health care provider to make sure he or she is not toxic or seriously ill.

Products must be kept away from children and pets. If children or pets accidentally swallow new or used patches, gum, or lozenges, the patient should immediately call a poison control center.

PATCH. The patch is the most commonly used type of NRT. It is convenient with few compliance problems, and no special skill is needed for its use. Patches are easily concealed under clothing and cause few side effects. However, the delivery of nicotine is slower than with other forms. Also, allergic reactions to the patch may occur.

The nicotine transdermal system is a multilayered unit that contains nicotine as the active agent that provides systematic delivery of nicotine for 16 to 24 hours. Determine the duration of action of the patch before using. Some patients find that wearing the patch for only 16 hours prevents bizarre dreams. If patients crave a cigarette when they wake up, they should wear a 24-hour patch. Do not underdose by wearing the same patch for longer than the 24-hour period. It is also necessary to use the patch for 8 to 12 weeks and to not stop the therapy prematurely.

Patches are available in 15 and 21 mg strengths for treatment initiation. The 21 mg patch is then tapered down to a 14 and a 7 mg patch; a 10 and a 5 mg patch follow the 15 mg patch. The NicoDerm CQ product stipulates that the patient should start with the highest-dose patch unless he or she is a light smoker (i.e., 10 or fewer cigarettes a day), weighs less than 100 lb, or has cardiac disease. Use this patch for 6 weeks, then transition to the patch of next lower strength for 2 weeks and the lowest-dose patch for another 2 weeks. Dosing of the Nicotrol product is similar to this (i.e., one patch daily for 6 weeks, then taper down for 2 weeks each). Table 71-2 provides the dosing schedule used for different brands.

GUM. The gum delivers nicotine faster than the patch and can be used for incidences of craving. It may satisfy the oral craving that smokers have. For some patients, gum chewing is a habit. It may delay weight gain because the patient chews instead of eating during an episode of craving. However, the potential for addiction to the gum is present. In gum chewing, the patient must use proper technique, which is different from normal gum chewing. The patient must chew the gum and then park it in the check for greater nicotine absorption. Some of the liabilities of using gum are that it is difficult to use with dentures, it is socially undesirable in certain situations, and the patient should not have food or drink 15 minutes before use. It also requires frequent dosing to control the craving.

Nicotine polacrilex contains nicotine bound to an ion exchange resin in a chewing gum base. The gum is available in two strengths: 2 mg for patients who should use a lower dose, and 4 mg for healthy patients who smoke 25 or more cigarettes a day. Patients chew a piece of gum every 1 to 2 hours for 6 weeks. They then taper the dose for the next 6 weeks. Duration of treatment is about 12 weeks. Usually, at least nine pieces of gum per day are required in the first 6 weeks, and the dose should not exceed 24 pieces per day. Gradually, patients should reduce the number of pieces of gum chewed per day, as well as the length of time that gum is chewed, after 6 weeks. Teach patients how to properly chew the gum. Many patients do not use enough gum, hoping to economize. They must be taught the importance of adequately suppressing their nicotine craving and methods that can be used to distract their attention.

LOZENGE. The nicotine polacrilex lozenge also delivers nicotine faster than the patch but has more flexible dosing and can be used in patients who smoke their first cigarette within 30 minutes of waking in the morning. Patients who use the lozenges complain of bad taste, mouth soreness, and dyspepsia. If the patient chews the lozenge, the rate of nicotine delivery is uneven. The lozenges come in 2 and 4 mg doses and deliver about 25% more nicotine than gum. The 4-mg dose is used for the patient who smokes within 30 minutes of rising; for others, use the 2 mg dose. Similar to the gum, lozenges are not tapered in terms of the strength used (e.g., 2 mg vs. 4 mg). Rather, the patient tapers the number of pieces used daily, while adhering to a schedule that is similar to that used for gum.

NASAL SPRAY. The nasal spray is useful for a patient with severe cravings who desires immediate relief. It has the fastest delivery of nicotine of the NRTs and more closely resembles the onset of the nicotinic effects of smoking. It has flexible dosing. However, it has the highest potential for prolonging nicotine addiction, when compared with other NRTs. Nasal irritation is the major limitation and is seen in 80% to 90% of patients. It may cause mouth and throat irritation. This product may prove too uncomfortable to use, and patients may take up to 2 weeks to adjust to this delivery route. Frequent dosing is needed; the patient must avoid contact with the skin and should wait 5 minutes before driving.

Each spray delivers 0.5 mg of nicotine. The patient should use one or two doses per waking hour for 3 to 6 months. Consider a tapering period by halving the number of doses used each week.

ORAL INHALER. The nicotine inhaler releases nicotine when the patients breathes through it and thus mimics the action of smoking. This dosage form may be useful for the patient who enjoys handling a cigarette. Patients with reactive airway disease generally are not candidates for this product because of the bronchoconstrictive effects of nicotine. A nicotine patch is preferable for these patients.

Inhaled nicotine is absorbed in the mouth—not in the lungs. Nicotine concentrations delivered by inhaler are approximately one third those provided by a cigarette. Therefore, nicotine serves to blunt cravings. Mouth and throat irritation is common and is a barrier to compliance. Frequent dosing is necessary. The cartridges must be stored between 59° and 86° F. Each cartridge contains 10 mg nicotine and delivers 4 mg. It also contains 1 mg menthol. The recommended dose is 6 to 16 cartridges per day for 3 months; these then are tapered for 6 to 12 months.

COMBINATION NRT THERAPY. Initial therapy for smoking cessation relies on one form of nicotine delivery, and patients are discouraged from using more than one product. For the patient who has difficulty finding the right dosage of nicotine but is still willing to try to stop smoking, combination therapy may be suggested. The following combinations have been shown to be effective: nicotine patch plus gum, spray, inhaler, or bupropion. These combination product schedules must be monitored to ensure that the patient is not overdosing.

BUPROPION. Bupropion as a systemic medication seems to reduce the craving for cigarettes or the urge to smoke. Its mechanism of action is not clear. Side effects include nausea, insomnia, tremor, and difficulty concentrating. Bupropion should be started 1 to 2 weeks before the quit date; 150 mg/day should be given orally for 3 days and then increased to 150 mg orally twice a day. Continue this dosage for 7 to 12 weeks. The dosage should not exceed 300 mg/day. Treatment for longer than 3 months usually is not necessary, and dose tapering is not needed. Bupropion can be used in addition to nicotine replacement products and may be especially useful for patients who are somewhat depressed because the chemicals are the same as for the depressant formulation. See Chapter 46 for additional information on bupropion.

VARENICLINE. This product is the newest drug in the smoking cessation arsenal. Safety and effectiveness in combination with other smoking cessation medications have not been established. Results from comparative trials with bupropion have shown similar efficacy, with a slight trend toward better outcomes with varenicline. Common side effects include nausea and abnormal dreams, which may limit acceptance by patients. The FDA has issued an alert to providers to monitor patients who are taking Chantix for depression, severe mood swings, abnormal dream states, and thoughts of suicide.

CLONIDINE. Clonidine has been used second line when patients refused or could not tolerate nicotine replacement, bupropion, or varenicline. Efficacy is considered limited after initial studies showed promise. Dosage is the same as for hypertension. Side effects such as sedation and dry mouth are common. See Chapter 15 for full information on clonidine.

NORTRIPTYLINE. Nortriptyline is a tricyclic antidepressant that has been shown in a limited number of trials to be effective for smoking cessation. Its effectiveness appears to be unrelated to its antidepressant effect. Start the medication 10 to 28 days before the stop date to allow it to achieve steady state. Start at 25 mg/day at bedtime. Increase slowly to a maximum dose of 75 to 100 mg/day. Common side effects reported in these trials were dry mouth (38%) and sedation (20%).

NICOTINE VACCINE. A phase 2 study of a nicotine vaccine has shown that the highest dose tested produced antibodies against nicotine and was associated with a higher rate of smoking cessation than placebo. Quit rates in the study were generally similar to those achieved with other smoking cessation aids; abstinence rates twofold to threefold higher than placebo were reported. The vaccine is in development by Nabi Biopharmaceuticals under the brand name NicVAX. It consists of a chemical derivative of nicotine linked to a protein to induce an immune response. The idea is that the antibodies produced will bind to nicotine in the bloodstream and prevent it from crossing the blood-brain barrier and entering the brain, thus preventing the positive-sensation stimulus of nicotine, which mediates its addictive properties. The manufacturer suggests that the vaccine may offer advantages over existing treatments because its effect is irreversible for potentially 6 to 12 months following vaccination, as antibodies to nicotine continue to be produced by the body's immune system. This is important in view of the high relapse rates associated with smoking cessation. The vaccine was generally well tolerated but was associated with injection site reactions, mild fever, and aches.

How to Monitor

- The first 2 weeks is a critical time. Monitor patients closely by telephone. Call within the first week to see how they are doing. Tell them to call the clinician if they are experiencing difficulty.
- Because most relapses occur within the first 3 months of cessation, the patient should be seen frequently in an effort to solve problems and prevent relapse.
- Because many patients relapse, check on smoking at each visit, and encourage patients to try again if they have relapsed.
- In older patients, monitor for cardiovascular effects, monitor blood pressure, and ask about angina.

Patient Variables

HOSPITALIZED PATIENTS. The hospital is an ideal place to have the patient stop smoking. Patients with cardiovascular disease should be given a decreased dose of the transdermal systems, to minimize the potential for adverse effects (asthenia, body aches, and dizziness) and cardiovascular complications (arrhythmias and MI).

GERIATRICS. Transdermal systems are found to be just as effective in geriatric patients.

PEDIATRICS. The safety and effectiveness of transdermal systems have not been tested in the pediatric population. Therefore, their use in children and adolescents is not recommended. Varenicline is not recommended for use in patients younger than 18 years.

PREGNANCY AND LACTATION

- *Category C:* bupropion, varenicline, nicotine gum
- *Category D:* Nicotine patch, nasal spray, inhaler
- Risks to the fetus include spontaneous abortion, low birth weight, anencephaly, cleft palate, and congenital heart disease (similar to smoking). Pregnant women should be encouraged to stop smoking because of the potential damage that smoking may do to their children. NRT should be used only when benefits outweigh risks. Nicotine passes freely into breast milk. Nicotine replacement therapy may be safer than smoking.

RACE/GENDER. The increase in smoking by women since 1950 is now showing up as a higher rate of death from lung disease among women. Cigarettes cause more damage to black women than to other populations. Black women show less likelihood of recovery after they quit smoking.

DRUG INTERACTIONS

- Numerous drug interactions occur with smoking, so smokers who are taking a medication that interacts with smoking may require higher dosages than nonsmokers. Polycyclic aromatic hydrocarbons (PAHs) are some of the major lung carcinogens found in tobacco smoke. PAHs are potent inducers of the hepatic cytochrome P450 (CYP450) isoenzymes 1A1, 1A2, and, possibly, 2E1. The primary pharmacokinetic interactions with smoking occur with drugs that are CYP1A2 substrates, such as caffeine, clozapine, fluvoxamine, olanzapine, tacrine, and theophylline. The pharmacokinetic profile of inhaled insulin is significantly affected; it peaks faster and reaches higher concentrations in smokers than in nonsmokers, achieving significantly faster onset and higher insulin levels.

> The primary pharmacodynamic drug interactions with smoking occur with hormonal contraceptives and inhaled corticosteroids. The most clinically significant interaction occurs with combined hormonal contraceptives. The use of hormonal contraceptives of any kind in women who are 35 years or older and who smoke 15 or more cigarettes daily is considered contraindicated because of the increased risk of serious cardiovascular adverse effects.

- The efficacy of inhaled corticosteroids may be reduced in patients with asthma who smoke. After a person quits smoking, an important consideration is how quickly the induction of CYP1A2 dissipates. Upon smoking cessation, smokers may require a reduction in the dosage of an interacting medication.

Patient Education

Patients need extensive education. All drug companies that supply NRT medications have patient information and support materials for patients who are trying to quit. See also

Text continued on page 758

TABLE 71-2 Comparison of Smoking Cessation Products

Product	Dosage Form	Dosing and Treatment Information	Approximate Cost	Nicotine Release Mechanism
Nicoderm CQ	Transdermal patch 16 or 24 hr (OTC)	>10 cig/day: 21 mg × 6 wk; 14 mg × 2 wk; 7 mg × 2 wk <10 cig/day: 14 mg × 6 wk; 7 mg × 2 wk May wear patch for 16 or 24 hr	7 mg (7), $28 14 mg (7), $50 21 mg (7), $50 21 mg (14), $50	Rate and diffusion controlling membrane
Nicotrol	Transdermal system 16 hr (OTC)	Steps 1, 2, and 3 deliver 15, 10, and 5 mg of nicotine, respectively. The patches are used once daily in a tapering manner: Step 1: weeks 1-6 Step 2: weeks 7-8 Step 3: weeks 9-10 Step 1 for >10 cig/day smokers Remove patch before sleep (only releases 16 hr) No tapering of dose <100 lb, <10 cig/day or cardiovascular disease: 14 mg × 6 wk; 7 mg × 2-4 wk	Patch $60 14 mg (30), $116 21 mg (30), $122	Adhesive containing rate-controlling membrane and concentration gradient
Habitrol	Transdermal 24-hr system (Rx)	>100 lb, >10 cig/day and NO cardiovascular disease: 21 mg × 6 wk; 14 mg × 2-4 wk; 7 mg × 2-4 wk <100 lb, <10 cig/day, or cardiovascular disease: 14 mg × 6 wk; 7 mg × 2-4 wk	7 mg (30), $110 14 mg (30), $116 21 mg (30), $122	Rate-limiting membrane and a concentration gradient
Nicorette and generic	Gum (OTC) in regular and mint flavors	2 mg: <25 cig/day 4 mg: >25 cig/day Weeks 1-6: 1 piece q1-2h Weeks 7-9: 1 piece q2-4h Weeks 10-12: 1 piece q4-8h Do not exceed 24 pieces/day. STOP ALL SMOKING. No acidic foods/beverages before and during use Chew, park gum between cheek and gum 1-5 min; repeat. Use one piece no longer than 30 min.	2-mg starter (48), $32; refill (100), $57 4-mg starter (48), $32; refill (110), $50	Ion exchange resin, releases when being chewed only, not when swallowed
Commit Nicotine Polacrilex Lozenge	2-mg, 4-mg lozenges	Patient should suck one lozenge q1-2h for weeks 1-6; one q2-4h for weeks 7-9; one q4-8h for weeks 10-12. Tapering is accomplished by reducing the number of lozenges per day.	$43 for 72 lozenges (2 and 4 mg)	Ion exchange resin
Nicotrol inhaler	Oral inhaler (Rx)	6-16 cartridges/day Best effects with continuous puffing for 20 minutes Individualize dosing. An open cartridge is good for only 1 day. Must use minimum of 6 cartridges/day for first 3-6 wk, then continue for 3 months; taper for next 6-12 wk. Do not exceed 6 months of use.	More expensive	Nicotine release mechanism
Nicotrol NS	Nasal spray (Rx)	One or two 0.5-mg sprays in each nostril/hr Gradually reduce rate over 6-8 wk. Do not exceed 5 sprays/hr or 40 sprays/day.	10 ml, $36	Information not applicable
varenicline (Chantix)	Oral tablet	Take 1 mg twice a day following a 1-wk titration as follows: Days 1 to 3: Take 0.5 mg once daily. Days 4 to 7: Take 0.5 mg twice daily. Day 8 through end of treatment (usually 12 wk): Take 1 mg twice daily. It patient cannot tolerate dose, lower temporarily. Continuing for 12 wk after smoking cessation helps patient to not relapse.		
bupropion SR (Zyban)	Oral sustained-release 150-mg tablet (Rx)	150 mg daily for 3 days, then increase to 150 mg bid Set quit date at 1-2 wk after beginning Zyban therapy, continue for 7-12 wk Not to exceed 200 mg/day Treatment >3 months generally NOT necessary Dose tapering NOT recommended Can be used with nicotine replacement products	60 150-mg tablets, $77.00	Not applicable

Cig, Cigarettes.

Patient Information Provided	Common Side Effects	Advantages	Disadvantages
Committed Quitters Program booklet, audiotape, tips for quitting, toll-free support	Local cutaneous reaction (erythema, pruritus, edema); dizziness; cutaneous itching or hypersensitivity; headache; sleep disturbances and abnormal dreams (with 24-hr use)		
Pathways to Change Program booklet, audiotape, tips for quitting, toll-free support number	Local cutaneous reactions: Erythema, pruritus, edema, hypersensitivity, headache Local cutaneous reactions: Erythema, pruritus, edema, hypersensitivity	Easily concealable Few compliance problems	
Patient Support Kit cassette, information booklet, guide for family/friends, prescription refill stickers	Sleep disturbances and abnormal dreams; headache Local cutaneous reactions: Erythema, pruritus, edema, hypersensitivity	Provides 24-hr steady concentration that may reduce morning cravings Easily concealable Few compliance problems	Allergic reactions to adhesive may occur.
Committed Quitters Program booklet, CD with tips for quitting, toll-free support number	Nausea/vomiting, jaw soreness, hiccups From incorrect chewing: headache, mouth/throat soreness, bad taste, indigestion	Use when prompted by cravings. May satisfy oral craving Dose easily titrated Gum chewing part of lifestyle for some people May delay weight gain	Must use proper chewing technique to lessen adverse effects and get benefits Difficult to use with dentures Gum may be socially inappropriate at times.
Go to Quit.com	Nausea, vomiting, bad taste, indigestion	For those who smoke more than 30 min after waking	May chew and not get even dosing
Pathways to Change materials, booklet, audiotape, tips for quitting, toll-free support number	Local irritation of throat and mouth; headache; dyspepsia; hiccups; coughing; rhinitis; bad taste in mouth	Mimics act of smoking Used to reduce cravings Dose easily titrated by patient	Cartridges should be stored between 59° and 86° F. May take up to 1 wk to get used to side effects Dependence to product may develop.
Pathways to Change materials, booklet, audiotape, tips for quitting, toll-free support number	Peppery/hot sensation in nose/throat; sneezing; coughing; runny nose; watery eyes	Used to suppress cravings Dose easily titrated by patient Immediate effect	Often found uncomfortable to use May take 2 wk to get used to delivery method Dependence on product may develop. Must avoid contact with skin Wait 5 minutes before driving.
Patients should take after eating and with a full glass of water. GETQUIT Support Plan is available to assist all patients who are taking varenicline.	Abnormal dreams, headache, insomnia, lethargy, abdominal pain, flatulence, nausea, and URI disorders are all common.	Continue to encourage patient to quit even if he or she relapses. Advise that most adverse effects are temporary.	Abnormal dreams are often most troubling and may cause patient to withdraw from using medicine.
Advantage Plan booklet, tips for quitting, toll-free support number	Risk of seizures increases to 1/1000 Nervousness, difficulty concentrating, rash, dry mouth, insomnia, constipation	No risk of nicotine toxicity if patient continues to smoke Ease of use; may be more beneficial in patients with subclinical depression Safer to use in pregnancy Can be used in combination with nicotine replacement	Seizure risk Increases cost of smoking cessation program

patient education materials in the reference section of this chapter.

ALL FORMS OF NRT
- No smoking while on NRT
- Dispose of used NRT properly. Patches are particularly hazardous to children.
- Keep out of reach of children and pets.

PATCH
- Place a new patch at the start of each day, and wear for 16 or 24 hours/day.
- Wear for 24 hours if patients crave cigarettes the minute they wake up.
- Wear for 16 hours if the patient has vivid dreams or sleep disruptions.
- Place on a new location that is relatively hairless between the neck and the waist.
- Dispose of used patch carefully: Fold sticky sides together, and insert in disposal tray.
- Wash hands after handling patches.
- Notify provider if the patient has skin reactions.

GUM
- Patients should use one piece at a time.
- They should begin chewing slowly and should avoid swallowing saliva immediately.
- They should chew until they experience a peppery taste or a tingle. This usually takes about 15 chews.
- Then they should stop chewing, park the gum between the cheek and gum, and leave it there.
- When the taste or tingle fades, usually after a minute or so, start to chew slowly again until taste or tingle returns.
- Stop chewing again. Park gum in a different place.
- Continue this until taste or tingle does not return; this usually takes about 30 minutes.
- Use gum at regular intervals.
- Do not consume acidic foods or beverages, alcohol, fruit, coffee, soft drinks, and so forth, for 15 minutes before and during use.

LOZENGE. Patient must allow the lozenge to dissolve slowly over 20 to 30 minutes, while swallowing as little as possible. The lozenge should not be chewed or swallowed. The patient should occasionally move the lozenge from one side of the mouth to the other. A warm feeling or tingling sensation may result.

SPECIFIC DRUGS
Nicotine Replacement Therapy

All NRT formulations share the following characteristics, except as noted.

CONTRAINDICATIONS. Not to be used in patients with hypersensitivity to nicotine or any component. Also should not be used in patients during the immediate post–myocardial infarction period or in patients with life-threatening arrhythmias or severe or worsening angina pectoris. Gum is contraindicated in active temporomandibular joint disease.

WARNINGS/PRECAUTIONS. Use with caution in patients with cardiovascular disease. Screen for CAD, arrhythmias, or vasospastic disease. Use in hypertensive patients only when benefit outweighs risk. Monitor BP closely.

Use cautiously in patients with hepatic or severe renal impairment, hyperthyroidism, pheochromocytoma, type 1 diabetes mellitus, active peptic ulcer disease, hypertension, or peripheral vascular and cardiovascular disease.

Patient MUST stop smoking completely when therapy is initiated. Many clinicians require patients to sign a form indicating that they have been told of the risks of continuing to smoke and of using NRT.

Transference of addiction from cigarette to patch or gum may occur. Patients should use NRT no longer than 3 months.
- *Patch:* Use with caution in certain dermatologic (atopic dermatitis) and eczematous conditions. Monitor all patients for contact allergy.
- *Gum:* Dental problems may be exacerbated.
- *Nasal spray:* Use is not recommended for patients with known chronic nasal disorders such as allergy, rhinitis, nasal polyps, sinusitis, asthma, bronchospasm, or reactive airway disease.
- *Inhaler:* Use with caution in patients with bronchospastic disease (other forms of nicotine replacement are preferred).

PHARMACOKINETICS. Transdermal systems deliver nicotine systemically through percutaneous absorption. After application to the skin, nicotine plasma concentrations usually peak and plateau within 2 to 4 hours. NicoDerm CQ onset is rapid and peaks between 2 and 4 hours; Habitrol onset is 1 to 2 hours, peaks between 6 and 12 hours, and slowly declines over the remaining period of patch application. The nicotine in gum is absorbed buccally. Onset and peak levels are dependent on the vigor, rapidity, and duration of chewing. The nasal inhaler has an onset of action of about 4 minutes and a half-life of 1 to 2 hours.

Nicotine has a large volume of distribution and is metabolized extensively in the liver, as well as in the kidney and lung. It has more than 20 metabolites. The main metabolite cotinine has a half-life of 15 to 20 hours. Ten percent is excreted unchanged in the urine.

ADVERSE EFFECTS
- Systemic effects of NRT include edema, flushing, hypertension, palpitations, tachyarrhythmias, tachycardia, dizziness, confusion, convulsions, depression, euphoria, numbness, paresthesia, syncope, tinnitus, weakness, headache, insomnia, dry mouth, nonspecific GI distress, nausea, vomiting, altered LFTs, constipation, diarrhea, difficulty breathing, cough, hoarseness, sneezing, and wheezing.
- Adverse effects of the patch are primarily seen as skin reactions and rash.
- Patch or gum may provide toxic levels of nicotine for young children who accidentally handle or chew product.
- Effects associated with gum are the mechanical effects of gum chewing, that is, traumatic injury to oral mucosa, jaw ache, and eructation caused by air swallowing. Oral mucosal changes include stomatitis, glossitis, gingivitis, pharyngitis, aphthous ulcers, and changes in taste perception.
- Nasal spray is irritating to nasal mucosa.
- Oral inhaler causes throat irritation.
- Monitor for depression, severe mood swings, abnormal dream states, and thoughts of suicide in those taking varenicline.

DRUG INTERACTIONS

- Nicotine increases general metabolism and lowers blood levels of the following drugs through enzyme induction: acetaminophen, caffeine, diazepam, chlordiazepoxide, β-blockers, olanzapine, clozapine, imipramine, pentazocine, propranolol, and theophylline.
- Nicotine increases circulating cortisol and catecholamines. Adjust doses of adrenergic agonists or blockers accordingly.
- Nicotine may reduce diuretic effects of furosemide, decrease subcutaneous insulin absorption, and decrease first-pass metabolism of propoxyphene.
- Gum interacts with food or drink in the mouth.

OVERDOSAGE

- *Symptoms:* Nausea and vomiting are early symptoms. Other symptoms include salivation, abdominal pain, headache, dizziness, confusion, weakness, hypotension, difficulty breathing, and tachycardia. Death may result from paralysis of respiratory muscles. Minimum oral lethal dose in adults is 40 to 60 mg. The lethal dose is much lower in children.
- *Treatment of overdosage of gum:* Empty stomach
- *Overdosage for patch:* Remove patch and flush skin with water; do not use soap.
- *Ingestion:* Refer to health care facility, administer activated charcoal, and provide supportive measures.

DOSAGE AND ADMINISTRATION. See Table 71-2.

NICOTINE RECEPTOR AGONIST

varenicline

CONTRAINDICATIONS. Hypersensitivity

WARNINGS

- Monitor for depression, severe mood swings, abnormal dream states, and thoughts of suicide in those taking varenicline
- Use caution in renal dysfunction; dosage adjustment required.
- Safety and efficacy of varenicline with other smoking cessation therapies have not been established.
- Increased adverse events when used concurrently with nicotine replacement therapy

- Safety and efficacy have not been established in children.
- Use caution in patients with renal insufficiency.
- Safety as combination therapy with other forms of NTR has not been confirmed and sole therapy is recommended.

PHARMACOKINETICS. Maximum plasma concentrations in 3 to 4 hours; steady state reached in 4 days. Absorption is complete and is unaffected by food with very low protein binding. Elimination half-life 24 hours, undergoes minimal metabolism, 92% excreted unchanged in urine. Dosage adjustment for elderly patients not required.

ADVERSE EFFECTS. Nausea is the most common adverse event (16% to 40%, dose related), and it may persist. Other effects include headache (15% to 19%), insomnia (18%), and abnormal dreams (9% to 13%).

<10%: Sedation (3%), nightmares (1% to 2%), lethargy (1% to 2%), malaise (7%), rash (3%), flatulence (6% to 9%), abdominal pain (6% to 7%), constipation (5% to 8%), dysgeusia (5% to 8%), xerostomia (5% to 6%), dyspepsia (5%), vomiting (1% to 5%), increased appetite (3% to 4%), anorexia (2%), gastroesophageal reflux (1%), dyspnea (2%), and rhinorrhea (1%)

DRUG INTERACTIONS. No known drug–drug interactions. However, cessation of smoking may alter the effects of concomitant drugs such as theophylline, warfarin, and insulin.

DOSAGE AND ADMINISTRATION. The medication is started 1 week prior to the patient's stop date. On days 1 to 3, give 0.5 mg once daily; on days 4 to 7, 0.5 mg bid; and thereafter, 1 mg bid. Treatment should be given for 12 weeks. An additional course of 12 weeks may be given to prevent relapse. Medication comes in packages that provide a proper dosing schedule.

See Chapter 46 for a full discussion of bupropion.

evolve A continually updated list of useful WebLinks may be found in the Evolve Resources at http://evolve.elsevier.com/Edmunds/NP/

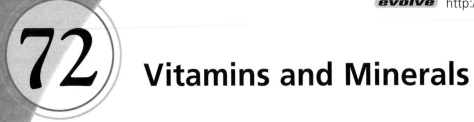

72 Vitamins and Minerals

DRUG OVERVIEW

Class	Generic Name	Trade Name
Multivitamins	General multivitamins	Various OTC
		Berocca Tablets
		Nephrocaps
		Nephro-Vite (Rx) Tablets
		Pro-Hepatone Capsules
		Renal Multivitamin Formula (Rx)
	Multivitamins with minerals	Various OTC
		Bacmin Tablets
		Berocca Plus Tablets
		Cezin-s Capsules
		Vicon Forte Capsules
		Vitamist Intra-Oral Spray Dietary Supplements
	Multivitamins with fluoride	Poly-Vi-Flor With Iron
		Vi-Daylin/F Chewable Multivitamin Tablets
		Vi-Daylin/F Multivitamin + Iron Chewable Tablets
	Parenteral multivitamins	Aquason A Parenteral
		Neurodep Injection
		Vicam Injection
	Prenatal vitamins (OTC)	Maturna Tablets
		Mynatal Capsules
		Natalins Tablets
		Nestabs FA Tablets
		Niferex-PN Tablets
	Prenatal Rx tablets	StuartNatal Plus Tablets
Other multivitamin formulations and products	Anti-folic acid antagonists	Leucovorin Calcium for Injection (Rx) Leucovorin Calcium Tablets
	Antioxidant combinations	Various
	Geriatric vitamin formulations	Various
	Pediatric vitamin formulations	Various
	Pediatric vitamins with fluoride	Various
	Iron combinations	Multiple
		Berocca Plus
		Fumatinic Capsules
		Iberet-Folic-500

DRUG OVERVIEW (Continued)

Class	Generic Name	Trade Name
		Hemocyte-F Tablets
		NephPlex Rx Tablets
		Nephro-Fer (Rx) Tablets
		Nephro-Vite (Rx) + Fe Tablets
		Nephron-A
		Niferex-150 Forte Capsules
		Niferex-PN Tablets
		Theragran Hematinic Tablets
		Vitafol Capsules
	Iron with vitamin B$_{12}$ and intrinsic factor	Chromagen Capsules
		Chromagen Tablets
		Fero-Grad-500 Filmtab
		Fero-Gradumet Filmtab
		Iberet
		Iberet-500 Filmtab
		Iberet-500 Liquid
		Iberet-Folic-500
		Pronemia Hematinic Capsules
Individual vitamins and minerals	Vitamin A	Aquasol A Drops, Capsules, Injection
	Vitamin B$_1$ (thiamine)	Thiamine HCl Injection
	Vitamin B$_3$ (niacin)	Nicotinic Acid Capsules, Nicobid, Nicolar, Slo-Niacin Controlled Release Tablets
	Vitamin B$_6$ (pyridoxine)	Pyridoxine Injection
	Vitamin B$_{12}$	Hydrocobalamin Injection
	Vitamin C (ascorbic acid)	Ascorbic Acid Injection
		Cenolate
	Vitamin D (calcitrol)	Calcijex Injection
		Rocaltrol Capsules
	Vitamin K	AquaMEPHYTON Injection (Rx)
		Mephyton Tablets
	Calcium	Calphron
		PhosLo
	Fluoride	Luride Drops
		Luride Lozi-Tabs Tablets
		Pediaflor Drops
	Folic acid ✸	Folvite Injection Folic Acid Tablets
	Phosphorus	K-Phos Neutral Tablets
		Neutra-Phos Tablets
		Neutra-Phos K Powder

Table continued on following page

DRUG OVERVIEW (Continued)

Class	Generic Name	Trade Name
		Uro-KP Neutral Tablets
	Zinc	Zincate

✹, Top 200 drug.

The integrity and health of the body are maintained through nutrients. Most commonly, these nutrients come from natural sources. With a poor diet or during times of stress or illness, supplementation may be required. Vitamins and minerals then may become important components of the therapeutic regimen. Additionally, new research findings confirm the role that some of these formulations play in improving or preventing some chronic diseases. Listed in this chapter are some of the prescription and OTC formulations of multivitamins that are currently available. Also included are prescription vitamins and minerals that are currently being marketed as individual therapies. Many nonprescription vitamin preparations and many other individual vitamins and minerals are sold OTC and are not discussed in this chapter. Prescriptions may be required for costs to be covered by insurance and by Medicare.

Vitamins and minerals are by definition essential for human life, and their role in basic metabolism has been well researched (Table 72-1). However, extensive new research documents their role in health promotion and disease prevention. This is a rapidly developing field, and it is necessary for the provider to keep current with the latest research. A number of nutrients have come onto the market after varying levels of research were conducted to support their use. These include lutein, phenols, date seed, and isoflavones. Some of these may prove helpful as additional studies define their usefulness in clinical practice; however, these trials and nutrients are not discussed here. Although these vitamins and minerals are discussed separately in this text, they are most commonly taken in multivitamin combinations, often including special formulations for pediatric or geriatric persons, or supplements that help to control hot flashes for menopausal women. Vitamin supplementation in correct doses requires inclusion of other vitamins and minerals as coenzymes, and so it is not only cheaper but more effective to package these products together.

In 2002, the American Medical Association made the recommendation for the first time that all Americans should take a general multivitamin daily (AMA, 2002). This reflects the failure of so many Americans to get all daily required nutrients through their diet, especially if they eat lots of processed and fast foods or are on weight loss diets. However, a standard multivitamin supplement does not come close to making up for an unhealthy diet. It provides a dozen or so of the vitamins known to maintain health—a mere shadow of what can be obtained from eating plenty of fruits, vegetables, and whole grains. Instead, a daily multivitamin provides a sort of nutritional safety net.

Although most people get enough vitamins to avoid the classic deficiency diseases, relatively few get enough of five key vitamins that may be important in preventing chronic disease. These include folic acid, vitamins B_6, B_{12}, D, and E. A standard, store brand, RDA-level multivitamin can supply enough of these vitamins for less than $40 a year. It may be difficult to find high-quality information about vitamins, minerals, and specific products because of the influence of the food industry. Information about nutrients should be obtained from reputable sources, such as the NIH Office of Dietary Supplementation (see http://dietary-supplements. info.nih.gov/), the Institute of Medicine, or agencies and associations that do not have products to sell.

Because no uniform manufacturing rules for supplements have been put forth, some research suggests that a multivitamin may not contain what the bottle claims, could be contaminated with something from the manufacturing plant, or might include tainted ingredients—all of which suggests that products should be bought from reputable companies.

Nutrients included in the diet affect numerous cellular metabolic mechanisms that are common in the pathogenesis of chronic disease. Unified dietary guidelines issued jointly by six national organizations (American Heart Association, American Cancer Society, American Dietetic Association, American Academy of Pediatrics, NIH, and American Society for Clinical Nutrition) have been proposed to help reduce the risk of cancer, atherosclerosis, obesity, and diabetes. These unified guidelines indicate that the simplest way to achieve a healthy diet would be to include less than 10% saturated fat and no more than 30% total fat, as measured in calories; 55% of total calories should be taken in the form of carbohydrates, no more than 300 mg of cholesterol should be consumed each day, and daily salt intake should be limited to less than 6 g. Twenty-five grams of dietary fiber should also be maintained; this approach is not only cardioprotective, it also helps to curb the tendency to eat more than is necessary by providing a feeling of fullness. The theory underlying the unified diet also suggests that total calories should be adjusted to achieve and maintain desirable weight. The simplest way to use the guidelines would be to have all people older than 2 years do the following:

- Eat a variety of foods.
- Choose most foods from plant sources.
- Eat at least five servings of fruits and vegetables every day (increases fiber).
- Eat at least six servings of whole grain foods each day (increases fiber and provides vitamins and minerals).
- Minimize the consumption of high-fat foods, especially those from animals.
- Limit the quantity of simple sugars in the diet, especially high fructose corn syrup.

Special concern has been expressed about the diet of certain groups of people. Problems are associated with (1) the increasing prevalence of obesity in children and women,

Text continued on page 768

TABLE 72-1   Summary of Important Information About Vitamins and Minerals

Nutrient	Major Function	Sources	RDA in IU
FAT-SOLUBLE VITAMINS			
Vitamin A	Essential for vision, especially in the dark Maintains epithelial tissue: Needed for proper functioning of the cornea, mucous membranes, GI tract, lungs, vagina, urinary tract, bladder, and skin By maintaining healthy epithelium, prevents infection and possibly cancer	Fat soluble: Stored for long periods in the liver Retinol sources: Liver, butter, fish oil, egg yolk, and fortified dairy products Beta carotene sources: Yellow and dark-green vegetables, orange fruits, watermelon, and cherries; the more intense the color, the more vitamin A the food contains	Dependent on body weight Infant 0-6 mo: 2100 IU Infant 6 mo-3 yr: 2000 IU Child 4-6 yr: 2500 IU Child 7-10 yr: 3300 IU Male 11+ yr: 5000 IU Female 11+ yr: 4000 IU Pregnancy: +1000 IU Lactation: +2000 IU
Vitamin D	Main function is calcium management; vitamin D makes sure enough calcium is readily available for retrieval. Promotes calcium absorption in the gut, pulls calcium out of bones, deposits calcium into bone, and monitors calcium excretion by the kidney	Sunlight is the best source of vitamin D. Fortified milk and milk products Other sources include seafood such as fish oils and oily fish (salmon, herring, sardines, mackerel).	Vitamin D RDAs are stable early in life, while bones are growing, but requirements decrease gradually with age. Infant and child to 18 yr: 400 IU Male and female to 22 yr: 300 IU Male and female 22+ yr: 200 IU Pregnancy and lactation: +200 IU Deficiency: Vitamin D 50,000 units weekly × 4, then monthly
Vitamin E	Potent antioxidant (prevents fats in cell membranes from oxidation or spoiling) Considered a possible cancer preventative because it protects cell walls from damage that can lead to tumor formation	Vegetable oils (corn, cottonseed, peanut) are the best sources; nuts (almonds, hazelnuts, safflower, sunflower, walnuts), wheat germ, and whole wheat flour are good sources. Vegetables (spinach, lettuce, onions) and fruits (blackberries, apples, pears) also contain vitamin E.	Vitamin E requirements are based on body size and fat intake; with increased polyunsaturated fat intake, vitamin E requirements increase (more fats to protect). Elderly people and alcoholics may require supplementation. The upper limit amount of vitamin E is 1000 IU; side effects from megadoses include an increased risk of hemorrhage damage due to its anticoagulant properties. Infant-12 mo: 9 to 12 IU Child 1-7 yr: 15 to 21 IU Child 11-18 yr: 24 IU Male 18+ yr: 22 IU of natural source vitamin E or 33 IU synthetic form Female 18+ yr: 22 IU of natural source vitamin E or 33 IU synthetic form Pregnancy: 22 IU Lactation: 28 IU
Vitamin K	Plays an essential role in blood clot formation	Two sources of vitamin K: K_1 is plant derived, and K_2 is produced by bacteria in the human intestine; 50% of each contributes to our daily supply. Synthetic vitamin K: K_3 has twice the potency. K_1 is found in dark-green leafy vegetables (brussels sprouts, spinach, cabbage, cauliflower) and is also found in oats, soybeans, egg yolks, and green tea.	There is a recommended "adequate and safe" range for this vitamin, rather than an official RDA.
WATER-SOLUBLE VITAMINS			
Vitamin B_1	B_1 (thiamine), similar to most B-complex vitamins, acts as a coenzyme or catalyst in the production of energy.	Most foods contain small amounts (if any) of this vitamin. Animal products that are relatively "rich" in thiamine are pork, beef, organ meats, and salmon. Some plant sources such as rye and whole wheat flours, rice bran, enriched cereals, nuts, and legumes (peas and beans in particular) are relatively rich. Brewer's yeast also contains significant amounts of thiamine.	Remember that thiamine deficiency is associated with alcoholism, and supplement accordingly.

IU - International unit.

Table continued on following page

TABLE 72-1   Summary of Important Information About Vitamins and Minerals (Continued)

Nutrient	Major Function	Sources	RDA in IU
Vitamin B$_2$	B$_2$ (riboflavin) is essential for the formation of two coenzymes, both of which play an important role in energy production; cellular growth cannot occur without B$_2$.	B$_2$ is present in both plant and animal products, but "excellent" sources are most often animals: Milk and milk products are probably the best, with liver being second. Other good sources are dairy products, chicken, leafy green vegetables, cereal, bread, wheat germ, brewer's yeast, and almonds.	Riboflavin is not stored in large amounts, so it must be taken in daily. Athletes (especially women) probably should consider supplementation.
Vitamin B$_3$	B$_3$ (niacin), one of the most stable B vitamins, performs tasks similar to riboflavin—taking part in multiple metabolic reactions related to energy production.	The best niacin sources are proteins such as meats, fish, poultry, nuts, legumes, milk, and eggs. Moderate sources include whole grain cereals and breads; highly processed grains have been stripped of much of their nutrient value, and unless they have been "fortified" are poor sources of niacin (and many other nutrients).	A water-soluble vitamin, B$_3$ needs to be constantly replenished.
Vitamin B$_6$	B$_6$ (pyridoxine) also assists in coenzyme reactions, helping the body process protein, fat, and carbohydrates. Stored in muscle tissue, it is readily available when energy is needed.	Vitamin B$_6$ is widely available from dietary sources. Animal products high in B$_6$ include meat and fish (salmon, shrimp, tuna). Plant products include whole grains (bran, whole wheat flour, wheat germ, rice), fruits and vegetables (bananas, avocados, carrots), and nuts (hazelnuts, soy, sunflower). Beer seems to be correlated with elevated serum levels of vitamin B$_6$.	Because excess vitamin B$_6$ can have toxic effects, limiting supplements to less than 200 mg/day is recommended. Used to treat peripheral neuropathy and mood swings on hormonal contraceptives; requires vitamin C, all B vitamins, magnesium, and zinc for optimal results
Vitamin B$_{12}$	The most chemically complex of the B vitamins, B$_{12}$ (cobalamin) plays a major role in energy production and growth, as well as in nervous system function and blood cell production.	B$_{12}$ is found primarily in animal protein (making strict vegetarians at risk for this deficiency). Good sources include fish (many types), dairy products, meats, and eggs.	
Folic acid	Critical for formation and activity of both DNA and RNA, thereby regulating growth and development; also plays a major role in red blood cell production Dietary folate has been found to reduce stroke risk by 20%. Folic acid deficiency has been related to an increase in congenital anomalies (neural tube defects); supplementation is strongly recommended in women of reproductive age, especially oral contraceptive users (more rapid depletion of this nutrient in these women).	Folic acid is found in plant products almost exclusively; best sources include green leafy vegetables (broccoli, spinach, romaine), fruit (oranges), nuts, grains (wheat germ, rice, barley), and legumes (beans, peas, lentils, soybeans). Because of problems with bioavailability, folic acid supplements and fortified cereals have been found to be more effective than a diet rich in naturally occurring folates in reducing total homocysteine levels. It is important to note that cooking these plant products significantly reduces the amount of available folic acid (heat fragile).	
Biotin	Another B vitamin Involved in enzymatic reactions related to protein, fat, and carbohydrate metabolism and energy production; also necessary to convert folic acid to its biologically active state	Biotin is produced largely by bacteria in the human intestine. Both animal and plant products are rich in biotin, with the best sources being liver and organ meats, molasses, and milk. Other sources include nuts (cashews, peanuts, walnuts, sunflower seeds), legumes (peas, lentils, soybeans), and whole grains (brown rice, bulgur, wheat, oats).	

TABLE 72-1 Summary of Important Information About Vitamins and Minerals (Continued)

Nutrient	Major Function	Sources	RDA in IU
Pantothenic acid	Pantothenic acid (another B vitamin) is converted to its biologic form—coenzyme A, which, similar to most B vitamins, is essential for energy production and protein, fat, and carbohydrate metabolism; it also plays roles in red blood cell formation and acetylcholine production.	The word *pantos* means everywhere, and that's where this B vitamin can be found—widely in dietary sources. The best sources are meat products (liver), but it is widely available in plant products (nuts, cereals, beans).	
Vitamin C	Major role is in collagen formation and stabilization. Vitamin C helps to repair damaged tissue and has antioxidant properties. Vitamin C also supports other nutrients, helping the body to activate folic acid and use iron.	Not present in animal products; vitamin C is available in a wide variety of fruits and vegetables. Sources include fruits (oranges and orange juice, lemons, grapefruit, tangerines, strawberries, tomatoes) and vegetables (broccoli, brussels sprouts, cabbage, green peppers, potatoes, spinach, hot peppers).	The upper intake level is 2000 mg/day for adults; high levels could cause adverse effects, including diarrhea. Adults older than age 55 and smokers may need vitamin C supplements.

MINERALS

Nutrient	Major Function	Sources	RDA in IU
Calcium	Main function is to grow, support, and maintain bone and tooth structures. Only 1% is free in serum, but that small amount is critical in nerve transmission, muscle contraction, and blood clotting.	Calcium is present in many foods, but not in large enough quantities to make the "average" diet adequate in calcium; people may require calcium supplementation to meet daily requirements of this mineral. Best food source is dairy products; bony fish (salmon, sardines) also have calcium, as do some green leafy vegetables, some nuts (Brazil, almonds), molasses, soybeans, and tofu.	Dietary requirements steadily increase through childhood, while bony matrix is being laid down, but even higher calcium intake should be considered with advancing age—especially in postmenopausal women at risk for osteoporosis.
Chromium	Chromium is insulin enhancing and may facilitate the binding of insulin to cell walls; it is therefore necessary for normal carbohydrate metabolism. Patients with adult-onset diabetes with normal chromium levels may require less exogenous insulin.	Similar to most minerals, water and soil content plays a role in dietary sources; in areas where chromium is present in drinking water, up to 70% of the average daily intake comes from this source. Other dietary sources include meats (beef, chicken, liver), shellfish (oysters), dairy products, eggs, fruits, and whole grains.	
Copper	Copper enhances the body's ability to store and use iron, as well as being a building block for various enzymes important in collagen formation, myelin sheath maintenance, and energy production.	Copper is present most often in plant products; the only nonplant products that include copper are shellfish (mussels, oysters) and bony fish (salmon). Plant sources that are particularly rich in copper include nuts (Brazil, cashews, hazelnuts, peanuts, walnuts), grains (barley, wheat germ, oats), natural sweeteners (honey, molasses), lentils, and mushrooms.	
Cobalt	Cobalt works with B_{12}, enhancing and supporting its function; without cobalt, B_{12} would be inactive; B_{12} functions include energy production, growth, nervous system functioning, and red blood cell production.	Cobalt is present in both animal and plant sources such as figs, shellfish (oysters, clams), milk, and buckwheat. Other, weak sources include cabbage, spinach, beet greens, lettuce, and watercress; strict vegetarians can become cobalt deficient.	No RDAs have been established for cobalt, but the average American diet contains about 5 to 8 mcg of cobalt per day.

Table continued on following page

TABLE 72-1   Summary of Important Information About Vitamins and Minerals (Continued)

Nutrient	Major Function	Sources	RDA in IU
Fluoride	Fluoride works with calcium to make bone and tooth matrixes harder and more resistant to decay, and it may help prevent osteoporosis.	Fluoridated water is the most common source of dietary fluoride. Fluoride occurs naturally in some drinking water and soil in many parts of the country, but in other areas, fluoride must be added to public drinking water. Food sources generally rich in fluoride (depending on soil and water concentrations of fluoride) include fish, tea, milk, and eggs.	
Iodine	Iodine functions as a building block of thyroid hormone and therefore is involved in cellular metabolism.	Ocean water contains iodine (people living near the oceans grew crops and ate foods with naturally high iodine levels and rarely suffered iodine deficiency; the farther away from the ocean people moved, the more problems they experienced with iodine deficiency). The most available source of iodine for Americans is fortified table salt. Other foods rich in iodine include seafood of all kinds (salmon is particularly high in iodine), sea salt, sunflower seeds, and seaweed.	Infant to 6 mo: 40 mcg Infant 6-12 mo: 50 mcg Child 1-3 yr: 70 mcg Child 4-6 yr: 90 mcg Child 7-10 yr: 120 mcg Child 11 + yr: 150 mcg Adult: 150 mcg Pregnancy: 220 mcg Lactation: 290 mcg Both inadequate and excessive iodine during pregnancy and lactation can be harmful to developing fetuses and infants.
Iron	Iron is an essential part of hemoglobin and is critical for oxygen transport.	Iron has many sources, both animal and plant; this abundance is vital because humans have trouble absorbing iron; they are able to use only about 10% of the iron that is available in the diet, except in pregnancy, when absorption increases to 15%. The best iron sources are animal—liver and other organ meats. Other good sources include dried fruits, beans, dark-green leafy vegetables, shellfish, enriched bread, grains (wheat germ, whole grains), nuts and seeds (cashews, pistachios, walnuts, pumpkin), and natural sweeteners (molasses).	Difficult to eat enough of any one of these foods for adequate supplementation. Do not take iron supplements with Ca^{++} or milk, which may block absorption.
Magnesium	Magnesium plays multiple roles: (1) promoting absorption of other minerals, (2) removing excessive amounts of other minerals, (3) assisting in nervous conduction, (4) enhancing protein metabolism, and (5) binding calcium to tooth enamel.	Magnesium is important in photosynthesis, so vegetables high in chlorophyll are good sources. Animal products contain small amounts of magnesium (amount varies depending on the animal's diet), although fish contains relatively high levels. Good sources include green leafy vegetables, seafood (many fish and shellfish), fruits and fruit juice, nuts and seeds (almonds, sunflower), molasses, soybeans, and wheat germ.	Pregnancy and lactation: Should come from dietary sources; supplementation during pregnancy and lactation is not recommended.
Manganese	Manganese is a "helper" nutrient—important in some biochemical reactions—but other minerals can perform these roles, so the presence of manganese is not critical. The main functions include energy production, glucose management, assistance with vitamin usage, and help in forming proper bone and collagen.	Manganese is available from both plant and animal sources. Good sources include organ meats, muscle meats, leafy green vegetables (spinach, tea, lettuce), nuts and beans, and whole grain cereals and breads.	Tolerable upper limit in adults is 11 mg/day; neurologic adverse effects, similar to symptoms caused by Parkinson's disease, have been observed in individuals who have consumed high amounts of manganese, and iron absorption by the body may be inhibited. Some glucosamine and chondroitin products have excessively high levels of manganese. Pregnancy and lactation: Supplementation is not recommended.

TABLE 72-1 Summary of Important Information About Vitamins and Minerals (Continued)

Nutrient	Major Function	Sources	RDA in IU
Molybdenum	Plays two major roles: (1) Assists in maintaining body iron reserves, (2) helps to use fat stores for energy	Similar to other minerals, concentrations in plant and animal foods depend on soil and water concentrations of this mineral; water alone (if rich in molybdenum) can provide more than 40% of the RDA. Good sources include dark-green leafy vegetables, organ meats, beans, and grains.	
Phosphorus	Phosphorus plays a major role in bone and tooth structure. It is also present in every cell in the body (appearing as part of cellular DNA) and is fundamental to body tissue growth, maintenance, and repair.	Because it is an essential part of cellular structure, meat is an excellent source of phosphorus. Good sources: All types of meat, seafood, milk and milk products, eggs Plant sources rich in phosphorus include nuts and seeds (almonds, peanuts, pumpkin, sunflower), legumes (beans, peas, and soybeans), and whole grains.	
Potassium	Almost 100% of the body's potassium stores are intracellular, creating a large concentration gradient across the cell membrane; this sets the stage for depolarization and nerve transmission. Potassium also does the following: • Helps maintain water balance • Governs acid-base balance • Helps with muscle contraction • Assists with protein and carbohydrate metabolism • Helps to form glycogen and catabolize glucose	Potassium is found in a wide assortment of foods, both animal and plant. Some of the best sources are plants; sources include fruits (avocado, banana, citrus, raisins, dried peaches, tomatoes), vegetables (spinach, parsnips, potatoes), nuts (almonds, Brazil nuts, cashews, peanuts, pecans, walnuts), dairy products, whole grain cereals, legumes, and molasses. Animal sources include lean meats and some seafood (sardines).	Dietary salt intake affects the body's levels of potassium inversely: Increased sodium intake = decreased potassium. Some experts suggest that minimum daily requirements should be 2000 to 2500 mg; the "average" American diet provides between 2000 and 6000 mg daily, so potassium deficiency is not common unless disease states or medications interfere with body stores.
Selenium	Selenium works together with vitamin E; it is a potent antioxidant and is found in high concentrations in the kidney, heart, spleen, and liver. Both selenium and vitamin E must be present in the body—selenium cannot take over the role of vitamin E, nor can vitamin E perform in place of selenium.	Again, food concentrations of selenium vary depending on selenium content in soil and water. Good sources include animal products such as liver, kidney, meats, eggs, milk, and seafood. Plant products vary widely, depending on the soil: Vegetables (broccoli, cabbage, celery, cucumbers, garlic, mushrooms, onions) and whole grains (bran, wheat germ)	The upper intake level is 400 mcg/day; side effects from higher doses could induce selenosis, a toxic reaction marked by hair loss and nail sloughing. Take with vitamin C.
Sodium	Similar to potassium, the major functions of sodium include nervous system conduction and acid-base regulation. Sodium is the major extracellular ion, creating another large concentration gradient for the nerve cell and thereby promoting nervous conduction. Other functions include the following: • Carbon dioxide transport • Assistance with muscle contraction • Amino acid transport • Prevention of excess water loss	Table salt is the major dietary source of sodium in American diets, but sodium is present in many foods—more frequently in animal than in plant sources; many processed foods have an extra high sodium content. Good sources include meat (bacon, beef, ham), seafood (clams, sardines), and dairy products. Other sources include grains, vegetables (green beans), and fruits (tomatoes).	In contrast to vitamins and minerals, sodium excess is more problematic for most people; staying below the upper limits can be a challenge. Infant-6 mo: 0.11-0.35 g Infant 6-12 mo: 0.25-0.75 g Child 1-3 yr: 0.32-1 g Child 4-6 yr: 0.45-1.35 g Child 7-10 yr: 0.6-1.8 g Child 11-17 yr: 0.9-2.3 g Adult: 1.1-3.3 g Pregnant and lactating: No restriction advised
Sulfur	Sulfur has two primary functions: (1) It serves as a building block of keratin (helps to maintain clear skin, healthy nails, and glossy hair), and (2) it assists in bile production, which aids in the digestion of fats.	Protein-containing foods are the best sources of sulfur; eggs are richest in this mineral. Other sources include meat, fish, milk, and a few plant sources (dried beans, cabbage, wheat germ).	No RDAs for sulfur exist; deficiency has not been reported.

Table continued on following page

TABLE 72-1   Summary of Important Information About Vitamins and Minerals (Continued)

Nutrient	Major Function	Sources	RDA in IU
Zinc	Zinc is important even though it is present in only tiny amounts. Zinc affects the following: • Insulin activity • Wound healing • Immune system response • Bone structure • Normal oil gland function • Normal fetal growth and development • Senses of taste and smell (these are preserved) Zinc has been found to prevent capsid protein formation in several viruses, including rhinoviruses, the most common cause of colds; zinc lozenges may help reduce the duration of symptoms of the common cold. Antioxidant/zinc combinations have been found to be the best treatment for slowing the progression of age-related macular degeneration.	Animal products are the best sources of zinc; particularly good sources are meats, seafood (oysters, herring), milk, and egg yolks. Vegetarians can get adequate zinc intake from whole grains (wheat bran, wheat germ), natural sweeteners (maple syrup, molasses), seeds (sesame, sunflower), and soybeans. Most fruits and vegetables are poor sources of zinc.	Lactating: Breast milk contains a zinc-binding protein, which improves absorption in the gut; infant formula is not as well absorbed.

(2) undernourishment among the elderly, (3) osteoporosis, iron deficiency, and folic acid intake in women, and (4) the special needs of various minority populations. The American College of Obstetrics and Gynecology maintains that vitamin supplementation is not required in the pregnant woman.

Eating a well-balanced diet, implementing an exercise program, replacing saturated fats with fish and nuts, and limiting salt and alcohol intake are other key components of a healthy lifestyle. Avoid extreme diets.

VITAMINS

Vitamins are organic materials essential for human survival that must be ingested on a regular basis because they are not synthesized by the body. Some are available in their active form; others are ingested as a "precursor" or "provitamin" that then is converted; two vitamins, vitamin K and biotin, are not ingested at all but are synthesized by bacteria inside the intestinal tract.

Thirteen essential vitamins have been identified to date, and more information about essential nutrients is being discovered every year. Only tiny quantities of vitamins are required on a daily basis, but chronic deprivation of even one vitamin will cause disease, and death can occur. The inverse is also true; some vitamins ingested in large quantities will cause illness and death. An "adequate" diet is one that includes an appropriate amount of each vitamin on a daily basis but does not include excessive amounts of any of them.

The body needs only small amounts of vitamins (that is why these are often referred to as *micronutrients*) because the body uses them without breaking them down, as happens to carbohydrates and other *macronutrients*. So far, 13 compounds have been classified as vitamins. Vitamins are classified into two types: fat soluble (will dissolve in oil) and water soluble (will dissolve in water). Vitamins A, D, E, and K—the four fat-soluble vitamins—tend to accumulate in the body. Vitamin C and the eight B vitamins—biotin,

folate, niacin, pantothenic acid, riboflavin, thiamine, vitamin B_6, and vitamin B_{12}—dissolve in water, so excess amounts are excreted.

Vitamins primarily serve regulatory functions and assist in the production of energy. They are not used in the body for structural purposes and cannot be used as an energy source. Vitamins are essential but differ markedly in their absorption and potential for toxicity.

Fat-Soluble Vitamins

Fat-soluble vitamins, which include vitamins A, D, E, and K ("DEAK" for short), are found primarily in various plant and animal oils or fats. Because these vitamins are stored in our body fat, daily ingestion is not required, but adequate body levels must be maintained over the long term. When ingested, these vitamins are transported through the body by the bloodstream. For these vitamins to remain dissolved in the blood, unique carrier proteins are required for each. Some people with particular metabolic and genetic diseases are unable to synthesize carrier proteins and can have extreme vitamin deficiency states despite adequate vitamin intake.

Fat-soluble vitamins have common properties—their ability to be stored, their mode of transport, and the severity of deficiency syndromes in young children—but each vitamin is unique in its function and in its physiologic effects of deficiency and toxicity. Development of fat-soluble vitamin deficiency can be gradual and the symptoms subtle, but toxicities can present suddenly and can be devastating in their effects. Overdosage is more of a problem with fat-soluble vitamins than with water-soluble vitamins because of their ability to be stored and accumulated.

Water-Soluble Vitamins

Water-soluble vitamins include all the B vitamins (B_1, B_2, B_3, B_6, B_{12}, folacin, biotin, and pantothenic acid) and vitamin C. With the exception of B_{12}, these vitamins are rapidly excreted from the body because the body has no way to store them. These vitamins must be ingested on a regular basis or deficiency symptoms will quickly appear. They are not particularly toxic, however, because high levels rarely develop. These products are readily available but are destroyed by heat. Because they are water soluble, the vitamins may leach out into water used for cooking and be discarded if the consumer is not aware of how to properly store and cook them. Overdosage may occur when large quantities are taken chronically and exceed the body's ability to excrete them.

The definition of a healthy daily intake of B vitamins is not set in stone and is likely to change over the next few years as data from ongoing randomized trials are evaluated. Because only a fraction of U.S. adults currently get the recommended daily intake of B vitamins through diet alone, use of a multivitamin supplement is becoming increasingly important.

MINERALS

Minerals are inorganic substances present in the body that work in combination with enzymes, hormones, and vitamins. Most human minerals are found in the skeleton and make up about 4% of total body weight. Calcium and phosphorus are by far the predominant minerals in the body.

Minerals, similar to vitamins, are essential for body function but are present in much smaller amounts. Both acute and chronic mineral deficiencies, as well as toxicities, can occur, because even though the daily intake may vary enormously, the average adult will consistently excrete several grams of minerals every day.

Minerals are classified as major or trace. Major minerals (calcium, phosphorus, magnesium, potassium, sodium, and chloride) must account for at least 0.01% of body weight. Trace minerals (arsenic, chromium, cobalt, copper, fluoride, iodine, iron, manganese, molybdenum, nickel, selenium, silicon, tin, vanadium, and zinc) fall below 0.01% but are still measurable and have metabolic impact, although the exact biologic significance of some of these trace minerals remains a mystery. The label applied to a particular mineral ("major" or "trace") does not imply significance; excess or deficiency of any of the minerals can be devastating.

Minerals are found in a variety of states as free ions or bound to many different substances (such as iron to hemoglobin or cobalt to vitamin B_{12}). This variety allows minerals to perform many different biologic roles within the body.

How to Monitor

Numerous tools are now available that provide noninvasive monitoring of dietary patterns or serve as computerized nutritional assessment tools. *MyPyramid Tracker* is an excellent resource for clinicians and laypersons to use in monitoring nutritional intake. Many of the commercial weight loss programs have a website at which the individual can complete a daily food and exercise log and receive feedback about dietary intake.

Blood studies to determine nutrient levels generally are not indicated. If a person presents with a particular set of physical symptoms that seem to be related to nutrient deficiencies or toxicities, blood and hair studies by specialists may provide the answers.

Patient Variables

Daily requirements of vitamins and minerals vary from person to person and with age, sex, physiologic state (e.g., pregnancy), and physical activity. The development of a completely com-

prehensive list is impossible, so the Food and Nutrition Board of the National Academy of Sciences, National Research Council, developed a list of RDAs that was first published in 1943 and is updated every few years. This RDA list was not intended to be comprehensive but attempts to define what amounts of each vitamin and mineral would be appropriate to meet the needs of normal, healthy people. In fact, the RDAs are deliberately set higher than the requirements for an "average" person, to compensate for dietary deficiencies or to offer a "safety zone."

A healthy individual who conscientiously adheres to the RDA will take in adequate amounts of essential vitamins and minerals. However, the RDA may be excessive or inadequate for a person in poor health or for someone who has a metabolic or genetic disorder. The U.S. Preventive Task Force is a good resource for current recommendations on vitamin and mineral supplements.

GERIATRICS. Elderly people may have highly variable nutritional needs depending on their state of health, but most may benefit from the use of daily multivitamins. Metabolic changes have slowed the digestive rate, increased the fat-to-muscle ratio, and decreased liver and renal functions; all of these events have an impact on digestion, absorption, and excretion of vitamins and minerals. Use of medication also can have a significant impact on absorption and utilization of nutrients.

Dietary deficiencies in the elderly can occur for many reasons, for example, because older persons may not eat sufficient food, may not eat the correct foods, or may not eat an adequate variety of foods. Vitamin B_{12} deficiency may result from decreased acidity of the stomach. The signs of vitamin deficiency may be subtle but always should be considered; for example, thiamine deficiency (associated with alcohol abuse) can cause Wernicke's encephalopathy or organic amnestic syndrome, folic acid deficiency is associated with dementia, and vitamin B_{12} deficiency can result in psychologic changes and peripheral neuropathy. Vitamin D deficiency is not uncommon among the elderly, especially in nursing home residents or others who do not get out in the sun. A vitamin D deficiency can contribute to osteoporosis.

PEDIATRICS. Pediatric RDAs for various vitamins and minerals vary widely; age and body weight are significant factors, and careful attention should be paid to children's diets throughout the growing years. Nutrient deficiency states are always quickly seen and often are more devastating in children than in adults. Some deficiencies can have lifelong effects as well; for example, vitamin D deficiency causes abnormalities in bone ossification, causing bones to become soft and bend in a disease called rickets. Vitamin D therapy will stop further damage but will not correct many existing bone deformities.

As children grow, their need for supplementation changes. Breastfed infants get almost all the nutrients they need from their mother. The only supplements these babies may need are fluoride (which is present in only small amounts in breast milk) and an iron supplement after 4 to 6 months of age. Bottle-fed infants receiving infant formula are receiving the RDA through the formula. Consider the use of iron-fortified formula after age 4 months.

As they start to eat solid foods, however, many children develop strong food preferences, and parents can struggle to maintain a balanced diet. Balance *over time* is the important point to remember. Not every meal has to include every nutrient; ensuring a balance for the day is sufficient. Caution parents to avoid food conflicts by frequently offering small portions of foods from many sources. Vitamin supplementation is not necessary for a child who is willing to eat from many food groups, but it may be helpful in the child who eats only a small variety of foods.

PREGNANCY AND LACTATION. In general, almost all vitamin and mineral RDAs increase during pregnancy, to support the increase in metabolic rate and the demands of a growing fetus. These nutritional needs, with the exception of iron, can be met by most women through diet. Iron requirements during pregnancy are nearly impossible to meet by diet alone, and iron deficiency anemia may result. Folic acid supplementation is being recognized increasingly as an essential pregnancy nutrient, and many physicians are recommending the use of iron and folic acid supplements by all pregnant women.

One potential problem in pregnancy is vitamin and/or mineral toxicity. Nutrients that are particularly harmful to a developing fetus if provided in excess (10 or more times the RDA) include iron, zinc, selenium, and vitamins A, B_6, C, and D. Although some vitamins taken in excess just pass through the system and are excreted in the urine, other vitamins may be stored in tissues, and toxicity may develop. When megadoses of vitamins such as A and C are consistently taken, the body develops a tolerance for the higher doses.

GENDER. Men's nutritional needs remain relatively stable from late adolescence into old age. With aging, illness, and injury, dietary needs must be reassessed, and supplementation might be considered. Elderly men (>80 years) are at risk for osteoporosis. Adequate calcium intake is essential in elderly men and women.

Women's needs vary widely throughout their lifetime. Until adolescence, children's needs are essentially the same, and a gradual increase in RDA is noted for most nutrients. During adolescence, however, women's dietary needs undergo striking changes.

With the onset of menses, dietary iron needs increase. Many women do not take in adequate amounts of dietary iron to compensate for monthly blood loss. This need decreases with the use of hormonal contraception. Adolescents and young women lower their risk of iron deficiency anemia when they use hormonal contraception.

It is certainly possible for an individual's diet to provide sufficient iron, but because many women diet to keep their weight down and men may engage in excessive exercise, and because many individuals do not develop good food habits (or do not learn them during adolescence), many American diets are inadequate, and iron supplementation should be considered.

Folic acid supplementation (400 mcg) should be taken by all women of reproductive age. A deficiency in this B vitamin has been shown to be related to an increase in neural tube defects in the developing fetus.

Appropriate calcium intake is a significant problem for American women. Chronic calcium deficiency often starts in young women and worsens with age. As adolescence begins, many women stop drinking milk. Many women become deficient in calcium just when they need it most for pregnancy, lactation, and menopause. Bone loss accelerates during the first 5 to 10 years after menopause and if not stopped can lead to devastating consequences. In a study on white women, it was estimated that 25% of women older than age 70 and 50% of those over age 80 will show evidence of vertebral fracture. By the age of 90, 33% of all white women will have sustained a hip fracture, and many of these women will die as a direct result of complications related to the fracture. Comparable data are not available for women of other races. Initiation of calcium supplementation by age 35 has been proposed by many scientists; it should continue through menopause and should be added as an adjunct to bisphosphonate treatment for osteopenia or osteoporosis (see Chapter 37).

Vitamin D is another critical bone-building nutrient that many women lack when they need it most—as they age. Vitamin D promotes calcium absorption, and one without the other is useless. Taking a calcium supplement without paying attention to vitamin D does not help bones. Many women become deficient in vitamin D because they stop drinking fortified milk and do not spend sufficient time outside to absorb UV radiation to make vitamin D. Many women, because they are worried about the risks of skin cancer, cover all exposed skin if they do go outside, again blocking vitamin D absorption.

Patient Education

All individuals should be counseled regarding their nutritional needs. Parents should be aware of the needs of growing children and should learn how to manage their children's diets. Young teenagers should be told about the importance of balance in the diet. This is particularly important for youth engaged in vigorous sports or types of dance such as wrestling or ballet when forced weight loss may be an issue, or when they are attempting to lose or gain weight. Older adolescents should be aware of typical "pitfalls," which include decreased calcium intake, increased alcohol and soda consumption, and fad and weight reduction diets. They also should be informed about the hazards of vitamin and mineral toxicities. Pregnant and lactating women, as well as young mothers, require frequent nutritional "updates" as they progress through the childbearing years. Older women should be encouraged to supplement their diet with calcium and vitamin D to prevent osteoporosis. Older people of both genders should receive periodic reminders about the importance of balance in the diet and, together with their care provider, should consider appropriate nutritional supplementation when illness or injury occurs.

For many years, RDAs were published. In 1997, dietary reference intakes were published as well. Since 2006, these terms have been further refined to include estimated average requirement, adequate intake, and tolerable upper intake level. These different levels are listed in common nutrition resources and in many pharmacology texts. Because of the overlap in these terms, for the purposes of this text, the term RDA will be used and will be specified for specific age groups and genders. RDAs are also available in small amounts for choline and chloride. These elements are not discussed in this text.

CONTROVERSY OVER ANTIOXIDANTS. The hypothesis that antioxidant vitamins might reduce the risk of many degenerative diseases is based on a large body of basic and human epidemiologic research. One of the most consistent findings in dietary research is that those who consume larger quantities of fruits and vegetables have lower rates of heart disease, stroke, and cancer. Attention has been focused recently on the antioxidant content of fruits and vegetables as a possible explanation for their apparent protective effects.

Increasing evidence suggests that free radical reactions are involved in early or later stages of development of human disease; it is therefore of particular importance for researchers to explore whether vitamin E and other antioxidants found in the human diet may be capable of lowering the incidence of disease. Low levels of antioxidants, which increase free radical activity, are clearly associated with an increased risk of these diseases. Put simply, the proposition is that if human diets are improved by an increase in the quantity of antioxidants included in them, it might be possible to use this approach to reduce the incidence of numerous degenerative diseases.

Antioxidant vitamins, which include beta carotene (provitamin A), vitamin E, and vitamin C, are hypothesized to decrease cancer risk by preventing tissue damage by trapping organic free radicals and/or deactivating excited oxygen molecules—a byproduct of many metabolic functions. These micronutrients may be reduced by smoking and passive smoking.

Over the past decade, extensive studies on the health effects of antioxidants have been conducted, many with inconclusive findings. The largest analysis of data on antioxidant vitamins ever conducted, which was published by Bjelakovic et al in 2007, shows that on the whole, antioxidant vitamins confer no health benefits. In fact, beta carotene, vitamin A, and vitamin E may actually increase mortality.

FAT-SOLUBLE VITAMINS

Vitamin A (Retinol, Beta Carotenes, Carotenoids)

As indicated by its name, vitamin A was the first vitamin discovered. It was identified in the early 1900s and occurs in three forms: retinols, beta carotenes, and carotenoids. Retinols are already active and are found in animal sources of food. The retinols are the most active form of vitamin A. Beta carotenes are provitamin A, which requires conversion to the active form. These are derived from plant sources; the carotenoids exist as free alcohol or in a fatty acyl-ester form. Because retinol is fat soluble and is stored in the liver, daily intake is not essential. Retinol is transported through the blood by retinol-binding protein. It stimulates the production and activity of white blood cells, takes part in remodeling bone, helps maintain the health of endothelial cells (those lining the body's interior surfaces), regulates cell growth and division, and enhances vision.

DEFICIENCY. Vitamin A deficiency ranks as the third most common nutritional deficiency in the world. It is rare in most industrialized countries. Vitamin A deficiency, which is the most common cause of blindness in children around the world, causes a decrease in visual acuity (especially night vision); without vitamin A supplementation, the corneal epithelium becomes dry, inflamed, and eventually keratinized, causing permanent scarring.

Epithelial tissue throughout the body is affected by a deficiency in vitamin A, which is manifested by keratin deposits. Early in the syndrome, deposition occurs around hair follicles, and hardened, pigmented "goose bumps" appear on the extremities. As the deficiency progresses, a larger portion of the body is involved, and skin peeling and scaling occur. Internal effects such as GI tract disturbances, oral and vaginal dryness, and keratinization are also seen.

Research is ongoing regarding the relationship between vitamin A and cancer. Vitamin A supplementation has not been shown to be helpful in curing existing cancers, but normal amounts of vitamin A in the diet may help to prevent the development of certain forms of cancer.

TOXICITY. Vitamin A (especially retinol) taken in excess can be hazardous and even life threatening. Signs of vitamin A toxicity include epithelial lining problems involving the GI tract (nausea, vomiting, and pain leading to weight loss and anorexia), mouth problems (cracking, drying, scaling, and bleeding lips and mouth corners), and scalp conditions (hair loss and itching). Other effects include amenorrhea, spleen and liver enlargement, transient hydrocephalus, and bone problems (joint pain, stunting of growth). Effects on the developing fetus have been noted in animals, and congenital malformations have been clearly documented. In humans, doses in excess of 31,000 to 36,000 IU have been related to an increase in birth defects and increase the risk of hip fracture. Too much preformed vitamin A interferes with the beneficial actions of vitamin D.

RECOMMENDED DAILY ALLOWANCES. The RDA requirements of vitamin A are based on retinol "equivalents" (RE) or micrograms of retinol. 1 RE = 1 mcg retinol. 1 RE of vitamin A = 3.33 units of retinol = 10 units beta carotene. RDA is 400 to 500 mcg/day (for infants <1 year), 300 mcg/day (1 to 3 years), 400 mcg/day (4 to 8 years), 600 mcg/day (for boys and girls 9 to 13 years), 900 mcg/day (for men, or 3000 IU* for those 14 to 70+ years), and 700 mcg/day (for women, or 2333 IU for 14 to 70+ years). The dose should be 770 mcg/day during pregnancy and 1200 to 1300 mcg/day during lactation.

Many juices, dairy products, breakfast cereals, and other foods are fortified with vitamin A. Many fruits and vegetables and some supplements also contain beta carotene and other vitamin A precursors, which the body can turn into vitamin A. In contrast to preformed vitamin A, beta carotene is not toxic even at high levels of intake. The body can make vitamin A from beta carotene as needed and there is no need to monitor intake levels, as there is with preformed vitamin A. It is therefore preferable to choose a vitamin supplement that provides all or the vast majority of its vitamin A in the form of beta carotene.

Vitamin D (Vitamin D_2, Ergocalciferol; D_3, Cholecalciferol)

Vitamin D acts as both a vitamin and a hormone. As a vitamin, it is present in food, and when ingested, it is immediately available for use. As a hormone, it is formed in one organ and has effects on another.

Vitamin D_3 is a steroid derivative. After irradiation by UV light, an inactive sterol converts to cholecalciferol. This is converted again within the liver, travels to the kidney, and is converted into the active form of vitamin D_3. D_3 travels to the bone and to the gut, where it exerts its effects, which are modified by positive and negative feedback loops.

---

*International units.

Vitamin D is easily obtained by 15 minutes of daily exposure to the sun. African Americans and others with dark skin tend to have much lower levels of vitamin D because little vitamin is formed through the action of sunlight on the skin. A study of people admitted to a Boston hospital, for example, showed that 57% were deficient in vitamin D.

Vitamin D helps to ensure that the body absorbs and retains calcium and phosphorus, which are critical for building bone. Laboratory studies also show that vitamin D keeps cancer cells from growing and dividing.

Preliminary studies indicate that insufficient intake of vitamin D is associated with an increased risk of fracture, and that vitamin D supplementation may prevent fracture. It also may help to prevent falls, a common problem that leads to substantial disability and death among older people. Other early studies suggest an association between low vitamin D intake and increased risks of prostate, breast, colon, and other cancers.

DEFICIENCY. Vitamin D deficiency was extremely common before the early 1900s and resulted in rickets (a childhood disease) and osteomalacia (the adult form of the disease). In both cases, the problem was inadequate bone ossification, which caused soft, pliable bones. Clinical symptoms included bowed legs, knock knees, contracted pelvis, skull malformations, and dental eruption delay. Adults experienced problems with bone fractures and, if the deficiency became severe enough, tetany resulted. During the early 1900s, it was discovered that lack of sunlight is the cause of rickets. Some countries in the Arctic Circle today regularly expose children to UV lamps to promote vitamin D absorption. Although many health care providers suggest limiting exposure of the skin to the sun to prevent skin cancer, vitamin D supplementation may be necessary to provide adequate vitamin D. Some research suggests that women who take vitamin D supplements have a 31% lower risk of death from heart disease compared with women who do not take supplements, regardless of whether they were taken with calcium. In addition to its influence on bones, vitamin D is involved in blood pressure regulation and acts as a tumor suppressant in some types of cancer. Some researchers urge higher doses for the entire population to prevent osteoporotic fractures. Vitamin D deficiency contributes to osteoporosis. Some recommend measuring vitamin D levels in the elderly and at risk persons, and supplementing as needed.

TOXICITY. Vitamin D is highly toxic in large doses because it is stored in fat cells and is not readily eliminated. After a large dose, vitamin D can be found circulating for months. Toxicity is more likely to occur in young children, and the consequences are more serious for them as well. Excess vitamin D leads to hypercalcemia; symptoms include confusion, muscle weakness, and anorexia. Calcium is deposited in many body tissues, and symptoms include serious GI tract disturbances, permanent kidney damage, aortic stenosis, and mental retardation.

RECOMMENDED DAILY ALLOWANCES. The current recommended intake of vitamin D is 5 micrograms up to age 50, 10 micrograms between the ages of 51 and 70, and 15 micrograms after age 70. Optimal intakes are higher though, with 25 micrograms (1000 IU) recommended for those over age 2. Few foods naturally contain vitamin D. Good sources include dairy products and breakfast cereals (which are fortified with

vitamin D), as well as fatty fish such as salmon and tuna. For most people, the best way to get the recommended daily intake is to take a multivitamin, but the level of vitamin D in most multivitamins (10 micrograms) is too low.

Vitamin E (Alpha-tocopherol)

Some experts consider vitamin E to be the most important antioxidant because it protects cell membranes and prevents damage to enzymes associated with them. Natural sources of vitamin E include vegetable oils such as sunflower oil, grains, oats, nuts, and dairy products. The value of vitamin E supplements is controversial. It has been suggested that vitamin E might be neuroprotective, with potential use in helping to prevent Alzheimer's disease in selected persons. Vitamin E also may shut down a critical enzymatic pathway to make platelets less sticky, thereby helping to prevent clogging of the arteries. Based on a variety of long-term national studies, the American Heart Association has concluded that "the scientific data do not justify the use of antioxidant vitamin supplements [such as vitamin E] for CVD risk reduction."

DEFICIENCY. Vitamin E deficiency is difficult to diagnose because it can be subtle, manifesting in many body systems or in only one. Vitamin E deficiency has been well documented in animals but has not been seen in healthy people who eat a varied diet. Again, children are more vulnerable to this deficiency, and most present with hematologic symptoms such as severe anemia and hemorrhage.

Because vitamin E absorption is dependent on pancreatic secretions and bile, biliary obstruction or pancreatic insufficiency can result in vitamin E deficiency.

TOXICITY. Megadoses of vitamin E are better tolerated than doses of many of the other fat-soluble vitamins, and toxicity is rarely seen. In animals given very high doses, growth retardation, poor bone calcification, and anemia are seen. Because of these effects in animals, large doses of vitamin E are not recommended in humans.

RECOMMENDED DAILY ALLOWANCES. Dosages are 4 mg/day for infants 0 to 6 months of age, 5 mg/day for infants 7 to 12 months, 6 mg/day for children 1 to 3 years, 7 mg/day for children 4 to 8 years, 11 mg/day for boys and girls 9 to 13 years, and 15 mg/day for men and women 14 to older than 70 years. These doses are the equivalent of 22 IU from natural source vitamin E or 33 IU of the synthetic form. Dosage during pregnancy and lactation is 19 mg/day. Although the data are sparse and conflicting, evidence from some observational studies suggests that at least 400 IU of vitamin E per day is needed for optimal health. Because standard multivitamins usually contain around 30 IU, a separate vitamin E supplement is needed to achieve this level. Current guidelines say that consuming more than 1000 mg of supplemental vitamin E per day is not considered safe; this is the equivalent of a supplement with 1500 IU of natural source vitamin E or 1100 IU of synthetic vitamin E.

Vitamin K (K_1, Phylloquinone; K_2, Menaquinone; Synthetic Vitamin K_3, Menadione)

Vitamin K helps to make six of the 13 proteins needed for blood clotting. Its role in maintaining the clotting cascade is so important that people who take anticoagulants such as warfarin (Coumadin) must be careful to keep their vitamin K intake stable. Vitamin K is also involved in building bone. Low levels of circulating vitamin K have been linked with low bone density, and supplementation with vitamin K leads to improvement in biochemical measures of bone health. A report from the Nurses' Health Study suggests that women who get at least 110 mcg of vitamin K a day are 30% less likely to break a hip than women who get less than that. Nurses who ate a serving of lettuce or another green leafy vegetable each day cut the risk of hip fracture in half compared with those who ate one serving a week. Data from the Framingham Heart Study also show an association between high vitamin K intake and reduced risk of hip fracture.

DEFICIENCY. Vitamin K deficiency is rare because vitamin K is so widely available from both dietary and internal sources. Deficiency can be a problem in newborn infants with sterile intestinal tracts, so synthetic vitamin K is given shortly after birth. Early feeding introduces bacteria into the gut so that newborns can start to make their own vitamin K.

Medications can interfere with vitamin K metabolism and absorption. Warfarin and the coumarins all decrease vitamin K effectiveness, usually by competing for biologically active receptor sites. Some antibiotics can alter the intestinal flora to the point that vitamin K–producing bacteria are significantly reduced. This can cause adverse bleeding events.

TOXICITY. Toxicity has rarely been seen with vitamin K, despite its fat-soluble nature. Hemolytic anemia from a variety of causes has been seen in newborns (especially in premature infants) and causes an increase in the breakdown of red blood cells. Allergic reactions to vitamin K_3 have also been reported.

RECOMMENDED DAILY ALLOWANCES. RDA is 2 mcg/day for infants 0 to 6 months, 2.5 mcg/day for infants 7 to 12 months, 30 mcg/day for children 1 to 3 years, 55 mcg/day for children 4 to 8 years, 60 mcg/day for boys and girls 9 to 13 years, 75 mcg/day for men and women 14 to 18 years, and 120 mcg/day for men 19 to older than 70 years. RDA is 90 mcg/day for women 19 to past 70 years and 90 mcg/day during pregnancy and lactation. This vitamin is found in many foods, especially green leafy vegetables and commonly used cooking oils. However, people who do not regularly eat a lettuce salad or green leafy vegetables are likely to be deficient in intake of vitamin K. According to a 1996 survey, a substantial number of Americans, particularly children and young adults, are not getting the vitamin K they need.

WATER-SOLUBLE VITAMINS

Vitamin B₁ (Thiamine)

DEFICIENCY. Vitamin B_1 deficiency was a common problem in the late nineteenth century that resulted in the disease beriberi. This disease is not commonly seen today except in special populations such as alcoholics. Physical symptoms of thiamine deficiency include fatigue, GI problems, muscle weakness and atrophy, bradycardia, and heart enlargement. Multiple peripheral nervous system problems (e.g., numbness, tingling, loss of reflexes) can occur, and more subtle central nervous system changes such as memory loss, decreased attention span, irritability, confusion, and depression appear as the

disease progresses. Prolonged thiamine deficiency can result in permanent damage to the nervous system.

Alcohol abusers are particularly prone to this disease for several reasons. Their diet is often inadequate, alcohol decreases intestinal absorption of thiamine, and thiamine is required to metabolize alcohol.

Wernicke's encephalopathy, a thiamine deficiency disease, is seen both in alcoholics and in people with pernicious vomiting. Symptoms can range from mild confusion to coma and death. If the person survives, permanent damage to the cerebral cortex may result in psychosis. Many of the symptoms of Wernicke's encephalopathy can be reversed with thiamine therapy.

TOXICITY. Vitamin B_1 toxicity is rare and the side effects are mild because thiamine is water soluble and is excreted readily from the body. People who ingest megadoses of thiamine may become drowsy, but hazardous effects have not been reported. Anaphylaxis after multiple thiamine injections has been reported and should be considered when this vitamin is administered in an injectable form.

RECOMMENDED DAILY ALLOWANCES. RDA is 0.2 mg/day for infants 0 to 6 months, 0.3 mg/day for infants 7 to 12 months, 0.5 mg/day for children 1 to 3 years, 0.6 mg/day for children 4 to 8 years, 0.9 mg/day for children 9 to 13 years, 1.2 mg/day for men 14 to older than 70 years, 1 mg/day for women 14 to 18, and 1.1 mg/day for women 14 to older than 70 years. The dosage increases to 1.4 mg/day during pregnancy and lactation.

Vitamin B₂ (riboflavin)

Riboflavin was discovered in the early 1900s as researchers were looking for growth factors in food. All identified foods shared a single common characteristic: They were yellow. Biochemists who were working at the same time kept running into a yellow enzyme that seemed to be strongly related to increases in metabolism. This yellow substance was riboflavin.

DEFICIENCY. Vitamin B_2 deficiency does not appear to occur in isolation; it occurs along with multiple nutrient deficiencies. However, symptoms resulting from inadequate B_2 intake have been isolated. These symptoms include cheilosis (cracks at the corner of the mouth) and inflammation of the oral mucosa accompanied by a purple-tinged glossitis, eye irritation, dermatitis (unusual in that symptoms include both dryness and greasy scaling), mood changes, depression and/or hysteria, growth retardation, and malformations.

TOXICITY. No symptoms of toxicity have been reported for riboflavin.

RECOMMENDED DAILY ALLOWANCES. RDA is 0.3 mg/day for infants 0 to 6 months, 0.4 mg/day for infants 7 to 12 months, 0.5 mg/day for children 1 to 3 years, 0.6 mg/day for children 4 to 8 years, 0.9 mg/day for children 9 to 13 years, 1.3 mg/day for men 14 throughout the life span, 1 mg/day for women 14 to 18 years, and 1.1 mg for women throughout the rest of their lives. During pregnancy, the dose goes to 1.4 mg/day, and during lactation, it increases to 1.6 mg/day.

Vitamin B₃ (Niacin, Nicotinic acid, Nicotinamide)

DEFICIENCY. Niacin deficiency causes cell destabilization that, if not corrected results in damage to and destruction of cells throughout the body. This disease is called *pellagra* (meaning "raw skin"). Symptoms are seen most clearly in body systems where cells divide rapidly, such as the skin, GI tract, and nervous system. Initially, persons report weakness, fatigue, anorexia, and indigestion. As the deficiency progresses, the classic symptoms of dermatitis, diarrhea, and dementia (the "three D's") develop. If uncorrected, a fourth D—death—may occur.

Niacin deficiency rarely occurs by itself and often is seen in multiple-nutrient deficiency states. Treatment of patients with pellagra with niacin supplementation alone usually is not sufficient or completely effective without consideration of other possible B-complex deficiencies.

Niacin is also used by some clinicians in the treatment of high cholesterol (see Chapter 22).

TOXICITY. Megadoses of nicotinic acid overdose cause skin irritation and flushing, as well as GI irritation, possible liver damage, and multiple enzyme changes. All symptoms are reversible if niacin doses are decreased. Nicotinamide does not seem to cause any symptoms of toxicity.

RECOMMENDED DAILY ALLOWANCES. RDA is 2 mg/day for infants 0 to 6 months, 4 mg/day for infants 7 to 12 months, 6 mg/day for children 1 to 3 years, 8 mg/day for children 4 to 8 years, and 12 mg/day for children 9 to 13 years. Throughout the rest of their lives, men should take 16 mg/day. Women should take 14 mg/day for the rest of their lives, except the rate should increase to 18 mg/day when they are pregnant and to 17 mg/day when they are lactating.

Vitamin B_6 (Pyridoxine)

Folic acid, vitamin B_6, and vitamin B_{12} work together to play key roles in recycling homocysteine into methionine, one of the 20 or so building blocks from which the body builds new proteins. Without enough folic acid, vitamin B_6, and vitamin B_{12}, this recycling process becomes inefficient, and homocysteine levels increase. Several observational studies have shown that high levels of homocysteine are associated with increased risks of heart disease and stroke. Increasing intake of folic acid, vitamin B_6, and vitamin B_{12} decreases homocysteine levels. This vitamin also is used as treatment for neuropathy and, as a precursor of serotonin, it works with other B vitamins to help mood swings for women on hormonal contraception. Vitamin B_6 works best in combination with vitamin C, magnesium, zinc, and other B vitamins.

DEFICIENCY. Because B_6 is involved in so many enzymatic reactions, deficiency presents in a wide array of symptoms. No particular disease is associated with pyridoxine deficiency, but symptoms similar to riboflavin and niacin deficiency are seen.

TOXICITY. High doses of vitamin B_6 have not been shown to be particularly harmful, although nervous system effects (e.g., numbness, clumsiness of the hands) have been reported. A water-soluble vitamin, B_6 is rapidly excreted in the urine.

RECOMMENDED DAILY ALLOWANCES. RDA is 0.1 mg/day for infants 0 to 6 months, 0.3 mg/day for infants 7 to 12 months, 0.5 mg/day for children 1 to 3 years, 0.6 mg for children 4 to 8 years, and 1 mg/day for children 9 to 13 years. Men should take 1.3 mg/day between the ages of 14 and 50, and the dose then should be increased to 1.7 mg/day throughout the rest of their lives. Women should take 1.2 mg/day from ages 14 to 18 years and 1.3 mg/day from 19 to 50 years; the dose then should be increased to 1.5 mg/day for the rest of their lives. During pregnancy, the dose should be 1.9 mg/day, and during lactation, 2 mg/day.

Vitamin B_12 (Cobalamin)

DEFICIENCY. Vitamin B_{12} deficiency can be caused by inadequate B_{12} intake or by lack of "intrinsic factor" in the gut, which helps to absorb vitamin B_{12} from foods. Any disruption of GI architecture (by surgery or disease) inhibits absorption, as does the development of antibodies to intrinsic factor or inheriting a disease that affects intrinsic factor formation or function.

The "classic" symptom of B_{12} deficiency is pernicious (or megaloblastic) anemia. Other deficiency problems include peripheral nervous system changes (numbness, tingling, ataxia), central nervous system changes (moodiness, confusion, agitation, delusions, hallucinations, and eventually, psychosis), and GI problems (loss of appetite, nausea, vomiting).

This deficiency often is found in geriatric populations and frequently is related to loss of intrinsic factor. The need for supplementation is increased by an increase in metabolic rate (hyperthyroidism), by GI tract disease, and by pregnancy. Because B_{12} is found in animal fat, vegetarians become deficient unless they supplement their diets. If B_{12} deficiency is caused by lack of intrinsic factor, then intrinsic factor must be replaced by injection.

A more common cause of deficiency often is diagnosed in older people who have difficulty absorbing vitamin B_{12} from unfortified foods; such individuals, however, typically can absorb vitamin B_{12} from fortified foods or supplements, providing yet another reason to take a multivitamin.

TOXICITY. Although B_{12} is stored in the liver in significant quantities, excretion of excess vitamin B_{12} is rapid, and symptoms of toxicity are not seen. Synthetic B_{12} (with its cyanide component) can be toxic and should be administered judiciously.

RECOMMENDED DAILY ALLOWANCES. RDA is 0.4 mcg/day for infants 0 to 6 months, 0.5 mcg/day for infants 7 to 12 months, 0.9 mcg/day for children 1 to 3 years, 1.2 mcg/day for children 4 to 8 years, and 1.8 mcg/day for children 9 to 13 years. Men and women should take 2.4 mcg/day for the rest of their lives. Dosage increases to 2.6 mcg/day during pregnancy and to 2.8 mcg/day during lactation.

Folacin (Folic Acid)

In addition to recycling homocysteine, folate plays a key role in building DNA, the complex compound that forms our genetic blueprint. Observational studies show that people who get higher than average amounts of folic acid from their diet or from supplements have lower risks of colon cancer and breast cancer. This could be especially important for those who drink alcohol because alcohol blocks the absorption of folic acid and inactivates circulating folate. An interesting observation from the Nurses' Health Study is that high intake of folic acid blunts the increased risk of breast cancer seen among women who have more than one alcoholic drink a day. A randomized, placebo-controlled trial has shown that daily folic acid significantly improves cognitive performance in older adults, specifically as it relates to memory and information processing. The relative reduction in homocysteine associated with folate treatment, especially when used to fortify wheat in bread may be associated by reduced risks of stroke although additional research is required to confirm this.

DEFICIENCY. Folic acid deficiency is one of the most common deficiencies in humans, and the symptoms are similar to B$_{12}$ deficiency. Intake of folic acid may disguise the symptoms of B$_{12}$ deficiency, so it may be important for the clinician to determine the patient's level of B$_{12}$ before treating him or her for folate deficiency.

Megaloblastic anemia is a worrisome complication. This deficiency is seen in pregnancy and often occurs during the third trimester. If megaloblastic anemia is present before conception, fetal neural tube defects such as spina bifida and anencephaly may result. Inadequate folic acid consumption (which also can occur without megaloblastic anemia) can lead to open neural tube defects. Inadequate folic acid intake will be evident in serum in as little as 1 month, and red blood cell and liver stores will be depleted in less than 3 months.

Deficiencies can result from inadequate intake, defective absorption, or abnormal metabolism.

TOXICITY. Even though folic acid is water soluble, symptoms of toxicity have occurred; the most severe among these is permanent nerve damage. Folic acid concentrations are restricted in OTC preparations to guard against inadvertent toxicity.

RECOMMENDED DAILY ALLOWANCES. RDA is 65 mcg/day for infants 0 to 6 months, 80 mcg/day for infants 7 to 12 months, 150 mcg/day for children 1 to 3 years, 200 mcg/day for children 4 to 8 years, and 300 mcg/day for children 9 to 13 years. Men and women should take 400 mcg/day for the rest of their lives. The dosage increases to 600 to 800/mcg per day during pregnancy and to 500 mcg/day during lactation.

Sufficient folic acid—at least 400 mcg a day—is not always easy to obtain from food. This is why women of child-bearing age are urged to take extra folic acid. This is also why the FDA now requires that folic acid be added to most enriched bread, flour, cornmeal, pasta, rice, and other grain products, along with the iron and other micronutrients that have been added for years.

Biotin

DEFICIENCY. Biotin deficiency is rare but can be induced by consuming large quantities of raw egg white. Avidin, a compound in egg white, binds with biotin and inhibits absorption. Symptoms include nonpruritic dermatitis, hypercholesterolemia, ECG changes, anemia, anorexia, nausea, fatigue, and muscle pain. Simply cooking the egg white destroys avidin.

Young infants can develop a biotin deficiency from poor absorption and can exhibit similar symptoms. Treatment with biotin provides prompt resolution of symptoms.

TOXICITY. Large doses of biotin have not produced any toxicity symptoms. Because of the water-soluble nature of this nutrient, it is easily excreted when taken in excess.

RECOMMENDED DAILY ALLOWANCES. RDA is 5 mcg/day for infants 0 to 6 months, 6 mcg/day for infants 7 to 12 months, 8 mcg/day for children 1 to 3 years, 12 mcg/day for children 4 to 8 years, 20 mcg/day for children 9 to 13 years, and 25 mcg/day for youth 14 to 18 years. Adults should take 30 mcg/day for the rest of their lives, including during pregnancy. Dosage increases to 35 mcg/day during lactation.

Pantothenic Acid (B$_5$, Pantetheine)

This B vitamin can be produced synthetically and is available in an injectable form.

DEFICIENCY. Deficiency of pantothenic acid has not been seen in humans because it is so readily available in food sources.

TOXICITY. Megadoses may cause GI upset (diarrhea), but no other toxicities have been reported. Because it is water soluble, pantothenic acid is readily excreted when ingested in excessive amounts.

RECOMMENDED DAILY ALLOWANCES. RDA is 1.7 mg/day for infants 0 to 6 months, 1.8 mg/day for infants 7 to 12 months, 2 mg/day for children 1 to 3 years, 3 mg/day for children 4 to 8 years, and 4 mg for children 9 to 13 years. Men and women should take 5 mg/day for the rest of their lives. Dosage increases to 6 mg/day during pregnancy and to 7 mg/day during lactation.

Vitamin C (Ascorbic Acid)

Vitamin C is a fragile vitamin that is readily destroyed by heat or exposure to air or to alkalis. It is the most common antioxidant found in vegetables and citrus fruits and is considered important in repairing damage caused by free radicals and in preventing them from becoming cancerous or accelerating the aging process. There is no question that vitamin C plays a role in controlling infection. It is also a powerful antioxidant that can neutralize harmful free radicals, and it helps to make collagen, a tissue needed for healthy bones, teeth, gums, and blood vessels. Although research has not confirmed that vitamin C prevents colds in most people, it does seem to prevent colds in select populations, such as individuals under heavy short-term physical stress.

DEFICIENCY. Vitamin C deficiency is called *scurvy*. Symptoms are related to a breakdown in or lack of repair of collagenous tissue, which causes muscle weakness, bleeding/swollen gums, tooth loss, rough skin, delayed wound healing, anemia, fatigue, and depression. This condition is not widespread in the United States but is still seen in some populations and should be considered when a person presents with these symptoms.

Children are at high risk for permanent damage when vitamin C deficiency persists. Damage to the epiphyseal junctions and thinning of the jawbone (causing loose teeth, spongy gums, and resorption of dentine) are among the most disturbing problems seen in children.

Some diseases and illnesses that affect collagen should be treated with vitamin C to facilitate healing. These include infections, burns, trauma, surgery, congestive heart failure, renal and hepatic disease, GI tract problems (e.g., gastroenteritis, diarrhea), and malignancies.

Low levels of vitamin C in the blood seem to be correlated with a higher incidence of clinical gallbladder disease. Individuals with higher levels of vitamin C have a significantly reduced risk of stroke.

TOXICITY. Because vitamin C is water soluble, it is easily excreted, up to a point. Once this renal "saturation point" has been reached, mild symptoms of toxicity have been seen. GI tract disturbances (e.g., diarrhea, nausea, vomiting, stomach cramps), facial flushing, headaches, dizziness, and faintness have all been reported.

RECOMMENDED DAILY ALLOWANCES. RDA is 40 mg/day for infants 0 to 6 months, 50 mg/day for infants 7 to 12 months, 15 mg/day for children 1 to 3 years, 25 mg/day for children 4 to 8 years, and 45 mg/day for children 9 to 13 years. Men should take 75 mg/day between the ages of 14 and 18 years, and then 90 mg/day for the rest of their lives. Women should take 65 mg/day between the ages of 14 and 18 years, and then 75 mg/day for the rest of their lives. The dose increases to 80 to 85 mg/day during pregnancy and to 115 to 120 mg/day during lactation.

As evidence continues to unfold, 200 to 300 mg of vitamin C a day appears to be a good target. This is easy to hit with a good diet and a standard multivitamin. Excellent food sources of vitamin C include citrus fruits or citrus juices, berries, green and red peppers, tomatoes, broccoli, and spinach. Many breakfast cereals are fortified with vitamin C.

MINERALS

Calcium

Calcium, the most abundant mineral in the human body, is found in the bone. Only 1% of the body's calcium supply is found outside the bony skeleton, but this 1% is critical for nerve transmission, muscle contraction, and blood clotting, to name only a few other roles. Other minerals such as magnesium, sodium, phosphorus, strontium, carbonate, and citrate combine with calcium to form the complete bone matrix. Calcium supplements have been shown to help maintain bone density. However, bone loss associated with aging climbs to pretherapy levels if calcium supplementation is discontinued. The calcium supplement formulation calcium citrate is 2.5 times more bioavailable than calcium carbonate, challenging the misperception that all calcium supplements are equal; however, only 20% of calcium as citrate is absorbed, along with 40% of calcium as carbonate. Calcium supplementation has been shown in randomized trials to decrease the risk of recurrence of colorectal adenoma, and calcium and vitamin D together may reduce the incidence of breast cancer. A new study has shown that calcium supplementation might increase vascular events in elderly women. The findings are somewhat unexpected, because previous trials have shown that calcium improves blood cholesterol levels. Further research is required.

DEFICIENCY. Calcium deficiency can occur at any time in life, although in the United States today, it is usually a disease of aging. Recent studies suggest that the amount of calcium an individual consumes may have an impact on the development of such diseases as hypertension and colon cancer. Decreased calcium levels definitely contribute to the development of osteoporosis. Yet the health benefits of taking calcium depend on the body's ability to absorb it, which may vary greatly among individuals. Large amounts of caffeine and protein and megadoses of vitamin A all decrease calcium absorption. Some individuals are lactose intolerant, making it difficult for them to use milk as a calcium source. Independent predictors of calcium absorption include dietary fat, fiber, alcohol intake, and serum concentrations of vitamin D. In particular, the amount of dietary fat consumed in relation to dietary fiber appears to play an important role in determining differences in calcium absorption. Fat may increase absorption of calcium by slowing its transit time through the intestines and by allowing longer contact with the absorptive surface.

If children have inadequate calcium intake, soft bones and weak teeth result. Adults who are deficient in calcium have a condition called *osteoporosis*. It has been seen in young adults who have certain diseases or are on certain medications (systemic steroids), but the most common osteoporosis sufferers are the postmenopausal woman and the elderly male. Bone density increases in childhood and young adulthood, peaking during the mid 20s. Very little new bone is laid down in the 30s and 40s, and with the onset of menopause and loss of estrogen from the circulation, women's bone densities plummet for 5 to 10 years before assuming a more gradual downward slope. If the postmenopausal woman had inadequate calcium intake, excessive calcium use (with multiple pregnancies), or a concomitant disease requiring systemic steroids during the bone-building years, bones could become dangerously fragile within the first few years after menopause.

Vitamin D is essential for calcium utilization. Even in the presence of adequate calcium intake, osteoporosis can result from vitamin D deficiency. The FDA has proposed a new health claim for foods and dietary supplements containing calcium plus vitamin D that would allow manufacturers to advertise their potential to reduce the risk for osteoporosis.

Calcium absorption is affected by need. If body requirements are low, calcium absorption from the gut will drop. During periods of increased calcium requirement (growth, pregnancy, or lactation), absorption from the intestinal tract increases markedly. Excretion of calcium from the gut and from the kidney, however, remains nearly constant, so a net negative calcium effect may be seen. Daily calcium intake of up to 700 mg may significantly reduce an individual's risk of distal colon cancer; 600 mg calcium from food or supplements lowers the risk of stroke in women by one third, probably by reducing cholesterol and possibly by inhibiting clot formation. Recommended amounts for individuals are based on the calculation of elemental Ca^{++} and must take into account the type of Ca^{++} used. Thus, the provider should calculate the exact amount needed by the individual for adequate supplementation.

Calcium interacts with phosphorus in attempting to maintain a phosphorus/calcium ratio of 1:1 or 1:1.5. The average American diet, however, provides two parts phosphorus/one part calcium daily, and the body compensates by excreting excess phosphorus. Unfortunately, calcium is always attached to the phosphorus, further decreasing body calcium levels. The body responds by pulling more calcium from storage; this process demineralizes the bones further.

Foods high in phosphorus include soda (regular and diet), processed foods, eggs, meat, and peanuts.

TOXICITY. Normally, calcium toxicity does not occur despite high oral intake of calcium. However, in the presence of other mineral imbalances, such as magnesium deficiency, soft tissue calcification can occur. Some disease states cause hypercalcemia and renal stones, but these seem to be related to internal management of calcium sources and not to excess intake.

RECOMMENDED DAILY ALLOWANCES. RDA is 210 mg/day for infants 0 to 6 months, 270 mg/day for children 7 to 12 months, 600 mg for children 1 to 3 years, 800 mg for children 4 to 8 years, and 1300 mg/day for youth 9 to 18 years. Both men and women should take 1000 mg/day between 19 and 50 years and should increase dosage to 1200 mg/day after age 51 and for the rest of their lives. Calcium requirements during pregnancy and lactation range from 1000 to 1300 mg/day, with younger women requiring more calcium during pregnancy and lactation. These recommendations are controversial because research undertaken to examine the amount of calcium required to balance that which is excreted suggests that less calcium should be taken per day.

Chromium

Chromium is a trace mineral, with serum containing only 20 parts per billion.

DEFICIENCY. The short-term symptoms of chromium deficiency are those of glucose intolerance; they include hypoglycemia and mood swings associated with rapid and large swings in blood glucose levels, especially after carbohydrate-rich meals. This is especially important if the carbohydrates involved have a high glycemic index. Over a longer term, the expected problems are those associated with diabetes, which is an almost inevitable consequence of chromium deficiency. High blood pressure, heart disease, stroke, and obesity all may occur. Symptoms are reversible when chromium is provided in the diet or in supplements.

TOXICITY. Chromium toxicity can occur. Excessive amounts can reverse the beneficial effects and actually cause a decrease in insulin activity.

RECOMMENDED DAILY ALLOWANCES. RDA is 0.2 mcg/day for infants 0 to 6 months, 5.5 mcg/day for infants 7 to 12 months, 11 mcg/day for children 1 to 3 years, 15 mcg/day for children 4 to 8 years, 25 mcg/day for boys 9 to 13 years, and 21 mcg/day for girls 9 to 13 years. Men require 35 mcg/day between the ages of 14 and 50 years and then should take 30 mcg/day for the rest of their lives. Women 14 to 18 years should take 24 mcg/day and should increase the dose to 25 mcg/day between ages 19 and 50 years, at which time the dose drops to 20 mcg/day for the rest of their lives. During pregnancy, the dose is 29 to 30 mcg/day, and during lactation, it increases to 44 to 45 mcg/day.

Cobalt

DEFICIENCY. This deficiency is identical to vitamin B_{12} deficiency.

TOXICITY. If excessive amounts of cobalt are ingested, polycythemia will develop because of the stimulating effect of cobalt on erythropoietin. This can lead to congestive heart failure in some individuals. Pericardial effusion, thyroid hyperplasia, and neurologic disorders also have been reported.

RECOMMENDED DAILY ALLOWANCES. Cobalt is a trace element; no RDAs are available.

Copper

Copper is another trace mineral that is found in almost all body tissues, although it is concentrated in the brain and liver.

DEFICIENCY. Clinical deficiency is rare but does occur in some disease states (kwashiorkor, chronic diarrhea), whereas subclinical deficiency is much more common and usually results from inadequate intake. Symptoms include anemia, collagen disorders, and nervous system conduction problems.

TOXICITY. Copper is toxic in large doses. Wilson's disease (genetically inherited) is a disease of excessive tissue copper and inadequate serum copper. Irreversible liver, kidney, and brain damage will result, along with nervous system damage and blindness, unless copper levels are lowered. Mild copper toxicity by ingestion usually leads to GI symptoms, headache, dizziness, weakness, and a copper taste in the mouth, whereas extreme toxicity can result in tachycardia, hypertension, jaundice, coma, and death.

RECOMMENDED DAILY ALLOWANCES. RDA is 200 mcg/day for infants 0 to 6 months, 220 mcg/day for infants 7 to 12 months, 340 mcg/day for children 1 to 3 years, 440 mcg/day for children 4 to 8 years, 700 mcg/day for children 9 to 13 years, 890 mcg/day for youth 14 to 18 years, and 900 mcg/day for men and women for the rest of their lives. The dose goes to 1000 mcg/day during pregnancy and to 1300 mcg/day during lactation.

Fluoride

An increasing number of townships and cities now add fluoride to their water supply, thus decreasing the need for fluoride supplementation in those areas. The American Academy of Pediatrics has issued recommendations on the use of fluoride supplementation in infants and children that are updated as new information becomes available.

DEFICIENCY. Deficiency was common until water began to be fluoridated, but the only symptom appeared to be weak dental structures and a marked increase in cavities.

TOXICITY. Fluoride toxicity can be significant and usually results from unusually high doses given over prolonged periods. A one-time dose 2500 times the RDA can be fatal but is rarely seen.

RECOMMENDED DAILY ALLOWANCES. RDA is 0.01 mg/day for infants 0 to 6 months, 0.5 mg/day for infants 7 to 12 months, 0.7 mg/day for children 1 to 3 years, 1 mg/day for children 4 to 8 years, 2 mg/day for children 9 to 13 years, 3 mg/day for boys 14 to 18 years, and then 4 mg/day for the rest of their lives. Women should have 3 mg/day beginning at age 14 and for the rest of their lives, including during pregnancy and lactation.

Iodine

Iodine, a trace mineral, is found in most parts of the body, with 50% in muscles, 7% in bones, 20% in the thyroid gland, 10% in the skin, and 13% in endocrine glands.

DEFICIENCY. Goiter, the classic symptom of iodine deficiency, can appear after several months of inadequate iodine intake. This enlargement of the thyroid gland is most often seen in areas of the world where the diet is iodine deficient. Although iodine deficiency was not common in the United States, it is on the rise here. The first National Health and Nutrition Examination Survey (NHANES I), which took place between 1971 and 1974, found that just 2.6% of U.S. citizens had iodine deficiency. The follow-up NHANES III survey, conducted between 1988 and 1994, found that 11.7% of citizens are iodine deficient. The October 1998 issue of the *Journal of Clinical Endocrinology and Metabolism* reported that over the previous 20 years, the percentage of Americans with low intake of iodine had more than quadrupled. Of particular concern is the fact that the percentage of iodine-deficient pregnant women has increased from 1% in 1974 to 7% in 1994. Maternal iodine deficiency is particularly dangerous to a developing fetus. Researchers have not identified a cause for the drop in iodine levels, although it is suspected that reduced salt in the diet, plus a reduction in the use of iodine as a food ingredient, may be responsible. This trend may necessitate concerted efforts to increase iodine levels in persons at risk of deficiency even in the United States.

The pituitary gland in the brain responds to a decrease in thyroid hormone and sends a signal to the thyroid gland—thyroid-stimulating hormone (TSH)—to produce more. If no iodine is available to make thyroid hormone, the gland is unable to secrete adequate amounts. The pituitary gland signals the thyroid with ever-increasing amounts of TSH, and over time, the thyroid grows larger, forming a goiter.

Iodine deficiency in pregnancy can be dangerous to a forming fetus. A condition called *cretinism* can result, with serious effects such as poorly formed bones, weak muscles, and severe mental retardation. Widespread use of iodized salt has substantially reduced the incidence of goiter.

TOXICITY. Iodine toxicity usually is not a problem for someone with a normal thyroid gland.

RECOMMENDED DAILY ALLOWANCES. RDA is 110 mcg/day for infants 0 to 6 months, 130 mcg/day for infants 7 to 12 months, 90 mcg/day for children 1 to 8 years, 120 mcg/day for children 9 to 13 years, and 150 mcg/day for adults for the rest of their lives. During pregnancy, the dose should be increased to 220 mcg/day and during lactation, to 290 mcg/day.

Iron (in Hemoglobin, Transferrin, and Ferritin)

Iron is available as a "recycled" mineral or is taken in the diet. Once taken in, iron is stored in the liver, spleen, and bone marrow, close to the sources of hemoglobin production. During pregnancy or as a result of chronic blood loss (menstruation, slow GI bleed), iron stores can be depleted at a rate of 10 to 40 mg/day. However, during pregnancy, the absorp-

tion of Fe^+ increases to 15% as the body's way of adapting to physiologic anemia of pregnancy. Iron supplementation has been found to provide relief for persons with angiotensin-converting enzyme inhibitor–induced dry cough, according to some research.

DEFICIENCY. Iron deficiency causes the most common form of anemia. Symptoms of anemia demonstrate the importance of oxygen to all living cells. Anemia causes dizziness, headache, drowsiness, fatigue, irritability, heart enlargement, and spoon-shaped nails.

Although anyone can be iron deficient, populations at highest risk for iron deficiency anemia include women of reproductive age, pregnant women, young children, the elderly, low-income populations, and any culture or individual whose diet may be low in meat.

TOXICITY. The body has no effective way to get rid of excess iron. Because the physiologic system is designed to recycle this mineral, iron toxicity is potentially fatal. Populations at risk include (1) young children who poison themselves with iron-fortified children's vitamins or their mother's iron-fortified vitamins (usually prescribed for pregnancy), (2) persons with hereditary hemochromatosis, who have a genetic condition that results in no excretion of iron, (3) alcoholics with chronic liver disease or pancreatitis (who have abnormally high iron absorption), and (4) elderly individuals who take iron-fortified vitamins needlessly.

RECOMMENDED DAILY ALLOWANCES. RDA is 0.27 mg/day for infants 0 to 6 months, 11 mg/day for infants 7 to 12 months, 7 mg/day for children 1 to 3 years, 10 mg/day for children 4 to 8 years, 8 mg/day for children 9 to 13 years, 11 mg/day for boys 14 to 18 years, and then 8 mg/day for the rest of their lives. Women should take 15 mg/day between 14 and 18 years, 18 mg/day between 19 and 30 years, and 8 mg/day for the rest of their lives. During pregnancy, the dose is increased to 27 mg/day, and during lactation, to between 9 and 10 mg/day. Do not take calcium with iron because the two products may bind and interfere with drug absorption.

Magnesium

Magnesium, which is considered a major mineral, accounts for only 1.75 oz in a 130-pound person. Bones contain 60% of the body's magnesium, with 27% found in muscle and serum containing only 3%. Only about 30% of dietary magnesium is absorbed, and this absorption is dependent on several intestinal factors, as well as on the presence or absence of dietary fat and other compounds that bind magnesium. Magnesium is a common ingredient in laxatives and antacids. Although the laxative action of magnesium is thought to be due to a local effect within the intestinal tract, it is also possible that released hormones such as cholecystokinin or activation of constitutive nitric oxide synthase might contribute to this pharmacologic effect. Magnesium may be given intravenously for suppression of ventricular ectopy, and in asthma or chronic lung disease when conventional treatment has failed. It may also have a role in the prevention and treatment of migraine or other primary headache disorders.

DEFICIENCY. Because magnesium is so important in cellular metabolism (moving sodium and potassium across the membrane), magnesium deficiency is most visible in the cardiovascular, neuromuscular, and renal systems. Symptoms of mild magnesium deficiency include mental status changes (confusion, personality changes, lack of coordination), GI tract problems (nausea, anorexia, vomiting), and musculoskeletal problems (weakness, muscle tremor). As deficiency worsens, more symptoms appear, such as tetany, bizarre muscle movements, dermatologic problems (alopecia, skin lesions), and cardiovascular changes (myocardial necrosis and lesions of the small arteries).

TOXICITY. Magnesium toxicity is rare because the kidneys are efficient at excreting excessive amounts of the mineral. Toxicity may occur in geriatric persons with renal insufficiency who use large quantities of milk of magnesia. When toxicity is acute, the symptoms can be dramatic and require immediate treatment. Symptoms include severe nausea and vomiting, extreme muscle weakness, occasionally progressing to paralysis, and difficulty breathing that may eventually lead to coma and death.

RECOMMENDED DAILY ALLOWANCES. RDA is 30 mg/day for infants 0 to 6 months, 75 mg/day for infants 7 to 12 months, 80 mg/day for children 1 to 3 years, 130 mg/day for children 4 to 8 years, and 240 mg/day for children 9 to 13 years. Boys 14 to 18 years should take 410 mg/day, which should be decreased to 400 mg/day between the ages of 19 and 30 years, and increased to 420 mg/day for the rest of their lives. Women should take 360 mg/day between the ages of 14 and 18 years, 310 mg/day between 19 and 30 years, and 320 mg/day for the rest of their lives. The dose should be changed to 350 to 400 mg/day during pregnancy and to 310 to 360 mg/day during lactation. Younger women should take higher doses.

Manganese

Manganese is another mineral that is present in only trace amounts and is concentrated in specific organs. It is found in measurable amounts only in the pituitary gland, liver, pancreas, kidney, intestinal mucosa, and bones. Little manganese is stored in the body. Total manganese does not usually measure more than 20 mg at any one time, and this mineral is excreted primarily through the bowel (via feces and bile). Little manganese is renally cleared.

DEFICIENCY. Deficiency has not been reported in humans, primarily because other minerals take over the biochemical roles that manganese usually plays. This could theoretically cause other types of nutrient deficiency, or more likely, could make other deficiencies worse.

TOXICITY. Manganese toxicity is possible because this mineral is not quickly excreted. Symptoms of toxicity include iron deficiency anemia (manganese interferes with iron absorption), depression, insomnia, impotence, leg cramps, headache, and speech impairment. In significant toxicity states, symptoms can resemble Parkinson's disease or viral encephalitis, with flat facial expression, muscle rigidity and spasms, and delusions or hallucinations.

RECOMMENDED DAILY ALLOWANCES. RDA is 0.003 mg/day for infants 0 to 6 months, 0.6 mg/day for infants 7 to 12 months,

1.2 mg/day for children 1 to 3 years, 1.5 mg/day for children 4 to 8 years, 1.9 mg/day for boys 9 to 13 years, and 2.2 mg/day for boys 14 to 18 years 2.3 mg/day is required for men for the rest of their lives. For women, RDA is 1.6 mg/day for girls between 9 and 18 years, then, 1.8 mg/day is required for the rest of their lives. During pregnancy, the dose increases to 2 mg/day, and during lactation, to 2.6 mg/day.

Molybdenum

Another trace mineral, molybdenum is found primarily in the liver and kidney, with small amounts noted in other body tissues (muscle, bone, brain, lung, and spleen).

DEFICIENCY. Molybdenum deficiency is both rare and mild. The effects of deficiency are seen in the blood (anemia) and in the teeth (decay). No other physiologic symptoms are observed.

TOXICITY. Toxicity is possible with molybdenum because, as for most minerals, excretion is slow and body requirements are low. Symptoms of excessive molybdenum intake include gout symptoms (painful, swollen joints), growth retardation and weight loss (especially in children), and copper deficiency (because molybdenum and copper compete for the same receptor sites in the intestine).

RECOMMENDED DAILY ALLOWANCES. RDA is 2 mcg/day for infants 0 to 6 months, 3 mcg/day for infants 7 to 12 months, 17 mcg/day for children 1 to 3 years, 22 mcg/day for children 4 to 8 years, and 34 mcg/day for children 9 to 13 years. For men and women, 43 mcg/day is required for youth 14 to 18 years, and then 45 mcg/day for the rest of their lives. During pregnancy and lactation, the rate is 50 mcg/day.

Phosphorus (Calcium Phosphate and Phosphoric Acid)

Phosphorus is a major mineral, second only to calcium in body requirements. Phosphorus and calcium are linked, that is, a decrease in one mineral causes a concomitant decrease in the other, as the kidney attempts to maintain a stable calcium/phosphorus ratio.

DEFICIENCY. Deficiency of phosphorus is not common because of the abundance of phosphorus in the American diet. Intake of phosphorus is almost universally higher than that of calcium, making the calcium/phosphorus ratio difficult to maintain, and possibly contributing to calcium deficiency syndromes and diseases (like osteoporosis).

TOXICITY. Because the kidneys closely regulate serum levels of phosphorus and calcium, phosphorous toxicity is uncommon, and direct symptoms are unlikely. The single largest problem that results from excess phosphorous intake is an imbalance in the calcium/phosphorus ratio.

RECOMMENDED DAILY ALLOWANCES. RDA is 100 mg/day for infants 0 to 6 months, 275 mg/day for infants 7 to 12 months, 460 mg/day for children 1 to 3 years, and 500 mg/day for children 4 to 8 years. The dose increases to 1250 mg/day for youth 9 to 18 years and then changes to 700 mg/day for the rest of their lives. During pregnancy and lactation, the rate is 700 mg/day, unless the woman is between 14 and 18 years, in which case the dosage should be 1250 mg/day.

Potassium

Potassium is a key cellular constituent involved in cellular metabolism, muscle contraction, and nerve conduction. Almost all body stores of this mineral are intracellular, creating a large concentration gradient across cell membranes.

DEFICIENCY. It is relatively easy to develop a potassium deficiency. Common causes include diuretic therapy, trauma (burns in particular), starvation, bulimia, gastroenteritis (especially with diarrhea and vomiting), and diabetic acidosis.

Symptoms of deficiency range from mild muscle weakness, impaired growth, bone fragility, and mental status changes to severe paralysis, decreased heart rate, and death.

TOXICITY. Potassium toxicity can be deadly, with symptoms ranging from confusion, fatigue, and intestinal tract changes to irregular or rapid heart rate, dropping blood pressure, and paralysis of arms and legs. Convulsions, coma, and cardiac arrest often occur before death.

Toxicity can be caused by excessive potassium supplement intake or by sudden increases in dietary potassium (as when switching to a salt substitute such as potassium chloride and using it excessively). Other medical conditions such as acute or chronic renal failure, adrenal insufficiency, severe acidosis (respiratory or metabolic), or systemic infection can cause potassium excesses.

RECOMMENDED DAILY ALLOWANCES. RDA is 0.4 g/day for infants 0 to 6 months, 0.7 g/day for infants 7 to 12 months, 3 g/day for children 1 to 3 years, 3.8 g/day for children 4 to 7 years, 4.5 g/day for children 9 to 13 years, and 4.7 g/day for individuals of both sexes for the rest of their lives, including during pregnancy. The dose is increased to 5.1 g/day during lactation.

Selenium

Selenium is a trace mineral that is closely related to sulfur in its behavior. It is found in higher concentrations in the kidney, heart, spleen, and liver but is present in all body tissues except fat. This mineral helps to protect the body from cancers, including skin cancer caused by sun exposure. It also preserves tissue elasticity and slows down the hardening of tissues associated with oxidation. Dietary sources of this mineral include whole grain cereals, seafood, garlic, and eggs.

DEFICIENCY. Selenium and vitamin E deficiencies often look alike, but selective selenium deficiencies have been seen, and the results can be devastating. In areas of the world that have poor selenium levels in soil, cardiomyopathy with resultant heart-related death has been seen, along with an increased risk of cancer death.

TOXICITY. Both the kidney and the lung excrete selenium, but toxicities have occurred. Individuals exposed to high selenium levels who are working in industrial settings have higher incidences of liver disease and cardiomyopathy. Persons who are exposed more gradually (from foods grown in selenium-rich soil) experience milder symptoms, such as dental decay, hair loss, fatigue, and occasionally paralysis.

RECOMMENDED DAILY ALLOWANCES. RDA is 15 mcg/day for infants 0 to 6 months, 20 mcg/day for infants 7 to 12 months, 20 mcg/day for children 1 to 3 years, 30 mcg/day for children 4 to 7 years, 40 mcg/day for children 9 to 13 years, and 55 mcg/day for men and women for the rest of their lives. During pregnancy, the dose is increased to 60 mcg/day, and during lactation, to 70 mcg/day.

Sodium

Sodium is essential in nerve conduction and cellular function; it accounts for 0.15% of body weight and is found in every cell of the body. Different from potassium, sodium is concentrated primarily in extracellular fluid, again creating a concentration gradient.

DEFICIENCY. Sodium deficiency is rare, and when it occurs, it is strongly associated with abnormalities in water management. Both dehydration and excess water intake cause a sodium imbalance. (Dehydration causes direct sodium loss, and water intoxication dilutes the normal serum sodium content.) Sodium deficiency is seen with diuretic use, starvation, GI tract problems (vomiting, diarrhea), profuse sweating, and excessive water intake.

Symptoms of sodium deficiency include muscle weakness, mental status changes, acidosis, and tissue atrophy.

TOXICITY. Sodium toxicity results in excessive water retention. If too much water is retained, edema and adverse cardiovascular effects such as hypertension, dizziness, stupor, and possibly coma are seen.

RECOMMENDED DAILY ALLOWANCES. RDA is 0.12 g/day for infants 0 to 6 months, 0.37 g/day for infants 7 to 12 months, 1 g/day for children 1 to 3 years, 1.2 g/day for children 4 to 8 years, 1.5 g/day for adults 9 to 50 years, 1.3 g/day for adults 50 to 70 years, and then 1.2 g/day for adults older than age 70. The dose of 1.5 g/day should continue during pregnancy and lactation. These recommendations are more restrictive than the USDA's 2005 Dietary Guidelines, which cite a maximum of 5 g of sodium per day.

Sulfur

Sulfur composes almost 0.25% of total body weight.

DEFICIENCY. Deficiency symptoms are unknown, although it is theoretically possible for deficiencies to develop.

TOXICITY. Sulfur toxicity has not been reported, and ingestion of excessive amounts has not been shown to be dangerous.

RECOMMENDED DAILY ALLOWANCES. None are posted.

Zinc

Zinc is a trace mineral that is present in only tiny amounts (2 to 3 g total). Zinc supplements are frequently ordered to aid in wound healing. Zinc is found in many foods that are part of a normal diet, including fortified cereals, meat, poultry, and whole grains. Anyone who is considering taking a zinc supplement should first consider whether his or her needs could be met through these dietary zinc sources.

DEFICIENCY. Because of the many roles that zinc plays in cellular integrity and defense, deficiency can produce widespread changes in skin and hair, growth retardation, anemia, poor wound healing, lethargy, and sterility.

Causes of zinc deficiency include poor dietary intake (especially protein-calorie malnutrition), acute or chronic infection (lots of zinc being used up), alcoholism and liver cirrhosis, renal disease, and malignancy. Populations at risk for zinc deficiency include children, pregnant women, hospitalized persons, low-income persons, elderly persons, athletes (increased loss through sweat), and strict vegetarians.

Zinc is critical in pregnancy for normal fetal growth and development. Inadequate zinc levels during pregnancy can cause congenital malformations (including changes in skeletal, brain, heart, GI tract, eye, and lung tissues) and growth retardation.

TOXICITY. Zinc toxicity is rare, and high zinc doses are required to produce toxic symptoms. The upper tolerable recommended dose of oral zinc in adults is 40 mg/day; higher levels have been associated with a decrease in copper absorption, resulting in anemia. Intranasal zinc may be associated with anosmia, and caution is recommended in its use. Chronic intake of zinc at levels over 450 mg daily can cause sideroblastic anemia; a 10 to 30 g intake of zinc sulfate can be lethal in adults. Toxic symptoms may include GI tract problems (nausea and vomiting), mental status changes (drowsiness, sluggishness, lightheadedness, and restlessness), and muscle coordination problems (difficulty writing or walking).

RECOMMENDED DAILY ALLOWANCES. RDA is 2 mg/day for infants 0 to 6 months, 3 mg/day for infants 7 to 12 months and up to 3 years, 5 mg/day for children 4 to 8 years, and 8 mg/day for children 9 to 13 years. Men should then have 11 mg/day for the rest of their lives. Women should have 8 mg/day for the rest of their lives. Dose increases to 11 to 12 mg/day during pregnancy and to 12 to 13 mg/day during lactation are combined with the higher doses given to younger women.

evolve A continually updated list of useful WebLinks may be found in the Evolve Resources at http://evolve.elsevier.com/Edmunds/NP/

73   Over-the-Counter Medications

Nonprescription medications or OTC medications are defined as drugs that are considered to be safe and effective without professional supervision, provided the required label directions and warnings are followed.

In general, consumers today are more educated about health treatment recommendations and are more likely to pursue OTC medications than ever before. Over-the-counter medications were a booming business in the United States in 2007, with Americans spending $17.8 billion on nonprescription remedies. Since 1976, 80 ingredients, dosages, or indications have been considered safe enough to be "switched" from prescription to OTC status (Consumer Health Care Products Association, 2006). Over-the-counter medicines are real drugs for real problems, and they augment prescriptions to improve well-being or treat maladies and illnesses.

EXTENT OF OTC MEDICATION USE

The OTC business in the United States is so large that it has been reported that people would rather choose a new car than be faced with the task of determining which OTC they should buy for a particular ailment (Consumer Health Care Products Association, 2006). The role of OTCs in today's health care market is growing because of the following: (1) a high number of uninsured who seek to treat themselves, (2) a more educated consumer, and (3) an active self-care movement.

The Nonprescription Drug Manufacturers Association (NDMA) estimates that more than 100,000 products now are available on an OTC basis—200 of these once were available only by prescription. These products contain one or more of about 700 active ingredients and are available in a variety of dosage forms, sizes, and strengths. OTC sales total more than $20 billion a year. The top-selling categories of OTCs include cough/cold remedies and headache remedies. It has been estimated that 77% of Americans take OTC medicines to treat common everyday ailments, with adults 65 years and older consuming 33% of all OTC medicines sold in the United States (Consumer Health Care Products Association, 2006).

In recent research on medications in nursing homes (Simoni-Wastila et al, 2006), study subjects were found to be high users of both prescription (Rx) (98%) and OTC (94%) medications. The average resident was administered 8.8 unique medications per month (5.9 Rx and 2.9 OTC medications). This study reported that 12 therapeutic classes accounted for 93.9% of OTC medications used by residents, but Rx use was also high in some of these same classes. For example:

- 70.3% of all subjects used nonopioid OTC analgesics, and 19.0% used nonopioid Rx analgesics.
- 13.8% used OTC antacids/antiulcer agents, whereas 35.8% used Rx products in this class.
- The highest overlap was in the category of cough and cold medications; 19.3% used OTCs and 20.1% used Rx drugs.

Prescription plans available to seniors do not usually cover OTC medications. OTCs represent an important component of the therapeutic regimen of nursing home residents, but even with people on fixed incomes, utilization rates are insensitive to drug coverage.

OTC products differ from prescription medications in the following ways (APC, 2007):

- A wider margin of safety is seen with OTC medications because most of these drugs have undergone rigorous testing before marketing and further refinement through years of OTC use by consumers.
- The distribution of OTCs makes them much more widely available than prescription drugs.

The most common categories of OTCs parallel the products available by prescription, essentially providing to the public access to medications without a health care provider's intervention. These include laxatives, acid-peptic disorder products (antacids, H_2-receptor antagonists), analgesics, cough/cold products (antihistamines, decongestants, expectorants, antitussives), vaginal antifungals, smoking cessation products, and topical steroids.

OTCs are sold at many sites; probably less than half of all OTC medications are sold in pharmacies. Because so many different names and reformulations of products are available, it is important for the provider to learn the drug name, not the product name. In addition, many of these products have multiple ingredients. The cost of buying multiple-ingredient products can be greater than the cost of buying ingredients singly, so it is important to check out commonly used products for price.

Surveys show that women are most likely to purchase OTC products; they also are more likely than men to read labels on medicines before taking them (APC, 2007). The FDA requires that OTC medication labels should present all important information in a manner that a typical consumer can read and understand. A standardized labeling format is used for all OTC medications marketed in the United States. Key information includes the active ingredients, followed by purpose(s), uses, warnings, and directions; these items are placed in the same order on all OTC packages in a readable format. The new label is based on FDA research that concluded that many consumers could not read the small print on labels, could not understand some of the complex words, and could not discern what information was most important to them because no standardized format was used.

One of the most important tasks involved in reading labels for OTC medications is to determine the presence of additional ingredients in a product that might pose risk to some patients. These hidden ingredients are included for different purposes and may be seen in the form of preservatives, color additives, delivery, or stabilizing products. If individuals have an allergy or intolerance to even small doses of these products, they may not be aware of the risks unless they read the label. Table 73-1 lists common ingredients present in a number of common OTC medications.

Health care providers should discuss with patients the basic principles of OTC products and should not assume that they can read the information, or that they know the information already. Many patient information handouts have been developed for OTC medications, but whether given verbally or in writing, the following are some basic principles that patients should be taught:

- Always read label instructions.
- Do not take OTC medicine in higher dosages or for a longer time than indicated on the label.
- If a symptom persists, stop self-treatment and talk with a health care professional.
- Side effects from OTCs are relatively uncommon, but know the potential side effects of the medicine to be taken.
- Each person is different, and reactions to medicines also may differ.
- All medicines have the potential to interact with other medicines, with food, or with preexisting conditions.
- If you do not understand label instructions, check with a pharmacist to have any questions answered.
- Discard medications after the expiration date.

Parents, in particular, should be aware of special information about using OTCs for children:

- Never guess at the amount of medicine to give a child. Half an adult dose may be too much or not enough to be effective. This is especially true of medicines such as Tylenol or Advil, in which several overdoses may actually lead to poisoning, liver destruction, or coma.
- Avoid making conversions. If the label says 2 teaspoons and you are using a dosing cup with ounces only, get another measuring device. (See *Medicines in My Home,* available at www.fda.gov/medsinmyhome/MIMH_consumers.htm, and the FDA website at www.fda.gov.)
- Always follow age limit recommendations. If the label says not to give a medicine to a child younger than age 2, do not do it.

- Always use the child-resistant cap, and relock the cap after use.
- Throw away old, discolored, or expired medicines or medicines that have lost their label instructions.
- Do not give children medicines that contain alcohol.

ADVANTAGES AND DISADVANTAGES OF OTC USE

The wide ability to acquire OTC medications from a variety of sources may mean that many consumers are not talking to health care providers about their symptoms. Patients may be selecting OTC medications without giving full consideration as to how these products interact with other medications or what their side effects may be. However, consumers also have taken to the Internet and other media outlets to learn more about common ailments, and they have become well informed regarding their bodies and ways to promote good health. As informed consumers, they are able to make reasonable decisions about how to use OTC medications safely.

The rate of product switching from prescription to OTC status appears to be increasing. From the mid 1980s to the mid 1990s, approximately one drug was switched annually. A flurry of activity began in 1995, with the reclassification of several drug classes, including H_2-receptor antagonists for heartburn, nicotine gum and patches, pediatric analgesics, and hair growth formulations.

Formerly, prescription-only drugs that were granted OTC approval were intended to treat acute or episodic conditions with recognizable symptoms. OTC medications were not designed for chronic conditions or diseases that required laboratory tests for either diagnosis or monitoring. Now, many OTC drugs are being used for chronic conditions. This movement gained popularity because research demonstrated that chronic health conditions are highly undertreated because of lack of health insurance for many Americans. Proponents argue that if drugs required to treat many conditions are available over the counter, they might be used more widely. Opponents suggest that many patients who self-diagnose their condition may go from undertreatment to

TABLE 73-1 Hidden Ingredients in Over-the-Counter Products

Hidden Drug	OTC Class That May Contain Drug
Alcohol (ethanol)	Cough syrups/cold preparations, mouthwashes
Antihistamines	Analgesics, asthma products, cold/allergy products, dermatologic preparations, menstrual products, motion sickness products, antiemetics, sleep aids, topical decongestants
Antimuscarinic agents	Antidiarrheals, cold/cough/allergy preparations, hemorrhoidal products
aspirin and other salicylates	Analgesics, antidiarrheals, cold/allergy preparations, menstrual products, sleep aids
caffeine	Analgesics, cold/allergy products, menstrual or diuretic products, stimulants, weight control products
Estrogens	Hair creams
Local anesthetics (usually benzocaine)	Antitussives; dermatologic preparations; hemorrhoidal products; lozenges; toothache, cold sore, and teething products; weight loss products
sodium	Analgesics, antacids, cough syrups, laxatives
Sympathomimetics	Analgesics, asthma products, cold/allergy preparations, cough syrups, hemorrhoidal products, lozenges, menstrual products, topical decongestants, weight control products

Modified from Katzung BG: *Basic and clinical pharmacology,* ed 8, Norwalk, Conn, 2000, Appleton & Lange.

inappropriate or harmful self-treatment, or that patients' conditions will worsen because of inaccurate treatment. Emergency contraception, antimicrobials, and statins are drugs for which great debate has arisen regarding the safety of moving them to OTC status.

The National Council on Patient Information and Education sponsored a survey in which one third of the sample reported that they take more than the recommended dose of nonprescription medicine, believing it will increase the effectiveness of the product. The survey also found that one third said that they are likely to combine OTC medications when they have multiple symptoms. About half of the respondents got their information about drugs from the mass media, and the other half obtained information from health professionals (New Drug Facts Label to Help Consumers, 2002).

Some products in OTC medications have fallen into disfavor over time. Phenylpropanolamine and ephedra alkaloids (such as ephedrine) are stimulants (sympathomimetic agents). As stimulants, they have a hypertensive effect that puts some patients at increased risk of heart attack or stroke, especially those with a history of cardiac and hypertensive disease. These adverse effects were the basis for the FDA requirement that these agents should be removed from products on the market.

Primary care providers should assume that most of their patients use OTC medications. In working with clients, the primary care provider should use basic principles guiding OTC use, including the following:
- Collect a good baseline of information built on a comprehensive drug history.
- Recommend nondrug therapies first, such as exercise, diet, fluids, and rest.
- Look at specific symptoms and treat each separately.

- Select the product that is simplest in formulation with regard to ingredients and dosage. Generally, single-ingredient formulations are preferred.
- Select products that contain therapeutically effective dosing. Watch out for combination products that may contain therapeutic doses of one ingredient and subtherapeutic doses of others.
- Read labels carefully. Products can change names and can change the doses of one or more ingredients. Many products contain extended-release properties that may or may not be of benefit to the patient.
- Be wary of advertising that claims the superiority of new products that are, in reality, only the old product in new packaging at higher prices.
- Watch for differences in prices, and recommend generic products when available.

HOW CAN THE PRIMARY CARE PROVIDER BE HELPFUL TO PATIENTS WHO ARE TAKING OTC MEDICATIONS?

Primary care providers have two major opportunities in which they may help patients navigate the confusing number of OTC medications currently available on the market. The first opportunity comes when providers recommend that patients take OTC medications as part of a therapeutic course that they are recommending for a problem. The second opportunity arises when providers see patients in their offices for acute or follow-up visits and take this opportunity to ask about OTC use. The primary care provider should use both of these opportunities to teach patients about the drugs they are taking.

OTC Product	Why You Should Ask Patients If They Are Taking This OTC	What You Should Teach Patients When You Recommend They Use This OTC
Vitamins and minerals	• Known dangers are associated with vitamin use, especially high-dose use. Megadoses of vitamins are rapidly excreted into the urine, with no additional benefit to the client. Occasionally, large doses of vitamin A may be stored in the tissues, producing a yellow hue to the skin. Most vitamin products can be toxic to children, and iron supplements can be deadly to small children. Folic acid can react adversely with anticancer treatment medications and mask signs of vitamin B_{12} deficiency. Sometimes the body becomes dependent on large doses of vitamin C when it is taken over a prolonged time; a period of deficiency may be noted with a return to normal doses. Clients with increased colon transit times may excrete some vitamin and mineral products unchanged in the stool. • Large amounts of calcium can limit the absorption of iron and other trace elements. They also can cause constipation and may impair kidney function.	• The marketing industry has suggested that natural products are better than synthetic vitamins. Not all claims for vitamins have been proved. Costs for some products have greatly increased based on product claims. • What is known is that vitamin and mineral supplements are useful when there are deficiencies, as in some young women and in the elderly. Benefits to the average healthy individual who consumes a variety of foods have not been proved. However, for the first time, the American Medical Association has suggested that individuals might benefit from a daily vitamin because of the generally poor nutrition of many Americans. • Vitamins are probably equivalent, whether they are natural or synthetic, costly or cheap. In fact, natural vitamins may contain other products or impurities that may make them less effective than synthetic or more standardized products. However, some preparations dissolve better than others or are given in amounts that facilitate the absorption of other coadministered vitamins and minerals.

OTC Product	Why You Should Ask Patients If They Are Taking This OTC	What You Should Teach Patients When You Recommend They Use This OTC
	• Although many major research studies have looked at antioxidants retrospectively and have suggested that major benefits are derived from increased utilization for many disease states, no intervention studies have determined conclusively that antioxidants prevent cancer. Epidemiologic evidence does indicate that those who eat fruits and vegetables regularly have a decreased risk of cancer. No conclusive evidence suggests that this is the result of antioxidants. Therefore, supplementation with vitamin antioxidants may be beneficial, but in certain populations, such as smokers, it may actually be harmful (see Chapter 72 for information on vitamins). • Supplements cannot make up for a poor diet or other unhealthful lifestyle practices such as smoking or lack of exercise. If patients do not eat a well-balanced diet and instead eat large amounts of high-fat or empty-calorie foods, they may want to consider taking a multivitamin/mineral. If patients cannot tolerate certain foods (e.g., dairy products), they may need to supplement their diet to ensure that they are getting the nutrients provided by that food group.	• National surveys have shown that those who least need supplements are most likely to take them, such as individuals who eat right, exercise, and do not smoke. No evidence indicates that clients who take vitamins live longer or have fewer cancers. Calcium is needed primarily in menopausal women and in older men, particularly those who are at risk for bone loss. Antioxidant vitamins occupy a large niche in the current literature on nutritional supplements. The major vitamin antioxidants are vitamin E or alpha-tocopherol, beta carotene or provitamin (precursor to vitamin A), vitamin C or ascorbic acid, and selenium. All of these are found in fruits and vegetables. • Most women in the United States 20 years of age or older consume about 1673 calories a day. Women who diet may eat fewer calories and must work harder to get the Recommended Dietary Allowances for essential vitamins and minerals. Recommended daily consumption of food guidelines remind people to balance what they are eating. Balance is important not only in ensuring consumption of essential nutrients daily, but in taking advantage of positive interactions among the different food groups. For example, vitamin C aids in iron absorption, so a slice of tomato on a turkey sandwich does more than look nice.
Aspirin	• The benefits of aspirin use in patients with prior occlusive cardiovascular disease are clear. In both men and women with a wide range of prior cardiovascular disease from a past heart attack or occlusive stroke to those with angina, coronary bypass surgery, or angioplasty, data from randomized trials demonstrate clear benefits of long-term aspirin therapy. • Research has not conclusively determined whether any benefits of aspirin for these individuals outweigh the risks, which include an increased tendency to bleed. One large-scale randomized trial, the Physicians' Health Study, showed conclusively that low-dose aspirin reduced the risk of a first heart attack by 44% in apparently healthy men.	• For those in the acute phase of an evolving heart attack, the net benefits of aspirin use are also clear: Immediate treatment of all such patients with aspirin will save lives as well as reduce the risk that the patient may experience another heart attack or a stroke. For those individuals without prior occlusive vascular disease, the side effects of aspirin are the same as for those who have had occlusive vascular events.
Smoking cessation products	• Smoking is the number one cause of preventable death and disease in the United States. • Ask how much patients are smoking and whether they have an interest in quitting. • See Chapter 71 for specifics of products.	• Safe and effective pharmacologic treatments are available to help smokers quit; almost 80% of treatments are available as medications that can be obtained without a doctor's prescription. • Recommend specific therapies of gum, lozenge, etc, and indicate that OTC nicotine replacement therapies may cost $200 to $350 for a full treatment course.
Products for heartburn or indigestion	• Ask what OTC product a patient is using and whether it is effective.	• Use of OTC antacids (pills, chewables, and liquids) and H_2-blockers can help to alleviate the symptoms of heartburn or GI distress. Recommend specific products based on symptoms.
Bowel products	• When a patient reports constipation, ask about fiber and fluid in the diet, and ask about laxatives, stool softeners, and enema products to determine whether there is overuse.	• Recommend specific products or that specific products not be used.
Analgesics	• By 2020, it is predicted that more than 60 million Americans will suffer from osteoporosis. Monitor what products the patient is using, the response, and other drugs the patient may be taking, and look for drug interactions. • PMS is a problem for many; in addition, an estimated 10% to 15% of American women of reproductive age suffer from endometriosis.	• Recommend use or not using specific products depending on patient comorbidities and whether the patient uses alcohol or other medications. • PMS requires regular therapy for many women. There is no cure for endometriosis, but OTC medicines such as acetaminophen, ibuprofen, and naproxen sodium help to reduce severe pain caused by endometriosis, particularly during menstruation.

Table continued on following page

OTC Product	Why You Should Ask Patients If They Are Taking This OTC	What You Should Teach Patients When You Recommend They Use This OTC
Antihistamines and decongestants	• Allergic diseases are a major cause of illness and disability in the United States, affecting 40 to 50 million Americans. An estimated 35 million Americans suffer from hay fever.	• OTC oral antihistamines and nasal sprays help to alleviate the symptoms of respiratory allergies; such topical treatments as hydrocortisone and diphenhydramine can be used to treat skin allergies.
Vaginal antifungals	• One of the most common problems treated with OTC medicines is vaginal yeast infection (candidiasis). Previously, women who were experiencing a recurrence of candidiasis were required to visit a doctor for a prescription to treat this common condition. Because of the availability of antifungals on a nonprescription basis, doctor visits from 1990 to 1994 were reduced by 15%, with an associated cost savings of $63.5 million for medical expenses and lost time from work.	• After a yeast infection has been documented, teach the patient about the possibility of recurrence, the symptoms to watch for, which products to use, and how to know whether or not they are successful. Give clear directions about when the patient should return to the health care provider for care.
Plan B emergency contraception	• For patients who may have been raped or who do not wish to be pregnant, ask whether they have used this product. Girls younger than 18 still require a prescription for this medication.	• Talk to all women about emergency contraception, so that they know it is an option should they need it. This product is kept behind the counter, and women over age 18 need to ask for it.

Consumer Health Care Products Association (CHPA), 2006. Available at www.CHPA.org.

SUMMARY

OTC preparations constitute a vast proportion of health care products and health care expenditures for individuals of many nations. As the results from research studies become more conclusive, it will continue to be the responsibility of health care providers to communicate with patients about the safety, effectiveness, and dangers inherent in these widely available products.

evolve A continually updated list of useful WebLinks may be found in the Evolve Resources at http://evolve.elsevier.com/Edmunds/NP/

Complementary and Alternative Therapies

BONNIE R. BOCK

The use of complementary and alternative medicine (CAM) has been increasing every year in the United States. In 1993, Dr. David Eisenberg of Harvard Medical School released a landmark study in *The New England Journal of Medicine* that showed one third of Americans were using unconventional medicine such as aromatherapy, acupuncture, and therapeutic touch. In May 2004, the National Center for Complementary and Alternative Medicine (NCCAM) and the National Center for Health Statistics (NCHS, part of the Centers for Disease Control and Prevention) released the results of the 2002 National Health Interview Survey (NHIS). This comprehensive report on the use of CAM in the United States concluded that as many as 62% of adults 18 years of age and older use some form of CAM. The most commonly used CAM modality in 2002 was herbal therapy (18.6%, representing more than 38 million U.S. adults), which was followed in frequency by relaxation techniques (14.2%, representing 29 million U.S. adults) and chiropractic medicine (7.4%, representing 15 million U.S. adults). Among CAM users, 41% had used two or more CAM therapies during the prior year. Factors associated with highest rates of CAM use were patient age 40 to 64 years, female gender, non-black/non-Hispanic race, and annual income of $65,000 or higher (Tindle et al, 2005).

Based on these statistics, this chapter is included in *Pharmacology for the Primary Care Provider,* third edition. Although a high level of scientific study and knowledge of all these products or techniques does not exist, and the information in this chapter must of necessity be somewhat brief, it is clear that primary care providers must have some exposure to the range of CAM practices because patients are using them. In general, not enough research has been done regarding CAM and various products to scientifically support or discredit their use, although European scientists have focused more attention on researching these products than have U.S. scientists. At this time, definitive conclusions cannot be drawn regarding the use of CAM, particularly the biologicals. Much of what appears in the literature continues to be based on observational reports and small studies.

DEFINING COMPLEMENTARY AND ALTERNATIVE THERAPIES

Complementary, alternative, nontraditional, unconventional, and *"Eastern" medicine* are terms that are used interchangeably to describe diverse medical and health care practices considered outside the realm of conventional or allopathic medical therapies that have yet to be validated by scientific methods (Straus, 2002). The term *complementary* describes therapy used to supplement more traditional medical care, and the term *alternative* suggests that therapy has taken the place of usual medical therapy. Complementary or alternative medicine is the term most frequently seen in the lay literature. *Integrative medicine* is a term that is used to describe the appropriate use of conventional and alternative methods to facilitate the body's innate healing response. Integrative medicine shifts the orientation of medicine to one of healing rather than disease and uses an approach that engages the body, mind, spirit, and community. It has also been defined as "the evidence-based combination of conventional with CAM for assuring the maximum therapeutic benefit for patients and practitioners" (Pelletier, 2007a). The NIH National Center for Complementary and Alternative Medicine (http://nccam.nih.gov) has identified five broad categories of CAM and integrative medicine for which a growing and substantial body of evidence about these techniques is based on research and clinical practice.

The current literature describes the following (Pelletier, 2007a):

- *Mind-body medicine:* Research about these approaches constitutes the largest body of CAM research. This research documents the efficacy of these types of interventions for the largest number of conditions for the greatest number of patients (Pelletier, 2004).
- *Acupuncture:* The Cochrane Library (www.cochrane.org) has 16 systematic reviews regarding the efficacy of this approach in conditions such as back pain, Bell's palsy, depression, dysmenorrhea, arthritis of the knee, and fibromyalgia (Kim, 2005; Martin et al, 2006).
- *Herbal medicine:* Information on herbal interventions (www.herbalgram.org) and drug–herb interactions (www.herbmed.org; www.healthyroads.com) is becoming increasingly sophisticated.
- *Traditional Chinese medicine (TCM):* This way of approaching diagnosis and treatment using ancient lore is now under study by several international NCCAM Centers of Excellence. Studies include research on irritable bowel syndrome, side effects of cancer treatment, and allergic asthma (AARP, 2007).
- *The National Institute of Health–NCCAM* annually has about 50 ongoing research studies (http://nccam.nih.gov). Among the many diverse areas under study are dietary practices and supplements, chiropractic, homeopathy, naturopathy, and electromagnetic effects, as well as Ayurvedic medicine, chelation, and spiritual healing (Bell, 2002; Kaptchuk & Miller, 2005; Merrell, 2006).

PRIMARY CARE PROVIDERS AND COMPLEMENTARY AND ALTERNATIVE THERAPIES

Patient interest has far outpaced the resources of the traditional health care system; standard texts and reference books do not cover herbs, supplements, and homeopathic remedies. Many patients believe that they know more than their health care providers, and their providers are not listening to them or respecting their choices. Responsible providers seek reliable information about the choices their patients are making, so they can provide better advice and treatment.

It is crucial for primary care providers to have up-to-date, balanced, and scientifically founded reference material to assist them in understanding nonconventional therapy, as they learn about the strengths, weaknesses, clinical indications, proper dosages, toxicities, and interactions of different therapies. It is important for primary care providers to be familiar with the many products available to patients that do not require a prescription. Many of these products contain ingredients that are useful in the treatment of common ailments. If primary care providers are familiar with these products and their ingredients, they can help patients choose the safest product for their ailment in the context of their present state of health or illness. It should be noted, however, that some of the active ingredients in these products may interact with prescribed medications or may even complicate existing medical conditions.

A growing body of knowledge is available to inform practitioners. Integrative medicine is part of a rapidly evolving face of health care that ushers in an era of genomics, international medicine, and evidence-based approaches (www.nap.edu/catalog/11182.html). Lack of knowledge about these techniques has caused practitioners to acknowledge and address the need for an adequate "evidence-based" foundation in conventional, CAM, and integrative medicine. The goal is to provide evidence-based standards by which all medicine should be judged and that will help both providers and patients as they consider new approaches to the treatment of old problems.

A good first approach regarding patient-initiated and controlled therapy is to obtain a thorough medication history because many patient-initiated alternative treatment remedies are purchased over the counter and patients often neglect to tell their providers about them. More than 70% of patients who use complementary therapies do not tell their providers of the use. Although easy availability of herbal and over-the-counter products makes many Americans consider these products safe, the fact is that not all herbal therapies are safe for all patients. General knowledge about patient-initiated products enables providers to evaluate specific regimens that their patients report taking; this decreases the potential for negative outcomes when products that may be harmful are used (Micozzi, 1998).

Even providers who take a drug history from patients may focus on prescription drug use and may fail to adequately document other product use. Questions regarding alternative treatments should be a routine part of the patient's medication history. Specific questions that may be asked include the following:

- Are you using any over-the-counter vitamins, herbs, or supplements?
- Why are you taking the product?
- What dosage are you taking?
- How long have you taken the medicine?

- Is it helping?
- Have you experienced any side effects?
- Are you being treated by an alternative therapist, that is, an herbalist, acupuncturist, naturopathic practitioner, or chiropractor?

It is also important to have patients bring in any products that they are using to each office visit, so an accurate record may be maintained. Original containers for these products provide additional information that assists the practitioner in evaluating their safety. These steps may be important in preventing dangerous drug interactions and complications.

When obtaining a history about complementary health measures, primary care providers should try to remain as nonjudgmental or neutral about alternate primary care remedies as possible. This approach is essential in earning patients' trust, so they will answer completely and honestly. Providers should understand that patients who use alternative therapies or complementary treatments do so for many reasons:

- Patients seek products that will maintain health, prevent disease, or provide treatment for existing health problems.
- They have tried conventional therapeutic options without success.
- Conventional therapies had undesirable side effects.
- No known therapy will relieve their problem.
- Other respected family or community members may have recommended the product.
- Conventional approaches have disregarded their religious or spiritual beliefs.
- Patients may be dissatisfied with the fragmentation of care provided by multiple medical specialties.
- Media reports and advertising promote alternative and complementary therapies as being more "natural" and therefore safe.
- Using complementary and alternative modalities gives patients power in controlling their treatment.
- Many complementary and alternative modalities focus on emotional and spiritual well-being.
- Complementary and alternative therapists generally provide three elements that often are not provided by conventional medicine: touch, talk, and time.
- Medical liability is an important issue as providers integrate complementary primary care practices or refer patients for alternative therapies. Standards of care for complementary and integrative therapies are developing as research and evidence-based guidelines are formulated. Providers who integrate CAM therapies into conventional care should determine whether evidence in the scientific and medical literature (1) supports both safety and efficacy, (2) supports safety but efficacy evidence is inconclusive, (3) supports efficacy but safety evidence is inconclusive, or (4) indicates serious risk or inefficacy.
- Strategies should be used to decrease the risk for potential malpractice liability when care providers counsel about or offer CAM therapies, and when they refer patients to other CAM providers (Cohen & Eisenberg, 2002). When counseling or offering CAM therapies, a provider should (1) determine clinical risk level by assessing evidence of safety and efficacy, (2) document literature that supports the therapeutic choice in the medical record and include a file of literature that supports the safety and efficacy of the treatment, (3) provide adequate informed consent by discussing the risks and benefits of CAM therapy,

including what is not known or cannot be evaluated, and (4) obtain written consent to use CAM treatment (or obtain written consent for the use of CAM treatment).

- When patients are referred to other CAM providers, similar strategies should be implemented: (1) Closely monitor the clinical risk level of the treatment that is being provided, (2) document the literature that supports the decision to refer, (3) provide adequate informed consent by discussing benefits and risks based on available medical literature, (4) document the patient's decision to visit a CAM provider, thereby establishing the patient's agreement to treatment, (5) continue to monitor the patient, and (6) inquire about the competence of the CAM provider by reviewing the licensing and scope of practice of the provider, understanding the care that is delivered, and inquiring about the provider's history of disciplinary action or malpractice litigation.

COMPLEMENTARY THERAPIES AND HERBAL MEDICINE

Complementary and alternative therapies in general have been somewhat mysterious, and the scientific basis for their therapeutic action is often uncertain. Over the past several years, as research and interest in this area have increased, more universities and medical schools are incorporating the use and teaching of complementary/alternative modalities, and many are conducting research in this area. In 2000, 64% of medical schools were offering courses that addressed complementary and alternative therapies. The number of CAM practitioners in the United States is projected to increase by 88% between 1994 and 2010, and the number of conventional physicians who incorporate CAM into their practices will increase by 16% (Breuner, 2006).

Because of the widespread use of complementary therapies, interest in the scientific study of various products is growing. In 1991, the Office of Alternative Medicine (OAM) was established within the NIH, and an Alternative Medicine Advisory Council was established in 1993. In November 1995, the NIH established the Office of Dietary Supplements to promote the scientific study of dietary supplements. In October 1998, Congress mandated the establishment of the OAM NIH center—the National Center for Complementary and Alternative Medicine. In February 1999, a charter creating NCCAM was signed, making it the 25th independent component of the NIH. In October 1999, NCCAM and the NIH Office of Dietary Supplements established the first Dietary Supplements Research Center, with an emphasis on botanical medicine. Since its inception, NCCAM has funded multiple studies. Results of these studies are available through NCCAM (http://nccam.nih.gov/health/herbsataglance.htm). Funding appropriated by Congress for NCCAM rose from $50 million in 1999 to $122.7 million in 2006. Major clinical trials conducted by NCCAM include the following:

- St. John's Wort and Depression—April 2002
- Acupuncture for Osteoarthritis of the Knee—December 2004
- Echinacea for the Prevention and Treatment of Colds in Adults—July 2005
- Glucosamine/Chondroitin Arthritis Intervention Trial (GAIT)—February 2006
- Black Cohosh and Menopause Symptoms—December 2006

Common Complementary and Alternative Practices

NCCAM has classified complementary and alternative modalities into five domains: alternate medical systems, mind–body interventions, manipulative and body-based methods, energy therapies, and biologically based therapies.

ALTERNATIVE MEDICAL SYSTEMS. Alternative medical systems are complete systems of theory and practice. Non-Western systems, such as traditional Chinese medicine and Ayurveda, are ancient systems that have been used for thousands of years, whereas systems developed in Western cultures such as naturopathic medicine and homeopathic and osteopathic systems have evolved apart from conventional allopathic medical practices used in the United States.

MIND–BODY INTERVENTIONS. Mind–body modalities use various techniques to enhance the mind's capacity to affect body functions and symptoms. Examples include meditation, prayer, hypnosis, yoga, biofeedback, and creative therapies such as music therapy, art therapy, and dance. Modalities such as patient support groups and cognitive-behavioral therapy were once considered CAM modalities but are now considered mainstream techniques.

MANIPULATIVE AND BODY-BASED METHODS. Body-based and manipulative methods are based on the manipulation and/or movement of one or more parts of the body. Modalities include chiropractic manipulation of the spine, and osteopathic treatments involve manipulation of the muscles and joints to treat illness. Massage, reflexology, and postural therapies are other modalities by which the provider's hands are used to treat the patient.

ENERGY THERAPIES. Energy therapies involve use of the following two types of energy fields:

1. Biofield therapies affect energy fields that purportedly surround and penetrate the human body. The existence of such fields has not yet been scientifically proven. Some forms of energy therapy, such as therapeutic touch, Reiki, and qi gong, manipulate biofields by applying pressure and/or manipulating the body by placing the hands in, or through, these fields.
2. Bioelectromagnetically based therapies involve the unconventional use of electromagnetic fields, such as magnetic fields, pulsed fields, and alternating current or direct current fields.

BIOLOGICALLY BASED THERAPIES. Biologically based therapies use substances that are found in nature to treat various conditions or to maintain health. Examples include botanical or herbal therapy, dietary supplements, orthomolecular medicine, and other "natural" therapies, which have yet to be scientifically proven (e.g., shark cartilage to treat lung cancer). Nonherbal biologics are discussed in Table 74-1.

The five domains are not mutually exclusive. Modalities may overlap domains. For example, acupuncture and acupressure are modalities that are used in traditional Chinese medicine, but they also may be considered forms of energy therapy.

Naturopathic medicine uses biologically based therapies, such as vitamins, herbs, and other natural remedies, to treat illness.

TABLE 74-1   Natural Remedies (Not Herbs or Vitamins)

Name	Source	Common Uses	Safety and Efficacy/Dosage	Drug Interactions
Chondroitin	Cattle cartilage	Eases aches and pains, protects and rebuilds cartilage	Safe and effective; 200-400 mg po bid-tid; 1000-1200 mg po daily	Antiplatelets, anticoagulants, ASA, NSAIDs
Coenzyme Q10	Produced in the body and formulated in soybean oil	Mitochondrial cytopathies, CHF, cardiovascular disorders, post-MI cardiac risk reduction, Alzheimer's, Parkinson's	Safe; dosage varies with use	Diabetes medications—hypoglycemic agents, insulins, warfarin, statins, β-blockers
Creatine	Muscle tissue or synthetic	Improving exercise performance and increasing muscle mass; ALS, CHF	Possibly unsafe in high doses 20 g/day for 5 days followed by a maintenance dose of 2 g or more per day	Gallium nitrate, aminoglycosides, nephrotoxic agents, tacrolimus
Glucosamine	Crab shells	Eases aches and pains, protects and rebuilds cartilage osteoarthritis, rheumatoid arthritis	Safe and effective if shells are not from polluted water; 500 mg po tid; 1500 mg po daily	Antiplatelets, anticoagulants, ASA, NSAIDs
DHEA	Androgen hormone synthesized from wild yams	Alleviates cancer, heart disease, and autoimmune disease; antiaging remedy	Believed to be safe, but all side effects not known Toxic to liver in sufficient quantities Efficacy not proven	Aromatase inhibitors, fulvestrant, tamoxifen
Melatonin	Hormone If from natural sources, it comes from the pineal glands of cattle	Cure for jet lag, helps the body's clock, sleep aid Antiaging	May inhibit sex drive in men 0.3-5 mg po every night (insomnia) 5 mg po every night × 7 days) for jet lag); start 3 days prior to flight	Immunosuppressants, corticosteroids, ginkgo biloba

Data from McPherson ML: *Over-the-counter medications: syllabus,* 1997 National Nurse Practitioner Conference, Washington, DC, November 1997, Nurse Practitioner Education Associates; Tyler VE: Herb/drug interactions, *Prevention,* 93-97, 1998, and Epocrates Rx Pro [database for PDA], Version 7.50, San Mateo (CA), 2002, Epocrates, Inc [updated 2006 Jan 19; cited 2006 Jan 26]. Available at www.epocrates.com.

Botanical therapies are discussed in this chapter. For additional information on vitamins and nutritional supplements, see Chapter 72.

Botanical Therapy

Herbal medicine (drugs from plant sources) has been used in most cultures since the beginning of time. In the United States, medicinal plants were the primary form of medication in nineteenth-century medicine. Today, herbal supplements often are used or prescribed as pharmaceuticals are, for a particular symptom or complaint. Approximately 38.2 million adults in the United States used herbs and supplements in 2002 (Kennedy, 2005). Many complementary and alternative modalities incorporate the use of herbal remedies. Traditional Chinese medicine, Ayurveda, naturopathy, and homeopathy make use of botanical therapies. Aromatherapy, often used in massage therapy, uses essential oils extracted from the petals, leaves, bark, resins, rinds, roots, stalks, seeds, and stems of aromatic plants to promote health and well-being. It is believed that these oils have medicinal properties that fight bacteria, viruses, bacterial toxins, and fungi. It has been suggested by researchers that the scents work by triggering the production of hormones that regulate physiologic functions.

A report (Kennedy, 2005) listed the top 10 herbal products taken by patients as echinacea to increase immunity; garlic to decrease cardiovascular problems; ginkgo biloba to fight dementia; St John's wort for depression; valerian, chamomile, ginger as calming agents; ginseng as a natural energy booster; saw palmetto for benign prostatic hyperplasia; and black cohosh for hot flashes. This article also listed the safety concerns and efficacy of these products.

Some clinicians and pharmacists have raised questions about the government's lack of regulation of complementary medicine practices, particularly those involving herbal products. Legislatively, few regulations are designed to oversee complementary therapies or herbal medicines. The Hatch-Richardson Bill of 1992 defines a dietary supplement as different from a food additive or a drug. Under this law, the manufacturer may make health claims without receiving approval from the government, if data are adequate to support the claim. In 1994, the Dietary Supplement Health and Education Act (DSHEA) defined a dietary supplement as a food and not as a drug or related item. Vitamins, minerals, amino acids, herbs, and enzymes all are used as dietary supplements and thus can be marketed under this law. The FDA considers a food to be a drug only when a medical claim is made for its use in curing a certain disease. Only when the claim is made that a product can be used to treat or cure an illness or disease must the manufacturer comply with the rigorous standards of safety and efficacy set forth by the FDA.

Although the FDA does not regulate herbal medicines, this agency took action on April 24, 1998, to protect consumers from misleading health claims by the booming herbal remedy industry. The goal of the FDA was to clarify for manufacturers what types of claims can and cannot be made on dietary supplement labels, so consumers can make more informed choices. FDA actions resulted from the agency's attempt to conform with the DSHEA of 1994, which distinguished health and disease claims from structure/function claims. The act says labels cannot make claims that a product cures a disease or has a special benefit or health effect without receiving special FDA approval. The act allows general statements about the product's function in the body. The new rules bar makers of vitamins and herbal remedies from claiming to cure, prevent, or alleviate cancer, acquired immunodeficiency syndrome, and other specific diseases. Companies are limited to making general claims about a product's ability to enhance the immune system. However, critics claim that most disease treatments can be described in terms of their effects on a structure or function of the body, so it is difficult to distinguish between allowable structure/function claims and prohibited disease claims.

ADVANTAGES AND DISADVANTAGES OF HERBAL THERAPY FOR PRIMARY CARE PRACTICE. Herbal preparations generally are thought to have three major advantages: lower cost, fewer side effects, and medicinal effects that tend to normalize physiologic function. When an herb is used effectively, its mechanism of action often corrects the underlying cause of a disorder or symptom. A synthetic pharmaceutical may be developed to alleviate a symptom without addressing the underlying cause. Research has suggested that the whole plant or crude extract of many plants often is much more effective than an isolated compound.

Herbal therapies have historical and cultural traditions that have created the impression that they are safe and natural. These impressions create a false sense of safety and efficacy for the consumer. Just because something is natural does not mean that it is safe or effective. Herbal preparations are not regulated anywhere in the world. Chinese medicine has used herbal products for centuries as a standard part of medical practice. These products are just beginning to be scientifically evaluated. The German Commission E, a panel that reviews the safety and efficacy of herbs, has done the most in terms of scientific research into the safety and efficacy of herbs. Although some of these studies have been small and do not begin to meet the scientific standard demanded by the FDA for prescription drugs, the German Commission E Monographs have been considered the gold standard in the field of herbal medicine for many years. Professional consensus is growing that if herbs are effective, they should be used under the supervision of a trained health care professional.

Safety, purity, and effectiveness are the primary issues to be considered when herbal products are evaluated. Important questions include the following:
- How much of the relevant herb does this product actually contain?
- What part of the plant was used to make the extract?
- What other chemicals does it contain?
- What are the active ingredients?
- What reliable information suggests that this herb is useful, and for what conditions?
- What herb–drug interactions may occur?

Consumers are using herbal remedies in record numbers, believing that these products are drugs that will prevent disease, treat illness, and improve health. Most publications on herbal therapies are written to sell products. As expensive new prescription drugs enter the market, cheaper nonprescription products reported to perform the same function also appear. For example, herbal preparations that purportedly have the same actions as the erectile dysfunction drug Viagra are being heavily marketed. Antiobesity products that contain ephedra were sold as herbal alternatives to fenfluramine and dexfenfluramine until ephedra was linked to serious adverse effects, including death, and was removed from the market. Herbs and natural products used to treat menopausal symptoms recently have increased in popularity, since questions have been raised about the safety of hormone replacement therapy.

The FDA does take action when warranted. In July 2002, the FDA advised consumers of the potential risk of severe liver injury associated with the use of dietary supplements that contain kava (also know as kava kava or *Piper methysticum*). The high-profile death of a baseball player led to restrictions on drugs containing ephedra. In response to dangers such as these, the FDA has removed some products from the market and posts information about high-risk products on the MedWatch homepage at www.fda.gov/medwatch. The Dietary Supplement and Nonprescription Drug Consumer Protection Act, which went into effect in December 2007, requires that serious adverse event reports be sent to the FDA, so that public safety concerns can be identified and addressed quickly.

Herbs can be used medicinally in many forms. They may be (1) consumed raw or in food as a garnish, spice, or main ingredient, (2) used in teas made by infusion or decoction, (3) taken as a tincture or extract in an alcohol or vinegar base, or (4) used topically in poultices and compresses. Herbal products are made by grinding parts of the plant and converting the ground material into pills, capsules, or liquid. Almost any part of the plant may be used, including stems, bark, leaves, flowers, roots, and seeds.

One of the major criticisms of herbal products is that concentration or dosage is highly variable because plants make different quantities of chemicals, depending on environmental conditions. The weight of a leaf may be the same as that of another, but the amount of biologically active chemical that is present varies according to the amount of sunlight to which the leaf has been exposed, the type of nutrition that has been provided by the soil, and the extent of dilution that nutrients have undergone. Some herbalists recommend that only herbs that have been standardized should be used. Manufacturers have developed standardization as a quality control measure. When a plant has been standardized, quantities of the plant and of one or more of the plant's phytochemicals are ensured; thus, investigators can use a standardized plant more easily than a raw, pulverized plant or simple extract when they conduct randomized trials. Standardization leads to consistent, measurable levels of one or more active ingredients. According to the particular standardization method used, however, levels of potentially useful compounds that are not among those measured and standardized may be reduced or eliminated. Therefore, although standardization of chemical compounds may facilitate replicability, the process may fail to provide reliable controls for assessment of pharmacologic activity (Rotblatt & Ziment, 2002).

No definitive standards or regulations can be used to judge the quality of herbal supplements; however, several helpful resources have been developed. In 2000, the United States Pharmacopeia (USP) created the Dietary Supplement Verification Program (DSVP) to inform and protect the growing number of consumers who use dietary supplements. This program assures the public that a dietary supplement product contains the ingredients listed on the product label. The USP is also preparing for the first time a United States Pharmacopeia that lists botanical products (USP-NF Botanical Monographs.)

which should make a contribution to the education of clinicians about products that are available.

The National Nutritional Foods Association (NNFA) has established a Good Manufacturing Practices (GMP) Certification Program for its members. This program mandates third-party inspections of manufacturing facilities to determine whether NNFA standards are being met. Manufacturers who meet the GMP of the NNFA are permitted to place a seal on all product labels that assures consumers of product quality. Companies that are members of the American Herbal Products Association (AHPA) are required to abide by strict policies and standards; membership generally indicates that a given company is committed to quality and integrity.

Another resource, Consumerlab.com, is a privately held company that independently tests vitamins, herbs, supplements, and nutritional products. Test results are published online (www.consumerlab.com) and provide helpful information for health care professionals and consumers to guide them in the selection of health, wellness, and nutrition products.

In April 2005, the FDA issued *A Dietary Supplement Labeling Guide*, for use by the dietary supplement industry. These nonbinding recommendations were established to ensure that dietary supplements sold in the United States are labeled properly.

DRUG–HERB INTERACTIONS

Herbal medicines were the only medicines used throughout history; however, concerns about drug interactions did not become a major issue until manufacturing companies began to supply them. In earlier days, practitioners of healing used a trial-and-error system to determine whether a particular herbal remedy would cure or kill. Today, with the predominant use of synthetic medications, many factors must be considered. Interactions between natural products and drugs are based on the same pharmacokinetic and pharmacodynamic principles as drug–drug interactions. Certain herbs may reduce or heighten the effects of synthetic medications; others may mimic these effects. Some may reduce bioavailability or alter cofactors; others act in an additive or complementary manner. Some herbs may be beneficial, others may have no effect on other medications, and the use of others may suggest that a synthetic drug did not work by virtue of the fact that the herb itself is exacerbating the disease. For example, echinacea, an immunostimulant, if taken by a patient with lupus, may increase symptoms of lupus even if the patient is taking immunosuppressants. Herbal medicines such as garlic, ginseng, and ginkgo are thought to interact with anticoagulant or antiplatelet therapy. Many patients who take these herbs in combination with anticoagulant medications do not reveal their use to their primary care provider (Saw et al, 2006). Generally, warfarin is the most commonly used drug, and St. John's wort is the herbal product most often reported to be involved in drug–herb interactions (Brazier, 2003). Table 74-2 lists herbs commonly used in NCCAM studies and potential drug interactions.

Despite concerns that have been expressed regarding drug–herb interactions, it is important that these interactions be viewed in perspective; it should be noted that drug–herb interactions generally are less severe than drug–drug interactions. Canadian researchers, while studying serious and fatal adverse drug reactions (ADRs) among hospitalized patients in the United States, observed that even when drugs are properly prescribed and administered, large numbers of ADRs may occur. In general, herbal products are less toxic than pharmaceuticals, and drug–drug interactions are much more common and severe than drug–herb interactions.

Herbal medicine information is now provided in books, monographs, pharmacopoeias, and newsletters, as well as on websites. The best resources are those that base efficacy or adverse effects claims on the primary clinical literature or on high-quality systematic reviews. The NCCAM *Herbs at a Glance* series of fact sheets on specific herbs, CAM on Pub Med, and the Cochrane Database of systematic reviews are recommended resources for evidence-based CAM and herbal information. Providers can check on herb–drug interactions by using several software programs that have been developed for use on computers and PDAs.

Beneficial Interactions

Many practitioners believe that botanical therapies should be used in conjunction with pharmaceuticals to enhance healing by strengthening the body's immune system to protect against infection and disease. An example of an enhanced combination is a blend of herbals with prescription antibiotics. Echinacea, a very popular herbal supplement, can be used as adjuvant therapy for relapsing infections of the respiratory and urinary tract. All blends of echinacea are designed to increase macrophage activity and levels of tumor necrosis factor and interleukin-2, thereby enhancing replication and phagocytosis of cytokine production by WBCs. Individual components of echinacea may exhibit antibacterial, antiviral, and antimycotic activities. Cranberry juice, which is also used as a preventative or adjunctive treatment for urinary tract infection, has been shown to be effective by preventing the adhesion of bacteria to the bladder wall.

Botanical remedies can be used to protect individuals from the side effects of pharmaceuticals. Milk thistle has been shown to protect the liver after exposure to hepatotoxins such as acetaminophen, ethanol, and halothane, and to restore liver function in patients with hepatitis and cirrhosis. Silymarin, one of the medicinal compounds included in this herb, has been shown to strengthen the outer surface of the liver and to encourage an enzymatic action that leads to cellular regeneration, thus allowing the liver to detoxify the bloodstream more efficiently.

Adverse Interactions

DETRIMENTAL EFFECTS. All medicines, whether natural or synthetic, have side effects or may interact with other substances. Herbs, as well as pharmaceuticals, may have both desirable and detrimental effects. Any substance that interferes with the absorption or excretion of a prescription medication can reduce bioavailability and have a deleterious effect on its intended action. Laxative and fiber-rich herbs (e.g., senna, aloe, marshmallow, slippery elm, psyllium) can decrease intestinal transit time and reduce drug absorption.

Herbs high in tannin precipitate alkaloids of medications such as atropine, ephedrine, codeine, and theophylline. Other herbs may exhibit antagonistic activity when taken with medication, or they may compromise the essential metabolism of a drug, especially if metabolized in the liver. Natural products such as drugs can affect CYP isozymes. The best-investigated

TABLE 74-2   Actions, Uses, and Drug Interactions of Commonly Used Herbs (Safety and Efficacy Not Confirmed)

Herb	Action	Common Clinical Uses	Drug Interactions
Black cohosh (*Cimicifuga racemosa, Actaea racemosa, Actaea macrotys*)	Menopausal symptoms, PMS	Action unknown—Does not exert estrogenic effect	None known
Chasteberry (*Vitex agnus-castus*)	Dopamine antagonist, reduction in prolactin secretion by pituitary gland	Menstrual irregularities, menopausal symptoms, PMS symptoms, mastalgia	Dopamine antagonists (antipsychotics, metoclopramide), dopamine receptor blocking agents, oral contraceptives, hormone replacement therapy (potential interaction)
Cranberry (*Vaccinium macrocarpon*)	Interferes with bacterial adherence to the urinary tract, epithelial cells, antibacterial	Prevention and treatment of UTIs and *Helicobacter pylori* infections, dental plaque prevention	Proton pump inhibitors—lansoprazole (Prevacid), omeprazole (Prilosec), and rabeprazole (AcipHex)—Might increase absorption of dietary vitamin B_{12}
Echinacea (*Echinacea angustifolia, Echinacea pallida, Echinacea purpurea*)	Immune system stimulatory effects, enhances phagocytosis; promotes wound healing—Promotes tissue regeneration and reduces inflammation	Common cold and upper respiratory infections; immune system stimulant; adjunct therapy in vaginal candidiasis (yeast infections) Topically: Wound healing, skin problems (acne, boils)	Immunosuppressants (potential interactions)
Feverfew (*Tanacetum parthenium*)	Antiinflammatory effects	Migraine prophylaxis, rheumatoid arthritis	Anticoagulants, antiplatelet drugs, aspirin (speculative interactions)
Garlic (*Allium sativum*)	Antihyperlipidemic, antithrombotic, antihypertensive, antimicrobial, anticancer, antiallergenic, antioxidant, immunomodulatory, hematologic (AGE)	Cardiovascular—Hypertension, hyperlipidemia, atherosclerosis; decreases platelet function; colon and stomach cancer prevention; treatment of URTIs	Anticoagulants, antiplatelet drugs, saquinavir (Fortovase, Invirase)
Ginger (*Zingiber officinale*)	Antiemetic, antiplatelet aggregation, antibacterial, antifungal, antirhinoviral, antischistosomal, antioxidant, antiatherosclerotic, antiinflammatory	Nausea—Due to surgery, motion sickness, chemotherapy, pregnancy, rheumatoid arthritis, osteoarthritis, joint and muscle pain	None known; cautious use with warfarin
Gingko (*Ginkgo biloba*)	Antioxidant, antiinflammatory, improves circulation by both decreasing blood viscosity and affecting vascular smooth muscle, increases cerebral and peripheral blood flow, microcirculation	Cerebral insufficiency—Alzheimer's disease/dementia, vertigo, tinnitus; vascular disease; multiple sclerosis; sexual dysfunction related to SSRI use; control of altitude sickness; hypoxia; insulin resistance	MAOIs (questionable evidence), anticoagulants, antiplatelet drugs, thiazide diuretics Antidepressant—Offsets sexual dysfunction with SSRIs; papaverine (potentiated effect); cyclosporine (helps prevent PAF-induced organ rejection)
Ginseng, panax (*Panax ginseng*)	Interferes with platelet aggregation and coagulation, analgesic, antiinflammatory, potential antiasthmatic, works against stress by affecting the hypothalamic-pituitary-adrenal (HPA) axis, affects immune function, may have anticancer effects	Adaptogen, general tonic, increases stamina, improves mental and physical performance; treatment of erectile dysfunction, hepatitis C, menopausal symptoms; lowers blood sugar, controls hypertension	Hypoglycemic agents, insulin, MAOI—phenelzine (possible interaction), antiplatelets (possible interaction), stimulants, caffeine Zidovudine (positive synergistic effect) Amoxicillin/clavulanic acid (potentiated effect)
Green tea (*Camellia sinensis*)	Antioxidant, antiviral (HPV)	Cancer prevention—Breast, stomach, skin, colon; improves mental alertness, weight loss, high cholesterol, sun damage; topical extract—Genital warts	Anticoagulants—warfarin (less effective), theophylline, alkaline medications; sulindac and/or tamoxifen (synergistic effect)
Hawthorn (*Crataegus laevigata*)	Improves cardiac insufficiency; increases cardiac work tolerance; decreases pressure/heart rate; increases ejection fraction; raises anaerobic threshold	Congestive heart failure, coronary artery disease	Digoxin, theophylline, caffeine, papaverine, sodium nitrate, adenosine, epinephrine (potentiate effects) Cardiovascular drugs

Table conitnued on following page

TABLE 74-2   Actions, Uses, and Drug Interactions of Commonly Used Herbs (Safety and Efficacy Not Confirmed) (Continued)

Herb	Action	Common Clinical Uses	Drug Interactions
Milk thistle *(Silybum marianum)*	Hepatoprotective; reduces triglycerides in serum; normalizes serum bilirubin and BSP retention; reduces malondialde-hyde concentration; increases superoxide dismutase activity in erythrocytes and lymphocytes; reduces cytotoxic lymphocytes; reduces procollagen-III peptide	Alcoholic liver disease, cirrhosis, infectious hepatitis, drug-induced hepatitis, gallbladder disorders, liver disease related to diabetes mellitus, *Amanita* mushroom poisoning	None known Psychopharmaceutical drugs (butyrophenones, phenothiazines)—Decrease lipid peroxidation damage to the liver (beneficial effect)
Saw palmetto *(Serenoa repens)*	Antiestrogenic; increases urinary flow rate; decreases residual urine; decreases dysuria; decreases nocturia; antiinflammatory properties	BPH	No confirmed drug interactions
St. John's wort *(Hypericum perforatum)*	Antidepressant, antiviral, antibiotic	Mild to moderate depression, SAD, OCD, menopause, fatigue, pediatric nocturnal incontinence, PMS; external uses—Acute and contused injuries, first-degree burns, myalgia	Antidepressants, oral contraceptives, anticoagulants, theophylline, HIV drugs—indinavir, cyclosporine, digoxin, irinotecan, drugs metabolized by CYP 450 3A4
Valerian *(Valeriana edulis, Valeriana jatamansii)*	Sedative-hypnotic, anxiolytic	Anxiety, insomnia, restlessness, and sleeping disorders; improving mood	Alcohol, barbiturates, benzodiazepines, sedatives (interactions not clinically proven)

Data from NCCAM: *Herbs at a glance,* available at http://nccam.nih.gov/health/herbsataglance.htm (accessed January 25, 2007); Blumenthal M, et al: *The ABC clinical guide to herbs,* Austin, Texas, 2003, American Botanical Council.

metabolic interactions are those involving St. John's wort. This herb, which is claimed to be effective in the treatment of mild to moderate depression, appears to be a potent inducer of isozyme CYP 3A4, and so the primary care provider who is considering its use must evaluate the impact of other drugs that the patients might be taking. Table 74-3 lists herbs that generally are considered unsafe.

ADDITIVE EFFECTS. Some herbs, when combined with pharmaceuticals that have similar or comparable actions, may have an additive effect. Additive effects may be beneficial or detrimental. In some cases, dosage of the herb or medication may be adjusted or reduced. In other cases, accentuated effects may result in overmedication and adverse effects. Many herbal weight loss and "herbal speed" products rely on the pharmacodynamic interaction between ephedra and caffeine or caffeine-containing herbs, such as cola nut (*Cola acuminata*), green tea (*Camellia sinensis*), guarana, and maté (*Ilex paraguariensis*). The two primary alkaloids contained in ephedra—ephedrine and pseudoephedrine—have additive cardiovascular effects when taken with caffeine. At higher doses, the ephedra–caffeine interaction has been cited as a cause of death. Another example of additive effects involves the use of botanicals such as ginkgo, garlic, ginseng, and ginger, which contain natural coumarins that can enhance the effects of the synthetic anticoagulants coumarin, warfarin, and even aspirin.

PATIENT VARIABLES

When treating the patient who uses herbal therapies, health care providers must consider factors that could affect the efficacy and safety of herbal use. As with prescribed medications,

herbal doses may have to be adjusted in the pediatric population according to weight or age. Until safety and efficacy in pediatric populations are studied, caution should be exercised when any herbal therapy is used in children. Pediatric studies funded by NCCAM include "A Randomized Controlled Trial of the Use of Craniosacral Osteopathic Manipulative Treatment and of Botanical Treatment in Recurrent Otitis Media in Children," "Treatment of Functional Abdominal Pain in Children: Evaluation of Relaxation/Guided Imagery and Chamomile Tea as Therapeutic Modalities," and "A Randomized Controlled Trial of Echinacea in Children."

Similarly, studies focused on the geriatric population have not been extensive. Geriatric patients often have multiple medical problems and may be taking one or more prescribed medications that could interact with herbal therapies. According to a survey conducted by AARP and the NCCAM in 2006, 69% of people 50 years of age or older do not talk to their doctors about their use of CAM. Nearly three fourths of respondents said that they take one or more prescription medications; in addition, 59% of respondents reported that they take one or more over-the-counter medications. Twenty percent of respondents stated that they take more than five prescription medications (AARP, 2007). Therefore, caution and careful assessment of medical and medication history are necessary when members of this population are treated.

As a general rule, herbs and most medications should be used during pregnancy and lactation only if absolutely necessary and only under the recommendation of a knowledgeable provider or herbalist. Little human research has explored the safety or harmfulness of herbs in pregnancy and lactation. In animal studies, many plants have been shown to stimulate uterine contractions, and, although not completely studied in

TABLE 74-3   Potentially Unsafe Herbs

Common Name	Toxic Constituents	Adverse Effects	Common Name	Toxic Constituents	Adverse Effects
Arnica	Flowers	Multiorgan toxicity	Jimsonweed	Seeds, leaves, flowers	Anticholinergic toxicity
Autumn crocus	Flowers, seeds	Multiorgan toxicity	Life root	Aerial parts	Hepatotoxicity
Belladonna	Leaves and roots	Anticholinergic toxicity	Lily of the valley	Roots, flowers, leaves	Cardiotoxicity
Bittersweet nightshade	Stems and berries	Anticholinergic toxicity	Lobelia	Leaves, seeds	Multiorgan toxicity
Black nightshade	Unripe berries	Anticholinergic toxicity	Mandrake	Roots	Anticholinergic toxicity
Bloodroot	Roots	GI toxicity	Marsh marigold	Flowers	GI toxicity
Broom (Scotch)	Aerial parts	Cardiotoxicity	Mayapple	Roots, resin	Multiorgan toxicity
Calabar bean	Seeds	Cholinergic toxicity	Mistletoe	Leaves, berries, branches	Multiorgan toxicity
Calamus	Roots	Hepatotoxicity	Monkshood	Roots, leaves, flowers	Cardiotoxicity
Canadian hemp	Aerial parts	Cardiotoxicity	Nux vomica	Seeds, bark	Neurotoxicity
Castor bean	Seeds	GI toxicity	Poison hemlock	Leaves, berries, flowers	Multiorgan toxicity
Chaparral	Leaves	Hepatotoxicity	Queen's delight	Roots	GI toxicity
Colton	Seeds, roots	Multiorgan toxicity	Waboo	Root bark, seeds, berries	Multiorgan toxicity
Comfrey	Roots, leaves	Hepatotoxicity	Wallflower	Seeds, flowers	Cardiotoxicity
Daffodil	Bulb, leaves, flowers	Multiorgan toxicity	Wild cherry	Leaves, seeds	Multiorgan toxicity
Foxglove	Seeds, leaves, flowers	Cardiotoxicity	Wormseed	Seeds, berries, aerial parts	Multiorgan toxicity
Germander	Aerial parts	Hepatotoxicity			
Hedge mustard	Aerial parts	Cardiotoxicity	Wormwood	Leaves, flowers	Neurotoxicity
Henbane	Leaves	Anticholinergic toxicity	Yellow jessamine	Roots	Multiorgan toxicity
Jalap	Roots	GI toxicity	Yohimbe	Bark	Multiorgan toxicity

Data modified from Swarbrick J: *Encyclopedia of pharmaceutical technology,* ed 2, New York, 2004, Dekker Encyclopedias–Taylor and Francis Group, Update Supplement, p 11-14.

humans, the fetotoxicity or teratogenicity of several herbs has been demonstrated conclusively enough to recommend that they should be avoided in pregnancy. These include mayapple and berberine-containing herbs such as goldenseal and barberry. Anthraquinone laxatives such as cascara sagrada, aloe latex, and rhubarb cross the blood–milk barrier, may cause infant diarrhea, and should not be used during lactation. Selected plants in human studies shown to be safe during pregnancy include echinacea root, licorice root, butcher's broom root, milk thistle seed, bilberry root, and ginger. Human studies have found that garlic, senna, and chaste tree are safe for use during lactation (Yarnell et al. 2003).

SUMMARY

Complementary and alternative modalities, along with botanical therapies, are gaining popularity in what is becoming a more integrative health care system. As scientific research tries to keep up with consumer use and demand, it is important that primary care providers become familiar with the most commonly used products and that they have access to information on unconventional modalities and products. As results reported by research studies become more conclusive, it will continue to be the responsibility of primary care providers to communicate with patients about the safety, effectiveness, and dangers of these widely available therapies.

evolve A continually updated list of useful WebLinks may be found in the Evolve Resources at http://evolve.elsevier.com/Edmunds/NP/

Readings and References

GENERAL

ACC/AHA/ESC 2006 Guidelines for the Management of Patients with Atrial Fibrillation: A report of the American College of Cardiology/American Heart Association Task Force on Practice Guidelines and the European Society of Cardiology Committee for Practice Guidelines, *J Am Coll Cardiol* 48(4):e149-e246, 2006.

Braunwald E et al: *Heart disease: a textbook of cardiovascular medicine*, ed 7, Philadelphia, 2005, Saunders.

Briggs GG et al: *Drugs in pregnancy and lactation: a reference guide to fetal and neonatal risk*, ed 7, Philadelphia, 2005, Lippincott Williams & Wilkins.

Burton LL et al, editors: *Goodman & Gilman's the pharmacological basis of therapeutics*, ed 11, New York, 2005, McGraw-Hill.

Calderwood SB: Overview of the beta-lactam antiinfectives. In Rose BD, editor *UpToDate*, Waltham, MA, 2007, UpToDate.

Chessare JB: Teaching clinical decision-making to pediatric residents in an era of managed care, *Pediatrics* 101(4, pt 2):762-766, 1998.

Chobanian AV et al: The seventh report of the Joint National Committee on Prevention, Detection, Evaluation, and Treatment of High Blood Pressure: The JNC 7 Report, *JAMA* 289:2560, 2003.

Chou R et al: Medications for acute and chronic low back pain: a review of the evidence for an American Pain Society/American College of Physicians clinical practice guideline, *Ann Intern Med* 147(7):505-514, 2007.

Colucci WS: Overview of the therapy of heart failure due to systolic dysfunction. In Rose BD, editor: *UpToDate*, Waltham, MA, UpToDate.

Drew RH: Emerging options for treatment of invasive, multidrug resistance *Staphylococcus aureus* infections, *Pharmacotherapy* 27(2):227-249, 2007.

Drug facts and comparisons, monthly update, St. Louis, 2008, Wolters Kluwer.

Edmunds MW: *Introduction to clinical pharmacology*, ed 5, St Louis, 2006, Mosby.

Gilbert DN et al: *The Sanford guide to antimicrobial therapy*, ed 36, Hyde Park, VT, 2006, Antimicrobial Therapy, Inc.

Goldstein, AO, Goldstein, BG: Dermatophyte (tinea) infections. In Rose BD, editor: *UpToDate*, Waltham, MA, 2007, UpToDate.

Groves KEM et al: Why physicians start or stop prescribing a drug: literature review and formulary implications, *Formulary* 37:186-194, 2002.

Hammer SM, Norrby SR: Principles of antiinfective therapy. In Cohen J, Powderly WG, editors: *Infectious diseases*, ed 2, St Louis, 2004, Mosby.

Hopper DC: Quinolones. In Mandell GL, et al, editors: *Principles and practice of infectious diseases*, ed 6, New York, 2005, Churchill Livingstone.

Hunt SA et al: ACC/AHA 2005 Guideline update for the diagnosis and management of chronic heart failure in the adult: a report of the American College of Cardiology/American Heart Association Task Force on Practice Guidelines: developed in collaboration with the American College of Chest Physicians and the International Society for Heart and Lung Transplantation: endorsed by the Heart Rhythm Society, *Circulation* 112:e154, 2005.

Kannam J et al: Overview of the management of stable angina pectoris. In Rose BD, editor: *UpToDate*, Waltham, MA, 2007, UpToDate.

Kaplan NM, Rose BD: Choice of therapy in essential hypertension: clinical trials. In Rose BD, editor: *UpToDate*, Waltham, MA, 2006, UpToDate.

Kaplan NM, Rose BD: Indications for use of specific antihypertensive drugs. In Rose BD, editor: *UpToDate*, Waltham, MA, 2007, UpToDate.

Katzung BG: *Basic and clinical pharmacology*, ed 10, Norwalk, CT, 2006, Appleton & Lange.

Kenred E et al: *Infectious disease epidemiology: theory and practice*, New York, 2006, Jones and Bartlett.

Lazarou J et al: Incidence of adverse drug reactions in hospitalized patients: a meta-analysis of prospective studies, *JAMA* 279:1200-1205, 1998. .

Long SS et al: *Principles and practice of pediatric infectious disease*, ed 3, New York, 2007, Churchill Livingstone.

Mandell GL et al, editors: *Principles and practice of infectious diseases*, ed 6, New York, 2005, Churchill Livingstone.

McKenry LM et al: *Mosby's pharmacology in nursing*, ed 22, St Louis, 2006, Mosby.

McPhee SJ et al: *Current medical diagnosis and treatment 2007*, ed 46, New York, 2006, McGraw-Hill.

McPhee SJ et al: *Current medical diagnosis and treatment 2008*, ed 47, New York, 2007, McGraw-Hill.

National Institutes of Health, National Heart, Lung, and Blood Institute, National High Blood Pressure Education Program: *Seventh report of the Joint National Committee on Prevention, Detection, Evaluation, and Treatment of High Blood Pressure*, NIH Publication No. 03-5233, Washington, DC, May 2003, U.S. Department of Health and Human Services.

Office of Technology Assessment (OTA), U.S. Congress: *Nurse practitioners, physician assistants, and certified nurse midwives: a policy analysis*. Health technology case study 37, Washington, DC, 1986, Author.

Saw JT et al: Potential drug-herb interaction with antiplatelet/anticoagulant drugs, *Comp Ther Clin Pract* 12(4):236-241, 2006.

Simoni-Wastila L et al: Over-the-counter drug use by Medicare beneficiaries in nursing homes: implications for practice and policy, *J Am Geriatr Soc* 54(10):1543-1549, 2006.

Talley NJ: American Gastroenterological Association medical position statement: evaluation of dyspepsia, *Gastroenterology* 129(5):1753-1755, 2005.

Woodwell DA: *National ambulatory medical care survey: 1996 summary. Advance data from vital and health statistics*, No. 295, Hyattsville, MD, 1997, National Center for Health Statistics.

Workowski KA, Berman SM: Sexually transmitted disease treatment guidelines, 2006, *MMWR Recomm Rep* 55(RR-11):1-94, 2006.

Yang YX et al: Long-term proton pump inhibitor therapy and risk of hip fracture, *JAMA* 296(24):2947-2953, 2006.

CHAPTER 1

Aiken KJ: *Direct to consumer advertising of prescription drug: physician survey preliminary results*, Division of Drug Marketing, Advertising and Communication, FDA, January 13, 2003. Available at www.fda.gov/cder/ddmac/globalsummit2003/sld001.htm.

Avorn G et al: The neglected medical history and therapeutics: choices for abdominal pain: a nationwide study of 799 physicians and 151 nurses, *Arch Intern Med* 151:694-698, 1991.

Burban GM et al: Influences on oncologists' adoption of new agents in adjuvant chemotherapy of breast cancer, *J Clin Oncol* 19:954-959, 2001.

Cherry DK, Woodwell DA: *National ambulatory medical care survey: 2000 summary*, U.S. Dept HHS, CDC, NCHS, Advance Data, Number 328, June 5, 2002.

Denig P, Haaijer-Ruskamp FM: Therapeutic decision making of physicians, *Pharm Week Scien Ed* 14:9-15, 1992.

DeNuzzo R: *25th Annual prescription survey: medical marketing and the media*, New York, 1981, Albany College of Pharmacy of Union University.

Freidson E: *Profession of medicine: a study of the sociology of applied knowledge*, New York, 1970a, Harper and Row.

Freidson E: *Professional dominance: the social structure of medical care*, Chicago, 1970b, Aldine.

Freidson E: *The professions and their prospects*, Beverly Hills, CA, 1971, Sage Publications.

Hing E et al: *National ambulatory medical care survey: 2004*, U.S. Dept HHS, NCHS, Advance Data, Number 374, June 23, 2006.

Knoben S, Wertheimer A: Physician prescribing patterns—therapeutic categories and age considerations, *Drug Intell Clin Pharm* 10:398-400, 1976.

Mahoney DF: Nurse practitioners as prescribers: past research trends and future study needs, *Nurse Pract* 17:44, 47-48, 50-51, 1992.

Mahoney DF: Appropriateness of geriatric prescribing decisions made by nurse practitioners and physicians, *IMAGE J Nurs Scholar* 26:41-46, 1994.

Medication therapy in ambulatory medical care: United States, 2003-2004. U.S. Department Health and Human Services, Centers for Disease Control and Prevention, National Center for Health Statistics. Series 13, No. 163, December 2006.

Miles D, Roland D: Prescribing patterns in a rural community, *Drugs Health Care* 2:187-194, 1975.

Miller R: Prescribing habits of physicians—a review of studies on prescribing of drugs. Parts IV-VI, *Drug Intel Clin Pharm* 7:557-564, 1973.

Miller R: Prescribing habits of physicians—a review of studies on prescribing of drugs. Parts VII-VIII, *Drug Intel Clin Pharm* 8:81-91, 1974.

Munroe D et al: Prescribing patterns of nurse practitioners, *Am J Nurs* 82:1538-1542, 1982.

National Center for Health Statistics (NCHS): *Drug utilization in general and family practice by characteristics of physicians and office visits, National ambulatory medical care survey, 1980*, Hyattsville, MD, March 18, 1983a, U.S. Public Health Service, No. 87 DHHS Pub. No (PHS) 83-1250.

National Center for Health Statistics (NCHS): *Drugs most frequently used in office-based practice: National ambulatory medical care survey, 1981*, Hyattsville, MD, April 1983b, U.S. Public Health Service, No. DHHS Pub. No. (PHS) 83-250.

Ramsey PG et al: History-taking and preventive medicine skills among primary care physicians: an assessment using standardized patients, *Am J Med* 104:152-158, 1998.

Rosenberg S et al: Prescribing patterns in the New York City Medicaid program, *Med Care* 12:138-151, 1974.

Rossiter L: Prescribed medicines: findings from the National Medical Care Expenditure Survey, *Am J Pub Health* 73:1312-1315, 1983.

Safreit B: Health care dollars and regulatory sense: the role of advanced practice nursing, *Yale J Reg* 99:417-488, Summer 1992.

Smith M: Drug product advertising and prescribing: a review of the evidence, *Am J Hosp Pharm* 34:1208-1224, 1977.

So AD: Free gifts: redundancy or conundrum? *J Gen Intern Med* 13:213-215, 1998.

Starr P: *The social transformation of American medicine*, New York, 1982, Basic.

Stolley P et al: The relationship between physician characteristics and prescribing appropriateness, *Med Care* 10:17-28, 1972a.

Stolley P et al: Drug prescribing and use in an American community, *Ann Intern Med* 76:537-540, 1972b.

Stolley P, Lasagna L: Prescribing patterns of physicians, *J Chronic Dis* 22:395-405, 1969.

Top drugs: Available at www.rxlist.com (lists the top 200 drugs prescribed each year, with a detailed database on prescriptions.

U.S. Department of Health and Human Services (USDHHS): *Medication therapy in ambulatory medical care: United States, 2003-2004*, Vital and Health Statistics, Series 13, Number 13, December 2006. DHHS Publication No (PHS) 2007-1734.

Vanselow NA et al: From the Institute of Medicine, *JAMA* 273:192, 1995.

CHAPTER 2

Accreditation Review Committee for the Physician Assistant (ARC-PA): *Standards for accreditation of educational programs for physician assistants*, ed 3, 2006.

Alexander BJ, et al: *Physician staffing for the VA, vol II, supplementary papers, nonphysician panel report*, Alexandria, VA, 1992, National Academies Press.

American Academy of Physician Assistants (AAPA): *Physician assistant prescribing and dispensing*, Alexandria, VA, 2006a, American Academy of Physician Assistants, Author.

American Academy of Physician Assistants (AAPA): *Physician assistants: state laws and regulations*, ed 10, Alexandria, VA, 2006, Author.

American Academy of Physician Assistants (AAPA): *Annual census on PAs*, Alexandria, VA, 2006, Author.

American Association of Colleges of Nursing (AACN): *The essentials of master's education for advanced practice nursing*, Washington, DC, 1996, 1998, Author.

American Association of Colleges of Nursing (AACN): *Position statement on the practice doctorate in nursing*, October 2004. Available at www.aacn.nche.edu.

American Association of Nurse Anesthetists (AANA): Annual Committee Reports of the AANA, 1989-1990, *AANA News Bull* 44(10)(Suppl):37-38, 1990.

American Association of Nurse Anesthetists (AANA): *Qualifications and capabilities of the certified registered nurse anesthetist*, Park Ridge, IL, 1992, Author.

American Association of Nurse Anesthetists (AANA): *Scope and standards for nurse anesthesia practice*, Park Ridge, IL, 1996, Author.

American Association of Nurse Anesthetists (AANA): *Nurse anesthetists: providing anesthesia into the next century: executive summary*, Park Ridge, IL, 1998, Author.

American College of Nurse -Midwives, Overview, http://acnm.org Accessed May 1, 2008 (ACNM): *Philosophy*, Washington, DC, 1989, Author.

American College of Nurse-Midwives (ACNM): *Accreditation of education programs*, Washington, DC, 1992, Author. American College of Nurse-Midwives.

American College of Nurse Midwives: *Code of ethics*, Washington, DC, 1997a, American College of Nurse Midwives.

American College of Nurse Midwives: *Core competencies for basic nurse-midwifery*,

Washington, DC, 1997b, American College of Nurse Midwives.

American College of Nurse Midwives: *Philosophy*, Washington, DC, 1989, American College of Nurse Midwives.

American College of Nurse Midwives (ACNM): *Standards for the practice of nurse-midwifery*, Washington, DC, 1992, Author.

American College of Nurse-Midwives (ACNM): *Code of ethics*, Washington, DC, 1997, Author.

American College of Nurse-Midwives (ACNM): *Core competencies for basic nurse-midwifery*, Washington, DC, 1997, Author.

American College of Nurse-Midwives (ACNM): *Midwifery education*, Washington, DC, 1997, Author.

American College of Nurse-Midwives (ACNM): *Nurse midwifery today; handbook on state legislation*, Washington, DC, 1997c, American College of Nurse Midwives, Author.

American College of Nurse Midwives: *Midwifery education*, Washington, DC, 1997d, American College of Nurse Midwives.

American Nurses Association (ANA): *Nursing: a social policy statement*, Kansas City, MO, 1980, The Association.

American Nurses Association (ANA): *Executive summary. Meta-analysis of process of care, clinical outcomes, and cost-effectiveness: nurse practitioners and certified nurse midwives*, Washington, DC; 1993.

Barclay L: AMA discloses master file physician data to pharmaceutical companies. Available at www.medscape.com/viewarticle/559704?src=mp.

Bell D: Writing of prescriptions through delegation, *Minn Med* 63:337-338, 1980.

Bosma J: Using nurse practitioner certification for state nursing regulation: an update, *Nurse Pract* 22:213, 1997.

Brown SA, Grimes DE: A meta-analysis of nurse practitioners and nurse-midwives in primary care, *Nurs Res* 44(6):332-339, 1995.

Bullough B: *The law and the expanding nursing role*, ed 2, New York, 1980, Appleton-Century-Crofts.

Buppert C: *Nurse practitioner's business practice and legal guide*, Gaithersburg, MD, 1999, Aspen.

Carr M: Merging advanced practice roles, *Nurse Pract* 21:160, 1996.

Cawley JF: The profession in 2002 and beyond, *J Acad Physician Assist* 10:7-15, 2002.

Cawley JF, Hooker, RS: The effects of resident work hour restrictions on physician assistant hospital utilization, *J Physician Assist Ed*, 17:41-43, 2006.

Cawley JF et al: Physician assistants and malpractice risk: findings from the national practitioner data bank, *Fed Bull*, 85(4):242-247, 1998.

Cipher DJ et al: Prescribing trends by nurse practitioners and physician assistants in the United States, *J Am Acad Nurse Pract* 18:291-296, 2006.

Clark S et al: Trends and characteristics of births attended byby midwives. Statistical Bulletin. Jan-Feb. 78:1, NY, 1997, Metropolitan Life Insurance Co.

Cohen H: *Physician assistant pursuit of prescribing authority: a five-state analysis*, master's thesis, Baltimore, MD, 1996, Johns Hopkins University.

Cooper R et al: Roles of non-physician clinicians as autonomous providers of patient care, *JAMA* 280(9):795-802, 1998.

Council on Certification of Nurse Anesthetists (CCNA): *1998 Recertification candidate handbook*, Park Ridge, IL, 1998, Author.

Davis A: Putting state legislative issues in context, *J Am Acad Physician Assist* 10:27-32, 2002.

Edmunds MW: Evaluation of nurse practitioner effectiveness: an overview of the literature, *Eval Health Prof* 1:69-82, Spring 1978.

Edmunds MW: Council's pursuit of national standardization for advanced practice nursing meets with resistance, *Nurse Pract* 17:81-83, 1992.

Edmunds MW: Nurse practitioners: remembering the past, planning the future, *Medscape Nurses* 2(1), 2000. Available at www.medscape.com/viewarticle/408388 (accessed May 1, 2008).

Edmunds MW, Scudder LC: *Annual descriptive survey of prescriptive practices of nurse practitioners*, National Conference for Nurse Practitioners, Washington, DC, 1996, 1997, 1998, NPA, Inc, Columbia, MD.

Fink JL: Drug prescribing by physician extenders, *Drugs Health Care* 2:195-199, 1975.

Ford LC: A nurse for all settings: the nurse practitioner, *Nurs Outlook* 27:516-521, 1979.

Gara N, Davis A: *The political process*. In Ballweg R et al, editors: *Physician assistant: a guide to clinical practice*, ed 3, Philadelphia, 2003, Saunders.

Grumbach K, Coffman J: Physicians and nonphysician clinicians: complements or competitors? *JAMA* 280:285-286, 1998.

Hansen C: *Access to rural health care: barriers to practice for nonphysician providers*, Bureau of Health Professions, Health Resources and Services Administration (HRSA-240-89-0037), Rockville, MD, November, 1992, Department of Health and Human Services.

Hanson CM, editor: Regulation and credentialing of advanced practice nurses, *Adv Pract Nurs Q4* (3), 1998.

Hooker RS, Berlin L: Trends in the supply of physician assistants and nurse practitioners in the United States, *Health Affairs* 21(5):174-81, 2002.

Hooker RS, Cawley JF: *Physician assistants in American medicine*, ed 2, New York, 2003, Churchill Livingstone.

Horrocks S et al: Systemic reviews of whether nurse practitioners working in primary care can provide equivalent care to doctors, *BMJ* 324(7341):819-823, 2002.

Houghland D: Final report to the legislature and the Healing Arts Licensing Boards: prescribing and dispensing pilot projects. Office of Statewide Health Planning and Development Division of Health Professional Development, State of California, 1982.

Hueston WJ, Rudy MA: A comparison of labor and delivery management between CNMs and family physicians, *J Fam Pract* 375:449-454, 1993.

Institute of Medicine (IM): *Crossing the quality chasm: a new health system for the 20th century*,

Washington, DC, 2001, National Academies Press.

Jones PE, Cawley JF: Physician assistants and health care reform, *JAMA* 271:1266-1272, 1994.

Kane RL et al: Effects of adding a Medex in practice costs and productivity, *J Commun Health* 3:216-226, 1978.

Kelly LY: Nursing practice acts, *Am J Nurs* 74:1311-1319, 1974.

Klein TA: Scope of practice and the nurse practitioner: regulation, competency, expansion, and evolution, *Top Adv Pract Nurs eJ* 5(2):2005. Available at www.medscape.com/viewprogram/4188.

Klein TA: Second licensure for NPs, *J Nurse Pract* 4(2):2007.

Kleinpell R, Gawlinski A: Assessing outcomes in advanced practice nursing practice: the use of quality indicators and evidence-based practice, *AACN Clin Issues* 16(1):43-57, 2005.

Knedle-Murray ME et al: Production process substitution in maternity care: issues of cost, quality, and outcomes by nurse-midwives and physician providers, *Med Care Rev* 50:91-112, 1993.

Lambing AV et al: Nurse practitioners and physicians' care activities and clinical outcomes with an inpatient geriatric population, *J Am Acad Nurse Pract* 16(8):343-352, 2004.

Laurant M et al: Substitution of doctors by nurses in primary care, *Cochrane Database Syst Rev* (2):CD001271, 2005.

Lenz E et al: Primary care outcomes in patients treated by nures practitioners or physicians: two-year follow up, *Med Care Res Rev* 61(3):332-351, 2004.

Lewis EP, editor: *The clinical nurse specialist*, New York, 1970, American Journal of Nursing.

Lugo NR et al: Ranking state NP regulation: practice environment and consumer healthcare choice, *Am J Nurse Pract* 11(4):18-24, 2007.

MacDorman MF, Singh GK: Midwifery care, social and medical risk factors and birth outcomes in the USA, *J Epidemiol Commun Health*, May, 1998.

Miller KP: Feeling the heat: nurse rpactitioners and malpractice liability, *J Nurse Pract* 3(1):24-26, 2006.

Mundinger MO et al: Primary care outcomes in patients treated by nurse practitioners or physicians: a randomized trial, *JAMA* 283:59-68, 2000.

National Council of State Boards of Nursing (NCSBN)et al (National Organization of Nurse Practitioner Faculties): *Curriculum guidelines and regulatory criteria for family nurse practitioners seeking prescriptive authority to manage pharmacotherapeutics in primary care, summary report, 1998*, HRSA 98-41, Washington, DC, 1998, U.S. Department of Health and Human Services.

National Council of State Boards of Nursing (NCSBN): *Changes in healthcare professions' scope of practice: legislative considerations*, 2006. Available at www.ncsbn.org.

National Council of State Boards of Nursing (NCSBN): *Vision paper: The future regulation of advanced practice nursing*. Available at www.ncsbn.org.

National Council of State Boards of Nursing (NCSBN): *Nurse licensure compact implementation*. Available at: www.ncsbn.org/nlc/rnlpvncompact_mutual_recognition_state.asp.

National Organization of Nurse Practitioner Faculties (NONPF): *Guidelines for family nurse practitioner curricular planning*, Washington, DC, 1980, Author.

National Organization of Nurse Practitioner Faculties (NONPF): *Model program standards for nurse practitioner programs*, Washington, DC, 1994, Author.

National Organization of Nurse Practitioner Faculties (NONPF): *Curriculum guidelines and criteria for evaluation of pharmacology content to prepare family nurse practitioners for prescriptive authority and managing pharmacotherapeutics in primary care*, Washington, DC, 1996, Author.

National Organization of Nurse Practitioner Faculties (NONPF): Curriculum guidelines and regulatory criteria for family nurse practitioners seeking prescriptive authority to manage pharmacotherapeutics in primary care, Washington, DC, 1999, Author.

National Organization of Nurse Practitioner Faculties (NONPF): *Advanced nursing practice: curriculum guidelines and program standards for nurse practitioner programs*, Washington, DC, 1995, Author.

National Organization of Nurse Practitioner Faculties (NONPF): *Domain and competencies for nurse practitioner practice*, Washington, DC, 2000, Author.

National Organization of Nurse Practitioner Faculties (NONPF): *Domain and competencies for nurse practitioner practice*, Washington, DC, 200, Author.

National Organization Nurse Practitioner Faculties (NONPF): *Nurse practitioner primary care competencies in specialty areas: adult, family, gerontological, pediatric, and women's health, USHHS: NONPF*. Available at www.nonpf.com/.

Nielsen JR: *Handbook of federal drug law*, ed 2, Philadelphia, 1992, Lea & Febiger.

Oakley D et al: Processes of care: comparisons of CNM and obstetricians, *J Nurs Midwifery* 40:399-409, 1995.

Pearson L: The Pearson report, *Am J Nurse Pract* 11(2):2007. Available at www.webnp.net/ajnp.html.

Phillips S: Annual update on how each state stands on legislative issues affected advanced nursing practice, *Nurs Pract* 32(1):14-17, 2007.

Riehl JP, McVay JW: *The clinical nurse specialist: interpretations*, New York, 1973, Appleton-Century-Crofts.

Robinson DDL et al: Second licensure for advanced practice: current status, *Nurs Pract* 21:71, 1996.

Rogers M: Nursing: to be or not to be? *Nurs Outlook* 20: 42-46, 1972.

Rosenblatt RA: Interspecialty differences in the obstetric care of low-risk women, *Am J Public Health* 87:344-351, 1997.

Safriet B: Health care dollars and regulatory sense: the role of advanced practice nursing, *Yale J Reg* 9:417-488, Summer 1992.

Safreit B: Impediments to progress in health care workforce policy: license and practice laws, *Inquiry* 31:310-317, 1994.

Scudder L: Prescribing patterns of nurse practitioners, *J Nurse Pract* 2(2):98-106, 2006.

Sekscenski E et al: State practice environments and the supply of physician assistants, nurse practitioners, and certified nurse midwives, *N Engl J Med* 331(19):1266-1271, 1994.

Sharp N: Regional or multistate licensure: Is it coming soon? *Nurs Pract* 22:10, 1997.

Simon AF, Link M: *Twenty-first annual survey of physician assistant educational programs in the United States 2005*, Alexandria, VA, 2006, Physician Assistant Education Association.

Sparacino PSA et al, editors: *The clinical nurse specialist: implementation and impact*, Norwalk, CT, 1990, Appleton & Lange.

Sullivan D: *Prescriptive privileges for nurse practitioners: a survey of pharmacists in Maryland*, master's thesis, Baltimore, 1988, University of Maryland School of Nursing.

Sutliff LS: Myth, mystique, and monopoly in the prescription of medicine, *Nurs Pract* 21:15, 1996.

Tobin MH: *Nurse anesthetists and prescriptive authority: what is it and do you need it?* Presentation at Fall Assembly of States, American Association of Nurse Anesthetists, 1991.

Tobin MH: Personal telephone interview by MW Edmunds on prescriptive status of CRNAs with American Association of Nurse Anesthetists director of State Government Affairs, January 2007.

Trandel-Korenchuk D, Trandel-Korenchuk K: How state laws recognize advanced nursing practice, *Nurs Outlook* 26:613-619, 1978.

U.S. Department of Health and Human Services (USDHHS), Health Resources and Services Administration, Agency for Health Care Policy and Research: *Curriculum guidelines & regulatory criteria for family nurse practitioners seeking prescriptive authority to manage pharmacotherapeutics in primary care: summary report, 1998*, Washington, DC, 1998, U.S. Government Printing Office, HRSA 98-41.

U.S. Department of Health and Human Services (USDHHS), Health Resources and Services Administration, Bureau of Health Professions, Division of Nursing: *Nurse practitioner primary care competencies in specialty areas: adult, family, gerontological, pediatric, and women's health*, Washington, DC, April 2002, U.S. Government Printing Office, HRSA 00-0532 [p].

Viens, DC: NONPF and quality NP education, *Top Adv Pract Nurs eJ* 3(3):2003.

Willis JB: Barriers to PA practice in primary care and rural medically underserved areas, *J Am Acad Physician Assist* 6:418-422, 1993.

Willis JB: Prescriptive practice patterns of physician assistants, *J Am Acad Physician Assist* 3:39-56, 1990.

Wing P et al: Changes in the legal practice environment of nure practitioners, *Am J Nurse Pract* 9(2):25-39, 2005.

Wing P et al: The changing professional practice of physician assistants, 1992-2000, *J Am Acad Physician Assist* 17:37-49, 2004.

Yeo TP, Edmunds MW: What to expect from medical liability tort reform, *Nurse Pract* 29(5):7, 2004.

Yocum C et al: *The curriculum guidelines and regulatory criteria for family nurse practitioners seeking prescriptive authority to manage pharmacotherapeutics in primary care*, National Organization of Nurse Practitioner Faculties, Washington DC, 1999.

CHAPTER 3

American Psychiatric Association: *Diagnostic and statistical manual of mental disorders*, ed 4, Washington, DC, 2000, The Association.

Aspden P et al, editors: *Preventing medication errors: quality chasm series*, Committee on Identifying and Preventing Medication Errors, Board on Health Care Services, Institute of Medicine of the National Academies, The National Academies Press, Washington, DC; 2006. Available at www.iom.edu/CMS/3809/22526/35939.aspx; prepublication copy (uncorrected proofs). Available at: www.nap.edu/catalog/11623.html#toc; press release (July 20, 2006). Available at: www8.nationalacademies.org/onpinews/newsitem.aspx?RecordID=11623.

Associated Press: Campaign on hospital errors saves lives, *New York Times*, June 15, 2006. Available at www.nytimes.com/2006/06/15/health/15hospitals.html.

Bates DW, et al: Incidence of adverse drug events and potential adverse drug events: implications for prevention, ADE Prevention Study Group, *JAMA* 274:29-34, 1995.

Bates DW, et al: The costs of adverse drug events in hospitalized patients, Adverse Drug Events Prevention Study Group, *JAMA* 277:307-311, 1997.

Bond CA, Raehl CL: Adverse drug reactions in U.S. hospitals, *Pharmacotherapy* 26(5):601-608, 2006.

Bourne, David: PHAR 4634 Biopharmaceutics/Pharmacokinetics, www.boomer.org/c/p1/ 2007 (accessed August 6, 2008).

Burton LL, Lazo JS, Parker KL, editors: *Goodman & Gilman's the pharmacological basis of therapeutics*, ed 11, New York, 2005, McGraw Hill .

Classen DC et al: Adverse drug events in hospitalized patients: excess length of stay, extra costs, and attributable mortality, *JAMA* 277:301-306, 1997.

Crossing the quality chasm: a new health system for the 21st century, Washington, DC, 2001, National Academies Press.

Cullen DJ et al: The incident reporting system does not detect adverse drug events: a problem for quality improvement, *Joint Comm J Qual Improv* 21:541-548, 1995.

DiPiro JT et al, editors: *Pharmacotherapy: a pathophysiologic approach*, ed 6, Norwalk, CT, 2005, McGraw-Hill, Appleton & Lange.

Dresser GK et al: Pharmaokinetic-pharmacodynamic consequences and clinical relevance of cytochrome P450 3A4 inhibition, *Clin Pharm* 38(1):41-57, 2000.

Esch AF et al: *WHO Tech Rep Ser*, Report No. 498, 1971.

Gholami K et al: Antiinfectives-induced adverse drug reactions in hospitalized patients, *Pharmacoepidemiol Drug Safe* 14(7):501-506, 2005.

Ginsberg G et al: Pharmacokinetics and pharmacodynamic factors that can affect sensitivity to neurotoxic sequelae in elderly individuals, *Environ Health Perspect* 113(9):1243-1249, 2005.

Gomes ER, Demoly P: Epidemiology of hypersensitivity drug reactions, *Curr Opin Allergy Clin Immunol* (4):309-316, 2005.

Hanlon JT et al.: Incidence and predictors of all and preventable adverse drug reactions in frail elderly persons after hospital stay. *J Gerontol A Biol Sci Med Sci* (5):511-515, 2006.

Institute for Healthcare Improvement: *Preventing adverse drug events through medication reconciliation, saving lives web & action programs*. Available at www.ihi.org/IHI/Programs/ConferencesAndTraining/WebandACTIONMedReconciliation.htm.

Kohn K et al: To err is human: building a safer health system, Washington, DC, 2000, National Academies Press. Available at www.nap.edu/catalog/9728.html.

Kvasz M et al: Adverse drug reactions in hospitalized patients: a critique of a meta-analysis, *Medscape Gen Med* 2(2):2000.

Lim HK et al: Automated screening with confirmation of mechanism-based inactivation of CYP3A4, CYP2C9, CYP2C19, CYP2D6, and CYP1A2 in pooled human liver microsomes, *Drug Metab Dispos* 33(8):1211-1219, 2005.

McCance KL, Huether SE: *Understanding pathophysiology*, ed 7, St Louis, 2007, Mosby.

McCannon CJ et al: Saving 100,000 lives in U.S. hospitals, *BMJ* 332:1328-1330, 2006.

Michalets EL: Clinically significant cytochrome P-450 drug interactions, *Pharmacotherapy* 18:84-112, 1998.

National Institute on Alcohol Abuse and Alcoholism (NIAAA): *Alert on alcohol and medication interactions*, No 27, PH 355, Washington, DC, January 1995, The Institute.

Osterberg L, Blaschke T: *Medication compliance and avoiding adverse drug reactions*. Available at www.medscape.com/viewprogram/5912_index.

Stringer JL: *Basic concepts in pharmacology*, ed 3, New York, 2005, McGraw-Hill.

U.S. Food and Drug Administration (FDA): *MedWatch Drug Reporting Program*, Washington, DC, 1990, FDA.

Weathermon R, Crabb DW: Alcohol and medication interactions. *Alcohol Res Health*. 1999;23(1):40-54.

Young LR et al: Adverse drug reactions: a review for healthcare practitioners, *Am J Manag Care* 3:1884-1906, 1997.

Zhou S et al: Therapeutic drugs that behave as mechanism-based inhibitors of cytochrome P450 3A4, *Curr Drug Metab* 5(5):415-442, 2004.

Zhou S et al: Mechanism-based inhibition of cytochrome P450 3A4 by therapeutic drugs, *Clin Pharmacokinet* 44(3):279-304, 2005.

CHAPTER 4

Abernathy AP et al: Palliative care pharmacotherapy literature summaries and analyses, *J Pain Palliat Care Pharmacother* 20(4):63-70, 2006.

American Pharmacists Association (APhA): *Medication compliance-adherence-persistence*

(CAP) digest, Washington, DC, 2003, American Pharmacists Association and Pfizer Pharmaceuticals.

Atkin PA et al: The epidemiology of serious adverse drug reactions among the elderly, Drugs Aging 14:141-152, 1999.

Baier MT: Pharmacotherapy for behavioral and psychological symptoms of dementia in the elderly, Am J Health Syst Pharm 64(2 Suppl 1): S9-S17, 2007.

Barry PJ et al: Inappropriate prescribing in the elderly: a comparison of the Beers criteria and the improved prescribing in the elderly tool (IPET) in acutely ill elderly hospitalized patients, J Clin Pharm Ther 31(6):617-626, 2006.

Beers MH: Explicit criteria for determining potentially inappropriate medication use by the elderly, Arch Intern Med 157:1531-1536, 1997.

Bigos KL et al: Population pharmacokinetics in geriatric psychiatry, Am J Geriatr Psychiatry 14(12):993-1003, 2006.

Boockvar KS et al: Medication reconciliation for reducing drug-discrepancy adverse events, Am J Geriatr Pharmacother 4(3):236-243, 2006.

Bourne D: Course in pharmacokinetics and biopharmaceutics (2007). Available at www.boomer.org/c/p4/index.php?Loc.Visitor.

Burton ME et al: Applied pharmacokinetics and pharmacodynamics: principles of therapeutic drug monitoring, ed 4, Baltimore, 2005, Lippincott Williams & Wilkins.

Chang CM et al: Use of the Beers criteria to predict adverse drug reactions among first-visit elderly outpatients, Pharmacotherapy 25(6):831-838, 2005.

Committee on Quality of Health Care in America: Institute of Medicine. To err is human: building a safer health system, Washington, DC, 2000, National Academies Press.

Cotrell V et al: Medication management and adherence among cognitively impaired older adults, J Gerontol Soc Work 47(3-4):31-46, 2006.

Cramer JA: Effect of partial compliance on the cardiovascular medication effectiveness, Heart 88(2):203-206, 2002.

Curtis LH et al: Inappropriate prescribing for elderly Americans in a large outpatient population. Arch Intern Med 164:1621-5, 2004.

Duthie EH et al: The practice of geriatrics, ed 4, Philadelphia, 2007, Saunders.

Egger SS et al: Prevalence of potentially inappropriate medication use in elderly patients: comparison between general medical and geriatric wards, Drugs Aging 23:823-838, 2006.

Egger T et al: Cytochrome p450 polymorphisms in geriatric patients: impact on adverse drug reactions—a pilot study, Drugs Aging 22:265-272, 2005.

Fick DM et al: Updating the Beers criteria for potentially inappropriate medication use in older adults: results of a U.S. consensus panel of experts, Arch Intern Med 163:2716, 2003.

Frankfort SV et al: Evaluation of pharmacotherapy in geriatric patients after performing complete geriatric assessment at a diagnostic day clinic, Clin Drug Invest 26:169-174, 2006.

Gallo JJ et al: Handbook of geriatric assessment, New York, 2006, Aspen.

Grady KL: Management of heart failure in older adults, J Cardiovasc Nurs 21(5 Suppl 1): S10-S14, 2006.

Gray SL et al: Benzodiazepine use and physical performance in community-dwelling elders, J Am Geriatr Soc 51:1563-1570, 2003.

Greene HA, Slattum PW: Resolving medication discrepancies, Consult Pharm 21(8):643-647, 2006.

Handler SM et al: Epidemiology of medication-related adverse events in nursing homes, Am J Geriatr Pharmacother 4:264-272, 2006.

Hartikainen S et al: Medication as a risk factor for falls: critical systematic review, J Gerontol A Biol Sci Med Sci 62(10): 1172-81, 2007.

Jacubeit T et al: Risk factors as reflected by an intensive drug monitoring system, Agents Actions 29:117-125, 1990.

Laroche ML et al: Impact of hospitalization in an acute medical geriatric unit on potentially inappropriate medication use, Drugs Aging 23:49-59, 2006.

Leape LL et al: Systems analysis of adverse drug events. ADE Prevention Study Group, JAMA 274(1):35-43, 1995.

Lindblad CI et al: Clinically important drug-disease interactions and their prevalence in older adults, Clin Ther 28:1133-1143, 2006.

Merle L et al: Predicting and preventing adverse drug reactions in the very old, Drugs Aging 22(5):275-291, 2005.

Molony S: Beers criteria for potentially inappropriate medication use in the elderly, Dermatol Nurs 16(6):547-548, 2004.

National Center for Health Statistics, http://www.cdc.gov/nchs/fastats/older_americans.htm Accessed May 1, 2008

Oo C, Hill G: Change in creatinine clearance with advancing age, J Am Geriatr Soc 50:1603, 2002.

Passarelli MC et al: Adverse drug reactions in an elderly hospitalized population: inappropriate prescription is a leading cause, Drugs Aging 22:767-777, 2005.

Quartarolo JM et al: Reporting of estimated glomerular filtration rate: effect on physician recognition of chronic kidney disease and prescribing practices for elderly hospitalized patients, J Hosp Med 2(2):74-78, 2007.

Ray RA, Street AF: Who's there and who cares: age as an indicator of social support networks for caregivers among people living with motor neuron disease, Health Soc Care Commun 13(6):542-552, 2005.

Sloane P et al: Inappropriate medication prescribing in residential care/assisted living facilities, J Am Geriatr Soc 50: 1001-1011, 2002.

Spina E, Scordo M: Clinically significant drug interactions with antidepressants in the elderly, Drugs Aging 19:299-320, 2002.

Troupin B: Conference report: update on family medicine—highlights from WONCA 2001, Medscape Family Medicine. Available at www.medscape.com/viewarticle/403641.

Williams CM: Using medication appropriately in older adults, Am Fam Physician 66(10): 1917-1924, 2002.

Wilson K et al: Antidepressant versus placebo for depressed elderly, Cochrane Database Syst Rev (2):CD000561, 2001.

Wynne H: Drug metabolism and aging, J Br Menopause Soc 11(2):51, 2005.

CHAPTER 5

American Academy of Pediatrics, Committee on Drugs: Alternative routes of drug administration advantages and disadvantages (subject review), Pediatrics 100:143-152, 1997. Available at http://pediatrics.aappublications.org/cgi/content/abstract/100/1/143 (accessed August 6, 2008).

American Academy of Pediatrics, Committee on Drugs: Guidelines for the ethical conduct of studies to evaluate drugs in pediatric populations, Pediatrics 95:286-294, 1995.

American Academy of Pediatrics, Committee on Drugs: The transfer of drugs and other chemicals into human milk, Pediatrics 108(3):776-779, 2001.

Bajcetic M et al: Off label and unlicensed drugs use in paediatric cardiology, Eur J Clin Pharmacol 61(10):775-779, 2005.

Banner W: Off label prescribing in children, BMJ 324(7349):1290-1291, 2002.

Burton LL, Lazo JS, Parker KL, editors: Goodman & Gilman's the pharmacological basis of therapeutics, ed 11, New York, 2005, McGraw Hill

Centers for Disease Control and Prevention (CDC): Related articles, infant deaths associated with cough and cold medications—two states, 2005, MMWR Morb Mortal Wkly Rep 56(1):1-4, 2007.

Connor DF, Meltzer BM: Pediatric psychopharmacology: fast facts, New York, 2006, Norton.

Cuzzolin L et al: Off-label and unlicensed prescribing for newborns and children in different settings: a review of the literature and a consideration about drug safety, Expert Opin Drug Saf 5(5):703-718, 2006.

Gilman JT: Therapeutic drug monitoring in the neonate and paediatric age group: problems and clinical pharmacokinetic implications, Clin Pharmacokinet 19:1, 1990.

Gupta A, Waldhauser LK: Adverse drug reactions from birth to early childhood, Pediatr Clin North Am 44:79-92, 1997.

Hale TW: Medication in mother's milk, ed 13, Amarillo, 2008, Pharmasoft.

Hansten PD, Horn JR: The top 100 drug interactions: a guide to patient management, ed 8, New York, 2007, H & H.

Horen B et al: Adverse drug reactions and off-label drug use in paediatric outpatients, Brit J Clin Pharmacol 54,665-670, 2002.

Kleigman RM et al: Nelson textbook of pediatrics, ed 18, Philadelphia, 2007, Saunders.

Koren G: Maternal-fetal toxicology: a clinician's guide, ed 3, New York, 2001, Informa Health Care.

Koren G, Cohen MS: Special aspects of perinatal and pediatric pharmacology. In Katzung BM: Basic and clinical pharmacology, ed 10, Norwalk, CT, 2006, McGraw-Hill.

Leeder JS et al: Pharmacogenetics in pediatrics: implications for practice, Pediatr Clin North Am 44:55-77, 1997.

Levine S et al: The essentials in pediatric dosing, Patient Care Nurse Pract 17: 48-75, 2000.

Li JS et al: Economic return of clinical trials performed under the pediatric exclusivity program, *JAMA* 297(5):480-488, 2007.

{McKenry & Salerno, 2005}

McKenry L, Tessier E, Hogan M: *Mosby's pharmacology in nursing,* ed 22, St. Louis, 2006, Mosby.

Nahata MC: Pediatrics. In DiPiro JTet al, editors: *Pharmacotherapy: a pathophysiologic approach,* ed 5, Norwalk, CT, 2002, McGraw-Hill, Appleton & Lange.

Nathan DG et al: *Hematology of infancy and childhood,* ed 6, Philadelphia, 2003, Lippincott.

Rakhmanina NY, van den Anker JN: Pharmacological research in pediatrics: from neonates to adolescents, *Adv Drug Deliv Rev* 20:58(1):4-14, 2006.

Rane A: Basic principles of drug disposition and action in infants and children. In Yaffe JF, Arandva JV, editors: *Neonatal and pediatric pharmacology,* ed 3, Philadelphia, 2004, Lippincott Williams & Wilkins.

Robertson J, Shilkofski N: *The Harriet Lane handbook: a manual for pediatric house officers,* ed 17, St Louis, 2005, Mosby.

Taketomo CK: *Pediatric dosage handbook,* ed 14, Hudson, OH, 2007, Lexi-Comp.

The Joint Commission: Preventing pediatric medication errors, Sentinel Event Alert Issue 39 April 11, 2008, Oakbrook Terrace, Il, 2008, The Joint Commission. Available at http://www.jointcommission.org/SentinelEvents/SentinelEventAlert/sea_39.htm.

U.S. Food and Drug Administration (FDA): *Specific requirements on content and format of labeling for human prescription drugs: revision of pediatric use subsection in the labeling: final rule,* December 13, 1994, Health and Human Services, FDA, 21 CFR Part 201.

Yaffe SY, Aranda JV: *Neonatal and pediatric pharmacology,* ed 3, Philadelphia, 2004, Lippincott Williams & Wilkins.

CHAPTER 6

Akus M, Bartick M: Lactation safety recommendations and reliability compared in 10 medication resources, *Ann Pharmacother* 10(6)1352-1360,): 2007.

Alwan Set al: Use of selective serotonin-reuptake inhibitors in pregnancy and the risk of birth defects, *N Engl J Med* 356:2684-2692, 2007.

American Academy of Family Physicians (AAFP): *Policy dtatement on breast-feeding,* 2002. Available at www.aafp.org/x6633.xml.

American Academy of Pediatrics Committee on Drugs: The transfer of drugs and other chemicals into human milk, *Pediatrics* 108:776-789, 2001.

American Academy of Pediatrics: Policy statement: use of psychoactive medication during pregnancy and possible effects on the fetus and newborn, *Pediatrics* 105:880-887, 2000.

American Academy of Pediatrics: Policy statement: breastfeeding and the use of human milk, *Pediatrics* 115:496-506, 2005.

American College of Obstetricians and Gynecologists and American College of Allergy Asthma and Immunology: The use of newer asthma and allergy medications during pregnancy, *Ann Allergy Asthma Immunol* 84:475-480, 2000.

American Diabetes Association (ADA): Standards of medical care in diabetes, 2006, *Diabetes Care* 29(1):S4-S42, 2006.

Amir LH: Medicines and breastfeeding: information is available on safe use, *Med J Aust* 186(9):485, 2007. (Erratum in June 4:186 [11]: 606.)

Anderson GD: Using pharmacokinetics to predict the effects of pregnancy and maternal-infant transfer of drugs during lactation, *Expert Opin Drug Metab Toxicol* 2(6):947-960, 2006.

August P: Management of hypertension in pregnancy. In Rose BD, editor: *UpToDate,* Waltham, MA, 2007, UpToDate.

Badell ML et al: Treatment options for nausea and vomiting during pregnancy, *Pharmacotherapy* 26(9):1273-1287, 2006.

Barkley L: Recommendations for screening, treatment of STIs during pregnancy. Available at www.medscape.com/viewarticle/560410 (accessed 8-06-08).

Bass J: Tuberculosis in pregnancy. In Rose BD, editor: *UpToDate,* Waltham, MA, 2007, UpToDate.

Bauer CR et al: Acute neonatal effects of cocaine exposure during pregnancy, *Arch Pediatr Adolesc Med* 159(9):824-834, 2005.

Benyamini L et al: The safety of amoxicillin/clavulanic acid and cefuroxime during lactation, *Ther Drug Monit* 27(4):499-502, 2005.

Briggs GG et al: Excretion of metformin into breast milk and the effect on nursing infants. *Obstet Gynecol* 105(1):1437-1441, 2005.

Chambers CD et al: Pregnancy outcome in women exposed to anti-TNF-alpha medications: the OTIS rheumatoid arthritis in pregnancy study [Abstract 1224], *Arthritis Rheum* 50(9):S479-S480, 2004.

Cone-Wesson B: Prenatal alcohol and cocaine exposure: influences on cognition, speech, language, and hearing, *J Commun Dis* 38(4):279-302, 2005.

Cooper WO et al: Major congenital malformations after first-trimester exposure to ACE inhibitors, *N Engl J Med* 354:2443-2451, 2006.

Dolan SM: Medication exposure during pregnancy: antidepressants, *Medscape Ob/Gyn Women Health* 10(1):2005.

Einarson A et al: The use of topical 5% imiquimod during pregnancy: a case series, *Reprod Toxicol* 21(1):1-2, 2006.

Friedman JM: ACE inhibitors and congenital anomalies, *N Engl J Med* 354:2498-500, 2006.

Friedman JM, Polifka JE: *Teratogenic effects of drugs: a resource for clinicians (TERIS),* ed 2, Baltimore, 2007, Johns Hopkins University Press.

Funai E: Hyperemesis gravidarum. In Rose BD, editor: *UpToDate,* Waltham, MA, 2007, UpToDate.

Gabbe SG et al: *Obstetrics—normal and problem pregnancies,* ed 5, New York, 2007, Churchill Livingstone.

Gentile S: SSRIs in pregnancy and lactation: emphasis on neurodevelopmental outcome, *CNS Drugs* 19(7):623-633, 2005.

Gentile S: Prophylactic treatment of bipolar disorder in pregnancy and breastfeeding: focus on emerging mood stabilizers, *Bipolar Disord* 8(3):207-220, 2006.

Gibson P: Hypertension and pregnancy. June, 2002. Available at www.emedicine.com/med/topic.3250.htm.

Greene MF: Teratogenicity of SSRIs—serious concern or much ado about little? *N Engl J Med* 356:2732-2733, 2007

Hale TW, Mcafee G: *A medication guide for breastfeeding moms,* New York, 2005, Pharmasoft.

Hale TW: *Medication in mothers' milk,* ed 13, Amarillo, TX, 2008, Pharmasoft.

Hooton T, Stamm WE: Urinary tract infections and asymptomatic bacteriuria in pregnancy. In Rose BD, editor: *UpToDate,* Waltham, MA, 2007, UpToDate.

Ilett K, Hale T: *Drug therapy and breastfeeding: from theory to clinical practice,* New York, 2002, Informa Healthcare.

Kallen BA et al: Maternal drug use in early pregnancy and infant cardiovascular defect, *Reprod Toxicol* 17(3):255-261, 2003.

Kallen BA et al: Is erythromycin therapy teratogenic in humans? *Reprod Toxicol* 20(2):209-214, 2005.

Koren G: *Medical safety in pregnancy and breastfeeding: the evidence-based, A to Z clinician's pocket guide,* New York, 2006, McGraw-Hill.

Lawrence RA, Lawrence RM: *Breastfeeding: a guide for the medical profession,* ed 5, St Louis, 1999, Mosby.

Lee RV et al, editors: *Medical care of the pregnant patient (women's health series),* Philadelphia, Washington DC, 2000, American College of Physicians.

Leslie KK et al: Chemotherapeutic drugs in pregnancy, *Obstet Gynecol Clin North Am* 32(4):627-740, 2005.

Linares TJ et al: Mental health outcomes of cocaine-exposed children at 6 years of age, *J Pediatr Psychol* 31(1):85-97, 2006.

Lo WY, Friedman, JM: Teratogenicity of recently introduced medications in human pregnancy, *Obstet Gynecol* 100:465-473, 2002.

Louik C et al: First-trimester use of selective serotonin-reuptake inhibitors and the risk of birth defects, *N Engl J Med* 356:2675-2683, 2007.

Magee L, Sadeghi S: Prevention and treatment of postpartum hypertension, *Cochrane Database Syst Rev* 25(1):CD004351, 2005.

Meadows M: Pregnancy and the drug dilemma, *FDA Consumer Magazine,* 2001. Available at www.fda.gov/fdac/features/2001/301_preg.html#categories. (Accessed 8-06-08)

Misri S: Depression in pregnant women. In Rose BD, editor: *UpToDate,* Waltham, MA, 2007, UpToDate.

Montouris G: Safety of the newer antiepileptic drug oxcarbazepine during pregnancy, *Curr Med Res Opin* 21(5):693-701, 2005.

Murphy HR et al: Improving outcomes of pregnancy for women with type 1 and type 2 diabetes, *Br J Diabetes Vasc Dis* 7(1): 38-42, 2007.

Nahum GG et al: Antibiotic use in pregnancy and lactation: what is and is not known about teratogenic and toxic risks, *Obstet Gynecol* 107(5):1120-1138, 2006.

Namazy JA, Schatz M: Treatment of asthma during pregnancy and perinatal outcomes,

Curr Opin Allergy Clin Immunol 5(3):229-233, 2005.

Nardiello S et al: Risks of antibacterial agents in pregnancy, *Infe Med* 10(1):8-15, 2002.

National Institutes of Health (NIH), National Heart, Lung, and Blood Institute, National Asthma Education Program: *Report of the working group on asthma and pregnancy: executive summary: management of asthma during pregnancy*, Bethesda, MD, March 1993, NIH (No. 93-3279A), pp. 1-20.

Nava-Ocampo AA et al: Use of proton pump inhibitors during pregnancy and breastfeeding, *Can Fam Physician* 52(7): 853-854, 2006.

Pack AM: Therapy insight: clinical management of pregnant women with epilepsy, *Nat Clin Pract Neurol* 2(4):190-200, 2006.

Pennell PB: 2005 AES annual course: evidence used to treat women with epilepsy, *Elipsia* 47 (Suppl 1):46-53, 2006.

Pickering TG: How should blood pressure be measured during pregnancy? *J Clin Hyperten* 7(1):46-49, 2005.

Report of the National High Blood Pressure Education Program Working Group on high blood pressure in pregnancy, *Am J Obstet Gynecol* 183(1):S1-S22, 2000.

Safari HR et al: Experience with oral methylprednisolone in the treatment of refractory hyperemesis gravidarum, *Am J Obstet Gynecol* 178:1054-1058, 1998.

Schardein JL, Macina OT: *Human developmental toxicants: aspects of toxicology and chemistry*, New York, 2006, CRC.

Schatz M, Weinberger SE: Management of asthma during pregnancy. In Rose BD, editor: *UpToDate*, Waltham, MA, 2007, UpToDate.

Schneider ME: *American College of Obstetricians and Gynecologists advises against paroxetine in pregnancy.* Available at www.internalmedicinenews.com/article/PIIS1097869007700215/fulltext.

Shephard TH, Lemire RJ: *Catalog of teratogenic agents*, ed 12, Baltimore, 2007, Johns Hopkins University Press.

Singer LTet al: Cognitive outcomes of preschool children with prenatal cocaine exposure, *JAMA* 291(2):2248-24546, 2004.

Substance Abuse and Mental Health Administration (SAMHA): Results from the 2005 National Survey on Drug Use and Health: National Findings, Office of Applied Statistics, NSDUH Series H-30, DHHS, Pub No. SMA 06-4194, Rockville, MD, 2006.

Tauscher AE et al: Psoriasis and pregnancy, *J Cutan Med Surg* 6(6):561-570, 2002.

U.S. Preventive Services Task Force: *Screening for gestational diabetes mellitus: recommendations and rationale*, Rockville, MD, February 2003, Agency for Healthcare Research and Quality (originally in *Obstet Gynecol* 101: 393-395, 2003). Available at www.ahrq.gov/clinic/3rduspstf/gdm/gdmrr.htm.

Weiner C, Buhimschi C: *Drugs for pregnant and lactating women*, New York, 2003, Churchill Livingstone.

Wokowski KA, Berman SM: Sexually transmitted diseases treatment guidelines, 2006, *MMWR Morb Mortal Wkly Rep* 55(30):1-94, 2006.

Working group report on high blood pressure in pregnancy: National High Blood Pressure Education Program. 00-3029. 2000. National Institutes of Health. Ref Type: Report.

Working group report on high blood pressure in pregnancy, *J Clin Hyperten* 3(2):75-88, 2001.

Yawn B, Knudtsen M: Treating asthma and comorbid allergic rhinitis in pregnancy: a review of the current guidelines, *J Am Board Fam Med* 20(3):289-298, 2007.

Zip C: A practical guide to dermatologic drug use in pregnancy, *Skin Therapy Lett* 11(4):1-4, 2006.

CHAPTER 7

Bagchi AD et al: Utilization of, and adherence to, drug therapy among medicaid beneficiaries with congestive heart failure, *Clin Ther* 29(8):1771-1783, 2007.

Bangalore S et al: Compliance and fixed-dose combination therapy, *Curr Hyperten Rep* 9(3):184-189, 2007.

Barker LR et al: *Principles of ambulatory medicine,* ed 7, Baltimore, 2006, Lippincott Williams & Wilkins.

Bezie Y et al: Therapeutic compliance: a prospective analysis of various factors involved in the adherence rate in type 2 diabetes, *Diabetes Metab* 32(6):611-616, 2006.

Briesacher BA et al: Patients at-risk for cost-related medication nonadherence: a review of the literature, *J Gen Intern Med* 22(6): 864-871, 2007.

Charles H et al: Racial differences in adherence to cardiac medications, *J Natl Med Assoc* 95:17-27, 2003.

Driscoll HC et al: Getting better, getting well: understanding and managing partial and non-response to pharmacological treatment of non-psychotic major depression in old age, *Drugs Aging* 24(10):801-814, 2007.

Frishman WH: Importance of medication adherence in cardiovascular disease and the value of once-daily treatment regimens, *Cardiol Rev* 15(5):257-263, 2007.

Gardiner P, Dvorkin L: Promoting medication adherence in children, *Am Fam Physician* 74(5):793-798, 2006.

Goeman DP, Douglass J: Optimal management of asthma in elderly patients: strategies to improve adherence to recommended interventions, *Drugs Aging* 24(5):381-394, 2007.

Graney MJet al: HIV/AIDS medication adherence factors: inner-city clinic patient's self-reports, *Tenn Med* 96:73-78, 2003.

Howland RH: Medication adherence, *J Psychosoc Nurs Ment Health Serv* 45(9):15-19, 2007.

Kraetschmer N et al: How does trust affect patient preferences for participation in decision-making? *Health Expect* 7(4): 317-326, 2006.

Marple BF et al: Keys to successful management of patients with allergic rhinitis: focus on patient confidence, compliance, and satisfaction, *Otolaryngol Head Neck Surg* 136(6 Suppl): S107-S124, 2007.

Mochari H et al: Cardiovascular disease knowledge, medication adherence, and barriers to preventive action in a minority population, *Prev Cardiol* 10(4):190-195, 2007.

Piette JD et al: The role of patient-physician trust in moderating medication nonadherence due to cost pressures, *Arch Intern Met* 165(15):1749-1755, 2005.

Rooney WR: Maintaining a medication list in the chart, *Fam Pract Manag* 10:52-56, 2003.

Simmons BB, Dubreuil AL: Case report: patient adherence to drug regimens vital to treatment, *Am Fam Physician* 76(6):769-770, 2007.

Simpson E et al: Drug prescriptions after acute myocardial infarction: dosage, compliance, and persistence, *Am Heart J* 145:438-444, 2003.

Steele RG, Grauer D: Adherence to antiretroviral therapy for pediatric HIV infection: review of the literature and recommendations for research, *Clin Child Fam Psychol Rev* 6:17-30, 2003.

Swanson J: Compliance with stimulants for attention-deficit/hyperactivity disorder: issues and approaches for improvement, *CNS Drugs* 27:117-131, 2003.

Turnbough L, Wilson L: "Take your medicine": nonadherence issues in patients with ulcerative colitis, *Gastroenterol Nurs* 30(3):212-217, 2007.

Wilson IB et al: Physician-patient communication about prescription medication nonadherence: a 50-state study of America's seniors, *J Gen Intern Med* 22(1):6-12, 2007.

CHAPTER 8

Aboff BM et al: Residents' prescription writing for nonpatients, *JAMA* 288(3):381-385, 2002.

Aspinall S et al: Medication errors in older adults: a review of recent publications, *Am J Geriatr Pharmacother* 5(1):75-84, 2007.

Bachynsky J et al: The practice of splitting tablets: cost and therapeutic aspects, *Pharmacoeconomics* 20:339-346, 2002.

Bernstein L et al: Medication reconciliation: Harvard Pilgrim Health Care's approach to improving outpatient medication safety, *J Health Qual* 29(4):40-45, 55, 2007.

Bridge L: Reducing the risk of wrong route errors, *Paediatr Nurs* 19(6):33-35, 2007.

Buppert C: *Prescribing: Preventing legal pitfalls for nurse practitioners*, Carolyn Buppert, 2006.

Cohen H: Reduce the risks of high-alert drugs, *Nursing 2007* 37(9):49-55, 2007.

Currie LM et al: Near-miss and hazard reporting: promoting mindfulness in patient safety education, *Stud Health Technol Inform* 129:285-290, 2007.

Dean B et al: Causes of prescribing errors in hospital inpatients: a prospective study, *Lancet* 359L:1373-1378, 2002.

Devine EB et al: Characterization of prescribing errors in an internal medicine clinic, *Am J Health Syst Pharm* 15; 64(10):1062-1070, 2007.

Edmunds MW: Advocating for NPs—go and do likewise, *Nurse Pract* 28:56, 2003a.

Edmunds MW: Warn patients of imported drug dangers, *Nurse Pract* 28:70, 2003b.

Esat A: NP invisibility: validation compliance supports advance practice nurses, *Nurse Pract* 28:52, 2003.

Grissinger M: Medication errors in long-term care: part 1, *Consult Pharm* 22(7):544-546, 549-552, 555-556, 2007.

Hirsch WR: E-SIGN paves the way for electronic signatures, *J Oncol Manag* 9(5): 8-9, 2000.

Hustey FM et al: Inappropriate prescribing in an older ED population, *Am J Emerg Med* 25(7):804-807 2007.

Institute of Medicine: *To err is human,* Washington, DC, 1999, Author.

Jayawardena S et al: Prescription errors and the impact of computerized prescription order entry system in a community-based hospital, *Am J Ther* 14(4):336-340, 2007.

Jolowsky C: *What rules govern presigned prescription refill orders? Ask the experts about pharmacotherapy* Available at www.medscape.com/viewarticle/549213 (accessed 08-06-08)

Koczmara C et al: Dangerous abbreviations: "U" can make a difference! *Dynamics* 16(3):11-15, 2006.

Kripalani M et al: Audit on inpatient prescription writing guidelines, *J Psychiatr Ment Health Nurs* 14(6):598-600, 2007.

Krohn R: Making E-prescribing work: a fresh approach, *J Health C Inf Manag* 17:17-19, 2003.

Madegowda B et al: Medication errors in a rural hospital, *Medsurg Nurs* 16(3):175-180, 2007.

Mann K et al: Adverse drug events and medication errors in psychiatry: Methodological issues regarding identification and classification, *World J Biol Psychiatry* 8:1-10, 2007.

Mills S: Legibility of doctors' signatures, *Ir Med J* 100(4):441, 2007.

Robinson CA et al: Discordance between ambulatory care clinic and community pharmacy medication databases for HIV-positive patients, *J Am Pharm Assoc* 47(5):613-615, 2007.

Rosenberg JM et al: Weight variability of pharmacist-dispensed split tablets, *J Am Pharm Assoc* 42:200-205, 2002.

Schelbred AB, Nord R: Nurses' experiences of drug administration errors, *J Adv Nurs* 60(3):317-324, 2007.

Shakib S, George A: Writing the prescription and informing the patient, *Aust Fam Physician* 32(9):702-704, 2003.

Slomski A: Could you read that? There's growing intolerance for lousy handwriting. Here's how to fix that indecipherable scrawl, *Med Econ* 6:84(7):68-70, 2007.

Subramanian S et al: Computerized physician order entry with clinical decision support in long-term care facilities: costs and benefits to stakeholders, *J Am Geriatr Soc* 55(9): 1451-1457, 2007.

Taylor BL et al: Prescription writing errors in the pediatric emergency department, *Pediatr Emerg Care* 21(12):822-827, 2005.

Teng J et al: Lack of medication dose uniformity in commonly split tablets, *J Am Pharm Assoc* 42:195-199, 2002.

U.S. Department of Justice, DEA: *Providers,* Washington, DC, 2006, US Department of Justice. Available at www.deadiversion. USDOJ.GOV/pubs/manuals/pract/pract_manual090506.pdf. (Accessed 8-06-08)

Varkey P et al: The effect of computerized physician-order entry on outpatient prescription errors, *Manag Care Interface* 20(3):53-57, 2007.

Vogus TJ, Sutcliffe KM: The impact of safety organizing, trusted leadership, and care pathways on reported medication errors in hospital nursing units, *Med Care* 45(10): 997-1002, 2007.

Zwarenstein MF et al: A cluster randomized trial protocol to evaluate electronic prescribing in an ambulatory care setting, *Trials* 8(1):28, 2007.

CHAPTER 9

(This reference list includes the older classical literature that is foundational to clinical decision making as well as current references.)

Allen GD et al: Reliability of assessment of critical thinking, *J Prof Nurs* 20(1):15-22, 2004.

Anderson LW et al: *Taxonomy for learning, teaching, and assessing: a revision of Bloom's taxonomy of educational objectives,* ed 2, New York, 2000, Allyn & Bacon.

Bandman EL, Bandman B: *Critical thinking in nursing,* Norwalk, CT, 1995, Appleton & Lange.

Bandura A: *Social foundations of thought and action,* Englewood Cliffs, NJ, 1986, Prentice-Hall.

Barry Y et al: Watchful waiting vs immediate transurethral resection for symptomatic prostatism: the importance of patients' preferences. , *JAMA* 259:3010-3017, 1988.

Benner P: *From novice to expert: excellence and power in clinical practice,* Menlo Park, CA, 1984, Addison-Wesley.

Benner P, Tanner C: Clinical judgment: how expert nurses use intuition, *Am J Nurs* 87(1)23-31, 1987.

Beyer BK: Critical thinking: what is it? *Soc Educ* 49 (4): 270-276, 1985.

Chessare JB et al: Impact of a medical school course in clinical epidemiology and health care systems, *Med Teach* 18:223-227, 1996.

Cockcroft PD: Clinical reasoning and decision analysis, *Vet Clin North Am Small Anim Pract* 37(3):499-520, 2007.

Crespo KE et al: Reasoning process characteristics in the diagnostic skills of beginner, competent, and expert dentists, *J Dent Educ* 68(12): 1235-1244, 2004.

Djulbegovic B et al: *Linking evidence-based medicine therapeutic summary measures to clinical decision analysis,* MedGenMed, January 13, 2000, Medscape, Inc.

Doig GS, Simpson F: Efficient literature searching: a core skill for the practice of evidence-based medicine, *Intens Care Med* 29(12):2199-2127, 2003.

Donald A: Evidence-based medicine: key concepts, *Medscape Psychiatry Ment Health eJ* 7(2):2002.

Eddy DM: Anatomy of a decision, *JAMA* 263:441-443, 1990.

Eddy DM: The challenge, *JAMA* 263:287-290, 1990.

Eddy DM: Evidence-based medicine: a unified approach, *Health Aff (Millwood)* 24(1):9-17, 2005.

Eddy DM: Reflections on science, judgment, and value in evidence-based decision making: a conversation with David Eddy by Sean R. Tunis, *Health Aff (Millwood)* 26(4): 500-515, 2007.

Edwards SL: Critical thinking: a two-phase framework, *Nurse Educ Pract* 7(5):303-314, 2007.

Ellermann CR et al: Logic models used to enhance critical thinking, *J Nurs Educ* 45(6):220-227, 2006.

Elstein A et al: Medical problem solving: a ten-year retrospective, *Eval Health Prof* 13: 5-36, 1990.

Evidence-based medicine working group: Evidence-based medicine: a new approach to teaching the practice of medicine, *JAMA* 268:2420-2425, 1992.

Flores-Mateo G, Argimon JM: Evidence-based practice in postgraduate healthcare education: a systematic review, *BMC Health Serv Res* 7:119, 2007.

Fox RC: Training for uncertainty. In Merton R et al, editors: *The student-physician: introductory studies in the sociology of medical education,* Cambridge, MA, 1957, Harvard University Press, pp 207-218, 228-241.

Fraenkel L, McGraw S: What are the essential elements to enable patient participation in medical decision making? *J Gen Intern Med* 22(5):614-619, 2007.

Groves M et al: Clinical reasoning: the relative contribution of identification, interpretation and hypothesis errors to misdiagnosis, *Med Teach* 25(6):621-625, 2003.

Hadley JA et al: Learning needs analysis to guide teaching evidence-based medicine: knowledge and beliefs amongst trainees from various specialities, *BMC Med Educ* 7:11, 2007.

Haynes B et al: Advances in evidence-based medicine resources for clinical practice, *Evid Based Med* 5:4-6, 2005.

Hayward R et al: User's guides to the medical literature VIII: how to use clinical practice guidelines: are the recommendations valid? *JAMA* 274:570-574, 2005.

Hirshfeld EB: Practice parameters versus outcome measurements: how will prospective and retrospective approaches to quality management fit together? *Nutr Clin Pract* 99:217-216, 1994.

Hobgood C et al: The influence of the causes and contexts of medical errors on emergency medicine residents' responses to their errors: an exploration, *Acad Med* 80(8):758-764, 2005.

Jacobs PM et al: An approach to defining and operationalizing critical thinking, *J Nurs Educ* 36:19-22, 1997.

Kassirer JP, Kopelman RI: Cognitive errors in diagnosis: instantiation, classification, and consequenes, *Am J Med* 86:433-441, 1989.

Kempainen RR et al: Understanding our mistakes: a primer on errors in clinical reasoning, *Med Teach* 25(2):177-178, 2003.

Lange LL et al: Use of Iliad to improve diagnostic performance of nurse practitioner students, *J Nurs Educ* 36:36-45, 1997.

Lipman TH, Deatrick JA: Preparing advanced practice nurses for clinical decision-making in specialty practice, *Nurse Educ* 22:47-50, 1997.

Mohler PJ: New drugs: how to decide which ones to prescribe, *Fam Pract Manag* 13(6): 33-35, 2006. Available at www.medscape.com/viewarticle/536092 (accesssed 8-06-08).

Mossler G: Half a dozen hobbling half-truths about practice guidelines, *Group Prac J* 46: 34-44, 1997.

Myrick F, Yonge O: Preceptor questioning and student critical thinking, *J Prof Nurs* 18: 176-181, 2002.

Norman GRet al: Knowledge and clinical problem-solving, *J Med Educ* 19:344-356, 1985.

Owens DK, Nease RF Jr: A normative analytic framework for development of practice guidelines for specific clinical populations, *Med Decis Making* 17:409-426, 1997.

Riddell T: Critical assumptions: thinking critically about critical thinking, *J Nurs Educ* 46(3):121-126, 2007.

Roberts SJ et al: Epigenesis of the nurse practitioner role revisited, *J Nurs Educ* 36: 67-73, 1997.

Schmidt NA, Brown JM: Use of the innovation-decision process teaching strategy to promote evidence-based practice, *J Prof Nurs* 23(3):150-156, 2007.

Scudder L: Using evidence-based information, *J Nurse Pract* 2(3):180-185, 2006.

Seldomridge LA, Walsh CM: Measuring critical thinking in graduate education: what do we know? *Nurse Educ* 31(3):132-137, 2006.

Shea B et al: A comparison of the quality of Cochrane reviews and systematic reviews published in paper-based journals, *Eval Health Prof* 25:116-129, 2002.

Shuval K et al: The impact of an evidence-based medicine educational intervention on primary care physicians: a qualitative study, *J Gen Intern Med* 22(3):327-331, 2007.

Steinberg EP, Luce BP: Evidence based? Caveat emptor! *Health Affairs* 24(1):80-82, 2005.

Stevens L: Evidence-based medicine, *Med Net* 4:5-11, 1998.

Terry R et al: The use of standardized patients to evaluate family medicine resident decision making, *Fam Med* 39(4):261-265, 2007.

Turner P: Critical thinking in nursing education and practice as defined in the literature, *Nurs Educ Perspect* 26(5):272-277, 2007.

Videbeck SL: Critical thinking: a model. *J Nurs Educ* 36:23-28, 1997.

Watson G, Glaser E: *Critical thinking appraisal manual*, New York, 1964, Harcourt & Brace.

Wimmers PF et al: Inducing expertise effects in clinical case recall, *Med Educ* 39(9):949-957, 2005.

Woolf SH: Practice guidelines: what the family physician should know, *Am Fam Physician* 51:1455-1463, 1995.

Young JS, et al: How residents think and make medical decisions: implications for education and patient safety, *Am Surg* 73(6):548-553, 2007.

CHAPTER 10

Aguirre AC et al: Performance of the English and Spanish S-TOFHLA among publically insured Medicaid and Medicare patients, *Patient Educ Couns* 56(3):332-339, 2005.

Andrus MR, Roth MT: Health literacy: a review, *Pharmacotherapy* 22:282-302, 2002.

Barker LR et al: *Principles of ambulatory medicine*, ed 7, Baltimore, Lippincott Williams & Wilkins, 2006.

Beranova E, Sykes C: A systematic review of computer-based software for educating patients with coronary heart disease, *Patient Educ Couns* 66(1):21-28, 2007.

Buchbinder R, et al: Functional health literacy of patients with rheumatoid arthritis attending a community-based rheumatology practice, *J Rheumatol* 33(5):879-886, 2006.

Bussey-Smith KL, Rossen RD: A systematic review of randomized control trials evaluating, *Ann Allergy Asthma Immunol* 98(6):507-516, 2007.

Chew LD et al: Brief questions to identify patients with inadequate health literacy, *Fam Med* 36(8):588-594, 2004.

Cotugna N et al: Evaluation of literacy level of patient education pages in health-related journals, *J Commun Health* 30(3):213-219, 2005.

Dandavino M et al: Why medical students should learn how to teach, *Med Teach* 27:1-8. 2007.

Davis TC et al: Low literacy impairs comprehension of prescription drug warning labels, *J Gen Intern Med* 21(8):847-851, 2006.

DeWalt DA et al: Development and pilot testing of a disease management program for low literacy patients with heart failure, *Patient Educ Couns* 55(1):78-86, 2004.

Dolan NC et al: Colorectal cancer screening knowledge, attitudes, and beliefs among veterans: does literacy make a difference? *J Clin Oncol* 1:22(13):2617-2622, 2004.

Evangelista LS et al: Developing a web-based education and counseling program for heart failure patients, *Prog Cardiovasc Nurs* 21(4):196-201, 2006.

Falvo DR: Effective patient education: a guide to increased compliance, ed 3, New York, 2004, Jones and Bartlett.

Georges CA et al: Functional health literacy: an issue in African-American and other ethnic and racial communities, *J Natl Black Nurses Assoc* 15(1):1-4, 2004.

Gresty K et al: Addressing the issue of e-learning and online genetics for health professionals, *Nurs Health Sci* (1):14-22, 2007.

Hironaka LK, Paasche-Orlow MK: The implications of health literacy on patient-provider communication, *Arch Dis Child*, Oct 4, 2006 epub.

Jackson R: Health literacy: an introduction to the literature, *J Indiana Dent Assoc* 84(4): 10-13, 2005-2006.

Jafri W et al: Improving the teaching skills of residents as tutors/ facilitators and addressing the shortage of faculty facilitators for PBL modules, *BMC Med Educ* 7(1):34, 2007.

Kerzman H et al: What do discharged patients know about their medication? *Patient Educ Couns* 56(3):276-282, 2005.

Koivunen M et al: A preliminary usability evaluation of web-based portal application for patients with schizophrenia, *J Psychiatr Ment Health Nurs* 14(5):462-469, 2007.

Kuhl EA et al: Using computers to improve the psychosocial care of implantable cardioverter defibrillator recipients, *Pacing Clin Electrophysiol* 29(12):1426-1433, 2006.

Lo S et al: Health literacy among English-speaking parents in a poor urban setting, *J Health Care Poor Underserved* 17(3): 504-511, 2006.

Lorig K: *Patient education: a practical approach*, ed 3, Thousand Oaks, CA, 2000, Sage.

Mackenzie SL et al: Patient and staff perspectives on the use of a computer counseling tool for HIV and sexually transmitted infection risk reduction, *J Adolesc Health* 40(6):572.e9-16, 2007.

Mann KV et al: Twelve tips for preparing residents as teachers, *Med Teach* 29(4): 301-306, 2007.

Morris NS et al: Literacy and health outcomes: a cross-sectional study in 1002 adults with diabetes, *BMC Fam Pract* 14(7):49, 2006.

Navarre M, et al: Influence of an interactive computer-based inhaler technique tutorial on patient knowledge and inhaler technique, *Ann Pharmacother* 41(2):216-221, 2007.

Nielsen-Bohlman L et al: *Health literacy: a prescription to end confusion*, Washington DC, 2004, National Academies Press.

Paasche-Orlow MK et al: The prevalence of limited health literacy, *J Gen Intern Med* 20(2):175-184, 2005.

Redman BK: *Advances in patient education*, 2004, Springer.

Reyes-Ortiz CA et al: The impact of education and literacy levels on cancer screening among older Latin American and Caribbean adults, *Cancer Control* 14(4):388-395, 2005.

Rogers ES et al: Misperceptions of medical understanding in low-literacy patients: implications for cancer prevention, *Cancer Control* 13(3):225-229, 2006.

Safeer RS, Keenan J: Health literacy: the gap between physicians and patients, *Am Fam Physician* 72(3):463-468, 2005.

Schillinger D et al: Does literacy mediate the relationship between education and health outcomes? A study of a low-income population with diabetes, *Public Health Rep* 121(3):245-254, 2006.

Schultz KW et al: Medical students' and residents' preferred site characteristics and preceptor behaviors for learning in the ambulatory setting: a cross-sectional survey, *BMC Med Educ* 6(4):12, 2004.

Shapiro J et al: "That never would have occurred to me": a qualitative study of medical students' views of a cultural competence curriculum, *BMC Med Educ* 26(6):31, 2006.

Shershneva MB et al: A model of teaching-learning transactions in generalist-specialist consultations, *J Contin Educ Health Prof* 26(3):222-229, 2006.

Teasdale TA, Shaikh M: Efficacy of a geriatric oral health CD as a learning tool, *J Dent Educ* 70(12):1366-1369, 2006.

U.S. Department of Health and Human Services (USDHHS), *Healthy People 2010*, ed 2, Washington, DC, 2002, U.S. Government Printing Office.

U.S. Public Health Service (USPHS), National Institute of Dental and Craniofacial Research, National Institute of Health, Department of Health and Human Services: The invisible barrier: literacy and its relationship with oral health. *J Public Health Dent* 5(3):174-182, 2005.

Waters BM et al: Effects of formal education for patients with inflammatory bowel disease: a randomized controlled trial, *Can J Gastroenterol* 19(4):235-244, 2005.

Weiss BD et al: Literacy education as treatment for depression in patients with limited literacy and depression: a randomized controlled trial, *J Gen Intern Med* 21(8): 823-828, 2006a.

Weiss BD et al: Quick assessment of literacy in primary care: the newest vital sign, *Ann Fam Med* 3(6):514-522, 2005. (Erratum in *Ann Fam Med* 4[1]:83, 2006b.)

Wolf MS et al: Health literacy and patient knowledge in a southern U.S. HIV clinic, *Int J STD AIDS* 15(11):747-752, 2004.

Wolf MS et al: Relation between literacy and HIV treatment knowledge among patients on HAART regimens, *AIDS Care* 17(7): 863-867, 2005.

Wolf MS et al: Misunderstanding of prescription drug warning labels among: patients with low literacy, *Am J Health Syst Pharm* 63(11): 1048-1055, 2006.

Wolf MS et al: Literacy, self-efficacy, and HIV medication adherence, *Patient Educ Couns* 65(2):253-260, 2007.

Wolf MS et al: To err is human: patient misinterpretations of prescription drug label instructions, *Patient Educ Couns* 67(3): 293-300, 2007a.

Wolf MS et al: Literacy, self-efficacy, and HIV medication adherence, *Patient Educ Couns* 65(2):253-60, 2007b.

CHAPTER 11

Giovino JM: Acne and related skin conditions in adolescence, *Clin Fam Pract* 5(3):609-626, 2003.

Goldstein, AO, Goldstein, BG: Pediculosis. In Rose BD, editor: *UpToDate*, Waltham, MA, 2007, UpToDate.

Goldstein, AO, Goldstein, BG: Scabies. In Rose BD, editor: *UpToDate*, Waltham, MA, 2007, UpToDate.

Gupta AK: Tinjea corporis, tinea cruris, tinea nigra, and piedra, *Dermatol Clin* 21(3): 395-400, 2003.

Habif TB: *Clinical dermatology*, ed 4, St Louis, 2004, Mosby.

Institute for Clinical Systems Improvement (ICSI): *Acne management*, Bloomington, MN, 2003, Author

Lipscomb A et al: *Recommendations for the treatment of pediculosis capitis (head lice) in children*, Austin, TX, 2002 May 13, University of Texas at Austin, School of Nursing.

The Medical Letter: Treatment guidelines: drugs for acne, rosacea and psoriasis, *Med Lett Drugs Ther* 3(35):49-54, 2005.

CHAPTER 12

Eye

Robert PY, Adenis JP: Comparative review of topical ophthalmic antibacterial preparations, *Drugs* 61:175-185, 2001.

American Academy of Ophthalmology: *Conjunctivitis*, 2003. Available at www.aao. org/aao/education/library/ppp/upload/Conjunctivitis_.pdf.

Distelhorst JS: Open-angle glaucoma, *Am Fam Physician* 67(9):1937-1944, 2003.

Greenberg MF, Pollard ZF: The red eye in childhood, *Pediatr Clin North Am* 50:105-124, 2003.

Lemp MA: Contact lenses and associated anterior segment disorders: dry eye, blepharitis, and allergy, *Ophthamol Clin North Am* 16(3):463-469, 2003.

Wirbelauer C: Management of the red eye for the primary care physician, *Am J Med* 119(4):302-306, 2006.

Yanoff M, Duker J: *Ophthalmology*, ed 2, St Louis, 2004, Mosby.

Ear, Throat, and Mouth

Haddad J Jr: Diseases of the external ear, In Behrman, editor: *Nelson textbook of pediatrics*, ed 17, Philadelphia, 2004, Saunders.

CHAPTER 13

Bolser D: Cough suppressant and pharmacologic protussive therapy: ACCP evidence-based clinical practical guidelines, *Chest* 129: 238S-249S, 2006.

Crisalida T et al, editors: *Allergy and asthma pocket guide*, New York, 2002, Adelphi.

Drug Enforcement Administration (DEA): General information regarding the combat methamphetamine epidemic act of 2005 [title VII of public law 109-177] page 8, 2006.

Goodkin J, editor: Treatment of allergic rhinitis and asthma, *Patient Care Nurse Pract* Fall 2001 (suppl).

Hay CM: Epidemiology and clinical manifestations of rhinovirus infections in adults. In Rose BD, editor: *UpToDate*, Waltham, MA, 2007, UpToDate.

Hay CM: Treatment and prevention of rhinovirus infections. In Rose BD, editor: *UpToDate*, Waltham, MA, 2007, UpToDate.

Hayden ML et al: *Diagnostic challenges in allergic rhinitis. The changing face of allergic rhinitis: new pieces in the clinical picture*, Monograph 1, Chicago, 2001, Pragmation Office of Medical Education.

Hayden ML et al: *Improving the outcomes of allergic rhinitis treatment. The changing face of allergic rhinitis: new pieces in the clinical picture*, Monograph 2, Chicago, 2001, Pragmation Office of Medical Education.

Institute for Clinical Systems Improvement (ICSI): Viral upper respiratory infection (VURI) in adults and children, Bloomington, MN, 2004, Author.

Lipworth B: Intranasal corticosteroids in allergic rhinitis: safety issues considered, *Respir Dig* 4:13-16, 2002.

Pratter MR et al: An empiric integrative approach to the management of cough: ACCP evidence-based clinical practice guidelines, *Chest* 129(1 Suppl):222S-231S, 2006.

Pratter MR: Cough and the common cold: ACCP evidence-based clinical practice guidelines, *Chest* 129(1 Suppl):72S-74S, 2006.

Ramey JT et al: Rhinitis medicamentosa, *J Invest Allergy Clin Immunol* 16(3):148-155, 2006.

Spector SL et al: Symptom severity assessment of allergic rhinitis: part 1, *Ann Allergy Asthma Immunol* 91(2):105-114, 2003.

University of Michigan Health System: *Allergic rhinitis*, Ann Arbor, 2002, Author.

CHAPTER 14

Adams NP, Jones PW: The dose-response characteristics of inhaled corticosteroids when used to treat asthma: an overview of Cochrane systemic reviews, *Respir Med* 100(8):1297-1306, 2006.

Akazawa M, Stempel DA: Single-inhaler combination therapy for asthma: a review of cost effectiveness, *Pharmacoeconomics* 24(10):971-988, 2006.

Akinbami LJ: *The state of childhood asthma*, United States, 1980-2005. USDHHS, CDC, National Center for Health Statistics, Advance Data Number 381, December 12, 2006.

Berger WE: The use of inhaled formoterol in the treatment of asthma, *Ann Allergy Asthma Immunol* 97(1):24-33, 2006.

Center for Drug Evaluation and Research: Public Health Advisory: Serevent Diskus, Advair Diskus, Foradil, Updated 5/2006. Available at www.fda.gov/cder/drug/advisory/LABA.htm.

Currie GP et al: Long-acting β_2-agonists in asthma: not so SMART? *Drug Saf* 29(8): 647-656, 2006.

Ducharme FM et al: Long-acting β_2-agonists versus anti-leukotrienes as add-on therapy to inhaled corticosteroids for chronic asthma, *Cochrane Database Syst Rev* (4):CD003137, 2006.

Fanta CH, Fletcher SW: An overview of asthma management. In Rose BD, editor: *UpToDate*, Waltham, MA, 2007, UpToDate.

Ferguson GT, Make B: Management of stable chronic obstructive pulmonary disease. In Rose BD, editor: *UpToDate*, Waltham, MA, 2007, UpToDate.

GINA Executive Committee: *Global strategy for asthma management and prevention*, Global Initiative for Asthma, 2006. Available at www.ginasthma.org. (Accessed 08-06-08)

GOLD Executive Committee: *Global strategies for the diagnosis, management, and prevention of chronic obstructive pulmonary disease*, Global Initiative for Chronic Obstructive Lung Disease, 2006. Available at www.goldcopd. com. (Accessed 08-06-08)

Joint Task Force on Practice Parameters: Attaining optimal asthma control: A practice parameter, *J Allergy Clin Immunol* 116(5): S3-S11, 2005. Available at www.guidelines. gov/summary/summary.wspx?doc_id=8394. (Accessed 08-06-08)

Lees GM: A hitchhiker's guide to the galaxy of adrenoreceptors, *BMJ* 283:173-178, 1981.

Li HT et al: Combination therapy with the single inhaler salmeterol/fluticasone proprionate versus increased doses of inhaled corticosteroids in patients with asthma, *Respiration* 2006, September.

National Asthma Education and Prevention Program Expert Panel Report 3: *Guidelines for the diagnosis and management of asthma*, NIH Publication No. 08-4051, Washington, DC, 2007, U.S. Government Printing Office. Available at www.nhlbi.nih.gov/guidelines/asthma/asthgdln.html. (Accessed 08-06-08)

National Asthma Education and Prevention Program Expert Panel Report 2: *Guidelines for the diagnosis and management of asthma*, NIH Publication No. 97-4051, Washington, DC, 1997, U.S. Government Printing Office.

National Asthma Education and Prevention Program Expert Panel Report: *Guidelines for the diagnosis and management of asthma—update on selected topics 2002,* NIH Publication No. 02-5075, Washington, DC, 2002, U.S. Department of Health and Human Services. Available at www.nhlbi.nih.gov/guidelines/asthma/index.htm.

National Asthma Education and Prevention Program Expert Panel Report 3: *Guidelines for the diagnosis and management of asthma,* NIH Publication No. 08-4051, Washington, DC, 2007, U.S. Government Printing Office. Available at www.nhlbi.nih.gov/guidelines/asthma/asthgdln.html.

Pedersen S: Clinical safety of inhaled corticosteroids for asthma in children: an update of long-term trials, *Drug Saf* 29(7):599-612, 2006.

Poole PJ, Black PN: Mucolytic agents for chronic bronchitis or chronic obstructive pulmonary disease, *Cochrane Database Syst Rev* 19(3):CD001287, 2006.

Rahimi R et al: Meta-analysis finds use of inhaled corticosteroids during pregnancy safe: a systematic meta-analysis review, *Hum ExperToxicol* 25(8):447-452, 2006.

Salo D et al: A randomized, clinical trial comparing the efficacy of continuous nebulized albuterol (15 mg) versus continuous nebulized albuterol (15 mg) plus ipratropium bromide (2 mg) for the treatment of acute asthma attack, *J Emerg Med* 31(4):371-376, 2006.

Salpeter SR, Buckley NS: Systematic review of clinical outcomes in chronic obstructive pulmonary disease: beta-agonist use compared with anticholinergics and inhaled corticosteroids, *Clin Rev Allergy Immunol* 31(2-3):219-230, 2006.

Sridhar AV, McKean M: Nedocromil sodium for chronic asthma in children, *Cochrane Database Syst Rev* 3:CD004108, 2006.

Tiner R, While A: Promoting quality of life for patients with moderate to severe COPD, *Br J Commun Nurs* 11(7):278-284, 2006.

Wallace LD, Troy KE: Office-based spirometry for early detection of obstructive lung disease. *J Am Acad Nurse Pract* 18(9):414-421, 2006.

Wood-Baker R et al: Systemic corticosteroids in chronic obstructive pulmonary disease: An overview of Cochrane systemic reviews, *Respir Med,* 2006, September.

CHAPTER 15

ALLHAT Officers and Coordinators for the ALLHAT Collaborative Research Group: Major outcomes in high-risk hypertensive patients randomized to angiotensin converting enzyme inhibitor or calcium channel blocker vs diuretic: Antihypertensive and Lipid-Lowering Treatment to Prevent Heart Attack Trial (ALLHAT), *JAMA* 288:2981-2997, 2002.

August P: Treatment of hypertension in pregnancy. In Rose BD, editor: *UpToDate,* Waltham, MA, 2007, UpToDate.

Domin, J, Kaplan N: Overview of hypertension in adults. In Rose BD, editor: *UpToDate,* Waltham, MA, 2007, UpToDate.

Flanigan JS, Vitberg D: Hypertensive emergency and severe hypertension: what to treat, who to treat, and how to treat, *Med Clin North Am* 90:439-451, 2006.

Frolich E: Innovative concepts of hypertension to understand and manage the disease, *Med Clin North Am* 88(1):xiii-xxi, 2004.

Grundy SM et al: Report of the National Heart, Lung, and Blood Institute/American Heart Association conference on scientific issues related to definition, *Circulation* 109:433-438, 2004.

Meigs J: The metabolic syndrome (insulin resistance syndrome or syndrome X). In Rose BD, editor: *UpToDate,* Waltham, MA, 2007, UpToDate.

Rosendorff C et al: Treatment of hypertension in the prevention and management of ischemic heart disease: a scientific statement from the American Heart Association Council for High Blood Pressure Research and the Councils on Clinical Cardiology and Epidemiology and Prevention, *Circulation* 115(21):2761-2788, 2007.

The fourth report on the diagnosis, evaluation, and treatment of high blood pressure in children and adolescents, NHLBI, August 2004.

Treatment guidelines: drugs for hypertension, *Med Lett Drugs Ther* 3(34):39-48, 2005.

CHAPTER 16

Awaty EH et al: Aspirin, *Circulation* 101:1206, 2000.

Burashnikov A et al: Atrium-selective sodium channel block as a strategy for suppression of atrial fibrillation: differences in sodium channel inactivation between atria and ventricles and the role of ranolazine, *Circulation* 116(13):1449-1457, 2007.

Dayspring TD: Coronary artery disease prevention in women, *Fem Patient* 26:47-53, 2001.

Eaton CB: Traditional and emerging risk factors for cardiovascular disease, *Prim Care Clin Office Pract* 32:963-976, 2005.

Fihn SD et al: Guidelines for the management of patient with chronic stable angina: treatment, *Ann Intern Med* 135:616, 2001.

Folsom AR et al: An assessment of incremental coronary risk prediction using C-reactive protein and other novel risk markers: The atherosclerosis risk in communities study, *Arch Intern Med* 166:1368-1373, 2006.

Gibbons RJ et al: American College of Cardiology/American Heart Association Task Force on Practice Guidelines (Committee on the Management of Patients with Chronic Stable Angina): ACC/AHA 2002 guideline update for the management of patients with chronic stable angina—summary article, *J Am Coll Cardiol* 41:159-168, 2003.

Kannam J et al: Nitrates in the management of stable angina pectoris. In Rose BD, editor: *UpToDate,* Waltham, MA, 2007, UpToDate.

Keleman MD: Angina pectoris: Evaluation in the office, *Med Clin North Am* 90:391-416, 2006.

Libby P: Current concepts of the pathogenesis of the acute coronary syndromes, *Circulation* 104:365, 2001.

Mehta MQ: Ranolazine: a novel agent that improves dysfunctional sodium channels, *Int J Clin Pract* 61(5):864-872, 2007.

Morrow DA et al, for MERLIN-TIMI 36 Trial Investigators: Effects of ranolazine on recurrent cardiovascular events in patients with non-ST-elevation acute coronary syndromes: the MERLIN-TIMI 36 randomized trial, *JAMA* 297(16):1775-1783, 2007.

Oberman A: Emerging cardiovascular risk factors, *Clin Rev* 33(Spring):33-38, 2000.

Rich MW et al: Safety and efficacy of extended-release ranolazine in patients aged 70 years or older with chronic stable angina pectoris, *Am J Geriatr Cardiol* 16(4):216-221, 2007.

Scirica BM: Ranolazine in patients with coronary artery disease, *Expert Opin Pharmacother* 8(13):2149-2157, 2007.

Scirica BM et al: Effect of ranolazine, an antianginal agent with novel electrophysiological properties, on the incidence of arrhythmias in patients with non ST-segment elevation acute coronary syndrome: results from the metabolic efficiency with ranolazine for less ischemia in non ST-elevation acute coronary syndrome thrombolysis in myocardial infarction 36 (MERLIN-TIMI 36) randomized controlled trial, *Circulation* 116(15):1647-1652, 2007.

White HD: Should all patients with coronary disease receive angiotensin converting enzyme inhibitors? *Lancet* 362:755-757, 2003.

Williams SVet al: Guidelines for the management of patients with chronic stable angina: diagnosis and risk stratification, *Ann Intern Med* 135:530, 2001.

CHAPTER 17

Adams KF et al: Executive summary. HFSA 2006 comprehensive heart failure practice guideline, *J Card Failure,* 12:10-38, 2006. Available online at www.HFSA.org (12:e1-e119).

Brunner HP et al: Management of elderly patients with congestive heart failure. Design of the trial of intensified versus standard medical therapy in elderly patients with congestive heart failure (TIME-CHF), *Am Heart J* 949:55, 2006.

Colucci WS: Clinical manifestations and evaluation of the patient with suspected heart failure. In Rose BD, editor: *UpToDate,* Waltham, MA, 2007, UpToDate.

Colucci WS: Use of digoxin in heart failure due to systolic dysfunction. In Rose BD, editor: *UpToDate,* Waltham, MA, 2007, UpToDate.

Dec GW: Digoxin remains useful in the management of chronic heart failure, *Med Clin North Am* 87:317-337, 2003.

Doust J et al: The role of BNP testing in heart failure, *Am Fam Physician* 74(11):1893-1898, 2006.

Hunt SAet al: ACC/AHA 2005 *guidelines for the evaluation and management of chronic heart failure in the adult: ACC/AHA Task Force,* Bethesda MD: American College of Cardiology Foundation (ACCF). Available at http://circ.ahajournals.org/cgi/content/full/112/12/1825.

Katz AM: Pathophysiology of heart failure: identifying targets for pharmacotherapy, *Med Clin North Am* 98:303-316, 2003.

Felker FMet al: Inotropic therapy for heart failure: an evidence-based approach, *Am Heart J* 142:393, 2001.

Francis GS: Pathophysiology of chronic heart failure, *Am J Med* 110(Suppl 7A):37S, 2001.

Goldberger AL: Basic approach to arrhythmias due to digitalis toxicity. In Rose BD, editor: *UpToDate,* Waltham, MA, UpToDate.

Guierrez C, Blanchard DG: Diastolic heart failure: challenges of diagnosis and treatment, *Am Fam Physician* 69(11):2609-2616, 2004.

Ismail N: Digitalis (cardiac glycoside) intoxication. In Rose BD, editor: *UpToDate*, Waltham, MA, 2007, UpToDate.

Medical Letter Drugs for Treatment of Heart Failure, *Treat Guide* 4(41):91-94, 2006.

Nesto RW: Heart failure in diabetes mellitus. In Rose BD, editor: *UpToDate*, Waltham, MA, UpToDate.

Rathore SS et al: Sex-based differences in the effect of digoxin for the treatment of heart failure, *N Engl J Med* 347:1403-1411, 2002.

Stuthers AD: The diagnosis of heart failure, *Heart* 84:334, 2000.

The Criteria Committee of the New York Heart Association: *Nomenclature and criteria for diagnosis of diseases of the heart and great vessels*, ed 9, Boston, 1994, Little, Brown.

CHAPTER 18

Arnsdorf MF: Antiarrhythmic drugs to maintain sinus rhythm in patients with atrial fibrillation: Clinical trials. In Rose BD, editor: *UpToDate*, Waltham MA.

Brophy JM et al: Beta-blockers in congestive heart failure, *Ann Intern Med* 134:550, 2001.

Cleland JG: Beta-blockers for heart failure: why, which, when, and where, *Med Clin North Am* 87(2):339-371, 2003.

Colucci WS: Use of beta blockers in heart failure due to systolic dysfunction. In Rose BD, editor: *UpToDate*, Waltham, MA, 2007, UpToDate.

Dei Cas L et al: Prevention and management of chronic heart failure in patients at risk, *Am J Cardiol* 91:10-17, 2003.

Ellicott WJ, Mayer PM: Incident diabetes in clinical trials of antihypertensives drugs: a network meta-analysis, *Lancet* 360:201-207, 2007.

Frigerio M et al: Prevention and management of chronic heart failure in management of asymptomatic patients, *Am J Cardiol.* 91:4-9, 2003.

Giardina EG: Clinical use and major side effects of sotalol. In Rose BD, editor: *UpToDate*, Waltham, MA, 2007, UpToDate.

Kannam JP et al: Beta blockers in the management of stable angina pectoris. In Rose BD, editor: *UpToDate*, Waltham, MA, 2007, UpToDate.

Khan N: Re-examining the efficacy of beta-blockers for the treatment of hypertension: a meta-analysis, *Can Med Assoc J* 174(12):1737-1742, 2006.

Klein L et al: Pharmacologic therapy for patients with chronic heart failure and reduced systolic function: review of trials and practical considerations, *Am J Cardiol* 91:18-40, 2003.

Podrid, PJ: Characteristics of beta blockers. In Rose BD, editor: *UpToDate*, Waltham, MA, 2007, UpToDate.

Rose BR, Kaplan NM: Indications for use of specific antihypertensive drugs: diaphragmatic pacing. In Rose BD, editor: *UpToDate*, Waltham, MA, 2007, UpToDate.

Rosenson RS et al: Beta blockers in acute myocardial infarction. diaphragmatic pacing. In Rose BD, editor: *UpToDate*, Waltham, MA, 2007, UpToDate.

Ross DS: Beta blockers in the treatment of hyperthyroidism. In Rose BD, editor: *UpToDate*, Waltham, MA, 2007, UpToDate.

Smith AJ et al: Current role of β-blockers in the treatment of chronic congestive heart failure, *Am J Health Syst Pharm* 58:140-145, 2001.

Tarsy D: Pharmacologic treatment of essential tremor. In Rose BD, editor: *UpToDate*, Waltham, MA, 2007, UpToDate.

Wink K: Are beta-blockers efficacious as first-line therapy for hypertension in the elderly? *Curr Hyperten Rep* 5:221-224, 2003.

CHAPTER 19

Black HR et al: Principal results of the controlled onset verapamil investigation of cardiovascular end points (CONVINCE) trial, *JAMA* 289:2073-2082, 2003.

Colucci, WS: Calcium channel blockers in heart failure due to systolic dysfunction. In Rose BD, editor: *UpToDate*, Waltham, MA, 2006, UpToDate.

Delehanty, JM: Variant angina. In Rose BD, editor: *UpToDate*, Waltham, MA, 2006, UpToDate.

Epstein M, Campese VM: Evolving role of calcium antagonists in the management of hypertension, *Med Clin North Am* 88:149-165, 2004.

Flack JM et al: Using angiotensin converting enzyme inhibitors in African-American hypertensives: a new approach to treating hypertension and preventing target-organ damage, *Curr Med Res Opin* 16:66-79, 2000.

Kannam, JP et al: Calcium channel blockers in the management of stable angina pectoris. In Rose BD, editor: *UpToDate*, Waltham, MA, 2006, UpToDate.

Kaplan NM, Rose BD: Treatment of hypertension in blacks In Rose BD, editor: *UpToDate*, Waltham, MA, 2006, UpToDate.

Kirpichnikov D, Sowers JR: Role of ACE inhibitors in treating hypertensive diabetic patients, *Curr Diab Rep* 2:251-257, 2002.

Saseen JJ et al: Treatment of uncomplicated hypertension: are ACE inhibitors and calcium channel blockers as effective as diuretics and beta-blockers? *J Am Board Fam Pract* 16:156-164, 2003.

Summaries for patients: Effects of blood pressure drugs in patients with diabetes and kidney disease, *Ann Intern Med* 138:542-549, 2003.

Where do calcium antagonists fit in the management of hypertension? *Drug Ther Perspect* 15:10-11, 2000.

CHAPTER 20

American Diabetes Association: Position statement: nephropathy in diabetes, *Diabetes Care* 27: S79-S83, 2004.

Antonelli Incalzi R et al: Trends in prescribing ACE inhibitors for congestive heart failure in elderly people, *Aging Clin Exp Res* 14:516-521, 2002.

August P: Angiotensin-converting enzyme inhibitors and receptor blockers in pregnancy. In Rose BD, editor: *UpToDate*, Waltham, MA, 2006, UpToDate.

Bingham III, CO: Overview of angioedema. In Rose BD, editor: *UpToDate*, Waltham, MA, 2006, UpToDate.

Burnier M et al: Angiotensin II type 1 receptor blockers, *Circulation* 103:904, 2001.

Lee VC et al: Meta-analysis: angiotensin-receptor blockers in chronic heart failure and high-risk acute myocardial infarction, *Ann Intern Med* 141(9):693-704, 2004.

Moore MA: Drugs that interrupt the renin-angiotensin system should be among the preferred initial drugs to treat hypertension, *J Clin Hypertens* 5:137-144, 2003.

Poole-Wilson PA: ACE inhibitors and ARBs in chronic heart failure: the established, the expected, and the pragmatic, *Med Clin North Am* 87:373-389, 2003.

Rahman M: Initial findings of the AASK: African Americans with hypertensive kidney disease benefit from an ACE inhibitor, *Cleve Clin J Med* 70:304-305, 309-310, 312, 2003.

Reeder GS: Angiotensin-converting enzyme inhibitors and receptor blockers in acute myocardial infarction: Recommendations for use. In Rose BD, editor: *UpToDate*, Waltham, MA, 2006, UpToDate.

Reeder GS et al: Angiotensin inhibition and blood pressure goal in patients at high risk for a cardiovascular event. In Rose BD, editor: *UpToDate*, Waltham, MA, 2006, UpToDate.

Rose BD, Bakris GL: Treatment and prevention of diabetic nephropathy. In Rose BD, editor: *UpToDate*, Waltham, MA, 2006, UpToDate.

Rose BD, Kaplan NM: ACE inhibitors in the treatment of hypertension. In Rose BD, editor: *UpToDate*, Waltham, MA, 2006, UpToDate.

Rose BD, Kaplan NM: Major side effects of ACE inhibitors. In Rose BD, editor: *UpToDate*, Waltham, MA, 2006, UpToDate.

Rose BD et al: Differences between angiotensin-converting enzyme inhibitors and receptor blockers. In Rose BD, editor: *UpToDate*, Waltham, MA, 2006, UpToDate.

Yusuf S et al: Effects of an angiotensin-converting-enzyme inhibitor, ramipril, on cardiovascular events in high-risk patients. The Heart Outcomes Prevention Evaluation Study Investigators, *N Engl J Med* 342:145, 2000.

CHAPTER 21

Arnsdorf MF: Atrial tachycardias in adults. In Rose BD, editor: *UpToDate*, Waltham, MA, 2007, UpToDate.

Arnsdorf MF: Myocardial action potential and action of antiarrhythmic drugs. In Rose BD, editor: *UpToDate*, Waltham, MA, 2007, UpToDate.

Arnsdorf MF, Podrid PJ: Overview of the presentation and management of atrial fibrillation. In Rose BD, editor: *UpToDate*, Waltham, MA, 2007, UpToDate.

Giardina EG, Zimetbaum PJ: Major side effects of amiodarone. In Rose BD, editor: *UpToDate*, Waltham, MA, 2007, UpToDate.

Kowey PR et al: Pharmacologic and nonpharmacologic options to maintain sinus rhythm:

guideline-based and new approaches, *Am J Cardiol* 91:33-39, 2003

Naccarelli GV et al: Old and new antiarrhythmic drugs for converting and maintaining sinus rhythm in atrial fibrillation: comparative efficacy and results of trials, *Am J Cardiol* 91:15-26, 2003.

Snow V et al: Management of newly detected atrial fibrillation: a clinical practice guideline from the American Academy of Family Physicians and the American College of Physicians, *Ann Intern Med* 139(12): 1009-1017, 2003.

CHAPTER 22

American Association of Clinical Endocrinologists (AACE): AACE lipid guidelines, *Endocr Pract* 6:162, 2000.

Betteridge JD, editor: *Lipids: current perspectives,* St Louis, 2000, Martin Dunitz.

Betteridge DJ, editor: *Lipids: Current perspectives,* St. Louis, 2000, Martin Dunitz.

Davis TM et al: Lipid-lowering therapy protects against peripheral sensory neuropathy in type 2 diabetes. American Diabetes Association 2007 Scientific Sessions Chicago, IL. June 22, 2007; Abstract 0004-OR.

Expert Panel on Detection, Evaluation, and Treatment of High Blood Cholesterol in Adults: Executive summary of the Third Report of the National Cholesterol Education Program (NCEP) Expert Panel on Detection, Evaluation, and Treatment of High Blood Cholesterol in Adults (Adult Treatment Panel III), *JAMA* 285:2486, 2001.

Farnier M: Ezetimibe in hypercholesterolemia, *IJCP* 56:611, 2002.

Gotto AM: *Contemporary diagnosis and management of lipid disorders,* ed 2, Newton, PA, 2001, Handbooks in Health Care.

Grundy SM et al: Implications of recent clinical trials for the national cholesterol education program adult treatment panel III guidelines, *Circulation* 110:227-239, 2004.

Jacobson TA: The safety of aggressive statin therapy: how much can low-density lipoprotein cholesterol be lowered? *Mayo Clin Proc* 81(9):1225-1231, 2006.

Kashyap ML et al: Long-term safety and efficacy of a once-daily niacin/lovastatin formulation for patients with dyslipidemia, *Am J Cardiol* 89:672, 2002.

Keenan JM: Treatment of patients with lipid disorders in primary care: treatment guidelines and their implications, *South Med J* 97: 266-276, 2003.

Krauss RM et al: AHA dietary guidelines: revision 2000: A statement for healthcare professionals from the Nutrition Committee of the American Heart Association, *Circulation* 102:2284, 2000.

Malloy MJ, Kane JP: Agents used in hyperlipidemia. In *Basic and clinical pharmacology,* ed 8, New York, 2001, McGraw-Hill.

Maron DJ et al: Current perspectives on statins, *Circulation* 101:207-213, 2000.

McEvoy GK, editor: *American hospital formulary service: drug information,* Bethesda, MD, 2001, American Society of Health-System Pharmacists.

McGowan MP: Lipid-lowering therapy in women: new treatment options, *Prev Cardiol Clin* 2002.

McKenney JM: New guidelines for managing hypercholesterolemia, *J Am Pharm Assoc* 41:596, 2001.

McKenney JM et al: Final conclusions and recommendations of the National Lipid Association Statin Safety Assessment Task Force, *Am J Cardiol* 97(Suppl):89C-94C, 2006.

Omega-3 poly unsaturated fatty acids (Omacor) for hypertriglyceridemia, *Med Lett Drugs Ther* 47:91-92, 2005.

Oregon Health Resources Commission: *HMG-CoA reductase inhibitors (STATINS)* Update 4, October 2006.

Pasternak RC et al: ACC/AHA/NHLBI clinical advisory on the use and safety of statins, *J Am Coll Cardiol* 40:567-572, 2002.

Plakogiannis R, Cohen H: Optimal low-density lipoprotein cholesterol lowering—morning versus evening statin administration, *Ann Pharmacother* 41:106-110, 2007.

Robins SJet al: VA-HIT Study Group, Veterans Affairs High-Density Lipoprotein Intervention Trial, relation of gemfibrozil treatment and lipid levels with major coronary events: VA-HIT: a randomized controlled trial, *JAMA* 285:1585, 2001.

Rosenson, RS: Lipid lowering with drugs other than statins and fibrates. In Rose BD, editor: *UpToDate,* Waltham, MA, 2007, UpToDate.

Rosenson, RS: Lipid lowering with statins. In Rose BD, editor: *UpToDate,* Waltham, MA, 2007, UpToDate.

Rosenson, RS: Lipoprotein classification; metabolism; and role in atherosclerosis. In Rose BD, editor: *UpToDate,* Waltham, MA, 2007, UpToDate.

Rosenson, RS: Overview of treatment of hypercholesterolemia. In Rose BD, editor: *UpToDate,* Waltham, MA, 2007, UpToDate.

Steinmetz KL: Colesevelam hydrochloride, *Am J Health Syst Pharm* 59:932, 2002.

Stevermer JJ, Meadows SE: What is the target for low-density lipoprotein cholesterol in patients with heart disease? *J Fam Pract* 51:893, 2002.

Teo KK, Burton JR: Who should receive HMG CoA reductase inhibitors? *Drugs* 62:1707, 2002.

CHAPTER 23

Ansell J et al: The pharmacology and management of the vitamin K antagonists: the seventh conference on antithrombotic and thrombolytic therapy, *Chest* 126:3 (Suppl), 2004.

Bates S et al: Use of antithrombotic agents during pregnanc: the seventh conference on antithrombotic and thrombolytic therapy, *Chest* 126:3 (Suppl), 2004.

Furie B: Oral anticoagulant therapy. In Hoffman R, et al, editors: *Hematology: basic principles and practice,* ed 3, Churchill Livingstone, 2000, New York.

Geerts W et al: Prevention of venous thromboembolism: the seventh conference on antithrombotic and thrombolytic therapy, *Chest* 126:3 (Suppl), 2004.

Hirsh J et al: The seventh conference on antithrombotic and thrombolytic therapy: evidence-based guidelines, *Chest* 126:3 (Suppl), 2004.

Hirsh J, Raschke R: Heparin and low-molecular weight heparin: the seventh conference on antithrombotic and thrombolytic therapy, *Chest* 126:3 (Suppl), 2004.

Jeffery S: Warfarin superior to aspirin for stroke prevention in AF: BAFTA trial published. Available at www.medscape.com/viewarticle/ 561301 (Accessed -8-06-08).

Leung LK: Overview of hemostasis. In Rose BD, editor: *UpToDate,* Waltham, MA, 2007, UpToDate.

Lexi-Drug: Coumadin. In Rose BD, editor: *UpToDate,* Waltham, MA, 2007, UpToDate.

Link MS: Warfarin: prescribe with care in the elderly, *Medscape J Watch Cardiol.* Available at www.medscape.com/viewarticle/559414.

Mandel J, Gaasch WH: Anticoagulation during pregnancy. In Rose BD, editor: *UpToDate,* Waltham, MA, 2007, UpToDate.

Paciaroni M et al: Efficacy and safety of anticoagulation treatment in acute cardioembolic stroke: A meta-analysis of randomized controlled trial, *Stroke* 38:423-430, 2007.

Ridker P et al: A randomized trial of low-dose aspirin in the primary prevention of cardiovascular disease in women, *N Engl J Med* 352:13, 2005.

Sacco R et al: Guidelines for prevention of stroke in patients with ischemic stroke or transient ischemic attack: a statement for healthcare professionals from the American Heart Association/American Stroke Association Council on Stroke, *Stroke* 37(2):2006.

Salem D et al: Antithrombotic therapy in valvular heart disease-native and prosthetic: the seventh conference on antithrombotic and thrombolytic therapy, *Chest* 126:3 (Suppl), 2004.

Shaughnessy K: Massive pulmonary embolism, *Crit Care Nurse* 27:1, 2007.

Singer D et al: Antithrombotic therapy in atrial fibrillation: the seventh conference on antithrombotic and thrombolytic therapy, *Chest* 126:3 (Suppl), 2004.

Valentine KA, Hull RD: Correcting excess anticoagulation after warfarin. In Rose BD, editor: *UpToDate,* Waltham, MA, 2007, UpToDate.

Weitz J et al: New anticoagulant drugs: the seventh conference on antithrombotic and thrombolytic therapy, *Chest* 126:3 (Suppl), 2004.

CHAPTER 24

Bytzer P: Goals of therapy and guidelines for treatment success in symptomatic gastroesophageal reflux disease patients, *Am J Gastroenterol* 98(Suppl):S31-S39, 2003.

Camilleri M et al: Prevalence and socioeconomic impact of upper gastrointestinal disorders in the United States: results of the U.S. Upper Gastrointestinal Study, *Clin Gastroenterol Hepatol* 3:543-552, 2005.

Cash BD: Latest from the literature on GERD and acid-related disorders: October 2006 Medscape, *Gastroenterology* 8(2):2006.

Available at www.medscape.com/
viewarticle/545597.

Gremse DA: Gastroesophageal reflux disease in
children: an overview of pathophysiology,
diagnosis, and treatment, *Am J Gastroenterol*
98(3 Suppl):S24-S30, 2003.

Kahrilas PJ: Medical management of gastroesophageal reflux disease in adults. In Rose BD,
editor: *UpToDate*, Waltham, MA, 2007,
UpToDate.

Kahrilas PJ: Clinical manifestations and
diagnosis of gastroesophageal reflux in adults.
In Rose BD, editor: *UpToDate*, Waltham,
MA, 2007, UpToDate.

Keady S: Update on drugs for gastroesophageal
reflux disease, *Arch Dis Child Educ Pract Ed*
92(4):ep114-ep118, 2007.

Richter JE: Gastroesophageal reflux disease
during pregnancy, *Gastroenterol Clin North
Am* 32:235-261, 2003.

Slyk MP: Treatment strategies for the
management of GERD in older adults,
Director 13(1):25, 27-32, 2005.

CHAPTER 25

Katz PO: Effectiveness of proton pump
inhibitors: beyond cost, *Rev Gastroenterol
Disord* (Suppl 4):S8-S15, 2004.

Katz PO: Putting immediate-release
proton-pump inhibitors into clinical
practice—improving nocturnal acid control
and avoiding the possible complications of
excessive acid exposure,
Aliment Pharmacol Ther 22 (Suppl 3):31-8, 2005.

Peura DA: Treatment regimens for *Helicobacter
pylori*. In Rose BD, editor: *UpToDate*,
Waltham, MA, 2007, UpToDate.

Ramakrishnan K, Salinas RC: Recommendations
for treating peptic ulcer disease, *Am Fam
Physician* 76:1005-1012, 2007

Robinson M: Proton pump inhibitors: update
on their role in acid-related gastrointestinal
diseases, *Int J Clin Pract* 59(6):709-715,
2005.

Soll, AH: Pharmacology of antiulcer medications. In Rose BD, editor: *UpToDate*,
Waltham, MA, 2007, UpToDate.

Soll, AH: Treatment of refractory or recurrent
peptic ulcer disease. In Rose BD, editor:
UpToDate, Waltham, MA, 2007,
UpToDate.

Wolfe, MW: Overview and comparison of
the proton pump inhibitors for the treatment of acid-related disorders. In Rose BD,
editor: *UpToDate*, Waltham, MA, 2007,
UpToDate.

CHAPTER 26

American College of Gastroenterology (ACG):
Guidelines for diagnosis and management
of chronic constipation and irritable bowel
syndrome: Chronic Constipation Task Force,
Am J Gastroenterol 100(Suppl 1):S1-S22,
2005.

Camilleri M et al: Pharmacological and
pharmacokinetic aspects of functional
gastrointestinal disorders, *Gastroenterology*
130(5):1421-1434, 2006.

Johnson DA: Treating chronic constipation: how
should we interpret the recommendations?
Clin Drug Invest 26:547-557, 2006.

Locke GR III: AGA technical review:
Constipation, *Gastroenterology* 119:1766,
2000. In Rose BD, editor: *UpToDate*,
Waltham, MA, 2007, UpToDate.

Locke GR, et al: American Gastroenterological
Association medical position statement:
guidelines on constipation, *Gastroenterology*
119(6):1761-1766, 2000.

Rome Foundation: Guidelines—Rome III
diagnostic criteria for functional
gastrointestinal disorders, *J Gastrointest Liver
Dis* 15(3):307-312, 2006.

Smith C et al: Patient and physician evaluation
of a new bulk fiber laxative tablet,
Gastroenterol Nurs 26:31-37, 2003.

Talley NJ: Functional gastrointestinal disorders
in 2007 and Rome III: something new,
something borrowed, something objective,
Rev Gatroenterol Disord 7(2):97-105, 2007.

Wald A: Treatment of chronic constipation in
adults. In Rose BD, editor: *UpToDate*,
Waltham, MA, 2007, UpToDate.

Wald A: Etiology and evaluation of chronic
constipation in adults. In Rose BD, editor:
UpToDate, Waltham, MA, 2007,
UpToDate.

Wanitschke R et al: Differential therapy of
constipation—a review, *Int J Clin Pharmacol
Ther* 41:14-21, 2003.

CHAPTER 27

Crum NF et al: New issues in infectious diarrhea, *Rev Gastroenterol Disord* 5 (Suppl 3):
S16-S25, 2005.

Elliott B et al: *Clostridium difficile*–associated
diarrhea, *Intern Med J* 37(8):561-568, 2007.

Isakow W et al: Probiotics for preventing and
treating nosocomial infections: review of
current evidence and recommendations,
Chest 132(1):286-294, 2007.

King CK et al: Managing acute gastroenteritis
among children: oral rehydration, maintenance,
and nutritional therapy, *MMWR Recomm Rep*
52(RR-16):1-16, 2003.

Marcos LA, Dupont HL: Advances in defining
etiology and new therapeutic approaches in
acute diarrhea, *J Infect* Sep 6 2007 (epub).

McMaster-Baxter NL, Musher DM: *Clostridium
difficile*: recent epidemiologic findings and
advances in therapy, *Pharmacotherapy*
27(7):1029-1039, 2007.

Minocha A: *Handbook of digestive diseases*,
Thorofare, NJ, 2004, Slack.

Nelson R: Antibiotic treatment for *Clostridium
difficile*–associated diarrhea in adults,
Cochrane Database Syst Rev (3):CD004610,
2007.

CHAPTER 28

American Gastroenterological Association
(AGA): Medical position statement: nausea
and vomiting, AGA Institute—Medical
Specialty Society, 2000 May 21. Available
at www.guideline.gov/summary/summary.
aspx?doc_id=3060&nbr=002286&string=na
usea+and+vomiting

American Society of Clinical Oncology:
Guideline for antiemetics in oncology: update
2006, American Society of Clinical
Oncology—Medical Specialty Society, 1999
Sep (revised 2006 Jun 20). Available at

www.guideline.gov/summary/summary.
aspx?doc_id=9372&nbr=005018&string=
nausea+and+vomiting (accessed 8-06-08).

Chinnery LW et al: American Society of
Clinical Oncology guideline for antiemetics
in oncology: update 2006, *J Clin Oncol*
24(18):1-16, 2006.

deCarvalo E et al: A pilot study of relaxation
techniques for management of nausea and
vomiting for patients receiving cancer
chemotherapy. *Cancer Nurs* 30(2):163-167,
2007.

Flake ZA et al: Practical selection of antiemetics, *Am Fam Physician* 69:
1169-1174,1176, 2004.

Hesketh, PJ: Pathophysiology and prediction of
chemotherapy-induced emesis. In Rose BD,
editor: *UpToDate*, Waltham, MA, 2007,
UpToDate.

Lexi-Comp: Antiemetics. In Rose BD,
editor: *UpToDate*, Waltham, MA, 2007,
UpToDate.

Longstreth GF et al: Characteristics of antiemetic drugs. In Rose BD, editor: *UpToDate*,
Waltham, MA, 2007, UpToDate.

Olver I et al: Nanomedicines in the treatment
of emesis during chemotherapy: focus on
aprepitant, *Int J Nanomedicine* 2(1):13-18,
2007.

Spinks A et al: Scopolamine (hyoscine) for
preventing and treating motion sickness,
Cochrane Database Syst Rev (3):CD002851,
2007.

Tipton JM et al: Putting evidence into practice:
evidence-based interventions to prevent,
manage, and treat chemotherapy-induced
nausea and vomiting, *Clin J Oncol Nurs*
11(1):69-78. 2007. (Erratum in: *Clin J Oncol
Nurs* 11[2]:18, 2007.)

Williams BA et al: Multimodal antiemesis
including low-dose perphenazine in an
ambulatory surgery unit of a university
hospital: a 10-year history. *ScienWorld
J* 7:978-986, 2007.

CHAPTER 29

Chun AB, Wald A: Treatment of irritable bowel
syndrome. In Rose BD, editor: *UpToDate*,
Waltham, MA, 2007, UpToDate.

Gershon MD, Tack J: The serotonin signaling
system: From basic understanding to drug
development for functional GI disorders,
Gastroenterology 131:397-414, 2007.

Gilkin RJ: The spectrum of irritable bowel
syndrome: a clinical review, *Clin Ther*
27(11):1969-1709, 2005.

Hadley Sk, Gaarder SM: Treatment of irritable
bowel syndrome, *Am Fam Physician* 72:
2501- 2506, 2005.

Kale-Pradhan PB, Wilhelm SM: Tegaserod
for constipation-predominant irritable
bowel syndrome, *Pharmacotherapy* 27:
267-77, 2007.

Lexi-Comp. IBS, In Rose BD, editor: *UpToDate*,
Waltham, MA, 2007, UpToDate.

The Medical Letter: Drugs for irritable bowel
syndrome, *Treatment Guidelines* 4(43):11-16,
2006.

Wald A: Treatment of irritable bowel syndrome.
In Rose BD, editor: *UpToDate*, Waltham,
MA, 2007, UpToDate.

CHAPTER 30

Adams KF et al: Executive summary: HFSA 2006 Comprehensive Heart Failure Practice Guideline, *J Cardiac Fail* 12:10-38, 2006. See total report at www.HFSA.org (12:e1-e119).

Appel LJ: The verdict from ALLHAT—thiazide diuretics are the preferred initial therapy for hypertension, JAMA 288(23):3039-3042, 2002.

Brater DC: Pharmacology of diuretics, *Am J Med Sci* 319(1):38-50, 2000.

Cohn JN et al: New guidelines for potassium replacement in clinical practice: a contemporary review by the National Council on Potassium in Clinical Practice, *Arch Intern Med* 160(16):2429-2436, 2000.

Doggrell SA, Brown H: The spironolactone renaissance, *Expert Opin Invest Drugs* 10(5):943-954, 2001.

Dumont L et al: Efficacy and harm of pharmacological prevention of acute mountain sickness: quantitative systemic review, *BMJ* 321:267-272, 2000.

Effectiveness of spironolactone added to an angiotensin-converting enzyme inhibitor and a loop diuretic for severe chronic congestive heart failure (the Randomized Aldactone Evaluation Study [RALES]), *Am J Cardiol* 78(8):902-907, 1996.

Hunt SA et al: ACC/AHA 2005 Guideline update for the diagnosis and management of chronic heart failure in the adult-summary article: a report of the American College of Cardiology/American Heart Association Task Force on Practice Guidelines, *J Am Coll Cardiol* 46:1116, 2005.

Juurlink DN et al: Rates of hyperkalemia after publication of the Randomized Aldactone Evaluation Study, *N Engl J Med* 351(6):543-551, 2004.

Kaplan NM, Rose BD: Treatment of isolated systolic hypertension. In Rose BD, editor: *UpToDate*, Waltham, MA, 2007, UpToDate .

Kelly J, Chambers J: Inappropriate use of loop diuretics in elderly patients, *Age Aging* 29:489-493, 2000.

Laragh JH, Sealey JE: K+ depletion and the progression of hypertensive disease or heart failure: the pathogenic role of diuretic-induced aldosterone secretion, *Hypertension* 37(part 2):806-810, 2001.

Major outcomes in high-risk hypertensive patients randomized to angiotensin-converting enzyme inhibitor or calcium channel blocker vs diuretic: The Antihypertensive and Lipid-Lowering Treatment to Prevent Heart Attack Trial (ALLHAT), JAMA 288(23):2981-2997, 2002.

Mattoo TK: Treatment of hypertension in children and adolescents. In Rose BD, editor: *UpToDate*, Waltham, MA, 2007, UpToDate.

Norris W: Potassium supplementation, diet vs pills: a randomized trial in postoperative cardiac surgery patients, *Chest* 125(2):404-409, 2004.

Pitt B et al: Eplerenone, a selective aldosterone blocker, in patients with left ventricular dysfunction after myocardial infarction, *N Engl J Med* 348:1309, 2003.

SHEP Cooperative Research Group: Prevention of stroke by antihypertensive drug treatment in older persons with isolated systolic hypertension. Final results of the Systolic Hypertension in the Elderly Program (SHEP), JAMA 265(24):3255-3264, 1991.

Rose BD: Clinical manifestations and treatment of hypokalemia. In Rose BD, editor: *UpToDate*, Waltham, MA, 2007, UpToDate.

Rose BD: Optimal dosage and side effects of loop diuretics. In Rose BD, editor: *UpToDate*, Waltham, MA, 2007, UpToDate.

Rose BD: Treatment of refractory edema. In Rose BD, editor: *UpToDate*, Waltham, MA, 2007, UpToDate.

Rose BD, Colucci WS: Use of diuretics in heart failure. In Rose BD, editor: *UpToDate*, Waltham, MA, 2007, UpToDate.

Rose BD, Post TW: Mechanism of action of diuretics. In Rose BD, editor: *UpToDate*, Waltham, MA, 2007, UpToDate.

Sica DA et al: Importance of potassium in cardiovascular disease, *J Clin Hyperten* 4(3):198-206, 2002.

The ALLHAT Officers and Coordinators for the ALLHAT Collaborative Research Group: major outcomes in high-risk hypertensive patients randomized to angiotensin-converting enzyme inhibitor or calcium channel blocker vs diuretic, JAMA 288(23):2981-2997, 2002.

CHAPTER 31

Benign Prostatic Hypertrophy

Lam JS et al: Changing aspects in the evaluation and treatment of patients with benign prostatic hyperplasia, *Med Clin North Am* 88:281-308, 2004.

Roehrborn CGet al: Sustained decrease in incidence of acute urinary retention and surgery with finasteride for 6 years in men with benign prostatic hyperplasia, *J Urol* 171:1194-1198, 2004.

USDHHS, PHS, AHCPR: *Guidelines on benign prostatic hyperplasia: diagnosis and treatment,* Clinical Practice Guideline No. 8. AHCPR Publication No, 94-0582, February 1994.

Erectile Dysfunction

Kostis JB et al: Sexual dysfunction and cardiac risk (the Second Princeton Consensus Conference), *Am J Cardiol* 96(2):313-321, 2005.

Cunningham GR, Kadmon D: Epidemiology and pathogenesis of benign prostatic hyperplasia. In Rose BD, editor: *UpToDate*, Waltham, MA, 2006, UpToDate.

Cunningham GR, Kadmon D: Medical treatment of benign prostatic hyperplasia. In Rose BD, editor: *UpToDate*, Waltham, MA, 2006, UpToDate.

Montague DK et al: Erectile dysfunction guideline update panel. The management of erectile dysfunction: an update, Linthicum, MD, 2006, American Urologic Association.

Sauer WH, Kimmel SE: Sexual activity in patients with heart disease. In Rose BD, editor: *UpToDate*, Waltham, MA, 2006, UpToDate.

Saper RB: Clinical use of saw palmetto. In Rose BD, editor: *UpToDate*, Waltham, MA, 2006, UpToDate.

Spark RF: Treatment of male sexual dysfunction. In Rose BD, editor: *UpToDate*, Waltham, MA, 2006, UpToDate.

CHAPTER 32

Baum N: Urinary incontinence in the geriatric patient, *Clin Geriatr* 14:35-38, 2006.

Bengtson J et al: Urinary incontinence: guide to diagnosis and management, Boston, 2004, Brigham and Women's Hospital.

Chapple C et al: A comparison of the efficacy and tolerability of solifenacin succinate and extended release tolterodine at treating overactive bladder-syndrome: results of the STAR Trial, *Eur Urol* 48:464-470, 2005.

DuBeau CE: Epidemiology, risk factors, and pathogenesis of urinary incontinence. In Rose BD, editor: *UpToDate*, Waltham, MA, 2007, UpToDate.

Epstein BJ et al: Newer agents for the management of overactive bladder, *Am Fam Physician* 74(12):2061-2068, 2006.

Fantyl JA et al: *Urinary incontinence in adults: acute and chronic management: clinical practice guideline*, No. 2, 1996 Update, Rockville, MD, U.S. Department of Health and Human Services, Public Health Service, Agency for Health Care Policy and Research; March 1996, AHCPR Publications Nl. 96-0682. Available at www.ahrq.gov. (accessed 8-06-08).

Hesch K: Agents for treatment of overactive bladder: a therapeutic class review, *Proc (Baylor Univ Med Cent)* 20(3):307-314, 2007.

Lexi-Comp: Urinary incontinence. In Rose BD, editor: *UpToDate*, Waltham, MA, 2007, UpToDate.

Papatsoris AG et al: An overview of stress urinary incontinence treatment in women, *Aging Clin Exp Res* 19(4):334-340, 2007.

Smith D: The bladder matters, *Women's Health Care* 4:17-25, 2005.

Smith PP et al: Current trends in the evaluation and management of female urinary incontinence, *Can Med Assoc J* 175(10):132-137, 2006.

Staskin DR: Overactive bladder in the elderly: a guide to pharmacological management, *Drugs Aging* 22(12):1013-1028, 2005.

The Medical Letter: Solifenacin and darifenacin for overactive bladder, *Med Lett Drugs Ther* 47(1204):234, 2005.

The Medical Letter: Trospium chloride (Sanctura): another anticholinergic for overactive bladder, *Med Lett Drugs Ther* 46(1188):63-64, 2004.

CHAPTER 33

Burns MJ et al: Acetaminophen (paracetamol) intoxication in adults. In Rose BD, editor: *UpToDate*, Waltham, MA, 2007, UpToDate.

Burns MJ et al: Pathophysiology and diagnosis of acetaminophen (paracetamol) intoxication. In Rose BD, editor: *UpToDate*, Waltham, MA, 2007, UpToDate.

Glass GG: Osteoarthritis, *Clin Fam Pract* 7:161-179, 2005.

Larson AM et al: Acute liver failure study group. Acetaminophen-induced acute liver failure, results of a United States multicenter, prospective study, *Hepatology* 42(6):1364-1372, 2005.

Mayhew MS: Acetaminophen toxicity, *J Nurse Pract* 3(3):186-188, 2007.

Porat R, Dinarello CA: Pathophysiology and treatment of fever in adults. In Rose BD, editor: *UpToDate*, Waltham, MA, 2007, UpToDate.

Rowden AK et al: Acetaminophen poisoning, *Clin Lab Med* 26(1):49-65, 2006.

Watkins PB et al: Aminotransferase elevations in healthy adults receiving 4 grams of acetaminophen daily, JAMA 296:87-93, 2006.

CHAPTER 34

Abrams CA: Platelet biology. In Rose BD, editor: *UpToDate*, Waltham, MA, 2007, UpToDate.

Aldandashi S et al: Combination treatment with dipyridamole, aspirin, and tPA in an embolic model of stroke in rats, *Exp Neurol* 205(2):563-568, 2007.

Dionne R: Relative efficacy of selective COX-2 inhibitors compared with over-the-counter ibuprofen, *Int J Clin Pract Suppl* (135):18-22, 2003.

Henry D, McGettigan P: Epidemiology overview of gastrointestinal and renal toxicity of NSAIDs, *Int J Clin Pract* Suppl (135): 43-49, 2003.

Hochberg MC: COX-2: where are we in 2003? Be strong and resolute: continue to use COX-2 selective inhibitors at recommended dosages in appropriate patients, *Arthritis Res Ther* 5(1): 28-30, 2003.

Katz WA: *Management of moderate chronic pain in osteoarthritis*, Medscape April 27, 2006. Available at www.medscape.com/viewprogram/5329.

Kong JS et al: Aspirin and nonsteroidal antiinflammatory drug hypersensitivity, *Clin Rev Allergy Immunol* 32(1):97-110, 2007.

Lamont EB et al: NSAIDs and colorectal cancer risk: do administrative data support a chemopreventive effect? *J Gen Intern Med* (8):1166-1171, 2007.

Lexi-Comp: NSAIDS. In Rose BD, editor: *UpToDate*, Waltham, MA, 2007, UpToDate.

Muluk V, Macpherson DS: Perioperative medication management. In Rose BD, editor: *UpToDate*, Waltham, MA, 2007, UpToDate.

Salzberg DJ, Weir MR: COX-2 inhibitors and cardiovascular risk, *Subcell Biochem* 42: 159-174, 2007.

Simon R, Namazy J: Adverse reactions to aspirin and nonsteroidal antiinflammatory drugs (NSAIDs), *Clin Rev Allergy Immunol* 24(3):239-252, 2003.

The Medical Letter: Do NSAIDs interfere with the cardioprotective effects of aspirin? *Med Lett Drugs Ther* (1188):61-62, August 2, 2004.

Wolfe MM: Risk factors associated with the development of gastroduodenal ulcers due to the use of NSAIDs, *Int J Clin Pract* Suppl (135):32-37, 2003.

CHAPTER 35

Adams MP et al: *Pharmacology for nurses: a pathophysiologic approach*, ed 2, New Jersey, 2008, Pearson/Prentice-Hall.

Chen YF et al: A systematic review of the effectiveness of adalimumab, etanercept and infliximab for the treatment of rheumatoid arthritis in adults and an economic evaluation of their cost-effectiveness, *Health Technol Assess* 10(42):iii-iv, xi-xiii, 1-229, 2006.

DeRuiter J, Riley T: How can adalimumab (Humira) be used to treat rheumatoid

arthritis? Available at www.uspharmacist.com/index.asp?show=article&page=8_1083.htm US Pharmacist Website (accessed 8-06-08).

Gaffo A et al: Treatment of rheumatoid arthritis, *Am J Health Syst Pharm* 63(24):2451-2465, 2006.

Harris ED, et al: Overview of the management of rheumatoid arthritis. In Rose BD, editor: *UpToDate*, Waltham, MA, 2007, UpToDate.

Hellmann DB, Stone JH: Arthritis and musculoskeletal disorders. In McPhee SJ et al, editors: *Current medical diagnosis and treatment 2008*, ed 47, New York, 2007, McGraw-Hill.

Hetland ML et al: Aggressive combination therapy with intraarticular glucocorticoid injections and conventional DMARDs in early rheumatoid arthritis twoyear clinical and radiographic results from the CIMESTRA study, *Ann Rheum Di* 67(6):815-822, 2007.

Lexi-Comp: DMARDS. In Rose BD, editor: *UpToDate*, Waltham, MA, 2007, UpToDate.

Rindfleisch JA, Muller D: Diagnosis and management of rheumatoid arthritis, *Am Fam Physician* 72(6):1037-1047, 2005.

Scott DL: Pursuit of optimal outcomes in rheumatoid arthritis, *Pharmacoeconomics* 22(2 Suppl 1):13-26, 2004.

Shanahan JC, St Clair EW: Rheumatoid arthritis. In Rakel RE, Bope ET, editors: *Conn's current therapy*, Philadelphia, 2007, Saunders.

Simon LS et al: Pain in osteoarthritis, rheumatoid arthritis and juvenile chronic arthritis, ed 2, Glenview (IL), American Pain Society (APS), 2002.

Van der Heijden JW et al: Drug insight: resistant to methotrexate and other disease-modifying antirheumatic drugs—from bench to bedside, *Nat Clin Pract Rheumatol* 3(1):26-34, 2007.

Venables PJW, Maini RN: Clinical features of rheumatoid arthritis. In Rose BD, editor: *UpToDate*, Waltham, MA, 2007, UpToDate.

CHAPTER 36

Arromdee E et al: Epidemiology of gout: is the incidence rising? *J Rheumatol* 29(11): 2403-2406, 2002.

Crowther CL: *Primary orthopedic care, ed 2*, St Louis, 2005, Mosby.

Becker MA: Clinical manifestations and diagnosis of gout. In Rose BD, editor: *UpToDate*, Waltham, MA, 2006, UpToDate.

Becker MA: Treatment and prevention of recurrent gout. In Rose BD, editor: *UpToDate*, Waltham, MA, 2006, UpToDate.

Becker MA: Treatment of acute gout. In Rose BD, editor: *UpToDate*, Waltham, MA, 2006, UpToDate.

Kamienski M: Gout: not just for the rich and famous! Every man's disease, *Orthop Nurs* 22(1):16-20, 2003.

Perez-Ruiz F et al: Effect of urate-lowering therapy on the velocity of size reduction of tophi in chronic gout, *Arthritis Rheum* 47(4):356-360, 2002.

Perez-Ruiz Fet al: Renal underexcretion of uric acid is present in patients with apparent high urinary uric acid output, *Arthritis Rheum* 47(6):610-713, 2002.

Saag KM, Teng GG: *Diagnosis and management of acute and chronic gout*, available at

www.medscape.com/viewarticle/550923 (accessesd July 5, 2007).

Schlesinger N, Schumacher HR Jr: Update on gout, *Arthritis Rheum* 47(5):563-565, 2002.

Shekarriz B, Stoller ML: Uric acid nephrolithiasis: current concepts and controversies, *J Urol* 168(4 pt 1):1307-1314, 2002.

Terkeltaub RA: Gout, *N Engl J Med* 349:17, 1647-1655, 2003.

Yamamoto T et al: A simple method of selecting gout patients for treatment with uricosuric agents, using spot urine and blood samples, *J Rheumatol* 29(9):937-941, 2002.

CHAPTER 37

Armstrong C: Practice guidelines: NAMS updates recommendations on diagnosis and management of osteoporosis in postmenopausal women, *Am Fam Physician* 74(9), 2006. Available at www.aafp.org/afp/20061101/practice.html#p1.

Campion JM, Maricie MJ: Osteoporosis in men, *Am Fam Physician* 67(7):1521-1526, 2003.

Davidson MR: Pharmacotherapeutics for osteoporosis prevention and treatment, *J Midwifery Womens Health* 48(1):39-54, 2003.

Eichner SF et al: Comparing therapies for postmenopausal osteoporosis prevention and treatment, *Ann Pharmacother* 37(5):711-724, 2003.

Genant HK, Jergas M: Assessment of prevalent and incident vertebral fractures in osteoporosis research, *Osteoporos Int* (epub): March 12, 2003.

Hulley SB, Grady D: The WHI estrogen-alone trial—do things look any better? JAMA 291(14):1769-1771, 2004.

Levine JP: Long-term estrogen and hormone replacement therapy for the prevention and treatment of osteoporosis, *Curr Womens Health Rep* 3(3):181-186, 2003.

Menostar: A low-dose estrogen patch for osteoporosis, *Obstet Gynecol* 105(2):432-433, 2005.

Placide J, Martens MG: Comparing screening methods for osteoporosis, *Curr Womens Health Rep* 3(3):207-210, 2003.

Position statement. Management of menopause in postmenopausal women, Menopause, *J North Am Menopause Soc* 13(3):338-339, 2006.

Rosen HN: Bisphosphonates in the management of osteoporosis in postmenopausal women. In Rose BD, editor: *UpToDate*, Waltham, MA, 2007, UpToDate.

Rosen HN, Drezner MK: Overview of the management of osteoporosis in postmenopausal women. In Rose BD, editor: *UpToDate*, Waltham, MA, 2007, UpToDate.

Rosen HN, Conzen S: Use of selective estrogen receptor modulators in postmenopausal women. In Rose BD, editor: *UpToDate*, Waltham, MA, 2007, UpToDate.

Sagraves R: Evaluating therapeutic modalities for prevention and treatment of postmenopausal osteoporosis, *Ann Pharmacother* 37(5):744-746, 2003.

Technical Appraisal 87 National Institute for Clinical Excellence: Bisphosphonates (alendronate, etidronate, risedronate), selective estrogen receptive modulators (raloxifene), and parathyroid hormone (teriparatide) for the secondary prevention of osteoporotic fragility fractures in postmenopausal women, January 2005. Available at www.nice.org.uk/download.aspx?o=TA087guidance (accessed 8-06-08).

Watts NB et al: Use of matched historical controls to evaluate the anti-fracture efficacy of once-a-week risedronate, *Osteoporos Int*, April 29 (epub), 2003.

CHAPTER 38

Caterino JM: Administration of inappropriate medications to elderly emergency department patients: results of a national survey, *Acad Emerg Med* 10(5):493-494, 2003.

Harris: *Kelley's textbook of rheumatology*, ed 7, Philadelphia, 2005, Saunders.

Harwood MI, Smith BJ: Low back pain: a primary care approach, *Clin Fam Pract* 7:279-304, 2005.

Institute for Clinical Systems Improvement (ICSI): *Adult low back pain*, Bloomington, MN, 2006, The Institute.

Lehrich JR, Sheon RP: Treatment of low back pain: initial approach. In Rose BD, editor: *UpToDate*, Waltham, MA, 2007, UpToDate.

Reeves RR, Mack JE: Possible dangerous interaction of OxyContin and carisoprodol, *Am Fam Physician* 67(5):941-942, 2003.

Reeves RR, Parker JD: Somatic dysfunction during carisoprodol cessation: evidence for a carisoprodol withdrawal syndrome, *J Am Osteopath Assoc* 103(2):75-80, 2003.

U.S. Preventive Services Task Force: Primary care interventions to prevent low back pain in adults: recommendation statement, *Am Fam Physician* 71(12):2337-2338, 2005.

van Tulder MW et al: Muscle relaxants for nonspecific low back pain: a systematic review within the framework of the Cochrane collaboration, *Spine* 28(17):1978-1992, 2003.

CHAPTER 39

Thibodeau GA, Patton KT: *Anatomy and physiology*, ed 6, St. Louis, 2007, Mosby.

CHAPTER 40

American Psychiatric Association (APA): *Diagnostic and statistical manual of mental disorders*, 4th Ed, Text Revision (DSM-IV-TR), Washington, DC, 2003, Author.

Biederman J et al: Long-term safety and effectiveness of mixed amphetamine salts extended release in adults with ADHD, *CNS Spectr* 10(12 Suppl 20):16-25, 2005.

Biederman J et al: A randomized, placebo-controlled trial of OROS methylphenidate in adults with attention-deficit/hyperactivity disorder, *Biol Psychiatry* 59:829-835, 2006.

Gibbins C, Weiss M: Clinical recommendations in current practice guidelines for diagnosis and treatment of ADHD in adults, *Curr Psychiatry Rep* (5):420-426, 2007.

Graydanus DE et al: Attention-deficit/hyperactivity disorder in children and adolescents: interventions for a complex costly clinical conundrum, *Pediatr Clin North Am* 50: 1049-1092, 2004.

Hazell P: Pharmacological management of attention-deficit hyperactivity disorder in adolescents: special considerations, *CNS Drugs* 21(1):37-46, 2007.

Hunt RD: *The neurobiology of AD/HD*, 2006. Available at www.medscape.com/viewarticle/541543_1 (accessed 8-06-08).

Jensen PS et al: Three-year follow-up of the NIMH MTA study, *J Am Acad Child Adolesc Psychiatry* 46(8):989-1002, 2007.

Kratochvil CJ et al: High-dose atomoxetine treatment of ADHD in youths with limited response to standard doses, *J Am Acad Child Adolesc Psychiatry* 46(9):1128-1137, 2007.

Lexi-Comp: ADHD. In Rose BD, editor: *UpToDate*, Waltham, MA, 2007, UpToDate.

Nutt DJ et al: Evidence-based guidelines for management of attention-deficit/hyperactivity disorder in adolescents in transition to adult services and in adults: recommendations from the British Association for Psychopharmacology, *J Psychopharmacol* 21(1):10-14, 2007.

Searight HR, Burke JM: Adult attention-deficit/hyperactivity disorder. In Rose BD, editor: *UpToDate*, Waltham, MA, 2007, UpToDate.

Swanson JM et al: Effects of stimulant medication on growth rates across 3 years in the MTA follow-up, *J Am Acad Child Adolesc Psychiatry* 46(8):1015-1027, 2007.

Weisler RH: Emerging drugs for attention-deficit/hyperactivity disorder, *Expert Opin Emerg Drugs* 12(3):423-434 2007.

Young D: Experts advise med guides for ADHD drugs, *Am J Health Syst Pharm* 63(9):794-797, 2006.

CHAPTER 41

American Psychiatric Association: *Treating Alzheimer's disease and other dementias of late life*. Available at www.psych.org/psych_pract/treatg/quick_ref_guide/AlzheimersQRG_04-15-05.pdf (accessed 8-06-08).

Bentue-Ferrer Det al: Clinically significant drug interactions with cholinesterase inhibitors: a guide for neurologists, *CNS Drugs* 17(13):947-963, 2003.

Birks J: Cholinesterase inhibitors for Alzheimer's disease, *Cochrane Database Syst Rev* Jan 25;(1):CD005593, 2006.

Cummings JL et al: Behavioral effects of memantine in Alzheimer's disease patients receiving donepezil treatment, *Neurology* 67:57-63, 2006.

DeLaGarza VW: Pharmacologic treatment of Alzheimer's disease: an update, *Am Fam Physician* 68(7):1365-1372, 2003.

Doody RS et al: Practice parameter: Management of dementia (an evidence-based review): Report of the quality standards subcommittee of the American Academy of Neurology, *Neurology* 56:1154-1166, 2001.

Gauthier S et al: Strategies for continued successful treatment of Alzheimer's disease: switching cholinesterase inhibitors, *Curr Med Res Opin* 19(8):707-714, 2003.

Hughes A et al: Gastrointestinal adverse events in a general population sample of nursing home residents taking cholinesterase inhibitors, *Consult Pharm* 19(8):713-720, 2004.

Ibah B, Haen E: Acetylcholinesterase inhibition in Alzheimer's disease, *Curr Pharm Des* 10(3):231-251, 2004.

Jonsson L: Pharmacoeconomics of cholinesterase inhibitors in the treatment of Alzheimer's disease, *Pharmacoeconomics* 21(14):1025-2037, 2003.

Knopman DS et al: Practice parameter: diagnosis of dementia (an evidence-based review): report of the quality standards subcommittee of the American Academy of Neurology, *Neurology* 56:1143-1153, 2001.

Lexi-Comp: Dementia. In Rose BD, editor: *UpToDate*, Waltham, MA, 2007, UpToDate.

Liston DR et al: Pharmacology of selective acetylcholinesterase inhibitors: implications for use in Alzheimer's disease, *Eur J Pharmacol* 486(1):9-17, 2004.

Lojkowska W et al: The effect of cholinesterase inhibitors on the regional blood flow in patients with Alzheimer's disease and vascular dementia, *J Neurol Sci* 216(1):119-126, 2003.

Pakrasi S: Clinical predictors of response to acetyl cholinesterase inhibitors: experience from routine clinical use in Newcastle, *Int J Geriatr Psychiatry* 18(10):879-886, 2003.

Palmer AM: Cholinergic therapies for Alzheimer's disease: progress and prospects, *Curr Opin Invest Drugs* 4(7):820-825, 2003.

Press D, Alexander M: Treatment of dementia. In Rose BD, editor: *UpToDate*, Waltham, MA, 2007, UpToDate.

Qaseem A et al: Current pharmacologic treatment of dementia: a clinical pracrice guideline from the American College of Physicians and the American Academy of Family Physicians, *Ann Intern Med* 148(5):370-378, 2008.

Ringman JM, Cumming JL: Current and emerging pharmacological treatment options for dementia, *Behav Neurol* 17(1):5-16, 2006.

Shadlen MF, Larson, EB: Evaluation of cognitive impairment and dementia. In Rose BD, editor: *UpToDate*, Waltham, MA, 2007, UpToDate.

U.S. Preventive Services Task Force: Screening for dementia: recommendation and rationale, *Ann Intern Med* 138:925-926, 2003.

Wu G et al: The cost-benefit of cholinesterase inhibitors in mild to moderate dementia: a willingness-to-pay approach, *CNS Drugs* 17(14):1045-1057, 2003.

CHAPTER 42

American Geriatrics Society Panel on Persistent Pain in Older Persons: The management of persistent pain in older persons, *J Am Geriatr Soc* 50:S205-S224, 2002.

American Pain Society (APS): *Principles of analgesic use in the treatment of acute pain and cancer pain*, Glenview, IL, 2003, Author.

Ardery G et al: Assessing and managing acute pain in older adults: a research base to guide practice, *MEDSURG Nurs* 12(1):7-18, 2003.

Bajwa ZH, Warfield CA: Pharmacologic therapy of cancer pain. In Rose BD, editor: *UpToDate*, Waltham, MA, 2007, UpToDate.

Bajwa ZH et al: Overview of the treatment of chronic pain. In Rose BD, editor: *UpToDate*, Waltham, MA, 2007, UpToDate.

Berry PH et al: *Pain: current understanding of assessment, management, and treatments*, Glenview, IL, 2006, American Pain Society.

Gruener D, Lande SD, editors: *Pain control in the primary care setting*, Glenview, IL, 2006, American Pain Society.

Guindon J et al: Recent advances in the pharmacological management of pain, *Drugs* 67(15):2121-2133, 2007.

Institute for Clinical Systems Improvement (ICSI): *Assessment and management of chronic pain*, Bloomington, MN, 2005, Author.

Institute for Clinical Systems Improvement (ICSI): *Assessment and management of acute pain*, Bloomington, MN, 2006, Author.

Lexi-Comp: Analgesics. In Rose BD, editor: *UpToDate*, Waltham, MA, 2007, UpToDate.

McMahon SB, Koltzenbur M: *Wall and Melzack's textbook of pain*, ed 5, Philadelphia, 2005, Saunders.

Nicholson AB: Methadone for cancer pain (review), *Cochrane Database Syst Rev* 1: CD003971, 2004.

Quigley C: Opioid switching to improve pain relief and drug tolerability (Review), *Cochrane Database Systc Rev* 3:CD004847, 2004.

Quigley C, Wiffen P: A systematic review of hydromorphone in acute and chronic pain, *J Pain Symp Manage* 25(2):169-178, 2003.

Regan JJ, Alderson A: OxyContin: maintaining availability and efficacy while preventing diversion and abuse, *Tenn Med* 96:88-90, 2003.

Wiffen PJ et al: Oral morphine for cancer pain (review). *Cochrane Database Syst Rev* 4: CD003868, 2003.

Zacny JP: Characterizing the subjective, psychomotor, and physiologic effects of a hydrocodone combination product (Hycodan) in non-drug-abusing volunteers, *Psychopharmacol* 165:146-156, 2003.

CHAPTER 43

Baos V et al: Use of a structured migraine diary improves patient and physician communication about migraine disability and treatment outcomes, *Int J Clin Pract* 59:281-286, 2005.

Becker WJ et al: Topiramate prophylaxis and response to triptan treatment for acute migraine, *Headache* 45(9):1424-1430, 2006.

Bigal ME, Lipton RB: When migraine progresses: transformed or chronic migraine, *Expert Rev Neurother* 6:297-306, 2006.

Brandes JL et al: Assessing the ability of topiramate to improve the daily activities of patients with migraine, *Mayo Clinic Proc* 81:1311-1319, 2006.

Diamond S et al: Patterns of diagnosis and acute and preventive treatment for migraine in the United States: results from the American Migraine Prevalence and Prevention study, *Headache* 47:355-363, 2007.

Diamond M et al: Topiramate improves health-related quality of life when used to prevent migraine, *Headache* 45:1023-1030, 2005.

Goalsby PJ et al: Drug therapy: migraine-current understanding and treatment, *N Engl J Med* 346:257-270, 2002.

Gunner JB et al: Practice guidelines for diagnosis and management of migraine headaches in children and adolescents: Part One, *J Pediatr Health Care* 21(5):327-332.

Headache impact test (HIT). Available at www.headachetest.com.

Leonardi M et al: The global burden of migraine: measuring disability in headache disorders with WHO's Classification of Functioning, Disability and Health (ICF), *J Headache Pain* 6:429-440, 2007.

Lewis D et al: Practice parameter: pharmacological treatment of migraine headache in children and adolescents: report of the American Academy of Neurology Quality Standards Subcommittee and the Practice Committee of the Child Neurology Society, *Neurology* 63(12): 2215-2224, 2004.

Linde K, Rossnagel K: Propranolol for migraine prophylaxis, *Cochrane Database Syst Rev* 2: CD003225, 2004.

Lipton RB et al: Migraine prevalence, disease burden, and the need for preventive therapy, *Neurology* 68:343-349, 2007.

Loder E, Biondi D: General principles of migraine management: the changing role of prevention, *Headache* 45(Suppl 1):S33-S47, 2004.

Lucas C: Strategies to improve migraine treatment results, *Drugs* 66 Suppl 3:9-16, 2006.

MacGregor EA et al: Impact of migraine on patients and their families: the Migraine and Zolmitriptan Evaluation (MAZE) survey— Phase III, *Curr Med Res Opin* 20:1143-1150, 2004.

Migraine Disability Assessment (MIDAS) Test: Available at www.migraine-disability.net.

Nachit-Ouinekh F et al: Use of the headache impact test (HIT-6) in general practice: relationship with quality of life and severity, *Eur J Neurol* 12:189-193, 2004.

National Headache Foundation (NHF) press release: *The NHF unveils migraine prevention consensus statement*. Available at www.headaches.org.

Ramadan M et al: Evidence-based guidelines for migraine headache in the primary care setting: pharmacological management for prevention of migraine, *Neurology* 2000. Available at www.aan.com.

Rothrock JF et al: Predictors of a negative response to topiramate therapy in patients with chronic migraine, *Headache* 45(7): 932-935, 2005.

Ruoff G, Urban G: Treatment of primary headache: patient education. In *Standards of care for headache diagnosis and treatment*, Chicago, 2004, National Headache Foundation.

Shattell M, Hogan B: Facilitating communication: how to truly understand what patients mean, *J Psychosoc Nurs Ment Health Serv* 43:29-32, 2004.

Silberstein SD: Practice parameter: evidence-based guidelines for migraine headache (an evidence-based review). Report of the quality standards subcommittee of the American Academy of Neurology (AAN), St Paul, MN, 2000, AAN.

Silberstein SD et al: Topiramate in migraine prevention: results of a large controlled trial, *Arch Neurol* 61:490-495, 2004.

Silberstein SD et al: The international classification of headache disorders, ed 2 (ICHD-II)—revision of criteria for 8.2 Medication-overuse headache, *Cephalalgia* 25:460-465, 2005.

Silberstein SD et al: The impact of migraine on daily activities: effect of topiramate compared with placebo, *Curr Med Res Opin* 22: 1021-1029, 2006.

Silberstein SD et al: Efficacy and safety of topiramate for the treatment of chronic migraine: a randomized, double-blind, placebo-controlled trial, *Headache* 47:170-180, 2007.

The Medical Letter: Drugs for migraine, treatment guidelines, *Med Lett Drugs Ther* 2(25):63-66, 2005.

CHAPTER 44

American Academy of Neurology: Practice parameter: evaluating a first nonfebrile seizure in children, Report of the Quality Standards Subcommittee of the American Academy of Neurology, the Child Neurology Society, and the American Epilepsy Society, *Neurology* 55:5, 2000.

American Academy of Neurology: Practice parameter: anticonvulsant prophylaxis in patients with newly diagnosed brain tumors, Report of the Quality Standards Subcommittee of the American Academy of Neurology, *Neurology* 54:10, 2000.

Deckers C et al: Selection criteria for the clinical use of the newer antiepileptic drugs, *CNS Drugs* 17:405-421, 2003.

Fishman MA: Febrile seizures. In Rose BD, editor: *UpToDate*, Waltham, MA, 2007, UpToDate.

French JA et al: Efficacy and tolerability of the new antiepileptic drugs I: treatment of new onset epilepsy: report of the Therapeutics and Technology Assessment Subcommittee and Quality Standards Subcommittee of the American Academy of Neurology and the AES, *Neurology* 62(8):1252-1260, 2004.

Friedman MJ, Sharieff GQ: Seizures in children, *Pediatr Clin North Am* 53:257-277, 2006.

King M: The new patient with a first seizure, *Aust Fam Physician* 32:221-228, 2003.

Lexi-Comp: Antiepileptics. In Rose BD, editor: *UpToDate*, Waltham, MA, 2007, UpToDate.

Marson AG et al: A randomized controlled trial examining the longer-term outcomes of standard versus new antiepileptic drugs. The SANAD trial, *Health Technol Assess* 11(37): 1-134, 2007.

Patsalos PN et al: The importance of drug interactions in epilepsy therapy, *Epilepsia* 43(4):365-385, 2002.

Perucca E: Marketed new antiepileptic drugs: are they better than old-generation agents? *Ther Drug Monit* 24:74-80, 2002.

Perucca E: Clinically relevant drug interactions with antiepileptic drugs, *Br J Clin Pharmacol* 61(3):246-255, 2006.

Prego-Lopez M, Devinsky O: Evaluation of a first seizure, *Postgrad Med* 111:1, 2002.

Schachter, SC: Pharmacology of antiepileptic drugs. In Rose BD, editor: *UpToDate*, Waltham, MA, 2007, UpToDate.

Schachter, SC: Risks associated with epilepsy and pregnancy. In Rose BD, editor: *UpToDate*, Waltham, MA, 2007, UpToDate.

Stecker MM: Status epilepticus in adults. In Rose BD, editor: *UpToDate*, Waltham, MA, 2007, UpToDate.

The Medical Letter: Drugs for epilepsy, treatment guidelines, *Med Lett Drugs Ther* 3(39):75-82, 2005.

Wilby J et al: Clinical effectiveness, tolerability and cost-effectiveness of newer drugs for epilepsy in adults: a systematic review and economic evaluation, *Health Technol Assess* 9(15):1-157, iii-iv, 2005.

Wilfong A: Epilepsy syndromes in children. In Rose BD, editor: *UpToDate*, Waltham, MA, 2007, UpToDate.

CHAPTER 45

Ebadi M et al: Therapeutic efficacy of selegiline in neurodegenerative disorders and neurologic diseases, *Curr Drug Targ* 7(11):1513-1529, 2006.

Hoehn MM, Yahr MD: Parkinsonism: onset, progression, and mortality. *Neurology* 57(10 Suppl 3):S11-S26, 2001

Massachusetts General Neurological Services: *Hoehn and Yahr staging scale for Parkinson's disease.* Available at http://neurosurgery.mgh.harvard.edu/Functional/pdstages.htm (accessed 8-06-08).).

Pahwa R et al: Quality Standards Subcommittee of the American Academy of Neurology, Practice parameter: treatment of Parkinson disease with motor fluctuations and dyskinesia (an evidence-based review): report of the Quality Standards Subcommittee of the American Academy of Neurology, *Neurology* 66(7):983-995, 2006.

Rao SS et al: Parkinson's disease: diagnosis and treatment, *Am Fam Physician* 74(12): 2046-2054, 2006.

Rasagiline (Azilect) for Parkinson's disease, *Med Lett Drugs Ther* 48:97-99, 2006.

Siderowf A, Stern M: Update on Parkinson disease, *Ann Intern Med* 138:651-658, 2003.

Tarsy, D: Pharmacologic treatment of Parkinson's disease. In Rose BD, editor: *UpToDate*, Waltham, MA, 2007, UpToDate.

Tarsy, D: Nonpharmacologic treatment of Parkinson's disease. In Rose BD, editor: *UpToDate*, Waltham, MA, 2007, UpToDate.

Tarsy, D: Motor fluctuations and dyskinesia in Parkinson's disease. In Rose BD, editor: *UpToDate*, Waltham, MA, 2007, UpToDate.

Weimerskirch PR, Ernst ME: Newer dopamine agonists in the treatment of restless legs syndrome, *Ann Pharmacother* 35:2001.

Weiner WJ: Meeting review: advances in the diagnosis, treatment, and understanding of Parkinson's disease and parkinsonism, *Rev Neurol Dis* 3(4):191-194, 2006.

CHAPTER 46

Cheung AH et al: Guidelines for Adolescent Depression in Primary Care (GLAD-PC): II. Treatment and ongoing management, *Pediatrics* 120(5):e1313-e1326, 2007.

Fave M et al: Comparison SSRI efficacy, *J Clin Psychopharmacol* 22:137, 2002.

Flockhart D: *Cytochrome P450 drug-interaction table*, Division of Clinical Pharmacology, Indiana University Department of Medicine, 2007. Available at http://medicine.iupui.edu/flockhart/table.htm.

Garland JE: Facing the evidence: Antidepressant treatment in children and adolescents, *Can Med Assoc J* 170:489-491, 2004.

Hirsch M, Birnbaum RJ: Antidepressant medication in adults: SSRIs and heterocyclics. In Rose BD, editor: *UpToDate*, Waltham, MA, 2007, UpToDate.

Hirsch M, Birnbaum RJ: Antidepressant medications in adults: MAO inhibitors and others. In Rose BD, editor: *UpToDate*, Waltham, MA, 2007, UpToDate.

Hirsch M, Birnbaum RJ: Sexual dysfunction associated with selective serotonin reuptake inhibitor (SSRI) antidepressants. In Rose BD, editor: *UpToDate*, Waltham, MA, 2007, UpToDate.

Hirsch M, Birnbaum RJ: Effect of SSRIs and other newer antidepressants on suicide risk in adults. In Rose BD, editor: *UpToDate*, Waltham, MA, 2007, UpToDate.

Hirshfeld RMA, Vornik LA: Newer antidepressants: review of efficacy and safety of escitalopram and duloxetine, *J Clin Psychiatry* 65 (Suppl 4):46-52, 2004.

Keller MB: Key considerations in choosing an antidepressant, *Postgrad Med [Special Report]*, November, 10-18, 2003.

Kent KJ, Boyer EW: Serotonin syndrome. In Rose BD, editor: *UpToDate*, Waltham, MA, 2007, UpToDate.

Lam RW: Review: antidepressants and psychotherapy may be equally effective for promoting remission in major depressive disorder, *Evid Based Ment Health* 6(2):45, 2003.

Lenzer J: FDA panel urges "black box" warning for antidepressants, *BMJ* 329:702, 2004.

Lyness JM: Depression: clinical manifestations and diagnosis. In Rose BD, editor: *UpToDate*, Waltham, MA, 2007, UpToDate.

McIntyre RS et al: What to do if an initial antidepressant fails? *Can Fam Physician* 49: 449-457, 2003.

Misri S, Lusskin SI: Depression in pregnant women. In Rose BD, editor: *UpToDate*, Waltham, MA, 2007, UpToDate.

Muldrow CD: *Treatment of depression: new pharmacotherapies, summary*, AHCPR Publication No. 99-E013, Washington, DC, 1999, Agency for Health Care Policy and Research.

Paulsen RH et al: Initial treatment of depression in adults. In Rose BD, editor: *UpToDate*, Waltham, MA, 2007, UpToDate.

Paulsen RH et al: Treatment of resistant depression in adults. In Rose BD, editor: *UpToDate*, Waltham, MA, 2007, UpToDate.

Ruhe H: Review: low dose tricyclic antidepressants may be effective for adults with acute depressive disorder, *Evid Based Ment Health* 6(2):46, 2003.

Stahl SM: *Antipsychotics and mood stabilizers (essential psychopharmacology)*, ed 3, London, 2008, Cambridge University Press.

To SE et al: The symptoms, neurobiology, and current pharmacological treatment of depression, *J Neurosci Nurs* 37(2): 02-107, 2005.

Vitiello B, Swedo S: Antidepressant medications in children, *N Engl J Med* 350:1489-1491, 2004.

Wong ICK et al: Use of selective serotonin reuptake inhibitors in children and adolescents, *Drug Saf* 27:991-1000, 2004.

Zuckerbrot RA et al, GLAD-PC steering group: Guidelines for Adolescent Depression in Primary Care (GLAD-PC): I. Identification, assessment, and initial management, *Pediatrics* 120(5):e1299-e1312, 2007.

CHAPTER 47

American Psychiatric Association: *Practice guideline for the treatment of patients with acute stress disorder and posttraumatic stress disorder*, Arlington, VA, 2004, Author.

Becker PM: Pharmacologic and nonpharmacologic treatments of insomnia, *Neurol Clin* 23: 1149-1163, 2005.

Brady K et al: Efficacy and safety of sertraline treatment of post traumatic stress disorder, *JAMA* 284:1837, 2000.

Carson WH et al: Drug development for anxiety disorders: new roles for atypical antipsychotics, *Psychopharmacol Bull* 38(Suppl 1):38-45, 2004.

Chokroverty, S: Evaluation and treatment of insomnia. In Rose BD, editor: *UpToDate*, Waltham, MA, 2007, UpToDate.

Ciechanowski P, Katon W: Overview of generalized anxiety disorder. In Rose BD, editor: *UpToDate*, Waltham, MA, 2007, UpToDate.

Ciechanowski P, Katon W: Overview of panic disorder. In Rose BD, editor: *UpToDate*, Waltham, MA, 2007, UpToDate.

Ciechanowski P, Katon W: Overview of phobic disorders. In Rose BD, editor: *UpToDate*, Waltham, MA, 2007, UpToDate.

Ciechanowski P, Katon W: Overview of post-traumatic stress disorder. In Rose BD, editor: *UpToDate*, Waltham, MA, 2007, UpToDate.

Gao K et al: Efficacy of typical and atypical antipsychotics for primary and comorbid anxiety symptoms or disorders: a review, *J Clin Psychiatry* 67(9):1327-1340, 2006.

Gorman JM: New molecular targets for antianxiety interventions, *J Clin Psychiatry* 64(Suppl 3): 28-35, 2003.

Maloney G: Antianxiety medications: A review of mechanisms and presentations of emergency-related emergencies, *JEMS* 29(12):70-71, 73-81, 2004.

Morgenthaler T et al: Practice parameters for the psychological and behavioral treatment of insomnia: An update. An American Academy of Sleep Medicine report, *J Sleep* 2007. Available at www.journalsleep.org/ViewAbstract.aspx?citationid=3076 (accessed 8-06-08).

Pimlott NJ et al: Educating physicians to reduce benzodiazepine use by elderly patients: a randomized controlled trial, *CMAJ* 168(7): 835-839, 2003.

The Medical Letter: Eszopiclone (Lunesta), a new hypnotic, *Med Lett Drugs Ther* 47(1203):17-19, 2005.

The Medical Letter: Ramelteon (Rozarem) for insomnia, *Med Lett Drugs Ther* 47(1221): 89-91, 2005.

Salzman C: Late-life anxiety disorders, *Psychopharmacol Bull* 38 Suppl 1:25-30, 2004.

Tonks A: Treating generalized anxiety disorder, *BMJ* 326(7301):700-702, 2003.

CHAPTER 48

Adachi N et al: Deja vu experiences in schizophrenia: relations with psychopathology and antipsychotic medication, *Compr Psychiatry* 48(6):592-596, 2007.

American Psychiatric Association (APA) Committee on Practice Guidelines: *Treating schizophrenia: a quick reference guide*, Washington DC, 2004, APA. Available with updates at www.psych.org/psych_pract/treatg/pg/Schizophrenia2ePG_05-15-06.pdf (accessed 8-06-08).

Buckley PF et al: First-episode psychosis: a window of opportunity for best practices, CNS Spectr 12(9 Suppl 15):1-12, 2007.

Citrome L: The effectiveness criterion: balancing efficacy against the risks of weight gain, J Clin Psychiatry 68(Suppl 12):12-17, 2007.

Craig TJ et al: Medication use patterns and two-year outcome in first-admission patients with major depressive disorder with psychotic features, Compr Psychiatry 48(6):497-503, 2007.

Gabbard GO: Gabbard's treatment of psychiatric disorders, ed 4, New York, 2007, American Psychiatric Publishing.

Goldberg TE, et al: Cognitive improvement after treatment with second-generation antipsychotic medications in first-episode schizophrenia: is it a practice effect? Arch Gen Psychiatry 64(10):1115-1122, 2007.

Haddad PM, Sharma SG: Adverse effects of atypical antipsychotics: differential risk and clinical implications, CNS Drugs 21(11):911-936, 2007.

Henderson DC: Weight gain with atypical antipsychotics: evidence and insights, J Clin Psychiatry 68 Suppl 12:18-26, 2007.

Hollis J, et al: Antipsychotic medication dispensing and risk of death in veterans and war widows 65 years and older, Am J Geriatr Psychiatry 15(11):932-941, 2007.

Jibson, MD: Overview of antipsychotic medications. In Rose BD, editor: UpToDate, Waltham, MA, 2007, UpToDate.

Kane JM: Treatment adherence and long-term outcomes, CNS Spectr 12(10 Suppl 17):21-26, 2007.

Lalonde P: Evaluating antipsychotic medications: predictors of clinical effectiveness. Report of an expert review panel on efficacy and effectiveness, Can J Psychiatry 48(3 Suppl 1):3S-12S.

Lehman AF et al: Practice guidelines for the treatment of patients with schizophrenia, ed 2, Washington, DC, 2004, American Psychiatric Association. Available with updates at www.psych.org/psych_pract/treatg/pg/Schizophrenia2ePG_05-15-06.pdf (accessed 8-06-08).

Lexi-Comp: Antipsychotics. In Rose BD, editor: UpToDate, Waltham, MA, 2006, UpToDate.

Mishra B et al: Atypicality in presentation of neuroleptic malignant syndrome caused by olanzapine, Indian J Med Sci 61(10):570-573, 2007.

Sharp B, Perdue C: Abnormal motor movements associated with combining psychostimulants and atypical antipsychotics in children, CNS Spectr 12(9):659-662, 2007.

Sink KM, et al: Pharmacological treatment of neuropsychiatric symptoms of dementia: a review of the evidence, JAMA 293:596-608, 2005.

Stern TA et al: Review Manual for Massachusetts General Hospital handbook of general hospital psychiatry, ed 5, St Louis, 2005, Mosby.

The Medical Letter: Choice of an antipsychotic, Med Lett Drugs Ther 45(1172):102-104, 2003.

The Medical Letter: Drugs for psychiatric disorders: treatment guidelines, Med Lett Drugs Ther 4(46):35-45, 2006.

Veterans Administration, Department of Defense: Management of persons with psychoses, Washington (DC), 2004, Department of Veterans Affairs, pp. 1-26.

Zaetta, JM et al: Indications for percutaneous interventional procedures in the patient with claudication. In Rose BD, editor: UpToDate, Waltham, MA, 2006, UpToDate.

Zhu B et al: Medication patterns and costs associated with olanzapine and other atypical antipsychotics in the treatment of bipolar disorder, Curr Med Res Opin 23(11):2805-2814, 2007.

CHAPTER 49

Anstey KJ et al: Prevalence, risk factors and treatment for substance abuse in older adults, Curr Opin Psychiatry. Available at www.medscape.com/viewprogram/6529 (accessed 8-06-08).

Anton R et al: Combined pharmacotherapies and behavioral interventions for alcohol dependence, the COMBINE study: a randomized controlled trial, JAMA (17):2003-2009, 2006.

Campral package insert, St Louis, 2005, Forest Pharmaceuticals.

Garbutt JC et al: Efficacy and tolerability of long-acting injectable naltrexone for alcohol dependence: a randomized controlled trial, JAMA 293(13):617, 625, 2005.

Gold MS, Aronson MD: Screening for and diagnosis of patients with alcohol problems. In Rose BD, editor: UpToDate, Waltham, MA, 2007, UpToDate.

Gold MS, Aronson MD: Treatment of alcohol abuse and dependence. In Rose BD, editor: UpToDate, Waltham, MA, 2007, UpToDate.

HPSSAT and the Robert Wood Johnson Foundation: Health professional students for substance abuse training diagnostic tools and resources. Available at www.hpssat.org/cirriculum/index.html (accessed 8-06-08).

HSTAT Health Services/Technology Assessment Text SAMHSA/CSAT treatment improvement protocols tip19 detoxification from alcohol and other drugs tip 24: a guide to substance abuse services for primary care clinicians. Available at www.ncbi.nlm.nih.gov/books/bv.fcgi?rid=hstat5.part.22441. (accessed 8-06-08).

Lexi-Comp: Alcohol dependence. In Rose BD, editor: UpToDate, Waltham, MA, 2007, UpToDate.

National Institute on Alcohol Abuse and Alcoholism: Helping patients who drink too much: a clinician's guide 2005 edition, U.S. Department of Health & Human Services, National Institutes of Health Publication 05-3769. Available at http://pubs.niaaa.nih.gov/publications/Practitioner/CliniciansGuide2005/clinicians_guide.htm, (accessed 8-06-08).

Resnick RB: Food and Drug Administration approval of buprenorphine-naloxone for office treatment of addiction, Drug Alcohol 69(1):1-7, 2003.

Screening and behavioral counseling interventions in primary care to reduce alcohol misuse: recommendation statement, Ann Intern Med 140(7):554-556, 2004.

Sullivan HT et al: Assessment of alcohol withdrawal: the revised clinical institute withdrawal assessment for alcohol scale (CIWA-Ar), Br J Addict 84:1353-1357, 1989.

Vivitrol Drug Package Insert, Cambridge, MA, 2006.

Weinhouse G, Manaker S: Alcohol withdrawal syndromes. In Rose BD, editor: UpToDate, Waltham, MA, 2007, UpToDate.

Willenbring ML, Wilkins JN: Identification and treatment of patients with alcohol dependence in your practice: pharmacotherapeutic and psychosocial intervention. Available at www.medscape.com/viewprogram/6694.

CHAPTER 50

Cruse LM et al: Prevalence of evaluation and treatment of glucocorticoid-induced osteoporosis in men, J Clin Rheumatol 12(5):221-225, 2006.

Goroll AH et al, editors: Primary care medicine, ed 5, Philadelphia, 2006, Lippincott Williams & Wilkins.

Hubner M et al: Comparative pharmacology, bioavailability, pharmacokinetics, and pharmacodynamics of inhaled glucocorticosteroids, Immunol Allergy Clin North Am 25(3):469-488, 2005.

Joos GF et al: Positioning of glucocorticosteroids in asthma and allergic rhinitis guidelines, Immunol Allergy Clin North Am 25:597-612, 2005.

Langer P et al: Survey of orthopaedic and sports medicine physicians regarding use of Medrol dosepak for sports injuries, Arthroscopy 22(12):1263-1269, 2006.

Lems WF et al: Positive effect of alendronate on bone mineral density and markers of bone turnover in patients with rheumatoid arthritis on chronic treatment with low-dose prednisone: a randomized, double-blind, placebo-controlled trial, Osteoporos Int 17(5):716-723, 2006.

Lexi-Comp: Glucocorticoids. In Rose BD, editor: UpToDate, Waltham, MA, 2007, UpToDate.

Maccari S et al: Prenatal stress and long-term consequences: implications of glucocorticoid hormones, Neurosci Biobehav Rev 27(102):119-127, 2003.

Regan TD et al: Taste comparison of corticosteroid suspensions, J Drugs Dermatol 5(9):835-837, 2006.

Summey BT, Yosipovitch G: Glucocorticoid-induced bone loss in dermatologic patients: an update, Arch Dermatol 142(1):82-90, 2006.

CHAPTER 51

AACE Thyroid Task Force: American Association of Clinical Endocrinologists medical guidelines for clinical practice for the evaluation and treatment of hyperthyroidism and hypothyroidism, Endo Pract 8(6):457-469, 2002.

American College of Obstetricians and Gynecologists (ACOG): Thyroid disease in pregnancy, Washington (DC), 2002, Author.

Bunevicius R, Prange AJ Jr: Psychiatric manifestations of Graves' hyperthyroidism: pathophysiology and treatment options, CNS Drugs 20(11):897-909, 2006.

Cassio Aet al: Treatment for congenital hypothyroidism: thyroxine alone or thyroxine plus triiodothyronine? *Pediatrics* 111 (5 Pt 1):1053-1060, 2003.

Greenspan FS, Dong BJ: Thyroid and antithyroid drugs. In Katzung BG, editor: *Basic clinical pharmacology*, ed 10, New York, 2007, McGraw-Hill.

Ineck BA, Ng TM: Effects of subclinical hypothyroidism and its treatment on serum lipids, *Ann Pharmacother* 37(5):725-730, 2003.

Lexi-Comp: Thyroid medications. In Rose BD, editor: *UpToDate*, Waltham, MA, 2007, UpToDate.

Ross D: Treatment of hypothyroidism. In Rose BD, editor: *UpToDate*, Waltham, MA, 2007, UpToDate.

Saxe JM: Thyroid diseases. In Winifred L et al, editors: *Women's primary health care*, San Francisco, 2004, UCSF Nursing Press.

Schindler AE: Thyroid function and postmenopause, *Gynecol Endocrinol* 17(1):79-85, 2003.

Thompson LDR: *Endocrine pathology: a volume in foundations in diagnostic pathology series*, New York, 2006, Churchill Livingstone.

Utiger RD: Thyroid hormone synthesis and physiology. In Rose BD, editor: *UpToDate*, Waltham, MA, 2007, UpToDate.

Wilson Net al: *Williams' textbook of endocrinology*, ed 10, Philadelphia, 2002, Saunders.

CHAPTER 52

American Diabetes Association: Clinical practice recommendations 2007, *Diabetes Care* 30(Suppl 1):S4–S41, 2007.

Bloomgarden, ZT: Aspects of type 2 diabetes and related insulin-resistant states, *Diabetes Care* 29(3):732-740, 2006.

Diabetes Control and Complications Trial (DCCT) research group: The effect of intensive treatment of diabetes on the development and progression of long-term complications in insulin-dependent diabetes mellitus, *N Engl J Med* 329:977-986, 1993.

Dungan K, Buse JB: Amylin and GLP-1-based therapies for the treatment of diabetes. In Rose BD, editor: *UpToDate*, Waltham, MA, 2007, UpToDate.

Dungan K, Buse JB: Glucagon peptide 1-based therapies for type 2 diabetes: a focus on Exenatide, *Clinical Diabetes* 23(2):56-62, 2005.

Fisher M, Kapustin, JF: A practical guide for the aggressive management of type 2 diabetes, *J Am Nurse Pract* 3(4):2007.

Fonseca VA: *Clinical diabetes: translating research into practice*, Philadelphia, 2006, Saunders.

Hainer TA: Managing older adults with diabetes, *J Am Acad Nurse Pract* 18(7):309-318, 2006.

Hirsch IB et al: A real-world approach to insulin therapy in primary care practice, *Clin Diabetes* 23(2):78-86, 2005.

LaSalle JR: New insulin analogs: Insulin detemir and insulin glulisine, *Pract Diabetol* 25(3):34-44, 2006.

Lexi-Comp: Antidiabetic agents. In Rose BD, editor: *UpToDate*, Waltham, MA, 2007, UpToDate.

McCulloch DK: Insulin secretion and pancreatic beta-cell function. In Rose BD, editor: *UpToDate*, Waltham, MA, 2007, UpToDate.

McCulloch DK: Sulfonylureas and meglitinides in the treatment of diabetes mellitus. In Rose BD, editor: *UpToDate*, Waltham, MA, 2007, UpToDate.

McCulloch DK: Thiazolidinediones in the treatment of diabetes mellitus. In Rose BD, editor: *UpToDate*, Waltham, MA, 2007, UpToDate.

Mentlein R: Therapeutic assessment of glucagon-like peptide-agonists compared with dipeptidyl peptidase IV inhibitors as potential antidiabetic drugs, *Expert Opin Invest Drugs* 14(1):57-64, 2005.

Prescribing inserts: *Byetta*. Available at http://pi.lilly.com/us/byetta-pi.pdf.

Prescribing inserts: *Januvia*. Available at www.merck.com/product/usa/pi_circulars/j/januvia/januvia_pi.pdf (accessed 8-06-08).

Prescribing inserts: *Symlin*. Available at www.symlin.com/PDF/HCP/SYMLIN-pi-combined.pdf.

UK Prospective Diabetes Study Group: Tight blood pressure control and risk of macrovascular and microvascular complications in type 2 diabetes (UKPDS 38), *BMJ* 317:703-713, 1998.

Uwaifo GI, Ratner RE: Novel pharmacologic agents for type 2 diabetes, *Endocrinol Metab Clin North Am* 34:155-197, 2005.

CHAPTER 53

Apgar B, Greenberg D: Using progestins in clinical practice, *Am Fam Physician*.

Berek JS: *Berek and Novak's gynecology*, ed 14, Philadelphia, 2007, Lippincott.

Bieber EJ et al: *Clinical gynecology*, Philadelphia, 2006, Saunders.

Hatcher RA et al: *Contraceptive technology*, ed 18 rev, New York, 2007, Ardent Media Trade.

Kim C et al: Oral contraceptive use and association with glucose, insulin, and diabetes in young adult women: The CARDIA study. Coronary artery risk development in young adults, *Diabetes Care* 25:1027-1032, 2002.

Levi F et al: Oral contraceptives and colorectal cancer, *Dig Liver Dis* 35:85-87, 2003.

Lexi-Comp: Contraceptives. In Rose BD, editor: *UpToDate*, Waltham, MA, 2007, UpToDate.

Rosen MP et al: A randomized controlled trial of second- versus third-generation oral contraceptives in the treatment of acne vulgaris, *Am J Obstet Gynecol* 188:1158-1160, 2003.

Shulman LP et al: Oral contraceptives and venous thromboembolic events, *J Reprod Med* 48:306-307, 2003.

Sicat BL: Ortho Evra, a new contraceptive patch, *Pharmacotherapy* 23:472-480, 2003.

The Medical Letter: Yasmin—an oral contraceptive with a new progestin, *Med Lett Drugs Ther* 44:55-57, 2002.

CHAPTER 54

American College of Obstetricians and Gynecologists (ACOG): *ACOG news release*, January 31, 2000. Available at www.acog.org.

American College of Obstetricians and Gynecologists (ACOG): *ACOG news release*, August 31, 2001. Available at www.acog.org.

American College of Obstetricians and Gynecologist (ACOG): *ACOG news release*, February 28, 2002. Available at www.acog.org.

American College of Obstetricians and Gynecologist (ACOG): *ACOG questions and answers on hormone therapy*, August 2002. Available at www.acog.org.

American College of Obstetricians and Gynecologist (ACOG): *ACOG news release*, November 29, 2002. Available at www.acog.org.

American College of Obstetricians and Gynecologists (ACOG): Vasomotor symptoms, *Obstet Gynecol* 104(4 Suppl): 106S-117S, 2004.

American Society of Reproductive Medicine (ASRM): ASRM statement on the release of data from the estrogen-only arm of the Women's Health Initiative, *ASRM Bull* 6(23):2004.

Anderson GL et al: Effects of conjugated equine estrogen in postmenopausal women with hysterectomy: the Women's Health Initiative randomized controlled trial, *JAMA* 291(14):1701-1712, 2004.

Farquhar CM et al: Long-term hormone therapy for perimenopausal and postmenopausal women, *Cochrane Database Syst Rev*, CD004143, 2005.

Hsia J et al: Conjugated equine estrogens and coronary heart disease: the Women's Health Initiative, *Arch Intern Med* 166(3):357-365, 2006.

Kravitz Het al: Sleep difficulty in women at midlife: a community survey of sleep and the menopausal transition, *Menopause* 10:10-28, 2003.

Lexi-Comp: Hormone replacement therapy. In Rose BD, editor: *UpToDate*, Waltham, MA, 2007, UpToDate.

MacLennan AH et al: Oral oestrogen and combined oestrogen/progestogen therapy versus placebo for hot flushes, *Cochrane Database Syst Rev* 4:CD002978, 2004.

Nelson HD et al: *Management of menopause-melated symptoms* (Rep. No. Pub. No. 05-E016-1), 2005, Agency for Healthcare Research and Quality.

Nelson HD et al: Nonhormonal therapies for menopausal hot flashes: systematic review and meta-analysis, *JAMA* 295(17): 2057-2071, 2006.

North American Menopause Society (NAMS): *Menopause: definitions and epidemiology*, Cleveland, 2002, Author. Available at www.menopause.org.

North American Menopause Society (NAMS): Estrogen and progestogen use in peri- and postmenopausal women: September 2003 position statement of the North American Menopause Society, *Menopause* 10(6): 497-506, 2003.

North American Menopause Society: *NAMS clinical guide*, Cleveland, 2003, Author.

North American Menopause Society (NAMS): Role of progestogen in hormone therapy for postmenopausal women: position statement of the North American Menopause Society, *Menopause* 10(2):113-132, 2003.

North American Menopause Society (NAMS): Treatment of menopause-associated vasomotor symptoms: Position statement of the North American Menopause Society, *Menopause* 11(1):11-33, 2004.

North American Menopause Society (NAMS): The role of testosterone therapy

in postmenopausal women: position statement of The North American Menopause
Society, *Menopause* 12(5):496-511, 2005.

North American Menopause Society (NAMS):
Management of osteoporosis in postmenopausal
women: 2006 position statement of the North
American Menopause Society, *Menopause*
13(3):340-367, 2006.

North American Menopause Societ (NAMS):
Estrogen and progestogen use in peri- and
postmenopausal women: March 2007 position
statement of the North American Menopause
Society, *Menopause* 14(2):168-182, 2007.

Rossouw JE et al: Risks and benefits of estrogen
plus progestin in healthy postmenopausal
women: principal results from the Women's
Health Initiative randomized controlled trial,
JAMA 288(3):321-33, 2002.

Rossouw JE et al: Postmenopausal hormone
therapy and risk of cardiovascular disease by
age and years since menopause, *JAMA*
297(13):1465-1477, 2007.

Salpeter SR et al. Mortality associated with
hormone replacement therapy in younger and
older women: a meta-analysis, *J Gen Intern
Med* 19(7):791-804, 2004.

Seibert C et al: Prescribing oral contraceptives
for women older than 35 years of age, *Ann
Intern Med* 138:54-64, 2003.

Shumaker SA et al: Estrogen plus progestin and
the incidence of dementia and mild cognitive
impairment in postmenopausal women: the
Women's Health Initiative Memory Study:
a randomized controlled trial, *JAMA*
289(20):2651-2662, 2003.

U.S. Food and Drug Administration: *Guidance
for industry: estrogen and estrogen/progestin drug
products to treat vasomotor symptoms and vulvar
and vaginal atrophy symptoms—recommendations
for clinical evaluation*, 2003. Available at
www.fda.gov/cder/guidance/5412dft.pdf.

U.S. Preventive Services Task Force:
*Recommendations and rationale—hormone
replacement therapy for primary prevention
of chronic conditions*, Washington, DC,
2002, Author.

U.S. Preventive Services Task Force: *Hormone
therapy for the prevention of chronic conditions
in postmenopausal women: recommendation
statement*, Washington, DC, 2005, Author.
Available at www.ahrq.gov/clinic.

Wattanakumtornkul S et al: Intranasal hormone
replacement therapy, *Menopause* 10:88-98,
2003.

Wysocki S et al: Individualized care for
menopausal women: Counseling women
about hormone therapy, *Womens Health Care*
2(12):8-16, 2003.

CHAPTER 55

Abeloff: *Clinical oncology*, ed 3, London, 2004,
Churchill Livingstone.

Buzdar AU: Preoperative chemotherapy
treatment of breast cancer—a review, *Cancer*
16:2007.

Cianfrocca M, Gradishar WJ: Counterpoint: the
argument for combination chemotherapy in
the treatment of metastatic breast cancer,
JNCCN 5(8):771-773, 2007.

Conlin AK, Seidman AD: Point: combination
versus single-agent chemotherapy: the

argument for sequential single agents,
JNCCN 5(8):766-770, 2007.

Ellis M, Hayes DF: Endocrine therapy of
metastatic breast cancer. In Rose BD, editor:
UpToDate, Waltham, MA, 2007, UpToDate.

Genetic risk assessment and BRCA mutation
testing for breast and ovarian cancer susceptibility: recommendation statement, *Ann Intern
Med* 143(5):355-361, 2005.

Goble S, Bear HD: Emerging role of taxanes in
adjuvant and neoadjuvant therapy for breast
cancer: The potential and the questions, *Surg
Clin North Am* 83:943-971, 2003.

Hayes DF: An overview of breast cancer and
treatment for early stage disease. In Rose BD,
editor: *UpToDate*, Waltham, MA, 2007,
UpToDate.

Lexi-Comp: Breast cancer. In Rose BD, editor:
UpToDate, Waltham, MA, 2007, UpToDate.

Moore A: Breast-cancer therapy—looking back
to the future, *N Engl J Med* 357(15):
1547-1549, 2007.

Rose C: Increasing protection after tamoxifen:
insights from the extended adjuvant aromatase
inhibitor trials, *J Cancer Res Clin Oncol* 134:1,
7-17, 2007.

Roukos DH: Prognosis of breast cancer in
carriers of BRCA1 and BRCA2 mutations,
N Engl J Med 357(15):1555-1556, 2007.

van der Hage JJ et al: Efficacy of adjuvant
chemotherapy according to hormone receptor
status in young patients with breast cancer:
a pooled analysis, *Breast Cancer Res* 11:9(5):
R70, 2007.

U.S. Preventive Services Task Force: Screening for
breast cancer: recommendations and rationale,
Ann Intern Med 137(5 Part 1):344-346, 2002.

CHAPTER 56

Gonzales R et al: Excessive antibiotic use for acute
respiratory infections in the United States,
Clin Infect Dis 33:757-762, 2001.

Steinman MA et al: Changing use of antiinfectives in community based outpatient practice,
1991-1999, *Ann Intern Med* 138(7):525-533,
2003.

CHAPTER 57

Aslam S, Musher DM: An update of diagnosis,
treatment and prevention of *Clostridium
difficile*–associated disease, *Gastroenterol Clin
North Am* 35:315, 2006.

Casey JR, Pichichero ME: Meta-analysis of
cephalosporin versus penicillin treatment of
group A streptococcal tonsillopharyngitis in
children, *Pediatrics* 113(4):866-882, 2004.

Cunha BA: *Infectious diseases in critical care
medicine*, ed 2, St Louis, Informa Health
Care, 2006.

Fisher TF et al: Reaction toward a new treatment
paradigm for acute otitis media, *Pediatr Emerg
Care* 21(3);170-172, 2005.

Gill JM et al: Use of antibiotics for adult upper
respiratory infections in outpatient settings: a
national ambulatory network study, *Fam Med*
38(5):349-354, 2006.

LaMont, JT: Pathophysiology and epidemiology
of Clostridium difficile infection. In Rose BD,
editor: *UpToDate*, Waltham, MA, 2007

Lexi-Comp: Antibiotics. In Rose BD, editor:
UpToDate, Waltham, MA, 2007, UpToDate.

Linder JA et al: Antibiotic treatment of children
with sore throat, *JAMA* 294(18):2315-2322,
2005.

Mandell LA et al: Update of practice guidelines
for the management of community-acquired
pneumonia in immunocompetent adults, *Clin
Infect Dis* 37(11):1405-1433, 2003.

Pappas PG et al: Guidelines for treatment of
candidiasis, *Clin Infect Dis* 38(2):161-189,
2004.

Riviello R, Lavelle K: Human and animal bites:
acute care and follow-up, *Consultant* 1091-1095,
2005.

Sexually transmitted diseases treatment guidelines, 2006, *MMWR Recomm Rep* 45(10):
1-94, 2006

Stevens DL, et al: Practice guidelines of the
diagnosis and management of skin and soft-
tissue infections, *Clin Infect Dis* 41(10):
1373-1406, 2005.

The Medical Letter: Treatment guidelines:
Antimicrobial prophylaxis fur surgery, *Med
Lett Drugs Ther* 2(20):27-32, 2004.

The Medical Letter: Treatment guidelines:
Choice of antibacterial drugs, *Med Lett Drugs
Ther* 2(19):13-17, 2004.

The Medical Letter: Antibacterial prophylaxis
for dental, GI and GU procedures, *Med Lett
Drugs Ther* 47(1213):59-60, 2005.

CHAPTER 58

Calderwood SB: Penicillins. In Rose BD, editor:
UpToDate, Walthan, MA, 2007, UpToDate.

Chambers HF: Penicillins. In Mandell GL et al,
editors: *Principles and practice of infectious
diseases*, ed 6, New York, 2005, Churchill
Livingstone.

Curtin-Wirt C et al: Efficacy of penicillin
vs amoxicillin in children with group A
β-hemolytic streptococcal tonsillopharyngitis,
Clin Pediatr (Phila) 42(3):219-225, 2003.

Holcomb, SS: Community acquired MRSA:
new guidelines for a new age, *Nurse Pract*
31(9):8, 11-12, 2006.

Jones RN et al: Influence of patient age on
the susceptibility patterns of *Streptococcus
pneumoniae* isolates in North America
(2000-2001): report from the SENTRY
Antimicrobial Surveillance Program, *Diagn
Microb Infect Dis* 46(1):77-80, 2003.

Lexi-Comp: Penicillin. In Rose BD, editor:
UpToDate, Waltham, MA, 2007, UpToDate.

Park MA, Li JT: Diagnosis and management of
penicillin allergy, *Mayo Clin Proc* 80(3):405,
2005.

Schrag S et al: Comparison of strategies to
prevent population-based, early-onset group B
streptococci disease in neonates, *N Engl
J Med* 347(4):233-239, 2002.

Uy IP et al: Changes in early-onset group B beta
hemolytic streptococcus disease with
changing recommendations for prophylaxis,
J Perinatol 22(7):516-22, 2002.

CHAPTER 59

Betts RF et al: *Reese and Betts' practical approach
to infectious diseases*, ed 5, Philadelphia, 2002,
Lippincott Williams & Wilkins.

Calderwood, SB: Cephalosporins. In Rose BD,
editor: *UpToDate*, Waltham, MA, 2007,
UpToDate.

Dancer SJ: The problem with cephalosporins, *J Antimicrob Chemother* 48(4):463-478, 2001.

Lexi-Comp: Cephalosporins. In Rose BD, editor: *UpToDate*, Waltham, MA, 2007, UpToDate.

Padmanabhan RA et al: What's new in antibiotics? *Dermatol Clin* 23:301-312, 2005.

Pichichero ME: A review of evidence supporting the American Academy of Pediatrics recommendation for prescribing cephalosporin antibiotics for penicillin-allergic patients, *Pediatrics* 115(4):1048-1057, 2005.

The Medical Letter: Cefditoren (Spectracef)—a new oral cephalosporin, *Med Lett Drugs Ther* 44(1122):5-8, 2006.

CHAPTER 60

Bassett J, Patrick B: Restoring tetracycline-stained teeth with a conservative preparation for porcelain veneers: case presentation, *Pract Proced Aesthet Dent* 16(7):481-486, 2004.

Chang TT, Nedorost ST: Esophagitis due to tetracycline and its derivatives in dermatology patients, *J Drugs Dermatol* 5(3):247-249, 2006.

Goulden V: Guidelines for the management of acne vulgaris in adolescents, *Paediatr Drugs* 5(5):301-313, 2003.

Lexi-Comp: Tetracyclines. In Rose BD, editor: *UpToDate*, Waltham, MA, 2007, UpToDate.

May DB: Tetracyclines. In Rose BD, editor: *UpToDate*, Waltham, MA, 2007, UpToDate.

Meyers B, Salvatore M: Tetracyclines and chloramphenicol. In Mandell GL et al, editors: *Principles and practice of infectious diseases*, ed 6, New York, 2005, Churchill Livingstone.

Wormser GP et al: Duration of antibiotic therapy for early Lyme disease: a randomized double-blind placebo-controlled trial, *Ann Intern Med* 138(9):697-704, 2003.

CHAPTER 61

Brown RB et al: Impact of initial antibiotic choice on clinical outcomes in community-acquired pneumonia: analysis of a hospital claims-made database, *Chest* 123(5):1503-1511, 2003.

Clay KD et al: Brief communication: severe hepatotoxicity of telithromycin: three care reports and literature review, *Ann Intern Med* 144:415-420, 2006.

Graziani AL: Azithromycin, clarithromycin, and telithromycin. In Rose BD, editor: *UpToDate*, Waltham, MA, 2007, UpToDate.

Lexi-Comp: Macrolides. In Rose BD, editor: *UpToDate*, Waltham, MA, 2007, UpToDate.

Lonks JR et al: Implications of antimicrobial resistance in the empirical treatment of community-acquired respiratory tract infections: the case of macrolides, *J Antimicrob Chemother* 50(Suppl S2):87-92, 2002.

Metlay JP et al: Macrolide resistance in adults with bacteremic pneumococcal pneumonia, *Emerg Infect Dis* 12(8):1223-1230, 2006.

Prunier AL et al: High rate of macrolide resistance in *Staphylococcus aureus* strains from patients with cystic fibrosis reveals high proportions of hypermutable strains, *J Infect Dis* 187(11):1709-1716, 2003.

Sivapalasingam S, Steigbigel NH: Macrolides, clindamycin, and ketolides. In Mandell GL et al, editors: *Principles and practice of infectious diseases*, ed 6, New York, 2005, Churchill Livingstone.

The Medical Letter: Azithromycin extended release for sinusitis and pneumonia, *Med Lett Drugs Ther* 47(1218):78-79 2006.

Waterer GW: Combination antibiotic therapy with macrolides in community-acquired pneumonia: more smoke but is there any fire? *Chest* 123(5):1328-1329, 2003.

CHAPTER 62

Croom KF, Goa KL: Levofloxacin: a review of its use in the treatment of bacterial infections in the United States, *Drugs* 63(24):2769-2802, 2003.

Hooper DC: Fluoroquinolones. In Rose BD, editor: *UpToDate*, Waltham, MA, 2007, UpToDate.

Lexi-Comp: Fluoroquinolones. In Rose BD, editor: *UpToDate*, Waltham, MA, 2007, UpToDate.

Poole M et al: A trial of high-dose, short-course levofloxacin for the treatment of acute bacterial sinusitis, *Otolaryngol Head Neck Surg* 134(1):10-17, 2006.

The Medical Letter: Gemifloxacin, *Med Lett Drugs Ther* 46(1192):78-79, 2004.

Washington CB et al: Pharmacokinetics and pharmacodynamics of novel extended release ciprofloxacin in healthy volunteers, *J Clin Pharmacol* 45(11):1236-1244, 2005.

CHAPTER 63

Bates DE: Aminoglycoside ototoxicity, *Drugs Today* 39(4):277-285, 2003.

Drew RH: Aminoglycosides. In Rose BD, editor: *UpToDate*, Waltham, MA, 2007, UpToDate.

Gilbert DN: Aminoglycosides. In Mandell GL et al, editors: *Principles and practice of infectious diseases*, ed 6, New York, 2005, Churchill Livingstone.

Gonzalez LS, Spencer JP: Aminoglycosides: a practical review, *Am Fam Physician*. Available at home.aafp.org/afp.981115ap/gonzalez.html.

Group A streptococcus. Available at www.cdc.gov/ncidod/diseases/bacter/strep_a.htm (accessed 8-06-08).

Lexi-Drug: AMO glycosides. In Rose BD, editor: *UpToDate*, Waltham, MA, 2007, UpToDate.

CHAPTER 64

Brackett CC et al: Likelihood and mechanisms of cross-allergenicity between sulfonamide antibiotics and other drugs containing a sulfonamide functional group, *Pharmacotherapy* 24(7):856-870, 2004.

Lexi-Comp: Sulfonamides. In Rose BD, editor: *UpToDate*, Waltham, MA, 2007, UpToDate.

Longworth DL: Microbial drug resistance and the roles of the new antibiotics, *Clev Clin J Med* 68(6):496-497, 501-502, 504, 2001.

Lu KCet al: Is combination antimicrobial therapy required for urinary tract infection in children? *J Microbiol Immunol Infect* 35(1):56-60, 2003.

Macejko AM: Treatment of UTIs, *Urol Clin North Am* 34(1):35-42, 2007.

Marion DW: Diaphragmatic pacing. In Rose BD, editor: *UpToDate*, Waltham, MA, 2007, UpToDate.

May DB: Trimethoprim-sulfamethoxazole: an overview. In Rose BD, editor: *UpToDate*, Waltham, MA, 2007

Nicolle L: Best pharmacological practice: urinary tract infections, *Expert Opin Pharmacother* 4(5):693-704, 2003.

Strom BL et al: Absence of cross-reactivity between sulfonamide antibiotics and sulfonamide nonantibiotics, *N Engl J Med* 349:1628-1635, 2003.

Zinner SH, Mayer KH: Sulfonamides and trimethoprim. In Mandell GL, et al, editors: *Principles and practice of infectious diseases*, ed 6, New York, 2005, Churchill Livingstone.

CHAPTER 65

AAP 2007 Red Book, Report of the Committee on Infectious Diseases, Washington, DC, 2007, American Academy of Pediatrics.

Agrawal S et al: Bioequivalence assessment of rifampicin, isoniazid and pyrazinamide in a fixed dose combination of rifampicin, isoniazid, pyrazinamide and ethambutol vs separate formulations, *Int J Clin Pharmacol Ther* 40(10):474-481, 2002.

American Thoracic Society: Treatment of tuberculosis, *Am J Respir Crit Care Med* 167:603, 2003.

Basgoz N: Clinical manifestations of pulmonary tuberculosis. In Rose BD, editor: *UpToDate*, Waltham, MA, 2007, UpToDate.

Bass JB: Epidemiology of tuberculosis. In Rose BD, editor: *UpToDate*, Waltham, MA, 2007, UpToDate.

Bass JB: General principles of the treatment of tuberculosis. In Rose BD, editor: *UpToDate*, Waltham, MA, 2007, UpToDate.

Bass JB: Treatment of latent tuberculosis infection in HIV-negative patients. In Rose BD, editor: *UpToDate*, Waltham, MA, 2007, UpToDate.

Bernardo J: Diagnosis of pulmonary tuberculosis. In Rose BD, editor: *UpToDate*, Waltham, MA, 2007, UpToDate.

Centers for Disease Control and Prevention (CDC): Treatment of tuberculosis in patients who are HIV positive, *MMWR Morb Mortal Wkly Rep* 49(09):5-189, March 10, 2000.

Centers for Disease Control and Prevention (CDC): Incidence of tuberculosis, *MMWR Morb Mortal Wkly Rep* 56(11):245-250, March 23, 2007.

Centers for Disease Control and Prevention (CDC): Treatment of tuberculosis, *MMWR Morb Mortal Wkly Rep* 52(RR11):1-77. June 20, 2003.

Cohen SM: Diagnosis and treatment of tuberculosis, *J Nurse Pract* 2(6):390-396, 2006.

Els, NV: Treatment of latent tuberculosis infection in HIV-infected patients. In RoseBD, editor: *UpToDate*, Waltham, MA, 2007, UpToDate.

Fountain FF et al: Isoniazid hepatotoxicity associated with treatment of latent tuberculosis infection: a 7-year evaluation from a public health tuberculosis clinic, *Chest* 128:116-123, 2005.

Lexi-Comp: Antitubercular drugs. In Rose BD, editor: *UpToDate*, Waltham, MA, 2007, UpToDate.

The Medical Letter: Treatment guidelines: drugs for tuberculosis, *Med Lett Drugs Ther* 2(28):83-88, 2004.

CHAPTER 66

Albougy HA, Naidoo S: A systematic review of the management of oral candidiasis associated with HIV/AIDS, *S Afr Dent J* 57(11): 457-466, 2002.

Bennett JE: Mycoses. In Mandell GL et al, editors: *Principles and practice of infectious diseases*, ed 6, New York, 2005, Churchill Livingstone.

Anstead GM, Graybill JR: Coccidioidomycosis, *Infect Dis Clin North Am* 20:621-643, 2006.

Chapman SW: Mycology, pathogenesis, and epidemiology of blastomycosis. In Rose BD, editor: *UpToDate*, Waltham, MA, 2007, UpToDate.

Chapman SW: Treatment of blastomycosis. In Rose BD, editor: *UpToDate*, Waltham, MA, 2007, UpToDate.

Goldstein AO, Goldstein BG: Tinea versicolor. In Rose BD, editor: *UpToDate*, Waltham, MA, 2007, UpToDate.

Kaufman CA: Endemic mycoses: blastomycosis, histoplasmosis, and sporotrichosis, *Infect Dis Clin North Am* 20:645-662, 2006.

Kauffman CA: Treatment of oropharyngeal and esophageal candidiasis. Diaphragmatic pacing. In Rose BD, editor: *UpToDate*, Waltham, MA, 2007, UpToDate.

Steinbach WJ, Walsh TJ: Mycoses in pediatric patients, *Infect Dis Clin North Am* 20: 663-678, 2006.

Luna B, Zaleznik DF: Triazoles. In Rose BD, editor: *UpToDate*, Waltham, MA, 2007,

Zhang AY et al: Advances in topical and systemic antifungals, *Dermatol Clin* 25: 165-183 2007.

CHAPTER 67

Busti AJ et al: Atazanavir for treatment of human immunodeficiency virus, *Pharmacotherapy* 24(12):1732-1747, 2004.

Bucciardini R, et al, on behalf of the INITIO Trial International Coordinating Committee: Health-related quality of life outcomes in HIV-infected patients starting different combination regimens in a randomized multinational trial: The INITIO-QoL Substudy, *AIDS Res Hum Retroviruses* 23(10):1215-1222, 2007.

Centers for Disease Control and Prevention (CDC): Reported HIV status of tuberculosis patients—United States, 1993-2005, *MMWR Morb Mortal Wkly Rep* 56(42):1103-1106, 2007.

Chen R et al: HIV-1 mutagenesis during antiretroviral therapy: implications for successful drug treatment, *Front Biosci* 10: 743-750, 2005.

Dolin R et al: *Aids therapy*, ed 3, New York, 2007, Churchill Livingstone.

Guidelines for antiretroviral agents in pediatric HIV infection, *MMWR Morb Mortal Wkly Rep* 47(RR-4):1-43, 1998. Available at www. hiatus.org (August 2001 update).

Hammer SM et al, for the International AIDS Society-USA panel: Treatment for adult HIV infection: 2006 recommendations of the

International AIDS Society-USA panel, *JAMA* 296(7):827-843, 2006.

Hanna GH, Hirsch MS: Antiretroviral therapy for human immunodeficiency virus infection. In Lazo M et al, editors: Patterns and predictors of changes in adherence to highly active antiretroviral therapy: longitudinal study of men and women, *Clin Infect Dis* 45(10):1377-1385, 2007.

Lexi-Comp: Antiretrovirals. In Rose BD, editor: *UpToDate*, Waltham, MA, 2007, UpToDate.

Masur H et al: Guidelines for preventing opportunistic infections among HIV-infected persons—2002. Recommendations of the U.S. Public Health Service and the Infectious Diseases Society of America, *Ann Intern Med* 137(5 Pt 2):435-478, 2002.

Mofenson LM: Antiretroviral treatment during pregnancy. In Rose BD, editor: *UpToDate*, Waltham, MA, 2007, UpToDate.

Orsega S: Treatment of adult HIV infection: antiretroviral update and overview, *J Nurse Pract* 3(9):612-614.

Ramadhani HO et al: Predictors of incomplete adherence, virologic failure, and antiviral drug resistance among HIV-infected adults receiving antiretroviral therapy in Tanzania, *Clin Infect Dis* 45(11):1492-1498, 2007.

Savarino A: A historical sketch of the discovery and development of HIV-1 integrase inhibitors, *Expert Opin Invest Drugs* 15(12):1507-1522, 2006.

Sánchez-Conde M et al: Efficacy and safety of a once daily regimen with efavirenz, lamivudine, and didanosine, with and without food, as initial therapy for HIV infection: the ELADI study, *AIDS Res Hum Retrovir* 23(10):1237-1241, 2007.

U.S. Department of Health and Human Services (USDHHS): *Guidelines for the use of antiretroviral agents in HIV-infected adults and adolescents*, Rockville, MD, 2006, DHHS.

Ward D: *Antiretroviral treatment—optimizing the management of highly treatment experienced patients with HIV*, 45th Annual Interscience Conference on Antimicrobial Agents and Chemotherapy—Treatment of HIV Infection, January, 2006. Available at www.medscape.com/viewarticle/522377 (accessed 08-06-08).

CHAPTER 68

Albrecht MA: Treatment and prevention of genital herpes simplex virus infection. In Rose BD, editor: *UpToDate*, Waltham, MA, 2007, UpToDate.

Gutierrez K, Arvin AM: Long term antiviral suppression after treatment for neonatal herpes infection, *Pediatr Infect Dis J* 22(4): 371-372, 2003.

Johnson RW, Dworkin RH: Treatment of herpes zoster and postherpetic neuralgia, *BMJ* 327(7392):748-750, 2003.

Juckett G: Avian influenza: preparing for a pandemic, *Am Fam Physician* 74(5): 783-790, 2006.

Lexi-Comp: Antivirals. In Rose BD, editor: *UpToDate*, Waltham, MA, 2007, UpToDate.

Pilcher H: Oseltamivir resistance raises bird flu concerns, *Lancet Infect Dis* 6(2):75, 2006.

Roberts CM: Genital herpes: evolving epidemiology and current management, *J Am Acad Physician Asst* 16(2):36-40, 2003.

The Medical Letter: Treatment guidelines: drugs for non-HIV viral infections, *Med Lett Drugs Ther* 3(32):23-32, 2005.

The Medical Letter: Antiviral drugs for prophylaxis and treatment of influenza, *Med Lett Drugs Ther* 48(1246):87-88, 2006.

Zachary KC: Acyclovir: An overview. In Rose BD, editor: *UpToDate*, Waltham, MA, 2007, UpToDate.

CHAPTER 69

Advisory Committee on Immunization Practices (ACIP): A comprehensive immunization strategy to eliminate transmission of hepatitis b virus infection in the United States, *MMWR* 55(RR16):1-25, 2006 Dec 87 (accessed 02/15/07).

Advisory Committee on Immunization Practices (ACIP): Notice to readers: updated recommendations of the Advisory Committee on Immunization Practices (ACIP) for the control and elimination of mumps, *MMWR* 55(Early Release)1-2, 2006 June 1. Available at http://www.cdc.gov/mmwr/preview/mmwrhtml/mm55e601a1.htm?s_cid=mm55e601a1_e (accessed 08-06-08).

Advisory Committee on Immunization Practices (ACIP): Prevention of hepatitis A through active or passive immunization, *MMWR* 55(RR07);1-23, 2006, May 19. Available at http://www.cdc.gov/mmwr/mmwrhtml/rr5507a1.htm?s_cid=rr5507a1_e (accessed 08-06-08). Advisory Committee on Immunization Practices (ACIP): Yellow fever vaccine recommendations of the ACIP, *MMWR Morb Mortal Wkly Rep* 51:1-10, 2002. Available at www.cdc.gov/mmwr/preview/mmwrhtml/rr5117a1.htm (accessed 08-06-08).

Advisory Committee on Immunization Practices (ACIP): A comprehensive immunization strategy to eliminate transmission of hepatitis B virus infection in the United States, *MMWR Morb Mortal Wkly Rep* 55:1-25, 2006.

Advisory Committee on Immunization Practices (ACIP): Notice to readers: updated recommendations of the ACIP for the control and elimination of mumps, *MMWR Morb Mortal Wkly Rep* 55:1-2, 2006. Available at www.cdc.gov/mmwr/preview/mmwrhtml/mm55e601a1.htm?s_cid=mm55e601a1_e.

Advisory Committee on Immunization Practices (ACIP): Prevention of hepatitis A through active or passive immunization, *MMWR Morb Mortal Wkly Rep* 55:1-23, 2006. Available at www.cdc.gov/mmwr/preview/mmwrhtml/rr5507a1.htm?s_cid=rr5507a1_e.

Advisory Committee on Immunization Practices (ACIP): Quadrivalent human papillomavirus vaccine, *MMWR Morb Mortal Wkly Rep* 6: 1-24, 2007. Available at www.cdc.gov/mmwr/preview/mmwrhtml/rr56e312a1.htm (accessed 08-06-08).

American Academy of Pediatrics Committee on Infectious Disease: *2006 red book: report of the committee on infectious diseases*, ed 27, Elk Grove Village, IL, 2006, the Academy.

American Academy of Pediatrics Committee on Infectious Disease: *Prevention of rotavirus disease: guidelines for use of rotavirus vaccine,*

2006, November 2. Available at www.cispimmunize.org/pro/pdf/Rotavirus-110306.pdf (accessed 08-06-08).

Centers for Disease Control (CDC): *Healthy People 2010*, Vol 1, ed 2, Washington, DC, 2001, Government Printing Office. Available at www.healthypeople.gov/Document/HTML/Volume1/14Immunization.htm (accessed 08-06-08).

Centers for Disease Control and Prevention (CDC): Update: Guillain-Barré syndrome among recipients of Menactra meningococcal conjugate vaccine—United States, June 2005–September 2006, *MMWR Morb Mortal Wkly Rep* 55(41);1120-1124, 2006. Available at www.cdc.gov/mmwr/preview/mmwrhtml/mm5541a2.htm (accessed 08-06-08).

Centers for Disease Control and Prevention (CDC): Update: Cardiac-related events during the civilian smallpox vaccination program—United States, 2003, *MMWR Morb Mortal Wkly Rep* 52(21):492-496, 2003. Available at www.cdc.gov/MMWR/preview/mmwrhtml/mm5221a2.htm (accessed 08-06-08).

Poland GA, et al: Standards for adult immunization practices, *Am J Prev Med* 25(2):144-150, 2003.

CHAPTER 70

Anderson JW et al: Low-dose orlistat effects on body weight of mildly to moderately overweight individuals: a 16 week, double-blind, placebo-controlled trial, *Ann Pharmacother* 40(10):1717-1723, 2006.

Blackburn GL et al: *Small steps and practical approaches to the treatment of obesity*, Medscape slide and audio presentation. Available at www.medscape.com/viewprogram/8204 (accessed 08-06-08).

Bray GA: Drug therapy of obesity. In Rose BD, editor: *UpToDate*, Waltham, MA, 2007, UpToDate.

Daniels SR et al: Overweight in children and adolescents: pathophysiology, consequences, prevention, and treatment, *Circulation* 111(15):1999-2012, 2005.

Derosa G et al: Efficacy and safety comparative evaluation of orlistat and sibutramine treatment in hypertensive obese patients, *Diabetes Obes Metab* 7(1):47-55, 2005.

Hutton B, Fergusson D: Changes in body weight and serum lipid profile in obese patients treated with orlistat in addition to a hypocaloric diet: a systematic review of randomized clinical trials, *Am J Clin Nutr* 80(6):1461-1468, 2004.

Institute of Medicine Committee on Prevention of Obesity in Children and Youth, Food and Nutrition Board, Board on Health Promotion and Disease Prevention. In Koplan JP, et al, editors: *Preventing childhood obesity: health in the balance*. Washington, DC, 2005, National Academies Press.

Lean M, Mullan A: Obesity: which drug and when? *Int J Clin Pract* 61(9):1555-1560, 2007.

Mannucci E et al: Orlistat and sibutramine beyond weight loss, *Nutr Metab Cardiovasc Dis* epub, Oct 8, 2007.

Miller JL, Silverstein JH: Management approaches for pediatric obesity, *Nat Clin Pract Endocrinol Metab* 3(12):810-818, 2007.

O'Meara S et al: A systematic review of the clinical effectiveness of orlistat used for the management of obesity, *Obes Rev* 5(1):51-68, 2004.

Padwal R et al: Long-term pharmacotherapy for obesity and overweight, *Cochrane Database Syst Rev* (4):D004094, 2003.

Padwal R et al: Long-term pharmacotherapy for overweight and obesity: a systematic review and meta-analysis of randomized controlled trials, *Int J Obes Relat Metab Disord* 27(12):1437-1446, 2003.

Sari R et al: Comparison of efficacy of sibutramine or orlistat versus their combination in obese women, *Endocr Res* 30(2):159-167, 2004.

Wadden TA et al: Lifestyle modification for the management of obesity, *Gastroenterology* 132(6):2226-2238, 2007. Erratum in: *Gastroenterology* 133(1):371, 2007.

CHAPTER 71

Coffay AO: Smoking cessation: tactics that make a big difference, *J Fam Pract* 56(10):817-824, 2007.

Fossati R et al: A double-blind, placebo-controlled, randomized trial of bupropion for smoking cessation in primary care, *Arch Intern Med* 167(16):1791-1797, 2007.

Garwood CL, Potts LA: Emerging pharmacotherapies for smoking cessation, *Am J Health Syst Pharm* 64(16):1693-1698, 2007.

Kroon LA: Drug interactions with smoking, *Am J Health Syst Pharm* 64(18):1917-1921, 2007.

Lexi-Comp: Smoking cessation. In Rose BD, editor: *UpToDate*, Waltham, MA, 2007, UpToDate.

Muramoto ML et al: Randomized, double-blind, placebo-controlled trial of 2 dosages of sustained-release bupropion for adolescent smoking cessation, *Arch Pediatr Adolesc Med* 161(11):1068-1074, 2007.

Naudi KB, Felix DH: Nicotine replacement lozenges: abuse-related hyperkeratosis of the lateral border of the tongue, A case report, *Br Dent J* 203(6):305-306, 2007.

O'Brien CP: A second varenicline trial, *Curr Psychiatry Rep* 9(5):346-347, 2007.

O'Brien CP: Varenicline as maintenance therapy, *Curr Psychiatry Rep* 9(5):347-348, 2007.

Okuyemi KS et al: Interventions to facilitate smoking cessations, *Am Fam Physician* 74(2):13, 2006.

Oncken C et al: Efficacy and safety of the novel selective nicotinic acetylcholine receptor partial agonist, varenicline, for smoking cessation, *Arch Intern Med* 166(15):1571-1577, 2006.

Oncken CA, Kranzler HR: Pharmacotherapies to enhance smoking cessation during pregnancy, *Drug Alcohol Rev* 22(2):191-202, 2003.

Rennard SI: *A randomized placebo-controlled trial of a conjugate nicotine vaccine (NicVAX) in smokers who want to quit: 12-month results*, Abstract 3712, Orlando, FL, November 4-7, 2007, American Heart Association.

Rennard SI, Daughton DM: Overview of smoking cessation. In Rose BD, editor: *UpToDate*, Waltham, MA, 2007, UpToDate.

Rezaishiraz H et al: Treating smokers before the quit date: can nicotine patches and denicotinized cigarettes reduce cravings? *Nicotine Tob Res* 9(11):1139-1146, 2007.

Stack NM: Smoking cessation: an overview of treatment options with a focus on varenicline, *Pharmacotherapy* 27(11):1550-1557, 2007.

The Medical Letter: Drugs for tobacco dependence: treatment guidelines, *Med Lett Drugs Ther* 1(10):65-68, 2003.

Thomas S: Smoking cessation. Part 2: nicotine replacement therapy, *Nurs Stand* 22(5):44-47, 2007.

U.S. Preventive Services Task Force: *Counseling to prevent tobacco use and tobacco-caused disease: recommendation statement*, Rockville, MD, 2003, Agency for Healthcare Research and Quality.

Yousey Y: Early attitudes about tobacco smoke exposure of young children at home, *Am J Matern Child Nurs* 32(3):178-183, 2007.

CHAPTER 72

American Heart Association (AHA) Nutrition Committee, et al: Diet and lifestyle recommendations revision 2006: a scientific statement from the AHA Nutrition Committee, *Circulation* 114(1):82-96, 2006.

Bischoff-Ferrari HA et al: Effect of vitamin D on falls: a meta-analysis, *JAMA* 291:1999-2006, 2004.

Bjelakovic G et al: Mortality in randomized trials of antioxidant supplements for primary and secondary prevention: systematic review and meta-analysis, *JAMA* 297:842-857, 2007.

Britten P, et al: Development of food intake patterns for the mypyramid food guidance system, *J Nutr Educ Behav* 38(Suppl 2):S78-S92, 2006.

By the way, doctor: does selenium interfere with other vitamins? *Harv Health Lett* 28:8, 2003.

Cook S, Gidding SS: Modifying cardiovascular risk in adolescent obesity, *Circulation* 115(17):2251-2253, 2007.

Cooper L et al: Vitamin D supplementation and bone mineral density in early postmenopausal women, *Am J Clin Nutr* 77:1324-1329, 2003.

Douglas RM et al: Vitamin C for preventing and treating the common cold, *Cochrane Database Syst Rev* CD000980, 2000.

Durga J et al: Effect of 3-year folic acid supplementation on cognitive function in older adults in the FACIT trial: a randomized, double blind, controlled trial, *Lancet* 369:208-216, 2007.

Gidding SS et al: Dietary recommendations for children and adolescents: a guide for practitioners: consensus statement from the American Heart Association, *Circulation* 112(13):2061-2075, 2005.

Glenville M: Nutritional supplements in pregnancy: commercial push or evidence based? *Curr Opin Obstet Gynecol* 18(6):642-647, 2006.

Greenwald P et al: Clinical trials of vitamin and mineral supplements for cancer prevention, *Am J Clin Nutr* 85(1):314S-317S, 2007.

Hercberg S, et al: The SU.VI.MAX study: a randomized, placebo-controlled trial of the health effects of antioxidant vitamins and minerals, *Arch Intern Med* 164:2335-2342, 2004.

Holick MF: Vitamin D: importance in the prevention of cancers, type 1 diabetes, heart disease, and osteoporosis, *Am J Clin Nutr* 9:362-371, 2004.

Jenkins KJ et al: Noninherited risk factors and congenital cardiovascular defects: current knowledge: a scientific statement from the American Heart Association Council on Cardiovascular Disease in the Young: endorsed by the American Academy of Pediatrics, *Circulation* 115(23):2995-3014, 2007.

Kris-Etherton PM et al: AHA science advisory: antioxidant vitamin supplements and cardiovascular disease, *Circulation* 110: 637-641, 2004.

Lee IM et al: Vitamin E in the primary prevention of cardiovascular disease and cancer: the Women's Health Study: a randomized controlled trial, *JAMA* 294:56-65, 2005.

Miller ER et al: Meta-analysis: high dosage vitamin E supplementation may increase all-cause mortality, *Ann Intern Med* 142(1):37-46, 2005.

MRC/BHF: Heart Protection Study of antioxidant vitamin supplementation in 20,536 high-risk individuals: a randomised placebo-controlled trial, *Lancet* 360(9326):23-33, 2002.

North American Menopause Society (NAMS): The role of calcium in peri- and postmenopausal women: 2006 position statement of the NAMS, *Menopause* 13(6):862-877, 2006.

Palacios C: The role of nutrients in bone health, from A to Z, *Crit Rev Food Sci Nutr* 46(8):621-628, 2006.

Papadimitropoulos E et al: Meta-analyses of therapies for postmenopausal osteoporosis; VIII: Meta-analysis of the efficacy of vitamin D treatment in preventing osteoporosis in postmenopausal women, *Endocr Rev* 23: 560-569, 2005.

Pazirandeh S et al: Overview of water-soluble vitamins. In Rose BD, editor: *UpToDate*, Waltham, MA, 2007, UpToDate.

Pazirandeh S et al: Overview of fat-soluble vitamins. In Rose BD, editor: *UpToDate*, Waltham, MA, 2007, UpToDate.

Timbo BB et al: Dietary supplements in a national survey: prevalence of use and reports of adverse events, *J Am Diet Assoc* 106(12):1966-1974, 2006.

Whelton PK et al: Clinical and public health advisory from The National High Blood Pressure Education Program, *JAMA* 288(15):1882-1888, 2002.

Yetley EA: Multivitamin and multimineral dietary supplements: definitions, characterization, bioavailability, and drug interactions, *Am J Clin Nutr* 85(1):269S-276S, 2007.

CHAPTER 73

American Pharmaceutical Council (APC): *Statistics on healthcare*, Washington, DC, 1998, APC.

Brass EP, et al: Potential impact on cardiovascular public health of over-the-counter statin availability, *Am J Cardiol* 97(6):851-856, 2006.

Consumer Health Care Products Association (CHPA), 2006. Available at www.CHPA.org.

Gemmell I, et al: Should we encourage over-the-counter statins? A population perspective for coronary heart disease prevention, *Am J Cardiovasc Drugs* 7(4): 299-302, 2007.

New drug facts label to help consumers, *Clinician News* July/August, 20, 2002.

Nordenberg T: New drug label spells it out simply, *FDA Cons Mag* 99:3232, July-August, 1999.

Reynolds T: Switching from prescription to over the counter, *Ann Intern Med* 135:177-180, 2002.

Strickland DS: Review: over-the-counter medications are effective for gastro-oesophageal reflux disease, *Evid Based Nurs* 10(3):76, 2007.

Waknine Y: *FDA proposes adding vitamin d to calcium claim for decreasing osteoporosis risk*, Medscape Medical News. Available at www.medscape.com/viewarticle/550774 (accessed 08-06-08).

CHAPTER 74

AARP Knowledge Management/National Center for Complementary and Alternative Medicine: *Complementary and alternative medicine research report*, January 2007.

American Association of Retired Persons (AARP) and National Center for Complementary and Alternative Medicine (NCCAM): *Complementary and alternative medicine: what people 50 and older are using and discussing with their physicians*, Washington, DC, 2007, AARP.

American Botanical Council: *FDA approves special green tea extract as a new topical drug for genital warts*, November 2006. Available at www.herbalgram.org.

Barnes PM et al: Complementary and alternative medicine use among adults: United States, 2002, *Advance data from vital and health statistics, no 343*, Hyattsville, Md, 2004, National Center for Health Statistics.

Bell IR et al: Integrative medicine and systematic outcomes research: issues in the emergence of a new model for primary health care, *Arch Intern Med* 162:133-140, 2002.

Blumenthal M: *The ABC clinical guide to herbs*, Austin, TX, 2003, American Botanical Council.

Brazier NC, Levine MA: Drug-herb interaction among commonly used conventional medicines: a compendium for health care professionals, *Am J Ther* 10(3):163-169, 2003.

Breuner C: Alternative and complementary therapies, *Adolesc Med Clin* 17(3):521-546, 2006.

Cohen M, Eisenberg DM: Potential physician malpractice liability associated with complementary and integrative medical therapies, *Ann Intern Med* 136(8):596-603, 2002.

Davidson RT et al: Hypericum Depression Trial Study Group. Effect of *Hypericum perforatum* (St. John's wort) in major depressive disorder: a randomized, controlled trial, *JAMA* 287:1807-1814, 2002.

Duke JA: *The green pharmacy*, Emmaus, PA, 1997, Rodale.

Duke JA: *Dr. Duke's essential herbs*, Emmaus, PA, 1999, Rodale.

Ezbianski, AA: Warfarin and herbal supplements: a volatile combination, *Adv Nurse Pract* 11(11):77-80, 2003.

Fontanarosa PB: *Alternative medicine: an objective assessment*, Chicago, 2000, American Medical Association.

Jellin JM et al: *Pharmacist's letter/prescriber's letter natural medicines comprehensive database*, ed 4, Stockton, CA, 2002, Therapeutic Research Faculty.

Kaptchuk TJ, Miller FG: What is the best and most ethical model for the relationship between mainstream and alternative medicine: opposition, integration, or pluralism? *Acad Med* 80:286-290, 2005.

Kemper K: Complementary and alternative medicine for children: does it work? *West J Med* 174:272-276, 2001.

Kennedy J: Herb and supplement use in the U.S. adult population, *Clin Thera* 27(11): 1847-1858, 2005.

Kim Y-K: Efficacy of acupuncture for treating knee osteoarthritis, *Altern Med J* 8:49-60, 2005.

Martin DP et al: Improvement in fibromyalgia symptoms with acupuncture: results of a randomized controlled trial, *Mayo Clin Proc* 81:749-757, 2006.

McDermott JH, Motyka TM: Expert column: assessing the quality of botanical preparations, *Medscape pharmacology*, 2000. Available at www.primarycare.medscape.com.

Merrell WC: The debate within integrative medicine, *J Alt Compl Med* 12:601-602, 2006.

National Center for Complementary and Alternative Medicine: *Expanding horizons of healthcare: five-year strategic plan, 2001-2005*, NIH Publication No. 01-5001, Washington, DC, 2002, U.S. Department of Health and Humans Services. Available at: http://nccam.nih.gov/.

Oldendick R et al: Population-based survey of complementary and alternative medicine usage, patient satisfaction, and physician involvement, *South Med J* 93:375-381, 2000.

Pelletier KR: *The best alternative medicine: what works? what does not?* New York, 2000, Simon & Schuster.

Pelletier KR: MindBody medicine in ambulatory care: an evidence based assessment, *J Amb Care Manage* 27:25-42, 2004.

Pelletier KR: Integrative medicine: sorting fact from fiction, *Medscape Gen Med* 9(4):26, 2007. Available at www.medscape.com/viewarticle/564560.

Pelletier KR: *New medicine—complete family health guide: integrating complementary, alternative, and conventional medicine for the safest and most effective treatment*, New York, 2007, Penguin.

Piscitelli SC et al: The effect of garlic supplements on the pharmacokinetics of saquinavir, *Clin Infect Dis*, electronic edition, December 3, 2001. Available at www.nih.gov.news/pr/dec2001/niaid-05.htm.

Pizzorno J, Murray M, editors: *Textbook of natural medicine*, New York, 1999, Churchill Livingstone.

Rotblatt M, Ziment I: *Evidence-based herbal medicine*, Philadelphia, 2002, Hanley & Belfus.

Scott GN, Elmer G: Update on natural product-drug interactions, *Am J Health Syst Pharm* 59:339-347, 2002. Available at www.medscape.com/viewarticle/429776.

Straus S: Exploring the Scientific Basis of Complementary and Alternative Medicine, *NIH Director's Wednesday Afternoon Lecture Series (Webcast)*, March 11, 2002. Available at http://nccam.nih.gov/news/2002/030802. htm (accessed 8-06-08)

Straus S: Exploring the scientific basis of complementary and alternative medicine, *NIH director's Wednesday afternoon lecture series (webcast)*, March 11, 2002..

Swarbrick J, editor: *Encyclopedia of pharmaceutical technology, 2004 update supplement*, ed 2, New York, 2004, Decker.

Tindle H et al: Trends in use of complementary and alternative medicine by U.S. adults 1997-2002, *Alt Ther Health Med* 11(1): 42-49, 2005.

Tyler V: *The honest herbal: a sensible guide to the use of herbs and related remedies*, Binghamton, NY, 1993, Hawthorn.

Yarnell E, et al: *Clincial botanical medicine*, Larchmont, NY, 2003, Mary Ann Liebert.

APPENDIX A

American Society of Hospital Pharmacists (ASHP): ASHP statement on the use of medications for unlabeled uses, *Am J Hosp Pharm* 49:2006, 1992.

Anonymous: Drug-approval pace remains brisk in 1997, *Am J Health Sys Pharm* 55:336-337, 1998.

Anonymous: FDA issues regulations on accelerated drug-approval process, *Clin Pharm* 12:253-254, 1993.

Anonymous: Investigational new drug, antibiotic, and biological drug product regulations; procedures for drugs intended to treat life-threatening and severely debilitating illnesses, *Fed Reg* 53:41516-41524, 1988.

Anonymous: Prescription practices and regulatory agencies. In Bennett DR, editor: *Drug evaluations, annual 1992*, Chicago, 1991a, American Medical Association.

Anonymous: Orphan drugs. In Bennett DR, editor: *Drug evaluations, annual 1992*, Chicago, 1991b, American Medical Association.

Barr J: Use of patient-reported outcomes in pharmaceutical economics and health policy, *Clin Ther* 28(10):1710-1711, 2006.

Bartling D, Hadamik H: *Development of a drug. It's a long way from laboratory to patient*, Darmstadt, Germany, 1982, Rhone-Poulenc.

Benzi G et al: Drugs trying to get to the parents: there will be incentives for the European scientific community to develop research in the field of the orphan drugs, *Pharmacol Res* 35:89-93, 1997.

Bootman JL et al: *Principles of pharmacoeconomics*, ed 2, Cincinnati, 1996, Harvey Whitney.

Briggs AH, Levy AR: Pharmacoeconomics and pharmacoepidemiology: curious bedfellows or a match made in heaven? *Pharmacoeconomics* 24(11):1079-1086, 2006.

Cimmons M: Moving closer to FDA reform, *Nat Med* 3:940, 1997.

Commission on Federal Drug Approval Process: *Final report*, Washington, DC, March 31, 1982.

Cote CJ: Unapproved uses of approved drugs, *Paediatr Anaesth* 7:91-92, 1997.

Data JL: Potential stifling effects of pharmacoeconomics and regulatory policies, *Am J Cardiol* 81:34F-35F, April 1998.

Davis M et al: Prescription drug costs for seniors, *J Gen Intern Med* 22(1):257-223, 2007.

D'Errico CC: Pharmacoeconomics analysis in a pediatric population, *Ann Thorac Surg* 65(6 Suppl):S52-S54, 1998.

Dervieux T, Bala MV: Overview of the pharmacoeconomics of pharmacogenetics, *Pharmacogenomics* 7(8):1175-1184, 2006.

Drug safety, pharmacoeconomics and pharmacoepidemiology, *J Hosp Med* 1(Suppl 1):66-67, 2006.

Drummond M: Pharmacoeconomics: friend or foe? *Ann Rheum Dis* 65(Suppl e):iii 44-iii47, 2006

Ensor PA: Projecting future drug expenditures 1992, *Am J Hosp Pharm* 49:140-145, 1992.

FDA's approved drug products with therapeutic equivalence evaluations: United States pharmaceutical drug information, Rockville, MD, 1997, Food and Drug Administration.

Fink JL III, Simonsmeier LM: Laws governing pharmacy. In Gennaro AR, editor: *Remington: the science and practice of pharmacy*, ed 19, Easton, PA, 1995, Mack.

Fox JL: Pharmacoeconomics: drug pricing's new guise, *Biotechnology* 13:435-436, May 1995.

Gwartney JD, Stroup R: *Microeconomics: private and public choice*, ed 8, New York, 1996, Academic Press.

Hogan GF: Repercussions on the Drug Price Competition and Patent Term Restoration Act of 1984, *Am J Hosp Pharm* 42:849-851, 1985.

Inglehart JK: The American health care system—expenditures, *N Engl J Med* 340(7): 576, 1999.

Johannesson M et al: Economics, pharmaceuticals, and pharmacoeconomics, *Med Dec Making* 18(2 Suppl):S1-S3, 1998.

Katz R: The introduction of new drugs. In Gennaro AR, editor: *Remington: the science and practice of pharmacy*, ed 19, Easton, PA, 1995, Mack.

Knoben JE et al: An overview of the FDA publication approved drug products with therapeutic equivalence evaluations, *Am J Hosp Pharm* 47:269-270, 1990.

Marwick C: Pharmacoeconomics: is a drug worth its cost? *JAMA* 272:1395, 1994.

Mathers CD, Loncar D: *Projections of global mortality and burden of disease from 2002 to 2030*, Medscape. Available at www.medscape.com/viewarticle/550284.

McNamee D: Different kind of drug-company freebie, *Lancet* 348:695, 1996.

Miller HI: FDA "reform"? *Science* 279:158-159, 1998.

Novarro L: Drugs and money: in the high-stakes hunt for blockbuster pharmaceuticals, companies are pouring billions each year into research and development with no guarantee that their products will ultimately pass FDA scrutiny, *Hosp Health Network* 71:54-56, 1997.

Pausjenssen AM et al: Guidelines for measuring the costs and consequences of adopting new pharmaceutical products: are they on track? *Med Decis Making* 18(2 Suppl):S19-S22, 1998.

Phillips PJ: Regulatory approval process, *ASAOP J* 43:881-882, 1997.

Poe DB: The giving of gifts: anthropological data and social psychological theory, *Cornell J Soc Relations* 12:47-63, 1977.

Postma MJ et al: Pharmacoeconomics in nephrology: considerations on cost-effectiveness of screening for albuminuria, *Nephrol Dial Transplant* 23(4):1216-1223, 2008.

Reh M: Changes at FDA may speed drug approval process and increase off-label use, *J Natl Cancer Inst* 90:805-807, 1998.

Richards JW: Community pharmacy economics and management. In Gennaro AR, editor: *Remington: the science and practice of pharmacy*, ed 19, Easton, PA, 1995, Mack..

Sano M et al for the Alzheimer Disease Cooperative Study Group: ADCS prevention instrument project: pharmacoeconomics: assessing health-related resource use among healthy elderly, *Alzheimer Dis Assoc Disord* 20(Suppl 3):S191-S202, 2006.

Schulman KA, Linas BP: Pharmacoeconomics: state of the art in 1997, *Annu Rev Public Health* 18:529-548, 1997.

Shah ND et al: Projecting future drug expenditures—2002, *Am J Health Syst Pharm* 59:131-142, 2002.

Stewart A: Choosing an antidepressant: effectiveness based pharmacoeconomics, *J Affect Disord* 48:125-133, 1998.

Thamer M et al: A cross-national comparison of orphan drug policies: implications for the US orphan drug act, *J Health Polit Policy Law* 23:265-290, 1998.

Troetel WM: How new drugs win FDA approval, *US Pharmacist* 57:54-66, November 1986.

Turpie AG: Burden of disease: medical and economic impact of acute coronary syndromes, *Am J Manag Care* 12(16 Suppl):S430-434, 2006.

United States Pharmacopeia: *Complete drug reference*, Rockville, Md, 1998, St Martin's.

Walley T et al: Pharmacoeconomics: basic concepts and terminology, *Br J Clin Pharmacol* 43:343-348, 1997.

Index

Notes: Entries followed by "b" indicate boxes; "f" figures; "t" tables. Page numbers in bold indicate primary drug discussions.

FDA PREGNANCY CATEGORIES

A   Controlled studies in humans

B   Human data reassuring (animal positive) OR animal studies show no risk

C   Human data lacking; animal studies positive OR not done

D   Human data show risk, benefit may outweigh

X   Animal or human data positive

DRUG SCHEDULING

I   High abuse potential

No currently accepted medical use

For research, instructional use, or chemical analysis only

II   High abuse potential

Currently accepted for medical use as narcotic, stimulant, or depressant drugs

May lead to severe psychologic and/or physical dependence

III   Less abuse potential than drugs in Schedules I and II

Currently accepted for medical use and includes compounds containing limited quantities of certain narcotic and nonnarcotic drugs

May lead to physical dependence or high psychologic dependence

IV   Low abuse potential relative to Schedule III substances

Currently accepted for medical use

May lead to limited physical or psychologic dependence

V   Low abuse potential relative to Schedule IV substances

Currently accepted for medical use; consists primarily of preparations of certain narcotic and stimulant drugs generally for antitussive, antidiarrheal, and analgesic purposes

Have less potential for physical or psychologic dependence